CLINICAL
CARDIAC
PACING

KENNETH A. ELLENBOGEN, MD
Director, Clinical Electrophysiology Laboratory
Medical College of Virginia
McGuire Veterans Affairs Medical Center
Virginia Commonwealth University
Richmond, Virginia

G. NEAL KAY, MD
Director, Clinical Electrophysiology Section
Division of Cardiology
University of Alabama at Birmingham
Birmingham, Alabama

BRUCE L. WILKOFF, MD
Director, Cardiac Pacing and Tachyarrhythmia Devices
Director, Cardiovascular Computing Services
The Cleveland Clinic Foundation
Cleveland, Ohio

CLINICAL CARDIAC PACING

W.B. SAUNDERS COMPANY
A Division of Harcourt Brace & Company

Philadelphia London Toronto Montreal Sydney Tokyo

W.B. SAUNDERS COMPANY
A Division of
Harcourt Brace & Company

The Curtis Center
Independence Square West
Philadelphia, Pennsylvania 19106

Library of Congress Cataloging-in-Publication Data

Clinical cardiac pacing / [edited by] Kenneth A. Ellenbogen, G. Neal Kay, Bruce L. Wilkoff.—1st ed.

p.   cm.

Includes index.

ISBN 0–7216–5462–2

1. Cardiac pacing.   I. Ellenbogen, Kenneth A.   II. Kay, G. Neal.   III. Wilkoff, Bruce L.

[DNLM: 1. Cardiac Pacing, Artificial.   2. Pacemaker, Artificial. WG 168 C6413 1995]

RC684.P3C54 1995   617.4′120645—dc20

DNLM/DLC   94–22692

CLINICAL CARDIAC PACING   ISBN 0–7216–5462–2

Printed in the United States of America.

Last digit is the print number: 9   8   7   6   5   4   3   2   1

To my parents, Roslyn and Leon,
who instilled in me a love of learning,
and my wife, Phyllis,
and children, Michael, Amy, and Bethany,
for their patience and support.

KAE

To my teachers, colleagues, and students
who have taught me about cardiac pacing.
I am also indebted to the many members of the industry
who have dedicated their professional careers
to the design and improvement of pacing technology.
These individuals have greatly improved the therapy
that clinicians can offer to their patients,
undoubtedly resulting in an improvement in their lives.
Perhaps most important,
this book is dedicated to my wife, Linda,
for her patience and understanding
during its preparation.

GNK

To my wife, Ellyn,
and children, Jacob, Benjamin, and Ephram,
for their godly and inspirational patience and support.
To Yeshua, the Messiah, and His
sustaining covenant, love.

BLW

CONTRIBUTORS

ECKHARD ALT, MD
Professor of Internal Medicine, V Medical Clinic, Technische Universität, Klinikum rechts der Isar, Munich, Germany
Accelerometers

P. S. ASTRIDGE, MB, MRCP
Registrar in Cardiology, Leeds General Infirmary, Leeds, England, United Kingdom
Clinical Trials and Experience

S. SERGE BAROLD, MB, BS, FRACP, FACC
Professor of Medicine, University of Rochester School of Medicine and Dentistry; Chief of Cardiology, The Genesee Hospital, Rochester, New York
Timing Cycles and Operational Characteristics of Pacemakers

PETER H. BELOTT, MD, FACC
Clinical Instructor of Medicine, University of California at San Diego School of Medicine, San Diego, California; Director, Pacemaker Center, El Cajon, California; Staff Cardiologist, Scripps East County, El Cajon, California; Alvarado Medical Center, San Diego, California; Grossmant Hospital, La Mesa, California
Permanent Pacemaker Implantation

DAVID G. BENDITT, MD
Professor of Medicine, University of Minnesota Medical School—Minneapolis, Minneapolis, Minnesota
Activity-Sensing, Rate-Adaptive Pacemakers

THOMAS D. BENNETT, PhD
Medtronic Inc., Minneapolis, Minnesota
Rate-Adaptive Pacing Controlled by Dynamic Right Ventricular Pressure (dP/dtmax)

ALAN D. BERNSTEIN, MSc, Eng, ScD
Adjunct Associate Professor, Department of Surgery, University of Medicine and Dentistry of New Jersey; Director of Technical Research, Department of Surgery, and Technical Director, Pacemaker Center, Newark Beth Israel Medical Center, Newark, New Jersey
Pacemaker and Defibrillator Codes

CHRISTOPHER A. BONNET, MD
Assistant Professor of Medicine, Medical College of Pennsylvania, Philadelphia, Pennsylvania; Director, Electrocardiography, and Electrophysiologist, Allegheny General Hospital, Pittsburgh, Pennsylvania
Clinical Experience with Antitachycardia Pacing

GENE A. BORNZIN, PhD
Senior Staff Scientist, Siemens Pacesetter, Inc., Sylmar, California
Rate-Modulated Pacing Controlled by Mixed Venous Oxygen Saturation

JEFFREY A. BRINKER, MD
Associate Professor of Medicine, Johns Hopkins University School of Medicine; Director of Interventional Cardiology, Johns Hopkins Hospital, Baltimore, Maryland
Pacing: FDA and the Regulatory Environment

CHARLES L. BYRD, MD
Clinical Professor of Surgery, University of Miami School of Medicine, Miami, Florida
Management of Implant Complications

FRANK J. CALLAGHAN, MS, MSEE
Director of Research and Development, Telectronics Pacing Systems, Miami, Florida
Evoked Potentials as a Sensor for Rate-Adaptive Pacing

A. JOHN CAMM, MD
Department of Cardiological Science, St. George's Medical School, London, England, United Kingdom
Overview of Ideal Sensor Characteristics

LON W. CASTLE, MD
Head, Section of Pacing and Electrophysiology, The Cleveland Clinic Foundation, Cleveland, Ohio
Carotid Sinus Hypersensitivity and Neurally Mediated Syncope; Pacemaker Radiography

DEREK T. CONNELLY, MB, CHB, MRCP
Senior Registrar in Cardiology, Broadgreen Hospital, Liverpool, England, United Kingdom
The Evoked QT Interval

SEBASTIAN COOK, MD
Associate Professor of Radiology, Ohio State University, Columbus, Ohio; Vice Chairman, Nuclear Medicine, and Staff, Radiology, The Cleveland Clinic Foundation, Cleveland, Ohio
Pacemaker Radiography

COLLEEN CREAMER, RN, MS, CCRN
Point Richmond, California
Follow-Up of the Paced Outpatient

ANN M. CRESPI, PhD
Manager, Tachy Battery Research and Development, Medtronic Inc., Brooklyn Center, Minnesota
Power Sources for Implantable Pacemakers

BARBARA J. DEAL, MD
Associate Professor of Pediatrics, Northwestern University Medical School; Director, Electrophysiology Service, and Attending Physician, Children's Memorial Hospital, Chicago, Illinois
Esophageal Pacing

MARIA DE GUZMAN, MD
Associate Professor of Medicine, University of Southern California School of Medicine; Director of Electrocardiography, Los Angeles County and USC Medical Center, Los Angeles, California
AV Node–His–Purkinje System Disease: AV Block (Acute)

KAREL DEN DULK, MD
Cardiologist, Department of Cardiology, Academic Hospital Maastricht, Maastricht, The Netherlands
Antitachycardia Pacing: Clinical Considerations

PARVIN C. DOROSTKAR, MD
Lecturer in Pediatric Cardiology, University of Michigan Medical School, Ann Arbor, Michigan
Pediatric Pacing

JAMES L. DUNCAN, MS
Director, Clinical Engineering, Siemens Pacesetter, Inc., Sylmar, California
Activity-Sensing, Rate-Adaptive Pacemakers

KENNETH A. ELLENBOGEN, MD
Associate Professor of Internal Medicine (Cardiology), and Clinical Assistant Professor of Surgery, Medical College of Virginia; Director, Clinical Electrophysiology Laboratory, Medical College of Virginia and McGuire Veterans Affairs Medical Center, Richmond, Virginia
Sensing; Atrioventricular Conduction System Disease; Special Clinical Applications and Newer Indications for Cardiac Pacing; Pacemaker Syndrome

ANDREW E. EPSTEIN, MD
Professor of Medicine, Division of Cardiovascular Disease, University of Alabama School of Medicine, University of Alabama at Birmingham, Birmingham, Alabama
Pacemaker-Defibrillator Interactions

NEAL E. FEARNOT, PhD
Adjunct Assistant Professor of Institute for Interdisciplinary Engineering Studies, Hillenbrand Biomedical Engineering Center, Purdue University, West Lafayette, Indiana
Temperature-Controlled Rate-Adaptive Pacing

RICHARD N. FOGOROS, MD
Associate Professor of Medicine, Medical College of Pennsylvania, Philadelphia, Pennsylvania; Director, Clinical Electrophysiology, Allegheny General Hospital, Pittsburgh, Pennsylvania
Clinical Experience with Antitachycardia Pacing

FETNAT M. FOUAD-TARAZI, MD
Associate Clinical Professor of Internal Medicine, Case Western Reserve University; Head, Research Cardiac Function Laboratory, Department of Cardiology, The Cleveland Clinic Foundation, Cleveland, Ohio
Carotid Sinus Hypersensitivity and Neurally Mediated Syncope

SEYMOUR FURMAN, MD
Professor of Surgery and Medicine, Albert Einstein College of Medicine; Attending, Cardiothoracic Surgery, Montefiore Medical Center, New York, New York
Foreword

NORA GOLDSCHLAGER, MD
Professor of Clinical Medicine, University of California, San Francisco, School of Medicine; Director, Coronary Care Unit, ECG Laboratory and Pacemaker Clinic, San Francisco General Hospital, San Francisco, California
Follow-Up of the Paced Outpatient

J. WARREN HARTHORNE, MD, FACC
Associate Professor of Medicine, Harvard Medical School; Director of Cardiac Pacemaker Laboratory, Massachusetts General Hospital, Boston, Massachusetts
Programmers for Cardiac Pacemakers

DAVID L. HAYES, MD
Associate Professor of Medicine, Mayo Medical School; Consultant, Cardiovascular Disease and Internal Medicine, and Director of Pacemaker Services, Mayo Clinic; Staff, Saint Mary's Hospital, Rochester Methodist Hospital, Rochester, Minnesota
Evaluation of Pacemaker Malfunction

JAN-PIETER HEEMELS, MS
Manager, Advanced Brady Development, Cardiac Pacemakers, Inc., St. Paul, Minnesota
Accelerometers

JOHN R. HELLAND, BS
Director, Leads Development, InControl, Inc., Redmond, Washington
Engineering and Clinical Aspects of Pacing Leads

JEFFREY R. IRELAND, BSEE
Product Development Manager, New Indications, Medtronic, Inc., Minneapolis, Minnesota
Pulse Generator Circuitry

FREDRICK J. JAEGER, DO
Assistant Staff, Department of Cardiology, The Cleveland Clinic Foundation, Cleveland, Ohio
Carotid Sinus Hypersensitivity and Neurally Mediated Syncope

DENISE L. JANOSIK, MD, FACC
Associate Professor of Medicine, Saint Louis University School of Medicine; Director, Electrophysiology and Pacemaker Services, Saint Louis University Medical Center, St. Louis, Missouri
Basic Physiology of Cardiac Pacing

DAVID T. KAWANISHI, MD
Associate Professor of Medicine, University of Southern California School of Medicine; Director, Cardiac Catheterization Laboratory, Los Angeles County and USC Medical Center; Director, Griffith Laboratories, Los Angeles, California
AV Node–His–Purkinje System Disease: AV Block (Acute)

G. NEAL KAY, MD
Director, Clinical Electrophysiology Section, Division of Cardiology, University of Alabama at Birmingham, Birmingham, Alabama
Artificial Electrical Cardiac Stimulation; Sensing; Pulse Generator Circuitry; Rate-Modulated Pacing Controlled by Mixed Venous Oxygen Saturation; Rate-Adaptive Pacing Based on Impedance-Derived Minute Ventilation

STEVEN P. KUTALEK, MD
Associate Professor of Medicine and Pharmacology, Hahnemann University School of Medicine; Director, Cardiac Electrophysiology, Hahnemann University Hospital, Philadelphia, Pennsylvania
Approach to Generator Change

ARTHUR J. LABOVITZ, MD, FACC
Professor of Medicine, Saint Louis University School of Medicine; Director, Echocardiography Laboratory and Noninvasive Hemodynamics, Saint Louis University Health Sciences Center, St. Louis, Missouri
Basic Physiology of Cardiac Pacing

CHU-PAK LAU, MD
Reader in Medicine and Chief, Division of Cardiology, Department of Medicine, University of Hong Kong, Queen Mary Hospital, Hong Kong
Overview of Ideal Sensor Characteristics

PAUL A. LEVINE, MD
Clinical Professor of Medicine, Loma Linda University School of Medicine, Loma Linda, California; Clinical Associate Professor of Medicine, University of California, Los Angeles, School of Medicine, Los Angeles, California; Staff Cardiologist, Loma Linda University Medical Center, Loma Linda, California; Consultant Cardiologist, Olive View Medical Center, Sylmar, California, and Veterans Administration Hospital, Sepulveda, California
Pacemaker Diagnostics: Measured Data, Event Marker, Electrogram, and Event Counter Telemetry

CHARLES J. LOVE, MD
Assistant Professor of Clinical Medicine, Ohio State University College of Medicine; Director, Pacemaker Services, Ohio State University Medical Center, Columbus, Ohio
Evaluation of Pacemaker Malfunction

PAUL LUDMER, MD, FACC
Clinical Instructor, University of California, San Francisco, School of Medicine, San Francisco, California; Codirector, East Bay Arrhythmia and Electrophysiology Center, Oakland, California, and Summit, Mt. Diablo, and John Muir Medical Centers, Alameda and Contra Costa Counties, California
Follow-Up of the Paced Outpatient

JAMES D. MALONEY, MD
Professor of Medicine, Baylor College of Medicine; Director, Center for Cardiac Arrhythmia Services and Electrophysiology, Baylor College of Medicine, The Methodist Hospital, Ben Taub General Hospital, Veterans Affairs Medical Center, Houston, Texas
Rate-Adaptive Pacing Based on Impedance-Derived Minute Ventilation

J. MARCH MAQUILAN, MD
Clinical Senior Instructor, Hahnemann University School of Medicine; Attending Cardiothoracic Surgeon, Hahnemann University Hospital, Philadelphia, Pennsylvania
Approach to Generator Change

H. TOBY MARKOWITZ, BSEE
Senior Scientist, Technical Fellow, Medtronic, Inc., Minneapolis, Minnesota
Pacemaker Diagnostics: Measured Data, Event Marker, Electrogram, and Event Counter Telemetry

JAY O. MILLERHAGEN, MS
Director, Bradycardia Marketing, Cardiac Pacemakers, Inc., St. Paul, Minnesota
Accelerometers

HARRY G. MOND, MD, FRACP, FACC
Physician, Clinical Tutor, University of Melbourne; Physician to Pacemaker Clinic, Royal Melbourne Hospital, Melbourne, Victoria, Australia
Engineering and Clinical Aspects of Pacing Leads

TIBOR NAPPHOLZ, BSc, BE
Vice President of Strategic Research, Telectronics, Englewood, Colorado
Rate-Adaptive Pacing Based on Impedance-Derived Minute Ventilation

SUSAN O'DONOGHUE, MD
Associate Director, Cardiac Arrhythmia Center, Washington Hospital Center, Washington, District of Columbia
The Use of Intracardiac Impedance-Based Indicators to Optimize Pacing Rate

LUIS E. PADULA, MD
Cardiology Fellow, Hartford Hospital, University of Connecticut School of Medicine, Hartford, Connecticut
Programmers for Cardiac Pacemakers

VICTOR PARSONNET, MD
Clinical Professor of Surgery, University of Medicine and Dentistry of New Jersey; Director of Surgery and Director of Pacemaker Center, Newark Beth Israel Medical Center, Newark, New Jersey
Pacemaker and Defibrillator Codes

E. J. PERRINS, BSc, MB, FRCP, FACC
Consultant Cardiologist, Leeds General Infirmary, Leeds, England, United Kingdom
Clinical Trials and Experience

EDWARD V. PLATIA, MD
George Washington University School of Medicine and Health Sciences; Director, Cardiac Arrhythmia Center, Washington Hospital Center, Washington, District of Columbia
The Use of Intracardiac Impedance-Based Indicators to Optimize Pacing Rate

SHAHBUDIN H. RAHIMTOOLA, MB, FRCP
Distinguished Professor; George C. Griffith Professor of Cardiology; Chairman, Griffith Center; Professor of Medicine, University of Southern California; Chief Physician I, Los Angeles County and USC Medical Center, Los Angeles, California
AV Node–His–Purkinje System Disease: AV Block (Acute)

DWIGHT W. REYNOLDS, MD
Professor of Medicine, and Director, Cardiology Fellowship Training Program, University of Oklahoma College of Medicine; Vice Chief, Cardiovascular Section; Director, Pacemaker Services, Interim Director, Cardiac Catheterization Laboratory, University Hospital, Oklahoma City, Oklahoma
Permanent Pacemaker Implantation

ANTHONY F. RICKARDS, FRCP, FESC, FACC
Senior Lecturer, Cardiothoracic Institute, University of London; Consultant Cardiologist, Royal Brompton National Heart and Lung Hospital, University of London, London, England, United Kindgom
The Evoked QT Interval

RODNEY SALO, MSc
Corporate Scientific Fellow, Cardiac Pacemakers, Inc., St. Paul, Minnesota
The Use of Intracardiac Impedance-Based Indicators to Optimize Pacing Rate

RICHARD SANDERS, MS
Vice President, Clinical Engineering, Intermedics, Inc., Angleton, Texas
Pacemaker Diagnostics: Measured Data, Event Marker, Electrogram, and Event Counter Telemetry

CRAIG L. SCHMIDT, PhD
Manager, Brady Battery Research and Development, Medtronic, Inc., Brooklyn Center, Minnesota
Power Sources for Implantable Pacemakers

MARK H. SCHOENFELD, MD, FACC
Associate Clinical Professor of Medicine, Yale University School of Medicine; Director, Cardiac Electrophysiology and Pacer Laboratory, Hospital of St. Raphael, New Haven, Connecticut
Programmers for Cardiac Pacemakers

T. DUNCAN SELLERS, MD
Staff, Electrophysiology, Memorial Hospital, Colorado Springs, Colorado
Temperature-Controlled Rate-Adaptive Pacing

GERALD A. SERWER, MD
Associate Professor of Pediatrics, University of Michigan Medical School; Director of Pediatric Pacing Service, C. S. Mott Children's Hospital at University of Michigan Medical Center, Ann Arbor, Michigan
Pediatric Pacing

MITCHELL J. SHEIN, MS
Electrical Engineer, Office of Device Evaluation, Pacing and Electrophysiological Device Branch, U.S. Food and Drug Administration, Rockville, Maryland
Pacing: FDA and the Regulatory Environment

RICHARD B. SHEPARD, MD
Professor of Surgery, University of Alabama School of Medicine, University of Alabama at Birmingham; Surgeon, Division of Cardiothoracic Surgery, University of Alabama Hospital, Birmingham, Alabama
Power Sources for Implantable Pacemakers

IGOR SINGER, MBBS, FRACP, FACP, FACC, FACA
Associate Professor of Medicine, University of Louisville School of Medicine; Chief, Arrhythmia Service, and Director, Electrophysiology and Pacing, University of Louisville Hospital, Louisville, Kentucky
Evoked Potentials as a Sensor for Rate-Adaptive Pacing

PAUL M. SKARSTAD, PhD
Director, Components Research and Development, Medtronic, Inc., Minneapolis, Minnesota
Power Sources for Implantable Pacemakers

HEIDI J. SMITH, PhD
Clinical Research and Medical Education Specialist, MED Institute, West Lafayette, Indiana
Temperature-Controlled Rate-Adaptive Pacing

BRUCE S. STAMBLER, MD
Assistant Professor of Medicine, Virginia Commonwealth University, Medical College of Virginia; Staff, Medical College of Virginia Hospital, McGuire Veterans Affairs Medical Center, Richmond, Virginia
Pacemaker Syndrome

KENNETH B. STOKES, BCHEM
Elk River, Minnesota
Artificial Electrical Cardiac Stimulation

NEIL F. STRATHMORE, MBBS, FRACP
Clinical Instructor, University of Melbourne; Cardiologist, Royal Melbourne Hospital, Melbourne, Victoria, Australia
Interference in Cardiac Pacemakers

RICHARD SUTTON, DScMED, FRCP, FACC, FESC
Consultant Cardiologist and Director of Cardiac Pacing and Electrophysiology, Royal Brompton National Heart and Lung Hospital, University of London, London, England, United Kingdom
Sinus Node Disease

DARREL F. UNTEREKER, PHD
Director of Technology, Medtronic, Inc., Minneapolis, Minnesota
Power Sources for Implantable Pacemakers

HEIN J. J. WELLENS, MD
Professor and Chairman, Department of Cardiology, Academic Hospital Maastricht, Maastricht, The Netherlands
Antitachycardia Pacing: Clinical Considerations

J. MARCUS WHARTON, MD
Associate Professor of Medicine, Duke University School of Medicine; Director, Clinical Cardiac Electrophysiology, Duke University Medical Center, Durham, North Carolina
Atrioventricular Conduction System Disease

BRUCE L. WILKOFF, MD
Associate Professor of Medicine, Ohio State University, Columbus, Ohio; Director of Cardiac Pacing and Tachyarrhythmia Devices, Director of Cardiovascular Computing Services, The Cleveland Clinic Foundation, Cleveland, Ohio
Cardiac Chronotropic Responsiveness; Pacemaker-Defibrillator Interactions

MARK A. WOOD, MD
Assistant Professor of Medicine, Virginia Commonwealth University, Medical College of Virginia; Cardiac Electrophysiology Laboratories, Medical College of Virginia and McGuire Veterans Affairs Medical Center, Richmond, Virginia
Temporary Cardiac Pacing

RAYMOND YEE, MD, FRCPC, FACC
Associate Professor of Medicine, University of Western Ontario Faculty of Medicine; Director, Arrhythmia Monitoring Unit, University Hospital, London, Ontario, Canada
Rate-Adaptive Pacing Controlled by Dynamic Right Ventricular Pressure (dP/dtmax)

FOREWORD

Medical books have different objectives. Some are handbooks, crammed with compressed but practical information, often only about clinical management. Others are intended to be tools for house staff in meeting the daily needs of patient care, while still others are brief guides to clinical management. Some are encyclopedic, intending to cover every known aspect of a discipline. Ellenbogen, Kay, and Wilkoff have written and edited a volume of the last category. It is an encyclopedia of the modern science and craft of cardiac pacing, basic and clinical. Little, if anything, that is of present interest in the large and rapidly growing field of clinical cardiac pacing for bradyarrhythmias has been omitted from this volume. This book may be the first to include a chapter on regulatory events in cardiac pacing. Not only is such a perspective valuable for manufacturers, industry scientists, and physicians and administrators, but also it demonstrates the growing importance of regulatory efforts and the participation of the profession, the industry, and the public in the development and introduction of modern implantable devices. Issues involving the interaction between a pacemaker and the implantable cardioverter defibrillator have been covered. In adhering substantially to cardiac pacing for bradycardia management, the authors have provided the most extensive exposition now available of what is known about this field.

This is a massive undertaking involving many capable authors. It is the result of a writing compilation by physicians and surgeons, clinical electrophysiologists, and, certainly not least, those industry scientists who have been, in large measure, creators of the modern technology of cardiac pacing. Each topic is presented by scholars in the field, and each presentation is likely to be a definitive statement about the topic. A benefit of that approach is that each of the contributing authors is allowed sufficient space to present the material that he or she has developed over a career, providing the reader with much that should be known about a topic, located in a single place. The references listed for each chapter are exhaustive, so the reader will have access to much of the supporting material that has been produced in recent years. The broad coverage that this format allows is demonstrated repeatedly in the text. An example is Chapter 26, Cardiac Chronotropic Responsiveness, which contains a major discussion of the entire field of exercise testing. In this chapter, the specific aspects of exercise testing to program a pacemaker sensor are presented within the broader context of what chronotropic responsiveness is normal and what is abnormal, and how to make that determination and distinction. The frequently published single- or double-chapter overview of cardiac pacing in textbooks of cardiology and medicine pale to inconsequence in comparison with this volume. The reader, even of the table of contents, will know that he or she can become a scholar by reading portions of this book. The reader of the table of contents will soon realize how much there was of which he or she was unaware. It is unlikely that anyone will read this book cover to cover, much more likely that specific chapters will be read when necessary and even that portions of chapters will be read when specific information is needed. The nature of this kind or writing and publishing effort is that a full presentation of a field is made so that the reader can select what is needed.

The encyclopedia conveys volumes about the evolution of the discipline itself. The first books about cardiac pacing were published during the 1970s. One- or two-hundred pages were then adequate. So slender a volume can no longer suffice. Even with this major volume, related topics of electrical stimulation, such as the implantable defibrillator for ventricular tachyarrhythmias and the fledgling field of atrial defibrillation, are covered only at their margins rather than in depth. This degree of expansion directs the growth of the parent discipline and the attendant scholarship required.

This volume is not only a book but also an indication of the maturation of the emerging specialty of electrical cardiac stimulation in one of its major limbs, bradycardia management. As the younger limb, tachycardia management, evolves, encyclopedias such as this will indicate the state of that maturity.

SEYMOUR FURMAN, MD

PREFACE

Cardiac pacing produced its greatest impact by treating the most profound cardiac arrhythmia, asystole. Since the first pacing system was implanted by Senning and Elmqvist in Sweden in 1958, the technology, indications, and physiology of cardiac pacing have dramatically evolved to the point where 300,000 cardiac pacemakers are implanted around the world each year. Over the intervening 37 years, cardiac pacing has become an everyday therapeutic option for millions of patients.

There are many consumers of pacemaker technology in addition to the patient. Besides pacemaker physicians, cardiologists, surgeons, internists, and family physicians examine and care for patients with pacemakers and need to evaluate the potential impact of pacing therapy on various medical conditions and treatments. In addition, many hospital technical and nursing personnel are exposed to pacemaker patients. The advances in the science and art of pacing have great importance for all personnel caring for patients with implanted pacemakers.

Cardiac pacing is an interdisciplinary field. Physicians primarily responsible for pacemaker therapy include not only cardiologists but also internists, cardiothoracic surgeons, vascular surgeons, general surgeons, and family practitioners. A wide variety of other personnel are involved in delivering care to pacemaker patients, including nurses, cardiovascular technicians, clinical engineers, and fellows in training. In addition to the diverse backgrounds of all these individuals caring for pacemaker patients, the practice of cardiac pacing has changed dramatically over the last 37 years. New advances in technology have aided the development of multi-programmable pacemakers, physiologic dual-chamber pacemakers, rate-responsive pacing, implantable defibrillators, antitachycardia pacemakers, new types of pacemaker leads, and new methods for extracting pacing leads.

The evolution of cardiac pacing has inspired the publishing of subspecialty journals, including PACE, StimuCoeur, and the European Journal of Cardiac Pacing and Electrophysiology, as well as several monographs and books. In addition, a variety of national and international societies of pacing and electrophysiology have been formed over the last two decades to promote the practice of clinical cardiac pacing. However, we believe that a comprehensive and contemporary exposition of the technical and clinical aspects of cardiac pacing was missing.

In order to meet the needs of clinicians, scientists, engineers, nurses, and technicians, a book that covers this vast subject in a comprehensive fashion and also provides practical information as well as relevant engineering and scientific information is necessary. We are excited about presenting the scientific basis for the practical and clinically useful axioms we rely on in our daily practice. To accomplish this task, we looked for experts in the field of cardiac pacing who could make their subject comprehensible and clinically relevant without ignoring its scientific or engineering principles. This often led to combining the talents of renowned clinicians with scientists and engineers from the pacing industry. Second, we wanted to have a truly comprehensive textbook, one that a surgeon, cardiovascular electrophysiologist, radiologist, or pediatric cardiologist could look to as a reference tool or as a guide to the daily care of pacemaker patients. In particular, we sought to make sure that each chapter was thorough, up to date, and well illustrated. The chapters are referenced extensively, allowing readers at any level to further their knowledge of any specific topic.

We gratefully acknowledge the invaluable assistance and encouragement of Richard Zorab, Editorial Manager, from W.B. Saunders Company for keeping us on track. Our colleagues at the Medical College of Virginia, The Cleveland Clinic Foundation, and the University of Alabama deserve kudos for their patience and for shouldering extra work to allow us to get our chapters and editing finished on time. The contributors to this text labored extensively, often combining the efforts of scientists, engineers, and physicians located in separate institutions, cities, and continents. Our medical media departments deserve a great deal of credit for the wonderful jobs they did with the illustrations. Finally, our secretaries Margaret Burchfield (Birmingham), Jody Karabinus (Cleveland), and Vera Wilkerson (Richmond) provided much of the effort that allowed us to complete this task.

It is hoped that this textbook will stand as a valuable tool for daily clinical decisions, reference, research, and the teaching of the many different individuals who care for pacemaker patients. We hope that this book proves to be a resource to all for many years to come.

KENNETH A. ELLENBOGEN

G. NEAL KAY

BRUCE L. WILKOFF

CONTENTS

BASIC CONCEPTS OF CARDIAC PACING

CHAPTER 1

ARTIFICIAL ELECTRIC CARDIAC STIMULATION

Kenneth B. Stokes
G. Neal Kay

The fundamental basis for cardiac pacing is myocardial stimulation, a complex biophysical process. An understanding of the factors that influence myocardial stimulation is important for all clinicians involved in the care of patients with implantable pacemakers. Thus, although this chapter focusing on artificial electrostimulation includes contributions from such diverse disciplines as cellular biology, cardiovascular physiology, electrode physics and chemistry, electrical and mechanical engineering, pharmacology, and pathology, the clinical relevance of these fields to patient care is emphasized. Electrostimulation is reviewed first on the cellular level. Next, the design and function of pacing electrodes is discussed, including the principles of strength-duration relationships and strength-interval relationships, constant-current versus constant-voltage pacing, anodal versus cathodal stimulation, unipolar versus bipolar stimulation, pacing impedance, pharmacologic and metabolic effects on stimulation threshold, and the practical aspects of pacemaker programming. Finally, the clinical relevance of each of these fundamental factors is discussed in the context of managing patients with implanted pacemakers.

Cellular Aspects of Myocardial Stimulation

THE PHOSPHOLIPID BIMEMBRANE

The property of biologic tissues such as nerve and muscle of responding to a stimulus with a self-regenerating electric response that is out of proportion to the strength of the stimulus is known as excitability.[1] Excitable tissues are characterized by a separation of charge across the cell membrane. Thus, it is the cell membrane that determines the fundamental property of excitability of the cardiac myocyte. The cell membrane of myocytes is composed principally of phospholipids, cholesterol, and proteins.[2] The membrane phospholipids have a charged polar headgroup and two long hydrocarbon chains arranged as shown in Figure 1–1. The cell membrane is arranged as two layers of phospholipids with their hydrophobic aliphatic chains oriented toward the center and their polar headgroup regions toward the peripheral, aqueous phase. Because the membrane is composed of two layers, the polar regions of the phospholipids interface with the polar aqueous environments inside and outside the cell. The lipid-soluble hydrocarbon chains are forced away from the aqueous phase to form a nonpolar interior. The close packing of the phospholipid molecules functions as a barrier, preventing the passive diffusion of charged ions and molecules through the membrane. The high density of charged polar headgroups determines the dielectric properties of the membrane. This allows a large voltage gradient to exist across the membrane, which is essential for maintenance of the myocyte resting potential and the property of excitability.

DETERMINANTS OF THE RESTING TRANSMEMBRANE POTENTIAL

There are relatively large gradients of individual ion concentrations across the cardiac cell membrane.[3] The extracellular/intracellular gradient for Na^+ is approximately 145 mM/10 mM, while that for K^+ is about 4.5 mM/140 mM. In the absence of a cell membrane, each cation moves rapidly in a direction determined by the concentration gradient. The diffusion force tending to move K^+ out of and Na^+ into the cell is proportional to their respective concentration gradients. The potential energy attributable to the diffusion force (PE_d) tending to move K^+ out of the cell is given by

Eq 1 $PE_d = RT \, ln \, [K^+]_i/[K^+]_o$

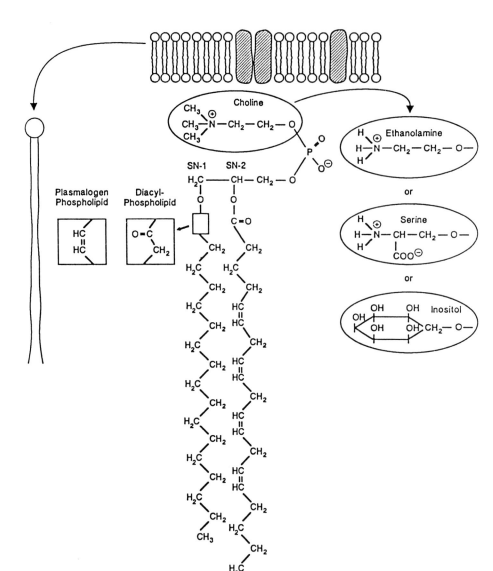

FIGURE 1–1. Sarcolemma structure and phospholipid composition. The lipid bilayer containing two membrane proteins is shown at the top of the figure. The detailed structure of the phospholipids is shown below. All of the aliphatic hydrocarbon groups on the sn-2 position are fatty acids that are covalently bound in the form of esters. The aliphatic hydrocarbon groups at the sn-1 position include either O-acyl esters or vinyl ethers. (From Creer MH, Dabmeyer DJ, Corr PB: Amphipathic lipid metabolites and arrhythmias during myocardial ischemia. *In* Zipes DP, Jalife J [eds]: Cardiac Electrophysiology: From Cell to Bedside. Philadelphia, WB Saunders, 1990, pp 417–432.)

where R is the gas constant, T is the absolute temperature, *ln* is the natural logarithm, $[K^+]_i$ is the concentration of potassium ion inside the cell, and $[K^+]_o$ is the concentration of potassium ion outside the cell. Thus, if the ratio of $[K^+]$ inside the cell to $[K^+]$ outside the cell is large, the potential energy across the membrane will increase. The separation of charged ions from the inside to the outside of the cell results in an electric potential across the membrane. In resting cardiac cells, the intracellular cytoplasm has a measured negative potential of about 90 mV compared to the extracellular fluid. This electric force tends to move positively charged ions, such as K^+ and Na^+, to the inside of the cell and negatively charged ions, such as chloride (Cl^-), to the outside of the cell in proportion to the potential gradient. The potential energy attributable to the electric force (PE_e) tending to move K^+ into the cell is expressed by

Eq 2 $PE_e = zFV_m$

where z is the valence (or the number of positive or negative electronic charges) of the ion, F is the Faraday constant

(96,500 coulombs(C)/equivalent), and V_m is the transmembrane potential difference (measured in millivolts). During equilibrium, the total of the potential energies due to diffusion and electric forces is zero, and no net ionic movement occurs. Thus, the sum of equations 1 and 2 set to zero yields the Nernst equation, which describes the potential that must exist for K^+ to be in equilibrium across the membrane of a resting cardiac cell:

Eq 3 $V_m(K^+) = -26.7 \; ln \; [K^+]_i/[K^+]_o$

or, in more familiar $\log_{10}$ terms, $V_m(K^+) = -61.5 \log [K^+]_i/[K^+]_o$. Using known values for intracellular and extracellular K^+, $V_m(K^+) = -90$ mV. When equation 3 is solved using Na^+ concentrations, a $V_m(Na^+)$ of $+50$ mV is obtained. Thus, it is the equilibrium potential of potassium ion (not sodium ion) that is the major factor responsible for the resting transmembrane potential. This suggests that the resting membrane is more permeable to K^+ than to Na^+. The Goldman constant field equation (modified by Hodgkin and Katz) describes how these and other ions contribute to V_m.[4]

Eq 4 $V_m =$

$$\frac{-RT}{F} \ln \frac{P_{K+}[K^+]_i + P_{Na+}[Na^+]_i + P_{Cl-}[Cl^-]_o + \ldots}{P_{K+}[K^+]_o + P_{Na+}[Na^+]_o + P_{Cl-}[Cl^-]_i + \ldots}$$

P_{K+}, P_{Na+}, and P_{Cl-} are the cell membrane permeabilities for the respective ions. Using physiologic concentrations, this equation yields a transmembrane potential of -90 mV (the equilibrium potential for K^+). Equation 4 describes how resting potentials vary as sodium and potassium ion concentrations are changed. Since there is a passive leak of charged ions through pores in the membrane, the resting potential is maintained by two active transport mechanisms that exchange Na^+ ions for K^+ and Ca^{2+} ions. The Na^+-K^+ ATPase "pump" moves 3 Na^+ ions out of the cell in exchange for 2 K^+ ions moved into the cell.[5-7] The basic unit of the Na^+-K^+ ATPase protein (pump) consists of one alpha and one beta subunit. The alpha subunit, with 1016 amino acids, is large, spanning the entire membrane, whereas the beta subunit is a smaller glycoprotein. There appear to be about 1000 pump sites per square micron of cardiac cell membrane. The fully activated pump cycles about 50 to 70 times per second (an interval of 15 to 20 msec/cycle). Similarly, the Na^+-Ca^{2+} pump moves 3 Na^+ ions out of the cell in exchange for 1 Ca^{2+} ion.[8, 9] Thus, both transport mechanisms result in the *net* movement of one positive charge out of the cell, producing polarization across the membrane. The function of both exchange mechanisms is dependent on the expenditure of energy in the form of high-energy phosphates and is susceptible to interruptions in aerobic cellular metabolism (such as occur during ischemia).

Propagation of an Electric Stimulus

When an electric current is applied to a cardiac cell membrane, the current propagates away from the site of the stimulus. This propagation of the stimulus occurs both passively (analogous to conduction of current along a low-resistance wire) and actively (with a self-regenerating wave of action potentials that are triggered within the myocardium). Both passive and active modes of propagation are important electric properties of the myocardium.

CABLE THEORY OF PASSIVE STIMULUS PROPAGATION

A cardiac myocyte can be thought of as a one-dimensional cable (Fig. 1–2).[10] The membrane can be conceptualized as a simplified circuit composed of a capacitor (with the ability to store charge) and a resistor (opposing the flow of current) in parallel. When a constant-current stimulus is applied at a site along the membrane, most of the charge initially flows into the capacitor. Eventually, the charge on the capacitor reaches a steady level. As current continues to be applied, it flows through the resistors across the membrane (R_m) and through the inside of the cell (R_i). In a simple resistance-capacitance circuit two constants determine passive conduction, the *time constant* and the *length constant*. In this model of passive electrotonic membrane conductance, the capacitor is charged

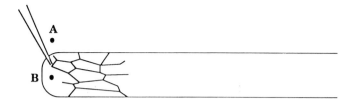

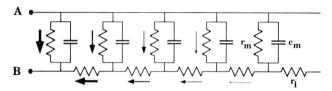

FIGURE 1–2. Equivalent circuit for a single fiber composed of electrically coupled single cells placed in an electrically conductive medium. A constant current is made to flow from A to B through the surface membrane and along the fiber core. Small voltage changes are produced so as to assure constant values of the resistors. (From Weidmann S: Passive properties of cardiac fibers. *In* Rosen MR, Jause MJ, Wit AL [eds]: Cardiac Electrophysiology: A Textbook. Mt. Kisco, NY, Futura, 1990, pp 29–35.)

along an exponential time course, 64% of the final charge being reached after time constant (T), assuming that there is no current flowing in the opposite direction. The change in voltage (V) across the membrane as a function of distance (X) will be:

Eq 5 $V_x = V_{x=0}(e^{-x/a})$

where a is the length constant of the fiber, the distance over which voltage drops by a factor of e, or about 37% of its original value at the site of stimulation. If r_m is the membrane resistance times unit length (ohm-cm) and r_i is the longitudinal resistance per unit length (ohm/cm), then the length constant (a) is defined by:

Eq 6 $a = \sqrt{\dfrac{r_m}{r_i}}$

In a cable, total membrane charge still changes exponentially, but the region near the site of the applied stimulus (X = 0) does so more quickly, and the region beyond this site (X = a) more slowly. The specific membrane capacity (C_m) is:

Eq 7 $C_m(F/cm^2) = T (sec)/R_m(ohm\text{-}cm^2)$

where R_m is the specific membrane resistance. A single Purkinje fiber typically has an internal resistance 2 to 3 times greater than that of blood. The specific membrane resistance of a Purkinje fiber is on the order of 10^4 ohm-cm^2. The time constant of the surface membrane is on the order of 10 msec and the membrane capacity is about 1 microfarad (μF)/cm^2.[11]

When a current is made to flow through a row of several different cells rather than through a single fiber, specialized regions of the membrane called gap junctions or intercalated discs provide low-resistance communication between cells. One square centimeter of junctional area has a resistance of approximately 0.1 ohm.[12, 13] Thus, in *normal* myocardium, these cell-to-cell contacts offer negligible resistance, the major part of the resistance being found in the cellular cytoplasm. Under pathologic conditions such as hypoxia or ischemia, however, the gap junctions become a major hindrance to axial current flow, preventing leakage of current to injured cells.[14, 15]

Active Electric Propagation in the Heart

ION CHANNELS

Artificial lipid membranes in their pure form are electric insulators. It is the presence of specialized protein molecules in the membrane that allows it to be conductive.[16, 17] These proteins determine the metabolic characteristics of the membrane and provide both active and passive transport of ions and molecules. The membrane proteins have numerous functions, including those of ion channels and signal transducers. The concept of ion channels was proposed in the early 1950s by Hodgkin and Huxley.[1] However, it was not until the introduction of the patch clamp technique by Neher and Sakmann in 1976 that the properties of these channels could be studied directly.[18, 19] Today it is known that there are basically two types of ion channels, distinguished by the factors that control whether the channel is in the open or closed configuration. For example, ion channels at muscle fiber endplates are *chemically* gated by specific transmitters (Fig. 1–3). The opening of these channels is triggered by the binding of acetylcholine, and their closing is induced by its unbinding. In neuronal axons conduction is mediated by faster *voltage*-gated channels. These channels respond to differences in electric potential across the membrane (between the inside and outside of the cell). Voltage-gated channels for sodium, potassium, and calcium appear to operate in similar ways, sharing many of the same structural features.

In addition, each type of channel can be subdivided into several subtypes with different conductive or gating properties.

Voltage-gated channels open in response to an applied potential. The source of this voltage can be an action potential propagated from an adjacent cell or the electric field of an artificial pacemaker. If depolarization of the membrane exceeds a threshold voltage, an action potential is triggered, resulting in a complex cascade of ionic currents flowing across the membrane into and out of the cell. As a result of this flow of charge across the membrane, the potential gradient across the membrane (Fig. 1–4) changes in a characteristic pattern of events that produce the cardiac action potential.

Selective membrane-bound proteins (ion channels) determine the passive transmembrane flux of an individual ion species. The transmembrane currents determine or influence cellular polarization at rest, action potential depolarization and repolarization, conduction, excitation-contraction coupling, and myofibril contraction. The channels that regulate transmembrane conduction of Na^+ and Ca^{2+} are voltage gated. The sodium channel is a large protein molecule composed of approximately 1830 amino acids.[20] It contains four internally homologous repeating domains. These are thought to be arranged around a central water-filled pore that is lined with hydrophilic amino acids. It is estimated that there are 5 to 10 Na^+ channels per square micron of cell membrane. When a change in the membrane potential to approximately -70 to -60 mV (the threshold potential) occurs, four to six positively charged amino acids move across the membrane under an electric field to cause a change in the conformation of the channel proteins, resulting in opening of the channel. Once a single Na^+ channel changes to the open conformation, it is estimated that approximately 10^4 Na^+ ions enter the cell. On depolarization of the membrane, the Na^+ channels remain open for less than 1 msec. Following rapid de-

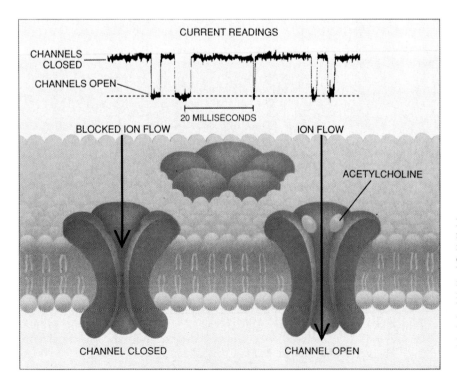

FIGURE 1–3. Receptor channels found at the neuromuscular endplate open in response to the transmitter acetylcholine. When no acetylcholine is present, effectively no current passes through a channel. When acetylcholine binds to the receptor, an elementary current of a few picoamperes flows. The measured durations of the current and the intervals between them vary because the interaction of acetylcholine molecules with the receptors is governed by probability. (From The patch clamp technique by E Neher and B Sakmann, March 1992. Copyright © 1992 by Scientific American, Inc. All rights reserved.)

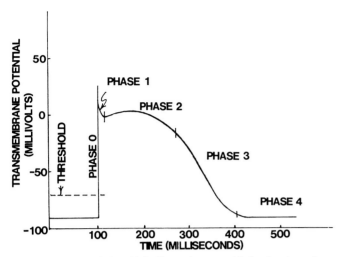

FIGURE 1–4. A typical Purkinje fiber action potential showing the various phases of depolarization and repolarization. In phase 0 (depolarization), Na⁺ rapidly enters the cell through fast channels. In phase 1, initial repolarization is primarily the result of activation of a transient outward K⁺ current and inactivation of the fast Na⁺ current. In phase 2 (plateau), the net current is very small, although the individual currents are about one order of magnitude larger. Phase 3 (final repolarization), in which the Na⁺-K⁺ pump brings the membrane potential to a stable point where inward and outward currents are again in balance, completes the cycle. (From Stokes K, Bornzin G: The electrode–biointerface (stimulation). *In* Barold S [ed]: Modern Cardiac Pacing. Mt. Kisco, NY, Futura, 1985, pp 33–78.)

applied stimulus. This abrupt change in the potential across the membrane is termed the *action potential.*[23] The cardiac action potential is an enormously complex event and consists of five phases.[24] These include phase 0, or rapid depolarization; phase 1, or initial rapid repolarization; phase 2, or the plateau phase; and phase 3, or rapid repolarization (see Fig. 1–4). Cells with spontaneous pacemaker activity are characterized by a phase of slow spontaneous depolarization of the membrane (phase 4) until the threshold potential is again reached and a new action potential is generated.

PHASE 0 (RAPID DEPOLARIZATION)

The upstroke of the action potential is triggered by a decrease in the potential gradient across the membrane to the threshold of -70 to -60 mV. On depolarization of the membrane to the less negative threshold voltage, the Na⁺ channels open, resulting in an influx of positively charged ions (the inward Na⁺ current) and a very rapid reversal of membrane polarity. The rate of depolarization in phase 0 ranges from 800 V/sec in Purkinje cells to 200 to 500 V/sec in atrial and ventricular myocytes. In these cells the inward Na⁺ current is primarily responsible for phase 0 of the action potential. In sinoatrial and AV nodal cells, in which the inward Ca²⁺ current predominates, the upstroke velocity of phase 0 is lower (20 to 50 V/sec).

PHASE 1 (INITIAL REPOLARIZATION)

Following voltage-dependent activation of the Na⁺ current in phase 0, the membrane potential rapidly changes from negative to positive. The increased conduction of Na⁺ is rapidly followed by voltage-dependent inactivation. The outward movement of K⁺ is a major contributor to the various repolarization phases. This process is very complex and has a number of discrete pathways.[25, 26] Most K⁺ currents demonstrate rectification, that is, decreased K⁺ conduction with depolarization. The K⁺ currents include the instantaneous inward rectifier K⁺ current, the outward (delayed) rectifier K⁺ current, the transient outward currents, and ATP-, Na⁺-, and acetylcholine-regulated K⁺ currents. The initial repolarization, however, is mainly the result of activation of a transient outward K⁺ current and inactivation of the fast inward Na⁺ current. The transient outward K⁺ current has two components. One component is voltage gated, and the other is activated by a local rise in Ca²⁺.[27]

PHASE 2 (PLATEAU PHASE)

The net current during the plateau phase is apparently very small, although the individual currents are about one order of magnitude larger.[28] There is a significant decrease in the K⁺ current. Among the inward currents are the slowly activating Na⁺ current, a Ca²⁺ current, and an Na⁺-Ca²⁺ exchange current. Outward currents include a slowly activating component of the transient (K⁺) current, a Cl⁻ current, a slowly activating K⁺ current, and the Na⁺-K⁺ electrogenic pump current. During phase 2 of the action potential the cardiac cell cannot be excited by an electric stimulus, regardless of its intensity.

polarization of the membrane, the Na⁺ channel again assumes the closed conformation. In addition to the Na⁺ channel, specialized proteins suspended in the cell membrane have different selectivities for K⁺, Ca²⁺, and Cl⁻ ions with markedly different time constants for activation and inactivation.

In contrast to Purkinje fibers, sinus and atrioventricular (AV) nodal cells are characterized by action potentials with slower rates of depolarization. In these structures, depolarization is primarily mediated by inward Ca²⁺ conduction through specialized Ca²⁺ channels. There are two types of Ca²⁺ channels in the mammalian heart, L- and T-type. The L-type channels are the major voltage-gated pathway for entry of Ca²⁺ into the myocyte, and they are heavily modulated by catecholamines.[21] The T-type channels contribute to spontaneous depolarization of the cell associated with automaticity (pacemaker currents). The pore of the Ca²⁺ channel has a functional diameter of approximately 0.6 nm, which is larger than the sodium channels (0.3 to 0.5 nm).[22] The selectivity for Ca²⁺ is very high, up to 10,000-fold greater than that for Na⁺ or K⁺. The key elements in this selectivity are high-affinity binding sites for Ca²⁺, positioned along a single file pore. "Elution" of a Ca²⁺ ion occurs when another Ca²⁺ ion enters and is selectively bound.

THE CARDIAC ACTION POTENTIAL

When the voltage gradient across the membrane of a myocyte decreases so that the inside of the cell becomes less negatively charged with respect to the outside of the cell, a critical voltage is reached (termed the threshold voltage) at which the cell membrane suddenly undergoes a further depolarization that is out of proportion to the intensity of the

PHASE 3 (FINAL REPOLARIZATION)

Deactivation of inward Na^+ and Ca^{2+} currents occurs faster than it does with the K^+ currents, favoring net repolarization of the membrane. When the membrane is sufficiently repolarized, an inward K^+ rectifier current is progressively activated, resulting in a regenerative increase in outward current and an increasing rate of repolarization. Repolarization is also accomplished by the function of the Na^+-K^+ ATPase pump. The membrane potential eventually becomes stable, so that inward and outward currents are again in balance, and the resting potential is reestablished. Between the end of the plateau phase and full repolarization the cell is partially refractory to electric stimulation. During this period, a greater stimulus intensity is required to generate an action potential than is needed following full recovery of the resting membrane potential.

PHASE 4 (AUTOMATICITY) AND THE CONDUCTION SYSTEM

It has been known for centuries that the heart can exhibit spontaneous contractions even when it is completely denervated. Leonardo da Vinci observed that the heart could "move by itself."[29] William Harvey reported that pieces of the heart could "contract and relax" separately.[30] However, not all parts of the heart possess the property of automaticity. In fact, cells in different areas of the heart have different transmembrane potentials, thresholds, and action potentials. Fast responses are characteristic of ordinary working ventricular muscle cells and His-Purkinje fibers (with resting membrane potentials of -70 to -90 mV with rapid conduction). Normal sinus and AV nodal cells have slow responses, with

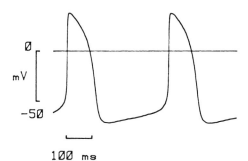

FIGURE 1–6. Spontaneous activity recorded in a single sinoatrial myocyte. The slow diastolic "pacemaker" depolarization extends from the maximum diastolic potential of -71 mV to the threshold for action potential onset, about -54 mV (ms = millisecond). (From DiFrancesco D: The hyperpolarization-activated current, I_f, and cardiac pacemaking. *In* Rosen MR, Jause ML, Wit AL [eds]: Cardiac Electrophysiology: A Textbook. Mt. Kisco, NY, Futura, 1990, pp 117–132.)

resting potentials of -40 to -70 mV and very slow conduction velocities. Automaticity is the property of certain cells that can initiate action potentials spontaneously. Many cells within the specialized conduction system have the potential for automaticity. Those cells or groups of cells with the fastest rate of spontaneous membrane depolarization during phase 4 are the first to reach threshold potential and initiate a propagated impulse. Thus, cells with the steepest slope of phase 4 become the heart's natural pacemakers. Ordinary working myocardial cells are usually not automatic. Normally, depolarization is initiated at the sinoatrial node (Fig. 1–5).[31, 32] Action potentials from an isolated sinoatrial node cell are shown in Figure 1–6.[33] Rather than maintaining a stable resting membrane potential, the repolarization of the action potential is followed by a slow depolarization from about -71 to -54 mV, at the threshold of initiation of another action potential. This slow, spontaneous depolarization drives cardiac automaticity. In the case of AV nodal cells, the fast upstroke is carried predominantly by an inward Ca^{2+} current. Repolarization is caused by delayed activation of the K^+ current. The balance of inward and outward currents determines the net "pacemaker" current and is finely regulated by both adrenergic and cholinergic neurotransmitters. In the presence of AV block or abnormal sinoatrial nodal function, AV junctional cells in the region of the proximal penetrating bundle usually assume the role of pacemaker at rates slower than that of the sinus node. In the absence of disease in the AV junction, the escape rhythm occurs with a frequency that is approximately 67% of the sinus rate.[34]

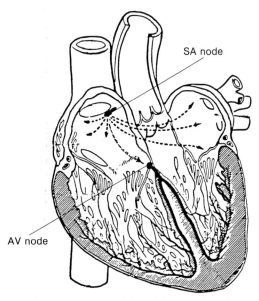

FIGURE 1–5. A schematic representation of the normal conduction system of the heart. The cycle begins at the sinoatrial node (SA), propagating a wave of depolarization across the atrium. As the stimulus enters the atrioventricular (AV) node, its conduction slows. This allows complete contraction of the atria before the impulse reaches the ventricles. As the impulse enters the His bundle, conduction velocity increases. The impulse is then transmitted through the left and right bundle branches and the Purkinje fibers throughout the right and left ventricular endocardial cells.

Artificial Induction of Self-Propagating Myocardial Currents

THEORIES OF ARTIFICIAL CARDIAC STIMULATION

For an electric stimulus to trigger a self-propagating wave of depolarization within the myocardium, an electric field of sufficient intensity must be applied between the two stimulating electrodes. There are two major theories about how an electric stimulus induces a self-propagating wavefront of depolarization within the myocardium. The *current density* theory maintains that the critical factor required to induce a regenerative wavefront of depolarization is the magnitude of current flowing through a given mass of myocardium between the stimulating electrodes. Thus, in this theory the stimulation threshold is a function of current density (A/cm³) in the excitable myocardium underlying the electrode.[35–38] The competing *electric field* theory holds that the critical factor affecting myocardial depolarization is the magnitude of the electric field (V/cm³ in viable tissue) that is induced in the myocardium beneath the stimulating electrode or between two electrodes.[39, 40] Ideally, these theories are related by Ohm's law:

Eq 8 $V = IR$

where V is the stimulus voltage, I is the current, and R is the total resistance to current flow. Thus, the greater the potential difference between two electrodes, the greater the current flow at the electrode-tissue interface. The total energy of a pacing stimulus is determined by the voltage and the current as well as by the duration of the stimulus:

Eq 9 $E = VI(t)$

where E is the stimulus energy, and t is the pulse duration. For a constant-voltage (CV) pulse generator, equation 9 can be expressed as:

Eq 10 $E = \dfrac{V^2 t}{R}$

The stimulation threshold of isolated cardiac myocytes has been shown to depend on their orientation within an electric field such that the threshold is lowest when the myocytes are oriented parallel to the field and highest when the axis of the myocytes is perpendicular to the field.[41] It is clear that myocardial stimulation may be induced by either anodal or cathodal stimulation, or both, though with somewhat different characteristics. Perhaps because of the absence of a generally accepted theory of electric stimulation, there is widespread confusion in the scientific literature about the measurement of stimulation threshold. Various investigators have used many different parameters to express stimulation threshold, including current (mA), potential (V), energy (microjoules [μC]), charge (microcoulombs), pulse width (msec), and voltage quantity (V-sec).[42–47] These controversies have been discussed in detail elsewhere and will not be resolved here.[48] For the purposes of this chapter, we will modify Furman's definition and state that stimulation threshold is *the minimum stimulus amplitude at any given pulse width required to consistently achieve myocardial depolarization outside the heart's refractory period.*[36] Thus, stimulation thresholds measured with a CV generator will be presented in volts and those of a constant-current (CI) generator will be presented in milliamperes.

Strength-Duration Relationships

CHRONAXIE, RHEOBASE, ENERGY, AND PULSE WIDTH THRESHOLDS

The intensity of an electric stimulus (measured in volts or milliamperes) that is required to capture the atrial or ventricular myocardium is dependent on the amount of time the

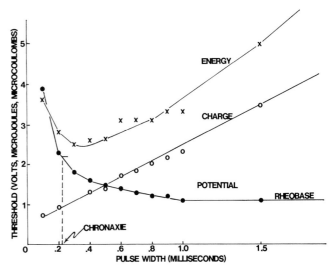

FIGURE 1–7. Relationships between chronic ventricular canine constant-voltage strength-duration curves expressed in terms of potential (V), charge (C), and energy (μJ) for a tined unipolar lead with an 8-mm² polished ring-tip electrode. Thresholds are measured at gain of capture. Rheobase is the current or voltage threshold to the right that is independent of pulse width. Chronaxie is the pulse width at twice rheobase. (From Stokes K, Bornzin G: The electrode–biointerface (stimulation). *In* Barold S [ed]: Modern Cardiac Pacing. Mt. Kisco, NY, Futura, 1985, pp 33–78.)

stimulus is applied, the pulse duration.[49, 50] This interaction of stimulus amplitude and pulse duration defines the strength-duration curve (Fig. 1–7). The voltage or current amplitude required for endocardial stimulation has an exponential relation to the pulse duration, with a relatively flat curve at pulse durations greater than 1 msec and a rapidly rising curve at pulse durations of less than 0.25 msec. Because of this fundamental property, a stimulus of very short pulse duration must be much more intense to capture the myocardium than a longer duration pulse. Conversely, increasing the pulse width more than 1 msec (along the flat portion of the curve) has little influence on the intensity of the stimulus that is required for capture. Thus, it is not acceptable to express the stimulation threshold accurately in terms of pulse amplitude without also defining pulse duration. The shape of the strength-duration curve is influenced by several factors, including the site of electric stimulation (transesophageal or endocardial), the type of stimulus used (constant-current versus constant-voltage), and the stimulation frequency.

In 1892, Hoorweg used a voltage source, a galvanometer, and low-leakage capacitors to conduct quantitative stimulation studies.[51] He found that the voltage at which a capacitor must be charged to cause a depolarization of nerves and muscles was an inverse function of capacitance:

Eq 11 $V(C) = aR + b/C$

where V(C) is the voltage (V) as a function of capacitance (C), R is resistance, and a and b are coefficients that vary with the specimen (tissue) tested. Hoorweg determined that there was one, and only one, specific capacitor for which energy at stimulation threshold was a minimum. He also determined that the threshold charge was a linear function "intersecting the y-axis above zero." It should be pointed out that Hoorweg apparently did not have the capability to measure thresholds at very short pulse widths because in reality the threshold charge increases toward infinity as the pulse width approaches zero. In 1901 Weiss tried to "make comparable the different methods of electrostimulation."[52] Building on Hoorweg's earlier work, he found a linear relationship between threshold charge and the duration of current flow. He called this relationship the "formule fondamentale," expressed as

Eq 12 $Q_{(t)} = \int^t I_t \, dt = at + b$

where $Q_{(t)}$ is the charge (Q) as a function of pulse width (t), I_t is the current during pulse width t, and a and b are coefficients depending on the specimen (type of tissue). Weiss also noted that the threshold energy varies as a function of the shape of the stimulus pulse while the quantity of electricity (charge) at threshold remains constant. In 1909, Lapique proposed giving the coefficients of the Weiss formula physiologic meanings.[53] He pointed out that at infinitely long pulse widths, there is a "fundamental threshold." He called this asymptote the *rheobase*. Thus, rheobase is defined as *the lowest stimulus current (or voltage) that results in capture of the heart at an infinitely long pulse duration.* Lapique also noted that the ratio a/b in the Weiss equation is a time constant that characterizes the tissue (that is, the time constant of the cell membrane). He called this *chronaxie*. He then redefined the Weiss equation as:

Eq 13 $I_t = a + \dfrac{b}{t} = I_{rheobase} \left(1 + \dfrac{t_{chronaxie}}{t} \right)$

where I_t is the current (I) during the pulse duration (t), $I_{rheobase}$ is the rheobase current (the lowest possible current threshold with t equal to infinity), and $t_{chronaxie}$ is the chronaxie time. Chronaxie is defined as *the threshold pulse width at twice rheobase amplitude,* as shown in Figures 1–7 and 1–8. Lapique also determined that stimulation at the chronaxie pulse width approaches the minimum threshold energy.[54] This appeared to be significant to Nernst, who developed the concept that the energy for stimulation is a constant.[55] As is clearly shown in Figure 1–7, this concept is not correct.

Lapique's modification of the Weiss equation can be further modified in terms of charge (Q) where[56]

Eq 14 $Q = I_{rheo}t + I_{rheo}\,t_{chron}$

At very short pulse widths, equation 14 approaches the limit of chronaxie times rheobase. The lower this product, the lower the charge necessary to stimulate the heart. Thus, the two most important reference points on a current or voltage strength-duration curve are rheobase and chronaxie. It must be pointed out, however, that in the modern literature, it is vanishingly rare to find strength-duration curves that extend to wide enough pulse widths to actually reach the true rheobase (typically requiring pulse widths of ≥ 10 msec). Thus, an *apparent* rheobase is usually measured at pulse widths of 1.5 to 2.0 msec. This means that the chronaxie obtained by finding the pulse width at twice the *apparent* rheobase is slightly low and represents an *apparent* chronaxie value. Nonetheless, it is these apparent values we usually work with clinically because most CV instrumentation does not allow measurements at pulse widths of more than 1.5 to 2.0 msec. From Figure 1–7 it is evident that the lowest practical pulse width is desirable to minimize charge drain (since the pulse generator's battery is a charge source). Too low a pulse width, however, puts thresholds close to the steeply ascending limb of the voltage or current curve where slight fluctuations could risk loss of capture. Irnich recommended that chronaxie, or the pulse width slightly to the left of chronaxie, is the most efficient for both pacing and defibrillation.[57, 58] In most cases, chronaxie appears to represent the best overall compromise between adequate safety and generator longevity. Irnich found that chronaxie varies as a function of stimulation mode, generator impedance, electrode size, shape, and material, and time following implantation.

To insist that thresholds can be measured in microjoules or milliseconds is to deny the fact that rheobase is a critical part of the strength-duration relationship. Regardless of the pulse width or energy used, one cannot stimulate unless the stimulus *amplitude* (either voltage or current) exceeds rheo-

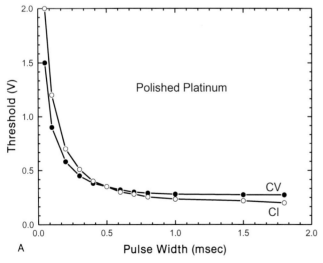

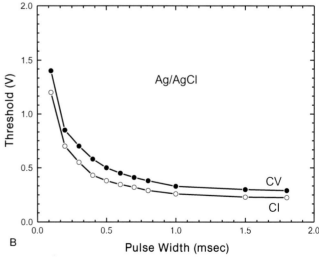

FIGURE 1–8. Constant-current compared with constant-voltage canine ventricular strength-duration curves for passively fixed, atraumatic electrodes. *A,* Polarizing, 8-mm² polished ring-tip electrode. *B,* Low-polarizing, platinized, microporous 8-mm² target-shaped electrode.

base.[59] For example, if rheobase is achieved with a pulse amplitude of 0.5 V and 10 msec, the pulse at this point on the strength-duration curve will have 5 µJ energy with a 500-ohm lead. A 0.4-V, 20-msec pulse on a 500-ohm lead has 6.4-µJ energy (28% greater than the ''threshold'' energy at 10 msec), but cardiac capture will not be achieved. A 100-msec pulse at 0.4 V has 32-µJ energy (540% greater than ''threshold'' energy at 10 msec) but still will not capture the heart. No matter how far we extend the pulse width (and increase the energy of the stimulus) we cannot capture the myocardium unless the stimulus amplitude is at least the rheobase value. Thus, there is probably no such thing as an energy threshold per se, although one can calculate the energy of the pulse at threshold.

PRACTICAL APPLICATION OF THE STRENGTH-DURATION RELATIONSHIP TO THRESHOLD MEASUREMENT

The strength-duration relationship requires the clinician to measure the stimulation threshold at a specific amplitude and pulse width. Clinically, the threshold can be measured by decreasing the amplitude of the CV stimulus at a constant pulse duration until loss of capture (voltage threshold) occurs or by decreasing the pulse width at a constant voltage (pulse width threshold). The stimulation threshold is defined clinically as the lowest voltage or pulse width that results in consistent capture of the myocardium, depending on whether the voltage or pulse width is decreased. It is important to keep in mind that the pulse width threshold is actually the pulse duration on the strength-duration curve when the programmed stimulus amplitude from the pulse generator is at threshold. If, however, the pulse voltage or current is less than rheobase, myocardial capture will not occur regardless of the pulse width. Thus, the term pulse width threshold is a misnomer for voltage or current threshold at a particular pulse width. Examination of the exponential strength-duration curve suggests that one must be very careful to consider its shape when programming an implantable pacemaker. For example, if the pulse width threshold is measured at 0.5 msec at an amplitude of 2.0 V, programming the pacemaker to a pulse width of 1.0 or even 1.5 msec provides a very small margin of safety (Fig. 1–9). In this individual, doubling the stimulus intensity to 4 V at a pulse duration of 0.5 msec would provide an adequate margin of safety. In contrast, consider another patient in whom the pulse width threshold was 0.15 msec at a pulse amplitude of 3.5 V. In this patient, increasing the pulse width to 0.45 msec would also provide an adequate safety margin. The reason why a threefold increase in pulse width is not adequate in the first example but is acceptable in the second is related to the location of the pulse width on the flat or ascending portion of the strength-duration curve. Thus, programming the pulse generator to twice the voltage threshold near the chronaxie pulse width usually provides an optimum output pulse with an adequate safety margin.

CAPTURE HYSTERESIS (WEDENSKY EFFECT)

The threshold stimulus amplitude that is measured by decreasing the voltage or current until loss of capture occurs has been noted by several authors to be less than that meas-

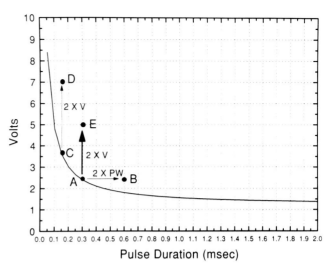

FIGURE 1–9. Programming of the pulse amplitude and pulse duration based on analysis of the strength-duration curve in an individual who was evaluated when the pulse generator was replaced (6 years following lead implantation). The rheobase voltage was 1.4 V, and the chronaxie pulse duration was 0.3 msec. Note that the stimulation threshold determined by decreasing the stimulus amplitude at a constant pulse duration of 0.5 msec was approximately 2.0 V (point A). Doubling of the pulse duration on the relatively flat portion of the strength-duration curve (point B) provides very little safety margin for ventricular capture. In contrast, consider a threshold value on the steeply ascending portion of the strength-duration curve (point C). Doubling the pulse amplitude adds very little safety margin on this portion of the curve (point D). An appropriate setting for a chronic pacing pulse might be achieved by doubling the pulse amplitude from point A to point E. Also note that a similar programmed setting could be obtained by tripling the pulse duration from point C. Thus, the shape of the strength-duration curve has an important influence on the choice of the amplitude and duration of the pacing pulse.

ured by increasing the stimulus intensity until capture occurs. This apparent hysteresis in threshold determined by increasing and decreasing the stimulus amplitude has been termed the Wedensky effect.[60] Although the mechanism for this observation was not clear until recently, this concept has enjoyed widespread acceptance. Langberg and colleagues used programmed stimulation with precisely timed stimuli to examine this phenomenon and noted no demonstrable capture hysteresis at pacing cycle lengths of greater than 400 msec.[61] These authors concluded that the Wedensky effect was related to asynchronous pacing in the relative refractory period when increasing the stimulus intensity compared to synchronous late diastolic stimulation when decreasing the stimulus amplitude until loss of capture. We have confirmed these observations using CV pacing in which asynchronous pacing was prevented while increasing stimulus intensity until capture was achieved (Fig. 1–10).

EFFECT OF PACING RATE ON STIMULATION THRESHOLD

Hook and associates reported a significant increase in ventricular pacing threshold in 10 of 16 patients at 400 msec and in 15 of 16 at 300 msec (relative to a pacing cycle length of 600 msec).[62] The phenomenon was not observed at every trial (12 of 72 trials at 400 msec, for example). The patients were all candidates for implantable defibrillators, and many (9 of 12) were receiving antiarrhythmic drugs. The leads

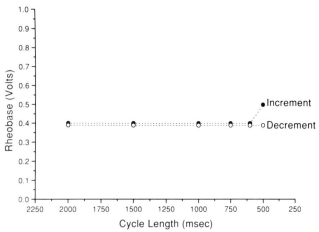

FIGURE 1–10. Pacing thresholds determined by gradually increasing and decreasing the pulse amplitude until gain and loss of capture, respectively, are demonstrated in a patient with complete atrioventricular (AV) block. The pacing threshold was determined at cycle lengths of 2000, 1500, 1000, 750, and 500 msec and a constant pulse duration of 2.0 msec. To prevent variation in cycle lengths during increments and decrements of pulse amplitudes, a backup pulse was delivered at 25 msec. Note that the threshold values determined in this manner are similar with increments and decrements of the stimulus amplitude. Thus, the Wedensky effect may be marginal when the pacing cycle length is maintained at a constant value.

were bipolar (a pair of epicardial corkscrews in 11 patients, an endocardial screw-in lead in 5 patients). These authors concluded that "the mechanisms responsible for the increase in thresholds at faster pacing rates in the majority of patients and the inconsistency in the observed thresholds over time have not been clearly defined." Some of the possible hypotheses presented to explain the phenomenon include the effects of electrode polarization (not having enough time to dissipate the postpulse potential completely before the next pulse), anodal stimulation, and intrusion into the refractory period.

The atrial stimulation threshold has also been shown to vary as a function of pacing rate.[63, 64] Katsumoto and colleagues reported that 29 of 36 patients exhibited atrial CI *current* and *energy* threshold variations as a function of pacing rate in the 60 to 120 bpm range.[65] All but two patients received "activated" vitreous carbon electrodes, which are known to have low polarization properties. In eight additional patients electrodes were secured to the endocardium during open heart surgery. These patients showed no statistically significant (defined as $p \le .05$) differences as a function of rate. The authors concluded that the rate-dependent changes were the result of small displacements of the electrode from the endocardium due to changes in atrial volume (in other words, the result of changes in impedance). Kay and coworkers also found significant human atrial threshold changes as a function of pacing rate (between 125 and 300 bpm) using CV stimulation.[66] They found a significant increase in rheobase voltage, chronaxie, and minimum threshold energy at pacing rates of more than 225 bpm using platinized (low polarizing) unipolar electrodes. They also measured strength-interval curves and found no correlation between atrial effective refractory period and rheobase voltage, chronaxie, or rate-dependent changes in either of these values. They concluded that the phenomenon is probably

related to the "opposing effects of decreasing cycle length on the action potential duration and the slope of the strength-interval curve. Thus, if the pacing interval shortens to a greater extent than the refractory period and pacing stimuli are delivered during the ascending limb of the strength-interval curve (the relative refractory period), the diastolic threshold will increase." The increase in stimulation threshold with increasing stimulation rate probably has minimal implications for pacing for bradycardia. It is important for antitachycardia pacing, however, because threshold must be measured at rates required to interrupt the arrhythmia. In addition, the safety factors used with antitachycardia pacemakers must be based on thresholds measured at the clinically appropriate rates rather than during pacing at resting rates.

A DIFFERENT WAY OF LOOKING AT STRENGTH-DURATION CURVES AND THEIR STABILITY

None of the relationships published in the last 100 years has exactly duplicated the capacitively coupled, CV strength-duration curves measured empirically with different types of electrodes. This may be due in part to the confounding effects of polarization, which varies significantly with electrode size, shape, surface finish, material, and so on. Another problem, however, is that the voltage and current strength-duration relationships, typically plotted on linear coordinates, are really exponential.[67] The strength-duration curve for CI thresholds is now seen as a straight line up to the point at which rheobase is reached (since polarization is not "seen" with CI pacing). The CV strength-duration curve for a polarizing polished platinum electrode is a straight line at pulse widths of less than 0.5 msec, before it is significantly distorted by polarization. The CV strength-duration curve for a modern, very low polarizing electrode approaches a straight line within pulse widths of clinical significance (≤ 1.0 msec [see Fig. 1–11]). This helps to demonstrate the distorting effects of polarization on strength-duration curves (and thus also on rheobase and chronaxie). It is important to note that, within the linear portion, all these curves have about the same slope (m) where

Eq 15 $I(CI) = Bt^m$

or

Eq 16 $V(CV) = At^m$

B is a CI constant and A is a CV constant that determines the location of the curve (on the Y axis). If we include the effects of electrode polarization, it is apparent that the strength-duration curve for CV pacing at pulse widths of less than rheobase must be:

Eq 17 $V = At^m + V_{pol}(t)$

where $V_{pol}(t)$ is the voltage due to polarization (V_{pol}) as a function of pulse width (t).

The slope of the strength-duration curves for passively fixed, atraumatic leads does not change with implant time (Fig. 1–12). The acute, peak, and chronic mean thresholds of five ventricular and three atrial passively fixed, atraumatic leads in 77 canines had a ($\log_{10}$) slope of about -0.60 ± 0.07 V/msec.[67] The correlation coefficient for these relationships is typically 0.99 or greater at pulse widths of 0.5 msec or

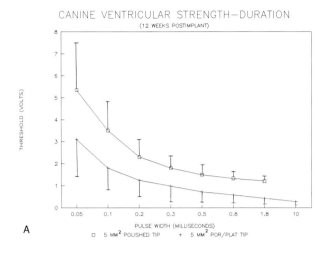

CANINE VENTRICULAR STRENGTH—DURATION
(12 WEEKS POSTIMPLANT)

A

□ 5 MM² POLISHED TIP + 5 MM² POR/PLAT TIP

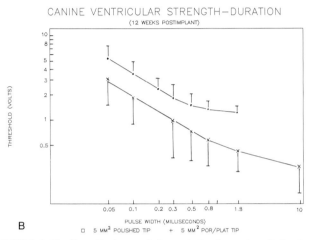

CANINE VENTRICULAR STRENGTH—DURATION
(12 WEEKS POSTIMPLANT)

B

□ 5 MM² POLISHED TIP + 5 MM² POR/PLAT TIP

FIGURE 1–11. Capacitively coupled constant-voltage strength-duration curves on linear *(A)* and logarithmic *(B)* coordinates for 5-mm² polished *(top line)* and porous platinized *(lower line)* platinum electrodes.

less for polished electrodes and 1.0 msec or less for low polarizing designs. Traumatic electrodes (such as those with active fixation) in our canine experience typically have a lower slope immediately after implantation, but this shifts to about the same −0.60 V/msec within days as the acute trauma to the electrode-tissue interface heals.

Since strength-duration curves are typically plotted on linear coordinates, voltage and current threshold changes with time following implantation are usually seen as a shift "upward" and "to the right." In most cases, chronaxie, being related to the slope of the curve (the tissue's time constant) does not change significantly with time. Of course, this assumes a normal evolution of the foreign body response, which may not be true in the presence of exaggerated pathologic changes. It also assumes no interference by drug therapy or electrolyte abnormalities. Today, it is generally recognized that because the CV strength-duration curve to the right of chronaxie begins to approach rheobase, there is little to be gained by wider pulse widths for the typical patient. In addition, at or below 0.5 msec, polarization is relatively small, so there is little wasted energy (charge, current, and so on). As a result, 0.5 msec has become the de facto standard used in the pacing community to measure and compare thresholds. However, new data are in the process of being

published that may change our understanding of the stability of chronaxie. Cornacchia and colleagues have shown that administration of propafenone shifts the strength-duration curve *and* chronaxie to the right.[67a] Thus, measurement of the strength-duration relationship may be required after administration of antiarrhythmic drugs together with reprogramming of an implantable pacemaker.

Several manufacturers have attempted to compensate for the gradual decline in stimulus voltage as a consequence of battery depletion by automatic "stretching" of the pulse duration to maintain the stimulus energy at a nearly constant value. Although this feature is designed to prevent loss of capture, increasing the pulse duration from a programmed value of 0.5 msec adds relatively little to the pacing safety margin because this approaches an essentially flat portion of the strength-duration curve. In fact, this automatic increase in pulse duration actually accelerates battery depletion.

Strength-Interval Relationships

In addition to the strength-duration relationship, voltage and current stimulation thresholds also vary as a function of the coupling interval of the stimulus to prior beats and to the stimulation frequency used for the basic drive train. A typical constant-current ventricular strength-interval curve is shown in Figure 1–13. At relatively long coupling intervals between the basic drive train and an extrastimulus (>270 msec), the intensity of the extrastimulus that is required for ventricular capture is relatively constant, approaching the rheobase value. However, at shorter extrastimulus coupling intervals (<250 msec), the intensity of the extrastimulus must be increased to elicit myocardial capture. The exponential rise at short intervals is the result of encroachment of the stimulus into the refractory period of the myocardium. During the *relative* refractory period (corresponding to the repolarization phase of the action potential), the myocardium can be induced to generate a new action potential if the stimulus has sufficient intensity. During the *absolute* refractory period

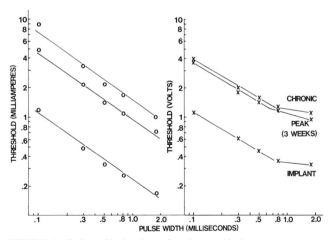

FIGURE 1–12. Logarithmic plots of canine ventricular constant-current *(left)* and constant-voltage *(right)* strength-duration curves for a passively fixed, atraumatic, unipolar lead with an 8-mm² polished platinum ring-tip at various implant times. (From Stokes K, Bornzin G: The electrode–biointerface (stimulation). *In* Barold S [ed]: Modern Cardiac Pacing. Mt. Kisco, NY, Futura, 1985, pp 33–78.)

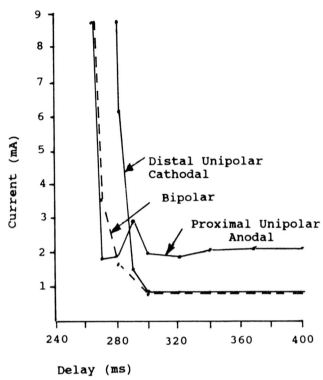

Delay (ms)

FIGURE 1–13. Strength-interval curves. Unipolar distal cathodal, unipolar proximal anodal, and bipolar strength-interval curves during an acute study in a patient with a temporary bipolar lead (equal sized cathode and anode). The bipolar and unipolar anodal refractory periods are equal and shorter than the refractory period of the unipolar cathodal curve (ms = millisecond). (From Mehra R, Furman S: Comparison of cathodal, anodal, and bipolar strength-interval curves with temporary and permanent pacing electrodes. Br Heart J 41:468, 1979.)

(corresponding to the plateau phase of the action potential), no depolarization can be effected regardless of the stimulus intensity. The strength-interval curve of atrial and ventricular myocardium is shifted to the left at shorter basic drive cycle lengths. Therefore, the *effective* refractory period, which is generally measured at a pulse duration of 2.0 msec and an amplitude that is twice that of the late diastolic threshold, decreases as a function of the pacing cycle length. At relatively slow pacing rates (less than 200 bpm), there is relatively little interaction between the strength-duration and strength-interval curves. However, as discussed earlier, at rapid pacing rates (over 225 bpm), pacing stimuli during the basic drive may encounter the relative refractory period. If the stimulus amplitude becomes subthreshold, 2:1 capture of the myocardium results.

Constant-Current Versus Constant-Voltage Stimulation

A CI generator delivers a (current) pulse that is usually a square wave. That is, the leading edge of the pulse (I_{le}) equals the trailing edge (I_{te}). The current delivered by a CI pulse generator is independent of pacing impedance to the limits of the power source (Fig. 1–14). If impedance decreases, the resultant voltage automatically decreases to keep current constant. In the presence of a high-resistance circuit such as with

a partial lead fracture, the limits of the power source are reached, and the battery is said to be "saturated." In this instance the battery cannot generate enough voltage to maintain a preset level of current, and this results in delivery of a lower current than that programmed. Although under normal operating conditions the current waveform is rectangular, the resultant voltage waveform is not. It starts out with an initial leading edge voltage (V_{le}) but increases as a function of pulse width to a larger trailing edge voltage (V_{te}, Fig. 1–15). At the end of the pulse an immediate drop in voltage equal to V_{le} is observed, followed by an exponential decay back to baseline. The voltage rise during the pulse (called the *overvoltage*) is caused by an increase in pacing impedance due to electrode polarization, and the afterpotential is caused by the gradual dissipation of that polarization.

Today, all implantable pulse generators are capacitively coupled, approximately CV devices. At the beginning of the pulse, the fully charged capacitor delivers a leading edge voltage that is constant regardless of impedance as long as the impedance is high enough (Fig. 1–16). The voltage drops during the pulse to the trailing edge value. This change in voltage over the pulse duration ("droop") is directly proportional to the total charge delivered (Q*, coulombs) and is inversely proportional to the capacitance of the pulse generator (C_{pg}, farads), or approximately:

Eq 18 $\quad V_{le} - V_{te} = Q*/C_{pg}$

Charge is also a function of impedance or resistance, where:

Eq 19 $\quad Q = It = \dfrac{Vt}{R}$

(in a simple resistive circuit) or $\dfrac{Vt}{Z_p}$ (in a complex nonlinear

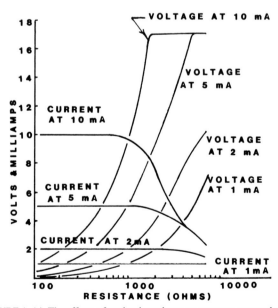

FIGURE 1–14. The effects of pacing impedance on constant-current leading edge waveform amplitudes using a Medtronic model 5880A external pulse generator. Current is independent of impedance until the battery is "saturated." Saturation occurs when the voltage cannot increase any more to keep current constant. (From Barold SS, Winner JA: Techniques and significance of threshold measurement for cardiac pacing. Chest 70:760, 1976.)

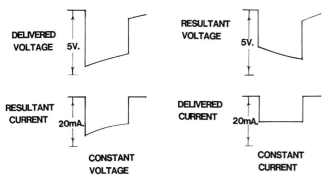

FIGURE 1–15. Voltage and current waveforms from a capacitively coupled, constant-voltage implantable pulse generator (Medtronic model 7000A, *left*) and the constant-current mode output of an external research stimulation device (Medtronic model 1356, *right*). A unipolar lead with a polished platinum 8-mm² ring-tip is used in conjunction with a 900-mm² titanium anode placed in 0.18% NaCl. The voltage across the lead is measured against a 100-mm² Ag/AgCl electrode to eliminate the anode's polarization from the waveform. (From Stokes K, Bornzin G: The electrode–biointerface (stimulation). *In* Barold S [ed]: Modern Cardiac Pacing. Mt Kisco, NY, Futura, 1985, pp 33–78.)

circuit such as a pacemaker). Therefore, the CV droop is also a function of pacing impedance (Z_p) where:

Eq 20 $$V_{le} - V_{te} = \frac{V^* t}{Z_p C_{pg}}$$

and V* is the total voltage applied (the area under the waveform bounded by V_{le} and V_{te}). With a very high impedance lead, therefore, the voltage pulse is almost rectangular ($V_{le} = V_{te}$). With a low pacing impedance, the droop is steeper because more current is drained from the output capacitor. Thus, the current begins with a high initial value in a CV generator but decreases to the trailing edge as a function of the pulse width. With very low impedances (<200 ohms), the battery may not be able to supply enough current to maintain a constant voltage. Leads for CV generators, therefore, are designed to have as high an impedance as is efficiently practical to minimize current drain.

Ideally, current (CI) thresholds are related to voltage (CV) thresholds by impedance. For example, if the pacing impedance really had a linear relationship between voltage and current (following Ohm's law), then for a 500-ohm system the current threshold should always be twice the voltage value. The reason that this relationship is usually not apparent is that impedance is not linear with pulse width and varies with time following lead implantation, electrolyte levels, and so on. The reason why impedance is not a simple linear function of pulse width is related to the phenomenon of electrode polarization, a topic to be discussed later in this chapter.

Constant-current strength-duration curves, therefore, can have slightly different shapes from CV curves. Irnich, for example, pointed out that (with polished electrodes) typical CI chronaxie values are almost twice those found with CV stimulation (see Fig. 1–8).[47] Today, most modern endocardial leads have relatively low polarizing electrodes (such as those with platinized or "activated" carbon surfaces). These tend to have a lower voltage rheobase and a somewhat higher chronaxie than polarizing (polished) electrodes (see Fig. 1–12).[68] Therefore, polarization affects the value of CV chron-

axie. This probably accounts for most, if not all, of the differences between the shape of CV and CI strength-duration curves.

Monophasic and Biphasic Waveforms

If we omit the postpulse recharge, most pacing stimuli are monophasic. However, abrupt reversal of polarity during the stimulus (biphasic waveform) has been demonstrated to decrease the voltage threshold required to defibrillate ventricular fibrillation.[69] Knisley and colleagues[70] studied the effect of biphasic and triphasic stimuli on excitation threshold in rabbit and frog ventricles (Fig. 1–17). At very long pulse durations (20 msec), there was no difference in the stimulation threshold between monophasic and biphasic stimulus waveforms. Thus, reversal of waveform polarity during the stimulus did not affect rheobase voltage. However, at shorter pulse durations (2.5 msec), the threshold voltage was significantly greater for biphasic than for monophasic waveforms. Thus, the chronaxie pulse duration was significantly increased by an intrastimulus polarity reversal. Although biphasic stimuli decrease the voltage required for defibrillation,

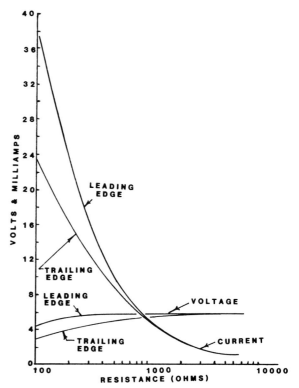

FIGURE 1–16. The effect of pacing impedance on capacitively coupled, constant-voltage leading and trailing edge waveform amplitudes using a Medtronic model 5950 pulse generator. The voltage of the leading edge remains constant as a function of pacing impedance of 200 ohms or more. The trailing edge of the voltage waveform, however, changes slightly with impedance of up to about 1000 ohms. Current falls rather significantly with increasing impedance. Any constant-voltage source may no longer be constant at very low pacing impedance values because the battery becomes unable to supply enough current to maintain a steady voltage. These very low impedance values are not likely to be encountered clinically in patients with a properly functioning pacing system. (From Barold SS, Winner JA: Techniques and significance of threshold measurements for cardiac pacing. Chest 70:760, 1976.)

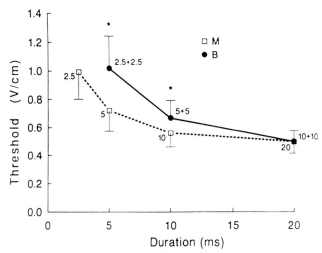

FIGURE 1–17. Monophasic (M) and biphasic (B) strength-duration curves obtained in strips of frog ventricular myocardium superfused with a solution containing 3 mmol/L of potassium. At a pulse duration of 20 msec there is no significant difference in the rheobase threshold. Note that the monophasic waveform produces a lower threshold than the biphasic waveform at pulse durations of 5 msec and less. Thus, although the monophasic and biphasic waveforms have a similar rheobase, chronaxie is less with monophasic than with biphasic stimuli (ms = millisecond). (From Knisely SB, Smith WM, Ideker RE: Effect of intrastimulus polarity reversal on electric field stimulation thresholds in frog and rabbit myocardium. J Cardiovasc Electrophysiol 3:239, 1992.)

the excitability threshold for bradycardia pacing at clinically relevant pulse durations appears to be increased with biphasic pulses. Thus, stimuli for bradycardia pacing are monophasic. This must not be confused with pre- or poststimulus "conditioning" or "fast-recharge" pulses, which are designed not to interfere with the pacing stimulus per se.

Anodal and Cathodal Stimulation

Generally speaking, anodal stimulation is associated with properties that are less desirable than cathodal stimulation. If the stimulating electrode is a unipolar cathode, the strength-interval curve has a shape that is very similar to that of a strength-duration curve. The shape of the typical anodal strength-interval curve is somewhat different from that of a cathodal curve (Fig. 1–18). Given equal sized electrodes, the anodal stimulation threshold is generally somewhat greater than that for cathodal stimulation at long coupling intervals. With progressively more premature coupling intervals, there is a dip in the anodal curve to threshold values that are less than those of the cathodal curve. At still more premature coupling intervals, the anodal curve rises steeply (as observed with cathodal stimulation).[71] The "dip" phenomenon is not always seen.[72] If the electrodes of a bipolar lead are of equal size or if the anode is smaller than the cathode, it is possible to achieve stimulation earlier in the cardiac cycle (in the relative refractory period) than with unipolar cathodal stimulation. This may occur because the threshold for anodal stimulation with electrodes of equal size is lower than that for cathodal stimulation in the strength-interval curve at shorter pulse widths.[71, 72]

That anodal stimulation can generate tachyarrhythmias in ischemic or electrolyte-unbalanced hearts is well documented.[73–76] This is one of several reasons why implantable bipolar leads are designed with anodes that are larger than cathodes. In fact, it is commonly thought that the bipolar anode needs to be big enough (50 mm^2) to prevent anodal stimulation. It is unlikely that this really prevents anodal stimulation, however, because most pulse generators are set at much higher outputs than threshold, such as 5.0 V and 0.5 msec with a 0.5-V, 0.5-msec cathodal stimulation threshold. A 50-mm^2 anode probably reaches threshold at a stimulus intensity well below 5 V and 0.5 msec. It is likely that with many bipolar leads delivery of the stimulation pulse actually results in capture of the myocardium at both the cathode and the anode. Thus, there is probably more to the size relationship between cathode and anode than is known.

It must be noted that bipolar pacing with equal sized electrodes is common in temporary pacing and implanted epicardial systems (in which two unipolar leads are often used for bipolar pacing). The clinician must keep the arrhythmogenic possibilities of such combinations in mind. Another reason why anodes should be relatively large is to preclude unacceptable corrosion rates. Platinum, for example, does not corrode under the cathodic current densities used in pacing, but anodic potentials can cause corrosion. The proximal electrode (anode) of a bipolar pacing lead, therefore, should be large enough to ensure that current density is too low to effect significant corrosion. Careful examination of explanted platinum polished distal tips (cathodes) often reveals rough surfaces that are the result of corrosion. Although this seems contradictory, it is easily explained. The distal tip is a cathode during its *stimulation* pulse. Some generators also have a fast recharge pulse following the stimulus to neutralize the afterpotential. Because the polarity of the fast recharge is reversed, this portion of the pulse is actually anodal. Thus, as the "cathode" size decreases, corrosion increases, eventually to unacceptable levels. Nonetheless, excellent canine performance has been reported with electrodes with as little as 0.6 mm^2 in geometric surface area.[77] How is excessive

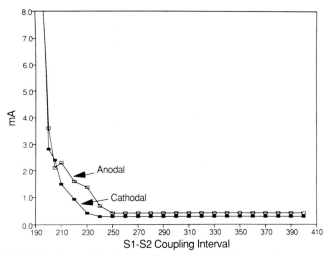

FIGURE 1–18. Anodal and cathodal ventricular strength-interval curves are demonstrated for an individual with AV block with unipolar constant-current stimuli. Note that the anodal threshold is slightly higher than the cathodal threshold at coupling intervals of greater than 250 msec. At coupling intervals of less than 210 msec, the anodal threshold is approximately equal to the cathodal threshold. In some individuals the anodal threshold may not decrease ("dip") to a value that is less than the cathodal threshold.

corrosion by the fast recharge prevented? When the electrode is made porous, the interfacing surface area is very large despite the very small volume encompassed by the geometric surface. This reduces the current density at the electrolyte-metal interface below that required for corrosion by the fast recharge pulse.

Unipolar and Bipolar Stimulation

All pacing systems require a negatively charged cathode and a positively charged anode to complete the electric circuit. Thus, in reality, all pacemakers are bipolar. The unipolar pacemaker has one electrode in the heart and a relatively large one remote from the heart, usually on the pulse generator can. In the bipolar pacemaker both the cathode and the anode are in (or on) the chamber of the heart to be paced and sensed. There has been a great deal of debate about the relative merits of unipolar versus bipolar pacing, most of which relates to issues other than stimulation per se. The effects of unipolar and bipolar configurations on sensing are profound and are covered in Chapter 2. The engineering aspects are equally important and are discussed in Chapter 3. At one time it was generally accepted that bipolar leads had higher stimulation thresholds than unipolar leads. This statement, based on old technology, is approximately true only if both electrodes are of equal size. In this case, the output voltage delivered by the pulse generator is divided equally between the two electrodes, causing the measured threshold to be higher. This situation can be corrected by making the cathode relatively small and the anode relatively large. This produces the largest potential difference across tissue adjacent to the cathode, reducing the stimulation threshold. It also makes the anode a relatively poor stimulating electrode, reducing the arrhythmogenic potential compared to a bipolar lead with equal sized electrodes.

How much larger than the cathode must the anode of a bipolar lead be to provide stimulation thresholds comparable to those of a unipolar system? Based on our canine studies, the answer is, as large as possible. In practical terms, the anode must be at least 3 times larger than the cathode to produce bipolar thresholds that are statistically equivalent to those of a unipolar system.[78] Based on the excellent long-term performance of leads such as the Medtronic model 6901 (11 mm^2 cathode, 48 mm^2 anode), it has become standard practice to ensure that the anode is at least 4.5 times larger than the geometric surface area of the cathode. The bipolar electrode spacing can also be important, especially for sensing (see Chapter 2). It is generally accepted, for example, that as the electrodes are moved closer together, the signal-to-noise ratio, resistance to crosstalk, and median frequency of the sensed signal increase, whereas signal amplitude may decrease. If the spacing is too close, transvenous electrode pairs may develop high stimulation thresholds because current can be shunted between the two electrodes, effectively producing a short circuit. In his classic thesis, De Caprio determined that the optimum bipolar spacing (for sensing) was about 8 mm.[79] In our limited canine ventricular work, we have found that an interelectrode spacing of approximately 8 to 10 mm produces the optimum trade-off.[77]

Design Features That Affect Performance of Pacing Electrodes

The performance of the pacing electrodes is the major determinant of the stimulus intensity required to produce a self-propagating wavefront in the myocardium. Therefore, the stimulation characteristics of the electrode determine the margin of safety between the stimulus intensity delivered by the output circuit of the pulse generator and the intensity required for stimulation. The electrodes also determine the pacing impedance, another factor that influences pulse generator longevity. In addition to providing myocardial stimulation, the electrodes determine the sensing characteristics of the pacing system.[80] In this section the size, surface structure, and biologic response to electrodes, which are critical factors in the design of pacing electrodes, will be discussed. Some secondary effects, including shape, spacing, fixation, and material, will also be reviewed.

SIZE OF THE STIMULATING ELECTRODE (GEOMETRIC SURFACE AREA)

It has been observed that the stimulation threshold varies as an inverse function of the size or geometric surface area of the stimulating electrode.[39, 40, 81, 82] Irnich argued that, in theory, the chronic stimulation threshold of a spherical electrode should decrease as its radius (geometric surface area) decreases to a minimum value.[39, 40] As the radius of the electrode decreases below this minimum value, chronic threshold should begin to increase. Irnich showed that the electric field strength (E) necessary for stimulation is a function of the potential (V) applied to a spherical electrode of radius r. Thus, for a given applied potential, the smaller the radius of the electrode, the more intense the electric field generated in the underlying myocardium. In this analysis, the strength of the electric field that is required to stimulate myocardium was assumed to be a universal constant (expressed in volts per centimeter). If the minimum field intensity required to initiate a depolarization is greater than that generated by the delivered stimulus, the applied voltage must be increased to achieve threshold. Conversely, if the electrode radius is increased, the field strength may not be sufficient to capture the heart without increasing the applied voltage.

It has long been recognized that the stimulation threshold increases during the first several weeks following lead implantation. This increase in threshold is related to the development of a conductive but nonexcitable fibrotic capsule with an approximate mean thickness (d) that forms around the electrode, separating it from normal, excitable myocardium.[83, 84] The fibrous capsule is a biologic response to the presence of a foreign body, in this case an electrode. It is not a response to the electric stimulus.[85] In reality, therefore, (r + d) describes the dimensions of the effective or "virtual" electrode as defined by Furman and associates.[36] If the stimulus voltage is held constant, the field strength varies as a function of the thickness of the inexcitable capsule. Thus, higher voltages must be applied to maintain the intensity of the field at the interface of the virtual electrode and the excitable myocardium (Fig. 1–19), so that chronic

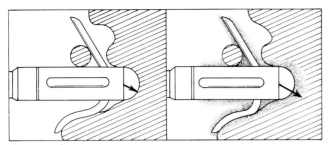

FIGURE 1–19. Schematic representation of simple collagenous capsule around the electrode that separates it from excitable tissue. In effect, the fibrous tissue now becomes a "virtual electrode" with radius r + d, where r is the (spherical) electrode's radius and d is the thickness of the fibrous tissue. (From Stokes K, Bornzin G: The electrode–biointerface (stimulation). *In* Barold S [ed]: Modern Cardiac Pacing. Mt. Kisco, NY, Futura, 1985, pp 33–78.)

thresholds (for steroid-free electrodes) must be higher than the implant values. This theory was modeled by Irnich[86] as:

$$\textbf{Eq 21} \quad E = \frac{V}{r}\left[\frac{r}{(r+d)}\right]^2$$

Holding everything else constant, the capsule thickness will be the same for electrodes with large or small radii. If, for example, two electrodes of different radii (r = 0.5 mm and 5 mm) develop a 1.0-mm thick capsule (d), the electrode with the smaller radius will be associated with a greater percentage increase in the radius of the virtual electrode (r + d) than will the larger electrode (300% versus 20%). This helps to explain the observation that smaller electrodes have lower acute thresholds but develop a greater rise in threshold over a period of time.[84, 87] As mentioned previously, there is a point (r = d) where the chronic threshold reaches a minimum. According to equation 21, when d is greater than r, the threshold increases. Therefore, there is a theoretical minimum spherical electrode radius at which the threshold must reach its minimum value. Irnich found this to be r equal to 0.72 mm with polished electrodes. In reality, because most electrodes are not spherical, the relationship between stimulation threshold and electrode radius is more complex. Therefore, electrode size is usually discussed in terms of geometric surface area.

RELATIONSHIP OF ELECTRODE SIZE AND SENSING PERFORMANCE

As discussed in Chapter 2, the amplitude of the electrogram sensed by the sensing amplifier of the pulse generator is less than the amplitude of the available signal in the myocardium. The magnitude of the electrogram is attenuated between the myocardium and amplifier in the pulse generator. The attenuation of the signal is related to the ratio of the source impedance (of the electrode-myocardial interface) and the input impedance of the sensing amplifier. The higher the source impedance, the more the signal amplitude is attenuated for a given input impedance. However, signal attenuation can be greatly minimized by increasing the input impedance of the sense amplifier so that the ratio of the source impedance to the input impedance is very small. In the early 1970s, a 5-mm² Eligoloy Microtip electrode was marketed. This electrode was later removed from the market because of poor sensing.[88] Although acceptable electrogram amplitudes were measured on an oscilloscope (with very high input impedance), there was a relatively high rate of sensing failure when this lead was implanted in combination with certain pulse generators. Although this electrode had good stimulation thresholds and about 1000 ohms pacing impedance, it also had about 5000 ohms sensing (source) impedance. Because the pulse generators of one manufacturer had a very low sensing amplifier input impedance (10,000 ohms), about one third of the actual electrogram amplitude was attenuated in the amplifier (see Chapter 2). Thus, the idea that "small electrodes do not sense well" was born, whereas in reality the problem lay in the design of the amplifier.[89] The significance of such an impedance mismatch was not generally recognized at the time, however. Given the sense amplifiers and electrode technology of the day, Furman and colleagues concluded that about 8 mm² provided the optimum compromise between a small surface area that allowed a low stimulation threshold and an acceptably high surface area for sensing.[36] The 8-mm² paradigm has remained the state of the art for electrode size until very recently. It is now recognized that small porous and microporous electrodes provide both excellent stimulation thresholds and sensing performance when combined with modern pulse generators that have a much higher input impedance than the earlier models.

ELECTRODE SURFACE STRUCTURE (INTERFACE SURFACE AREA)

Based on animal studies, it has been claimed that electrodes with pores that allow tissue ingrowth have thinner fibrous capsules and somewhat lower chronic thresholds than solid or polished surfaces.[90–93] These claims have been somewhat controversial when they are applied to humans.[94–97] Pore structures of certain dimensions are known to promote rapid tissue ingrowth.[98] It has been argued that this ingrowth provides rapid stability of the electrode at its interface with the myocardium and prevents electrode motion that otherwise may result in tissue irritation and high chronic stimulation thresholds. On the other hand, properly designed tines and myocardial screws provide immediate stability and good chronic threshold performance. Activated carbon electrodes are reported to have porosity on the order of 10 nm (Fig. 1–20).[99] The endocardial Target Tip electrode, introduced in 1983, has several grooves in a hemispherical, 8-mm² electrode that provide regions of high electric field strength and promote endocardial stability.[100] The surface is platinized to produce submicron-sized surface microporosity (see Fig. 1–20). Although fibrotic tissue cannot grow into such small structures, these microporous electrodes have significantly lower chronic thresholds than their otherwise equivalent porous and polished counterparts.[99–104] For example, Breivik and colleagues found that the acute stimulation thresholds of the Target Tip and the polished ring-tip were equivalent.[105] In contrast, the chronic human stimulation thresholds 3 months after implantation were 83% lower for platinized electrodes. Heinemann and associates found a mean pulse width threshold of 0.11 ± 0.05 msec at a 2.5-V pulse amplitude 2 weeks after implantation of the Target Tip electrode compared with 0.38 ± 0.22 msec for a polished ring-tip electrode.[106] After 6 months, the mean thresholds dropped to 0.08 ± 0.03 msec at 2.5 V for the Target Tip lead. A platin-

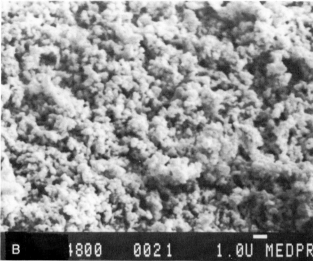

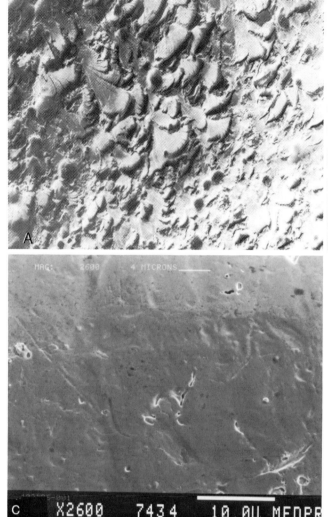

FIGURE 1–20. Electron micrographs of microporous electrode surfaces. *A,* Activated carbon surface of lead of Siemans model 412S/60 at about 8000 magnifications. *B,* Platinized surface of Medtronic model 4011 at 6900 magnifications. *C,* Polished platinum surface of Medtronic model 6971 at 7000 magnifications. The polished platinum surface has little microstructure. Its actual microscopic surface area is similar to its apparent or geometric surface area (8 mm²). The platinized platinum surface is composed of particles so small that they absorb visible light and the surface appears black. The true surface area of the interface, therefore, must be many orders of magnitude greater than the geometric surface area. (*A* from Seeger W: A scanning electron microscopic study on explanted electrode tips. *In* Aubert AE, Ector H [eds]: Pacemaker Leads. Amsterdam, Elsevier Science Publishers, 1985, pp 417–432.)

ized myocardial 10-mm² "fishhook" electrode has also produced excellent results in children, suggesting that a complex microscopic surface structure is also applicable to active fixation electrodes.[107] Thus, it appears that the chronic thresholds of porous and microporous electrodes are superior to those of polished surfaces. However, the argument that ingrowth of tissue into the electrode prevents motion and results in a less irritating interface with the myocardium remains unproved.

MULTIVARIANT EFFECTS OF ELECTRODE SIZE, SHAPE, MATERIAL, AND SURFACE STRUCTURE

Irnich's optimum (spherical) electrode radius and Furman's 8-mm² compromise were based on observations of the performance of *polished* electrodes, which were all that were available in the early and mid 1970s. If we add the effects of electrode shape, surface structure, size, location, and chemical composition, the number of permutations becomes excessive for a typical scientific analysis of each factor. The combined effects of a wide range of platinum electrode geometric surface areas, shapes, and surface structures on chronic (12-week) unipolar canine ventricular thresholds have been stud-ied, allowing us to evaluate their individual effects.[108, 109] As shown in Figure 1–21, the correlation between threshold and geometric surface area for polished electrodes of 85, 53, and 26 mm² is fair (r = 0.83), with threshold decreasing as a function of decreasing size. The slope of the curve is about 0.02 V/mm². Between about 4.5 mm² (the smallest tested) and 26 mm², however, the size-threshold correlation for polished electrodes is negligible, and no statistically significant differences can be demonstrated regardless of electrode shape. The correlation coefficient between chronic thresholds and electode size for *porous* electrodes ranging in geometric surface area from 10 mm² (the largest tested) to about 1.5 mm² is only 0.083 (no correlation) (Fig. 1–22). We were unable to discriminate to a statistically significant level between porous and microporous surfaces in this analysis. Surface areas below 1.5 mm² produced dramatically increasing thresholds. In the *porous, steroid-eluting* population of electrodes (Fig. 1–23) we also found no significant relationship between geometric electrode surface area and chronic threshold between 14 mm² (the largest tested) and about 0.6 mm². The correlation coefficient between surface area and threshold for this group of electrodes was only 0.041 (no correlation). Stimulation thresholds rose dramatically as a function

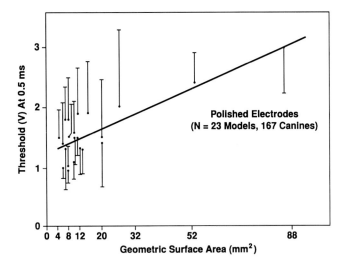

FIGURE 1–21. Chronic (12-week) canine ventricular (gain of capture) thresholds (V) at 0.5 msec as a function of geometric surface area of *polished* platinum electrodes (n = 23 models, 167 animals). The correlation is fair at about 0.82. The slope is about 0.02 V/mm². There are no significant differences in threshold for (geometric) electrode surface areas between 26 mm² and 4.5 mm² (the smallest tested). The thresholds of 53- and 85-mm² polished (endocardial) electrodes were significantly higher than those of the rest of the group. There were no significant differences between endocardial and myocardial electrodes as a function of electrode shape (ms = millisecond). (From Stokes K: The effects of ventricular electrode surface area on pacemaker lead performance. *In* Adornato E, Galarsi A [eds]: The '92 Scenario on Cardiac Pacing. Rome, L. Pozzi, 1992, pp 505–514.)

of geometric surface area for electrodes of less than 0.6 mm². All three curves relating stimulation threshold to geometric electrode surface area are shown in Figure 1–24 on the same scale (without error bars) for comparison. Within the limits defined earlier, these three populations of electrodes are significantly different from one another. Thus, it is clear that the major determinant of chronic stimulation threshold within clinically useful ranges is not so much the electrode's size, geometric surface area, or shape as its surface structure (the interface surface area) and the property of steroid elution. This analysis strongly suggests that the reason these factors have a significant influence on chronic stimulation threshold is related to their effects on inflammation at the myocardial interface (the foreign body response). This analysis also supports the relationships suggested earlier by Irnich, Furman, and others, but new technology has changed the boundaries of these relationships.

Threshold Changes as a Function of Time Following Lead Implantation

It is well known that stimulation thresholds change with time following implantation, typically rising to a peak after

several weeks.[110–113] With older polished electrodes, thresholds in some patients evolved over longer periods (as long as 6 months).[114] Luceri and coworkers observed that after the acute rise in stimulation threshold, 43% of 120 patients had stable chronic thresholds for up to 8 years.[115] Seventeen percent of patients had decreasing chronic thresholds at a rate of 5% decrease per year, and 19% had rising thresholds at a rate of 14% per year. Twenty percent of patients had thresholds that varied widely about a stable mean. Some typical acute-to-chronic changes as a function of time in the canine are shown in Figure 1–25 for passively fixed 8-mm² ventricular and for 11-mm² atrial polished platinum electrodes. Atrial thresholds typically rise to a peak within 1 week and then decrease substantially. The chronic atrial threshold is often substantially lower than the chronic ventricular value. The ventricular thresholds have a lower peak value, and in many cases this peak may not be apparent for 3 or 4 weeks. It is clear that there is a wide range of variability in chronic stimulation thresholds between patients with this type of electrode. Therefore, one cannot assume that the threshold course will be typical for any given individual.

Polished electrodes are still used, primarily for transvenous screw-in and epicardial-myocardial leads. In addition, there are still many patients in whom the older polished electrodes

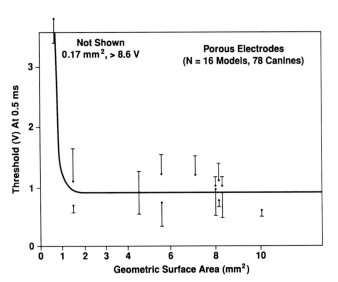

FIGURE 1–22. Chronic (12-week) canine ventricular (gain of capture) thresholds (V) at 0.5 msec as a function of geometric surface area of *porous* electrodes. This series includes 16 designs (n = 78 animals). The term porous refers to totally porous, porous surface, microporous, and differential current density (DCD) electrodes. The correlation coefficient in the geometric surface area range of 10 mm² (the largest tested) and about 1.5 mm² is only 0.083 (no correlation). The slope of the curve at 1.5 mm² or more is 0.006 V/mm². Surface areas below 1.5 mm² produced dramatically increasing thresholds (ms = millisecond). (From Stokes K: The effects of ventricular electrode surface area on pacemaker lead performance. *In* Adornato E, Galassi A [eds]: The '92 Scenario on Cardiac Pacing. Rome, L. Pozzi, 1992, pp 505–514.)

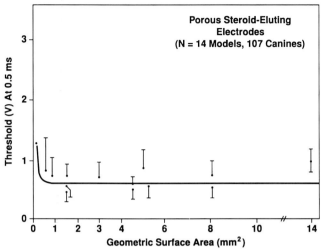

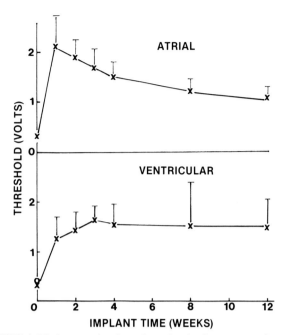

FIGURE 1–23. Chronic (12-week) canine (gain of capture) ventricular thresholds (V) at 0.5 msec as a function of geometric surface area of *porous steroid-eluting* electrodes. The curve includes 14 designs (107 animals). No significant relationship (correlation 0.041) was found between the electrode surface area and a chronic threshold of between 14 mm^2 (the largest tested) and about 0.6 mm^2. The slope of the curve at 0.6 mm^2 or greater was only 0.017 V/mm^2. Thresholds rose dramatically as a function of geometric surface area of less than 0.6 mm^2 (ms = millisecond). (From Stokes K: The effects of ventricular electrode surface area on pacemaker lead performance. *In* Adornato E, Galassi A [eds]: The '92 Scenario on Cardiac Pacing. Rome, L. Pozzi, 1992, pp 504–515.)

FIGURE 1–25. Acute-to-chronic canine gain of voltage capture threshold changes at 0.5 msec as a function of implant time for unipolar leads with passively fixed, atraumatic, polished platinum 11-mm^2 atrial *(upper)* and 8-mm^2 ventricular *(lower)* electrodes.

are implanted. Thus, the preceding discussion is still useful today. For passively fixed leads, however, polished electrodes are obsolete. It is reasonable to assume that in the future this will be true of all leads. Modern passively fixed electrodes have a porous or microporous surface structure. Many passively fixed leads implanted today also elute a glucocorticosteroid. As shown in Figures 1–26 and 1–27, the technologic progression from polished to porous to microporous to steroid-eluting electrodes has significantly reduced the evolution of stimulation threshold as a function of time

following implantation.[106] In fact, as can be determined from the follow-up data available to date, the thresholds of porous and microporous steroid-eluting leads do not change significantly with time following implantation.[101, 116–118] The reasons for threshold changes as a function of time and electrode design are to be found in the foreign body response to the electrodes.

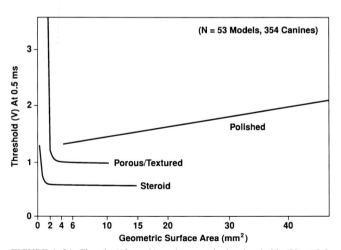

FIGURE 1–24. Chronic (12-week) canine ventricular thresholds (V) at 0.5 msec as a function of geometric surface area from Figures 1–21, 1–22, and 1–23, shown without data points or error bars for clarity (53 unipolar ventricular lead models, n = 354 canines). These three populations are significantly different from each other (ms = millisecond). (From Stokes K: The effects of ventricular electrode surface area on pacemaker lead performance. *In* Adornato E, Galassi A [eds]: The '92 Scenario on Cardiac Pacing. Rome, L. Pozzi, 1992, pp 505–514.)

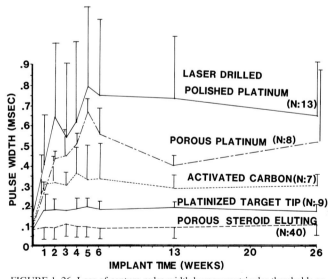

FIGURE 1–26. Loss of capture pulse width human ventricular thresholds as a function of implant time on a series of unipolar leads with similar geometric surface area electrodes.[106] These threshold values appear to be typical of this type of electrode and are not unique to the particular manufacturer. The top curve is that of a polished electrode with holes drilled in it by a laser. Its performance appears to be similar to that of polished electrodes in general. The second curve is that of porous surface platinum, next is microporous carbon, then microporous platinized platinum (with grooves) and, last, platinized porous platinum with steroid.

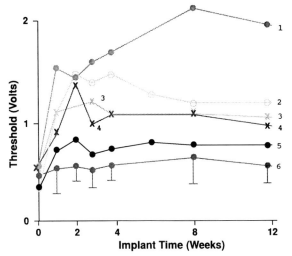

FIGURE 1–27. Canine ventricular voltage thresholds of 8-mm² unipolar, transvenous, tined leads at 0.5 msec as a function of implant time. 1, Polished platinum ring-tip (manufacturer A). 2, Polished platinum ring-tip (manufacturer B). 3, Porous surface platinum hemisphere (manufacturer C). 4, Porous surface titanium hemisphere (manufacturer B). 5, Platinized Target Tip (manufacturer B). 6, Steroid-eluting titanium porous surface electrode (manufacturer B).

The Electrode-Tissue Interface and the Foreign Body Response

PASSIVELY FIXED LEADS WITH STEROID-FREE POLISHED ELECTRODES

The body's response to an implanted device is relatively well characterized.[119, 120] Figure 1–28 shows schematically what ordinarily happens at an implant site as a function of time. If one analyzes the tissues adjacent to canine ventricular endocardial atraumatic electrodes as a function of time following implantation, the evolution depicted in Figure 1–28 is typically observed with one exception. The classic view of inflammation holds that the initial event is dilation of blood vessels and alteration in the vascular endothelium, resulting in increased permeability. This increased perfusion and permeability of the blood vessel walls allows plasma to leak into the surrounding tissue, producing edema. Because plasma and serum are more conductive than myocardium, pacing impedance decreases almost immediately following lead implantation. In the first 1 to 3 days, there is no evidence of cellular inflammation, and thresholds do not change significantly.

The lack of a cellular response in the first few days is an exception to the classic view of surgical wound inflammation. In a surgical wound, polymorphonuclear leukocytes (PMNs) normally are present during this period to scavenge necrotic debris, bacteria, and so on. The lack of PMNs adjacent to atraumatic endocardial electrodes is explained only by the fact that the electrode is placed very far from the surgical wound. After approximately 2 to 3 days, a mixed cellular inflammation begins to appear in the tissues surrounding the electrode, and the stimulation threshold begins to rise. Tissue inflammation reaches its peak in about a week, with interstitial edema and cellular necrosis clearly evident. Pacing impedance typically reaches its minimum value at the inflammatory peak (about 1 week), after which it increases as inflammation subsides. The stimulation threshold may or may not reach its peak at the same time as the nadir of pacing impedance.

Following the early mixed cellular reaction, the inflammatory response is characterized by a gradual accumulation of macrophages that reach the electrode surface, adhere, and become activated. The major function of the macrophage is phagocytosis of dead or foreign cells and particles by the process of endocytosis (Fig. 1–29A).[121] In the case of a very large foreign object such as a pacing electrode, the process of endocytosis is impossible. In this case, the macrophage tries to destroy the large foreign body by means of exocytosis, the extracellular release of enzymes and oxidants (Fig. 1–29B). Macrophages spread over the electrode surface, often differentiating into foreign body giant cells. Their lysosomes migrate to the membrane surface, releasing hydrolytic enzymes and oxidants into the surrounding tissue and onto the electrode surface. Myocytes adjacent to the electrode-tissue interface are bathed in a soup of inflammatory mediators resulting from exocytosis. These mediators of the inflammatory response dissolve the subcellular collagen beams, struts, and nets that hold the myocytes in the normal orderly array of myocardium.[122]

After 3 to 4 weeks (for a stable, biocompatible device), the more global inflammatory response has essentially resolved with a collagenous capsule surrounding the electrode. If the electrode is biocompatible and stable relative to the

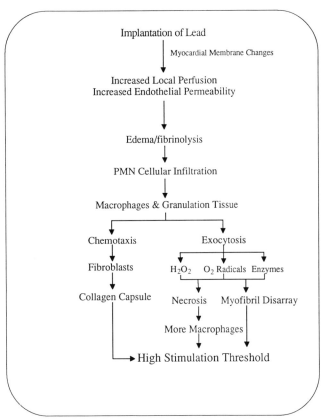

FIGURE 1–28. Schematic representation of the inflammatory process and foreign body response to lead implantation. These events have been approximately correlated with time following the implant of a cardiac pacemaker lead, based on our histologic studies of canine electrode-tissue sites.

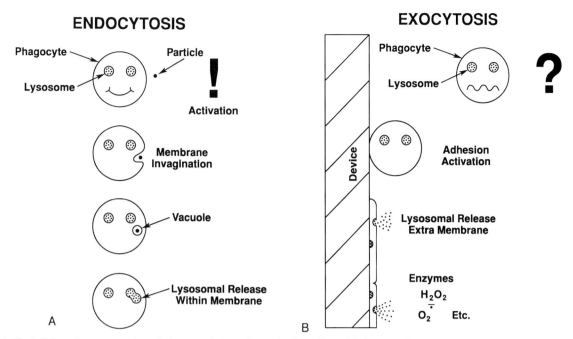

FIGURE 1–29. *A*, Schematic representation of phagocytosis by endocytosis. A small particle is attached to the macrophage's membrane. The membrane invaginates, encapsulating the particle in a membrane-lined vesicle. The vesicle and a lysosome migrate toward each other, and their membranes fuse. The particle is then destroyed by lysosomal enzymes or oxidants. *B*, Schematic representation of the process of "frustrated phagocytosis" by exocytosis—the acute foreign body response on the surface of the device resulting in lysosomal release of inflammatory mediators on the device surface and into the adjacent tissue.

myocardium, there are few further significant visible histologic changes in the adjacent tissues after this period. The stimulation threshold of a polished electrode may still be at or just past the peak phase in the ventricle, however. Thresholds may subsequently decrease, remain stable, or increase, depending on the intensity of the chronic foreign body response at the electrode-tissue interface.

Chronic atraumatic polished electrodes (Fig. 1–30*A*) typically have a layer of foreign body giant cells on their surface. These are covered by a layer (or layers) of macrophages that can be surprisingly thick. This cellular component of the capsule is not an acute, transient phenomenon but has been observed on electrodes up to 13 years following implantation in our canine studies. These cells are covered by a layer of collagen that is oriented along the surface of the electrode. The myocytes adjacent to the collagen layers are disarrayed and interspersed with collagen fibers that are radially oriented with respect to the surface of the electrode. There may also be circular "holes" in this layer of disoriented myocytes that appear to be infiltrated with fatty material. We have observed groups of macrophages with fused membranes (foreign body giant cells) enveloping bundles of myocardial fibers adjacent to the electrode 1 to 4 weeks following implantation. Based on our unpublished work, the presence of this fatty infiltration and its location and severity depend on the stability, myocardial location, and shape of the electrode relative to the vector of myocardial contraction. Outside the disarrayed myofiber zone, one finds normally oriented myocardium. Thus, it is clear that the concept of a simple fibrous capsule (Irnich's "d") separating the electrode surface from viable myocardium does not completely describe this complex biologic response and its effect on pacing.

PASSIVELY FIXED LEADS WITH POROUS AND MICROPOROUS ELECTRODES

Electrodes with pores on the order of 10 to 100 μm in size allow the ingrowth of collagen as a result of chronic inflammation. Thus, in a sense, macroporous electrodes promote inflammation. In addition, the chronic capsule surrounding porous electrodes can be associated with significant myofibrillar disarray (see Fig. 1–30*B*). Despite these factors, porous electrodes are associated with a relatively thin collagenous capsule. Histologic study of the chronic tissue reaction surrounding porous electrodes has shown that inflammatory cells are usually not found on the surface of the electrode. Rather, the active cellular component of the fibrous capsule is located *within* the pores and is removed with the device during the tissue-trimming operation. Similarly, microporous electrodes tend to have few cells on their surfaces in the presence of well-healed interfaces (see Fig. 1–30*C*). We have found that the chronic tissue interface of electrodes with the Target Tip design has an active cellular component deep in the grooves of the electrode (see Fig. 1–30*D*). The smooth, outer surface, however, interfaces directly with collagen.

PASSIVELY FIXED LEADS WITH STEROID-ELUTING ELECTRODES

It has long been recognized that systemically administered glucocorticosteroids decrease both acute and chronic stimulation thresholds. Indeed, the administration of oral or parenteral glucocorticosteroids to patients with exit block may allow the stimulation threshold to decrease to a level that maintains effective pacing. Initially it was believed that the

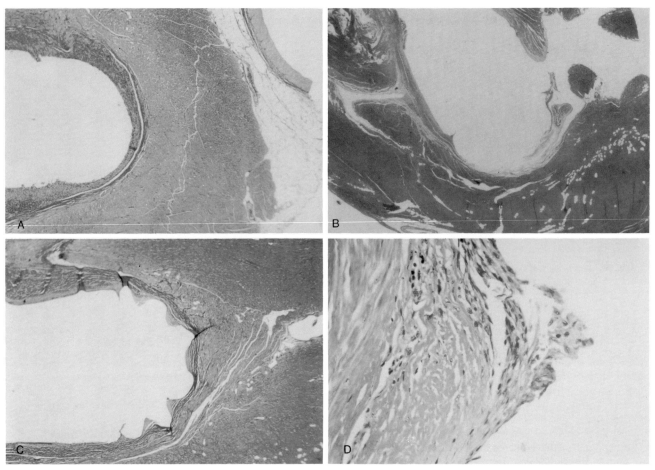

FIGURE 1–30. Optical micrographs of chronic electrode-tissue interfaces. *A,* The capsule surrounding a polished electrode *(upper left)* has a relatively thick layer of activated phagocytic cells including foreign body giant cells on the surface, with macrophages further ''out.'' Collagenous material encapsulates these cells, and fibrous ''stringers'' extend ''outward'' into the myocardium. *B,* Myofibrillar disarray is seen between the collagenous capsule and the normal myocardium. The capsule surrounding a porous electrode *(upper right)* appears to be thinner. The active cellular component of the capsule and some of the collagen, however, have been removed with the electrode to facilitate trimming the tissues. *C,* A microporous (Target Tip) electrode-tissue interface is shown in the lower left section of the micrograph. Note the thin fibrous capsule over the external surfaces and at the ridges. *D,* Some macrophages are seen deep in the Target Tip electrode's grooves at higher magnification.

threshold-lowering effect of systemic glucocorticoid therapy resulted from effects on the myocyte membrane and from sodium and potassium ''retention.''[123] Steroid-eluting leads, in which a dexamethasone sodium phosphate or acetate is gradually released from a reservoir within or around the electrode, have been developed. It has been conclusively demonstrated that steroid elution decreases chronic thresholds. Despite the clear clinical benefits of steroid elution on the evolution of stimulation thresholds, the mechanism of this effect is less well understood. Although steroid-eluting porous electrodes tend to have thinner capsules than polished platinum electrodes, the capsule surrounding a steroid-eluting lead can be difficult to differentiate from porous electrodes in blind analyses. The capsule surrounding a steroid-eluting lead is characterized by minimal cellularity between the collagen and the electrode surface and minimal myofibrillar disarray.

WHY THRESHOLDS EVOLVE AND THE EFFECT OF GLUCOCORTICOSTEROIDS

Although it is commonly accepted that chronic thresholds are higher than the implant value (because a fibrous capsule separates the electrode from viable tissue), the role of the cellular component of the fibrous capsule and its effect on adjacent viable myocytes is less well recognized. Acutely, the release of inflammatory mediators from lysosomes results in dissolution of the normal myocardial microstructure. Certainly the membranes and intercalated discs of myocytes exposed to these proteolytic enzymes and oxidants must be affected to some degree, causing their electric properties to change. Although the acute cellular inflammatory response subsides over several weeks, it appears that the chronic cellular component of the capsule, even in a well-healed situation, continues to leak mediators of inflammation. Undoubtedly, this chronic leakage occurs at a significantly reduced level compared to that in the acute and subacute phases. We propose that it is this chronic leakage that causes the chronic increase in the stimulation thresholds of the adjacent myocytes, in addition to the effect resulting from an increase in the radius of the ''virtual electrode.''

Glucocorticosteroids are known to stabilize the membranes of phagocytes such as macrophages through interaction with surface receptors, inhibiting release of lysosomal contents.[124] It has been shown, however, that dexamethasone and its derivatives have no significant electric effects on myocyte membranes.[125, 126] It is probable that the salutary effect of systemic glucocorticoids on stimulation threshold is the result of inhibition of the release of inflammatory mediators from the cellular components of the fibrous capsule. When steroid therapy is discontinued, the release of inflammatory mediators resumes, and stimulation thresholds once again increase. The same phenomenon minimizes inflammation (foreign body response) on and adjacent to the surface of a steroid-eluting electrode. Acute stabilization of macrophage membranes on the electrode surface reduces or minimizes lysosomal release, thereby minimizing myofibrillar disarray and myocyte membrane damage. Chronic steroid elution suppresses the slow, insidious leakage of inflammatory mediators, thereby preventing threshold increase, without the risk of systemic side effects.

PATHOLOGIC CHANGES DUE TO MECHANICAL INSTABILITY AT THE MYOCARDIAL-ELECTRODE INTERFACE

Mechanically unstable electrodes can provoke a significant pathologic response in the myocardium. Consider, for example, a transvenous corkscrew electrode that "rocks" at the interface with the endocardium because the lead behind it is too stiff. In some cases, large pockets of activated macrophages may develop on either side of the helix, resulting in formation of a "preabscess." In other cases, very thick collagenous capsules form and then differentiate into cartilage and, if the instability is severe enough, into bone. Since active fixation myocardial electrodes interfere with the contractile motion of the adjacent myofibers, myocardial degeneration with fatty infiltration may result in patterns that are clearly related to this mechanical interference. For example, the center of a myocardial helix may fill in with fatty "cells." A myocardial pin may provoke myocardial degeneration and fatty infiltration as well. Thus, it is clear that mechanical instability at the electrode-myocardial interface may produce marked histologic and physiologic effects that result in deterioration of stimulation threshold.

Some Second-Order Effects of Electrode Design

SPATIAL AND SIZE RELATIONSHIPS BETWEEN ELECTRODE PAIRS

It was established previously that, within clinically relevant limits, porous and microporous electrode size and shape per se have no significant effect on the chronic stimulation thresholds (at least with steroid-free electrodes). Nonetheless, the size and shape of the electrode may still be important factors under certain circumstances. For example, a small displacement can affect the performance of a smaller electrode because its high-density field influences relatively few cells.[39, 40] A larger electrode is not as threshold efficient, but perforation is less likely, and small displacements have less effect on lead performance. The ring-tip electrode design is essentially a small electrode made into a large shape.[127] This allows high electric field strength coverage of a larger number of myocardial cells while affording a lower probability of perforation than a lead with a smaller tip. Although myo-

cardial screws, barbs, hooks, and so on are traumatic to the underlying myocardium, these electrodes all have points that serve as sources of high field strength. Thus, myocardial electrodes can perform well chronically, assuming that the lead is not so stiff as to apply undue forces on the electrode-myocardial interface.

ELECTRODE FIXATION

The most efficient electrode design will provide poor long-term performance if it is mechanically unstable, resulting in both high stimulation thresholds and histopathologic evidence of excessive trauma. However, for chronically stable, steroid-free electrodes in canines we have found no correlation between the mechanism of fixation and the chronic stimulation threshold (Table 1–1). Given similar geometric surface areas, we found comparable chronic canine ventricular thresholds with tined, flanged, screw, and hook-in polished electrodes, whether endocardial or myocardial. These results have been confirmed by human studies in both the atrium and the ventricle.[128–130] Thus, the hypothesis that fixation remote from the polished electrode stimulation site is necessary for low chronic thresholds does not appear to be valid.[131, 132] It has not been established whether this is also true for steroid-eluting electrodes.

ELECTRODE MATERIALS

To minimize inflammation and its subsequent effects on stimulation threshold, electrodes for permanent pacing should be biocompatible and resistant to chemical degradation. Many materials, such as platinum, titanium, titanium oxide, titanium nitride, carbon, tantalum pentoxide, iridium, and iridium oxide, have been shown to be acceptable for use as pacing electrodes.[133–135] Even silver, which is toxic in neurologic tissue and certainly not very corrosion resistant, has been used successfully in the heart as an electrode.[133] Titanium and tantalum have been known to acquire a surface coating of oxides, which, it has been argued, may impede charge transfer at the electrode interface. To prevent this, titanium has been coated with platinized platinum or vitreous carbon. Others accept the concept that the oxide layer acts as the dielectric of a capacitor such that no charge is transferred across the dielectric during stimulation. In any case, titanium oxide electrodes are highly corrosion resistant, and these combinations have been found to provide excellent long-term performance as pacing electrodes.[136–140] Some theories have held that the foreign body reaction is a response to the electrode material per se.[99, 141] Therefore, many attempts have been made to improve thresholds through the use of more biocompatible materials. For example, it has been claimed that pyrolytic carbons are more biocompatible and produce lower chronic thresholds than platinum.[99, 102, 103, 136] It should be recognized that, besides having a different composition, these electrodes are also microporous. When similar electrodes are polished, we have found that the chronic canine thresholds are not significantly different from those occurring with polished platinum. There can be no doubt that proper electrode material selection is necessary to prevent unacceptable toxic responses or corrosion. At this point, however, there does not appear to be a biocompatible electrode composition per se that significantly improves thresholds.

TABLE 1–1. CHRONIC (12-WEEK) UNIPOLAR CANINE (CONSTANT-VOLTAGE) THRESHOLDS (V_{thr}) OF POLISHED PLATINUM ELECTRODES AT 0.5 msec VERSUS FIXATION MECHANISM

MODEL NO.	INSERTION FIXATION	ELECTRODE LOCATION SHAPE	SURFACE AREA (mm²)	STIMULATION THRESHOLD (V_{thr})	n	p vs 6971[a]
6901	Endocardial flange	Endocardial cylinder	11	1.9 ± .77	11	.2
6950	Endocardial long tines	Endocardial cylinder	11	1.6 ± .48	4	>.5
6961	Endocardial short tines	Endocardial ring	8	1.8 ± .69	9	.35
6971	Endocardial medium tines	Endocardial ring	8	1.5 ± .57	8	—
4016	Endocardial helix	Myocardial helix	10	1.1 ± .30	6	.1
6959	Endocardial helix	Endocardial ring	13	1.3 ± .42	8	.4
6955	Endocardial helix	Myocardial helix	10	1.6 ± .51	10	>.5
4951	Epicardial hook	Myocardial hook	10	1.5 ± .44	10	>.5
6917	Epicardial helix	Myocardial helix	12	1.4 ± .53	17	>.5

[a]$p < .05$ considered statistically significant.
From Stokes K, Bornzin G: The electrode–biointerface (stimulation). *In* Barold S (ed): Modern Cardiac Pacing. Mt. Kisco, NY, Futura, 1985, pp 33–78.

Of course, not all conductive materials are suitable for use as electrodes. Certain materials such as zinc, copper, mercury, nickel, and lead are associated with toxic reactions in the myocardium and are unsuitable for use in permanent pacing leads.[133] Stainless steels are highly variable in composition and microstructure, and there is great variability between production lots. Electrodes made from one lot may be acceptable, whereas those made from another lot may corrode unacceptably. Because some of the corrosion products may be inflammatory or toxic, high thresholds may occasionally occur with these materials. Thus, stainless steel electrodes are no longer used for implantable electrodes. The polarity of the electrode may also have an important influence on its corrosion resistance. For example, Eligoloy, a non-noble and highly polarizing metal alloy, has been adequate as a cathode. However, when used as an anode, this alloy is susceptible to a significant degree of corrosion. As a result, Eligoloy is only rarely used as an electrode today.

The materials presently used for permanent pacing electrodes include platinum-iridium, titanium (oxide), platinum- or carbon-coated titanium, platinized platinum, vitreous carbon, and iridium oxide. The platinized platinum, ''activated'' carbon, and iridium oxide electrodes are associated with a reduced degree of polarization. A negligible degree of corrosion occurs with these materials. The vitreous carbon electrodes have been improved by roughening the surface, a process known as ''activation'' that increases the interface surface area, thereby reducing polarization.

ELECTRODE LOCATION (EPICARDIAL, ENDOCARDIAL, MYOCARDIAL)

As shown previously in canine ventricles for electrodes without steroid elution, the site of fixation has no effect on stimulation thresholds. Similarly, epicardially applied corkscrews, transvenous corkscrews, and passively fixed endocardial electrodes all tend to have about the same chronic thresholds in canines (Table 1–1). Nonetheless, it is generally agreed that epicardial or myocardial electrodes without steroid elution have a less desirable threshold performance than endocardial leads in humans. Certainly, the development of the steroid-eluting lead has produced endocardial electrodes that have superior performance compared with steroid-free transvenous active fixation devices and epicardial or myocar-

dial devices. It is also true that most epicardial or myocardial leads today are used in pediatric pacing, patients in whom threshold complications are relatively frequent.[142, 143] One reason why modern endocardial, passively fixed lead performance is superior today may be that their electrodes incorporate newer innovations. For example, state-of-the-art passively fixed, endocardial electrodes are porous, microporous, and steroid-eluting. Because of the mechanical limitations involved, transvenous active fixation and epicardial or myocardial leads are significantly more complex and more difficult to design with all the attributes needed to produce low chronic stimulation thresholds. There is, however, no inherent reason why transvenous active fixation or myocardial electrodes should not perform as well as or better than endocardial systems. Thus, high expectations that low-threshold, highly efficient, transvenous active fixation devices and epicardial or myocardial leads will become available in the reasonably near future are reasonable.[142–146]

Pacing Impedance

Impedance (Z) is a complex phenomenon that is poorly understood in the pacing community and is often confused with resistance (R). Indeed, resistance is usually a good first approximation of impedance. Nonetheless, a reasonable understanding of the fundamental concepts in pacing requires a basic understanding of impedance. Impedance is defined as the *sum of all forces opposing the flow of current in an electric circuit*. In most circuits, impedance is defined as

Eq 22 $$Z = \sqrt{R^2 + (A_i - A_c)^2}$$

where R is the sum of the resistances that follow Ohm's law (R = V/I) and A_i is the inductive reactance where

Eq 23 $$A_i = 2\pi f L$$

and A_c is the capacitive reactance,

Eq 24 $$A_c = \frac{1}{2\pi f C}$$

The frequency of the signal (f) is measured in Hertz, the inductance (L) in Henrys, and the capacitance (C) in farads. In pacing, however, the inductance is usually considered to be too small to be of significance. Some argue that there can be no such entity as impedance in a direct current (DC) circuit because frequency is (by definition) zero. Pacing stimuli, however, are not exactly DC signals. They do have significant frequency components when analyzed by fast Fourier transform, as shown in Figure 1–31. Thus, the term ''impedance'' is correctly applicable to the pacing stimulus. Pacing impedance (Z_p), therefore, is typically represented as

Eq 25 $\quad Z_p = \sqrt{R^2 + \left(\frac{1}{2\pi fC}\right)^2}$

Although impedance can be very complicated, we will try to simplify it by examining its components separately. This is facilitated by referring to a simplified equivalent circuit for pacing impedance shown in Figure 1–32.

PACING RESISTANCE

There are a number of resistances in the total pacemaker circuit, including the resistances of the conductor wires, the tissue between the electrodes, and the electrode-tissue interfaces (remember, there are always two electrodes). The resistance of the conductor wire leading to the stimulating electrode (R_w) is usually a significant value, typically in the range of 50 to 150 ohms. The resistance of the conductor wire leading to the anode (R_w) may be significant, as with a bipolar lead (typically 50 to 150 ohms), or insignificant, as with a unipolar pacing system, approaching zero. The resistance of the tissue (R_t) can vary, depending on the electrode spacing. It is relatively low for a bipolar lead (approximately 50 ohms) but significantly higher for a unipolar system (approximately 150 ohms). The resistance of the electrode-tissue interface depends on the geometric surface area of the electrodes. Because efficient cathodes are relatively small, the resistance at the cathode-tissue interface (R_c) can be relatively high (for example, roughly 250 ohms for an 8-mm^2 hemispherical electrode), whereas that of the anode (R_a) should be much less (such as 100 ohms for a bipolar lead and 5 ohms for a unipolar pacemaker).

When the pacing pulse is turned on, several events occur

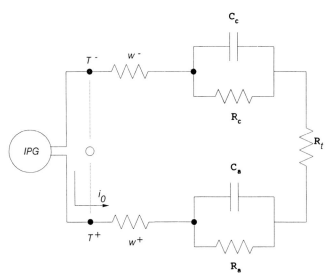

FIGURE 1–32. A simplified equivalent circuit for a cardiac pacemaker. T^- and T^+ are the negative (cathode) and positive (anode) terminals of the pulse generator (in a unipolar device, T^+ is inside the can). R_{w-} is the resistance of the conductor wire leading to the distal tip of the lead (cathode), and R_{w+} is the resistance of the wire leading to the bipolar lead's proximal ring electrode or the unipolar pulse generator's can. R_t is the resistance of the tissue between the bipolar lead's two electrodes, or that of the lead tip to the pulse generator in a unipolar system. R_c is the ohmic polarization of the cathode, and R_a is that of the bipolar anode or unipolar generator can. C_c is the capacitance of the cathode, and C_a is that of the anode (can). The equivalent circuit is the same for unipolar and bipolar systems, but the values for some of the components differ.

almost immediately. Unless the electrode is a perfect capacitor, electrochemical reactions must occur at the electrode surface–electrolyte interface to allow charge to be transferred from an electronic to an ionic medium. As the stimulus is initiated, majority carriers such as Na^+ and Cl^- rapidly conduct charge away from the interface. This is observed as the initial fast rise or leading edge (l_e) of the pulse waveform, where $R = V_{le}/I_{le}$, as shown in Figure 1–33. The leading edge resistance occurring at the cathode is R_c (Fig. 1–33), and that at the anode is R_a. Sometimes this leading edge resistance is referred to as *ohmic polarization.*

ELECTRODE CAPACITANCE

When one places a metal in an electrolyte solution, a potential is developed at the electrolyte-metal interface. This can be observed by placing a pacing lead in a saline-filled beaker. If the electrode is tapped against the glass, surprisingly large voltage spikes can be seen on an oscilloscope connected to the lead terminal and a reference electrode in the beaker. In 1879 Helmholtz suggested that a layer of ions exists on the surface of an electrode, which is surrounded by a layer of oppositely charged ions in the solution.[147] This theory is thermodynamically inadequate, however, so the diffuse double layer was proposed by Stern in 1924.[147, 148] A more recent model of the double layer was described by Devanathan and associates.[148] In this model, a layer of water molecules adsorbs to the surface of the electrode. A second layer of hydrated ions and more water is formed (Fig. 1–34). In physiologic electrolytes, these ions include Na^+ and Cl^- in major concentrations *(majority carriers).* Other ions pres-

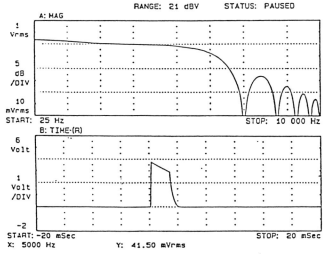

FIGURE 1–31. Frequency analysis of a stimulating pulse. *Bottom,* A capacitively coupled constant-voltage pacing pulse (about 1.8 V, leading edge) in the time domain. *Top,* A fast Fourier transformation of the same pulse in the frequency domain. (From Schaldach M: The stimulating electrode. *In* Electrotherapy of the Heart. Berlin, Springer-Verlag, 1992, p 153.)

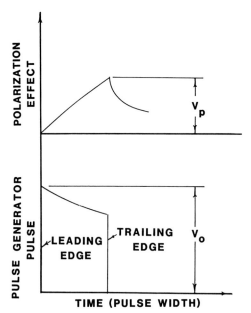

FIGURE 1–33. The effect of polarization *(upper diagram)* has been separated from the capacitively coupled constant-voltage pacing pulse *(lower diagram)* to help clarify the electrical manifestations of electrode polarization. At the leading edge of the pulse, polarization is essentially zero. With time (pulse width) the voltage due to polarization (sometimes called polarization overvoltage, V_p) increases. When the pacing pulse is shut off, polarization overvoltage decays exponentially as a result of diffusion. (From Stokes K, Bornzin G: The electrode–biointerface (stimulation). *In* Barold S [ed]: Modern Cardiac Pacing. Mt. Kisco, NY, Futura, 1985, pp 33–78.)

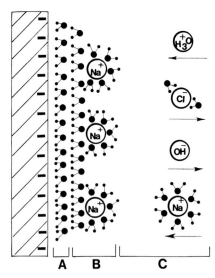

FIGURE 1–34. Hypothesized structure of the double layer at an uncharged *(left)* and charged *(right)* cathodic electrode interface. Region A contains a layer of surface hydration. Region B contains a second, more loosely held hydration layer with hydrated ions. Based on electrostatic considerations, layer B has a high dielectric constant, approaching that of pure water. It has a thickness of less than 10 Angstrom units (1.0 nm). Region C is bulk solution. (From Stokes K, Bornzin G: The electrode–biointerface (stimulation). *In* Barold S [ed]: Modern Cardiac Pacing. Mt. Kisco, NY, Futura, 1985, pp 33–78.)

equal in magnitude to the leading edge of the pulse. A slow decay of potential occurs, as shown in Figures 1–34 and 1–36. This slow decay is the result of the diffusion of the polarized ions back to electroneutrality.

ent in lower concentrations *(minority carriers)* include hydronium (H_3O^+), hydroxyl (OH^-), and phosphate (HPO_4^{2-}). These layers have relatively high dielectric constants and form an interface that behaves electrically like a capacitor (C_c and C_a in Figure 1–33). Thus, the commonly used and simplified model of pacing impedance (Z_p) includes a capacitor and a resistor in parallel, both in series with resistances.

ELECTRODE POLARIZATION

When the pulse is turned on, majority carriers are rapidly depleted near the electrode surface. Minority carriers must then carry charge across the capacitive double layer. Because the minority carriers are rapidly depleted, more ions must diffuse into the region from relatively remote areas.[149] As the pulse width increases, the voltage required to push current past the capacitive barrier also increases. This phenomenon is presented in schematic form in Figure 1–33 and in graphic form in Figure 1–35. Because the voltage rise is dependent on the concentration of majority and minority carriers, this phenomenon is known as concentration polarization (CP). Mindt and Schaldach reported that the magnitude of CP may be as large as 5 to 20 f/cm² for polished electrodes.[150]

As a result of CP, there are local accumulations and depletions of ionic species such as H_3O^+, OH^-, Cl^-, Na^+, and so on, which are slightly separated from their counter ions. It should be noted that a large force (voltage) is required to separate ions very slightly without precipitation. Thus, a significant increase in potential that is a function of pulse width (termed overvoltage) can occur during a constant-current pulse. When the pulse is turned off, the ohmic polarization instantaneously disappears, as shown by a trailing edge drop

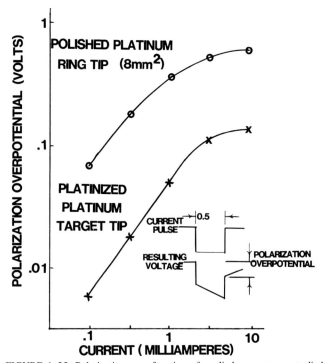

FIGURE 1–35. Polarization as a function of applied current was studied using an 8-mm² platinized Target Tip electrode and an 8-mm² polished platinum ring-tip in a 0.18% saline solution. Polarization overvoltage was defined as shown in the lower right inset. (From Stokes K, Bornzin G: The electrode–biointerface (stimulation). *In* Barold S [ed]: Modern Cardiac Pacing. Mt. Kisco, NY, Futura, 1985, pp 33–78.)

OPTIMIZING IMPEDANCE

The effects of impedance on the pacing system are quite significant. On the positive side, high impedance reduces current drain from the battery, increasing its longevity. From this standpoint, the higher the pacing impedance, the better. On the negative side, electrode polarization during the pulse contributes nothing to stimulation. More potential must be applied to overcome the effects of polarization, raising the measured stimulation threshold. In addition, the afterpotential resulting from electrode polarization can interfere with sensing. Therefore, the ideal pulse would have no polarization and would be all resistance. The way in which the resistance is distributed in the system, however, can also have markedly different effects, making the stimulating pulse either efficient or inefficient with an unnecessarily higher threshold and a lower safety factor. To clarify these issues, we need to examine the electrode-tissue interface impedance and conduction losses.

OPTIMUM IMPEDANCE AT THE ELECTRODE-TISSUE INTERFACE

The resistance (ohmic polarization) of the stimulating electrode is inversely and exponentially proportional to the geometric surface area of the electrode and the temperature and conductivity of the tissue.[151, 152] Because for all practical purposes we can assume that in vivo temperature and conductivity are essentially constant, maximizing the resistance may be accomplished simply by decreasing the geometric surface area of the electrode as illustrated in Figure 1–36. A simple reduction in size alone, however, has the negative effect of increasing polarization impedance. Thus, the way in which electrode size is reduced is critically important.

Electrode polarization is represented mathematically as the capacitive reactance $1/2\pi fC$ (equation 24). At any given frequency, therefore, the ideal electrode has very high capacitance, so that the reactance (polarization) approaches zero.

For a given electrode material, capacitance (C) is essentially a function of the interface surface area (A_i):

Eq 26 $$C = \frac{eA_i}{d}$$

where e is the dielectric constant of the double layer and d is its thickness. Since e and d are essentially constants in vivo, the capacitance of the electrode varies as a function of its *interface* surface area (A_i). How does one make a very large surface area into a small geometric volume? Initially, this was accomplished by making the electrodes porous.[90–93] Microporous electrodes such as activated carbon or platinized platinum have an even higher real surface area.[67, 99, 153] This is equivalent to taking a very large sheet of paper and crumpling it into a small ball. Thus, we find that the polarization overvoltage of polished electrodes is greater than that of porous, which is greater than that of microporous electrodes because the capacitance of microporous surfaces is greater than that of porous surfaces and still greater than that of polished surfaces.

Another approach to the problem of decreasing polarization is to use a material that supplies its own majority charge carriers. An example is the silver-silver chloride electrode in chloride solution. The majority carrier, in this case chloride, cannot be depleted. Chloride evolves at the cathode and is formed at the anode. Thus, voltage across the electrode interface has a waveshape essentially identical to that of the applied constant current, and the electrode is said to be "nonpolarizing." Unfortunately, there does not appear to be a suitable nonpolarizing (charge carrier–supplying) electrode material available for permanent implantation. Silver-silver chloride electrodes, for example, are not used for permanent pacing because the anode erodes and the AgCl eventually dissolves from the cathode.[153, 154] Thus, the ideal, practical stimulating electrode is made of a corrosion-resistant, biocompatible material with a small geometric size and a very high interface surface area, thereby affording a very high capacitance.

CONDUCTOR RESISTANCE AND CONDUCTION LOSSES

A very simple and commonly used method of increasing the system impedance without adding electrode polarization is to use higher resistance lead conductors. On the positive side, this process reduces current drain from the battery. However, increasing resistance in the wire also increases the stimulation threshold and reduces the safety factor. Based on Kirchhoff's law, the current in a circuit (assuming 100% efficiency) must be the same in every resistive element at any given instant. Therefore, according to Ohm's law, the voltage must be divided at points in the circuit proportional to the resistance. When we use the word *voltage* we really mean a potential *difference* between the cathode compared with the anode. A pulse generator programmed to deliver a 5.0-V output pulse really develops a −5.0-V potential at the cathode relative to the anode. That being the case, the voltage available at the stimulating cathode must be less than that which the generator is actually programmed to deliver by an amount proportional to the resistance of the conductor wire

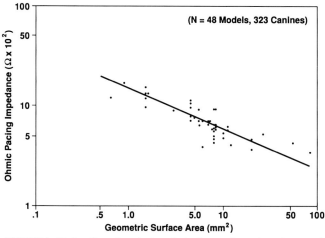

FIGURE 1–36. Leading edge ohmic polarization or electrode resistance of chronic (12 weeks after implant) canine ventricular leads measured with a Medtronic model 5311 PSA as a function of the (unipolar) cathode's geometric surface area. Each data point is a population of canines in which one lead design was tested. The study includes 323 animals and 48 lead models.

(R_{cw}). The voltage divider principle as applied to the cathode of a unipolar pacemaker system can be reduced to:

Eq 27 $\quad V_c = V_o \left(1 - \dfrac{R_w}{Z_p} \right)$

where V_c is the voltage between the cathode and the anode, V_o is the voltage output of the pulse generator, R_w is the resistance of the conductor wire, and Z_p is the total pacing impedance.[155] If the total pacing impedance in a hypothetical unipolar pacemaker circuit is 500 ohms and the resistance of the conductor to the cathode (R_w) is zero, then the potential between the cathode and the unipolar anode, the pulse generator can, will be the same as the output voltage of the pulse generator. If the conductor resistance is 150 ohms and all other factors in the circuit are held constant, the total impedance will increase to 650 ohms. This will reduce current drain, prolonging the longevity of the pulse generator battery compared to the 500-ohm system. It will also reduce the voltage between the cathode and the anode by $^{150}/_{650}$, or 23%. Thus, if the clinician sets the pulse generator output pulse at 5 V, in reality only 3.8 V is produced between the electrodes. In this case, the safety factor may be less than the clinician believes.

Voltage division also affects stimulation threshold. Again, consider the hypothetical unipolar pacemaker in which the resistance of the conductor wire joining the pulse generator to the stimulating electrode is zero, the total impedance is 500 ohms, and the stimulation threshold is 1 V. If the conductor resistance is increased to 150 ohms, thereby increasing the total pacing impedance to 650 ohms, the measured threshold would increase by 30% (1.3 V). At first, this may not seem significant. In some situations, however, it could cause the clinician to program the device to higher outputs, resulting in unnecessarily higher current drains and reduced battery longevity. If one accepts the current density theory of pacing or uses a CI generator, the effect of the conductor wire resistance cannot be dismissed. The resistance in a conductor causes some of the current to be wasted as heat. This is expressed as the power (P) loss, which is expressed by:

Eq 28 $\quad P = I^2R$

The energy (E) wasted as heat due to conductor resistance is:

Eq 29 $\quad E = Pt$

where t is the time that the pulse is applied (the pulse duration). In fact, these equations give exactly the same percentage losses as voltage division.[155] Therefore, regardless of how one views the basic mechanism of myocardial stimulation, increased resistance in the lead conductor represents a waste of energy. Thus, it is clear that although high pacing impedance may be desirable, impedance should be maximized at the electrode-tissue interface, not as resistance in the lead conductors. The ideal lead has as low resistance as practical in its conductors. It does not matter whether the system is unipolar or bipolar—the principles are the same.

Pharmacologic Effects on Cardiac Stimulation

ANTIARRHYTHMIC DRUGS

Several types of antiarrhythmic drugs have been demonstrated to increase stimulation thresholds, both in humans and in animals. Type 1 drugs decrease Na^+ conductance and decrease the rate of rise of the action potential. Thus, it should be no surprise that these agents may increase the threshold for pacing. Type 1A drugs such as quinidine[156] and procainamide[157] may result in increased thresholds, especially when administered in high doses.[158] Type 1C drugs (encainide, flecainide, and propafenone) have all been associated with increased pacing thresholds.[159–163] The increase in stimulation threshold seen with these drugs correlates with the change in QRS duration. In addition to type 1 agents, propranolol has been demonstrated to result in an increase in pacing threshold when administered intravenously.[164] Amiodarone, lidocaine, tocainide, and verapamil have been reported to have minimal effects on pacing threshold.[165]

Metabolic Effects on Cardiac Stimulation

Stimulation thresholds may rise during sleeping or eating, factors associated with withdrawal of sympathetic tone and increased vagal tone.[165, 170] In contrast, factors associated with increased sympathetic tone such as exercise or assumption of the upright posture are associated with a decrease in threshold. The myocardial stimulation threshold is increased by several metabolic abnormalities, including hypoxemia, hypercarbia, metabolic alkalosis, and metabolic acidosis. Hughes and colleagues noted an increase in pacing threshold of more than 70% with either metabolic acidosis or alkalosis.[166] In the presence of respiratory or cardiac arrest the pacing threshold may increase by well over 100%, resulting in loss of capture despite the use of a conventional safety margin. Because of this observation, antitachycardia pacing devices such as pacemakers or implantable cardioverter-defibrillators are often designed to deliver high-intensity stimuli during antitachycardia pacing or following a high-energy shock. In patients undergoing implantation of a cardioverter-defibrillator, Khastgir and colleagues were unable to demonstrate an increase in pacing threshold at 10 and 60 seconds following defibrillation.[167] It should be emphasized that defibrillation was performed promptly and under controlled circumstances in this study population. In the presence of primary respiratory arrest, pacing stimuli may not capture the myocardium until adequate ventilation and pH balance are restored. Thus, careful attention to respiration and pH must be maintained during anesthesia in patients with implanted pacemakers to ensure continued myocardial capture. Ischemia produces variable effects on stimulation threshold, depending on the location of the pacing electrode relative to the ischemic myocardium. In the presence of acute myocardial ischemia, the resting membrane potential decreases (cells become partially depolarized), the action potential upstroke velocity decreases, and the duration of the action potential dramatically shortens. In the presence of metabolic blockade with 2,4-dinitrophenol, Delmar noted an upward shift in the strength-duration curve, indicating an increase in the current required for capture at all pulse durations.[168] Thus, if the stimulating electrode is located in an ischemic region, the stimulation threshold would be expected to increase. With further ischemia and infarction, the myocardial threshold may rise dramatically. However, if the stimulating electrode is located in a nonischemic region (such as the right ventricle) during activation of the sympathetic nervous system as a consequence of ischemia in a remote zone (such as the left ventricle), the stimulation threshold may be expected to decrease.

Hyperkalemia has been shown to increase the stimulation threshold when the serum K^+ concentration exceeds 7.0 mEq/L.[169, 170] In contrast, in the presence of hypokalemia, intravenous K^+ may decrease the pacing threshold and restore capture of a subthreshold pulse.[171] In addition, the reduced excitability that occurs during hyperkalemia can be corrected by the intravenous administration of calcium.[172] Hyperglycemia in the range of 600 mg/dL may increase stimulation thresholds by as much as 60%.[173] Thus, patients with diabetes or renal failure, conditions associated with the potential for altered glucose metabolism and electrolyte abnormalities, may need a larger safety margin than other patients. Hypothyroidism has been demonstrated to increase pacing thresholds, an effect that is reversible with thyroxine replacement.[174, 175] As stated previously, glucocorticosteroids have been shown to decrease stimulation thresholds and have been used to treat exit block in both acute and chronic situations.[176] Endogenous and synthetic catecholamines are effective in lowering pacing thresholds.[177, 178] The effect of intravenous epinephrine and isoproterenol is an initial decrease in stimulation threshold followed by an increase. Intravenous and sublingual isoproterenol reverses high pacing thresholds related to antiarrhythmic drug toxicity.[179]

Calculating Battery Longevity and Programming Generators for Optimum Performance

A pacemaker battery is a source of electric charge (measured in coulombs). Current (measured in amperes) is the rate at which charge flows in a circuit where:

Eq 30 $\quad 1 \text{ Ampere} = 1 \dfrac{\text{Coulomb}}{\text{Second}}$

Pacemaker batteries are rated in terms of their quantity of charge (current $\times$ time) or in units of ampere-hours. The longevity (L) of the battery is the *deliverable* charge capacity (Q_c) divided by the rate at which charge is consumed.

Eq 31 $\quad \text{Longevity (yr)} = \dfrac{Q_c \times 10^6}{8760 \ (\text{hr/yr})(I_c + I_l)}$

where I_c is the current drained by the pulse generator circuitry and I_l is the current drained through the lead to the patient.[155] Note that I_c and I_l are "continuous" measures of current, not the current per each pacing pulse. The current drained by the circuit is a function of the circuit design and is not programmable by the clinician. The deliverable battery capacity is also a fixed parameter and is not clinically adjustable. Thus, the clinician has only one parameter that can be adjusted to affect battery longevity, the current being transmitted through the lead (I_l). The lead current is given by:

Eq 32 $\quad I_l = \dfrac{V_o^2 t}{Z_p V_b CL \times 10^{-6}}$

where V_o is the generator output voltage, t is the pulse duration, Z_p is the pacing impedance, V_b is the battery voltage, and CL is the cycle length (msec).[155] The pacing impedance

and the battery voltage are also not clinically adjustable. Thus, the only parameters of the output pulse that the clinician may adjust to optimize battery longevity are V_o (amplitude in volts) and t (pulse duration in milliseconds). In addition, a significant improvement in battery longevity can be made by decreasing the frequency with which pacing pulses are delivered, such as by programming the upper and lower pacing rates, the AV delay, hysteresis, and pacing mode.

ADEQUATE MARGIN OF SAFETY

A pacemaker must be operated within a reasonable safety factor that ensures capture of the myocardium by the delivered pulse. Because the output pulse is a fixed value, the safety margin must change with spontaneous variation in stimulation threshold. We need to know, therefore, how much the stimulation thresholds actually change in the acute-to-chronic period, and chronically on an hour-to-hour and day-to-day basis. The safety factor (SF) for pacing has been defined as a function of the output voltage of the pulse generator (V_o) divided by the stimulation threshold voltage (V_{thr}), where:

Eq 33 $\quad SF = V_o / V_{thr}$

Alternatively, we can think of safety factors as a percentage, where:

Eq 34 $\quad SF = \dfrac{(V_o - V_{thr})}{V_{thr}} \times 100$

Thus, if V_o is 2.5 V and V_{thr} is 1.0 V, then the SF = 2.5:1 or 150%. Both of these indices are valid, although the simple ratio (equation 33) is easier to use. In present medical practice the clinician often sets the pulse generator output pulse to 5 V and 0.5 msec at implant and then measures the stimulation threshold approximately 6 weeks later. The chronic output pulse is then programmed based on these results. In adults, settings of 5 V and 0.5 msec at implant appear to ensure capture for a very large majority of patients with any modern lead. This is not necessarily the situation in children, who experience a higher rate of exit block owing to their very active inflammatory responses. Because of the unique inflammation-suppressing properties of steroid-eluting electrodes, these devices are indicated for pediatric pacing whenever possible.[116, 180, 181] The safety factors provided during the peak threshold phase are highest for steroid-eluting porous electrodes and less for (in descending order) microporous electrodes, porous electrodes, and polished-tip electrodes, based on data in Figures 1–25 and 1–26. There may also be situations in which the patient's pacemaker must be left at the maximum output at implantation (for example, if the patient will not be available for follow-up). In these cases, an acceptable balance of safety margin and battery longevity is achieved with a setting of 2.5 V and 0.5 msec with a steroid-eluting electrode, or 5 V and 0.5 msec with other leads.

Most of today's perception of the range of chronic circadian threshold variation is based on the work of Sowton and Norman (published in the mid 1960s), Preston and colleagues (the late 1960s), and Westerholm (1971).[182–184] The first two studies used CI generators and reported thresholds in terms of energy. Because the computed energy "thresholds" could have been a reflection of changes in impedance, the actual variation in voltage threshold cannot be determined from these studies. Westerholm, who reported both voltage and energy data, noted substantial circadian variation in both parameters. In all of these studies, the leads were primarily epicardial-myocardial with polished electrodes. Based on our own canine results, these human data may be of marginal relevance to modern CV generators and porous, steroid-eluting electrodes. We have found no significant threshold changes in adult canines using modern chronic atrial or ventricular leads as a function of eating, sleeping, exercise, and so on.[185] This finding is supported by Kadish and colleagues, who found no changes in chronic human pacing thresholds over a 24-hour period in four of five patients studied.[186] Although in one patient threshold at 0.6 msec changed from 1.0 to 1.5 V between 3 and 6 PM, Kadish and colleagues concluded that "ventricular pacing thresholds do not show substantial diurnal variability." Grendahl and Schaanning also found minimal variation in pacing threshold during the day, after meals, or during sleeping or physical activity.[187] Shepherd and associates reported large transient increases in stimulation threshold in a child during two successive summers that were presumed to be related to a summer cold.[188] The effects of various drugs on thresholds have been reported, but neither the test protocols nor the results have been consistent.[189] Thus, there appears to be little in the literature to support the statistical validity of any particular safety factor.

Based on the earlier report of Preston and colleagues, Barold and coworkers suggested that V_o/V_{thr} must be 1.75 or more to ensure an adequate safety margin, assuming a ± 50% change in energy at threshold throughout the day.[190] Ohm and his colleagues studied threshold evolution as a function of implant duration for an 8-mm² polished platinum ring electrode and found that this lead had a peak threshold of 2.2 ± 0.75 V at 0.5 msec pulse duration 2 weeks after implant.[191, 192] Assuming an output setting of 5 V and 0.5 msec pulse duration, the average patient had a V_o/V_{thr} of 2.3 during threshold peak. The 98th percentile patient (the mean + 2 standard deviations) had 5 V/(2.2 + 2 × 0.75 V), or about a 1.35 safety margin at peak threshold. To the best of our knowledge, exit block with that lead at a 5-V, 0.5-msec output setting 2 weeks after implant was extremely rare. Therefore, it seems reasonable that even safety margins as low as 1.35 may be acceptable for many patients. Nonetheless, unusual and unpredictable situations may happen that may justify higher values.[188] The presently accepted chronic safety factor is at least 2:1. This seems to be adequate for the great majority of patients. In patients who are highly dependent on the pacemaker, an even higher safety margin may be appropriate. In other situations, as in patients who are not pacemaker dependent, lower values, even as low as 1.35:1, may be acceptable.

PROGRAMMING VOLTAGE VERSUS PULSE WIDTH FOR MAXIMUM PULSE GENERATOR LONGEVITY

A common clinical concern with programming the pulse generator to optimize battery longevity relates to whether it is more useful to program the amplitude or the duration of the output pulse. Based on equation 32 and on examination of the strength-duration relationship, it is more efficient to reduce the voltage output of the pulse (V_o) because the cur-

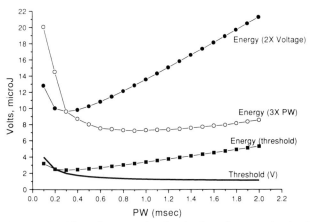

FIGURE 1–37. Effect of programming the stimulus voltage to twice threshold (at a constant pulse width [PW]) or programming the pulse width to 3 times threshold value (at constant voltage) on current drain and safety margin. See text for discussion.

rent drain varies as the square of voltage. Figure 1–37 illustrates the effect of doubling the threshold voltage (at a constant pulse width) or tripling the threshold pulse width (without changing the voltage) on current drain. In this example, the rheobase voltage was determined to be 1.0 V and the chronaxie duration was 0.3 msec. The stimulation threshold was measured at 4.0 V at a pulse duration of 0.1 msec or 2 V at 0.3 msec. Tripling the pulse duration at 4.0 V to 0.3 msec provides an adequate (2:1) safety margin with a current of 8 mA/pulse (4.8 μA continuous current) and a stimulus energy of 9.6 μJ. Similarly, doubling the threshold voltage at a pulse duration of 0.3 msec from 2.0 to 4.0 V gives an identical current drain (8 mA/pulse, or 4.8 μA) and safety factor. If the patient has a higher threshold, for example, 2 V at 1.0 msec, doubling the voltage or tripling the pulse width would still give the same current drain (12 μA). The safety factor, however, would be significantly different. Tripling the pulse width would provide a marginal (at best) safety margin because threshold is approaching rheobase on the flat portion of the strength-duration curve. It is necessary to double the voltage in this case to ensure a 2:1 safety margin. The foremost consideration in programming voltage and pulse duration is the factor of patient safety.

Summary

Perhaps the most important concept needed for programming an implantable pacing system is a thorough understanding of the strength-duration relationship. Modern pulse generators allow the clinician to program both the pulse amplitude (in volts) and the pulse duration (in milliseconds). It must be recognized that the stimulation threshold is a function of both these parameters. The exponential shape of the strength-duration curve must always be considered when programming the output pulse to ensure an adequate margin of safety between the delivered stimulus and the capture threshold. For example, pulse durations of 1.0 msec and greater are located on the flat portion of the strength-duration curve, whereas pulse durations of less than 0.15 msec are on the steeply rising portion of the curve. The practical importance of this can be appreciated by considering two points on the strength-duration curve shown in Figure 1–9. If the clinician determines that the threshold occurs at point A (2.0 V and 0.5 msec) by decreasing the stimulus voltage at a constant pulse duration, programming the pulse duration to 1.0 msec (point B) provides very little margin of safety. Similarly, if the threshold is determined to be at point C (3.5 V and 0.15 msec) by decreasing the pulse duration at a constant voltage, doubling the stimulation voltage to 7.0 V (point D) also provides a poor safety margin. When one considers the shape of the strength-duration curve, a more appropriate programmed setting would be provided by doubling the threshold voltage at a pulse duration of 0.5 msec (point E, 4 V and 0.5 msec). As a general rule, if the threshold is determined by decreasing the stimulus voltage, an adequate margin of safety can be assumed by doubling the voltage if the pulse duration used is greater than 0.3 msec.

The two most important points on the strength-duration curve (rheobase and chronaxie) are easily estimated with modern pulse generators (see Fig. 1–9). Rheobase can be estimated by decreasing the output voltage at a pulse duration of 1.5 to 2.0 msec. Chronaxie can then be estimated by determining the threshold pulse duration at twice the rheobase voltage. If the threshold is determined by decreasing the pulse duration, an adequate safety margin can be assumed by tripling the pulse duration only if the threshold is 0.2 msec or less. If rheobase and chronaxie are measured, doubling the threshold voltage at the chronaxie pulse duration provides an excellent method for programming a pacing system. Although programming the output of a pulse generator must first ensure patient safety, conservation of battery life is also an important consideration. As a general rule, in the choice between decreasing pulse width or decreasing voltage, it is more energy efficient (charge efficient) to reduce the voltage output of the pulse because the current drain varies as the square of voltage. As stated earlier, doubling the pulse amplitude quadruples the current drain, whereas doubling the pulse width only doubles the current drain.

The clinician must also consider the acute-to-chronic evolution of the stimulation threshold when programming the pulse generator at the time of implantation. Because there is typically an acute rise in threshold during the first several weeks following lead implantation, the voltage and pulse duration may need to be programmed to higher values than needed for chronic pacing. The physician is wise to reevaluate the stimulation threshold following the acute rise (and subsequent fall) that may occur following implantation. For most patients, the pacing system can be programmed to chronic output settings at a follow-up evaluation approximately 6 weeks after lead implantation. Although these recommendations may not be applicable to patients receiving a steroid-eluting lead, a degree of caution is probably warranted. The importance of drug and electrolyte effects on the strength-duration curve should also be appreciated. For patients requiring antiarrhythmic drug therapy, the stimulation threshold should be measured following drug initiation to ensure an adequate margin of safety for pacing. Similarly, individuals who are more likely to experience alterations in electrolyte concentration (such as patients with renal failure) may require programming of their pacemaker with a greater margin of safety. Perhaps most important, the degree to which the heart is dependent on pacing to sustain life or

prevent severe symptoms must be factored into the choice of a programmed margin of safety. For pacemaker-dependent individuals, a pacing pulse that is at least 2.5 times the chronic capture threshold is generally recommended. In contrast, patients who are unlikely to experience severe symptoms should failure to capture occur may have the pacemaker programmed to a lower margin of safety (approximately 2 times threshold). The effect of pacing rate on the stimulation threshold should also be considered in patients requiring antitachycardia pacing. For patients requiring pacing rates of more than 250 bpm, the pacing threshold should be measured at all rates likely to be used for antitachycardia pacing to ensure capture.

Modern implantable pulse generators use a CV output circuit. Because the current resulting from a CV pulse is inversely related to pacing impedance, a high (conductor) resistance lead decreases the current drain on the pulse generator battery, but it also reduces the margin of safety. Thus, in the presence of a very high resistance (such as with a conductor fracture), the current (and voltage) between the electrodes will decrease, often resulting in failure of the pulse to capture the myocardium. In contrast, in the presence of a lead insulation failure, the impedance of the pacing circuit decreases, resulting in an increase in current and little change in the stimulation threshold (depending on the size of the breach versus the electrode size). Pacing impedance is determined by four factors: (1) resistance in the conductor wire; (2) polarization at the electrode-tissue interface; (3) resistance (or ohmic polarization) at the electrode-tissue interface; and (4) resistance of the tissues between the electrodes. The first two of these factors are energy inefficient, decreasing current available for stimulation, whereas the third factor decreases current drain without decreasing the efficiency of stimulation. Thus, the ideal electrode would have high resistance at the electrode-tissue interface but low resistance in the conductor wire and low polarization.

This chapter has covered a variety of factors that influence the most basic aspect of pacing, myocardial stimulation. All clinicians involved in the management of patients with an implanted pacemaker must have a basic understanding of these factors, which contribute to patient safety, battery longevity, and proper function of the pacing system.

REFERENCES

1. Hodgkin AL, Huxley AF: A quantitative description of membrane current and its application to conduction and excitation in nerve. J Physiol (Lond) 117:500, 1952.
2. Corr PB: Contribution of lipid metabolites to arrhythmogenesis during early myocardial ischemia. In Rosen MR, Janse MJ, Wit AL (eds): Cardiac Electrophysiology: A Textbook. Mt. Kisco, NY, Futura, 1990, pp 720–722.
3. Kleber AG: Sodium-potassium pumping. In Rosen MR, Janse MJ, Wit AL (eds): Cardiac Electrophysiology: A Textbook. Mt. Kisco, NY, Futura, 1990, pp 37–54.
4. Hodgkin AL, Katz B: The effect of sodium ions on the electrical activity of the giant axon of the squid. J Physiol (Lond) 108:37, 1949.
5. Thomas RC: Electrogenic sodium pump in nerve and muscle cells. Physiol Rev 52:563, 1972.
6. Glitsch HG: Electrogenic Na pumping in the heart. Ann Rev Physiol 44:389, 1982.
7. Gadsky DC: The Na/K pump of cardiac cells. Ann Rev Biophys Bioeng 13:373, 1984.
8. Mullins IJ: The generation of electric currents in cardiac fibers by Na/Ca exchange. Am J Physiol 236:C103, 1979.

9. Hilgemann DW: Numerical approximations of sodium-calcium exchange. Prog Biophys Mol Biol 51:1, 1988.
10. Weidmann S: Passive properties of cardiac fibers. *In* Rosen MR, Janse MJ, Wit AL (eds): Cardiac Electrophysiology: A Textbook. Mt. Kisco, NY, Futura, 1990, pp 29–35.
11. Mobley BA, Page E: The surface of sheep cardiac Purkinje fibres. J Physiol (Lond) 220:547, 1972.
12. Metzger P, Weingart R: Electric current flow in cell pairs isolated from adult rat hearts. J Physiol (Lond) 366:1177, 1985.
13. Stewart JM, Page E: Improved stereological techniques for studying myocardial cell growth: Application to external sarcolemma, T system, and intercalated disks of rabbit and rat hearts. J Ultrastr Res 65:119, 1978.
14. Hofmann H: Interaction between a normoxic and a hypoxic region of guinea pig and ferret papillary muscles. Circ Res 56:876, 1985.
15. Kleber AG, Riegger CB, Janse MJ: Electrical uncoupling and increase of extracellular resistance after induction of ischemia in isolated, arterially perfused rabbit papillary muscle. Circ Res 61:271, 1987.
16. Bean RC: Protein-mediated mechanisms of variable ion conductance in thin lipid membranes. Membranes 2:409, 1973.
17. Haydon DA, Hladky SB: Ion transport across thin lipid membranes: A critical discussion of mechanisms in selected systems. Q Rev Biophys 5(2):187, 1972.
18. Neher E, Sakmann B, Steinbach JH: The extracellular patch clamp: A method for resolving currents through individual open channels in biological membranes. Pflügers Arch Eur J Physiol 375:219, 1978.
19. Neher E, Sakmann B: The patch clamp technique. Sci Am 266(3):44, 1992.
20. Ebihara L: The sodium current. *In* Rosen MR, Janse MJ, Wit AL (eds): Cardiac Electrophysiology: A Textbook. Mt. Kisco, NY, Futura, 1990, pp 63–74.
21. Hartel HC, Duchatelle-Gourdon I: Structure and neural modulation of cardiac calcium channels. J Cardiovasc Electrophysiol 3:567, 1992.
22. Tsien RW: Calcium channels in the cardiovascular system. *In* Rosen MR, Janse MJ, Wit AL (eds): Cardiac Electrophysiology: A Textbook. Mt. Kisco, NY, Futura, 1990, pp 75–89.
23. Carmeliet E: The cardiac action potential. *In* Rosen MR, Janse MJ, Wit AL (eds): Cardiac Electrophysiology: A Textbook. Mt. Kisco, NY, Futura, 1990, pp 55–62.
24. Hoffman BF, Cranefield PF: Electrophysiology of the Heart. New York, McGraw Hill, 1960.
25. Binah O: The transient outward current in the mammalian heart. *In* Rosen MR, Janse MJ, Wit AL (eds): Cardiac Electrophysiology: A Textbook. Mt. Kisco, NY, Futura, 1990, pp 93–106.
26. Joho RH: Toward a molecular understanding of voltage-gated potassium channels. J Cardiovasc Electrophysiol 3:589, 1992.
27. Coraboeuf E, Carmeliet E: Existence of two transient outward currents in sheep cardiac Purkinje fibers. Pflügers Arch 392:352, 1982.
28. Cohen IS, Datyner N: Repolarizing membrane currents. *In* Rosen MR, Janse MJ, Wit AL (eds): Cardiac Electrophysiology: A Textbook. Mt. Kisco, NY, Futura, 1990, pp 107–116.
29. Bottazzi F: Leonardo as physiologist. *In* Leonardo da Vinci. London, Leisure Arts, 1964, pp 373–387.
30. Harvey W: De Motu Cordis [The Movement of the Heart and Blood 1628]. Translated by D. Whitteridge. Oxford, Blackwell, 1900.
31. Keith A, Flack M: The form and nature of the muscular connections between the primary divisions of the vertebrate heart. J Anat Physiol 41:172, 1907.
32. Irisawa H: Comparative physiology of the cardiac pacemaker mechanism. Physiol Rev 58:461, 1978.
33. DiFrancesco D: The hyperpolarization-activated current, I_f, and cardiac pacemaking. *In* Rosen MR, Janse ML, Wit AL (eds): Cardiac Electrophysiology: A Textbook. Mt. Kisco, NY, Futura, 1990, pp 117–132.
34. Urthaler F, Isobe JH, James TN: Comparative effects of glucagon on automaticity of the sinus node and atrioventricular junction. Am J Physiol 227:1415, 1974.
35. Furman S, Parker B, Escher DJW: Decreasing electrode size and increasing efficiency of cardiac stimulation. J Surg Res 11:105, 1971.
36. Furman S, Hurzler P, Parker B: Clinical thresholds of endocardial cardiac stimulation: A long-term study. J Surg Res 19:149, 1975.
37. Angello DA, McAnulty JH, Dobbs J: Characterization of chronically implanted ventricular endocardial pacing leads. Am Heart J 107(6):1142, 1984.
38. Geddes LA, Bourland JD: The strength-duration curve. IEEE Trans Biomed Eng BME 32(6):458, 1985.
39. Irnich W: Considerations in electrode design for permanent pacing. *In* Thalen HJT (ed): Cardiac Pacing, Proceedings of the IVth International Symposium on Cardiac Pacing. Assen, The Netherlands, Van Gorcum, 1973, p 268.
40. Irnich W: Engineering concepts of pacemaker electrodes. *In* Schaldach M, Furman S (eds): Advances in Pacemaker Technology. New York, Springer-Verlag, 1975, p 241.
41. Bardou AL, Chenais J-M, Birkui PJ, et al: Directional variability of stimulation threshold measurements in isolated guinea pig cardiomyocytes: Relationship with orthogonal sequential defibrillating pulses. PACE 13:1590, 1990.
42. Preston TA, Fletcher RD, Lucchesi BR, Judge RD: Changes in myocardial thresholds. Physiologic and pharmacologic factors in patients with implanted pacemakers. Am Heart J 74:235, 1967.
43. Katsumoto K, Niibori I, Takamatsu T, Kaibara M: Development of glassy carbon electrode (dead sea scroll) for low energy cardiac pacing. PACE 9(6, pt II):1220, 1986.
44. Mond H, Stokes K, Helland J, et al: The porous titanium steroid eluting electrode: A double blind study assessing the stimulation threshold effects of steroid. PACE 11(2):214, 1988.
45. Hill WE, Murray A, Bourks JP, et al: Minimum energy for cardiac pacing. Clin Phys Physiol Meas 9(1):41, 1988.
46. Breivik K, Ohm O-J, Engedal H: Acute and chronic pulse-width thresholds in solid versus porous tip electrodes. PACE 5:650, 1982.
47. Irnich W: The chronaxie time and its practical importance. PACE 3:292, 1980.
48. Stokes KB, Barold SS, McVenes R, Byrd CL: Thresholds vs longevity: A requiem for energy parameters. In press.
49. Dressler L, Gruse G, von Knorre GH, et al: The optimization of the pulse delivered by the pacemaker. PACE 2:282, 1979.
50. Chaptal AP, Ribot A: Statistical survey of strength-duration threshold curves with endocardial electrodes and long-term behavior of these electrodes. *In* Meere C (ed): Proceedings of the VIth World Symposium on Cardiac Pacing. Montreal, PACESYMP, 1979, pp 21–22.
51. Hoorweg JL: Condensatorentladung und Auseinandersetzung mit du Bois-Reymond. Pflügers Arch 52:87, 1892.
52. Weiss G: Sur la possibilité de render comparable entre les appareils cervant à l'excitation electrique. Arch Ital Biol 35:413, 1901.
53. Lapique L: Definition experimentale de l'excitabilité. C R Soc Biol 67:280, 1909.
54. Lapique L: La Chronaxie et Ses Applications Physiologiques. Paris, Hermann, 1938.
55. Nernst W: Zur Theorie des elektrischen Reizes. Pflügers Arch 122:275, 1908.
56. Ripart A, Mugica J: Electrode-heart interface: Definition of the ideal electrode. PACE 6(pt II):410, 1983.
57. Irnich W: Elektrotherapie des Herzens. Berlin, Fachverlag Schiele, 1976.
58. Irnich W: The chronaxie time and its practical importance. PACE 3:292, 1980.
59. Bernstein AD, Parsonnet V. Implications of constant energy pacing. PACE 6(6):1229, 1983.
60. Wedensky NE: Über die beziehungzwischen Reizung und Erregung im Tetanus. St. Petersburg, Ber Akad Wiss 54:96, 1887.
61. Langberg JJ, Sousa J, El-Atassi R, et al: The mechanism of pacing capture hysteresis in humans [Abstract]. PACE 15:577, 1992.
62. Hook BC, Perlman RL, Callans JD, et al: Acute and chronic cycle length dependent increase in ventricular pacing threshold. PACE 15:1437, 1992.
63. Plumb VJ, Karp RB, James TN, Waldo AL: Atrial excitability and conduction during rapid atrial pacing. Circulation 63:1140, 1981.
64. Buxton AE, Marchlinski FE, Miller JM, et al: The human atrial strength-interval relation: Influence of cycle length and procainamide. Circulation 79:271, 1989.
65. Katsumoto K, Niibori T, Watanabe Y: Rate dependent threshold changes during atrial pacing: Clinical and experimental studies. PACE 13:1009, 1990.
66. Kay GN, Mulholland DH, Epstein AE, Plumb VJ: Effect of pacing rate on human atrial strength-duration curves. J Am Coll Cardiol 15(7):1618, 1990.
67. Stokes K, Bornzin G: The electrode–biointerface (stimulation). *In* Barold S (ed): Modern Cardiac Pacing. Mt. Kisco, NY, Futura, 1985, pp 33–78.
67a. Cornacchia O, Maresta A, Nigro P, et al: Effect of propafenone on chronic ventricular pacing threshold in patients with steroid-eluting

(capsure) and conventional leads. Eur J Cardiac Pacing Electrophysiol 2:A88, 1992.

68. Garberoglio B, Inguaggiato B, Chinaglia B, Cerise O: Initial results with an activated pyrolytic carbon tip electrode. PACE 6:440, 1982.

69. Jones JL, Jones RE, Balasky G: Improved cardiac cell excitation with symmetrical biphasic defibrillation waveforms. Am J Physiol 253:H1418, 1987.

70. Knisley SB, Smith WM, Ideker RE: Effect of intrastimulus polarity reversal on electric field stimulation thresholds in frog and rabbit myocardium. J Cardiovasc Electrophysiol 3:239, 1992.

71. Mehra R, Furman S: Comparison of cathodal, anodal, and bipolar strength-interval curves with temporary and permanent pacing electrodes. Br Heart J 41:468, 1979.

72. Kay GN: Basic aspects of cardiac pacing. In Ellenbogen KA (ed): Cardiac Pacing. Cambridge, MA, Blackwell Scientific, 1992.

73. Preston TA: Anodal stimulation as a cause of pacemaker-induced ventricular fibrillation. Am Heart J 86:366, 1973.

74. Wiggers CJ, Wegria R, Pinera B: Effects of myocardial ischemia on fibrillation threshold: Mechanism of spontaneous ventricular fibrillation following coronary occlusion. Am J Physiol 131:309, 1940.

75. Mehra R, Furman S, Crump JF: Vulnerability of the mildly ischemic ventricle to cathodal, anodal and bipolar stimulation. Circ Res 41:159, 1977.

76. Bilitch M, Cosby RS, Cafferry EA: Ventricular fibrillation and competitive pacing. N Engl J Med 276:598, 1967.

77. Stokes K, Bird T, Taepke R: A new low threshold, high impedance microelectrode. In Antonioli GE, et al (eds): Pacemaker Leads. Amsterdam, Elsevier, 1991, pp 543–548.

78. Bird T, Stokes K: Ventricular electrode spacing and anode size [Abstract 205]. Rev Eur Technol Biomed 3(12):63, 1990.

79. De Caprio V: Endocardial electrograms from transvenous pacemaker electrodes. Thesis, Polytechnic Institute of New York, 1977.

80. Ripart A, Fletcher R: Sensing. In Ellenbogen KA, Kay GN, Wilkoff B (eds): Clinical Cardiac Pacing. Philadelphia, WB Saunders, 1992.

81. Barold SS, Ong LS, Heinle RA: Stimulation and sensing thresholds for cardiac pacing: Electrophysiologic and technical aspects. Prog Cardiovasc Dis 24:1, 1981.

82. Smyth NPD, Tarjan PP, Chernoff E, et al: The significance of electrode surface area and stimulating thresholds in permanent cardiac pacing. J Thorac Cardiovasc Surg 71:559, 1976.

83. Parsonnet V, Zucker IR, Kannerstein ML: The fate of permanent intracardiac electrodes. J Surg Res 6:285, 1966.

84. Thalen HJT, Van den Berg JW: Threshold measurements and electrodes of the cardiac pacemaker. Acta Pharmacol Nederl 14:227, 1966.

85. Akyurekli Y, Taichman GC, White DL, et al: Myocardial responses to sutureless epicardial lead pacing. In Meere C (ed): Proceedings of the VIth World Symposium on Cardiac Pacing. Montreal, PACESYMP, 1979, Chap 33–3.

86. One notes that this equation lacks a critical parameter required by the strength-duration nature of thresholds, time. According to W. Irnich, all measurements were made at 1.0 msec (personal communication).

87. Adamec R, Lasserre B, Simonet F, et al: Behaviour of epimyocardial stimulation threshold after heart pacemaker implantation using sutureless electrodes. In Meere C (ed): Proceedings of the VIth World Symposium on Cardiac Pacing. Montreal, PACESYMP, 1979, Chap 33–1.

88. Hughes H, Brownlee R, Tyres G: Failures of demand pacing with small surface area electrodes. Circulation 54:128, 1976.

89. Antonioli EG, Baggioni FG, Grassi G: Intracardiac electrogram parameters, electrode surface area and pacer input impedance: Their correlations. J Ital Cardiol 10(5):536, 1980.

90. Wilson GJ, MacGregor DC, Bobyn JD, et al: Tissue response to porous-surface electrodes: Basis for a new atrial lead design. In Moore C (ed): Proceedings of the VIth World Symposium on Cardiac Pacing. Montreal, PACESYMP, 1979, Chap 29–12.

91. Amundson D, McArthur W, MacCarter D, et al: Porous electrode-tissue interface. In Moore C (ed): Proceedings of the VIth World Symposium on Cardiac Pacing. Montreal, PACESYMP, 1979, Chap 29–16.

92. Amundson DC, McArthur W, Moshaffafa M: The porous endocardial electrode. PACE 2:40, 1979.

93. MacGregor DC, Wilson GJ, Lixfeld W, et al: The porous surface electrode: A new concept in pacemaker lead design. J Thorac Cardiovasc Surg 78:281, 1979.

94. Breivik K, Ohm O-J, Engedahl H: Acute and chronic pulse-width thresholds in solid versus porous tip electrodes. PACE 5:650, 1982.

95. Berman ND, Dickson SE, Lipton IM: Acute and chronic clinical performance comparison of porous and solid electrode design. PACE 5:67, 1982.

96. Freud GE, Chinaglia B: Sintered platinum for cardiac pacing. Int J Artif Organs 4:238, 1981.

97. MacCarter DM, Lundberg KM, Corstjens JP: Porous electrodes: Concept, technology and results. PACE 6:427, 1983.

98. MacGregor DC, Pilliar RM, Wilson GJ, et al: Porous metal surfaces: A radical new concept in prosthetic heart valve design. Trans Am Soc Artif Intern Organs 22:646, 1976.

99. Elmqvist H, Schuller H, Richter G: The carbon tip electrode. PACE 6:436, 1983.

100. Bornzin GA, Stokes KB, Wiebusch WA: A low-threshold, low-polarization platinized endocardial electrode [Abstract]. PACE 6:A–70, 1983.

101. Heineman F, et al: Clinical comparison of available "low threshold leads" [Abstract]. Vienna, Tenth Congress of European Society of Cardiology, August, 1988.

102. Beck-Jansen P, Schuller H, Winther-Rasmussen S: Vitreous carbon electrodes in endocardial pacing. In Meere C (ed): Proceedings of the VIth World Symposium on Cardiac Pacing. Montreal, PACESYMP, 1979, Chap 29–9.

103. Richter GJ, Weidlich E, Sturm FV, et al: Non-polarizable vitreous carbon pacing electrodes in animal experiments. In Meere C (ed): Proceedings of the VIth World Symposium on Cardiac Pacing. Montreal, PACESYMP, 1979.

104. Midel MG, Jones BR, Brinker JA: A comparison of platinized grooved electrode performance with ring-tip electrodes. PACE 12:752, 1989.

105. Breivik K, Hoff P-I, Tronstad A, et al: Promising new pacemaker lead. PACE 7:465, 1984.

106. Heinemann F, Davis M, Helland J: Clinical performance of a pacing lead with a platinized "target tip" electrode [Abstract]. PACE 7:471, 1984.

107. Karpawich PP, Hakimi M, Arciniegas E, et al: A new low threshold platinized epicardial pacing electrode: Initial experience in children. Abstract, 39th Annual Scientific Session of the ACC, New Orleans, March 18–23, 1990. J Am Coll Cardiol 15:68A, 1990.

108. Stokes K: The effects of ventricular electrode surface area on pacemaker lead performance. In Adornato E, Galassi A (eds): The '92 Scenario on Cardiac Pacing. Rome, Luigi Pozzi, 1992, pp 505–514.

109. Stokes KB, Bird T, Gunderson B: The mythology of threshold variations as a function of electrode surface area. PACE 14(11):1748, 1991.

110. Pearce JA, Bourland JD, Neilsen W, et al: Myocardial stimulation with ultrashort duration current pulses. PACE 5:52, 1982.

111. Meyers GH, Parsonnet V: Engineering in the Heart and Blood Vessels. New York, Wiley-Interscience, 1989.

112. Hurzeler P, Furman S, Escher DJW: Cardiac pacemaker current thresholds versus pulse duration. In Silverman HT, Miller IF, Salkind AJ (eds): Electrochemical Bioscience and Bioengineering. Princeton, Electrochemical Society, 1973, p 124.

113. Barold SS, Winner JA: Techniques and significance of threshold measurement for cardiac pacing. Chest 70:760, 1976.

114. Brownlee WC, Hirst R: Six years experience with atrial leads. PACE 9(6 pt II):1239, 1989.

115. Luceri RM, Furman S, Hurzeler P, et al: Threshold behavior of electrodes in long-term ventricular pacing. Am J Cardiol 40:184, 1977.

116. Mond H, Stokes K: The electrode-tissue interface: The revolutionary role of steroid elution. PACE 15(1):95, 1992.

117. Ohm O-J, Breivik K: Pacing leads. In Gomez FP et al (eds): Cardiac Pacing. Electrophysiology. Tachyarrhythmias. Madrid, Grouz, 1985, pp 971–985.

118. Hoff PI, Breivik K, Tronstad A, et al: A new steroid-eluting electrode for low-threshold pacing. In Gomez FP et al (eds): Cardiac Pacing. Electrophysiology. Tachyarrhythmias. Mt. Kisco, NY, Futura, 1985, pp 1014–1019.

119. Anderson JM: Inflammation, wound healing and foreign body response. In Biomaterial Science, An Introductory Text. Society for Biomaterials, 1990.

120. Anderson JM: Inflammatory response to implants. ASAIO Trans 11(2):101, 1988.

121. Henson PM: Mechanisms of exocytosis in phagocytic inflammatory cells. Am J Pathol 101:494, 1980.

122. Robinson TF, Cohen-Gould L, Factor SM: Skeletal framework of mammalian heart muscle: Arrangement of inter- and pericellular connective tissue structures. Lab Invest 29(4):482, 1983.

123. Preston TA, Judge RD: Alteration of pacemaker threshold by drug and physiologic factors. Ann NY Acad Sci 167:686, 1969.

124. Sibille Y, Reynolds HY: Macrophages and polymorphonuclear neutrophils in lung defense and injury. Am Rev Respir Dis 141:471, 1990.

125. Benditt DG, Kriett JS, Ryberg C, et al: Cellular electrophysiologic effects of dexamethasone sodium phosphate: Implications for cardiac stimulation with steroid-eluting electrodes. Int J Cardiol 22(1):67, 1989.

126. Stokes KB, Kriett JM, Gornick CA, et al: Low-threshold cardiac pacing electrodes. In Frontiers of Engineering in Health Care—1983. Proceedings of the Fifth Annual Conference of the IEEE Engineering in Medicine and Biology Society, New York, 1983.

127. Mond H, Sloman JG, Cowling R, et al: The small tined pacemaker lead—absence of displacement. In Meere C (ed): Proceedings of the VIth World Symposium on Cardiac Pacing. Montreal, PACESYMP, 1979, Chap 29-5.

128. Baker JH, Shepard RB, Plumb VJ, Kay GN: Effects of fixation mechanism and electrode material on atrial stimulation threshold: Long-term evaluation in 338 patients [Abstract]. PACE 15:54, 1992.

129. Cornacchia D, Jacopi F, Fabbri M, et al: Comparison between active screw-in and passive leads for permanent transvenous ventricular pacing [Abstract]. PACE 6:A56, 1983.

130. El Gamal M, Van Gelder L, Bonnier J, et al: Comparison of transvenous atrial electrodes employing active (helicoidal) and passive (tined J-lead) fixation in 116 patients [Abstract]. PACE 6:205, 1983.

131. Kay GN, Anderson K, Epstein AE, Plumb VJ: Active fixation atrial leads: Randomized comparison of two lead designs. PACE 12:1355, 1989.

132. Rasor NS, Spickler JW, Clabaugh JW: Comparison of power sources for advanced pacemaker applications. In 7th Intersociety Energy Conversion Engineering Conference, Washington DC, American Chemical Society, 1972, p 752.

133. Hirshorn MS, Holley LK, Hales JR, et al: Screening of solid and porous materials for pacemaker electrodes. PACE 4:380, 1981.

134. Schaldach M: New pacemaker electrodes. Trans Am Soc Artif Intern Organs 17:29, 1971.

135. Helland J, Stokes K: Nonfibrosing cardiac pacing electrode. US Patent 4033357, February 17, 1976.

136. Elmqvist H, Schuller H, Richter G: The carbon tip electrode. PACE 6:436, 1983.

137. Thuesen L, Jensen PJ, Vejby-Christensen H, et al: Lower chronic stimulation threshold in the carbon-tip than in the platinum-tip endocardial electrode: A randomized study. PACE 12:1592, 1989.

138. Bornzin GA, Stokes KB, Wiebush WA: A low threshold, low polarization, platonized endocardial electrode. PACE 6:A-70, 1983.

139. Mugica J, Duconge B, Henry L, et al: Clinical experience with new leads. PACE 11:1745, 1988.

140. Djordjevic M, Stojanov P, Velimirovic D, et al: Target lead—low threshold electrode. PACE 9:1206, 1986.

141. Timmis GC, Helland J, Westveer DC, et al: The evolution of low threshold leads. Clin Prog Pacing Electrophysiol 1:313, 1983.

142. Stokes KB: Preliminary studies on a new steroid eluting epicardial electrode. PACE 11:1797, 1988.

143. Hamilton R, Gow R, Bahoric B, et al: Steroid-eluting epicardial leads in pediatrics: Improved epicardial thresholds in the first year. PACE 14:2066, 1991.

144. Stokes K, Frohlig G, Bird T, et al: A new bipolar low threshold steroid eluting screw-in lead [Abstract 336]. Eur J Cardiac Pacing Electrophysiol 2(2):A89, 1992.

145. Brinker J, Crossley G, Hurd H, et al: Multicenter randomized controlled study of a new bipolar steroid eluting active fixation lead. PACE 16:946, 1993.

146. Crossley GH, Kay GN, Ferguson B, et al: Performance of a steroid-eluting active fixation lead in patients with a prior history of exit block. Submitted to NASPE, 1993.

147. Moor WJ: Physical Chemistry. Englewood Cliffs, NJ, Prentice-Hall, 1972, p 510.

148. Conway BE: Theory and Principles of Electrode Processes. New York, Ronald Press, 1965, p 33.

149. Kahn A, Greatbatch W: Physiologic electrodes. In Ray C (ed): Medical Engineering. Chicago, Year Book, 1974, p 1073.

150. Mindt W, Schaldach M: Electrochemical aspects of pacing electrodes. In Schaldach M, Furman S (eds): Advances in Pacemaker Technology. New York, Springer-Verlag, 1975, p 297.

151. Lindemans FW, Denier van der Gon JJ: Current thresholds and luminal size in excitation of heart muscle. Cardiovasc Res 12:477, 1977.

152. Irnich W, Gebhardt U: The pacemaker-electrode combination and its relationship to service life. In Thalen HJT (ed): To Pace or Not to Pace, Controversial Subjects in Cardiac Pacing. The Hague, Martin Nijhoff, 1978, p 209.

153. Piersma BJ, Calhoon SW Jr, Greatbatch W: Some comparisons of Pt and Ti physiological electrodes. In Silverman HT, Miller IF, Salkind AJ (eds): Electrochemical Bioscience and Bioengineering. Princeton, Electrochemical Society, 1973, p 133.

154. Greatbatch W: Metal electrodes in bioengineering. CRC Crit Rev Bioeng 5:1, 1981.

155. Stokes K, Bird T, Taepke R: High pacing impedance: Efficient or wasteful [Abstract 452]. PACE 14:730, 1991.

156. Wallace AG, Cline RE, Sealy WC, et al: Electrophysiologic effects of quinidine. Circ Res 19:960, 1966.

157. Gay RJ, Brown DF: Pacemaker failure due to procainamide toxicity. Am J Cardiol 34:728, 1974.

158. Moss AJ, Goldstein S: Clinical and pharmacological factors associated with pacemaker latency and incomplete pacemaker capture. Br Heart J 31:112, 1969.

159. Hellestrand KJ, Burnett PJ, Milne JR, et al: Effect of the antiarrhythmic agent flecainide acetate on acute and chronic pacing thresholds. PACE 6:892, 1983.

160. Salel AF, Seagren SC, Pool PE: Effects on encainide on the function of implanted pacemakers. PACE 12:1439, 1989.

161. Montefoschi N, Boccadamo R: Propafenone induced acute variation of chronic atrial pacing threshold: a case report. PACE 13:480, 1990.

162. Huang SK, Hedberg PS, Marcus FI: Effects of antiarrhythmic drugs on the chronic pacing threshold and the endocardial R wave amplitude in the conscious dog. PACE 9:660, 1986.

163. Bianconi L, Boccadamo R, Toscano S, et al: Effects of oral propafenone therapy on chronic myocardial pacing threshold. PACE 15:148, 1992.

164. Kubler W, Sowton E: Influence of beta-blockade on myocardial threshold in patients with pacemakers. Lancet 2:67, 1970.

165. Preston TA, Fletcher RD, Lucchesi BR, Judge RD: Changes in myocardial threshold. Physiologic and pharmacologic factors in patients with implanted pacemakers. Am Heart J 74:235, 1967.

166. Hughes HC, Tyers GFO, Torman HA: Effects of acid-base imbalance on myocardial pacing thresholds. J Thorac Cardiovasc Surg 69:743, 1975.

167. Khastgir T, Lattuca J, Aarons D, et al: Ventricular pacing threshold and time to capture postdefibrillation in patients undergoing implantable cardioverter-defibrillator implantation. PACE 14:768, 1991.

168. Delmar M: Role of potassium currents on cell excitability in cardiac ventricular myocytes. J Cardiovasc Electrophysiol 3:474, 1992.

169. Gettes LS, Shabetai R, Downs TA, et al: Effect of changes in potassium and calcium concentrations on diastolic threshold and strength-interval relationships of the human heart. Ann NY Acad Sci 167:693, 1969.

170. Lee D, Greenspan K, Edmands RE, et al: The effect of electrolyte alteration on stimulus requirement of cardiac pacemakers. Circulation 38:124, 1968.

171. Walker WJ, Elkins JT, Wood LW, et al: Effect of potassium in restoring myocardial response to a subthreshold cardiac pacemaker. N Engl J Med 271:597, 1964.

172. Surawicz B, Chelbus H, Reeves JT, et al: Increase of ventricular excitability threshold by hyperpotassemia. JAMA 191:71, 1965.

173. Westerholm CJ: Threshold studies in transvenous cardiac pacemaker treatment. Scand J Thorac Cardiovasc Surg (Suppl) 8:1, 1971.

174. Schlesinger Z, Rosenberg T, Stryjer D, et al: Exit block in myxedema, treated effectively by thyroid hormone replacement. PACE 3:737, 1980.

175. Basu D, Chatterjee K: Unusually high pacemaker threshold in severe myxedema: Decrease with thyroid hormone therapy. Chest 70:677, 1976.

176. Nagatomo Y, Ogawa T, Kumagae H, et al: Pacing failure due to markedly increased stimulation threshold 2 years after implantation: Successful management with oral prednisolone: A case report. PACE 12:1034, 1989.

177. Haywood J, Wyman MG: Effects of isoproterenol, ephedrine, and potassium on artificial pacemaker failure. Circulation (Suppl) 32:II-110, 1965.

178. Katz A, Knilans TK, Evans JJ, Prystowsky EN: The effects of isoproterenol on excitability, supranormal excitability and conduction in the human ventricle [Abstract]. PACE 14:710, 1991.

179. Levick CE, Mizgala HF, Kerr CR: Failure to pace following high-dose

anti-arrhythmic therapy—reversal with isoproterenol. PACE 7:252, 1984.

180. Stokes KB, Church T: The elimination of exit block as a pacing complication using a transvenous steroid-eluting lead [Abstract 475]. PACE 10(3):748, 1987.
181. Till JA, Jones S, Rowland E, et al: Clinical experience with a steroid eluting lead in children [Abstract]. Circulation 80:389, 1989.
182. Sowton E, Norman J: Variations in cardiac stimulation thresholds in patients with pacing electrodes. Digest of the 7th International Conference on Medical and Biological Engineering. Stockholm, Ljungi ofs, Litografiska AB, 1967.
183. Preston TA, Fletcher RD, Lucchesi BR, et al: Changes in myocardial threshold: Physiologic and pharmacologic factors in patients with implanted pacemakers. Am Heart J 74:235, 1967.
184. Westerholm C-J: Threshold studies in transvenous cardiac pacemaker treatment. Scand J Thorac Surg Suppl 8:1, 1971.
185. McVenes R, Lahtinen S, Hansen N, Stokes K: Physiologic and drug induced changes in cardiac pacing and sensing parameters [Abstract 324]. Eur J Cardiac Pacing Electrophysiol 2(2):A86, 1992.
186. Kadish A, Kong T, Goldberger J: Diurnal variability in ventricular stimulation threshold and electrogram amplitude [Abstract]. Eur J Cardiac Pacing Electrophysiol 2(2):A86, 1992.
187. Grendahl H, Schaanning CG: Variations in pacing threshold. Acta Med Scand 187:75, 1970.
188. Shepherd R, Kim J, Colvin E, et al: Pacing threshold spikes months and years after implant [Abstract 308]. PACE 14:694, 1991.
189. Barold S: Effect of drugs on pacing thresholds. In Antonioli GE, et al (eds): Pacemaker Leads 1991. New York, Elsevier, 1991, pp 73–86.
190. Barold SS, Ong LS, Heinle RA: Stimulation and sensing thresholds for cardiac pacing: Electrophysiologic and technical aspects. Prog Cardiovasc Dis 24:1, 1981.
191. Ohm O-J, Breivik K: Pacing leads. In Gomez FP, et al (eds): Cardiac Pacing. Electrophysiology. Tachyarrhythmias. Madrid, Editorial Grouz, 1985, pp 971–985.
192. Hoff PI, Breivik K, Tronstad A, et al: A new steroid-eluting electrode for low-threshold pacing. In Gomez FP, et al (eds): Cardiac Pacing. Electrophysiology. Tachyarrhythmias. Mt. Kisco, NY, Futura, 1985, pp 1014–1019.
193. Creer MH, Dobmeyer DJ, Corr PB: Amphipathic lipid metabolites and arrhythmias during myocardial ischemia. In Zipes DP, Jalife J (eds): Cardiac Electrophysiology: From Cell to Bedside. Philadelphia, WB Saunders, 1990, pp 417–432.
194. Seeger W: A scanning electron microscopic study on explanted electrode tips. In Aubert AE, Ector H (eds): Pacemaker Leads. Amsterdam, Elsevier, 1985, pp 405–410.
195. Schaldach M: The stimulating electrode. In Electrotherapy of the Heart. Berlin, Springer-Verlag, 1992, p 153.
196. Stokes K, Anderson J: Low threshold leads: The effect of steroid elution. In Antonioli GE (ed): Pacemaker Leads. Amsterdam, Elsevier, 1991, pp 537–542.

CHAPTER 2

SENSING

G. Neal Kay
Kenneth A. Ellenbogen

Normal pacemaker operation requires coordination between the pulse generator and the heart's own intrinsic electric activity. The ability of the pulse generator to appropriately sense electric signals that originate in the myocardium is dependent on the electrophysiologic properties of the underlying myocardium, the characteristics of the electrode within or in contact with the heart, the conductors within the lead, and the sensing amplifier in the pulse generator. Each of these components has an important influence on the sensing performance of the pacing system. In addition to these components that must detect electric events in the myocardium, the timing circuits in the pulse generator must reject unwanted electric signals such as far-field cardiac events, skeletal myopotentials, or interference that originates in the environment. This chapter focuses on the fundamental factors of myocardial sensing and their clinical application to cardiac pacing systems.

Components of the Intracardiac Electrogram

ORIGIN OF THE INTRACARDIAC ELECTROGRAM

A fundamental property of excitable tissues such as myocardium is the ability to maintain a resting electric potential across the cell membrane. In the case of a normal ventricular myocyte, the interior of the cell is electrically negative with respect to the outside with a resting potential gradient of approximately -90 mV across the membrane (see Chapter 1). In the absence of electric currents within the myocardium, two electrodes placed on the outside of a cardiac myocyte in its resting state would record the same electric potential ($+90$ mV) with respect to the inside of the cell. *Relative to each other* there would be no net potential difference between the electrodes (Fig. 2–1). Thus, in the resting state this pair of electrodes would record no electric signal. However, in addition to the property of separation of charge across the cell membrane, the normal myocardium is characterized by

the ability to generate self-propagating action potentials that result from a complex cascade of precisely timed electric currents that flow across the membrane through specialized ion channels and between cells through intercalated discs. Consider the sequence of electric events recorded by a pair of electrodes placed at separate endocardial sites as a depolarizing wave of action potentials sweeps through the underlying myocardium (Fig. 2–2). As the wave of action potentials moves from left to right in this figure, electrode 1 suddenly shifts from recording the positively charged outside of the underlying cell to recording a potential that is approximately 0 mV relative to the inside of the cell (Fig. 2–2A).

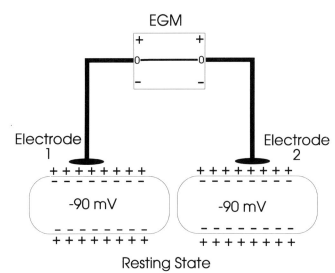

FIGURE 2–1. Schematic representation of two electrodes recording from two myocytes in the resting polarized state. Both cells have a gradient of 90 mV across the membrane, and the interior of the cell is electrically negative with respect to the outside of the cell. Although both electrode 1 and electrode 2 record from the electrically positive outside of the cell, with respect to one another they record the same charge. Thus, because both electrodes record the same charge, the electrogram (EGM) recorded between these electrodes shows no deflection from neutral.

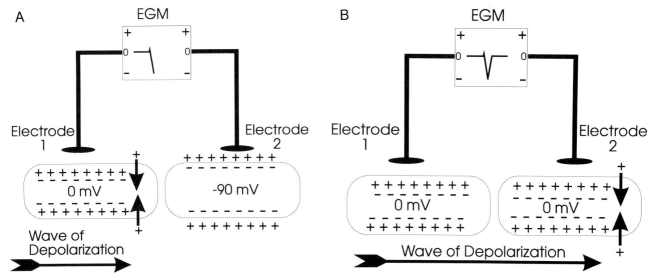

FIGURE 2–2. *A,* The effect of a wave of action potentials is demonstrated as it travels from left to right in this figure. Note that as the wave of depolarization progresses, positively charged Na^+ ions move from the outside to the inside of the cell, causing the inside of the cell to become charged to approximately 0 mV with respect to the outside. Although the cell under electrode 1 is depolarized and shows no separation of charge across the membrane, it is electrically negative relative to the cell under electrode 2. Because the two electrodes record different charges, there is a potential difference between them, and a negative (downward) deflection is recorded in the electrogram (EGM). *B,* The wave of depolarization advances over the cell on the right causing the same transmembrane potential (0 mV) in the cells under both electrode 1 and electrode 2. The electrogram records no difference in potential between electrodes 1 and 2, and the deflection returns to baseline.

Although the inside and outside of the myocardial cells underlying this electrode are approximately electrically neutral, electrode 1 has suddenly become electrically negative relative to electrode 2. The electrogram recorded between these electrodes at this precise moment inscribes a brisk downward (negative) deflection. As the depolarizing wave continues to advance so that the myocardium under electrode 2 also becomes depolarized (see Fig. 2–2B), the two electrodes record similar absolute voltage, and the electrogram returns briskly to the baseline. Thus, as this diagram illustrates, it is the

difference in electric potential between two electrodes produced by electric currents within the myocardium that generates the intracardiac electrogram.

Figure 2–3 illustrates how the orientation of two electrodes relative to a wavefront of depolarization can have a dramatic influence on the intracardiac electrogram. In Figure 2–3A, if the interelectrode axis is oriented parallel to the wavefront of depolarization, a brisk electrogram is inscribed. In contrast, if the two electrodes are oriented exactly perpendicular to the wavefront (see Fig. 2–3B), both electrodes record from the

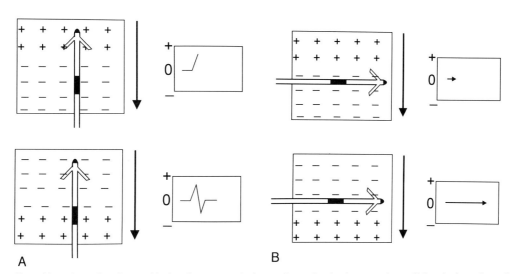

FIGURE 2–3. The effect of interelectrode axis on a bipolar electrogram. *A,* A wavefront of activation spreads parallel to the interelectrode axis of a bipolar lead. Note that as the wave of positive charges advances toward the tip electrode (*top*), a brisk positive deflection is inscribed in the electrogram. As the wave of activation spreads past the ring electrode, the electrogram shifts abruptly from positive to negative before returning to baseline. *B,* The interelectrode axis is perpendicular to the spread of activation. Note that the wave of activation reaches the tip and ring electrodes simultaneously, with no net difference between the electrodes at any point (*top* and *bottom*). Therefore, the electrogram does not show a deflection from baseline. This diagram illustrates the importance of interelectrode axis on the morphology of the intracardiac electrogram.

electrically positive outside of the resting myocytes. As the wavefront of depolarization passes directly under both electrodes, the electric potential of the myocardium suddenly shifts to approximately 0 mV. However, *relative to each other,* there is *no difference in electric potential* between the electrodes. Thus, if two electrodes record precisely the same electric charge at all times, no intracardiac electrogram is generated.

UNIPOLAR VERSUS BIPOLAR ELECTROGRAMS

So far we have considered only the electric signals recorded from a pair of electrodes in contact with the myocardium, that is, the bipolar sensing configuration. Unipolar pacing systems use one electrode in contact with the myocardium (usually the cathode) and another electrode typically in contact with the pulse generator case (usually the anode). Although there are clinically important differences between bipolar and unipolar sensing, the same principles of sensing apply to both configurations. The only difference is that a unipolar electrogram records the difference in potential between a more widely spaced pair of electrodes. As the depolarizing wave advances toward the electrode in contact with the myocardium, this electrode becomes slightly positive relative to the electrode on the pulse generator case (Fig. 2–4A). As the depolarizing wave passes directly under the electrode in contact with the myocardium, this electrode suddenly becomes negatively charged relative to an electrode that is remote from the heart, and a brisk negative deflection is inscribed in the electrogram (see Fig. 2–4B). As the wavefront passes away from the intracardiac electrode, the electrogram returns to baseline. Because electrograms are the graphic representation of a difference in potential between two electrodes over time, the unipolar sensing configuration is also influenced by other electric signals that are nearer to the other electrode that is not in contact with the heart. For example, unipolar atrial electrograms are more likely to record large far-field cardiac signals such as R waves than are bipolar electrograms. Events nearer the extracardiac electrode such as skeletal myopotentials affect this electrode more than the intracardiac electrode and also inscribe their electric signals in the unipolar electrogram. Thus, unipolar sensing has the potential disadvantages of greater susceptibility to unwanted far-field intracardiac signals and skeletal myopotentials. However, a bipolar electrogram is really the instantaneous difference in potential between two unipolar electrograms recorded from each electrode and a remote indifferent electrode. In mathematical terms, the bipolar electrogram is equal to the unipolar electrogram from electrode 1 minus the unipolar electrogram from electrode 2: $BiEGM = UniEGM_1 - UniEGM_2$. This relationship explains the diminished susceptibility of bipolar recordings to extracardiac signals because the two electrodes in close proximity are likely to record simultaneously similar extraneous potentials, which are then canceled. Because of this fact, unipolar electrograms may also be less susceptible to the orientation of the interelectrode axis in some cases than are bipolar electrograms. For example, Figure 2–5A illustrates unipolar electrograms recorded from the tip and ring electrodes of a

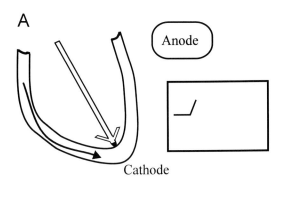

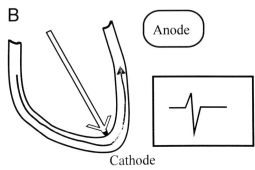

FIGURE 2–4. *A,* Demonstrates the concept of unipolar sensing. Note that there are actually two electrodes, one located within the heart (cathode) and one located outside the heart in contact with the pulse generator case (anode). As a wavefront of activation advances toward the intracardiac electrode *(arrow),* the electrogram records a positive deflection. At the moment the wavefront passes the cathode *(B),* the electrogram suddenly shifts from positive to negative before returning to baseline as the wave spreads away.

bipolar pacing lead. The unipolar tip electrogram has an amplitude that is equal to twice the unipolar ring electrogram. However, there is a phase shift in the moment of activation (the intrinsic deflection) as the wave of depolarization travels beneath the electrodes in which the tip electrode is activated slightly earlier than the ring electrode. The bipolar electrogram is equal to the difference in potential at each point in time between the tip and ring electrodes. However, if the unipolar tip and ring electrograms have similar amplitude and timing, the difference in potential between the electrodes is small, and the bipolar electrogram may be of much lower amplitude than either unipolar electrogram alone (see Fig. 2–5B).

When unipolar and bipolar electrograms are studied in a population of patients, there is usually no significant difference in the mean amplitude between these configurations. For example, DeCaprio and colleagues reported that the mean unipolar ventricular electrogram was 12.2 ± 5.2 mV in amplitude among 49 patients, whereas the bipolar configuration was a mean of 11.8 ± 6.0 mV ($p = $ NS).[1] However, these authors reported considerable intraindividual variability with the bipolar electrogram smaller than the unipolar electrogram in 49% of patients, larger than the unipolar electrogram in 43%, and equal in 8%. Other studies have similarly reported that, on average, bipolar atrial and ventricular electrograms have amplitudes that are approximately equal to those of simultaneously recorded unipolar electrograms.[2]

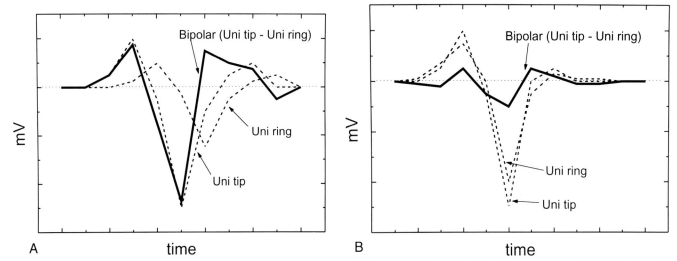

FIGURE 2–5. The relationship between unipolar and bipolar electrograms recorded between the tip and ring electrodes of a bipolar pacing lead is shown. *A,* The unipolar ring electrogram is equal to exactly half the amplitude of the unipolar tip electrogram. Note that there is a phase shift in the timing of activation, the tip electrogram being activated earlier than the ring electrode. The bipolar electrogram is equal to the unipolar tip electrogram minus the unipolar ring electrogram at all times. Because there is a difference in the amplitude and timing of the unipolar tip and ring electrograms, the bipolar electrogram has acceptable amplitude. *B,* The unipolar ring electrogram has an amplitude that is only slightly less than that of the unipolar tip electrogram. In addition, there is essentially no phase shift. Although both unipolar electrograms demonstrate acceptable amplitude for sensing, the bipolar electrogram shows both diminished amplitude and diminished slew rate.

ELECTROGRAM WAVEFORMS, AMPLITUDE, AND SLEW RATE

The *intrinsic deflection* of an electrogram is the rapid downstroke of the electrogram as the myocardium underlying the electrode suddenly becomes electrically negative during depolarization. Furman and colleagues noted that 58% of unipolar endocardial electrograms at lead implantation had an intrinsic deflection that was biphasic, with an initial upstroke followed by a downstroke such that the R and S waves were roughly equal.[2] In 30% of cases the electrogram was predominantly monophasic negative, and in 12% it was monophasic positive. The acute ventricular electrogram may demonstrate a current of injury with an elevated ST segment that later disappears.[2] The intracardiac electrogram is characterized in clinical practice in terms of its amplitude (measured in millivolts) and its slew rate (measured in volts/second). Both factors are important determinants of whether an electric event will be sensed by the pacemaker. Figure 2–6 illustrates the minimum amplitude and slew rate that should be accepted at lead implantation to ensure appropriate sensing. The amplitude of an electrogram depends on several factors, including the mass of myocardium underlying the electrode, the contact of the electrode with the myocardium, the orientation of the electrode with respect to the axis of depolarization, and the presence of any inexcitable tissue between the myocytes and the electrode. Since the right ventricle typically has a much greater mass of myocytes than the right atrium, the ventricular electrogram usually has a much greater amplitude than the atrial electrogram. Electrodes that are located within infarcted myocardium or that become encapsulated with a thick layer of fibrotic tissue typically demonstrate a lower amplitude than electrodes directly in contact with healthy myocytes.

The slew rate represents the maximal rate of change of the electric potential between the sensing electrodes. Mathemat-ically, the slew rate is the first derivative of the electrogram (dV/dt) and is a measure of the change in electrogram voltage over time. The slew rate is thus directly linked to the electrogram amplitude and duration. In general, an electrogram with an acceptable amplitude usually has an acceptable slew rate. Nevertheless, there are exceptions to this rule, so that both parameters should be measured with a pacing system analyzer at the time of lead implantation. Figure 2–7 demonstrates the interaction of electrogram amplitude, slew rate, and sensitivity threshold with respect to whether or not an electrogram is sensed by the sensing amplifier of a pacemaker. Note that electrograms of very low amplitude are not

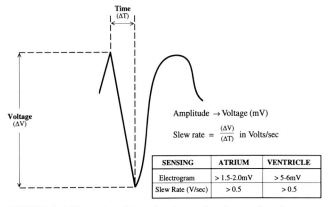

SENSING	ATRIUM	VENTRICLE
Electrogram	> 1.5-2.0mV	> 5-6mV
Slew Rate (V/sec)	> 0.5	> 0.5

Amplitude → Voltage (mV)

Slew rate = $\dfrac{(\Delta V)}{(\Delta T)}$ in Volts/sec

FIGURE 2–6. The major clinical descriptors of an intracardiac electrogram are illustrated. The amplitude of the electrogram is the difference in voltage recorded between two electrodes and is measured in millivolts. The slew rate is equal to the first derivative of the electrogram (dV/dt) and is a measure of the sharpness of the electrogram. Slew rate is measured in volts per second. In general, the amplitude of the electrogram should be greater than 1.5 to 2.0 mV in the atrium and at least 5 to 6 mV in the ventricle at the time of lead implantation to ensure adequate sensing. The slew rate should be at least 0.5 V/sec in both the atrium and the ventricle.

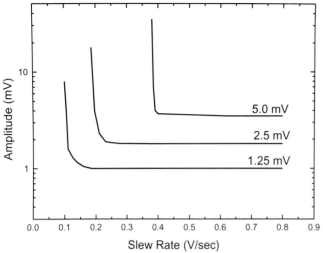

FIGURE 2–7. This figure demonstrates the interaction of electrogram amplitude (mV) and slew rate (V/sec) at three sensitivity settings for the Medtronic Spectrax sensing amplifiers. Note that with a programmed sensing threshold of 1.25 mV, electrograms with an amplitude of more than 1 mV will be sensed provided that the slew rate is at least 0.15 V/sec. If the slew rate is less than 0.1 V/sec, the amplitude must be greater to allow the electrogram to be sensed. At higher sensitivity threshold settings, greater amplitudes and slew rates are required for sensing by an electrogram.

sensed, regardless of the slew rate. On the other hand, electrograms with an amplitude that exceeds the sensitivity threshold are not sensed if the slew rate is inadequate. There is a further interaction between the programmed sensitivity threshold and the adequacy of the slew rate, with greater slew rates required for appropriate sensing when the sensitivity threshold is programmed to a higher value.

Furman and colleagues reported that unipolar and bipolar ventricular electrograms were similar in amplitude (12.19 vs. 11.75 mV) and slew rate (2.82 vs. 2.82 V/sec), although the unipolar electrogram is characterized by a greater current of injury (2.62 vs. 1.64 mV) and T-wave amplitude (2.41 vs. 1.60 mV) than the bipolar configuration.[2] As would be expected from the greater mass of the left ventricle compared with the right ventricle, the mean amplitude of the epicardial unipolar ventricular electrogram was greater for the left than for the right ventricle (18.0 vs. 11.2 mV). These authors found that atrial unipolar endocardial electrograms had a mean amplitude of 4.83 ± 2.21 mV with a slew rate of 1.18 V/sec. The far-field R wave of the unipolar atrial electrogram measured 2.21 mV in amplitude with a slew rate of only 0.13 V/sec. Respiratory variation in ventricular electrogram amplitude was a mean of $\pm 9.7\%$ for unipolar atrial electrograms and $\pm 11.5\%$ for bipolar atrial electrograms. The effect of respiration on ventricular electrograms was less, although the unipolar configuration was somewhat less susceptible to respiratory changes than the bipolar configuration ($\pm 5.3\%$ unipolar and $\pm 9.4\%$ bipolar).

The effect of exercise on the atrial electrogram has been studied by Frohlig and colleagues in 33 patients with dual-chamber pacemakers.[3] In this study involving bicycle exercise with telemetered atrial electrograms, 29 of the pacemakers were unipolar and 4 were bipolar, and all leads were of the active-fixation, screw-in variety. Six of 33 patients developed atrial undersensing during exercise at sensitivity

values that were adequate at rest. There was a decline in the mean atrial electrogram amplitude from 6.4 ± 1.9 mV at rest to 5.6 ± 1.9 mV during exercise, whereas the slew rate decreased from 1.35 ± 0.45 V/sec to 1.18 ± 0.45 V/sec ($p < .001$). The decrease in atrial electrogram amplitude ranged up to 41%, and the slew rate decreased by up to 51%. In general, the frequency content of the atrial electrogram was characterized by an increase in low-frequency and a decrease in high-frequency signals. Thus, a complete evaluation for suspected inappropriate sensing may require the use of exercise or ambulatory electrocardiographic monitoring.

EVOLUTION OF ELECTROGRAMS OVER TIME

Like stimulation thresholds, intracardiac electrograms typically demonstrate changes during the first several weeks following lead implantation. The amplitude of the intracardiac electrogram usually declines to a nadir during the first several days to weeks following lead implantation before increasing to a chronic value that is slightly lower than that noted at implantation.[4, 5] This decrease in electrogram amplitude is related to the development of a layer of inexcitable tissue surrounding the electrode in contact with the myocardium. This fibrotic capsule effectively increases the distance between the surface of the electrode and the excitable myocardium in which the electric signals arise. Platia and Brinker reported that the mean atrial unipolar electrogram amplitude decreased from 3.5 mV at implant to 2.2 mV at 1 month before returning to a chronic value of 3.2 mV at 13 months.[6] For ventricular unipolar electrograms, there was a slight decrease in the amplitude from 13.5 mV at implant to 10.1 mV at 1 month before a chronic value of 13.0 mV was recorded at 13 months. DeCaprio and colleagues reported that unipolar ventricular electrograms showed a reduction in amplitude from a mean of 12.4 ± 5.2 mV at implant to 12.1 ± 5.3 mV during chronic follow-up.[1] The change in slew rate was more significant, with a reduction from 3.5 V/sec at implant to 2.3 V/sec at chronic follow-up. Bipolar electrograms demonstrated similar evolutionary changes, with a decrease in amplitude from 13.4 to 10.5 mV and a decrease in slew rate from 3.6 V/sec to 2.2 V/sec. The evolution of electrogram amplitude is often more dramatic with active fixation leads, in which atrial undersensing may occur during the first several days following lead implantation despite quite adequate electrogram amplitudes recorded acutely. To account for these changes in electrogram amplitude over time, the filtered electrogram recorded at lead implantation should be at least twice the sensitivity threshold that will be programmed in the pulse generator. This is especially true for electrodes with relatively traumatic active-fixation mechanisms. The addition of corticosteroid elution to pacing leads tends to attenuate the evolution of electrograms over time.[7] Because of this, it may be possible to accept a somewhat lower margin between the sensitivity setting in the pulse generator and the filtered electrogram amplitude at lead implantation if passive-fixation, corticosteroid-eluting leads are used.

FREQUENCY SPECTRA OF INTRACARDIAC ELECTROGRAMS

The electrogram that is recorded between two electrodes may register changes in voltage from sources other than the underlying myocardium such as skeletal muscles and environmental interference. In addition to a characteristic timing of electric events within the heart (e.g., the P wave occurs before the R wave, which is followed by the T wave), intracardiac electrograms have a characteristic frequency spectrum that often differs from the frequencies of unwanted signals (Fig. 2–8). The spectrum of frequencies of an intracardiac electrogram can be studied by fast Fourier transformation, a technique that transforms the waveform into a series of sine waves and plots the energy content of the signal as a function of frequency. Myers and associates studied the bandwidth of intracardiac ventricular electrograms in 30 patients using a physiologic recorder and electrodes of varying size.[5] They defined the bandwidth of the signal as the point at which the amplitude spectrum has decreased to one fourth of its peak value. The bandwidth of the ventricular electrogram ranged from as narrow as 5 Hz to as wide as 116 Hz, depending on the size of the electrode and the loading conditions of the sense amplifier (see later discussion under the section on sensing impedance). In general, small electrodes demonstrated a wider electrogram bandwidth than large electrodes at a low input impedance of the sensing amplifier but little difference at high input impedances.

Kleinert and colleagues reported that ventricular unipolar electrograms contained R waves with maximal energy in the frequencies ranging from approximately 10 to 50 Hz.[8] The peak energy of the intracardiac R wave was centered at approximately 25 to 30 Hz. The T wave in the intracardiac ventricular electrogram has a much lower range of frequencies, the peak energies being located below 3 Hz. Atrial electrograms are characterized by a frequency spectrum that is similar to that of the ventricular electrogram, with typical energies in the range of 10 to 50 Hz. The peak energies are centered at approximately 20 to 30 Hz. The far-field R wave in the unipolar atrial electrogram is typically composed of lower frequencies, ranging from 5 to 20 Hz. It is therefore possible for pacemaker sensing circuits to attenuate the low frequencies that are characteristic of the T wave by filtering without interfering with P-wave or R-wave sensing (see following section). Myopotentials typically have a higher frequency spectrum than P waves or R waves, with maximal energies in the range of 50 Hz. However, although myopotentials contain more high-frequency components, there is considerable frequency overlap between R waves and P waves and signals generated by the pectoralis muscle. In general, myopotentials have a lower amplitude than ventricular electrograms. This is not true for P waves, however. Therefore, although some components of myopotentials can be effectively filtered, unipolar pacing systems remain susceptible to myopotential inhibition.

FILTERING OF INTRACARDIAC SIGNALS

To improve the signal-to-noise ratio of intracardiac signals, sensing amplifiers incorporate filters that are intended to reject unwanted signals while allowing appropriate sensing of P waves and R waves. Ideally, the filter would allow the intrinsic deflection in the atrium and ventricle to pass while removing T waves, far-field cardiac events such as R waves in the atrial electrogram or P waves in the ventricular electrogram, skeletal myopotentials, or afterpotentials. Figures 2–9 and 2–10 illustrate the effect of different filtering frequencies on the waveform of right atrial and right ventricular electrograms. Note that as the high-pass filter (designed to attenuate frequencies lower than this setting while allowing higher frequencies to "pass") is increased, there is a decrease in the amplitude of the electrogram. Klitzner and Stevenson studied the effect of high-pass filters on the ventricular electrogram in patients with right ventricular catheters and noted that an increase in the high-pass filter from 1 to 10 Hz had little effect on the electrogram amplitude (from 9.0 mV to 11.2 mV) or duration (from 35 msec to 39 msec).[9] However, a high-pass filter of 30 Hz decreased the ventricular electrogram amplitude to 8.2 mV and the duration to 34 msec. An increase in the high-pass filter to 100 Hz further decreased the amplitude to 4 mV and the duration to 24 msec (Fig. 2–11). Decreasing the low-pass filter (designed to attenuate signals with high frequencies, allowing lower frequencies to "pass") from 2500 Hz to 100 Hz had no effect on electrogram amplitude or duration.

Permanent pacemakers use analog filters that have a *center frequency* at which the signal is least attenuated (Fig. 2–12). At frequencies above and below the center frequency, the signal amplitude is decreased. In other words, for any programmed sensitivity threshold setting signals above or below the center frequency must have a greater amplitude to be sensed than signals in the center frequency range. The center frequency of the sensing amplifier that is measured is markedly dependent on the waveform used for testing. Several different types of test signals are used, including square waves, sine waves, sine squared waves, and triangular waves. The filters are evaluated by varying the duration of these test waveforms with the duration of the wave being inversely related to its frequency. The sine squared test waveform has been most commonly used for evaluating sensing ciruits, although manufacturers have not agreed on a consistent approach. The effect of using different test waveforms to determine the amplitude of a signal that will be sensed by the pulse generator at any given sensitivity setting is the presence of a variance of as much as 100% in the sensing threshold for an electrogram between manufacturers. Because of this, the same ventricular electrogram may be measured very dif-

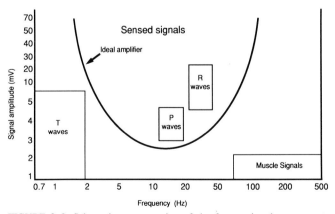

FIGURE 2–8. Schematic representation of the frequencies that are most typical of T waves, P waves, R waves, and myopotentials. An ideal sensing amplifier would have maximum sensitivity to signals with frequencies ranging from 10 to 40 Hz (typical of P waves and R waves) and decreased sensitivity to signals with very low (T waves) or very high (myopotentials) frequencies. In reality, there is often an overlap between the frequencies of myopotentials and the desired P waves and R waves.

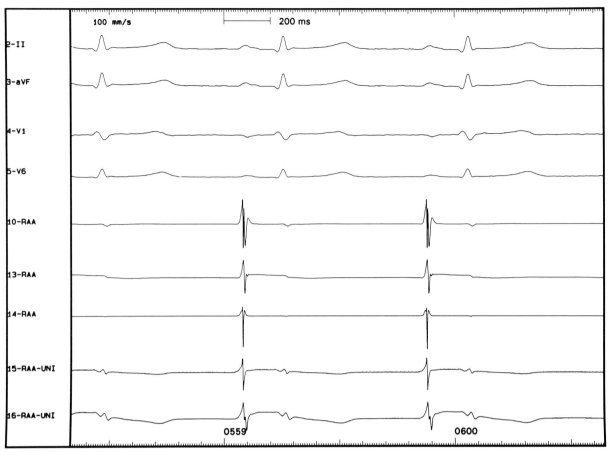

FIGURE 2–9. The effect of filtering on the electrogram recorded from the right atrial appendage (RAA). From top to bottom, surface electrocardiographic leads II, aVF, V₁, and V₆ are recorded simultaneously with bipolar electrograms filtered at 30 to 500 Hz (10-RAA), 0.05 to 100 Hz (13-RAA), and 100 to 2000 Hz (14-RAA). A notch filter designed to remove 60-Hz alternating current (AC) signals is used for the uppermost RAA electrogram. The two bottom tracings illustrate unipolar recordings with filter settings of 0.05 to 100 Hz and 0.05 to 1000 Hz (15-RAA-UNI and 16-RAA-UNI, respectively).

ferently by the pulse generator of different manufacturers. In addition, the ability of a pulse generator to reject unwanted signals is influenced by the test waveform that is used. Thus, skeletal myopotentials that are effectively rejected by one pulse generator may result in inappropriate inhibition of another. In response to this lack of tight correlation between the electric signals generated in the myocardium and the sensitivity measurements made by different pulse generators, Irnich[7a] proposed a new sensitivity test signal for unipolar application that is 20 msec in duration with a 4-msec downstroke followed by a 16-msec upstroke (Fig. 2–13). Such an asymmetrical waveform is more likely to reflect the range of conduction velocities within human myocardium and the shape of endocardial electrograms.

This discussion of filtering has important clinical implications at the time of pacemaker implantation. One cannot assume that an electrogram that is recorded on a physiologic recorder with a wide bandpass filter and high input impedance will accurately reflect the filtered electrogram that is actually sensed by the pulse generator. For example, Steinhaus and colleagues found that the amplitude of atrial electrograms recorded with a physiologic recorder, the pacing system analyzer (PSA) of different manufacturers, the atrial or ventricular channels of the same PSA, or those telemetered from the pulse generator correlated poorly with a wide range

of values measured by these devices for the same cardiac signal.[10] Therefore, the electrogram should be measured by a PSA that uses the same sensing amplifier as the pulse generator that is to be implanted. Because ventricular electrograms usually have a far greater amplitude and slew rate than atrial electrograms, the matching of PSA and pulse generator is less critical for ventricular than for atrial leads.

AFTERPOTENTIALS

Following delivery of a stimulation pulse, the myocardium in contact with the stimulating electrode becomes electrically charged as current is transferred from the electrode to the myocardium. For a cathodal pulse, the negatively charged electrode in contact with the endocardium becomes surrounded by positively charged ions (such as Na^+ and H_3O^+) while negatively charged ions (such as Cl^-, HPO_4^{2-}, and OH^-) are electrotonically repelled from the electrode. This *polarization* at the electrode-tissue interface begins at the start of the pacing pulse and increases to the end of the stimulus. Following the pacing stimulus, the degree of polarization gradually dissipates as ions reestablish electric neutrality. Polarization thus represents a voltage source in the tissues that will be sensed as an electric signal of opposite polarity to the stimulation waveform (Fig. 2–14). Polariza-

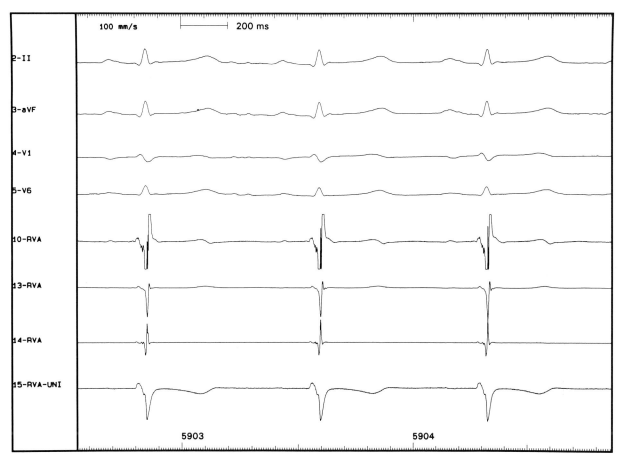

FIGURE 2–10. Effect of filtering on the right ventricular apex (RVA) electrogram. From top to bottom four surface electrocardiographic leads (leads II, aVF, V₁, and V₆) are displayed with intracardiac electrograms recorded at the RVA. Filter settings for the RVA electrograms (*top* to *bottom*) are: bipolar, 30 to 500 Hz with notch filtering (10-RVA); bipolar, 0.05 to 100 Hz without notch filtering (13-RVA); bipolar, 100 to 2000 Hz without notch filtering (14-RVA); and unipolar, 0.05 to 1000 Hz (15-RVA-UNI).

tion is related to several factors, including the amplitude and duration of the stimulation pulse, and the radius, surface area, and geometry, surface structure, and chemical composition of the electrode. The magnitude of afterpotentials depends on the polarization properties of the electrode, decreasing with increasing microscopic surface area. The chemical content of the electrode also has a major impact on polarization, afterpotentials being reduced with materials that have low polari-

zation properties. The materials presently used for permanent pacing electrodes include platinum-iridium, titanium (oxide), platinum- or carbon-coated titanium, platinized platinum, vitreous carbon, and iridium oxide. The platinized-platinum, ''activated'' carbon, and iridium oxide electrodes are especially associated with a reduced degree of polarization. The vitreous carbon electrodes can be manufactured by a process known as ''activation,'' which increases the electrode surface

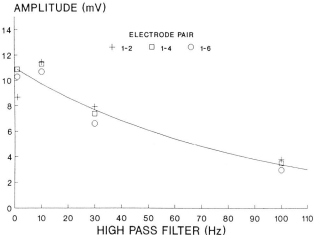

FIGURE 2–11. The effect of high-pass filtering on the amplitude of right ventricular intracardiac electrograms in humans. Note that as the high-pass filter is increased in frequency from 0.05 to 100 Hz, the amplitude of the electrogram is progressively reduced. (From Klitzner TS, Stevenson WG: Effects of filtering on right ventricular electrograms recorded from endocardial catheters in humans. PACE 13:69, 1990.)

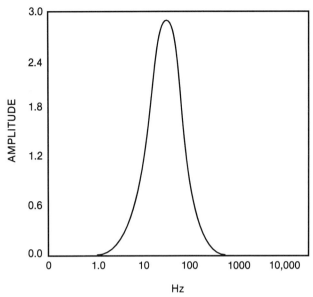

FIGURE 2–12. Effect of filtering on the amplitude of an intracardiac electrogram that will be sensed for a modern permanent pulse generator. The size of the signal actually sensed by the sensing amplifier is shown on the ordinate as a function of signal frequency on the abscissa. Note that the signal frequency for which the amplifier is most sensitive (*center*) is approximately 30 to 40 Hz.

area by roughening the surface, thereby reducing polarization. To reduce afterpotentials and prevent loss of stimulation efficiency related to polarization at rapid pacing rates, manufacturers have introduced "rapid recharge" circuits following pacing stimuli. For example, Medtronic Inc. has used a recharge period following delivery of the pacing stimulus in which the output capacitor is allowed to recharge from the accumulated polarization in the myocardium over a period of 8 msec.[11] This allows the polarization to dissipate at the electrode-tissue interface and reduces afterpotentials. In some older pulse generator models (Medtronic Spectrax SX and SX-HT), rapid recharging of the output capacitor also oc-

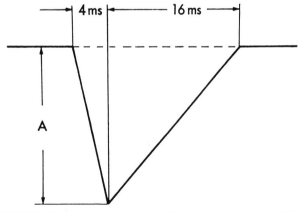

FIGURE 2–13. Proposed test signal waveform for testing sensing amplifiers. A 20-msec test signal with a 4-msec initial downward deflection and a 16-msec upward deflection was found by Irnich to best reflect the characteristics of intracardiac electrograms. The 4/16 msec test signal proposed to Irnich was changed by ISO, CENELEC to 2/13 msec. (From Irnich W: Intracardiac electrograms and sensing test signals: Electrophysiological, physical, and technical considerations. PACE 8:870, 1985.)

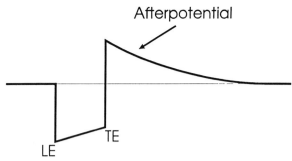

FIGURE 2–14. Diagram of a constant-voltage pacing pulse (downward deflection) with leading edge (LE) and trailing edge (TE) voltage and a resultant afterpotential of opposite polarity. Afterpotentials may interfere with sensing, especially if the stimulus is of high amplitude and duration.

curred following sensed events. Such recharge pulses could sometimes be identified on the surface electrocardiogram and were misinterpreted as attenuated pacing stimuli that ranged from 3% to 20% of the amplitude of a unipolar pacing stimulus (Fig. 2–15).[12] Rapid recharge after sensing has been eliminated from more recent pulse generator models.

Unless suitable blanking of the sense amplifiers is employed, afterpotentials can be sensed by the pulse generator and can inappropriately inhibit pacing output. If a high stimulation amplitude is used, afterpotentials may also be sensed by the sense amplifier in the opposite chamber. For example, afterpotentials resulting from atrial stimulation may be sensed by the ventricular sense amplifier of a dual-chamber pacemaker and may inappropriately inhibit ventricular output, a phenomenon known as crosstalk (Fig. 2–16). Crosstalk is more likely to occur with a wide interelectrode distance and is much more common with unipolar than with bipolar sensing configurations. Thus, the combination of an atrial stimulus with high amplitude and a ventricular sense amplifier programmed to a low sensitivity threshold value (more sensitive) is especially likely to generate crosstalk. To avoid crosstalk, the ventricular sense amplifier is blanked (made insensitive to electric signals) immediately following delivery of the atrial pacing stimulus. For many manufacturers, the duration of the ventricular blanking period is a programmable parameter, although values of 25 to 50 msec are most commonly used. The phenomenon of "reverse crosstalk," in which the atrial sense amplifier detects far-field electric

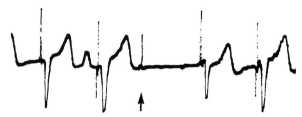

FIGURE 2–15. Surface electrocardiographic tracing made from a patient with a Medtronic Spectrax pulse generator that incorporates a rapid recharge pulse after sensed ventricular events. The first two complexes represent VVI pacing stimuli. The third complex demonstrates an attenuated stimulus artifact (*arrow*) that is the result of a rapid recharge pulse delivered synchronously with a sensed ventricular event. This artifact could easily be mistaken for noncapture of a pacing stimulus. (From Barold SS, Kulkarni H, Thawani AJ, et al: Electrocardiographic manifestations of the rapid recharge function of pulse generators after sensing. PACE 11:1215, 1988.)

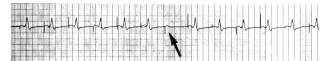

FIGURE 2–16. Crosstalk in a patient with a DDD pacemaker. In this patient, the ventricular blanking period had been shortened with an atrial stimulus amplitude of 7.5 V and a pulse duration of 2.0 msec because of a high stimulation threshold. The first six complexes show atrial pacing followed by ventricular pacing. The seventh complex from the left shows an atrial pacing stimulus and an inhibited ventricular pacing stimulus due to sensing of afterpotentials from the atrial lead by the ventricular sensing channel. Crosstalk is most likely to occur in the presence of an atrial stimulus of high amplitude and duration combined with a sensitive ventricular sensing setting.

events in the ventricle, may also occur.[13] In most cases, reverse crosstalk is the result of sensing far-field R waves in the atrial electrogram rather than ventricular afterpotentials. Reverse crosstalk may become clinically manifest with dual-

chamber pacemakers that offer automatic mode reversion algorithms designed to switch from the DDD or DDDR mode to the VVI or VVIR mode in response to atrial tachyarrhythmias (Fig. 2–17). In the presence of a low programmed atrial sensing threshold value, the far-field R wave in the atrial electrogram could result in inappropriate mode switching of the Telectronics Meta DDDR model 1250 pulse generator from the DDDR to the VVIR mode, even with bipolar atrial sensing. Such occurrences have largely been rectified by increasing the atrial blanking period from 100 msec to 150 msec following the ventricular pacing stimulus in more recent iterations of these devices (Telectronics model 1254).

Since pacing systems that sense the evoked intracardiac electrogram have been developed as a sensor for rate-adaptive pacing (the paced depolarization integral, or PDI), afterpotentials can produce difficulties in accurately measuring this parameter. Measurement of the evoked intracardiac electrogram may be most useful as a method for detecting myocardial capture following delivery of a pacing stimulus. How-

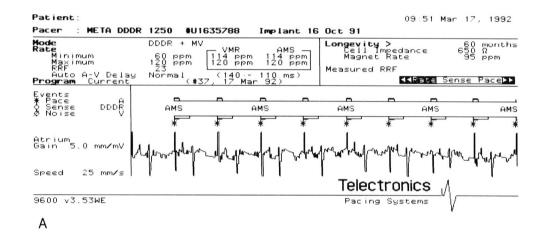

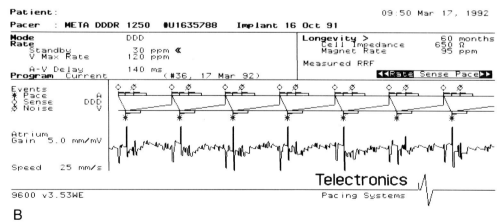

FIGURE 2–17. Inappropriate automatic mode switching (AMS) demonstrated by sensing of the far-field ventricular electrogram with the Meta DDDR model 1250 pulse generator. There is bipolar atrial and ventricular sensing. *A,* DDDR pacing with programmer printouts showing simultaneous tracings of the events recorded by the pacemaker and the intracardiac atrial electrogram. AMS occurred during the events recorded in *A.* The atrial electrogram shows prominent voltage corresponding to the ventricular stimulus artifact. Following this are the smaller voltages of the far-field paced ventricular electrogram. Soon after this appear the larger voltages of the retrograde atrial electrogram, another potential cause of AMS. *B,* When the pacemaker is reprogrammed to the DDD mode, AMS does not occur because the sensed far-field paced ventricular electrogram is beyond the 2-msec AMS window and is interpreted as noise. Sensing in the postventricular atrial refractory period (PVARP) with resetting of the atrial refractory period now occurs, but there is no retrograde atrial deflection in the atrial electrogram. This fact confirms that the far-field paced ventricular electrogram was responsible for the AMS and not the retrograde P wave (VMR, ventricular maximum rate or upper tracking rate; RRF, rate response factor). (From Mond H, Barold SS: Dual-chamber, rate-adaptive pacing in patients with paroxysmal supraventricular tachyarrhythmias: Protective measures for rate control. PACE 16:2168, 1993.)

ever, since afterpotentials are produced by pacing stimuli that do not capture the myocardium as well as by those that do, these polarization-related artifacts have presented a significant technologic challenge for manufacturers attempting to design algorithms that automatically detect capture. Low polarization electrodes are especially important for accurate capture detection.

BLANKING AND REFRACTORY PERIODS

As the preceding discussion demonstrates, it is not possible to distinguish the desired components of an electrogram from unwanted signals by filtering alone. Therefore, pulse generators use the expected timing of atrial and ventricular activation as a means of improving signal discrimination. To ignore afterpotentials induced by atrial or ventricular pacing stimuli, the atrial and ventricular sensing amplifiers are blinded for a brief period following the pacing stimulus. This period is generally about 20 to 50 msec in duration. Thus, if an electric event occurs within this *blanking* period, it will not be sensed. For dual-chamber pacing systems, the ventricular sense amplifier is also blanked immediately following an atrial pacing stimulus (Fig. 2–18). To avoid sensing of T waves by the ventricular sense amplifier, a programmable refractory period is employed (Fig. 2–19). During the refractory period, the pulse generator will not respond to electric signals that exceed the programmed sensitivity threshold value. Combined with filtering, refractory periods have greatly reduced the incidence of T-wave sensing. Nevertheless, programming of the refractory period to an inappropriately short duration may allow T-wave sensing, especially if a very sensitive sensing threshold value is programmed. In addition, patients with a prolonged QRS duration or a prolonged QT interval may need a longer refractory period to be programmed to avoid sensing of T waves. Recognition of T-wave sensing is accomplished by ensuring consistent prolongation of the pacemaker escape interval by an amount that coincides with the T wave. Thus, if the T wave is consistently oversensed, the apparent lower pacing interval of a VVI pacemaker prolongs to a value that is equal to the programmed escape interval plus the stimulus-to-T interval. For example, if a lower pacing interval of 1000 msec (60 bpm) is programmed with a T wave that is consistently oversensed 250 msec following the pacing stimulus, the ac-

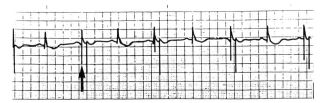

FIGURE 2–18. Loss of atrial sensing with apparent ventricular undersensing and ventricular pacing. Note that in the second complex an atrial pacing stimulus follows the P wave because of undersensing in the atrium. The atrial pacing stimulus occurs at the start of the ventricular QRS complex. The ventricular electrogram is not sensed because of blanking in the ventricular sensing amplifier immediately following an atrial pacing stimulus. This sequence is repeated in the fourth, sixth, and eighth complexes. Atrial undersensing may lead to apparent ventricular undersensing because the ventricular blanking period does not permit sensing of electric signals for a period of 10 to 40 msec following an atrial output pulse.

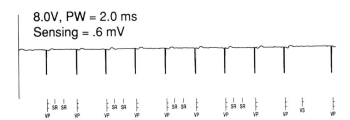

8.0V, PW = 2.0 ms
Sensing = .6 mV

FIGURE 2–19. The importance of a programmable refractory period to prevent inappropriate sensing of afterpotentials and T waves in a patient with a unipolar VVI pacemaker programmed to 8 V and a 2.0-msec pulse width (PW) with a high ventricular sensitivity (0.6 mV). Following the pacing stimulus, the marker channel identifies three events: ventricular pacing stimulus (VP), sensed event during the refractory period due to either sensing of the afterpotential or the T wave (SR). The refractory period prevents the pacemaker from responding inappropriately to these unwanted electric signals.

tual pacing interval would be 1250 msec (48 bpm). Similarly, intermittent T-wave oversensing results in pauses equal to the programmed lower pacing interval plus the stimulus to sensed T-wave interval.

The programmed refractory period is especially important for proper function of AAI pacemakers in which far-field R waves or even T waves may be sensed by very sensitive programmed sensing threshold values that are commonly used in the atrium. Thus, the atrial refractory period must be longer than the paced PR interval as measured by the intracardiac atrial electrogram. This interval must include the entire intracardiac R wave to avoid far-field sensing. The atrial refractory period of an AAIR pacemaker is usually in the range of 325 to 450 msec. For unipolar AAIR pacemakers, an even longer refractory period may be necessary to avoid oversensing of far-field T waves. If a far-field signal is oversensed, the actual pacing rate prolongs in the same manner as described earlier for VVI pacemakers. This situation can be even more complex with AAIR pacing systems because the PR interval may prolong with excessively rapid atrial pacing rates, especially if the rate-adaptive sensor is programmed overly aggressively. Rate-adaptive pacemakers have the additional complication of increasing the lower pacing rate in response to output of the sensor. Thus, if the refractory period is longer than the pacing interval at the upper programmed pacing rate, asynchronous pacing may occur at high sensor-indicated rates.

Refractory and blanking periods are required in both the atrial and ventricular sensing amplifiers of dual-chamber pacemakers. Following the atrial pacing stimulus, the atrial and ventricular sensing amplifiers are blanked for a period to avoid sensing afterpotentials. The atrial channel is blanked for the entire duration of the AV delay. Following the post-atrial blanking period in the ventricular channel, the ventricular sense amplifier is alert for the occurrence of an intrinsically conducted QRS complex. Delivery of a ventricular pacing stimulus or the occurrence of an intrinsic ventricular beat activates a refractory period in the ventricular sensing amplifier to avoid afterpotentials and T-wave oversensing. The atrial sense amplifier also enters a postventricular atrial blanking period of 100 to 160 msec as well as a *postventricular atrial refractory period* (PVARP) after the ventricular pacing stimulus or an intrinsic ventricular complex. The atrial blanking period is designed to avoid oversensing of

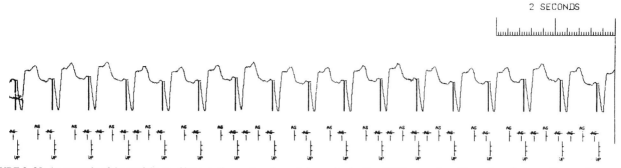

2 SECONDS

FIGURE 2–20. An example of the usefulness of intracardiac marker channels in a patient with a DDD pacemaker. The surface electrocardiogram demonstrates ventricular pacing at the upper rate limit during atrial flutter. The atrial marker channel demonstrates atrial events that were sensed within PVARP (A̶S̶) and atrial events sensed outside PVARP (AS). Note that following a ventricular pacing stimulus (VP), some atrial electrograms are not sensed, resulting in apparent electrogram dropout because the atrium is blanked for a period following delivery of a ventricular pacing stimulus. Only atrial signals recorded outside PVARP (AS) are tracked.

far-field R waves, whereas the PVARP is designed to avoid tracking of retrogradely conducted atrial beats that may follow ventricular activation or ventricular premature depolarizations (VPDs). The net result is a period of refractoriness in the atrial sense amplifier known as the *total atrial refractory period* (TARP), which is equal to the AV delay plus the PVARP: (TARP = AV delay + PVARP).

The duration of the total atrial refractory period has profound implications for atrial sensing and tracking of the atrium at high sinus rates (Fig. 2–20) (see Chapter 31). To allow appropriate recognition of very rapid atrial signals associated with pathologic arrhythmias such as atrial fibrillation, many newer dual-chamber pacemakers with mode-switching algorithms allow electric signals that occur after the atrial blanking period but within the PVARP to be logged into atrial rate counters without tracking.[14] Such sensing within the PVARP may also avoid the occurrence of asynchronous atrial pacing at high sensor-indicated pacing rates. Since the AV delay of most recent generations of dual-chamber pacemakers shortens in response to increasing atrial rates or sensor input, the TARP also shortens. Several manufacturers now offer dual-chamber pacemakers that also shorten PVARP with increasing atrial or sensor-indicated rates, further reducing the TARP during exercise. The result of these newer algorithms is that the programmed upper tracking rate can be more safely increased while providing protection from retrogradely conducted atrial beats and pacemaker-mediated tachycardia. Appropriate recognition of pathologic atrial arrhythmias is also enhanced, improving the sensitivity of mode-switching algorithms.

SENSING IMPEDANCE

As discussed previously, the intracardiac electrogram originates from electric currents in the underlying myocardium. However, the electric signal may become distorted as it is transmitted by the pacing lead to the sensing amplifier. The theoretical model for understanding pacemaker sensing has been described as a voltage source (the myocardium) in series with a resistor and a capacitor that are in parallel (Fig. 2–21). The three components of sensing impedance include tissue resistance (R_t), Faraday resistance (R_F), and Helmholtz capacitance (C_H). The total sensing impedance (Z_S) is approximated by:

$$\textbf{Eq 1} \quad Z_s \cong R_t + \frac{R_F}{(1 + C_H R_F)}$$

The tissue resistance (R_t) can be measured in the standard manner as the ratio of current to voltage: $R_t = \frac{I}{V}$. Tissue resistance is related to the ohmic resistance of the lead conductor and the resistance of the myocardium; it typically ranges from 300 to 1000 ohms for a permanent pacing lead. The Faraday resistance represents the impediment to current flow across the tissue-electrode interface and is indirectly related to the surface area of the electrode. Ohm measured the Faraday resistance at the tissue-electrode interface and found it to range from as low as 7.7 kOhms (kΩ) for the large surface area ring electrode of a bipolar lead (48 mm²) to as high as 87 kΩ for a tip electrode measuring 11 mm².[15] The Helmholtz capacitance (C_H) is the polarization capacitance at the tissue-electrode surface and is related to the frequency content of the signal. Capacitance (C) is the ratio

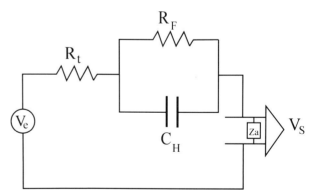

FIGURE 2–21. Schematic representation of sensing impedance. The electric signal in the myocardium is a voltage source (V_e). The tissue resistance (R_t) represents the impediment to flow of current through the myocardium, the electrode, and the lead conductor(s). The Faraday resistance (R_F) is related to the transfer of charge from the myocardium to the electrode. The tissue-electrode interface is also capable of storing charge, represented by a Helmholtz capacitor (C_H). Thus, sensing impedance is represented by a resistor (R_t) in series with a resistor (R_F) and a capacitor (C_H) that are in parallel. The current then flows through the input impedance of the sensing amplifier (Z_a). The amplitude of the signal that is actually sensed by the sense amplifier (V_s) is somewhat less than the amplitude of the electrogram at its source in the myocardium (V_e). The greater the input impedance of the sense amplifier in relation to the sensing impedance, the less the electrogram is attenuated.

of charge (Q) to voltage (V) (C = Q/V). Therefore, for a high-capacitance electrode, a large amount of charge can be stored on the electrode without generating a significant voltage. Capacitance is directly related to the surface area of the electrode and generally ranges from 1 to 10 mF. The greater the polarization capacitance of the electrode, the lower the sensing impedance (Z_s). As discussed in Chapter 1, polarization capacitance is dependent on the surface area of the electrode, the surface structure, and the electrode materials. Electrodes with low polarization properties have a high Helmholtz capacitance.

The higher the frequency of the signal, the lower the capacitance (and the higher the sensing impedance). A resistance-capacitance circuit may also introduce electrogram distortion such that the electrogram is effectively filtered. The lower frequency limit (f) of such a filtering effect of an electrode is determined by the formula:

$$\text{Eq 2} \quad f = \frac{1}{2\pi RC}$$

where R is the Faraday impedance and C is the Helmholtz capacitance. Ideally, the low-frequency filtering effect of an RC circuit should be less than the range of frequencies expected for P waves and R waves (10 to 40 Hz). For low-capacitance electrodes, f is increased compared with high-capacitance electrodes and may result in effectively filtering frequencies within the desired range of R waves and P waves. For example, Fischler found that the lower frequency cutoff of low-capacitance electrodes (Eligoloy) may be as high as 15 Hz in the presence of a low input impedance of the sensing amplifier (20 kW).[16] Therefore, to avoid distortion of the electrogram, the electrode should have a high capacitance.

Sensing impedance is important to understand because it relates to the amplitude of the electrogram that is actually sensed by the pulse generator. The voltage of the signal that is sensed by the pulse generator (V_s) is directly related to the input impedance of the sense amplifier (Z_A) and inversely related to the sensing impedance (Z_s) by the formula:

$$\text{Eq 3} \quad V_s = \left(\frac{Z_A}{Z_A + Z_s} \right) \times V_E$$

where V_E is the voltage of the electrogram at its source in the myocardium. Thus, if Z_A is equal to Z_s, then V_s would be equal to $\frac{1}{2} V_E$. In other words, if the sensing impedance is equal to the input impedance of the amplifier, the electrogram sensed by the pulse generator would be only half the amplitude of the electrogram in the myocardium. Such an attenuation of the electrogram amplitude by an input impedance that is too low or a sensing impedance that is too high is referred to as *impedance mismatch*. To minimize the attenuation of the electrogram by impedance mismatch, the input impedance of the sensing amplifier must be increased to a value that is far greater than the sensing impedance. If the input impedance is infinite, no attenuation of the electrogram would occur. Physiologic recorders usually have an input impedance of 500 to 1000 kΩ and produce very little attenuation of the electrogram. The input of sense amplifiers of modern pulse generators is typically 25,000 to 40,000 W, thus minimizing impedance mismatch and electrogram distortion. Since electrodes with a small surface area have a

higher Faraday resistance and a lower Helmholtz capacitance than larger electrodes (and therefore a higher sensing impedance), it has been suggested by several investigators that small electrodes have poor sensing characteristics.[16] However, if the input impedance of the sense amplifier is made appropriately high, small electrodes provide both excellent stimulation and sensing characteristics. Thus, sensing performance can be influenced by amplifier design to maximize the benefits of a small electrode.

ELECTRODE SIZE, INTERELECTRODE DISTANCE, AND ORTHOGONAL ELECTRODES

The radius of an electrode has important effects on stimulation threshold, pacing impedance, sensing impedance, and polarization characteristics (see Chapter 1). Despite higher Faraday impedance, lower Helmholtz capacitance, and higher total sensing impedance, small electrodes provide electrograms that are equivalent in amplitude and slew rate to larger electrodes, provided that the input impedance of the sensing amplifier is high.[15] The interelectrode distance of a bipolar pacing lead has little effect on the amplitude and slew rate of the intracardiac electrogram but has a major impact on the duration of the electrogram.[1] The greater the separation of electrodes, the longer the duration of the electrogram. This is primarily a function of greater far-field signals with wider electrode separation. Very small electrodes with close interelectrode distances produce electrograms with a short duration and attenuated far-field signals. To further minimize far-field signals and improve signal-to-noise discrimination, Goldreyer and colleagues developed an orthogonal pacing lead that incorporated a pair of platinum-iridium electrodes placed perpendicular to the long axis of the catheter (Fig. 2–22).[17, 18] The orthogonal electrodes float freely within the atrium without necessarily contacting the atrial endocardial surface. The mean P-wave amplitude recorded from a pair of orthogonal electrodes in the high right atrium was 2.4 ± 1.7 mV with a far-field R wave that was only 0.07 mV. The surface area of the orthogonal electrodes had an important effect on the amplitude of the atrial electrogram, with a mean P wave of 2.0 ± 0.77 mV for electrodes with a 0.8-mm² surface area and 1.32 ± 0.27 mV for 10-mm² surface area electrodes. The duration of the bipolar orthogonal electrogram was only 15 to 20 msec. Thus, the advantage of orthogonal electrodes is the excellent signal-to-noise discrimination provided by the rejection of far-field events, which allows very low sensitivity thresholds to be used with sensing amplifiers. Orthogonal atrial electrodes have been used successfully for VDD pacemakers that provide atrial synchronous pacing with a single ventricular lead.[19–22] The only apparent disadvantages of such lead designs are the inherent complexity of a multiconductor lead with its attendant concerns about reliability and an inability to stimulate the atrium with free-floating orthogonal electrodes in many individuals.

EFFECT OF LEAD MALFUNCTION ON SENSING PERFORMANCE

Sensing is frequently impaired in the presence of either lead fracture or insulation failure. Fractured lead conductors result in high ohmic resistance. In the case of a complete conductor fracture the resistance becomes so high that the

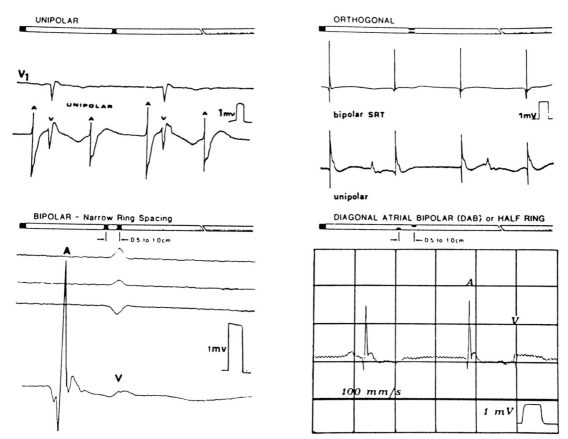

FIGURE 2–22. The effect of sensing configuration and interelectrode distance on the atrial electrogram is shown for four different sensing configurations. Note that the unipolar atrial electrogram (*top left*) is characterized by a large far-field R wave (V) that may approximate the size of the atrial deflection (A). A bipolar electrode configuration with close electrode spacing (*bottom left*) records a far-field R wave (V) that is much smaller than the atrial deflection (A). An orthogonal lead configuration (*top right*) uses electrodes placed half-circumferentially on the lead at right angles to the lead body and records an atrial deflection that is of short duration and has minimal far-field ventricular R waves. A diagonal atrial bipolar electrode configuration with the electrodes on opposite sides of the lead body but separated by several millimeters provides a sharp atrial deflection with a small far-field R wave (*bottom right*). (From Antonioli GE, Ansani L, Barbieri D, et al: Single-lead VDD pacing. *In* Barold SS, Mugica J [eds]: New Perspectives in Cardiac Pacing 3. Mt. Kisco, NY, Futura, 1993.)

resulting sensing impedance completely attenuates the electrogram. Partial or intermittent lead fractures may result in a sensing impedance that is elevated, leading to impedance mismatch and both attenuation of the electrogram amplitude and distortion of the electrogram waveform as a result of RC filtering (see previous discussion). Intermittent lead fractures may also produce artifacts in the electrogram as the fractured ends of the conductor wires make and break contact. These artifacts are often referred to as "make-and-break" potentials (Fig. 2–23). Lead fractures are thus characterized by failure of both stimulation and sensing. Insulation failure is a more

common clinical problem, especially with coaxial bipolar leads. In the case of an inner insulation failure, in which the inner and outer conductor coils intermittently contact one another, spurious signals are often recorded (Fig. 2–24). These sensing artifacts can result in inhibition of the pacing pulse if they exceed the threshold sensing amplitude programmed for the pulse generator. If such sensing artifacts are recorded in the atrial channel of a DDDR pacing system, inappropriate tracking may result. If both conductors are in continuous contact, the sensed electrogram potential may be shorted between the wires, resulting in undersensing. In many cases of insulation failure, oversensing is the first clinical manifestation. Insulation failures may also become clinically manifest by inappropriate rate-adaptive sensor function for pacing systems that measure dynamic lead impedance such as minute ventilation sensors. Indeed, we have recorded pacing at the upper rate limit of a VVIR pacemaker sensing minute ventilation as the first clinical manifestation of a polyurethane insulation failure.

Clinical Aspects of Pacemaker Sensing

For clinicians involved in the care of patients with permanent pacemakers, evaluation of sensing begins at the time of

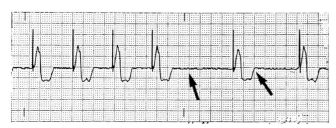

FIGURE 2–23. Ventricular oversensing related to make-and-break potentials resulting from inner insulation failure of a coaxial bipolar, polyurethane-insulated ventricular lead. The patient has a VVI pacing system with chronic atrial fibrillation. Note the irregular ventricular pacing stimuli with pauses caused by inhibition of the pulse generator by artifactual signals.

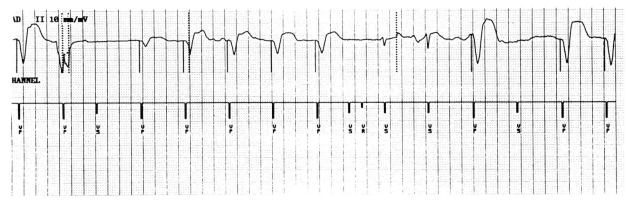

FIGURE 2–24. Oversensing of artifactual signals from a lead with insulation failure. A surface electrocardiographic lead with a ventricular marker channel in a patient with a VVIR pacing system is shown. Note that ventricular signals (VS, ventricular sensed signal; VR, ventricular sensed signal during the refractory period) are sensed by the pacemaker in the absence of QRS complexes on the surface electrocardiogram. Ventricular pacing stimuli are marked by the symbol VP.

pacemaker implantation. Measurement of a sensing threshold is typically performed using a PSA. Ideally, the PSA used to obtain these measurements has filter settings identical to those found in the pulse generator being implanted. Therefore, the PSA and pulse generator should be manufactured by the same company. In most cases, however, accurate ventricular sensing thresholds can be obtained using a PSA from a different manufacturer than that of the implanted pulse generator. However, the margin for error in determining atrial sensing thresholds is generally lower, and the PSA should mimic the sensing circuits found in the pulse generator to be implanted whenever possible. Some physicians additionally record electrograms on a physiologic recorder at the time of lead implantation to assess an "injury current" (Fig. 2–25). The current of injury is a "mountain-like" elevation of the electric potential immediately following the intrinsic deflection (typically in the ST segment for a ventricular electrogram). The injury current is thought to result from damage produced by contact or pressure from the pacing lead on the endocardial surface. The presence of an injury current is thought to ensure adequate contact between the lead and the endocardium, making lead dislodgment a less likely occurrence.

To avoid future problems with oversensing or undersensing in the implanted pacing system, it is necessary to obtain the best possible intracardiac signal. The ventricular electrogram at the time of implantation should be larger than 6 mV and should have a slew rate greater than 0.5 V/sec. The atrial electrogram should ideally be greater than 1.5 mV and should also have a slew rate of at least 0.5 V/sec. An electrogram of borderline amplitude may be adequate for sensing if the slew rate is satisfactory. However, an electrogram with inadequate amplitude will not be sensed regardless of slew rate. It is important to remember that the amplitude and frequency spectrum of the electrogram can be expected to change with time, particularly with active-fixation leads. A 15% to 20% decrease in R-wave amplitude and a 25% to 50% decrease in R-wave slew rate may be seen as the electrode-tissue interface of the lead matures.[1, 2] de Buitleir and colleagues recorded P-wave and R-wave amplitudes during the first 30 minutes after implantation of active- and passive-fixation Medtronic leads.[25] There was a significant increase

in both P-wave and R-wave amplitude with screw-in (active) fixation leads immediately after implantation that peaked 20 minutes later (Fig. 2–26). By 30 minutes following lead implantation, the peak P-wave and R-wave amplitudes were greater than those recorded immediately after the leads were screwed in. For example, the P-wave amplitude increased from 3.7 ± 2.2 mV immediately after implantation to 5.2 ± 3.1 mV at 30 minutes ($p < .001$ vs. baseline). In their study there was no significant difference between P-wave or R-wave amplitude between the active-fixation leads and the passive-fixation (tined) leads. P-wave and R-wave amplitudes were similar for tined fixation leads and screw-in (active) fixation leads. There was no significant change in P-wave or R-wave amplitude with the passive-fixation, tined leads during the first 30 minutes following lead implantation. The increase in R-wave and P-wave amplitude was also noted in patients with marginal electrode amplitude on the first measurement. Data on long-term stability (years) of P-wave and R-wave amplitude with active- versus passive-fixation atrial leads are lacking. For optimal long-term sensing, physicians performing implantation should use the type of lead with which they feel most comfortable until definitive data become available.

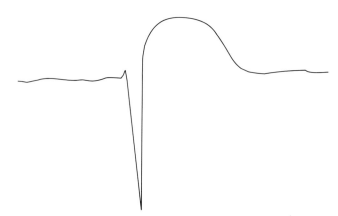

FIGURE 2–25. Current of injury pattern following implantation of a unipolar pacing lead. Note the marked ST segment elevation indicating pressure of the electrode against the endocardium.

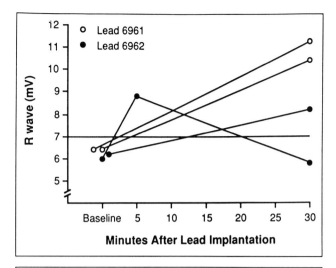

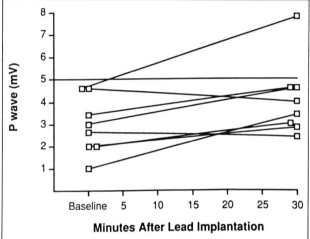

FIGURE 2–26. Effect of time on amplitudes of R waves (*top*) and P waves (*bottom*) immediately following implantation of active-fixation pacing leads. Note that R-wave amplitudes in four patients that were less than 7 mV immediately after lead implantation showed increases by 30 minutes after implantation. Also note that the atrial electrogram amplitude in most patients increased from baseline to a higher level 30 minutes following implantation of the lead. (From de Buitleir M, Kou WH, Schmaltz S, et al: Acute changes in pacing threshold and R- or P-wave amplitude during permanent pacemaker implantation. Am J Cardiol 65:999, 1990.)

UNIPOLAR VERSUS BIPOLAR SENSING PERFORMANCE

Another important decision to be made prior to lead implantation is the choice of unipolar or bipolar leads. The relative advantages of unipolar compared with bipolar pacing and sensing are summarized in Table 2–1.[1, 26–28] It is important for the physician to consider the relative merits of each factor when deciding which type of lead to implant. During the last decade, most physicians have switched to implanting greater numbers of bipolar systems. There are, however, a number of circumstances in which unipolar systems may have an advantage. Unipolar leads have historically been associated with a lower incidence of lead failure due to insulation failure or conductor fracture than comparable bipolar leads. This fact is probably related to the much simpler construction of unipolar leads. In addition, because of their

smaller diameter, it is theorized that unipolar leads may be less likely to induce subclavian vein thrombosis than the larger diameter bipolar leads. Unipolar leads are more easily repaired than bipolar leads, and the unipolar pacing stimulus artifact tends to be larger than bipolar stimuli, making electrocardiographic (ECG) interpretation less difficult. Despite these advantages of unipolar leads, bipolar leads have several important clinical advantages. These include the lower likelihood that myopotentials or other extracardiac signals will be sensed. Oversensing of far-field intracardiac signals, such as P waves or R waves, is much less common with bipolar than with unipolar pacing systems. Bipolar leads allow the implanting physician more programming flexibility during follow-up evaluations because many pulse generators allow sensitivity polarity to be programmed (e.g., either bipolar or unipolar from either the tip or ring electrodes). With bipolar leads and pulse generators, the pulse generator may be buried under the pectoralis or rectus abdominis muscles because muscle stimulation by the pacemaker is not a clinical concern with the bipolar pacing configuration.

CLINICAL EVALUATION OF SENSING

It should be remembered that the amplitude, slew rate, and frequency spectrum of electrograms may change from the time of lead implantation to chronic follow-up (Fig. 2–27). Sensing can be evaluated using a number of different techniques in most patients at any time after implantation of a modern pacing system. However, in the presence of an unreliable escape atrial or ventricular rhythm, sensing of intrinsic cardiac signals may be difficult or impossible. In patients with a stable intrinsic atrial or ventricular rhythm, sensing can be tested by monitoring the surface electrocardiogram for the presence of atrial or ventricular demand pacing stimuli during the patient's spontaneous rhythm. To assess the amplitude of the intrinsic intracardiac electrogram measured by the sensing amplifier, the lower pacing rate is programmed to a value less than the patient's intrinsic rate. The sensitivity threshold value is then increased (to a less sensitive setting) until normal inhibition of the pacing stimuli is

TABLE 2–1. **ADVANTAGES OF UNIPOLAR AND BIPOLAR LEADS**

UNIPOLAR	BIPOLAR
Smaller lead diameter	Offers programmable polarity of pacing and sensing
Improved long-term reliability	Improved rejection of far-field signals
Simpler design and construction Easier to repair	Reduced crosstalk
Increased stimulus artifact amplitude improves ECG interpretation	Reduced myopotential oversensing
Slightly lower stimulation threshold	Reduced T-wave sensing
	Reduced electromagnetic interference susceptibility
	Muscle stimulation not a problem
	Can be implanted submuscularly in thin or asthenic individuals
	Allows measurement of transthoracic impedance

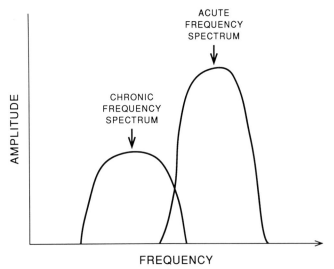

FIGURE 2–27. The effect of lead evolution on the amplitude and frequency spectrum of intracardiac electrograms. The amplitude of the electrogram can be expected to decrease between implantation and chronic follow-up, and a shift will occur in the frequency spectrum to lower frequencies. These changes in the electrogram may lead to undersensing in some individuals despite adequate electrogram characteristics at the time of lead implantation.

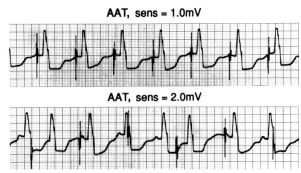

FIGURE 2–29. Usefulness of the AAT pacing mode to determine atrial sensing. In the upper panel, an atrial sensitivity setting of 1.0 mV is programmed. Note that atrial pacing stimuli are delivered simultaneously with sensed P waves. Note also that the P wave begins slightly prior to the pacing stimulus, indicating that the stimuli are triggered by sensed atrial events occurring after onset of the surface electrocardiographic P wave. In the lower panel, the atrial sensitivity has been reprogrammed to 2.0 mV. Atrial pacing stimuli are now delivered asynchronously, indicating that the intrinsic P-wave amplitude must be less than the programmed value of 2.0 mV.

lost, as noted by inappropriate demand pacing at a rate less than the intrinsic rate. In some pulse generators sensitivity threshold testing is automated, with the programmer displaying the surface ECG while decreasing the sensitivity of the sensing amplifier after a fixed number of beats. For patients with complete atrioventricular (AV) block who have DDD pacemakers, the atrial sensing threshold is most easily tested by programming the lower rate and AV delay to values that ensure atrial tracking and ventricular pacing. The atrial sensitivity threshold is then programmed to less sensitive values until atrial tracking is lost, indicating that the intrinsic atrial electrogram is less than the programmed atrial sensing threshold (Fig. 2–28).

Sensing can also be effectively evaluated by programming the pulse generator to the triggered mode (e.g., VVT, AAT, or DDT) and observing the electrocardiogram for the timing of pacing stimuli relative to intrinsic electric events such as P waves, R waves, or T waves. In Figure 2–29, AAT pacing shows atrial spikes coincident with P waves at a programmed sensitivity of 1.0 mV. As the sensitivity threshold is in-

creased (to a less sensitive value), the atrial pacing stimuli occur randomly, indicating failure to sense the intrinsic P wave at the programmed value. In the presence of apparent ventricular oversensing, the triggered VVT pacing mode allows recognition of T-wave sensing (manifested by pacing stimuli synchronous with the T wave), or random make-and-break potentials (manifested by pacing stimuli that are randomly distributed throughout the cardiac cycle). Indeed, in the presence of lead insulation failure, VVI pacing may be dangerous because the ventricular stimuli can be repetitively inhibited by electric artifacts from the lead. The VVT mode, in contrast, provides pacing at a programmed minimum rate and also marks the artifactual signals with pacing stimuli. The AAT mode is especially helpful for evaluating suspected far-field R-wave sensing, which can be identified by atrial pacing stimuli delivered synchronously with both the P waves and the R waves.

The clinical evaluation of pacemaker sensing has been greatly simplified by the introduction of telemetered intracardiac electrograms and sensing markers (known as marker channels, main timing events, and so on) (Fig. 2–30). The capability to simultaneously display the surface electrocardiogram, intracardiac electrograms recorded from the pulse generator (Fig. 2–31), and sensing markers on the programmers allows the clinician to know exactly which signals the pacing system is sensing and the nature of the pulse generator's interpretation of the recorded electric events. The intracardiac electrogram can be calibrated and measured, and the sensitivity threshold value can be approximated from the measured amplitude of the signal. It should be stressed, however, that the amplitude of the electrogram that is telemetered by the programmer and the amplitude of the signal that is sensed by the sensing amplifier may be somewhat different. The filtered, processed, and displayed waveforms do not exactly correspond to the processing of the pulse generator's sensing amplifiers. Marker channels or event markers denote what the pacemaker circuitry is "seeing" and how it responds. Marker channels, intracardiac electrograms, and programming to the triggered mode provide additional information to the physician about where the intracardiac signal is

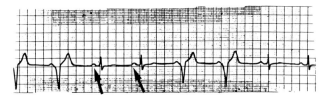

FIGURE 2–28. Atrial undersensing in a patient with a bipolar DDD pacemaker. In the first two complexes ventricular pacing stimuli are delivered with a short atrioventricular (AV) interval following P waves. The third and fourth complexes show no ventricular pacing stimuli with intrinsically conducted QRS complexes because atrial sensing has failed. For patients with bipolar pacemakers, programming the atrial sensitivity to progressively less sensitive settings may allow determination of the atrial sensing threshold despite small pacing stimuli that are difficult to recognize on the surface electrocardiogram.

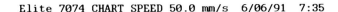

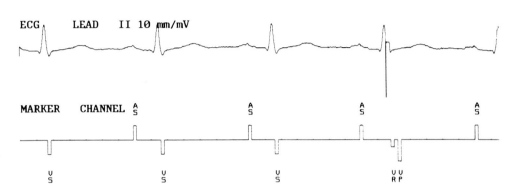

FIGURE 2–30. Simultaneous recording of the surface electrocardiogram and a marker channel in a patient with a DDDR pacemaker. Note that ventricular sensing (VS) by the pacemaker occurs late relative to the surface QRS complex. The fourth complex demonstrates a ventricular pacing stimulus within the QRS that produces no identifiable change in the QRS morphology. This represents pseudofusion (VP, ventricular pacing stimuli; VR, sensed ventricular event in the refractory period).

sensed relative to the surface ECG (see Chapter 32 for details).

CLINICAL EVALUATION OF MYOPOTENTIAL OVERSENSING

In the 1970s Wirtzfeld and others reported the clinical manifestations of skeletal muscle interference and its potential effects on pacemaker function.[29–33] Because myopotentials are more commonly sensed by unipolar pacing systems, myopotential oversensing limited the widespread acceptance of early DDD pacemakers, most of which were unipolar. Myopotential interference is generally manifested in any of three ways. First, and by far the most common, is myopotential inhibition, which refers to the inappropriate inhibition of pacing stimuli in either the atrial or the ventricular channel (or both) owing to sensing of myopotentials (Figs. 2–32 to

2–34). Second, DDD pulse generators that sense myopotentials by the atrial sensing amplifier may demonstrate ventricular tracking of these artifactual signals (Fig. 2–35). Third, the pulse generator may revert to an asynchronous or noise reversion mode in response to skeletal myopotentials. This occurs when continuous sensing of myopotentials during the noise-sampling period leads the pulse generator to diagnose interference and initiate asynchronous pacing to prevent inappropriate inhibition of pacing.

Various groups have reported that skeletal myopotential interference occurs in 11% to 85% of individuals with unipolar pacemakers.[30–33] Myopotential interference may be clinically diagnosed by the recording of pauses in the paced cardiac rhythm during ambulatory ECG (Holter) monitoring or during certain muscular exercises.[34, 35] In patients with pulse generators implanted in the pectoral region, exercises that may be used to provoke myopotential inhibition include

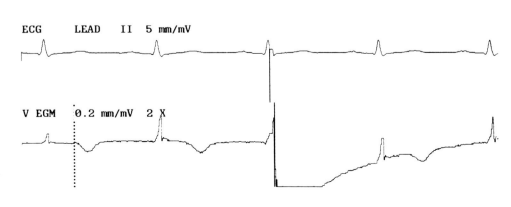

FIGURE 2–31. Recordings from the same patient shown in Figure 2–30. The intracardiac ventricular electrogram (V EGM) is shown with simultaneous tracings from the surface electrocardiogram (ECG). Note that the intrinsic deflection of the ventricular electrogram occurs late relative to the surface QRS. The third complex demonstrates a ventricular pacing stimulus just prior to the intrinsic deflection in the electrogram (pseudofusion). This illustrates that the pacemaker uses the intrinsic deflection to determine the occurrence of a ventricular event.

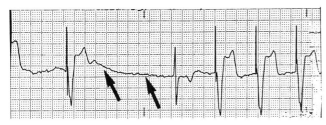

FIGURE 2–32. Myopotential inhibition in a patient with a VVI pacemaker and atrial fibrillation with slow ventricular response. The lower pacing rate was 80 bpm (last three complexes). A pause between the second and third complexes is related to myopotentials that were sensed by the pulse generator.

pushing or pulling the hands together with maximum strength, pressing the patient's hands against those of the clinician or against a wall, or performing an isometric handgrip (Fig. 2–36). Other exercises include adduction and abduction of the arm against resistance. Another maneuver is to ask the patient to use the arm ipsilateral to the pulse generator to scratch the chest, neck, or back. Treadmill exercise can also be used as an additional testing maneuver to diagnose myopotential oversensing. Daily activities that may elicit pectoral muscle myopotential inhibition include raking leaves, shoveling snow, or performing isometric arm exercises. Testing for myopotential oversensing with an abdominal pulse generator (implanted above the rectus abdominis muscle) involves lifting the legs several inches off the table with the patient in the supine position or having the patient recline backward from the sitting to the supine position. In addition to oversensing myopotentials arising from the pectoralis or rectus abdominis muscles, diaphragmatic myopotentials can be oversensed during deep inspiration, coughing, straining, or sneezing. Myopotential inhibition should be tested at multiple programmed sensitivity thresholds.

Secemsky and colleagues reported that myopotential interference could be detected by the combined use of ambulatory electrocardiographic monitoring and exercise testing in 39% of patients with unipolar pacing systems.[36] In patients with ECG-documented myopotential inhibition, 14% had symptoms ranging from mild dizziness to syncope. DeBoer and colleagues reported myopotential inhibition in 9 of 10 patients when the unipolar atrial sensitivity value was programmed to 0.5 mV.[37] Fetter and colleagues studied unipolar pulse generators made by three manufacturers in 77 patients and found myopotential inhibition in 47%.[38] There was a wide range of clinical manifestations, with pauses ranging from 0.3 to 3.9 seconds. They noted that the incidence of myopotential inhibition varied from 33% to 78%, depending

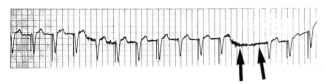

FIGURE 2–33. Myopotential inhibition in a patient with a unipolar DDD pacemaker. Note a pause near the end of the tracing coincident with "noise" on the surface electrocardiogram produced by muscular activity. Such motion artifacts on the surface electrocardiogram are often seen at the time of myopotential sensing and may serve as a clue to the diagnosis.

Mode: DDD   Rate: 60 ppm   A-V Delay: 165 msec
Magnet: OFF

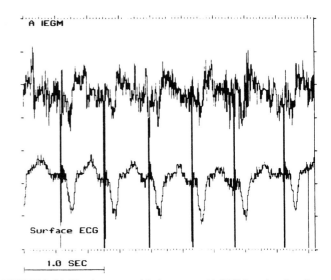

ECG/IEGM PARAMETERS	
Surface ECG	ON
Surface ECG Gain	1.0 mv/div
Surface ECG Filter	ON
Intracardiac EGM	A IEGM
Intracardiac EGM Gain	1 mv/div
Chart Speed	25.0 mm/sec

FIGURE 2–34. Simultaneous atrial electrogram (A IEGM, *top*) and surface electrocardiogram (ECG, *bottom*) in a patient with myopotential tracking with a unipolar DDD pacemaker. Note that the myopotentials may exceed 1.5 mV in the atrial electrogram.

on the manufacturer of the pulse generator. Silastic-coated pulse generators had a lower incidence of myopotential inhibition than noncoated generators. Brevik and associates noted that the incidence of myopotential inhibition depended greatly on how it is measured.[39] For example, at a programmed atrial sensitivity of 2.5 mV, myopotential inhibition was present on ambulatory monitoring in 25% of patients but could be demonstrated by provocative exercise testing in 40% of these individuals. Myopotential inhibition persisted in some patients until the atrial sensitivity threshold was programmed as high as 3.5 mV. Other groups have reported that a sensitivity threshold of approximately 3.0 to 4.5 mV may be required to eliminate myopotential inhibition.[33] In contrast to unipolar sensing, skeletal myopotential inhibition is rare in patients with bipolar pulse generators.

Although less common with bipolar pacing systems, myopotential oversensing is not limited to unipolar and "older" pulse generators. For example, Barold and coworkers and el Gamal and colleagues reported pacemaker inhibition due to diaphragmatic myopotentials in patients with bipolar pacemakers.[40, 41] Myocardial perforation was probably not present in these patients because both groups reported no diaphragmatic or intercostal stimulation with the highest programmable stimulus amplitude. Barold and colleagues also reported on the incidence of oversensing from diaphragmatic myopotentials during maximal inspiration in the supine po-

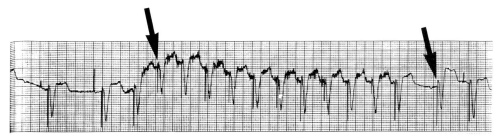

FIGURE 2–35. Myopotential tracking in a patient with a unipolar DDD pacemaker. The first two complexes demonstrate atrial and ventricular pacing at the lower rate limit. Coincident with the occurrence of motion artifact on the surface electrocardiogram (third complex) the ventricular pacing rate increases to the upper tracking limit. Following cessation of muscular activity (second complex from right), normal atrial tracking is restored.

sition with varying programmed sensitivities in 119 patients with pulse generators from six manufacturers.[42] Diaphragmatic myopotential inhibition was observed in 8.7% of bipolar and 20% of unipolar systems. Myopotential inhibition was observed in all but two cases at programmed sensitivity values that were more sensitive than nominal. The incidence of myopotential inhibition varied depending on the manufacturer of the pulse generator. Clinically, oversensing of diaphragmatic myopotentials was almost never a serious clinical problem because the related pauses were usually short. This problem was corrected by appropriate programming of the

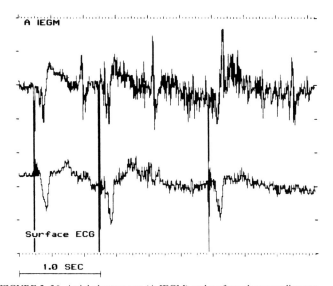

Mode: VVI   Rate: 75 ppm

Magnet: OFF

ECG/IEGM PARAMETERS

Surface ECG	ON	
Surface ECG Gain	1.0	mv/div
Surface ECG Filter	ON	
Intracardiac EGM	A IEGM	
Intracardiac EGM Gain	1	mv/div
Chart Speed	25.0	mm/sec

A IEGM

Surface ECG

1.0 SEC

FIGURE 2–36. Atrial electrogram (A IEGM) and surface electrocardiogram (ECG) are recorded during muscular activity in a patient with complete AV block and a DDD pacemaker that had been programmed to the VVI mode. Note that the myopotentials in the atrial electrogram may approach the amplitude of the intracardiac P wave.

sensitivity value. Myopotential inhibition from the rectus abdominis has been reported by some investigators to occur in up to 40% of generators implanted above the abdominal wall, whereas others report a lower incidence.[43, 44] Myopotentials sensed from the pectoralis and rectus abdominis muscles may act synergistically, accounting for inhibition of pulse generators located in either the pectoral or abdominal region.[42] Intercostal muscles may also contribute to myopotential inhibition or triggering of unipolar atrial generators during deep inspiration.

Newer pulse generators have used sensing amplifiers with refined atrial and ventricular filtering characteristics to avoid myopotential sensing. Nevertheless, myopotential inhibition, tracking, and stimulation remain a clinical problem for some patients with unipolar pacemakers. For example, Lau and colleagues and Volosin and associates have both reported myopotential inhibition with newer unipolar rate-adaptive pacemakers.[45, 46] Volosin and associates reported a patient with a temperature-sensitive, rate-adaptive pacemaker who developed sufficient myopotential inhibition with exercise to prevent an increase in heart rate.[46] This patient had to be programmed to the VOOR pacing mode to allow appropriate rate modulation. Lau and colleagues reported myopotential oversensing in 22 patients with activity-sensing, QT-sensing, respiratory rate–sensing, and dP/dt-sensing pacemakers.[45] The duration of the pauses resulting from myopotential inhibition was variable but tended to be less during rate-adaptive pacing. In two of five patients with the Biorate device (Biotec, S.p.A., Bologna, Italy) the respiratory rate–sensing pacemaker had to be explanted because of uncontrolled myopotential inhibition. The problem was corrected in the remainder of patients by reprogramming ventricular sensitivity or programming to the VVT mode. Myopotential inhibition has been reported to occur less frequently in children than in adults by Michalik and colleagues.[47] Only 6% of children with unipolar pacemakers demonstrated myopotential inhibition, with most cases occurring in larger children.

Myopotential inhibition can usually be corrected by reprogramming. The most common correction for this problem is modifying the atrial or ventricular sensitivity threshold to a less sensitive setting. In some patients it may not be possible to eliminate myopotential oversensing without incurring the development of intermittent or constant undersensing, particularly of the P wave. Another method of eliminating inhibition is to program the pacemaker to the triggered mode. This may allow sensing of the P wave or R wave but will also lead to tracking of myopotentials, resulting in periods of increased pacing rate. An additional disadvantage of this approach is that constant pacing and increased battery drain occur. Other, less desirable options include reprogramming to an asynchronous pacing mode (e.g., VOO, AOO), avoiding upper body exercise, performing reoperation with implantation of a bipolar lead, placing a Silastic boot around the pulse generator, replacing the pulse generator with one incorporating a sensing amplifier that is less sensitive to myopotentials, or repositioning the pulse generator to a site where it is less likely to be stimulated by myopotentials.

ELECTROMAGNETIC INTERFERENCE

Electromagnetic interference and the response of the pacemaker to this phenomenon (noise reversion) are described in detail in Chapter 40. The effects of these extracorporeal energy sources on the pulse generator are worth mentioning because they may lead to sensing problems. These disorders of sensing may be of clinical significance, especially in patients who are pacemaker dependent or have unipolar pacemakers that are more likely to sense these extraneous signals. Electromagnetic interference may lead either to inhibition of pacing stimuli or to reversion to an asynchronous pacing mode, depending on the number of impulses that are sensed by the pulse generator during the noise-sampling portion of the refractory period.

FAR-FIELD SENSING

There are a number of clinical situations in which the atrial sensing amplifier may detect signals that originate in the ventricle or in which the ventricular sensing amplifier may detect signals that arise in the atrium. These electric signals that arise remote from the pacing electrode are known as far-field signals. Far-field sensing may occur under many circumstances. Particularly well described is the phenomenon referred to as crosstalk (Fig. 2–37) (see Chapter 31), which occurs when the atrial stimulus is sensed by the ventricular sensing amplifier, leading to potential inhibition of the ventricular output and possibly asystole in a patient with heart block. Conditions that predispose to crosstalk include unipolar pacing and sensing, high amplitude or pulse width of the atrial stimulus, a short AV interval, and a highly sensitive ventricular sensitivity setting. Griffin and others have shown that unipolar atrial sensing is associated with far-field ventricular electrograms that are at least three times the amplitude of those recorded with bipolar atrial leads in the right atrial appendage.[48] Coombs and colleagues carefully evaluated the conditions for crosstalk and questioned whether ad-

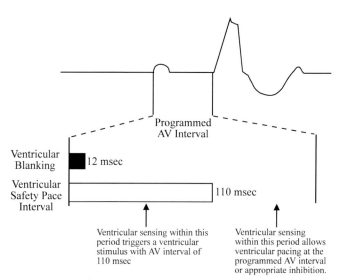

FIGURE 2–38. Ventricular safety pacing.

ditional factors may contribute to this phenomenon.[49] These additional factors were identified as short blanking periods and the residual polarization voltage on the atrial pacing lead. They noted that crosstalk can occur with bipolar pacemakers and was more likely to occur with a bipolar system when the pacing rate was high (ranging from 110 to 130 bpm). Modern pulse generators have programmable features for managing crosstalk including programmable ventricular blanking periods, rapid recharge pulses in the atrial output circuit, and nonphysiologic AV delay (*ventricular safety pacing*) (Fig. 2–38).

The nonphysiologic AV delay feature is designed to prevent inhibition of ventricular pacing by crosstalk. This feature provides a shortened paced AV interval when an electric event is sensed by the ventricular amplifer outside the ventricular blanking period but within the first 110 msec of the AV delay. When an electric event is sensed within this window in the ventricle, the nonphysiologic AV delay feature results in delivery of a ventricular pacing stimulus with a shortened AV paced interval (110 msec) rather than inhibition of the ventricular pacing output. This is essentially a safety feature and has been termed safety pacing by one manufacturer. It can be recognized by a paced AV delay that is shorter than the programmed interval.

Far-field sensing has been reported to occur with T waves in patients with VVI pacemakers, R waves in patients with AAI and AAIR pacemakers, afterpotentials from the ventricular paced complex in VVI pacemakers, and R waves in patients with DDD pacemakers. Van Gelder and colleagues, Mond and associates, and Barold have all described patients in whom the ventricular output was inhibited by far-field sensing of P waves.[50–52] This occurs most frequently in patients with a dislodged ventricular lead when the pacing bipole is close enough to the tricuspid valve to sense atrial activity (Fig. 2–39). Interestingly, the patient described by Van Gelder and colleagues did not have any evidence of lead dislodgement.[50] Brandt and coworkers studied 119 patients with DDD pacemakers and programmed the atrial sensitivity of the atrial sense amplifier to various settings to determine the threshold for far-field QRS sensing.[53] In their patients the TARP and AV delay were programmed to minimal values to

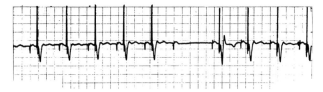

FIGURE 2–37. Oversensing due to "chatter" of an active-fixation ventricular lead that inhibits ventricular pacing. This patient had an active-fixation lead known to be associated with artifactual signals related to instability of the active-fixation mechanism. Note that the sixth complex is associated with atrial pacing without a subsequent ventricular pacing stimulus. Reprogramming to the DOO mode was done in this patient prior to reoperation, which confirmed artifacts in the ventricular electrogram.

2 SECONDS

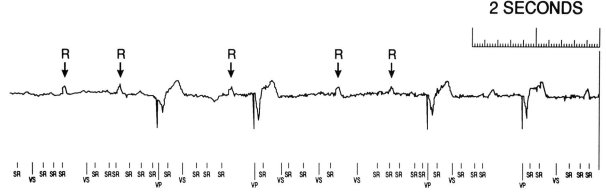

FIGURE 2–39. Oversensing of atrial fibrillation in a patient in whom the ventricular lead had become dislodged to near the tricuspid annulus. Note that the marker channel demonstrated multiple sensed events (VS), most of which occurred within the refractory period (SR). The ventricular lead was sensing ventricular R waves as well as atrial activity (P waves) during atrial fibrillation.

facilitate far-field sensing. Thirty-five percent of patients had far-field sensing of the QRS complex. In 27 of 42 patients with far-field R-wave sensing this problem was eliminated by reprogramming of atrial sensitivity. The remainder of their patients needed reprogramming of other parameters to avoid far-field sensing. No particular clinical or electrophysiologic variables predicted the problem of far-field R-wave sensing. Shandling and colleagues described a patient with far-field R-wave sensing by the atrial channel of the ventricular depolarization.[57] Possible reasons for this occurrence suggested by the authors include prolonged intraventricular conduction defect due to drugs, prolonged ventricular depolarization, and prolonged spike to ventricular depolarization due to latency. Far-field R-wave sensing usually occurs in patients with no evidence of atrial lead dislodgment. The authors have tried to explain this occurrence by suggesting that the atrial and ventricular leads are anatomically close or the heart is relatively small.[50–53] Barold and associates have also described two cases of patients with an antitachycardia pacemaker implanted in the atrium (Intermedics CyberTach 60) in whom double sensing of the P waves and QRS complexes led to inappropriate delivery of burst pacing during sinus rhythm.[54] The same phenomenon could occur when antitachycardia pacing is delivered in the ventricle. Another and less common cause of far-field sensing is sensing of T waves or afterpotentials.[55, 56] Both are unusual occurrences with modern pulse generators and appear to be more common with unipolar pacemakers. T-wave oversensing and afterpotential inhibition are more likely to occur with high pacing stimulus amplitudes, long pulse widths, and short refractory periods. In some cases, it may be very difficult to differentiate T-wave oversensing from afterpotential inhibition. Oversensing due to T-wave and afterpotential sensing is corrected by decreasing the sensitivity of the ventricular sense amplifier, lengthening the programmable refractory period, or decreasing the pulse generator stimulus amplitude and duration.

The management of far-field R-wave oversensing depends on its clinical recognition.[57] The options for corrective action include decreasing ventricular sensitivity, decreasing atrial stimulus voltage or pulse width, prolonging the ventricular refractory period, or lengthening the ventricular blanking interval. One study of atrially implanted, activity-sensing pacemakers showed that the average atrial sensitivity for reliable discrimination of P waves from far-field R waves was 3.0 mV.[58] Thus, programming of the atrial sensitivity threshold to a less sensitive value cannot always be used to eliminate far-field R-wave sensing. In some cases, stopping an antiarrhythmic drug that causes significant conduction delay[57] and programming or upgrading the patient to a bipolar sensing configuration may be necessary. If these maneuvers are unsuccessful, the patient can be programmed to a VDD or DAT mode. A less ideal solution to this problem is to program the pacemaker to the DVI or VVI mode.

FUSION, PSEUDOFUSION, AND PSEUDOPSEUDOFUSION

Triggered pacing modes (e.g., VVT, AAT), intracardiac electrograms, and marker channels may indicate where, relative to the surface ECG, the intracardiac signal is sensed.[59, 60] Fusion is defined as depolarization of the ventricle resulting from electric activation occurring at two or more sites. Ventricular fusion usually results when ventricular activation simultaneously occurs by conduction over the specialized AV node–His-Purkinje conduction system as well as from a wave of depolarization that propagates away from the site of the ventricular pacing stimulus. Fusion is manifested on the electrocardiogram as a QRS complex that is wider than that seen during normal intrinsic ventricular activation. Pseudofusion (Fig. 2–40) refers to the electrocardiographic appearance of an *ineffectual* pacemaker stimulus that fails to capture the ventricle that is superimposed on a QRS complex originating from normal atrioventricular conduction. In pseudofusion, although the pacing stimulus is of sufficient amplitude to capture the ventricle, it does not contribute to ventricular activation because it is delivered after the majority of the ventricles have been depolarized by normal AV conduction. Thus, pseudofusion typically occurs in patients with a right ventricular endocardial lead and right bundle branch block conduction. Pseudofusion may also occur in patients with underlying left bundle branch block and a left ventricular epicardial pacing lead(s). It is more likely to occur in patients with intraventricular conduction delay to the site of the sensing lead, so that the pacing site is activated late in the QRS complex. Pseudofusion can be simply considered "late sensing."

Pseudopseudofusion is a term used to indicate the electro-

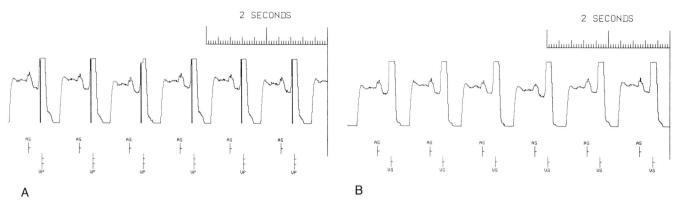

A   B

FIGURE 2–40. *A,* Marker channel annotation in a patient with a DDD pacemaker and pseudofusion. This patient had an intrinsic QRS complex with right bundle branch block (RBBB) with a programmed AV delay of 175 msec. The atrial signal (AS) is sensed appropriately and is followed by a ventricular pacing stimulus (VP) near the end of the QRS complex, suggesting the possibility of ventricular undersensing. Ventricular pacing was observed at all ventricular sensitivity levels (from 4 mV to 0.6 mV) in this individual. *B,* The AV delay has been reprogrammed to 250 msec, and the marker channel demonstrates ventricular sensing (VS) near the end of the surface QRS. Pseudofusion is most commonly observed in patients with an intrinsic QRS complex with RBBB morphology who have right ventricular endocardial pacing leads, because the right ventricular apex is activated late relative to other areas of the ventricle.

cardiographic appearance of an atrial pacing stimulus that occurs at or near the onset of the QRS complex, thereby resulting in the initiation of a ventricular blanking period with failure to sense the QRS and delivery of a ventricular pacing stimulus in the terminal portion of the QRS complex (or ST segment). The term pseudopseudofusion indicates that the pacing stimulus is not capable of directly contributing to ventricular activation. Pseudopseudofusion is seen with committed DVI pacing or ventricular safety pacing and does not imply pulse generator malfunction (Fig. 2–41). Pseudopseudofusion may also occur in DDD pacemakers with loss of atrial sensing.

DIFFERENTIAL DIAGNOSIS OF UNDERSENSING

The causes of undersensing are summarized in Table 2–2 and are discussed in more detail in Chapter 33. Undersensing can result from a variety of causes including R waves or P waves with low amplitude and slew rate at the time of lead implantation, fibrosis at the site of electrode-endocardial contact, micro- or macrodislodgment of the lead, misprogramming of the pacemaker to an asynchronous mode or an insensitive sensitivity setting, eccentricities of a particular pulse generator, inadequate amplitude or slew rate of an ectopic depolarization (premature atrial contraction [PAC] or ventric-

COMMITTED AV SEQUENTIAL (DVI) PACING

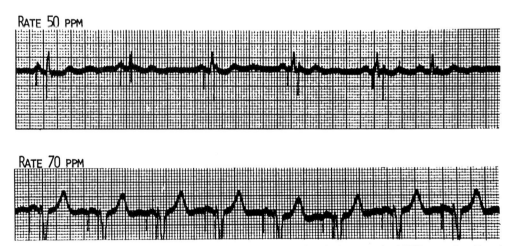

FIGURE 2–41. Pseudopseudofusion. *Top,* Repeated pseudopseudofusion from a normally functioning committed DVI pacemaker. Note that there is no atrial sensing in the DVI mode. In a committed DVI pacemaker, the ventricular pacing stimulus is delivered after every atrial pacing stimulus. Note that a pacing rate of 50 ppm is similar to the intrinsic sinus rate with atrial pacing stimuli in the middle of the P wave. The ventricular pacing stimulus is delivered within the QRS in the first two complexes and after the QRS in the third, fourth, and fifth complexes. In the bottom tracing appropriate atrial and ventricular capture are demonstrated during pacing at 70 ppm. Thus, committed DVI pacing may superficially resemble pseudofusion if the intrinsic heart rate is similar to the programmed lower pacing rate. (From Levine PA, Mace RC: Ventricular pacing. *In* Leving P, Mace R [eds]: Pacing Therapy. Mount Kisco, NY, Futura, 1983, p 97.)

TABLE 2–2. **ETIOLOGIES OF UNDERSENSING**

Micro- or macrodislodgment of pacing lead
Temporary reversion to an asynchronous mode
Lead conductor fracture
Lead insulation failure
Pulse generator component failure, jamming of magnetic reed switch
Eccentricities of individual pulse generator (e.g., Medtronic Activitrax)
Factors that can affect electrogram amplitude
   Myocardial infarction or fibrosis near electrode site
     Antiarrhythmic drug toxicity
     Marked electrolyte disturbances, particularly of potassium
Premature ventricular or atrial beats (despite adequate signals during sinus rhythm)
Transient aftercardioversion or defibrillation
PSEUDO "UNDERSENSING"
   Late sensing of intrinsic depolarization at the lead interface (pseudofusion)
   Reprogramming to an asynchronous mode or inappropriate programming to a decreased sensitivity setting or prolonged refractory period

ular premature depolarization [VPD]), and delayed sensing due to intrinsic deflection occurring late relative to the P wave or QRS in the surface ECG. Perhaps the most common cause of undersensing is lead dislodgment, especially with atrial leads (Fig. 2–42). An example of a "pacemaker eccentricity" causing undersensing is the Medtronic Activitrax (Medtronic Inc., Minneapolis, MN), which could deliver a single output pulse at the programmed maximal activity rate when a sensed ventricular event occurred within 8 msec after

the activity sensor circuit was triggered.[61] This resulted in an output pulse on the ECG at intervals of 400, 480, or 600 msec after the sensed event corresponding to the programmed maximal upper rate for the VVIR mode of 150, 125, or 100 bpm, respectively. Other causes of undersensing include alteration of the intracardiac electrogram by the effects of antiarrhythmic drug toxicity or electrolyte imbalance. Transient undersensing may occur following repeated defibrillation or cardioversion, particularly with unipolar pacemakers.

DIFFERENTIAL DIAGNOSIS OF OVERSENSING

The many causes of oversensing are summarized in Table 2–3 and are discussed in Chapter 33. Oversensing can result from the sensing of extraneous signals originating within or outside the heart. Extraneous cardiac signals include environmental noise or interference such as signals generated by medical devices, and myopotentials. Intracardiac signals that can cause oversensing include far-field signals, T waves, afterpotentials, and concealed extrasystoles (Fig. 2–43). Other intracardiac causes include artifactual "chatter" from an inactive screw on an active-fixation electrode, lead fracture (Fig. 2–44), insulation failure (Fig. 2–45), or a loose-set screw on the pulse generator (Fig. 2–46). An uncommon cause of oversensing that occurs during pacemaker implantation or in the immediate postoperative period is the presence of a temporary pacemaker. Pacing stimuli delivered from the pulse generator may inhibit the newly implanted

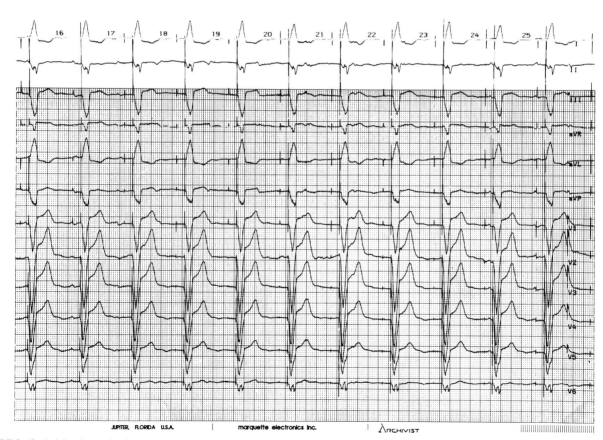

FIGURE 2–42. Atrial undersensing in a patient with a DDD pacemaker. Note that atrial and ventricular pacing stimuli are delivered by the pulse generator at the lower pacing rate without synchronization to the intrinsic P wave. The most common cause of atrial undersensing is lead dislodgment, as was the case in this example.

DDD 50/150/125

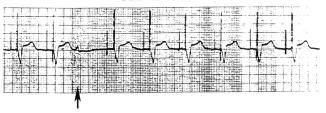

FIGURE 2–43. Apparent oversensing in the ventricular channel of a DDD pacemaker. However, on close inspection of the surface electrocardiogram a very small signal can be identified (*arrow*). This was a premature ventricular contraction that was relatively isoelectric in this lead. This tracing highlights the importance of using multiple electrocardiographic leads to identify atrial and ventricular events.

permanent pulse generator.[62] Rarely, electric signals generated within the implantable pulse generator itself may inhibit output of the device. This was reported to occur in one patient with the Telectronics Meta MV in which impedance pulses were sensed, leading to inhibition of pacing pulses.[63] Table 2–4 lists a number of clinical findings that should suggest a potential problem with sensing due to lead-related malfunction.

OTHER CLINICAL ISSUES RELATED TO SENSING PERFORMANCE

ANTITACHYCARDIA PACING

The requirements of antitachycardia pacemakers for sensing is a subject that has received inadequate attention. Sensing requirements for ventricular tachycardia, ventricular fibrillation, atrial flutter, paroxysmal atrial tachycardia, and atrial fibrillation are all clinically important issues. Timmis and associates and Klementowicz and Furman compared the amplitude of the atrial electrogram during antegrade and retrograde conduction.[64, 65] Timmis and colleagues analyzed multiple features of atrial electrograms that may be of value in the discrimination of anterograde from retrograde depolarization, including peak-to-peak amplitude, duration, maximum slew rate, mean slew rate, square root of energy, maximum frequency, half-power frequency, and Fourier transformation. They reported a significant difference between anterograde and retrograde signals for all of these variables. In seven of nine patients, at least one variable was sufficiently different to differentiate anterograde from retrograde signals reliably. However, no individual variable was capable of discriminating anterograde from retrograde conduction in more than four patients. At least three variables were needed to make this discrimination in seven patients.

TABLE 2–3. ETIOLOGIES OF OVERSENSING

EXTRACARDIAC SIGNALS
Electromagnetic interference
  Radio or television transmitters, radar, arc welding equipment, power-generating plants
  Household appliances (rare)—direct contact with electric razors or toothbrushes
  Medical equipment—electrocautery, diathermy, transcutaneous electrical neurostimulation stimulator, magnetic resonance imaging device, lithotripsy device
Myopotential inhibition—pectoral muscles, intercostal muscles, diaphragm, rectus abdominis
INTRACARDIAC SIGNALS
Lead problems
  Lead fracture
  Insulation failure
  Loose-set screw in generator head
  Chatter in active-fixation lead
Far-field sensing of P waves, R waves, T waves
T-wave sensing
Afterpotential sensing
Sensing of both atrial and ventricular activity
Concealed extrasystoles
Interaction with temporary pacemakers or another pacing catheter
Autointerference—sensing of signal originating from pulse generator itself

Thus, it appears that there is a large degree of overlap between anterograde and retrograde atrial signals with both time and frequency domain measurements. Klementowicz and Furman studied 34 patients (31 with unipolar systems, 3 with bipolar systems) and found a measurable difference in amplitude of anterograde compared with retrograde atrial electrograms.[65] Differences of at least 0.25 mV were found in 30 of 31 patients with unipolar atrial electrograms and in all 3 patients with bipolar atrial electrograms. Slew rate differences were present in 30 patients with unipolar systems and in 2 patients with bipolar systems. The discrimination of anterograde from retrograde atrial signals is an important issue in patients with paroxysmal atrial tachycardias such as AV nodal reentry or AV reentry due to a concealed bypass tract. In patients who have antitachycardia pacemakers, atrial signals must be adequate during sinus rhythm as well as during tachycardia, in which the atrial signal is a retrograde depolarization and its amplitude may decrease by up to 75% compared with sinus rhythm. A patient with an atrial electrogram that is of marginal amplitude sensed during sinus rhythm may have an inadequate atrial electrogram amplitude during tachycardia.

Sensing of atrial flutter and atrial fibrillation represents an additional important clinical issue. Atrial amplitudes can vary widely during atrial fibrillation, with signals varying in am-

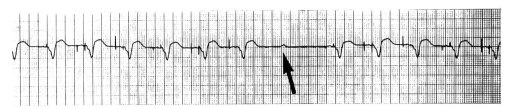

FIGURE 2–44. Oversensing in a patient with a DDD pacemaker. Following the seventh QRS complex a P wave is seen without subsequent ventricular pacing. In this case oversensing was found to be due to a lead fracture with intermittent loss of electrical contact and multiple episodes of ventricular inhibition.

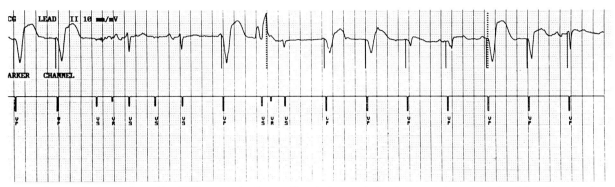

FIGURE 2–45. Oversensing in a patient with a VVIR pacemaker from artifacts in the ventricular electrogram due to insulation failure. Note that the marker channel identifies sensed events (VS) that are synchronous with the surface QRS as well as events that cannot be identified on the surface electrocardiogram. Oversensing of such artifactual signals is a very common clinical presentation of lead insulation failure. (VP, ventricular pacing stimulus; VR, ventricular sensing during ventricular refractory period.)

plitude 2 to 8 fold over consecutive beats. Fixed-gain amplifiers with atrial sensitivity settings limited to 0.5 to 0.75 mV may have intermittent undersensing of the atrial signal, leading to signal dropout and failure to activate mode-switching algorithms (see later discussion). Wood and coworkers (preliminary communication) have reported that atrial flutter is associated with minimal variability in atrial electrogram amplitude. In contrast, atrial fibrillation is associated with widely varying electrogram amplitudes. It is likely that atrial filters will need sensitivities in the 0.1 to 0.2 mV range to sense 90% of electrograms during atrial fibrillation.

Sensing of ventricular tachycardia with fixed-gain amplifiers may be associated with undersensing. Leitch and col-

leagues and Ellenbogen and associates have prospectively measured ventricular electrogram amplitude during sinus rhythm and during ventricular tachyarrhythmias in patients undergoing defibrillator implantation.[66, 67] During ventricular tachycardia, there is relatively little beat-to-beat variation in electrogram amplitude. In addition, the ventricular electrogram amplitude is generally only mildly decreased compared to sinus rhythm. During polymorphic ventricular tachycardia and ventricular fibrillation, ventricular electrogram amplitude can vary by as much as 500% on a beat-by-beat basis. The average ventricular electrogram amplitude generally decreases markedly during polymorphic ventricular tachycardia and fibrillation compared with sinus rhythm. Clinically, de-

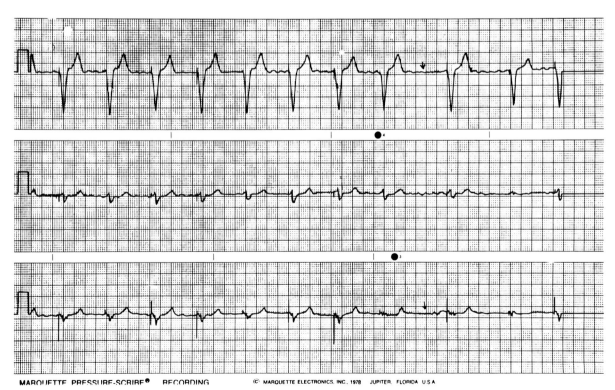

MARQUETTE PRESSURE-SCRIBE® RECORDING   © MARQUETTE ELECTRONICS, INC., 1978   JUPITER, FLORIDA U.S.A.

FIGURE 2–46. Intermittent oversensing due to a loose screw at the lead connector–pulse generator header block. Following the eighth QRS complex there is a pause (arrow) due to oversensing from artifacts in the electrogram caused by mechanical movement of the lead connector within the header of the pulse generator.

TABLE 2–4. CLINICAL FINDINGS SUGGESTING A POSSIBLE LEAD-RELATED SENSING PROBLEM

Change in stimulation threshold
Sudden decrease in amplitude or slew rate for P wave or R wave measured by telemetry or invasively
Change in pacing impedance
  Decreased impedance (<250 ohms) suggests insulation failure
  Increased impedance (>2000 ohms) suggests conductor fracture
Change in stimulus waveform
  >25% increase in leading to trailing edge voltage droop
  Absence of stimulus artifact
Radiograph demonstrating conductor fracture or loose connector-pin connection
Sudden occurrence of pectoral muscle stimulation
  Especially with bipolar lead
Sudden onset of phrenic nerve or diaphragmatic stimulation
Syncope or presyncope
Sensation of pauses in paced rhythm
Palpitations

fibrillators with fixed-gain sensitivities have to be carefully evaluated for evidence of undersensing during ventricular tachycardia and ventricular fibrillation. We have reported two patients with Telectronics Guardian 4202 and 4210 defibrillators with maximal sensitivity of 0.5 to 1.0 mV who had episodes of undersensing during monomorphic and polymorphic ventricular tachycardia, despite having adequate sensing and ventricular electrograms larger than 4 to 5.7 mV during sinus rhythm (Fig. 2–47).[68] Singer and colleagues also reported a patient with a third-generation implantable cardioverter-defibrillator with fixed-gain sensing that demonstrated undersensing of ventricular fibrillation.[69] Singer and colleagues emphasized that the dynamic nature of the QRS signal during ventricular fibrillation probably leads to undersensing more frequently than is suspected with fixed-gain devices just from inspection of stored electrograms or RR intervals. A fundamental requirement of antitachycardia devices that are intended to sense ventricular fibrillation or atrial fibrillation is therefore the ability to accommodate changes in signal amplitude during the arrhythmia. These arrhythmias typically may change from high-amplitude signals during sinus rhythm to a low-amplitude signal, then to asystole, and back again to high-amplitude signals in sinus rhythm. This necessitates the presence of amplifiers that are not easily saturated by high-amplitude signals and will not clip the signals, which could lead to double sensing if the refractory periods are programmed inappropriately. On the

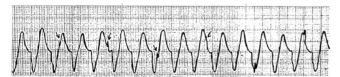

FIGURE 2–47. Electrocardiogram demonstrating sustained ventricular tachycardia at a rate of 130 bpm in a patient with an implantable cardioverter-defibrillator (ICD). The ICD was programmed to a sensitivity of 1.0 mV. During ventricular tachycardia there is undersensing, and ventricular pacing occurs at a rate of 45 bpm (*arrows*). During sinus rhythm the R wave measured greater than 5.7 mV, and during ventricular tachycardia the ventricular electrogram measured less than 0.7 mV. (From Sperry RE, Ellenbogen KA, Wood MA, et al: Failure of a second- and third-generation implantable cardioverter-defibrillator to sense ventricular tachycardia: Implications for fixed-gain sensing devices. PACE 15:749, 1992.)

other hand, amplifiers that are very sensitive may have more problems with noise. As a result of the large dynamic sensing range required by implantable cardioverter-defibrillators, most devices incorporate automatic adjustment of sensing gain within their algorithms.

In addition to sensing problems of antitachycardia devices, bradycardia pacemakers may undersense during tachyarrhythmias. For example, if ventricular tachycardia is appropriately sensed by a VVI pacemaker, pacing should be inhibited. However, if the signal is of insufficient amplitude, ventricular pacing will continue during the ventricular arrhythmia. In other patients, even when the ventricular signal is sensed, the rate of ventricular tachycardia may be so high that the ventricular electrogram is sensed during the noise-sampling period of the ventricular refractory period.[70] This may lead to the pacemaker reverting to its "noise reversion mode" and pacing asynchronously (VOO). These reports emphasize the importance of sensing algorithms and sensing amplifiers for implantable antitachycardia devices that have very low maximal sensing threshold (0.1 to 0.3 mV) and are able to sense signals with widely varying amplitudes.

MODE SWITCHING IN RESPONSE TO ATRIAL FIBRILLATION

The use of DDD and DDDR pacemakers in patients with paroxysmal atrial fibrillation has become more widespread as the advantages of AV synchrony and the potential proarrhythmic effects of VVIR pacing have become clear (see Chapter 18). Patients with sick sinus syndrome and intermittent episodes of atrial tachycardia are more frequently undergoing implantation of dual-chamber devices. In these patients, especially if they have concomitant AV nodal conduction disease, spontaneous AV block, or previous AV nodal ablation, atrial tracking may occur at or close to the upper rate limit during atrial tachyarrhythmias. This has been a significant limitation to dual-chamber pacing for patients with paroxysmal atrial tachyarrhythmias. Recently, automatic mode conversion algorithms have been introduced for DDDR pacing by Telectronics with the Meta DDDR (model 1250 and now 1254) (Fig. 2 48).[13, 71] When programmed to a dual-chamber, rate-adaptive pacing mode (e.g., DDDR, DDIR, or VDDR), the pacemaker detects and monitors the atrial electrogram during a designated window within the PVARP that immediately follows the nonprogrammable atrial blanking period. Automatic mode conversion occurs in the model 1250 when atrial activity is sensed during the PVARP, beyond an atrial blanking window that is 100 msec in duration. Following detection of atrial activity during the PVARP, the pacing mode switches from DDDR to VVIR mode, with the rate being controlled by the sensor. The newer algorithm allows the physician to program mode switching on and off and also allows mode switching during DDD or VDD pacing to the VVI mode. If a P wave is sensed within a window of 2 msec after the blanking period, the device automatically switches from the DDD to the VVI mode (model 1250). In the newer generation of these devices (model 1254), mode switching during DDD pacing is identical to that in the algorithm during DDDR pacing. In the first mode-switching algorithm (model 1250), a single P wave that fell into the PVARP sensing window would trigger a mode switch. The newer mode-switching algorithm allows the physician to pro-

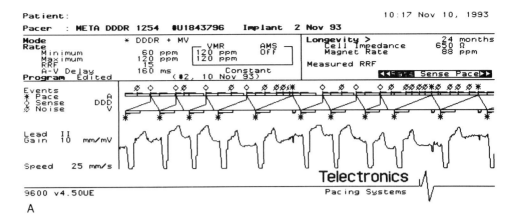

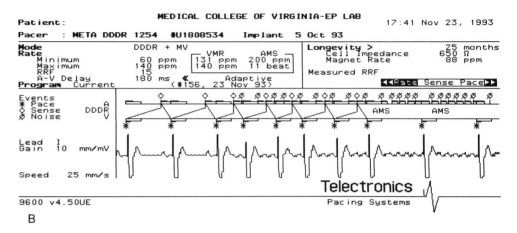

FIGURE 2–48. *A,* A telemetry printout from a Telectronics model 1254 pulse generator during atrial fibrillation in the DDD mode without automatic mode switching (AMS). Note that during atrial fibrillation frequent sensed atrial events occur that are rapid and irregular (*upper tracing*), resulting in pacemaker Wenckebach behavior in the surface electrocardiogram (*lower tracing*). *B,* The AMS feature is shown in a patient with paroxysmal atrial fibrillation and complete AV block. The first three complexes represent sinus rhythm with normal DDDR tracking function. Following the third complex atrial fibrillation develops that is sensed by the atrial sense amplifier and noted as "noise" in the annotated main timing events. Following the seventh ventricular complex, the mode is automatically switched from DDDR to VVIR (AMS). (VMR, ventricular maximum rate or upper tracking rate.)

gram the number of beats that are required to trigger a mode switch (5 or 11) and the required atrial rate. The newer algorithm also provides for extension of the atrial blanking period after a ventricular paced beat. Since an atrial blanking period of 100 msec is too short to avoid detection of far-field R waves in many patients, the model 1254 devices incorporate a blanking period that has been extended to 150 msec. These newer algorithms avoid some of the older limitations of the algorithm, including inappropriate mode switching during sinus tachycardia, following single PACs, and single PVCs with retrograde VA conduction[14] and far-field paced QRS complexes. Many additional companies are incorporating sophisticated mode-switching algorithms into future generations of DDDR pacemakers. In addition to providing more programmability with respect to the number of beats and atrial rate required to trigger mode switching, data storage capabilities will become available to allow assessment of the atrial rhythm.

An important consideration in the design of mode-switching algorithms is the need to ensure atrial sensing during atrial fibrillation. For mode switching to be reliable, the atrial electrogram must be sensed during both sinus rhythm and atrial fibrillation or flutter. For example, if a P wave measures 2 mV during sinus rhythm but varies from 0.1 to 1.0 mV during atrial fibrillation, sufficient signal dropout may occur to lead to intermittent atrial undersensing and tracking of the atrial rate instead of mode switching (Fig. 2–49). In addition, some atrial tachycardias may develop at a rate that leads to every other P wave occurring within the atrial blanking pe-

riod, so that the sensed atrial rate will be only half the actual rate. This can be corrected in some cases by programming the mode-switching algorithm to trigger this feature at a lower atrial rate. In addition, programming a relatively slow upper tracking rate will allow the device to develop pacemaker Wenckebach behavior, thereby changing the ventricular rate (and the atrial blanking period) so that such aliasing of P waves does not occur.

ATRIAL SENSING WITH SINGLE-PASS VDD PACING

Single-pass leads for patients with complete heart block and normal sinus node function in whom VDD pacing would be appropriate are currently used in Europe for selected patients. VDD pacing is discussed in more detail in Chapter 19. In the mid 1970s, it was noted that closely spaced, floating electrodes in the mid right atrium consistently recorded an atrial electrogram that could be appropriately sensed.[72, 73] In an early study by Antonioli and colleagues, atrial electrograms were recorded from 25 unipolar ventricular pacing leads with the atrial electrode floating in the midatrium.[73] The mean minimum and maximum values of the atrial electrogram varied from 1.11 ± 0.67 to 2.16 ± 1.07 mV, and the slew rate varied from a mean minimum of 0.15 ± 0.09 to 0.29 ± 0.15 V/sec. The frequency content of the signal was calculated to obtain information about the center frequency of the bandbass amplifier that would be necessary to record this signal. Based on several studies, investigators were able to determine that atrial sensing depends on the distance of

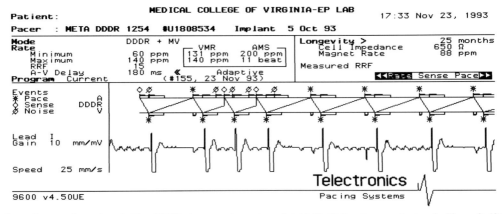

FIGURE 2–49. Failure of automatic mode switching (AMS) due to undersensing of atrial fibrillation (same patient as in Figure 2–48). Note that there is occasional sensing of the atrial signal during atrial fibrillation with failure to satisfy the criteria for mode switching (200 ppm for 11 beats) at an atrial sensitivity of 2.0 mV. Thus, failure to sense the atrial electrogram during atrial fibrillation may be a problem for devices designed to switch pacing modes in response to paroxysmal atrial arrhythmia because of varying amplitude in the electrogram.

the atrial sensing electrode from the myocardial wall, orientation of the dipole, spacing between electrodes, electrode size, gain of the atrial differential sense amplifier, interference patterns, and phase imbalance (Table 2–5).[17–20, 74] Measurement of atrial signal amplitude and electrogram amplitude showed that a dipole spacing of 1 to 2 cm gave optimal signal amplitude. Phase imbalance studies showed that if the dipole was too widely spaced or if the electrode surface area was too large, the two electrodes would record signals that could cancel each other out. In early designs, the unipolar atrial floating electrode proved to be too sensitive to myopotentials, electromagnetic fields, and ventricular far-field signals. There was considerable overlap between atrial and ventricular signals in terms of amplitude, but the slew rate for the atrial signal (0.19 ± 0.09 V/sec) was considerably greater than that for the ventricular signal (0.06 ± 0.02 V/sec). Other difficulties included the need to use a prior chest radiograph to determine the optimal distance between the ventricular and atrial electrodes. This early lead had a 60-mm^2 floating ring electrode located 12 to 18 cm from the tip.

TABLE 2–5. **FACTORS INFLUENCING SENSING PERFORMANCE**

Electrode size
Electrode surface area
Electrode surface structure
Electrode chemical composition
Electrode-tissue contact
Fibrotic capsule surrounding electrode
Steroid elution
Active- versus passive-fixation mechanism
Orientation of interelectrode axis
Interelectrode distance
Unipolar vs. bipolar devices
Orthogonal electrodes
Programmed polarity (tip vs. ring)
Respiration
Exercise
Catecholamines
Body position
Antiarrhythmic drugs
Sensing amplifier input impedance
Amplifier filtering characteristics
Blanking and refractory period timing

In the 1980s, bipolar atrial configuration single-pass leads were shown to have improved signal-to-noise selectivity with an optimal bipolar spacing of 0.5 to 1 cm. Multiple configurations were tested for sensing. These included a bipolar atrial lead with wide ring spacing (3 cm), a bipolar atrial lead with narrow ring spacing (0.5 to 1 cm), a dipole orthogonal to the longitudinal axis of the lead, and two diagonal half-ring electrodes with 0.5 to 1 cm spacing. Optimal sensing with respect to atrial electrogram amplitude and slew rate was achieved uniformly with orthogonal leads and bipolar leads with a narrow ring spacing of 0.5 to 1.0 cm. The diagonal atrial bipolar or half-ring configuration with 0.5- to 1.0-cm spacing generally produced adequate atrial electrograms but had a slightly lower amplitude than the orthogonal and bipolar leads. The AV ratios detected with a 1-cm spaced electrode are good in almost all positions except on the atrial floor. Placement of the atrial dipole close to the atrial wall and in the mid to high right atrium seems to be ideal in terms of rejecting ventricular far-field signals and optimizing the amplitude and frequency content of the atrial signal.

Several single-pass VDD pacing systems are now commercially available. They consist of a triaxial lead in which the distal tip is a unipolar ventricular electrode and two atrial partially circumferential (half-ring) electrodes with areas of greater than 6 mm^2. These electrodes are located 180 degrees apart (Fig. 2–50) and are called a diagonal atrial bipolar configuration. Another system in clinical use has a bipolar ventricular electrode and two atrial ring electrodes separated by 5 mm, with a 25-mm^2 surface area placed proximally on the lead. The lead is manufactured with atrial electrodes positioned 11, 13, and 15 cm from the ventricular electrode. The orthogonal electrode system initially consisted of a pair of small electrodes (1 mm^2) oriented at 90 degrees to each other at the same level on the lead. Various iterations of this lead have been tested, including ones with three and four electrodes in circumferential arrangements. In a version of the orthogonal lead that was implanted with a VDD pulse generator (model RS4-SRT, Cardiac Pacemakers Inc, St. Paul, MN),[75] atrial sensing was adequate in only 58% of patients and resulted in longer implantation times than conventional leads.

Practical aspects of implanting and programming VDD pacing systems are discussed in more detail in Chapter

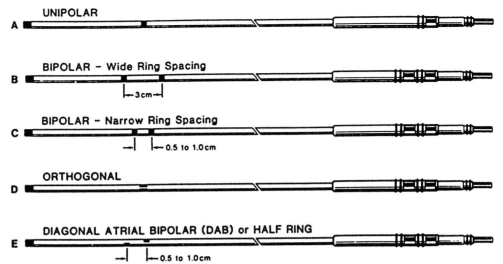

FIGURE 2–50. Comparison of electrode configurations for a standard unipolar pacing lead (*A*), a bipolar lead with 3-cm spacing (*B*), a bipolar lead with narrow spacing of 0.5 cm (*C*), a lead with orthogonal electrodes placed directly opposite one another (*D*), and diagonally opposed electrodes with a half-ring design (*E*). (From Furman S, Hayes DL, Holmes DF: A Practice of Cardiac Pacing, 3rd ed. Mt. Kisco, NY, Futura, 1993, p 104.)

19.[21, 22] It is important to highlight the fact that VDD pacing systems have been in clinical use for over a decade. Clinical experience with these systems has been largely limited to Europe and Japan, but whether these systems become widely accepted for use in this country or not, they illustrate important principles and limitations of sensing small intracardiac electric signals.

Summary

The ability of a pacing system to detect intrinsic cardiac electric signals and to distinguish these signals from unwanted cardiac and extracardiac signals is an important aspect of the design and function of cardiac pacemakers. Sensing is dependent on the biophysical properties of the voltage source within the myocardium and the electrode-tissue interface. The size, shape, surface structure, and chemical composition of the electrodes used for sensing have important effects on sensing performance. In addition to amplifying cardiac electric signals, sensing amplifiers must distinguish desired from extraneous signals using filtering of the electrogram as well as blanking the period of sensing based on the expected sequence of cardiac signals. As more sophisticated algorithms for managing tachyarrhythmias and storing diagnostic information are developed, the basic principles of sensing performance will continue to assume an important role in cardiac pacing.

REFERENCES

1. DeCaprio V, Hurzeler P, Furman S: A comparison of unipolar and bipolar electrograms for cardiac pacemaker. Circulation 56:750, 1977.
2. Furman S, Hurzeler P, DeCaprio V: Cardiac pacing and pacemakers III. Sensing the cardiac electrogram. Am Heart J 93:794, 1977.
3. Frohlig G, Schwendt H, Schieffer H, Bette L: Atrial signal variations and pacemaker malsensing during exercise: A study in the time and frequency domain. J Am Coll Cardiol 11:806, 1988.
4. Parsonnet V, Myers GH, Kresh YM: Characteristics of intracardiac electrograms II. Atrial endocardial electrograms. PACE 3:406, 1980.
5. Myers GH, Kresh YM, Parsonnet V: Characteristics of intracardiac electrograms. PACE 1:90, 1978.
6. Platia EV, Brinker JA: Time course of transvenous pacemaker stimulation impedance, capture thresholds, and intracardiac electrogram amplitude. PACE 9:620, 1986.
7. Mond HG, Stokes KB: The electrode-tissue interface: the revolutionary role of steroid elution. PACE 15:95, 1992.
7a. Irnich W: Intracardiac electrograms and sensing test signals: Electrophysiological, physical, and technical considerations. PACE 8:870, 1985.
8. Kleinert M, Elmqvist H, Strandberg H: Spectral properties of atrial and ventricular endocardial signals. PACE 2:11, 1979.
9. Klitzner TS, Stevenson WG: Effects of filtering on right ventricular electrograms recorded from endocardial catheters in humans. PACE 13:69, 1990.
10. Steinhaus DM, Foley L, Knoll K, Markowtiz T: Atrial sensing revisited: Do bandpass filters matter? [abstract] PACE 16:946, 1993.
11. Medtronic, Inc: Spectrax SX 5984, 5984 LP, 5985 Technical Manual. Minneapolis, Medtronic, Inc., 1984.
12. Barold SS, Kulkarni H, Thawani AJ, et al: Electrocardiographic manifestations of the rapid recharge function of pulse generators after sensing. PACE 11:1215, 1988.
13. Mond HG, Barold SS: Dual chamber, rate adaptive pacing in patients with paroxysmal supraventricular tachyarrhythmias: Protective measures for rate control. PACE 16:2168, 1993.
14. Lau CP, Tai YT, Fong PC, et al: Atrial arrhythmia management with sensor controlled atrial refractory period and automatic mode switching in patients with minute ventilation sensing dual chamber rate adaptive pacemakers. PACE 15:1504, 1992.
15. Ohm O-J: The interdependence between electrogram, total electrode impedance, and pacemaker input impedance necessary to obtain adequate functioning of demand pacemakers. PACE 2:465, 1979.
16. Fischler H: Polarization properties of small-surface-area pacemaker electrodes—implications on reliability of sensing and pacing. PACE 2:403, 1979.
17. Goldreyer BN, Olive AL, Leslie J, et al: A new orthogonal lead for P synchronous pacing. PACE 4:638, 1981.
18. Goldreyer BN, Knudson M, Cannom DS, Wyman MG: Orthogonal electrogram sensing. PACE 6:464, 1983.
19. Wainwright RJ, Crick JCP, Sowton E: Clinical evaluation of a single-pass electrode for all modes of pacing. PACE 6:210, 1983.
20. Antonioli GE, Ansani L, Barbieri D, et al: Single-lead VDD pacing. *In* Barold SS, Mugica J (eds): New Perspectives in Cardiac Pacing, 3. Mt. Kisco, NY, Futura, 1993, pp 359–381.
21. Varriale P, Pilla AG, Tekriwal M: Single-lead VDD pacing system. PACE 13:757, 1990.
22. Curzio G and the Multicenter Study Group: A multicenter evaluation of a single pass lead VDD pacing system. PACE 14:434, 1991.
23. Hurzeler P, DeCaprio V, Furman S: Endocardial electrograms and pacemaker sensing. Med Inst 10(4):178, 1976.
24. Angello DA: Principles of electrical testing for analysis of ventricular endocardial pacing leads. Prog Cardiovasc Dis 27:57, 1984.
25. de Buitleir M, Kou WH, Schmaltz S, et al: Acute changes in pacing threshold and R- or P-wave amplitude during permanent pacemaker implantation. Am J Cardiol 65:999, 1990.
26. Nielsen AP, Cashion R, Spencer WH, et al: Long-term assessment of unipolar and bipolar stimulation and sensing thresholds using a lead

configuration programmable pacemaker. J Am Coll Cardiol 5:1198, 1985.

27. Furman S: Bipolar pacing. PACE 9:619, 1986.
28. Scalhorn R, Markowitz T: Bipolar dual chamber pacemakers: Is myopotential sensing still a problem? PACE 11:852, 1988.
29. Wirtzfeld S, Lampadius M, Ruprecht EO: Unterdruckung von Demand-Schrittmachern durch Muskelpotentials. Dtsch Med Wochenschr 97:61, 1972.
30. Levine PA, Klein MD: Myopotential inhibition of unipolar pacemakers. A disease of technologic progress. Ann Intern Med 98:101, 1983.
31. Watson WS: Myopotential sensing in cardiac pacemakers. In Barold SS (ed): Modern Cardiac Pacing. Mt. Kisco, NY, Futura, 1985, pp 813–837.
32. Berger R, Warren J: Myopotential inhibition of demand pacemakers: Etiologic, diagnostic, and therapeutic considerations. PACE 2:596, 1979.
33. Fetter J, Hall DM, Hoff GL, Reeder JT: The effect of myopotential interference on unipolar and bipolar dual chamber pacemakers in the DDD mode. Clin Prog Electrophysiol Pacing 3:368, 1985.
34. Brevik K, Ohm OJ: Myopotential inhibition of unipolar QRS-inhibited (VVI) pacemakers assessed by ambulatory Holter monitoring of the electrocardiogram. PACE 3:470, 1980.
35. Halpern JL, Camunas JL, Stern EH, et al: Myopotential interference with DDD pacemakers. Endocardial electrographic telemetry in the diagnosis of pacemaker-related arrhythmias. Am J Cardiol 54:97, 1984.
36. Secemsky SI, Hauser RG, Denes P, et al: Unipolar sensing abnormalities: Incidence and clinical significance of skeletal muscle interference and undersensing in 228 patients. PACE 5:10, 1982.
37. DeBoer H, Kofflard M, Scholtes T, et al: Differential bipolar sensing of a dual chamber pacemaker. PACE 11:158, 1988.
38. Fetter J, Bobeldyk GL, Engman FJ: The clinical incidence and significance of myopotential sensing with unipolar pacemakers. PACE 7:871, 1984.
39. Brevik K, Ohm OJ, Engedal H: Long-term comparison of unipolar and bipolar pacing and sensing, using a new multiprogrammable system. PACE 6:592, 1983.
40. Barold SS, Ong LS, Falkoff MD: Inhibition of bipolar demand pacemaker by diaphragmatic myopotentials. Circulation 56:679, 1977.
41. el Gamal M, Van Gelder B: Suppression of an external demand pacemaker by diaphragmatic myopotentials: A sign of electrode perforation? PACE 2:191, 1979.
42. Barold SS, Falkoff MD, Ong LS, et al: Diaphragmatic myopotential inhibition in myopotential inhibition in multiprogrammable unipolar and bipolar pulse generators. In Steinbach K (ed): Cardiac Pacing. Proceedings of the VIIIth World Symposium on Cardiac Pacing. Darmstadt, Germany, Steinkopff Verlag, 1983, p 537.
43. Rosenqvist M, Nordlander R, Andersson M, et al: Reduced incidence of myopotential pacemaker inhibition by abdominal generator implantation. PACE 9:417, 1986.
44. Gialafos J, Maillis A, Kalogeropoulos C, et al: Inhibition of demand pacemakers by myopotentials. Am Heart J 109:984, 1985.
45. Lau CP, Linker NJ, Butrous GS, et al: Myopotential interference in unipolar rate responsive pacemakers. PACE 12:1324, 1989.
46. Volosin KJ, Rudderow R, Waxman HL: VOOR-Nondemand rate modulated pacing necessitated by myopotential inhibition. PACE 12:421, 1989.
47. Michalik RE, Williams WH, Hatcher CR Jr: Myopotential inhibition of unipolar pacing in children. PACE 8:25, 1985.
48. Griffin JC: Sensing characteristics of the right atrial appendage electrode. PACE 6:22, 1983.
49. Coombs WJ, Reynolds DW, Sharma AD, et al: Cross talk in bipolar pacemakers. PACE 12:613, 1989.
50. Van Gelder LM, El Gamal MIH, Tielen CHJ: P-wave sensing in VVI pacemakers: Useful or a problem? PACE 11:1413, 1988.
51. Mond HG, Sloman JG: The malfunctioning pacemaker system. Part II. PACE 4:168, 1981.
52. Barold SS, Gaidula JJ: Evaluation of normal and abnormal sensing functions of demand pacemakers. Am J Cardiol 28:201, 1971.
53. Brandt J, Fahraeus T, Schuller H: Far field QRS complex sensing via the atrial pace-maker lead. II. Prevalence, clinical significance and possibility of intraoperative prediction in DDD pacing. PACE 11:1546, 1988.
54. Barold SS, Falkoff MD, Ong LS, et al: Double sensing by atrial automatic tachycardia terminating pulse generator. PACE 10:58, 1987.
55. Warnowicz MA, Goldschlager N: Apparent failure to sense (undersensing) caused by oversensing: Diagnostic use of a noninvasively obtained intracardiac electrogram. PACE 6:1341, 1983.
56. Hauser RG, Susmano A: After-potential oversensing by a programmable pulse generator. PACE 4:391, 1981.
57. Shandling AH, Castellanet MJ, Messenger JC, et al: Utility of the atrial endocardial electrogram concurrent with dual-chamber pacing in the determination of a pacemaker mediated arrhythmia. PACE 11:1419, 1988.
58. Shandling AH, Castellanet MJ, Thomas L, et al: Impaired activity rate responsiveness of an atrial activity triggered pacemaker. The role of differential atrial sensing in its prevention. PACE 12:1927, 1989.
59. Barold SS, Falkoff MD, Ong LS, et al: Interpretation of electrocardiograms produced by a new unipolar multiprogrammable "committed" AV sequential demand (DVI) pulse generator. PACE 4:692, 1981.
60. Levine PA, Brodsky SJ: Fusion, pseudofusion, pseudopseudofusion and confusion. Clin Prog Pacing Electrophysiol 1:70, 1983.
61. Lindemans FW, Rankin IR, Murtaugh R, et al: Clinical experience with an activity sensing pacemaker. PACE 9:978, 1986.
62. Waxman HL, Lazzara R, El-Sherif N: Apparent malfunction of demand pacemaker due to spurious potentials generated by contact between two endocardial electrodes. PACE 1:531, 1978.
63. Wilson JH, Lattner S: Apparent undersensing due to oversensing of low amplitude pulses in a thoracic impedance sensing, rate responsive pacemaker. PACE 11:1479, 1988.
64. Timmis GC, Westveer DC, Bakalyar DM, et al: Discrimination of anterograde from retrograde atrial electrograms for physiologic pacing. PACE 11:130, 1988.
65. Klementowicz PT, Furman S: Selective atrial sensing in dual chamber pacemakers eliminates endless loop tachycardia. J Am Coll Cardiol 6:1338, 1986.
66. Leitch JW, Yee R, Klein GJ, et al: Correlation between the ventricular electrogram amplitude in sinus rhythm and ventricular fibrillation. PACE 13:1105, 1990.
67. Ellenbogen KA, Wood MA, Stambler BS, et al: Measurement of ventricular electrogram amplitude during intraoperative induction of ventricular tachyarrhythmias. Am J Cardiol 70:1017, 1992.
68. Sperry RE, Ellenbogen KA, Wood MA, et al: Failure of the second and third generation implantable cardioverter defibrillator to sense ventricular tachycardia: Implications for fixed-gain sensing devices. PACE 15:749, 1992.
69. Singer I, Adams L, Austin E: Potential hazards of fixed gain sensing and arrhythmia reconfirmation for implantable cardioverter defibrillators. PACE 16:1070, 1993.
70. Fontaine JM, Alma-Perri CA, El-Sherif N: DDD pacemaker pseudomalfunction during supraventricular tachycardia. PACE 11:1380, 1988.
71. Barold SS, Mond HG: Optimal antibradycardia pacing in patients with paroxysmal supraventricular tachyarrhythmias: Role of fallback and automatic mode switching mechanisms. In Barold SS, Mugica J (eds): New Perspectives in Cardiac Pacing 3. Mt. Kisco, NY, Futura, 1993, pp 483–518.
72. Curry PVL, Raper DA: Single lead for permanent physiological cardiac pacing. Lancet 2:757, 1978.
73. Antonioli GE, Grass G, Baggioni FG, et al: New method for atrial triggered pacemaker. G Ital Cardiol 10:679, 1980.
74. Flammang DF, Renirie L, Begemann M, et al: Amplitude and direction of atrial depolarization using a multipolar floating catheter: Principles for a single lead VDD pacing system. PACE 14:1040, 1991.
75. Ramsdale DR, Charles RG: Rate-responsive ventricular pacing: Clinical experience with the RS4-SRT pacing system. PACE 8:378, 1985.

CHAPTER 3

ENGINEERING AND CLINICAL ASPECTS OF PACING LEADS

Harry G. Mond
John R. Helland

The implantable cardiac pacemaker is an integrated, highly sophisticated system comprising a lead and a pulse generator. The leads are the only link between the sophisticated electronics in the pulse generator and the heart. Thus, the leads play the critical role of delivering the output pulse from the pulse generator to the myocardium and transferring the intracardiac electrogram from the myocardium to the sensing circuit of the pulse generator. With rate-adaptive cardiac pacing, the lead may also be an integral part of the artificial sensor. Despite marked advances in the technology of pulse generators and sensors, concomitant advances in pacing leads have occurred relatively slowly. Perhaps the most significant developments in pacing leads have occurred in the design of electrodes. Problems still exist with lead conductors, insulation, and fixation mechanisms that need to be solved to achieve the reliability and ease of use that are required for creating the fully automatic pacing systems of the future. This chapter addresses the engineering and clinical aspects of cardiac pacing leads. When relevant, a historical perspective of the evolution of modern pacing leads is discussed.

Lead Polarity

A controversy has continued unabated for more than 30 years about which cardiac pacing system, unipolar or bipolar, is superior.[1] Compared with their unipolar counterparts, early bipolar leads were large, cumbersome, and difficult to implant. Today, with major technologic and engineering advances, bipolar leads approximate unipolar designs in size and ease of insertion. By strict definition, all electric circuits, including those of a pacemaker, are bipolar. To complete the circuit, electrons flow from the cathode to the anode. When applied to transvenous leads, the terms unipolar and bipolar simply indicate *the number of electrodes in contact with the heart* (Fig. 3–1). A unipolar lead has only one electrode (the cathode), which is located at the tip. Current flows from the negatively charged cathode to the heart and returns to the anode (the pulse generator) to complete the circuit. In contrast, in a bipolar lead both electrodes are a short distance from each other at the distal end. The tip electrode is usually the cathode, and a ring electrode proximal to this serves as the anode. If the voltage gradient (or current density) in the myocardium in contact with the cathode is of sufficient intensity, myocardial stimulation and cardiac contraction result (see Chapter 1).

In reality, the differences between unipolar and bipolar pacing are relatively minor. Both configurations are reliable for long-term pacing in both the atrium and the ventricle. Unipolar and bipolar leads have seen waves of popularity that have reflected the state of the art at the time, the local availability of leads and pulse generators, and individual physician preferences. Today, however, there is a growing worldwide trend toward the increased use of bipolar leads. The principal differences between these two electrode configurations are discussed here.

SIZE

Historically, bipolar transvenous leads were thicker and stiffer than unipolar leads. This made them more difficult to insert at the venous entry site and more cumbersome to manipulate through the cardiac chambers. There was also fear that these thicker, stiffer leads would obstruct venous

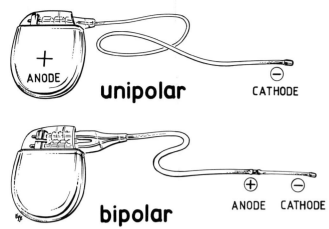

FIGURE 3–1. Diagram demonstrating differences between unipolar and bipolar lead systems. See text for details.

channels, compromise tricuspid valve function, or perforate the heart. The original designs had two parallel conductors individually encased in a large, dual-lumen insulated tube. At the proximal end of the lead was a rather bulky bifurcated bipolar connector. Today, bipolar pacing leads have become almost as thin as their unipolar counterparts because the conductors are wound around one another. The evolution of bipolar leads is discussed later in this chapter.

REPAIR AND REDUNDANCY

In general, there is little difficulty in repairing a standard unipolar lead, particularly one that is insulated with silicone rubber. The extravascular section of the lead can be cut short and a new connector attached by using the connector replacement kit that is supplied by most lead manufacturers. Repair is not so simple with bipolar leads. With a bifurcated connector, one pole can be capped if the other is suitable for unipolar pacing. The repair, however, becomes more complicated or impossible with modern coaxial bipolar leads, especially if the insulation is made of polyurethane.

STIMULATION THRESHOLD

In general, the larger the size of the anode, the lower the total pacing impedance. In the unipolar pacing system an indifferent plate with a large surface area is used as the anode, usually the pulse generator casing. Because the size of the anode in a unipolar pacing system (the pulse generator case) can be made larger than that in a bipolar system (the proximal electrode), the total impedance in the unipolar system is less. Theoretically, unipolar leads should also have a lower pacing impedance than bipolar leads because only one conductor coil is required. Thus, with unipolar pacing, the lower resistance to current flow in the conductor results in a lower voltage drop across the lead. With a constant-voltage generator, unipolar leads should have a lower voltage threshold than bipolar leads. However, modern pacing leads have a small, lower-polarization cathode that plays a much more important role in determining overall pacing impedance than the larger anode. Because of this, bipolar leads offer only a slightly higher impedance than unipolar leads, a difference

that is mostly attributable to the resistance of the extra conductor coil.[2] Modern leads, whether unipolar or bipolar, also have very low stimulation thresholds.[2] On a practical basis, there is essentially no difference between the stimulation thresholds of unipolar and bipolar pacing leads.

SENSING OF INTRACARDIAC ELECTROGRAMS

For many years there has been a widely held view that unipolar pacing systems were superior to bipolar systems with respect to the sensing of intracardiac signals. This idea was suggested by early studies with temporary leads, usually in the situation of an acute myocardial infarction or following open heart surgery.[3, 4] With its larger interelectrode distance, the unipolar system ''sees'' more of the heart and has more ''space'' in which to detect a spontaneous intracardiac electric event. In contrast, the small interelectrode distance of a bipolar system restricts the sensing zone to a limited area of myocardium. Modern implantable pacing systems are very different with respect to sensing of spontaneous intracardiac signals than earlier designs. Recent comparative studies of unipolar and bipolar sensing configurations show comparable ventricular electrogram amplitudes and slew rates.[5–8] These studies also show that, regardless of the sensing mode, ventricular electrogram amplitudes and slew rates usually exceed the standard limits of the sensing circuit by a comfortable margin. In contrast, atrial potentials may have very low amplitudes, particularly in elderly patients, who are the main recipients of cardiac pacemakers. Despite this, in comparative studies bipolar atrial sensing has not been inferior to unipolar sensing[9, 10] and on occasion may actually be superior.[11]

FAR-FIELD SENSING

The atrial sense amplifier of a dual-chamber (or AAI) pacemaker may demonstrate apparent inappropriate sensing that is related to far-field signals arising in the ventricles. Although such far-field R waves usually have a small amplitude in the atrial electrogram, in the presence of high atrial sensitivity settings such signals may be inappropriately interpreted as atrial depolarizations. Generally, this is more likely to occur if the tip of the atrial lead is positioned near the tricuspid valve. Because all leads sense the difference in electric potential between the anode and the cathode, a bipolar lead with closely spaced electrodes is less likely to record far-field electric signals than a unipolar lead, in which the electrodes are widely spaced. Bipolar leads positioned within the right atrial appendage have been shown to sense significantly smaller far-field ventricular signals than unipolar leads in the same atrial position.[12] This occurred despite the similar size of the atrial component of the unipolar and bipolar electrograms. Thus, with respect to decreasing the size of far-field cardiac signals, bipolar leads have a clear advantage. It should be emphasized that bipolar atrial sensing decreases the amplitude of far-field R waves, although these potentials can still be recorded.

CROSSTALK

Crosstalk is an alteration in pacemaker timing induced by the sensing in one chamber of a signal originating in the opposite cardiac chamber.[13] The most commonly described model of crosstalk is the inappropriate sensing of the atrial pacing stimulus by the ventricular channel in dual-chamber pacing. The resulting inhibition of ventricular output may be either intermittent or persistent and can be life threatening in the pacemaker-dependent patient. Because of the larger amplitude of the pacing stimulus, crosstalk is far more common with unipolar than with bipolar dual-chamber pacing systems.[13–22] Crosstalk with bipolar dual-chamber systems is very rare and when present is probably related to residual polarization afterpotentials and noise in the sensing circuit.[16–19]

SKELETAL MUSCLE MYOPOTENTIAL OVERSENSING

Unipolar pacing systems are far more susceptible to oversensing and inhibition from skeletal myopotentials adjacent to the implanted pulse generator than are bipolar systems. In fact, skeletal myopotential inhibition represents the most common source of unipolar oversensing, although its clinical importance in terms of patient symptoms and well-being remains controversial.[23–32] Because of the proximity of the anode (the pulse generator can) to the pectoral or abdominal muscles in patients with unipolar pacemakers, it is not surprising that inappropriate sensing occurs with ipsilateral muscular contraction. This is less likely to occur if the pulse generator is separated from the muscle by a silicone boot or coating.[33, 34] Because of the frequent need to use high atrial sensitivity settings, the problem of skeletal myopotential inhibition is more commonly observed with atrial pacing systems, making bipolar sensing highly desirable in the atrium. With unipolar dual-chamber systems, inappropriate sensing of skeletal myopotentials may result in inhibition of atrial and ventricular output,[35–37] or inappropriate triggering of the ventricle may result in loss of atrioventricular (AV) synchrony and pacemaker-mediated tachycardia.

EXTRACORPOREAL OVERSENSING

Electromagnetic interference (EMI) from an external source outside the body may enter a pacemaker-sensing circuit either directly into the pulse generator or through the lead. Because the pulse generator is shielded by a metal case, direct penetration by electromagnetic interference is uncommon. The antenna effect of the lead remains a potential problem, although serious cases of oversensing of EMI are rare today and are limited to a small number of environmental situations. In theory, unipolar pacing leads should be more sensitive to EMI than bipolar leads because they are associated with a larger interelectrode distance, which amplifies the antenna effect.[38, 39]

This problem may be of greatest significance with the more highly sensitive settings that are often required for atrial sensing. With DDD pacing, inappropriate atrial sensing will not lead to serious bradycardia. Rather, EMI is more likely to result in pacemaker-mediated tachycardias, which, although annoying, are usually transient and benign.

RIGHT VENTRICULAR PERFORATION

Because of their stiffness, bipolar leads (especially the earlier models) may be more prone to right ventricular per-

foration.[40] This problem became evident when physicians performing implantations who were comfortable leaving a generous curve of a unipolar lead in the ventricle used the same technique with a bipolar lead. The stiff distal end of the lead may damage the endomyocardium and in some cases may result in ventricular penetration or perforation. Factors that influence the forces transmitted to the heart include the interelectrode distance, the cathode design (size and shape), the lead conductor, and the insulation materials. As discussed later in this chapter, certain leads with polyurethane insulation are very stiff and are more prone to right ventricular penetration or perforation. The problem of right ventricular perforation with bipolar leads can be overcome by using careful implantation techniques and the newer silicone rubber–insulated leads that have more flexible tips.[40]

SKELETAL MUSCLE STIMULATION

The proximity of adjacent skeletal muscle to the anode of a unipolar pulse generator may result in undesirable stimulation of this skeletal muscle. The resultant muscle twitching can usually be prevented at the time of implantation by positioning the pulse generator housing toward the subcutaneous tissues, away from the muscle. Minor but nevertheless annoying skeletal muscle stimulation may still occur with unipolar pacing systems, especially if high stimulation voltages are used. Skeletal muscle stimulation is not a problem with bipolar pacing systems unless there is an insulation break in the lead that allows the current to stimulate nearby muscle tissue.

DEPTH OF THE PULSE GENERATOR POCKET

Because of the potential for local skeletal muscle stimulation from the anode, unipolar pulse generators cannot be buried deep to skeletal muscle. This may be a problem in elderly patients with very little subcutaneous tissue or in young patients in whom the cosmetic result is especially important. Bipolar pacemakers are not prone to such problems and must be used if a submuscular pocket is planned.

STIMULUS ARTIFACT SIZE

The unipolar stimulus artifact that is recorded on the surface electrocardiogram (ECG) is significantly larger than a bipolar stimulus of equal intensity (Fig. 3–2). Because of this difference, bipolar pacemakers can be difficult to test by electronic means that depend on surface ECG electrodes to measure the pacing rate and pulse width from the stimulus. Occasionally it may be difficult to determine from the ECG whether a rhythm is bipolar pacing or a spontaneous rhythm propagated by a wide QRS complex. This problem in interpretation may arise during routine testing, ECG monitoring, or analysis of a Holter monitor recording. In these situations, temporary programming to the unipolar configuration can be very helpful in interpreting the ECG recordings.

POLARITY PROGRAMMING FLEXIBILITY

A bipolar lead connected to a pulse generator that offers programming of lead polarity allows noninvasive switching between either unipolar or bipolar pacing and sensing. Dif-

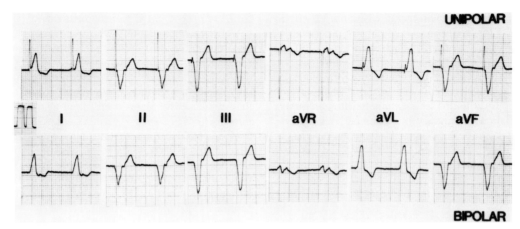

FIGURE 3–2. Twelve-lead electrocardiograms demonstrating differences between unipolar and bipolar pacing. There is a large stimulus artifact with unipolar pacing.

ferent degrees of programming flexibility are available, the most sophisticated systems offering separately selectable polarities for pacing and sensing in both the atrium and the ventricle.[1] The ability to switch from bipolar to unipolar pacing and sensing may be especially important in patients with failure of the outer lead insulation or fracture of the anode conductor, in whom bipolar pacing may be abnormal while unipolar function is usually at least temporarily intact. The ability to program the polarity configuration separately for pacing and sensing also allows one to exploit the advantages of either configuration while minimizing its disadvantages.

VULNERABILITY TO VENTRICULAR ARRHYTHMIAS

There is a theoretical risk of ventricular fibrillation whenever a pacemaker stimulus is delivered in the vulnerable period of the ventricle. Experimentally, the ventricular fibrillation threshold is lower with anodal or bipolar stimulation than with conventional unipolar cathodal stimulation.[41] Despite these laboratory observations, no clinical differences between permanent unipolar and bipolar systems have been reported with respect to the risk of inducing ventricular arrhythmias.

SPECIAL PACING SYSTEMS: IMPLANTABLE CARDIOVERTER-DEFIBRILLATOR INTERACTIONS

Because of the specific sensing requirements of automatic antitachycardia pacemakers and implantable cardioverter-defibrillators (ICD) with pacing capability, these systems must be bipolar to minimize inappropriate sensing of far-field and extracardiac signals. Combined implantation of a pacemaker and an ICD is almost always best accomplished with a bipolar pacemaker to minimize the chances of oversensing of pacing stimuli by the ICD. Unipolar pacemakers can inhibit detection of ventricular fibrillation if the pacing stimuli decrease the automatic sensitivity of the sensing circuit in the ICD. In addition, oversensing of pacing stimuli by the ICD can result in double or even triple counting, resulting in delivery of inappropriate shocks. With combined implantation of a pacemaker and an ICD, delivery of an appropriate shock from an ICD may result in switching of the pulse generator from bipolar to unipolar pacing if this function is present. Consequently, nonpolarity programmable bipolar pulse generators are recommended when a dual-chamber pacing system is implanted in a patient with an ICD.[1]

A number of sensor-driven pacing systems such as those using impedance measurements (i.e., minute ventilation) require a bipolar lead. In others, such as the evoked QT-interval sensor, unipolar pacing is preferred.[42]

RELIABILITY

Perhaps the most important reason for choosing a unipolar pacing lead concerns the issue of long-term reliability. Theoretically, the more complex a lead design, the more components are required for its manufacture and the greater the chances for its failure. Unipolar leads, which may have only six to eight components, are easier to fabricate than bipolar leads, which have more than twice as many components. Some newer lead designs that incorporate a rate-adaptive sensor or transvenous defibrillation leads that also provide pacing and sensing capabilities have more than 40 components. Not surprisingly, unipolar leads have a track record of fewer mechanical failures than comparable bipolar leads.

As a result of the trend toward greater use of conventional bipolar leads, there has been a growing incidence of insulation failure due to a variety of mechanisms. One manufacturer, Medtronic Inc. (Minneapolis, MN), publishes comprehensive periodic updates on lead performance and the causal mechanisms of lead malfunction. With comparable leads there is a marked trend toward improved long-term reliability for unipolar compared with bipolar configurations. For example, the bipolar version of one polyurethane-insulated lead (model 4012 Target Tip) has a cumulative survival at 8 years of $80.2 \pm 4.5\%$. This compares with an 8-year survival of $96.7 \pm 1.9\%$ for the unipolar equivalent (model 4011). A newer version of a polyurethane-insulated lead demonstrates a similar trend, with a $95.6 \pm 2.9\%$ survival at 4 years for the bipolar model and a $99.2 \pm 1.6\%$ survival for the unipolar model.[43] Despite these data, excellent long-term survival has been documented with other types of polyurethane[44, 45] and silicone rubber, although the data on the latter are still preliminary.[43]

The reliability of pacing leads is also influenced by the

implantation technique used. For example, use of the subclavian vein puncture for lead insertion exposes it to the risk of crush injury as the lead passes between the clavicle and the first rib, particularly with bipolar leads.[46, 47] Using the cephalic vein as the lead entry site avoids the clavicle–first rib failure mechanism but does not completely protect the lead from failure possibly related to the sutures on the anchoring sleeve.[48] This problem is discussed in detail later in the section, Lead Insulation.

As new lead designs are developed, improvements in reliability must clearly be a goal, particularly with the more complex bipolar or multipolar varieties. Ideally, all leads should perform reliably during the lifetime of the patient.

SUMMARY OF DIFFERENCES BETWEEN BIPOLAR AND UNIPOLAR LEADS

A summary of the differences between bipolar and unipolar pacing systems is shown in Table 3–1. If reliability were comparable, bipolar leads would appear to be preferable in most respects.

The Pacing Electrode

ELECTRODE SIZE

The earliest transvenous pacing leads had large stimulating electrodes that had surface areas of approximately 100 mm^2.[49] Such electrodes presented a very large surface area to the endocardium, which resulted in a very low pacing impedance, generally on the order of 250 ohms. Because current flow is inversely related to impedance, a large amount of current was drained from the power source with these leads. In addition, because the current was dispersed over a large surface area, there was a high stimulation threshold. By reducing the cathodal surface area, high current densities and lower stimulation threshold levels were obtained, together

TABLE 3–1. POLARITY PREFERENCE: UNIPOLAR VERSUS BIPOLAR

	BIPOLAR	UNIPOLAR
Lead size		+
Lead repair		+ +
Redundancy	+	
Stimulation threshold	0	
Cardiac myopotential sensing	0	
Far-field sensing	+ +	
Crosstalk	+ + +	
Skeletal myopotential oversensing	+ + +	
Extracorporeal (EMI) oversensing	+ +	
Right ventricular perforation		+ +
Local skeletal muscle stimulation	+ + +	
Depth of pulse generator pocket	+ + +	
Stimulus artifact size		+ + +
Programming flexibility	+ + +	
Vulnerability to ventricular arrhythmias		+
Special pacing systems/ICD interactions	+ + +	
Reliability		+ +

0, No significant difference.
+, Not significant but preferable.
+ +, Significant but not an important preference.
+ + +, Significant and important preference.

with more acceptable current drain and increased longevity of the power source.[50–54] By the late 1970s, most pacing leads had cathodes with surface areas of approximately 8 to 12 mm^2 that produced impedance measurements of 400 to 800 ohms. At that time, further reductions in cathode size were thought to be potentially unsafe because of the effects of microdislodgment on tissue contact. Nevertheless, leads with 6-mm^2 or even 4-mm^2 electrodes were introduced and were found to be safe for long-term pacing and sensing.[55, 56] Today, serious consideration is being given to electrodes with surface areas of less than 2 mm^2 that provide acute and chronic impedance measurements of over 1000 ohms.[57]

There are possible limits to the reduction of electrode surface area. For example, with a small geometric surface area, there is increased polarization, at least for polished electrodes. As the surface area decreases, the polarization impedance may become so high that for a constant-voltage stimulus, current flow may become insufficient to capture the heart. Sensing of cardiac myopotentials may also be compromised by an electrode with an extremely small surface area if the input impedance of the sense amplifier is too low. Marked attenuation of an intracardiac signal may occur as a result of high sensing (source) impedance associated with small-surface-area electrodes.[58] Extremely small electrodes, depending on their design, may be more likely to penetrate or perforate the myocardial wall. This problem may be exacerbated when the distal portion of the lead is relatively stiff.[40] The net result may be a high stimulation threshold, exit block, loss of sensing, or cardiac tamponade.

POLARIZATION AND ELECTRODE POROSITY

Although the reduction in cathodal surface area significantly reduces current drain, this does not necessarily produce a low stimulation threshold. As discussed in Chapter 1, impedance is related to three major factors: (1) impedance at the electrode-tissue interface; (2) ohmic resistance of the lead conductor(s); and (3) polarization on the electrode surface. The last two of these factors result in decreased efficiency of the lead with wasting of stimulus energy. Thus, the ideal lead should have high electrode-tissue impedance but low ohmic resistance of the conductor and low polarization. A lead with a small cathodal surface area may result in increased energy losses from polarization, although this effect is not as pronounced as the opposite changes that occur with large cathode size.[59]

The term polarization refers to an electrochemical impedance generated at the electrode-tissue interface. Electric current within metal conductors is ohmic, or due to the flow of electrons. However, in body tissues current flow is due to the movement of charged molecules or ions. At the electrode-tissue interface ohmic energy is transferred to ionic energy and thus an intense chemical reaction occurs. The polarization that develops is due to the alignment of oppositely charged particles at this interface and is a capacitance effect. It explains the change in impedance that occurs during delivery of the pacing stimulus. At the leading edge of the constant-voltage stimulus, the capacitance is zero. During the stimulus, the capacitance increases to reach its maximum at the trailing edge of the stimulus. The capacitance gradually decreases after the stimulus owing to the dissipation of ions back to electric neutrality. The accumulation of ions in the myocardium gives rise to the afterpotential that is typically recorded following a pacing stimulus. This electrochemical polarization effect increases as the geometric electrode surface area is reduced. Polarization impedance also depends on the time that has elapsed since lead implantation, the electrode materials, the electrode surface structure, the current that is delivered (increases with increasing current), the pulse duration (increases with extended pulse durations), the tissue chemistry, and the stimulation polarity.[54, 59] The polarization effect can represent as much as 30% to 40% of the total pacing impedance, but this contribution may be as high as 70% for some smooth-surface, small-area electrodes.[54]

In an early attempt to produce a low-polarization electrode the differential current density (DCD) electrode was designed. This device used a small insulating or dielectric, saline-filled container that was composed of silicone rubber or Teflon with a hole or holes at the distal end that allowed an enveloped electrode with a large surface area to contact the endocardium.[60–62] The current density at the hole(s) was high, but there was no direct electrode-tissue interface and thus virtually no polarization effect. Because of design problems, these electrodes did not gain clinical acceptance. The trade-off between low stimulation thresholds resulting from electrodes with a small radius and the effects of polarization was effectively addressed by electrodes designed with a complex surface structure. During the late 1970s it was recognized that a porous electrode was, in a sense, an extension of the DCD electrode concept and had low-polarization properties.[63] With porous electrodes, the geometric electrode radius can be made small while the real electrode surface area is very large because it includes the internal spaces within the electrode pores. Thus, the net effect of a small electrode with a complex surface structure is the creation of a relatively large, low-polarization, true electrolytic surface area.

The original porous electrode consisted of sintered platinum-iridium fibers, giving the appearance of a fine wire mesh (Fig. 3–3). Because the whole electrode was composed of these fibers, it was referred to as a "totally porous" electrode.[64] The other form of porous electrode involved surface treatment of a solid electrode, and this was called a "porous surface" electrode. The pores can be created in a number of ways such as by sintering a metal powder or microspheres onto a solid metal substrate. The result is an interconnecting network of pores uniformly distributed throughout the coating.[65] Depending on the surface porosity, such electrodes may be macroporous (constructed with small spheres) or microporous (created by using a fine metal powder). Platinum electroplating using platinum powder is another way of producing a microporous surface on an electrode. The electrode appears black because the surface particles are smaller than the wavelength of visible light, which is therefore absorbed (Fig. 3–4). Large microsurface areas can also be created by coating the electrode with platinum iridium,[66] titanium nitride[67] (Fig. 3–5), or iridium oxide thermally bonded onto a titanium substrate.[68]

Totally porous and porous surface electrodes have been compared in dogs, and the average stimulation threshold and sensing impedance were found to be significantly lower with a porous surface electrode.[69] Studies comparing porous electrodes with solid-tip electrodes generally show superior stimulation thresholds and sensing characteristics with the porous designs.[70–75] A porous surface cathode can also be incorporated into an active-fixation lead. The screw, which passes through the center of the porous electrode, is used for lead fixation but not for stimulation or sensing.[76] It is also possible to create a microporous surface on the screw of an epimyocardial electrode; this has been shown to produce improved stimulation thresholds and sensing in myocardial leads.[77]

In a variation of the porous surface design pores are drilled with a laser into a mushroom-shaped or dish-shaped electrode (Fig. 3–6). Again, the pores create both areas of low polarization and zones of high current density. Clinical studies of both of these electrodes have shown lower chronic stimulation thresholds,[78] although the thresholds are higher

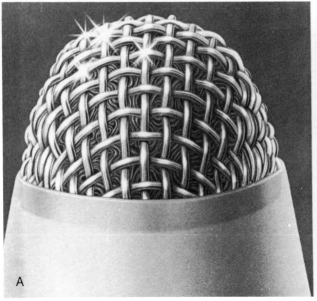
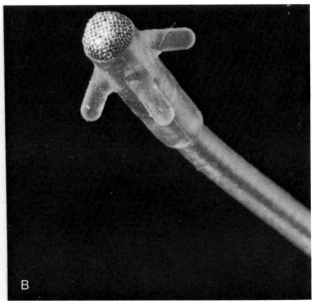

FIGURE 3–3. Totally porous electrode, CPI model 4131 (Courtesy of Cardiac Pacemakers Inc., St. Paul, MN).

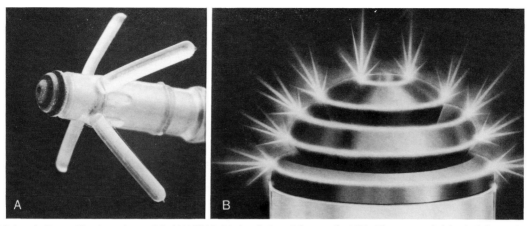

FIGURE 3–4. Medtronic Target Tip electrode, models 4011/4012 (Medtronic Inc., Minneapolis, MN). The porous platinized platinum electrode is shaped like a target with zones of high current density. (Courtesy of Medtronic Inc.)

than those seen with some other porous designs.[79] Low-polarization leads can also be created by etching or texturizing the electrode surface.[80, 81]

ELECTRODE COMPOSITION

The composition of the electrode is also critical to its long-term function. Of particular importance is the degree of corrosion or degradation of the electrode material that occurs over time. Some metals, such as stainless steel[82] and zinc,[83] are clearly unacceptable because corrosion is excessive and metal ions released at the electrode-tissue interface can cause an excessive foreign body reaction in the surrounding tissues. This results in a thick, perielectrode fibrous capsule. Platinum is relatively unreactive but acts as a catalyst for the breakdown or reformation of water, depending on whether electrons are consumed (anode) or given up (cathode). Alloying platinum with 10% iridium increases its mechanical strength without altering its electric performance.[82] Consequently,

either pure platinum or a platinum-iridium alloy has been commonly used in the cathode position. Platinum powder can be very effectively sintered onto platinum to create a low-polarization porous electrode. Another cathode material that was widely used in the past is Eligoloy (Elgin National Watch Company, Elgin, IL), an alloy of cobalt, iron, chromium, molybdenum, nickel, and manganese.[82] Eligoloy, however, cannot be used as the anode in bipolar leads owing to its potential for excessive corrosion. Both platinum-iridium and Eligoloy cathodes show very minor corrosion over time, although no adverse clinical effects have been documented.[84]

In Europe and the United States carbon has been extensively used as a material for cathodes because of its low stimulation thresholds and low polarization properties. Normal carbon or graphite is mechanically weak, brittle, and has poor wear resistance.[85] In contrast, vitreous carbon, a highly purified pyrolytic form of carbon, has excellent mechanical strength, biocompatibility, and complete inertness to body

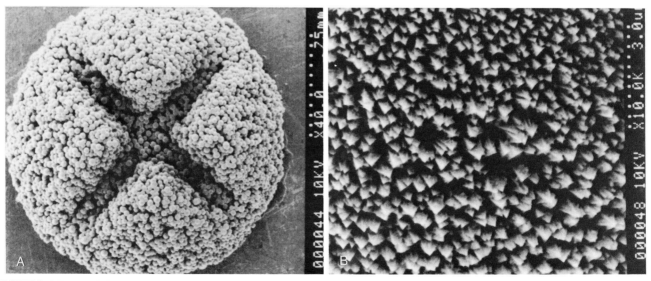

FIGURE 3–5. Porous-platinum electrode with a titanium nitride–coated surface. *A,* At 40× the grooves and platinum particles promoting tissue ingrowth are visible. *B,* High-power electron microscopic photograph shows the porous surface (10,000× magnification).

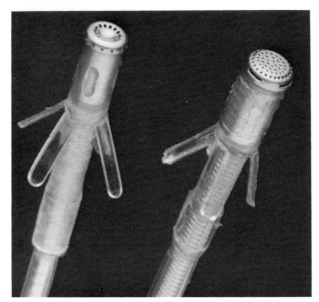

FIGURE 3–6. Electrodes with laser-drilled pores made by Telectronics Pacing Systems (Denver, CO). *Left*, Dish shape, Telectronics Laserdish 030–281. *Right*, Mushroom shape, Telectronics Laserpore 030–240. (Courtesy of Telectronics Pacing Systems.)

tissues.[86, 87] A disadvantage of vitreous carbon is excessive polarization loss,[88] which can be overcome by treating the surface with an oxidation process called *surface activation*.[85, 86, 88, 89] Animal studies have shown only minor tissue reactions with vitreous carbon compared with that surrounding platinum-iridium electrodes.[62, 85, 88–90] Numerous short- and long-term studies have testified to the excellent stimulation thresholds achieved with activated carbon electrodes, particularly when compared to those achieved with polished platinum-iridium electrodes.[86, 90–93] The *glassy carbon electrode* is also microporous but differs from other commercially available carbon electrodes by having a smooth glassy luster.[94] Other materials such as titanium, titanium oxide, titanium

alloys, coated titanium, and especially titanium nitride are also suitable for use as electrode materials, both as anodes and cathodes.[62, 66, 95–98] Although titanium is extremely popular used as the anode in unipolar pacing systems (the pulse generator's housing), cathodal use of titanium has been limited to a platinum-coated titanium, steroid-eluting electrode. However, the low chronic stimulation thresholds obtained with this electrode are due to the properties of steroid elution rather than to the electrode's configuration or materials.[99]

ELECTRODE-TISSUE INTERFACE

The rise in stimulation threshold that normally occurs after lead implantation is a direct result of inflammation at the electrode-tissue interface (Fig. 3–7).[100] The magnitude of this rise in stimulation threshold is unpredictable and in some cases excessive. In these situations, it is necessary and common to use relatively high voltage outputs, at least for the first 2 to 4 months after implantation. As the inflammatory process subsides and a fibrous capsule is formed, the stimulation threshold usually falls to a chronic plateau level that is often considerably higher than that measured at implantation. The critical factor that must be controlled to achieve consistently low stimulation thresholds after implantation is the suppression of inflammation.[100]

In the design of pacing electrodes, a number of basic bioengineering principles that influence the stimulation threshold are important. As already discussed, the cathode should be small enough to allow the stimulation pulse to produce high current density and electric field strength. However, electric field strength decreases as a function of the square of the distance between the electrode surface and the tissue to be stimulated. Consequently, the electrode radius should optimally be equal to or less than the thickness of the fibrous capsule that inevitably envelops it. If the electrode is smaller than the fibrous capsule, the stimulation thresholds will actually increase.[98] To ensure good clinical performance, the lead must also provide adequate fixation for the electrode. The development of fixation mechanisms such as tines has

STIMULATION THRESHOLD MEASUREMENTS POST IMPLANTATION

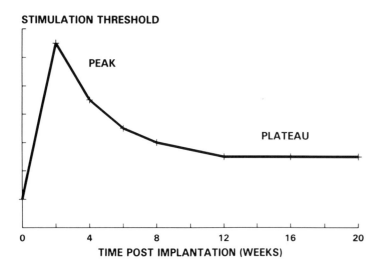

FIGURE 3–7. Typical stimulation threshold rise for a standard electrode after implantation. The acute peak rise in stimulation threshold is unpredictable, and the chronic plateau level is higher than that documented at implantation.

greatly reduced the risk of electrode dislodgment.[101] In addition, tissue ingrowth into porous and grooved electrodes may also enhance mechanical stability and ensure intimate electrode contact with the endocardium at the electrode-tissue interface.

The mechanical design of the lead is also important for control of the inflammation and reduction of fibrosis at the electrode-tissue interface. The electrode should be stable and should lie gently against the endocardium, causing as little physical irritation as possible. A lead design that allows excessive pressure to be imparted to the distal electrode can cause excessive trauma to the endomyocardium and provoke an accelerated inflammatory response. In some cases, lead stiffness can result in myocardial ischemia and even ventricular perforation.[40] Because of this effect of lead stiffness on chronic stimulation thresholds, the mass of the distal portion of the lead should be as small as possible but not too small to act as a penetrating needle point. To further prevent trauma at the electrode-tissue interface, softer forms of silicone or polyurethane have been used for the distal portion of the leads made by some manufacturers. Physical methods aimed at preventing irritation at the electrode-tissue interface should also be considered. Ripart and Mugica have suggested interposing an inert biocompatible conducting material such as a hydrogel between the electrode and the endocardium to reduce mechanical irritation.[102] It is even possible to impregnate these materials with drugs such as anti-inflammatory agents. It should be recognized, however, that hydrogel-coated pacing electrodes could introduce new problems involving gel hydration and lead sterilization.

The use of local pharmacologic agents is a novel and highly effective way to counter the inflammatory reaction occurring at the electrode-tissue interface. For research purposes, drug delivery systems that dispense controlled doses of pharmacologic agents directly at the electrode-tissue interface have been developed and used in animal studies.[103, 104] The agents that have been studied include anti-inflammatory drugs, anticoagulants, and agents that prevent the formation of an extracellular matrix. Apart from glucocorticosteroids, no consistent improvement in stimulation threshold has been found, and in some cases significant deterioration in stimu-

lation threshold has occurred. For example, heparin inhibits fibrin formation and prevents the development of a protective fibrous barrier during acute inflammation, thus allowing more physical damage to occur.[103] Other agents that prevent extracellular matrix formation without altering the inflammatory response, namely, tunicamycin and *cis*-hydroxyproline, also cause an elevation in stimulation threshold,[104] indicating that prevention of inflammation is the most important consideration in reducing the chronic stimulation threshold. Based on these studies, it is not surprising that glucocorticosteroid-eluting electrodes, because of their potent anti-inflammatory action, significantly reduce both peak and chronic stimulation threshold levels.[103, 104] Glucocorticosteroids are believed to limit both the early and late stages of inflammation. For implantable pacing leads, dexamethasone sodium phosphate has been found to be much more effective than prednisolone.[103] Prednisolone, unlike dexamethasone, has a high affinity for proteins, rendering the protein-bound drug pharmacologically inactive. The early edema at the electrode-tissue interface is protein-rich, and therefore minute amounts of prednisolone released by a drug-eluting device may be immediately inactivated.[103]

Dexamethasone sodium phosphate has now been used clinically in a number of pacing leads that have steroid-eluting electrodes. The original design included a platinum-coated titanium electrode.[105] The porous electrode is hemispherical in shape and has a geometric surface area of about 8 mm[2] (Fig. 3–8). Immediately behind the electrode lies a plug of silicone rubber impregnated with dexamethasone sodium phosphate. This plug is referred to as a ''monolithic controlled release device'' (MCRD), and the amount of elutable drug is less than 1 mg. Extensive experience with the steroid-eluting electrode, both in experimental animals and in humans, has demonstrated very low acute and chronic stimulation thresholds in both the atrium and the ventricle and has virtually eliminated the early postoperative peak.[99, 106–114] In particular, excellent results have been obtained in children[115] (a group known to have a high incidence of elevated stimulation thresholds) and in patients with a previous history of high-threshold exit block.[116, 117]

The precise role of dexamethasone sodium phosphate in

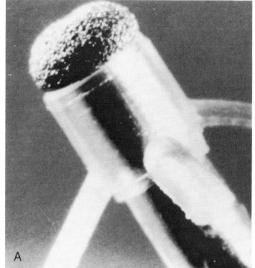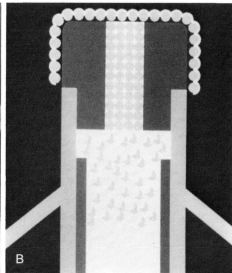

FIGURE 3–8. *A*, Porous surface, steroid-eluting electrode (Medtronic Capsure 4003). The electrode is platinum-covered titanium. *B*, Cross-sectional diagram of the same electrode showing the silicone rubber plug impregnated with dexamethasone sodium phosphate lying immediately behind the electrode. (*A* and *B* courtesy of Medtronic Inc.)

this first-generation electrode was initially uncertain. It was considered possible that the unique design and materials of the electrode may have been responsible for the favorable results. However, it has now been demonstrated conclusively that it is the steroid that prevents the rise in stimulation threshold.[99, 118] Histologically, the chronic inflammatory reaction is diminished by steroid[119, 120] despite the fact that the drug is not present in sufficient quantity to prevent or significantly reduce inflammation, as measured by the presence and numbers of phagocytic cells. However, it does appear to be present in sufficient concentration to prevent or minimize the release of the damaging inflammatory mediators, both acutely and chronically, thereby attenuating formation of the fibrous capsule.[100]

The ability of glucocorticosteroids to lower stimulation thresholds has been shown to persist for at least 8 years of clinical follow-up (Fig. 3–9). It is probable that once the initial inflammation subsides, minimal further chronic inflammation occurs, thus allowing the stimulation threshold to remain stable and low under the influence of steroid elution. A thin fibrous capsule may help to prevent mechanical irritation of the endocardium by the electrode surface and may also act as a physical barrier, which is believed to retard but not stop excessive elution of steroid from the electrode. Sufficient steroid can still find its way into the electrode-tissue interface to maintain a chronic anti-inflammatory effect. The rate of elution in vivo has been shown to decrease exponentially with time. Analysis of explanted steroid-eluting leads has shown that about 20% of the steroid still remains in the silicone plug after 4 years.[121] Based on this knowledge, it is more than likely that the steroid will last the life of the great majority of patients who receive pacing leads with this capability. Uncertainty still remains, however, about whether steroid is necessary only during the acute inflammatory phase. Studies need to be conducted to confirm this hypothesis.

Steroid-eluting electrodes are associated with excellent sensing properties as well. The long-term sensing performance has been investigated in several studies, which have shown excellent R-wave amplitudes measured at lead implantation, coupled with long-term sensing thresholds and telemetered ventricular electrograms.[106, 108, 112, 113, 122–124] Other studies have shown that R-wave sensing with steroid-eluting electrodes is superior to that achieved with standard electrodes.[125, 126] This improvement in sensing is probably a result of the steroid-mediated reduction of the inflammatory response. Steroid-eluting electrodes have also shown superior P-wave sensing compared with platinized porous-platinum (Medtronic Target Tip) electrodes.[112] However, from the data that are available, it is not possible to determine whether the differences in sensing are due to the steroid or to the electrode design.

The original steroid-eluting electrode was composed of platinum-coated titanium. Without steroid elution, this electrode is associated with relatively high and unpredictable stimulation thresholds, which are appreciably higher than those achieved with the platinized porous-platinum Target Tip electrode.[99] When the mean chronic stimulation thresholds from a standard platinized porous-platinum electrode were compared with those of the steroid-eluting platinized porous-platinum electrode, only minor differences were noted, particularly 3 years after implantation.[100] There was, however, a small, somewhat attenuated peak with the platinized porous-platinum electrode and a slight but persistently higher stimulation threshold.[122, 127] These results contrast with the data obtained from the polished platinum ring electrode, which mimics results obtained from the steroid-free titanium electrode as well as from other designs of polished and porous-platinum electrodes.[122, 128] The platinized porous-platinum electrode is, therefore, far superior to the polished platinum or porous-titanium electrode without steroid. Controversy remains about whether a steroid-eluting electrode is really necessary when almost comparable chronic data can be achieved with electrodes composed of microporous carbon or platinized porous platinum. All steroid-free electrodes still tend to develop an unpredictable acute peak stimulation threshold, which makes it necessary to program pulse generators at implantation to a 5-V output and 0.5-msec pulse width to ensure an adequate margin of safety. Despite the low mean chronic stimulation thresholds seen with platinized porous-platinum electrodes, unpredictable rises in chronic stimulation threshold still occur.[129] With steroid-eluting electrodes, significant chronic stimulation threshold rises have not been reported providing that mechanical causes such as myocardial penetration, perforation, or lead dislodgment have been excluded. Patients receiving a steroid-eluting electrode at implantation coupled with a good lead design and implantation technique can be safely paced from the day of implantation at 2.5 V. When stimulation threshold is measured regularly, the majority of patients with steroid-eluting electrodes can be safely paced at 1.6 V.[130] The ability to use these low-current drains safely has important ramifications for pulse generator longevity and size, especially in patients with dual-chamber and rate-responsive systems. As discussed earlier, steroid-eluting electrodes are clearly superior to other electrodes in patients with previously documented exit block, and they should be used whenever such patients are encountered.

With the technical and clinical information currently avail-

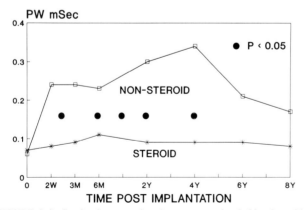

STEROID (4003) Vs NON STEROID (4003)
Mean Autothreshold Pulse Width(1.5V)

FIGURE 3–9. Graphs demonstrating the mean autothreshold pulse width reduction values (msec) at 1.5-V output from two series of identical Medtronic Capsure 4003 electrodes, one with steroid and one without steroid. From 2 weeks post implantation, the lead containing steroid had statistically superior stimulation threshold levels. From 3 to 8 years post implantation, the stimulation threshold values remained markedly different but not statistically significant because of the small numbers of patients remaining in the study. W, weeks; M, months; Y, years.

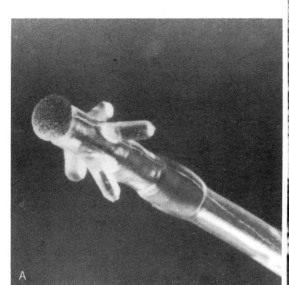
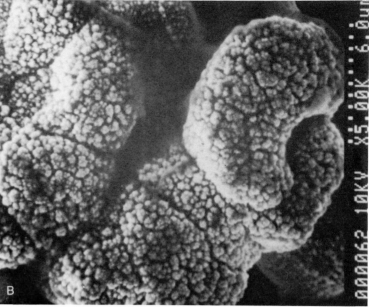

FIGURE 3–10. *A*, The platinized porous-platinum, steroid-eluting electrode of the Medtronic Capsure SP 5023 device has a 5.8-mm² surface area. *B*, Scanning electron microscopic photograph of the same electrode at 5000× magnification. (*A* and *B* courtesy of Medtronic Inc.)

able about stimulation threshold and polarization, a number of new leads have been designed with more advanced electrodes. A steroid-eluting, platinized microporous-platinum electrode with a 5.8-mm² surface area (Fig. 3–10) has completed clinical trials[131–133] and has been found to have lower stimulation thresholds than the original platinum-coated titanium design.[134] It also provides improved or higher lead impedances than its predecessor. A steroid-eluting epicardial lead has also been described.[135] Unlike other permanent pacing leads implanted using a transthoracic approach, the electrode is not a helical screw. Therefore, this lead is not myocardial. The electrode is a platinized porous-platinum button-shaped configuration that can be duplicated in a bipolar design (Fig. 3–11). As in the original transvenous steroid-eluting electrode, there is a silicone rubber plug impregnated with dexamethasone sodium phosphate behind the electrode. The mechanism of steroid elution and its effects on the inflammatory response are believed to be similar to those in the endocardial lead design. Early animal data comparing models with and without steroid and implanted in both the atrium and the ventricle have shown very encouraging results,[136] as have the initial implant data in the pediatric age group.[137] This suggests that such an electrode can be placed on the epicardium and that the steroid can adequately inhibit inflammation, fibrosis, and the associated rise in stimulation threshold. Such a lead would be particularly helpful in pediatric patients.[138, 139]

A silicone rubber plug within the electrode is not the only method by which steroid can be delivered to the electrode-tissue interface. Another electrode design makes use of a porous-ceramic or silicone rubber collar impregnated with dexamethasone sodium phosphate. This drug-eluting collar is positioned immediately proximal to the tip electrode. Human studies have shown a significant reduction in stimulation thresholds in patients with these electrodes with both unipolar[140–145] and bipolar[146] leads. There may be a significant advantage in placing the steroid-eluting device outside the elec-

trode. For example, the steroid-eluting collar could be incorporated into an active-fixation screw-in lead (Fig. 3–12). Animal studies using such leads have shown significantly lower stimulation thresholds than those seen with comparable leads without steroid.[147, 148]

Another steroid-eluting lead has a titanium nitride–coated, 3.5-mm² hemispherical electrode. This electrode is further coated with an ion-exchange membrane impregnated with

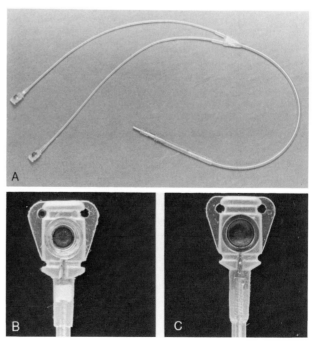

FIGURE 3–11. *A*, Bipolar, platinized porous-platinum, steroid-eluting electrodes designed to be sutured to the epicardium (Medtronic investigational model 10366). *B* and *C*, Detailed views of the electrodes showing the cathode on the left and the anode on the right. See text for details. (*A–C* courtesy of Medtronic Inc.)

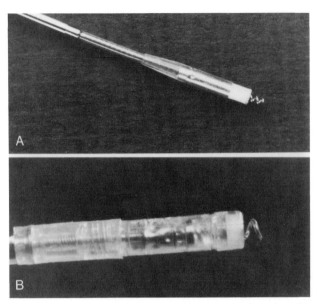

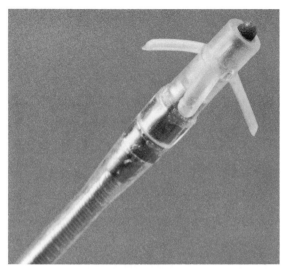

FIGURE 3–13. Medtronic's Nanotip electrode (investigational model 10331). (Courtesy of Medtronic Inc.)

FIGURE 3–12. *A*, Active-fixation lead with a porous electrode and an electrically inert screw. Surrounding the electrode is a silicone rubber collar impregnated with dexamethasone sodium phosphate. (Courtesy of Telectronics Pacing Systems.) *B*, Active-fixation lead with an electrically active screw. There is a steroid-eluting collar surrounding the screw. (Courtesy of Medtronic Inc.)

dexamethasone sodium phosphate. Canine and early human clinical studies have shown very low stimulation thresholds at implantation with almost no elevation in stimulation thresholds through follow-up to 1 year.[149]

To date very little clinical work has been done on pacing electrodes smaller than 3 mm² because of theoretical concerns about exit block and undersensing of R waves and P waves. Using various electrode configurations with surface areas as small as 1.0 mm², animal studies have confirmed that excellent stimulation thresholds and higher pacing impedances can be obtained with both steroid-eluting and steroid-free electrodes (Fig. 3–13).[57] These 1000-ohm electrodes employ microporous coatings to increase the actual surface area, thus improving intracardiac sensing. Such electrodes are now undergoing clinical trials.

Lead Fixation

Transvenous leads may be attached to the endocardium either actively or passively. Active-fixation leads incorporate devices that invade the endomyocardium, whereas passive-fixation leads promote fixation by indirect means. When correctly implanted, both fixation mechanisms result in an extremely low incidence of lead dislodgment.

PASSIVE FIXATION

The first attempt to attach a fixation device to a lead was made by using a wedge or flange at the tip. Although this device probably reduced the incidence of lead dislodgment, carefully controlled studies were never performed.[150] Other early passive-fixation designs included the Helifix electrode[151] (Vitatron Medical B.V., Dieren, the Netherlands) and the balloon-tip lead[152] (Siemens Elema, Solna, Sweden [now

Siemens Pacesetter]), neither of which was commercially successful because difficulties were encountered with implantation and a high incidence of operative and postoperative complications was reported.[143, 153] In the late 1970s small tines positioned immediately behind the electrode were introduced, and within a few years these leads had revolutionized implantation techniques and resulted in a very low incidence of lead dislodgment (see Figs. 3–3, 3–4, and 3–6).[154] A variety of other passive-fixation designs have been introduced including wings, cones, and fins (Fig. 3–14). Tines and other devices are extensions of the insulation material that are designed to become entrapped within the trabeculae of the right atrial appendage and right ventricle. Today, tined leads remain the most popular method of lead fixation, particularly in the right ventricle.[155]

ACTIVE FIXATION

Most transvenous active-fixation leads are composed of an electrically active (cathode) screw at the distal end of the

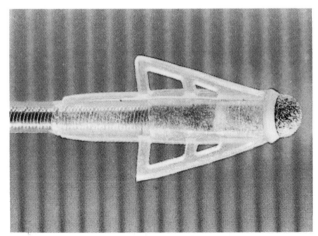

FIGURE 3–14. Telectronics steroid-eluting tined lead (Encor Dec 033–301). Behind the porous electrode is a silicone rubber collar impregnated with dexamethasone. (Courtesy of Telectronics Pacing Systems.)

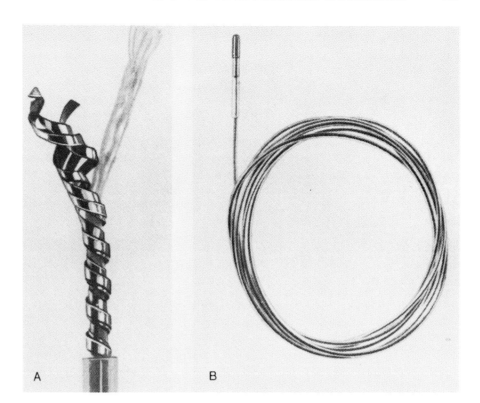

FIGURE 3–15. Elema-Schonander (now Siemens Pacesetter) EM 588. *A*, Conductor showing the stainless steel ribbons wrapped around the central terylene core. *B*, Lead with a 100-mm² electrode and no fixation device. The insulator is polyethylene. (*A* and *B* courtesy of Siemens Pacesetter.)

A   B

lead. The original designs had a fixed, unprotected screw that could damage the venous and intracardiac structures during lead insertion. Newer designs with retractable screws have become popular, particularly for atrial use.[156] Unlike tined leads, active-fixation leads traumatize the endomyocardium and result in significant elevations of stimulation thresholds after implantation.[157] In one attempt to improve these stimulation thresholds, the screw was electrically insulated from the conductor and protruded centrally from a porous ring-shaped cathode. Although the electrode itself was passive, continual rubbing against the endocardium resulted in even higher stimulation thresholds than occurred with the electrically active screw design.[157] A steroid-eluting collar immediately behind the screw may decrease the stimulation thresholds in these active-fixation leads (see Fig. 3–12).

Lead Conductors

The conductor of a pacing lead is the coil of wire that conducts the electric current from the pulse generator to the stimulating electrode. Unipolar leads require one conducting coil, whereas bipolar leads require two. The conductors are also responsible for conducting the sensed cardiac signals (intrinsic or evoked) from the electrodes to the sensing amplifier of the pulse generator. One of the original and most reliable conductors was a design commonly used in the 1960s that was composed of four tinsel ribbons of stainless steel wrapped around a central terylene core (Fig. 3–15). Such a multistrand lead provided redundant current pathways and had immense flexibility and a low incidence of conductor fracture. Transvenous implantation of this lead was very difficult because there was no method for stiffening the lead to guide the tip to the apex of the right ventricle. A major

advance in pacemaker implantation occurred with the introduction of helically coiled conductors. Originally these consisted of a single strand of tightly coiled wire wound with an empty core, which allowed the passage of a stainless steel stylet to the tip electrode. The introduction of stylets for stiffening the lead greatly improved the ease of implantation. Such leads were relatively prone to fracture, however, particularly at stress points such as sites where anchoring ligatures were applied, where the conductor entered a lead connector, or where the lead was encased in an endocardial bridge within the heart. In these situations, the point of fracture was a fulcrum in which one side of the conductor moved differently from the other. Thus, one side of the conducting wire was in tension while the other was in compression. To make the conductor more flexible and more resistant to fracture, two or more wires were combined in a multifilar coil arrangement (Fig. 3–16). This created a system of redundancy if a fracture occurred in one of the conductor wires and greatly reduced the clinical occurrence of lead fracture.

The original conductor materials were stainless steel and platinum. These materials were later replaced by more corrosion-resistant alloys with improved fatigue resistance such as MP35N, an alloy of nickel, chromium, cobalt, and molybdenum. To further reduce resistance to current flow, specialized conductors were designed, including the drawn brazed strand (DBS)[158] and the drawn filled tube (DFT)[143] designs. These wires were composed of a central core of highly conductive material such as silver surrounded by a more durable corrosion-resistant material such as MP35N (see Fig. 3–16). The direct current (DC) resistance of such leads may be only several ohms, less than 10% of MP35N alone. Modern conductors undergo intense fatigue and fracture testing by continual bending of the lead to a specific angle or over a specified radius. With bipolar leads, conductor fractures have

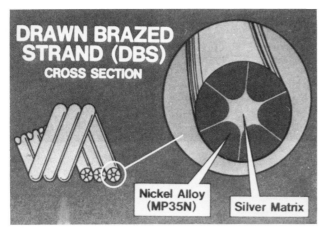

FIGURE 3–16. Cross-section of a drawn brazed strand lead conductor showing the silver matrix surrounded by MP35N. (Courtesy of Medtronic Inc.)

been responsible for a large proportion of chronic lead complications, although a variety of design changes have improved conductor strength, flexibility, and resistance to fatigue.

Bipolar transvenous leads obviously require two conductors. In the original configuration a parallel arrangement of dual-lumen insulation tubing was used with a single insulator surrounding both conductors. The coaxial design allows the creation of a much smaller circumference of the body of the lead with a single inner lumen for stylet control and an even distribution of insulating material around the outer conductor. The inner coil connects to the cathodal tip and is separated from the outer coil by an inner insulating tube. Such leads are only slightly thicker than unipolar designs. As discussed previously, despite the considerable advantages of the coaxial lead design, the long-term reliability of these leads appears to be less than that of unipolar leads.

The recent development of *coated wire technology* has allowed the manufacture of thin bipolar leads whose outside diameter is nearly as small as that of unipolar leads. This technique involves coating single strands of conductor wire with a very thin layer of insulation. Two or more conductors can be grouped together into a multifilar single coil, which is then placed within another insulated tube to form a lead body that has virtually the same flexibility and handling characteristics as a unipolar lead (Fig. 3–17). For example, with a quadrifilar coil, two of the insulated wires can be connected to the cathodal electrode, while the other two are attached to the anodal electrode of a bipolar lead. With such a lead, stylet passage to the tip may be difficult owing to the friction of the stylet against the insulating coating on the wires. However, because it is so thin, it is hoped that the design will eliminate the complications seen with traditional bipolar leads including the occurrence of subclavian crush injury and the problems associated with stiffness that were discussed earlier. Because it is multifilar, there is virtually no limit to the number of conductors that can be used in such a lead, thus extending its use to sensor technology.

Nonmetals such as plastics or carbon can also be used as the conductors in pacing leads. For example, a carbon fiber conductor has been suggested in which as many as 3000 fibers in two bundles are placed around a central insulated core for stylet insertion. Short-term animal studies have

shown that this design has adequate strength, duration, and biocompatibility.[159] Because of the problems of conductor fracture, a *fail-safe* lead has been suggested by Green, in which a standard primary conductor is surrounded by a secondary conductor medium such as a liquid gel or paste.[160] Because such materials are not readily available and because the leads could be very difficult to manufacture and sterilize, lead manufacturers have opted to stay with and improve the reliability of the proven coil conductors.

Unlike endocardial leads, epimyocardial leads do not require a stylet for implantation. Thus, there is considerably more flexibility in the design of epicardial conductors. Most epimyocardial leads use a tinsel wire conductor. Despite this, lead conductor fractures remain a significant problem with epimyocardial leads because of the greater stresses imposed by the movement of the heart, diaphragm, and abdominal muscles. In addition, because these types of conductors are not stretchable, it is possible that the higher stimulation thresholds that occur with epimyocardial leads may be due in part to the inability of the lead to adapt to the vigorous movements within the chest. Epimyocardial leads with stretchable conductor coils are now being designed.[130]

Lead Insulation

One of the earliest insulating materials used for permanent pacemaker leads was polyethylene (see Fig. 3–15). This material had excellent biocompatibility and reasonable biostability. However, as an insulator for pacing leads, polyethylene was stiff, thick, difficult to bond, and abraded by nonpolished metals, and it was found to have poor long-term performance.[161] During the 1960s silicone rubber (MDX4-4515-50A) became very popular as an insulating material for pacing leads. Although highly biocompatible and biostable, this material has relatively low tear strength and could be easily damaged during surgery by sharp instruments or tight ligatures. To compensate for the relatively low tear strength of silicone rubber, a thick layer of insulation was required, making the lead diameter considerably larger than leads designed with polyethylene. Another disadvantage of silicone rubber is its high coefficient of friction, which makes it difficult to pass one lead over another during implantation of two leads for dual-chamber pacing. This potential disadvantage of silicone rubber has recently been overcome by the

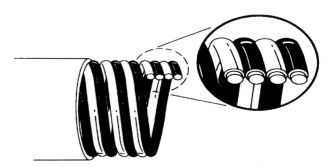

FIGURE 3–17. Schematic representation of single-coil multiconductor technology. Each conductor strand is individually coated with a very thin layer of insulator, and the multiconductor single helical coil is then insulated again with a thicker conventional insulator. (Courtesy of Telectronics Pacing Systems.)

technique of surface polishing or coating the lead with a highly lubricious material called *fast-pass coating*.[103] During the late 1970s a stronger and tougher high-performance silicone rubber insulator (ETR Q747-50A) was introduced that allowed manufacture of thinner leads. Lead manipulation, however, could be difficult because the insulator tended to stretch or elongate if the lead was pulled back after it was entrapped in the trabeculae or chordae. The stiffening stylet was then not able to reach the tip of the lead to allow remanipulation.

Polyurethane, a generic name for a very large family of synthetic polymers, was first used clinically as an insulator for transvenous pacing leads in 1978.[162] As a group, the polyurethanes have very high tensile and tear strengths, good flexibility, and a low coefficient of friction when wet with blood.[163] Polyurethanes have over 18 times the friction coefficient of silicone rubber, making them much easier to insert and pass along venous channels.[164] Other advantages include properties of biocompatibility and noncarcinogenicity much like those of silicone rubber. Its low thrombogenicity is comparable to that of silicone rubber.[165] Unfortunately, many polyurethanes degrade rapidly in the body as a result of enzymatic activity. Others cannot be extruded and injection-molded into insulation tubing suitable for pacing leads. One group, the Pellethanes 2363 (Upjohn Co., CPR Division, Torrance, CA), was found to be biostable and suitable for pacing lead insulation.

The properties of polyurethanes vary according to the *soft* and *hard* segments of the polymer molecular chain used. The soft segments are composed of polyether or polyesther chains, and the hard segments are made of urea or urethanes. Structurally, segmented polyurethanes are composed of a core of hard segments surrounded by soft skin composed of soft segments. The hard and soft segments are thermodynamically immiscible, thus tending to separate. It is this structural feature that determines the mechanical and surface properties of polyurethane.[166]

Because it was possible to manufacture very thin polyurethane insulating tubing for pacing leads, polyurethane leads became extremely popular. By 1983, however, a number of disturbing reports appeared questioning the long-term integrity and reliability of this insulating material. These reports described in vivo degradation of implanted polyurethane with surface cracking and subsequent insulation failure.[167–172] It soon became clear that polyurethane insulation failures were in part related to specific manufacturing processes in certain leads using the polyurethane insulating material Pellethane 80A.

The tendency of the hard and soft segments to separate, as described earlier, creates inherent stresses in segmented polyurethanes.[166] These in turn can be intensified during manufacture and in particular during the cooling process following extrusion. In this step the molten polymer is forced through a die or into a mold, after which it is rapidly cooled. Polyurethane tubing manufactured by the extrusion technique causes the surface molecules to cool quickly and contract and results in surface tension. However, the core molecules remain hot and therefore in compression. A zero stress boundary or neutral axis remains between the surface and the core, the depth of which depends on the manufacturing processes used.[169] This results in surface cracking or crazing, which can be further exacerbated by ongoing lead manufacturing proc-

esses such as expansion and shrinking of the insulator during insertion of the conductor coil,[173] stretching and bonding, and surface trauma during and following implantation. In a corrosive biologic environment, lipid and protein absorption may be deposited onto the damaged surface, causing swelling, which disrupts the surface organization.[169] The resultant insulation degeneration, referred to as *environmental stress cracking (ESC)*, may lead to insulation failure when the cracking propagates through the full thickness of the insulator to the conductor.

Explanted leads using Pellethane 80A insulation have demonstrated varying degrees of ESC. The most minor change, which is very common, is referred to as *surface frosting* and consists of a whitish haze that does not result in functional clinical insulation failure (Fig. 3–18). The depth of the crack is typically 2.5 to 30 μm and is worst in areas subjected to applied strains during either manufacture or implantation.[169] With time and in the presence of environmental stresses, this process may progress to insulation failure. The more significant ESC changes seen in explanted leads occur in areas where excessive strains are applied during manufacture or at implantation, particularly with ligatures around the lead.[48] They may also occur where the lead insulation lies between the clavicle and the first rib when a lead is introduced by subclavian puncture.[46, 47]

Clinical insulation failures reported in leads implanted using the cephalic vein approach are an interesting group.[174] A high incidence of insulation failure in leads made of Pellethane 80A has been noted by one of the authors (HM). In all cases, the cephalic vein approach was used, and visual inspection of the lead entry and collar ligation sites demonstrated surface frosting only. In other cases, leads extracted for other reasons showed patches of marked frosting near the electrode (see Fig. 3–18) and where the lead turns to enter the right ventricle from the right atrium. In these areas, endocardial tunnels may form around the lead where contact

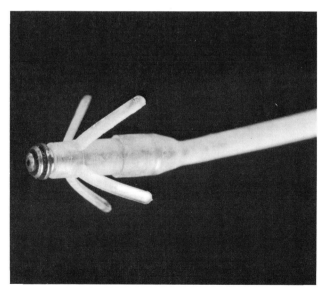

FIGURE 3–18. Medtronic Target Tip lead insulated with polyurethane showing crazing around the proximal portion of the lead where the polyurethane has been stretched around the terminal portion of the lead. This portion of the lead was buried beneath and between trabeculae and was subjected to extra forces related to cardiac movement at the apex of the right ventricle.

with the endocardium is made, resulting in excessive stresses on the insulation. It is possible, therefore, that intracardiac sites may also be responsible for insulation failures.

Metal-induced oxidation (MIO) is another reported mechanism of insulation failure. MIO is an oxidative degradation of the polyurethane insulation and involves a reaction of the polymer with oxygen that is believed to be released by hydrogen peroxide, which comes from inflammatory cells on the outer surface of the lead (Fig. 3–19).[175] A catalyst is required for the reaction to occur. These catalysts are probably metallic corrosion products from the conductor that result following ingress of body fluids onto the lead.[173] Although this fluid may result from breakdown of the insulation, fluid ingress has also been reported with breakdown of the bonding at the electrode-insulation junction and with stylet perforation during implantation.[176] Clinically, there may be failure of the outer insulation of unipolar and bipolar leads or of the inner insulation of bipolar leads. To minimize MIO, conductors can be barrier coated.[43] The objective is to cover the conductor coil with a submicroscopic layer of platinum, which is inert and minimizes the potential for metal ion release and thus interaction with the insulation materials.[177]

As a result of information gathered on the causes and mechanisms of ESC and MIO, manufacturing changes were instituted to overcome the problems encountered with Pellethane 80A.[178] Despite this, questionable long-term implant performance continues to plague some of the more recent generations of bipolar leads that use the same Pellethane 80A polyurethane, in particular, the Medtronic models 4012 and 4004 bipolar tined leads.[43, 174, 179–182] Unipolar leads have not shown an increased incidence of insulation problems apart from those caused by trauma at surgery or at ligature sites.[183–185]

Some currently available polyurethane-insulated leads are composed of Pellethane 55D. This polyurethane is stiffer and harder than Pellethane 80A owing to the presence of significantly fewer polyether segments.[186] Pacing leads using Pellethane 55D insulation are consequently much stiffer than those of a similar size composed of Pellethane 80A and may therefore be more prone to perforate the right ventricle.[40] The long-term clinical results of Pellethane 55D have shown much better biostability than Pellethane 80A.[44, 187, 188]

New versions of polyurethanes currently being tested do not use polyether segments and are soft and flexible but just as strong as the current polyurethanes. These polymers do not seem to suffer from the degradation mechanisms noted earlier. The results of early testing indicate a very promising future for lead insulation.[189]

Questions remain about whether a controversy about polyurethane still exists. A number of early-model Pellethane 80A-insulated leads have demonstrated unacceptable clinical

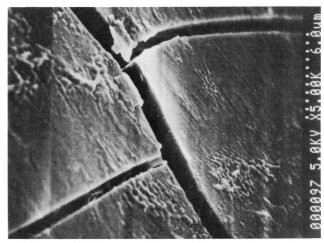

FIGURE 3–19. Scanning electron microscopic photograph of a polyurethane lead showing insulation cracking due to metal-induced oxidation.

failure rates owing to well-recognized problems with the insulation. Whether these problems with Pellethane 80A have now been corrected only time will tell. Some investigators believe that there is no current controversy about polyurethane insulation.[178, 190, 191] Pellethane 55D-insulated leads, however, although free of the degradation problems of Pellethane 80A-insulated leads, are difficult to implant and prone to right ventricular perforation owing to the stiffness of the lead. A comparison of the physical parameters of silicone rubber and polyurethanes used as insulators for pacing leads is shown in Table 3–2.

New varieties of polyurethane are being investigated, and combinations of silicone rubber and polyurethane may be clinically acceptable. The major part of the body of the lead may be made of polyurethane, but at the distal end, where the lead lies inside the ventricle, the insulation may be made of a softer silicone rubber. Another alternative is to use insulating tubing composed of a thin but tough protective outer coating of polyurethane over thin, high-performance silicone rubber in a coaxial arrangement.[178] Silicone rubber remains a popular insulating material for pacing leads. It requires a thicker layer to protect the conductor, and long-term results are excellent.[192] In addition, the insulator is soft, and perforation of the right ventricle is very rare when the lead is correctly implanted.[40]

Lead Connectors

The connector is the portion of the lead used to connect the lead to the pulse generator. The original pacing leads had

TABLE 3–2. **LEAD INSULATION COMPARISONS**

	COMMON INSULATION TYPES			
PHYSICAL PARAMETERS	POLYURETHANE PELLETHANE 2363-80A	POLYURETHANE PELLETHANE 2363-55D	SILICONE RUBBER MDX4-4515-50A	SILICONE RUBBER ETR Q747-50A
Durometer hardness	82A	55D	52A	50A
Ultimate tensile strength (psi)	4500	6900	1350	1300
Ultimate elongation (%)	550	390	450	900
Tear strength (psi)	470	650	80	230

no specialized connector. A small area of conductor at the proximal end was exposed and attached directly to the pulse generator using a small set-screw.[193] On occasion, the set-screw had a sharp cutting end, and exposure of the conductor was not necessary. This was tedious, time-consuming, and unreliable. Consequently, a proliferation of unique connectors developed. Eventually, two similar and very reliable unipolar connector designs emerged, one 5 mm in diameter and the other 6 mm. Both had to be used with a pulse generator that had the appropriate connector port, although the smaller size could be adapted to fit the larger. For bipolar pacing, two unipolar connectors were necessary. A major improvement in lead connectors was the low-profile, in-line bipolar design. An in-line connector places both electric terminals on a single lead pin with an insulating barrier separating the anode from the cathode. Because it was critical to prevent short circuiting between the terminals, a number of unique designs were introduced during the early 1980s. These designs were not always low in profile and in some cases were quite cumbersome (Fig. 3–20). With unique in-line designs, it is difficult or impossible to modify the connector to suit a pulse generator for which it is not designed. The connector–pulse generator compatibility problem has been a major clinical concern, especially at the time of pulse generator replacement. In some cases adapters can solve this problem, although occasionally a new lead is required. Not surprisingly, numerous pleas for standardization were made.[194–196]

With the initial impetus coming from the German pacing group, a meeting was held with a group of pacemaker manufacturers to plan development of a low-profile, in-line connector standard that would be suitable for both unipolar and bipolar leads.[197] Early progress was slow because the initial committee was multidisciplinary and represented only some of the pacemaker manufacturers. There was concern that a connector standard would be enforced without regard to future evolutionary developments, thus restricting innovation in lead and pulse generator design rather than enhancing it. Actually, this concern was probably justified because marked changes in pacemaker design were occurring during the early to late 1980s.[198]

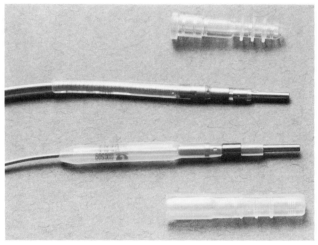

FIGURE 3–21. *Above,* Medtronic VS-1B bipolar 3.2-mm connector (long lead pin and no sealing rings) and 5-mm unipolar conversion sleeve. *Below,* Telectronics low-profile, unipolar 3.2-mm connector with a 5-mm upsizing sleeve. From external appearances the connectors appear to be similar, although the Telectronics ring is anodized (blue) to indicate that it is a protection sleeve and not an anode.

By late 1985, there was a low-profile 3.2-mm unipolar and bipolar pacemaker lead connector designated Voluntary Standard 1, or VS-1.[199] Pacemaker manufacturer rivalry, however, resulted in three variations of lead connector and pulse generator–connector cavity designs—the VS-1, VS-1A, and VS-1B. Sadly and not surprisingly, these variations were not totally interchangeable. The differences were mainly related to bipolar leads and concerned the length of the lead connector pin and the presence or absence of sealing rings on the connector (Fig. 3–21). The size of the connector pin is critical for bipolar leads. Although a long connector pin (VS-1A and VS-1B) will fit into the short receiving port of the VS-1 pulse generator, the proximal anodal ring contact of the connector may not mate correctly with the anodal terminal of the pulse generator. As a consequence, bipolar pacing and sensing may not be possible. To many pacemaker implanters, these subtle differences are not obvious until they are confronted with lead and pulse generator incompatibility either at surgery or postoperatively during pacemaker testing. Such errors are expensive and potentially very risky for the patient.

Sealing rings are an integral part of the insulating mechanism of low-profile in-line connectors. They do not, however, need to be on the lead connector itself because they can also reside within the receiving port of the pulse generator. Engineering principles usually demand that any sealing rings reside on the component to be replaced, in most cases, the pulse generator. This is because sealing rings may be damaged during replacement of the pulse generator, potentially compromising a pacing system if they are not part of the replaced hardware.

With these controversies in mind, a joint IEC/ISO International Pacemaker Standards Working Group (ISO TC150/SC2/WG2 and IEC62D/WG6) set about to define a formal international standard for lead connectors. The VS-1 lead connector design was adopted by the group to yield a standard that called for a low-profile connector with sealing rings on the lead, with the option of additional sealing rings inside

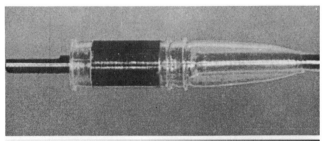

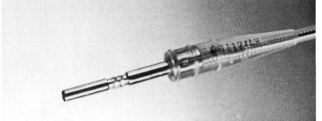

FIGURE 3–20. Early models of high-profile in-line bipolar connectors.

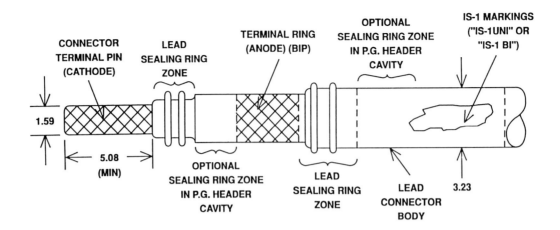

(NOMINAL DIMENSIONS SHOWN IN MM)

FIGURE 3–22. Schematic representation of an IS-1 standard lead connector.

the pulse generator–connector cavity. This final standard has been designated the IS-1 UNI for unipolar leads and IS-1 BI for bipolar leads and has now been adopted as the official international standard for lead connectors (see Fig. 3–15).

To help with the problem of VS-1–IS-1 incompatibility, there is flexibility for manufacturers of pulse generators with respect to the length of the bore for the lead pin within the connector cavity and the presence or absence of sealing rings in the connector cavity. It is imperative, therefore, that prior to pulse generator replacement the implanter check the compatibility of the implanted lead and the proposed pulse generator.

In addition, the similarity of unipolar and bipolar leads can also be a potential problem in that the IS-1 standard calls for these lead connectors to be interchangeable. To prevent a unipolar lead from being inadvertently attached to a bipolar pulse generator that does not have polarity programming, the labeling for both lead and pulse generator must be carefully inspected. To prevent damage to a unipolar IS-1 lead connector from the anode set-screw of a bipolar connector cavity, a protective ring may be assembled by the manufacturer over the lead connector at the appropriate position (Fig. 3–22). This ring, however, may be mistaken for a true anode terminal, and the lead may be thought to be bipolar. Although the manufacturer's intentions are good, the results at surgery may be potentially disastrous should a unipolar lead be implanted with a bipolar pulse generator.

In terms of backward compatibility of IS-1 leads to older pulse generators, unipolar and bipolar low-profile connectors can be easily converted to the standard 5-mm unipolar design by the use of a sleeve (see Fig. 3–22). This capability will be very useful during the transition phase when IS-1 and VS-1 leads are used with older style connector pulse generators.

Summary

In recent years remarkable advances have been made in the design of pacing leads. The most important change has been the development of small porous electrodes that provide extremely low chronic stimulation thresholds and low polar-ization characteristics. It is important not to forget the less heralded advances in conductor and insulator technology. These advances have resulted in safer and more reliable leads. In addition, the remarkable international and intercompany cooperation that resulted in the development of the IS-1 lead connector standard has effected a major improvement in the clinical practice of cardiac pacing.

REFERENCES

1. Mond HG: Unipolar versus bipolar pacing—poles apart. PACE 14:1411, 1991.
2. Mond H, Strathmore N, Hunt P, et al: Bipolar and unipolar permanent pacing leads—which is superior? PACE 12:678, 1989.
3. Barold SS, Gaidula JJ: Failure of demand pacemaker from low-voltage bipolar ventricular electrograms. JAMA 215:923, 1971.
4. Yates JD, Preston TA: Failure of demand function in temporary epicardial bipolar pacemaker systems. Ann Thorac Surg 15:135, 1973.
5. Breivik K, Ohm O-J, Engedal H: Long-term comparison of unipolar and bipolar pacing and sensing, using a new multiprogrammable pacemaker system. PACE 6:592, 1983.
6. Czermin J, Kaliman J, Laczovics A, et al: Unipolar versus bipolar pacing—a prospective, intrapatient, long-term study. PACE 10:663, 1987.
7. Binner L, Richter P, Wieshammer S, et al: Bipolar versus unipolar mode in dual-chamber pacing: Comparison of myopotential interference, acute and long-term pacing, and sensing thresholds. PACE 10:646, 1987.
8. DeCaprio V, Hurzeler P, Furman S: A comparison of unipolar and bipolar electrograms for cardiac pacemaker sensing. Circulation 56:750, 1977.
9. Klementowicz P, Andrews C, Furman S: Superior bipolar sensing: A prospective study. J Am Coll Cardiol 9:31A, 1987.
10. Masterson M, Yuzcu EM, Maloney JD, et al: Atrial pacing and sensing: Unipolar versus bipolar. Seven different leads compared. PACE 10:435, 1987.
11. De Boer H, Kofflard M, Scholtes T, et al: Differential bipolar sensing of a dual-chamber pacemaker. PACE 11:158, 1988.
12. Griffin JC: Sensing characteristics of the right atrial appendage electrode. PACE 6:22, 1983.
13. Levine PA, Venditti FJ, Podrid PJ, et al: Therapeutic and diagnostic benefits of intentional crosstalk-mediated ventricular output inhibition. PACE 11:1194, 1988.
14. Young TE, Byrd CL, Winn CM, et al: Crosstalk update in state-of-the-art-pacemakers. PACE 8:791, 1985.
15. Irwin M, Cameron D, Louis C, et al: Crosstalk-stimulation of the ventricle in the implanted dual unipolar system. PACE 11:508, 1988.

16. Reynolds D, Combs W, Bennett T: "Crosstalk" in bipolar DDD pacemakers. PACE 10:734, 1987.
17. Midei MG, Levine JH, Walford GD, et al: Incidence of myopotential interference and crosstalk inhibition in unipolar and bipolar dual-chamber pacemakers. PACE 10:1010, 1987.
18. Sweesy MW, Batey RL, Forney RC: Crosstalk during bipolar pacing. PACE 11:1512, 1988.
19. Combs WJ, Reynolds DW, Sharma AD, et al: Cross-talk in bipolar pacemakers. PACE 12:1613, 1989.
20. Byrd CL, Schwartz SJ, Gonzales M, et al: Rate-responsive pacemakers and crosstalk. PACE 11:798, 1988.
21. Barold SS, Falkoff MD, Ong LS, et al: Arrhythmias caused by dual-chambered pacing. *In* Steinbach K, Glogar D, Laszkovics A, et al (eds): Cardiac Pacing. Proceedings of the VIIth World Symposium on Cardiac Pacing. Darmstadt, Steinkopff Verlag, 1983, pp 505–510.
22. Barold SS, Falkoff MD, Ong LS, et al: Timing cycles of DDD pacemakers. *In* Barold SS, Mugica J (eds): New Perspectives in Cardiac Pacing. Mt. Kisco, NY, Futura, 1988, pp 69–119.
23. Mymin D, Cuddy TE, Sinha SN, et al: Inhibition of demand pacemakers by skeletal muscle potentials. JAMA 223:527, 1973.
24. Ohm O-J, Bruland H, Pederson OM, et al: Interference effect of myopotentials on function of unipolar demand pacemakers. Br Heart J 36:77, 1974.
25. Redd R, McAnulty J, Phillips S, et al: Demand pacemaker inhibition by isometric skeletal muscle contraction. Circulation 50 (Suppl 49):III-241, 1974.
26. Gribbin B, Abson CP, Clarke LM: Inhibition of external demand pacemakers during muscular activity. Br Heart J 36:1210, 1974.
27. Anderson ST, Pitt A, Whitford JA: Interference with function of unipolar pacemaker due to muscle potentials. J Thorac Cardiovasc Surg 71:698, 1976.
28. Jacobs LJ, Kerzner JS, Diamond MA, et al: Myopotential inhibition of demand pacemakers: Detection by ambulatory electrocardiography. Am Heart J 101:346, 1981.
29. Jacobs LJ, Kerzner JS, Diamond MA: Pacemaker inhibition by myopotentials detected by Holter monitoring. PACE 5:30, 1982.
30. Furman S: Electromagnetic interference. PACE 5:1, 1982.
31. Hauser RG: Bipolar leads for cardiac pacing in the 1980s: A reappraisal provoked by skeletal muscle interference. PACE 5:34, 1982.
32. Secemsky SI, Hauser RG, Denes P, et al: Unipolar sensing abnormalities: Incidence and clinical significance of skeletal muscle interference and undersensing in 228 patients. PACE 5:10, 1982.
33. Berger R, Jacobs W: Myopotential inhibition of demand pacemakers: Etiologic, diagnostic, and therapeutic considerations. PACE 2:596, 1979.
34. Hurvitz RJ, Meyer BW, Lindesmith GG, et al: Skeletal muscle potential (myopotential) inhibition of demand pacemakers. PACE 2:A-105, 1979.
35. Echeverria HJ, Luceri RM, Thurber RJ, et al: Myopotential inhibition of unipolar AV sequential (DVI) pacemaker. PACE 5:20, 1982.
36. Fetter J, Hall D, Hoff GL, et al: The effects of myopotential interference on unipolar and bipolar dual-chamber pacemakers in the DDD mode. Clin Prog Electrophysiol Pacing 3:368, 1985.
37. Zimmern SH, Clark MF, Austin WK, et al: Characteristics and clinical effects of myopotential signals in a unipolar DDD pacemaker population. PACE 9:1019, 1986.
38. Exworthy KW: Electromagnetic compatibility of pacemaker systems. *In* Meere C (ed): Proceedings of the VIth World Symposium on Cardiac Pacing. Montreal, Pacesymp, 1979, Chap 35–7.
39. Reis R: Potential interference with medical electronic devices. Bull NY Acad Med 55:1216, 1979.
40. Cameron J, Ciddor G, Mond H, et al: Stiffness of the distal tip of bipolar pacemaker leads. PACE 13:1915, 1990.
41. Merx W, Han J, Yoon M: Effects of unipolar cathodal and bipolar stimulation on vulnerability of ischemic ventricles to fibrillation. Am J Cardiol 35:37, 1975.
42. Molajo AO, Burgess L: Comparison of paced evoked response sensing of transvenous porous platinum ventricular leads during unipolar and bipolar pacing. PACE 12:678, 1989.
43. Medtronic Inc: Product performance report, February 1993. Minneapolis, Medtronic Inc, 1993.
44. Furman S, Benedek ZM, and the Implantable Lead Registry: Survival of implantable pacemaker leads. PACE 13:1910, 1990.
45. Hayes DL: Pacemaker polarity configuration—what is best for the patient? PACE 15:1099, 1992.
46. Jacobs DM, Fink AS, Miller RP, et al: Anatomical and morphological evaluation of pacemaker lead compression. PACE 16:434, 1993.
47. Magney JE, Flynn DM, Parsons JA, et al: Anatomical mechanisms explaining damage to pacemaker leads, defibrillator leads, and failure of central venous catheters adjacent to the sternoclavicular joint. PACE 16:445, 1993.
48. Sweesy MW, Forney CC, Hayes DL, et al: Evaluation of an in-line bipolar poyurethane ventricular pacing lead. PACE 15:1982, 1992.
49. Mond H: The Cardiac Pacemaker: Function and Malfunction. New York, Grune & Stratton, 1973, pp 60–66.
50. Furman S, Parker B, Escher DJW: Decreasing electrode size and increasing efficiency of cardiac stimulation. J Surg Res 11:105, 1971.
51. Smyth NPD, Tarjan PP, Chernoff E, et al: The significance of electrode surface area and stimulating thresholds in permanent cardiac pacing. J Thorac Cardiovasc Surg 71:559, 1976.
52. Lindesmans FW, Zimmerman ANE: Cardiac current, voltage, charge and energy thresholds as functions of electrode size and impulse duration. *In* Meere C (ed): Proceedings of the VIth World Symposium on Cardiac Pacing. Montreal, Pacesymp, 1979, Chapter 3.2.
53. Furman S, Garvey J, Hurzeler P: Pulse duration variation and electrode size as factors in pacemaker longevity. J Thorac Cardiovasc Surg 69:382, 1975.
54. Barold SS, Ong LS, Heinle RA: Stimulation and sensing thresholds for cardiac pacing: Electrophysiologic and technical aspects. Prog Cardiovasc Dis 24:1, 1981.
55. Mond H, Holley L, Hirshorn M: The high impedance dish electrode—clinical experience with a new tined lead. PACE 5:529, 1982.
56. Schuchert A, Kuck KH: Benefits of smaller electrode surface area (4 mm^2) on steroid-eluting leads. PACE 14:2098, 1991.
57. Stokes K, Bird T: A new efficient nanotip lead. PACE 13:1901, 1990.
58. Mond H: The Cardiac Pacemaker. New York, Grune & Stratton, 1983, pp 37–41.
59. Tyers GFO, Torman HA, Hughes HC Jr: Comparative studies of "state of the art" and presently used clinical cardiac pacemaker electrodes. J Thorac Cardiovasc Surg 67:849, 1974.
60. Parsonnet V, Gilbert L, Lewin G, et al: A nonpolarizing electrode for endocardial stimulation of the heart. J Thorac Cardiovasc Surg 56:710, 1974.
61. Hein F, Blaser R, Thull R, et al: Electrochemical aspects of pacing electrodes (discussion). *In* Watanabe Y (ed): Cardiac Pacing. Proceedings of the Vth International Symposium, Tokyo. Amsterdam, Excerpta Medica, 1977, pp 510–515.
62. Timmis GC, Helland J, Westveer DC: The evolution of low-threshold leads. Clin Prog Pacing Electrophysiol 1:313, 1983.
63. Amundson DC, McArthur W, Mosharrafa M: The porous endocardial electrode. PACE 2:40, 1979.
64. MacCarter DJ, Lundberg KM, Corstjens JPM: Porous electrodes: Concept, technology, and results. PACE 6:427, 1983.
65. MacGregor DC, Wilson GJ, Lixfeld W, et al: The porous-surfaced electrode: A new concept in pacemaker lead design. J Thorac Cardiovasc Surg 78:281, 1979.
66. Skalsky M, McMichael A, Maddison D, et al: Evaluation of a new low-polarisation, high-impedance Pt/Ir-coated porous 6-mm^2 dish electrode. PACE 8:788, 1985.
67. Kreyenhagen P, Helland J: Evaluation of a titanium nitride–coated tip electrode. *In* Antonioli GE, Aubert AE, et al (eds): Pacemaker Leads 1991. Proceedings of the Second European Conference on Pacemaker Leads. Ferrara, Elsevier, 1991, pp 451–458.
68. Adler S, Spehr P, Allen J, et al: Chronic animal testing of new cardiac pacing electrodes. PACE 13:1896, 1990.
69. Bobyn JD, Wilson GJ, Mycyk TR, et al: Comparison of a porous-surfaced with a totally porous ventricular endocardial pacing electrode. PACE 4:405, 1981.
70. Breivik K, Ohm O-J, Dregelid E, et al: Electrophysiological characteristics of porous electrodes versus solid ones. PACE 4:A-5, 1981.
71. Tayler D, Oakley D, Rowbotham D, et al: Comparison of a porous-tipped with a conventional endocardial pacing lead. PACE 4:A-76, 1981.
72. Bobyn JD, Wilson GJ, Mycyk TR, et al: Improved electrophysiological performance using a new porous-surfaced ventricular endocardial pacing electrode. PACE 4:A-82, 1981.
73. Powell L, McEachern M, Elrod P, et al: Atrial endocardial porous and nonporous electrodes: A comparative study. Clin Prog Electrophysiol Pacing 4:41, 1986.

74. Heinemann F, Davis M, Helland J: Clinical performance of a pacing lead with a platinized target-tip electrode. PACE 7:471, 1984.

75. Djordjevic M, Stojanov P, Velimirovic D: Target lead—low-threshold electrode. PACE 9:1206, 1986.

76. Ormerod D, Walgren S, Berglund J, et al: Design and evaluation of a low-threshold, porous-tip lead with a mannitol coated screw-in tip ("sweet tip"). PACE 11:496, 1988.

77. Karpawich PP, Stokes KB, Helland JR, et al: A new low-threshold platinized epimyocardial pacing electrode: Comparative evaluation in immature canines. PACE 11:1139, 1988.

78. McMichael A, Wilson A, Mond H, et al: A two-year evaluation of two laser-porous electrodes. PACE 10:743, 1987.

79. Heinemann F, Coppess M, Stokes K, et al: Clinical comparison of "high tech" pacemaker leads. Clin Prog Electrophysiol Pacing 4(Suppl):43, 1986.

80. Hirshorn MS, Holley LK, Skalsky M, et al: Characteristics of advanced porous and textured surface pacemaker electrodes. PACE 6:525, 1983.

81. Window B, Thompson A, Sharples F, et al: Sputter technology—a technique for producing low-polarisation surfaces. PACE 10:743, 1987.

82. Thalen HJTH, van den Berg JW, van der Heide JN, Nieven J: The Artificial Cardiac Pacemaker. London, William Heinemann, 1969, pp 161–168.

83. Hirshorn MS, Holley LK, Hales JRS, et al: Screening of solid and porous materials for pacemaker electrodes. PACE 4:380, 1981.

84. Parsonnet V, Villanueva A, Driller J, et al: Corrosion of pacemaker electrodes. PACE 4:289, 1981.

85. Richter GJ, Weidlich E, Sturm FV, et al: Nonpolarizable vitreous carbon pacing electrodes in animal experiments. In Meere C (ed): Proceedings of the VIth World Symposium on Cardiac Pacing. Montreal, Pacesymp, 1979, Chapter 29.13.

86. Elmqvist H, Schueller H, Richter G: The carbon-tip electrode. PACE 6:436, 1983.

87. BeckJansen P, Schuller H, Winther-Rasmussen S: Vitreous carbon electrodes in endocardial pacing. In Meere C (ed): Proceedings of the VIth World Symposium on Cardiac Pacing. Montreal, Pacesymp, 1979, Chapter 29.9.

88. Gargeroglio B, Inguaggiato B, Chinaglia B, et al: Initial results with an activated carbon-tip electrode. PACE 6:440, 1983.

89. Ripart A, Mugica J: Electrode-heart interface: Definition of the ideal electrode. PACE 6:410, 1983.

90. Mugica J, Henry L, Attuel P, et al: Clinical experience with 910 carbon-tip leads: Comparison with polished platinum leads. PACE 9:1230, 1986.

91. Pioger G, Ripart A: Clinical results of low-energy unipolar or bipolar activated carbon-tip leads. PACE 9:1243, 1986.

92. Pioger G, Mugica J: Five years' experience with 1527 carbon-tip leads: Comparison with polished platinum-tip leads. PACE 9:283, 1986.

93. Thuesen L, Jensen PJ, Vejby-Christensen H, et al: Lower chronic stimulation threshold in the carbon-tip than in the platinum-tip endocardial electrode: A randomized study. PACE 12:1592, 1989.

94. Katsumoto K, Niibori T, Takamatsu T, et al: Development of glassy carbon electrode (Dead Sea scroll) for low-energy cardiac pacing. PACE 9:1220, 1986.

95. Moracchini PV, Cappelletti F, Melandri PF, et al: Titanium oxide–tip electrode: A solution to minimize polarization and threshold increase. PACE 8:A-85, 1985.

96. Greatbatch W: Implantable Active Devices. 3. Electrodes and Leads. Clarence, New York, Greatbatch Enterprises, 1983, pp 1–37.

97. Schaldach M, Hubman M, Weikl A, et al: Sputter-deposited TiN electrode coatings for superior sensing and pacing performance. PACE 13:1891, 1990.

98. Irnich W: Engineering concepts of pacemaker electrodes. In Schaldach M, Furman S (eds): Advances in Pacemaker Technology. New York, Springer-Verlag, 1975, pp 241–272.

99. Mond H, Stokes K, Helland J, et al: The porous titanium steroid-eluting electrode: A double-blind study assessing the stimulation threshold effects of steroid. PACE 11:214, 1988.

100. Mond H, Stokes KB: The electrode-tissue interface: The revolutionary role of steroid elution. PACE 15:95, 1992.

101. Mond H, Sloman G: The small tined pacemaker lead—absence of dislodgement. PACE 3:171, 1980.

102. Ripart A, Mugica J: Electrode-heart interface: Definition of the ideal electrode. PACE 6:410, 1983.

103. Stokes K, Bornzin G: The electrode-biointerface: Stimulation. In Barold SS, Magica J (eds): Modern Cardiac Pacing. New York, Futura, 1985, pp 33–77.

104. Brewer G, McAuslan BR, Skalsky M, et al: Initial screening of bioactive agents with potential to reduce stimulation threshold. PACE 11:509, 1988.

105. Stokes KB, Bornzin GA, Wiebusch WA: A steroid-eluting, low-threshold, low-polarizing electrode. In Steinbach K, Glogar D, Laszkovics A, et al (eds): Cardiac Pacing. Proceedings of the VIIth World Symposium on Cardiac Pacing, Vienna. Darmstadt, Steinkopff Verlag, 1983, pp 369–376.

106. Kruse I, Terpstra B: Clinical experience with a steroid-eluting electrode for atrial and ventricular pacing. In Aubert AE, Ector H (eds): Pacemaker Leads. Amsterdam, Elsevier Science, 1985, pp 255–260.

107. Hoff PI, Breivik K, Tronstad A, et al: A new steroid-eluting lead for low-threshold pacing. PACE 8:A-4, 1985.

108. Kruse IM: Long-term performance of endocardial leads with steroid-eluting electrodes. PACE 9:1217, 1986.

109. Church T, Martinson M, Rueter J, et al: A multi-center clinical trial of unipolar steroid-eluting electrodes. PACE 10:659, 1987.

110. Cuddy TE, Rabson JLR, Bucher DR, et al: A comparison of threshold performance in bipolar and unipolar steroid-eluting electrodes. PACE 10:434, 1987.

111. Aonuma K, Iesaka Y, Nogami A, et al: Long-term improvement of atrial-pacing threshold and sensitivity with steroid-tip leads: A comparative study between steroid and target tip leads. PACE 11:510, 1988.

112. Pirzada FA, Moschitto LJ: Steroid-eluting electrodes: Four-year experience. PACE 14:695, 1991.

113. Pirzada FA, Moschitto LJ, DiOrio D: Long-term follow-up of steroid-eluting electrodes. Cardiostim 90. RBM 12:105, 1990.

114. Helloco A, Lelong B, Leborgne O, et al: Clinical experience with steroid endocardial lead in permanent atrial pacing. Cardiostim 90. RBM 12:105, 1990.

115. Till JA, Jones S, Rowland E, et al: Clinical experience with a steroid-eluting lead in children. Circulation 80:II-389, 1989.

116. Stokes K, Church T: The elimination of exit block as a pacing complication using a transvenous steroid-eluting lead. PACE 10:748, 1987.

117. Petitot JC, Metivet F, Lascault G, et al: What improvement with the Medtronic steroid eluting lead 4003? Cardiostim 90. RBM 12:108, 1990.

118. Tronstad A, Hoff PI, Ohm O-J: Myocardial excitability thresholds of a new steroid lead compared to two nonsteroid leads: A double-blind study. PACE 10:754, 1987.

119. Radovsky AS, Van Vleet JF: Effects of dexamethasone elution on tissue reaction around stimulating electrodes of endocardial pacing leads in dogs. Am Heart J 117:1288, 1989.

120. Radovsky AS, Van Vleet JF, Stokes KB, et al: Paired comparisons of steroid-eluting and nonsteroid endocardial pacemaker leads in dogs: Electrical performance and morphologic alterations. PACE 11:1085, 1988.

121. Stokes K: Controlled release of steroid to enhance pacemaker performance [review]. Proceedings of the 13th Annual Meeting of the Society for Biomaterials, New York, 1987, p 52.

122. Greve H, Heuer H, Peters W: Intra- and postoperative data of the Medtronic electrodes target tip 4011–58 and steroid 4003. Clin Prog Electrophysiol Pacing Suppl:42, 1986.

123. Vardas PE, Kenny RA, Ingram A: Acute and chronic performance of new technology versus conventional endocardial pacing leads. Clin Prog Electrophysiol Pacing Suppl:38, 1986.

124. Schuchert A, Hopf M, Kuck KH, et al: Chronic ventricular electrograms: Do steroid-eluting leads differ from conventional leads? PACE 13:1879, 1990.

125. Bucking J, Schwartau M: The effect of localized steroid elution from a pacemaker electrode on the pacing threshold and intracardiac R wave amplitude [translated]. Herzschrittmacher 5:27, 1985.

126. Timmis GC: "Meet the Experts" presentation at the North American Society of Pacing and Electrophysiology meeting, May 1986. In Medtronic Inc. Think System, MC 871503, September 1987; and Capsure Leads: The Drug, Technology, and Benefits Abstracted, MC 870675, 1987.

127. Gillis AM, Rothschild JM, Fudge W, et al: A randomized comparison of a bipolar steroid-eluting lead and standard porous titanium lead. Cardiostim 90. RBM 12:62, 1990.

128. Wish M, Fletcher R, Cohen A, et al: Steroid tipped and porous platinum permanent pacemaker leads. Cardiostim 90. RBM 12:63, 1990.

129. Jones BR, Midei MG, Brinker JA: Does the long-term performance of the target-tip electrode justify reducing a pacemaker's nominal output? PACE 9:299, 1986.
130. Hiller K, Rothschild JM, Fudge W, et al: A randomized comparison of a bipolar steroid-eluting lead and a bipolar porous platinum-coated titanium lead. PACE 14:695, 1991.
131. Hoff PI, Breivik K, Tronstad A, et al: A new steroid-eluting electrode for low-threshold pacing. In Gomez FP (ed): Cardiac Pacing: Electrophysiology. Tachyarrhythmias. Mt. Kisco, NY, Futura, 1985, pp 1014–1079.
132. Schallhorn R, Oleson K: Multi-center clinical experience with an improved steroid-eluting pacemaker lead. PACE 11:496, 1988.
133. Llewellyn M, Bennett D, Heaps C, et al: Limitation of early pacing threshold rise using a silicone insulated, platinised, steroid-eluting lead. PACE 11:496, 1988.
134. Mond H, Hunt P, Hunt D: A second-generation steroid-eluting electrode. Cardiostim 90. RBM 12:62, 1990.
135. Stokes KB: Preliminary studies on a new steroid-eluting epicardial electrode. PACE 11:1797, 1988.
136. Kugler JD, Fetter J, Fleming W: A new steroid-eluting epicardial lead: Experience with atrial and ventricular implantation in the immature swine. PACE 13:976, 1990.
137. Johns JA, Fish FA, Burger JD, et al: Steroid-eluting epicardial pacing leads in pediatric patients: Encouraging early results. J Am Coll Cardiol 20:395, 1992.
138. Hamilton R, Bahoric B, Griffiths J, et al: Steroid-eluting epicardial leads in pediatrics: Improved epicardial thresholds in the first year. PACE 14:633, 1991.
139. Johns JA, Fish FA, Burger JD, et al: Steroid-eluting epicardial pacing leads in pediatric patients: Encouraging early results. PACE 14:633, 1991.
140. Wilson A, Cowling R, Mathivanar R, et al: Drug-eluting collar—a new approach to reducing threshold. Cardiostim 90. RBM 12:61, 1990.
141. Brewer G, Mathivanar R, Skalsky M, et al: Composite electrode tips containing externally placed drug-releasing collars. PACE 11:1760, 1988.
142. Mathivanar R, Anderson N, Harman D, et al: In vivo elution of drug-eluting ceramic leads with a reduced dose of dexamethasone sodium phosphate. PACE 13:1883, 1990.
143. Crossley GH, Bubien R, Dailey SM, et al: Chronic stimulation threshold with a drug-eluting collar electrode: Long-term follow-up. PACE 14:628, 1991.
144. Wilson A, Kay N, Padeletti L, et al: A multicentre study of steroid-eluting collar leads. PACE 14:629, 1991.
145. Schuchert A, Kuck KH: Benefits of smaller electrode surface area (4 mm^2) on steroid-eluting leads. PACE 14:2098, 1991.
146. Skalsky M, Mathivanar R, Anderson N, et al: Threshold performance of bipolar leads with a drug-eluting collar (DEC). Cardiostim 90. RBM 12:108, 1990.
147. Anderson N, Mathivanar R, Skalsky M, et al: Active fixation leads—long-term threshold reduction using a drug-infused ceramic collar. PACE 14:639, 1991.
148. Anderson N, Skalsky M, Ng M, et al: Active fixation leads—threshold reduction using dexamethasone acetate. Cardiostim 90. RBM 12:109, 1990.
149. Guerola M, Lindegren U, Hagel P: One-year clinical evaluation of new porous titanium nitride electrodes coated with steroid and a layer of ion-exchange membrane. Eur J C P E 2:A90, 1992.
150. Mond H: The Cardiac Pacemaker. New York, Grune & Stratton, 1983, pp 75–76.
151. Bergdahl L: Helifix, an electrode suitable for transvenous and ventricular implantation. J Thorac Cardiovasc Surg 80:794, 1980.
152. Sloman JG, Mond HG, Bailey B, et al: The use of balloon-tipped electrodes for permanent cardiac pacing. PACE 2:579, 1979.
153. Bennett D, Bray C, Ward C, et al: Comparison of 2 types of active fixation electrodes. PACE 4:A-32, 1981.
154. Mond H, Sloman G: The small tined pacemaker lead—absence of dislodgement. PACE 3:171, 1980.
155. Mond H, Kertes P, Strathmore N, et al: Endocardial screw-in lead: Clinical experience in the atrial position. PACE 10:719, 1987.
156. Bisping HJ, Kreuzer J, Birkenheier H: Three-year clinical experience with a new endocardial screw-in lead with introduction protection for use in the atrium and ventricle. PACE 3:424, 1980.
157. Mond H, Ong TW, Strathmore N, et al: Atrial pacing leads: Active or passive fixation. Abstract presented at the Vth Asian-Pacific Symposium on Electrophysiology (APSPE), Makuhari, Japan, Aug. 1–4, 1993. PACE 16:1619, 1993.
158. Upton JE: New pacing lead conductors. In Meere C (ed): Proceedings of the VIth World Symposium on Cardiac Pacing. Montreal, Pacesymp, 1979, Chapter 29.6.
159. Chisholm AW, Cameron JR, Froggart GM, et al: A new long-life electrode. PACE 4:A-85, 1981.
160. Green GD: Pacemaker Leads. Impulse. St. Paul, MN, Cardiac Pacemakers Inc, June 1976.
161. Dolezel B, Adamirova L, et al: In vivo degradation of polymers. Biomaterials 10:96, 1989.
162. Stokes K, Cobian K, Lathrop T: Polyurethane insulators, a design approach to small pacing leads. In Meere C (ed): Proceedings of the VIth World Symposium on Cardiac Pacing. Montreal, Pacesymp 1979, Chapter 28.2.
163. Guerin P: Use of synthetic polymers for biomedical application. PACE 6:449, 1983.
164. Scheuer-Lesser M, Irnich W, Kreuzer J: Polyurethane leads: Facts and controversy. PACE 6:454, 1983.
165. Stokes K: The biostability of polyurethane leads. In Barold SS, Mugica J (eds): Modern Cardiac Pacing. New York, Futura, 1985, pp 173–198.
166. Pande GS: Thermoplastic polyurethanes as insulating materials for long-life cardiac pacing leads. PACE 6:858, 1983.
167. Parins DJ, Black KM, McCoy KD, Horvath NJ: In Vivo Degradation of a Polyurethane. St. Paul, MN, Cardiac Pacemakers Inc, 1981.
168. Stokes K: The long-term biostability of polyurethane leads. Stimucoeur Med 10:205, 1982.
169. Byrd CL, McArthur W, Stokes K, et al: Implant experience with unipolar pacing leads. PACE 6:868, 1983.
170. Scheuer-Leeser M, Irnich W, Kreuzer J: Polyurethane leads: Facts and controversy. PACE 6:454, 1983.
171. Timmis GC, Westveer DC, Martin R, et al: The significance of surface changes on explanted polyurethane pacemaker leads. PACE 6:845, 1983.
172. Round Table Discussion: The polyurethane controversy. PACE 6:459, 1983.
173. Phillips R, Frey M, Martin RO: Long-term performance of polyurethane pacing leads: Mechanisms of design-related failures. PACE 9:1166, 1986.
174. Irwin M, Graham KJ, Hayes D, et al: Does the venous route used for lead placement affect the incidence of lead failure? PACE 15:571, 1992.
175. Stokes K, Urbanski P, Upton J: The in vivo auto-oxidation of polyether polyurethanes by metal ions. J Biomater Sci Polymer 1:207, 1990.
176. Davis M, Stokes K: Polyurethane cardiac pacing—six years' experience. Cardiostim 84. RBM 6:256, 1984.
177. Medtronic Report: Ensuring and evaluating pacing lead performance. Medtronic News 20:21, 1992.
178. Stokes KB, Church T: Ten-year experience with implanted polyurethane lead insulation. PACE 9:1160, 1986.
179. Woscoboinik JR, Maloney JD, Helguera ME, et al: Pacing lead survival: Performance of different models. PACE 15:1991, 1992.
180. Fletcher R, McManus C, Keung E, et al: The Veterans Affairs Lead Registry—10-year follow-up. PACE 15:512, 1992.
181. Hayes DL, Graham KJ, Irwin M, et al: A multicenter experience with a bipolar tined polyurethane ventricular lead. PACE 15:1033, 1992.
182. Sweesy MW, Forney CC, Hayes DL, et al: Evaluation of an in-line bipolar polyurethane ventricular pacing lead. PACE 15:1982, 1992.
183. Pirzada FA, Seltzer JP, Blair-Saletin D, et al: Five-year performance of the Medtronic 6971 polyurethane endocardial electrode. PACE 9:1173, 1986.
184. Hayes DL, Stokes KB, Helland J: Clinical survivorship and failure mechanisms of polyurethane pacing leads. PACE 8:779, 1985.
185. Beyersdorf F, Kreuzer J, Schmidts L, et al: Examination of explanted polyurethane pacemaker leads using the scanning electron microscope. PACE 8:562, 1985.
186. Stokes KB, Frazer AW, Carter EA: The biostability of various polyether polyurethanes under stress. ANTEC'84 84:1073, 1984.
187. Telectronics Lead Performance Report. Denver, Telectronics Pacing Systems Inc, 1991.
188. Byrd CL, Schwartz SJ, Wettenstein E: Chronic analysis of polyurethane leads. PACE 8:A-83, 1985.
189. Szycher M, Stokes K, Anderson J (eds): Sixth Annual Seminar on Biostability of Polyurethanes, Boston. Lancaster, PA, Technomic Publishing, 1992.

190. Mugica J, Daubert JC, Lazarus B, et al: Is polyurethane lead insulation still controversial? PACE 15:1967, 1992.

191. Stokes KB: Recent advances in lead technology. *In* Barold SS, Mugica J (eds): New Perspectives in Cardiac Pacing. Mt. Kisco, NY, Futura, 1988, pp 222–223.

192. Aubert AE, Arkens O, Ector H, et al: Permeability of silicone insulation and corrosion of conductor wires in pacemaker leads. PACE 8:A-54, 1985.

193. Mond H: The Cardiac Pacemaker: Function and Malfunction. New York, Grune & Stratton, 1983, pp 71–75.

194. Furman S: Lead connectors [editorial]. PACE 12:1, 1989.

195. Irnich W: Pacemaker standards [editorial]. PACE 12:269, 1989.

196. Furman S: Connectors [editorial]. PACE 13:567, 1990.

197. Executive Committee of the German Working Group on Cardiac Pacing: Communication to Professor K Steinbach, European Working Group on Cardiac Pacing, June 1985.

198. Doring J, Flink R: The impact of pending technologies on a universal connector standard. PACE 9:1186, 1986.

199. Calfee RV, Saulson SH: A voluntary standard for 3.2-mm unipolar and bipolar pacemaker leads and connectors. PACE 9:1181, 1986.

CHAPTER 4

POWER SOURCES FOR IMPLANTABLE PACEMAKERS

Darrel F. Untereker
Richard B. Shepard
Craig L. Schmidt
Ann M. Crespi
Paul M. Skarstad

This chapter provides the clinician with information about power sources used in implantable pacemakers and defibrillators. The purpose is to communicate background information about galvanic cells that is related to the practical choices about batteries that must be made by engineers in designing pacemakers and defibrillators and by implanting physicians in managing patients. The chapter first describes the basic principles and terminology of batteries. It then discusses the important factors to be considered in the design of batteries and how these relate to the clinical characteristics of pulse generator performance.

The battery is conceptually different from the other components of an implantable pacing system. In principle, although not always in practice, the other components of pacing systems are designed to last indefinitely. However, the available chemical energy of the battery is consumed during its normal use. Thus, the battery has a finite service life because a battery contains a fixed amount of the active chemicals that furnish its energy. As the pacemaker or defibrillator is used, the battery's remaining energy supply is reduced. Eventually, the output voltage falls to a level that is insufficient to operate the device within the limits specified by the clinical needs of cardiac pacing. By this time, the battery is no longer useful and must be replaced. At present, the only practical way of producing a reliable device is to build the power source into the pulse generator can. Thus, the entire pulse generator must be replaced to replace the battery.

Definitions

Some basic definitions relating to batteries are listed here. They are listed to provide a common ground for the purposes of this chapter. The reader may wish to refer to these definitions at times when the terminology seems contradictory or becomes obscure.

Oxidation: Any process that increases the positive charge or decreases the negative charge of an atom, ion, radical, or compound (the loss of electrons by an atom or a compound).

Reduction: Any process that decreases the positive charge or increases the negative charge of an atom, ion, radical, or compound (the gain of electrons by an atom or compound).

Anion: A negatively charged ion. It is attracted to positively charged ions and repelled by negatively charged ions.

Cation: A positively charged ion. It is attracted to negatively charged ions and repelled by positively charged ions.

Conduction: The movement of charge under the influence of an electric field. There are two fundamental forms of conduction—electronic, in which electrons are the charge carriers, and ionic, in which a charged chemical species (ions) are the charge carriers. Usually metals are electronic conductors, whereas solutions and some non-metallic substances are ionic conductors.

Anode: (a) The electrode at which oxidation occurs in an electrochemical cell; (b) The material that undergoes oxidation in an electrochemical cell; (c) The electrode that furnishes electrons to the external circuit, thus the negative terminal of a galvanic cell discharging spontaneously.

Cathode: (a) The electrode at which reduction occurs in an electrochemical cell; (b) The material that undergoes reduction in an electrochemical cell; (c) in a spontaneously discharging galvanic cell, the positive terminal that attracts electrons from the external circuit.

Galvanic cell: A device that is capable of spontaneously transforming chemical energy into electric energy.

Battery: A group of one or more galvanic cells connected in series, in parallel, or a combination of the two for the purpose of increasing their voltage or current capability.

Half-cell potential: A numerical value expressed as a voltage (vs. an arbitrary reference electrode) that characterizes a substance's tendency to either give up or take on electrons compared to its present state.

Stoichiometry: The numerical relationship between atoms or molecules that will exactly react with one another.

Rate: Refers to current in battery terminology (i.e., rate capability means the ability to deliver a sustained current of a certain magnitude; this should not be confused with pacing rate).

Basic Function and Electrochemistry of Batteries

ENERGY STORAGE IN BATTERIES

A battery converts chemical energy into electric energy. The source of this energy is the electrochemical reactions that occur within the battery. The amount and type of the materials participating in these reactions are the primary factors that determine the deliverable energy content of a battery.

CHEMICAL REACTIONS

When a typical chemical reaction occurs, one chemical substance interacts directly with another to form a reaction product. For example, in burning, the fuel combines with oxygen from the air to form combustion products, which usually include water, carbon dioxide, and perhaps other species. The original fuel is oxidized during this process. Oxygen from the air is reduced. The exact amounts of each material that react with one another are determined by the stoichiometry of the reaction. Equations 1 to 4 are examples of different types of oxidation-reduction reactions. These are called redox reactions and show the stoichiometric relationship between the reactants.

Eq 1 $2 H_2 + O_2 \rightarrow 2 H_2O$ (the formation of water)
Eq 2 $2 C_6H_6 + 15 O_2 \rightarrow 12 CO_2 + 6 H_2O$ (the burning of benzene)

Eq 3 $2 Fe + 3 O_2 \rightarrow Fe_2O_3$ (the rusting of iron)
Eq 4 $Li + \frac{1}{2} I_2 \rightarrow 2 LiI$ (the discharge of a lithium-iodine pacemaker battery)

Chemical reactions like these occur spontaneously because the products are in a lower energy state than the reactants. The difference in energy appears as heat in the case of combustion or rusting. A battery or galvanic cell is designed to convert part of this energy difference into electric energy rather than heat.

ELECTRON TRANSFER

A battery operates because the electrons transferred during a redox reaction are channeled from one terminal of the battery through the device to be powered and back to the battery through its other terminal. The maximum work these electrons can do outside the battery is the difference in the energy of the reactants and products in the spontaneous discharge reaction of the battery. Chemical reactions such as those shown in equations 1 to 4 show reactants on the left side of the equation and products on the right side. In concept, these reactions can be thought of as the sum of two partial or half reactions. Half reactions are written so that two half reactions are added together to describe a complete chemical reaction. For example, equation 4 shows the chemical reaction that describes the discharge of the most common battery system used to power pacemakers. Equations 5a and 5b show the two half reactions that, when added together, describe the principal part of the electrochemical reaction that occurs during discharge of a lithium-iodine battery. In this case the total reaction also includes the two ions that combine to form a solid material, LiI.

Eq 5a $Li \rightarrow Li^+ + e^-$
Eq 5b $\frac{1}{2}I_2 + e^- \rightarrow I^-$

HALF-CELL POTENTIALS

Half-cell equations, like 5a and 5b, indicate what reactions can occur. However, half-reaction equations give no information about the likelihood that any reaction will actually occur. The thermodynamic tendency for a reaction to occur is measured by its half-cell potential (see definitions at the beginning of the chapter). Table 4–1 shows the potentials associated with some half-cell reactions used in battery systems. The most positive values are substances that easily give up electrons and become more positively charged (oxidized). These materials are typically metals. Substances with negative half-cell potentials have a tendency to accept electrons. These materials gain electrons and become more negatively charged (reduced).

Major Chemical and Electrical Components of Batteries

A battery must convert the potential energy of its component chemicals to electric energy in a controlled, predictable, and long-lasting manner. Figure 4–1 shows a very simple battery. The major parts are the anode, the cathode, and the electrolyte.

TABLE 4–1. STANDARD OXIDATION POTENTIALS OF SOME COMMON SUBSTANCES

REDOX REACTION		HALF-CELL POTENTIAL
Li	$\rightarrow Li^+ + e^-$	3.05
Na	$\rightarrow Na^+ + e^-$	2.71
Mg	$\rightarrow Mg^{+2} + 2\,e^-$	2.37
Al	$\rightarrow Al^{+3} + 3\,e^-$	1.66
Zn	$\rightarrow Z^{+2} + 2\,e^-$	0.76
Co	$\rightarrow Co^{+2} + 2\,e^-$	0.28
H_2	$\rightarrow 2\,H^+ + 2\,e^-$	0.00
Ag	$\rightarrow Ag^{+2} + e^-$	-0.79
I^-	$\rightarrow \frac{1}{2}I_2 + e^-$	-0.54
2 Br$^-$	$\rightarrow Br_2 + 2\,e^-$	-1.07
2 H_2O	$\rightarrow O_2 + 2/H^+ + 4\,e^-$	-1.23
2 F$^-$	$\rightarrow F_2 + 2\,e^-$	-2.65

ANODE AND CATHODE

The two major battery components involved in the electrochemical reaction during discharge of a galvanic cell are the anode and the cathode. The anode, which is oxidized, is often a metal and is converted to a cation during the discharge process. It furnishes electrons to the external circuit. The second major component, the cathode, picks up electrons from the external circuit during the discharge of the battery. Typically, the cathode is not a metallic substance, although cathodes exist that have metallic characteristics.

The terms anode and cathode may seem to be the opposites of the conventions used for pacing leads. For example, note that the anode of the battery is the terminal that gives off electrons. This battery terminal is connected via the pulse generator circuitry to the cathode of the pacing lead (tip electrode), the negatively charged electrode in contact with the myocardium. The cathode of the battery accepts electrons from the anode of the lead (or pulse generator can in the case of a unipolar pacemaker). This apparent inconsistency is actually correct when one considers that the anode material within the battery becomes positively charged as a consequence of losing electrons while the cathode material within the battery becomes negatively charged by accepting electrons.

ELECTROLYTE

Notice that the anode and the cathode are separated by the electrolyte. If the anode and the cathode were not separated, the battery would not function because the chemical reaction could occur without passing current through the external circuit.

The battery furnishes electrons at one terminal, pushes them through an external circuit, and receives them at a second terminal. If this were all that happened in a battery, the discharge process would not occur for very long. The reason is that a large positive charge would quickly develop on the anodal side of the battery, and a large negative charge would develop on the cathodal side. The negative charge accumulating on the cathodal terminal would repel additional electrons coming through the external circuit from the anode and soon suppress this reaction. On the anodal side, an equal number of positive charges building up on that terminal would also suppress further oxidation until that process also stopped. It is the electrolyte that prevents this from happening, allowing the chemical reaction to continue in a sustainable manner. The electrolyte allows the mobility of ions but not of electrons. Thus, as positive and negative charges build up on the anode and cathode, the electrolyte, which is in contact with both electrodes, allows ions to migrate toward these electrodes to neutralize the internal charge. The electrolyte cannot be an electronic conductor or the battery would be internally shorted just as it would if the positive and negative terminals were directly connected by a wire.

DISCHARGE PRODUCT ACCUMULATION

The discharge product accumulates at either electrode interface or within the electrolyte. Just where it collects depends on the relative mobility of the migrating ions and the solubility of the discharge product in the electrolyte.

ELECTROLYTE COMPOSITION

In many battery systems the electrolyte is a salt dissolved in a liquid. This is the case with common flashlight batteries, in which the electrolyte is zinc chloride dissolved in water.

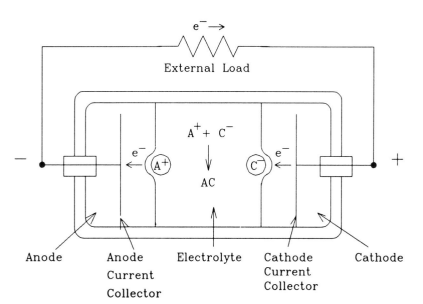

FIGURE 4–1. Schematic representation of simple sealed battery. The anode material is labeled A, the cathode material C, and the discharge reaction A + C → AC. In this example both A$^+$ and C$^-$ are mobile ions, and the discharge product, AC, is insoluble and precipitates in the electrolyte solution.

However, the batteries used for implantable medical devices that contain a liquid electrolyte solution do not use water but nonaqueous solvents instead. This is true because water reacts with many of the energetic materials that are used in implantable medical batteries.

SOLID ELECTROLYTES

Not all electrolyte materials are liquid. The electrolyte material in some important batteries are solids. One example is lithium iodide, which is the electrolyte in the lithium-iodine battery. The role of lithium iodide as a solid electrolyte is extremely important and determines many of this battery's major characteristics. This particular battery system is fairly unique because the lithium iodide is both the discharge product and the electrolyte.

BALANCED CELLS; STOICHIOMETRIC RELATIONSHIPS

Separation of the anode and cathode is required for a battery to be functional. The left side of Figure 4–1 shows the anode, which will lose electrons to form A^+ ions; the right side shows the cathode, which will gain electrons to form C^- ions as the battery discharges. These processes occur in concert; the electrons generated on the anodal side of the battery are consumed on the cathodal side. This stoichiometric relationship must be maintained whether the discharge product is formed chemically or electrochemically. Thus, there is a specific ratio of the anode and cathode that reacts to form the discharge product. A cell that contains exactly the required ratio of anodal and cathodal materials is a balanced cell. Most batteries are not designed with the stoichiometric ratio of the active cathodal and anodal materials. This is done for several reasons. Two reasons are basic safety and the provision of controllable and gradual end-of-service characteristics.

The maximum energy content of a battery is fixed by the amount of anodal or cathodal materials. This energy may appear as heat or electricity, depending on the specific battery chemistry, the design of the battery, and the manner in which it is discharged; however, the total amount of energy delivered is invariant. Thus, the more energy that appears as heat, the less that will be available as electricity to power an electric device.

Cell Thermodynamics and Kinetics

The operation of any battery is dependent on both thermodynamic and kinetic processes. Thermodynamics, in this context, refers to whether a chemical reaction can or is likely to occur. Chemical kinetics, on the other hand, refers to how fast the reaction actually proceeds. In general, thermodynamic properties relate to the theoretical limits of battery operation, whereas kinetics often determine how much of the energy can be delivered and at what current.

CELL VOLTAGE AND CURRENT

The voltage of a single cell can be calculated from fundamental thermodynamic quantities. The theoretical voltage is calculated from the half-cell potentials for the anodal and cathodal reactions. This is the voltage that is measured in a cell when there are no kinetic limitations, a condition that occurs only when an insignificant amount of current is being drawn from the battery. The terminology for this is open-circuit voltage. In practice, the open-circuit voltage is measured using a high-impedance (resistance) digital voltmeter.

CHEMICAL KINETIC LIMITATIONS

As soon as current is drawn from the battery, chemical kinetic limitations are observed. With the onset of current flow, for example, the voltage at the battery terminals is diminished compared with the open-circuit value. At the extreme, the current that flows from the battery into a complete short circuit is limited by the cell kinetics. The relationship between load-circuit voltage and open-circuit voltage is determined by both the chemistry and the design of the battery. A typical relationship is shown in Figure 4–2.

OPEN- AND SHORT-CIRCUIT VOLTAGES AND CURRENTS

In Figure 4–2 the load-circuit voltage approaches the open-circuit voltage because the current approaches zero. At the other extreme, the short-circuit current is observed when the load-circuit voltage approaches zero. How rapidly the curve in Figure 4–2 changes with current depends on the particular battery chemistry and how the battery is designed. For example, a lead-acid battery for automotive use is constructed of very conductive materials and is designed with high surface area electrodes (anode and cathode) so that extremely high currents can be drawn from it to run the car's starter. On the other hand, a transistor radio battery is designed with small electrodes to manage the relatively low currents that are typical of small, portable electronic devices.

For any specific battery, the output voltage and the current are closely related; the output voltage is a function of the load current. However, there is no fundamental relationship between voltage and current that holds for all batteries. Even for the same chemical components, the shape of a battery's current-voltage curve, like the one shown in Figure 4–2, is mainly dependent upon the design of the battery.

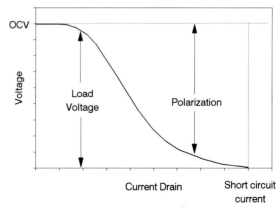

FIGURE 4–2. Typical load voltage–current drain plot for a battery. The load voltage is always less than the open-circuit voltage. Current drain increases toward the right. The exact shape of the plot depends on the chemistry and design of the battery.

TEMPERATURE EFFECTS ON BATTERY FUNCTION

The characteristics of a battery change with temperature. For many applications, battery specifications must be developed to cope with the entire range of temperatures in which the battery is expected to operate. In general, battery performance deteriorates rapidly with decreasing temperature. A battery's voltage is lower in cold temperatures than in warmer ones. Also, kinetics are generally slower under colder conditions; thus, the ability of a battery to supply current is also diminished at low temperatures. Fortunately, implantable devices operate within the physiologic range, approximately 37°C. However, even for implantable medical devices, there are situations during manufacturing, shipping, delivery, and sterilization in which the power source may be exposed to temperatures that are quite different from body temperature. Engineers must take these into account when designing and choosing power sources.

Battery Terminology

CAPACITY

The fundamental unit of battery capacity is the coulomb (C), which is the amount of charge delivered by 1 ampere (A) of current in 1 second. In the context of implantable devices, a more practical unit of capacity is the ampere-hour (Ah), which represents the charge carried by a current of 1 A flowing past the measurement site for 1 hour. A battery for an implantable medical device usually has a capacity rating of between 0.5 and 2 Ah.

Many papers have been written about the proper way of determining and specifying the capacity of a medical battery.[1–3] No one method is uniquely correct. What is important to the physician who is interested in comparing the battery capacities of different pacemakers is to pay careful attention to the assumptions and methods that were used to estimate the capacity. The various methods produce numbers ranging from theoretical values that can never be achieved in the field to very realistic values that are based on detailed models or accelerated testing. In general, more optimistic numbers are obtained from theoretical calculations based only on the amount of active materials in the battery. More sophisticated methods take into account known limitations or limited use of the components within the battery. For example, most batteries are not able to use up all of their active components before they cease to function in a clinically useful manner. A prediction that does not take this into account is too optimistic. In addition, other limitations come into play. For example, the load-circuit voltage decreases as the battery is used. Because the electronic circuits of the pulse generator must operate above a specified minimum voltage, the cell capacity that generates a voltage below this minimum value is not usable. This further limits the capacity that can be delivered in practical use.

Estimating the deliverable capacity of medical batteries is made especially difficult because of their long service life. The time frame for the operation of most implantable medical devices is so long (several years) that real-time measurements of capacity are not practical. Therefore, accelerated tests and models are usually used to estimate the amount of deliverable capacity in these batteries before they are put into clinical use. Fortunately, technology has improved a great deal in this area, and it is now possible to make quite accurate projections of battery capacity.[4–6]

ENERGY DENSITY

The fundamental unit of energy is the joule (J). This is the energy given to 1 C of charge that is accelerated by a difference in potential of 1 V. One joule is also the energy transferred by 1 W of power for 1 second. Just as battery capacity is often measured in ampere-hours, battery energy is often expressed in watt-hours (Wh) instead of joules. The battery parameter of interest is energy density, a factor that can be expressed on either a weight or a volume basis. For medical applications volume is usually more important than weight, so ratings based on volumetric energy density are most commonly used. The time integral of the product of voltage and current divided by the total volume of the battery is its energy density. The energy density of a battery can be approximated by the product of average voltage and nominal capacity divided by volume. Modern batteries for pacemakers have energy densities as high as 1 Wh/cm^3, including the exterior case.

The deliverable energy density of a battery also depends on the type of battery and how it is constructed. Theoretically, the energy density is maximized when all extraneous materials in the battery are minimized and the amount of active anodal and cathodal materials are the stoichiometric ratio for the discharge reaction. However, a battery designed for maximum energy density would in most instances not meet other important requirements including optimum reliability and longevity. A medical battery designer attempts to make energy density as large as possible while still meeting all other requirements.

Battery Structure and Related Functional Characteristics

CURRENT COLLECTOR

The current collector makes the connection between the positive or negative terminal of the battery and its respective active electrode inside the cell. A current collector is usually a wire, screen, or grid that is embedded in the anode or cathode material of the battery. The current collector often also serves as a structural member of the battery to provide physical integrity and strength to that portion of the cell. The size of the current collector can also be used to limit the maximum current that can be drawn from a cell, minimizing the risks from an inadvertent short of the cell during its manufacture or assembly into a pulse generator. Many medical batteries use the exterior case of the battery as the current collector for the cathode. These batteries are termed case-positive designs.

SEPARATOR

The separator is often confused with the electrolyte. The electrolyte is the medium that conducts ions within the battery, whereas the separator is a physical structural member of the cell that keeps the anode and cathode materials apart, preventing shorting of the cell. All batteries need an electrolyte, but not all batteries require a separator. A separator is usually needed in batteries that contain liquid electrolytes. Without a separator, there would be little to stop the anode from shorting to the cathode if the cell were squeezed or if there were any internal movement of the electrodes during use (which can result from volume changes during discharge). The separator is made of a material that has a porous structure so that the electrolyte solution can fill the pores and communicate between the anodal and cathodal sides of the battery. The ions in the electrolyte move through the pores as they maintain electric neutrality in the cell. Flashlight batteries use paper separators. Medical batteries with liquid electrolytes use porous polymer films that do not react with other components of the battery system.

CELL INTERNAL IMPEDANCE

Cell internal impedance (resistance) is an important battery property that plays a crucial role in the clinical performance of many implantable devices. Cell internal impedance and internal resistance are often used interchangeably, though impedance is calculated using a time-varying current, whereas resistance is calculated from steady state behavior. The difference between cell resistance and impedance is important to the designer of a pulse generator when considering the overall effects of voltage drops related to sudden changes in load on the battery such as may occur during programming, telemetry, or any event requiring the battery to deliver large current pulses.

BATTERY TERMINALS

As discussed previously, the nomenclature for the terminals of a battery may seem confusing. The anode is often mistakenly called the positive terminal. Actually, the anode is (connected to) the negative terminal, and the cathode is the positive battery terminal. The reason is that oxidation occurs at the anode, where an excess of electrons is generated. The electrons flow out of the battery through the anode current collector. Similarly, electrons that have dissipated their energy in an external device are attracted to the positive battery terminal, which is (connected to) the cathode, where reduction occurs. Keeping in mind that the anode is the source of electrons and the cathode is the sink for electrons is useful for remembering the terminology.

HERMETIC SEAL

Many batteries need to be sealed, but few batteries other than those used for implantable medical devices and aerospace applications need to be so well sealed that they are truly hermetic (i.e., gas tight). Hermeticity implies the use of welded construction and feedthroughs to make electric connections between the outside and the inside of the battery. This is necessary to prevent slow interchanges of materials in or out of the battery. For example, batteries using lithium electrodes must be sealed to prevent water from entering the case. In addition, some of the components used inside medical lithium batteries are volatile and could be corrosive or damaging if they leaked out. Medical batteries are typically considered hermetically sealed if the leak rate for a test gas (helium) through the battery case is less than 1×10^{-7} cm^3/sec at 1 atmosphere helium pressure difference between the inside and the outside of the cell.

Nonideal Battery Behavior

The previous discussion has focused on the principles and the nomenclature of battery operation. It is also important to understand some of the things that limit battery operation. Several important nonideal processes are discussed in the following paragraphs.

POLARIZATION

Polarization is any process that causes the voltage at the terminals of a battery to drop below the open-circuit value when it is providing current. Internal resistance is one cause. Another cause is the development of a concentration gradient within the battery. As a battery discharges, the ions in the electrolyte must move to maintain electric neutrality. If they cannot move quickly enough, concentration gradients develop within the battery. These gradients limit the rate at which the battery can discharge. A concentration gradient also lowers the load voltage because the half-cell potentials at the anode and cathode are logarithmically related to the ratio of the reactant and product concentrations.

Similarly, the electron transfer during a redox reaction may not be able to occur as rapidly as the external demand requires. In such cases, the maximum rate of discharge of the battery becomes governed by the rates at which the redox reactions can occur. When current is drawn from a battery, all of these processes occur to some extent. The net effect of these kinetic limitations is observed as a decrease in the voltage at the terminals of the battery.

SELF-DISCHARGE

Self-discharge is the spontaneous discharge of a cell or battery by an internal chemical reaction rather than through useful electrochemical discharge. We have all seen the effects of self-discharge at one time or other. The flashlight that does not work when needed after prolonged lack of use is a good example. One mechanism by which this can occur involves a slow direct reaction between the anode and the cathode. Other self-discharge processes usually involve reactions between either the anode or the cathode and another substance in the battery, such as the solvent in the electrolyte. A typical example would be a reaction between the anode and the electrolyte solvent that forms a passive film or a gas. The zinc-mercuric oxide batteries used to power pulse generators in the past generated hydrogen gas by such a process. These reactions are usually very slow, but because medical batteries are expected to operate for many years, the accumulated effects can be appreciable. Although it is very hard to measure the very slow rate of self-discharge reactions, microcalorimetry, which can detect the small amounts of heat that are involved, has been used for this purpose.[7, 8] The rate of heat generation can then be used to calculate the rate of self-discharge by thermodynamic principles and equations.

Classification of Batteries

Batteries may be classified in many ways. For example, they are often categorized by application, functional characteristics, chemistry, or the physical state of some component. One fundamental distinction is that between primary and secondary batteries.

PRIMARY BATTERIES

Primary batteries are designed to be used only until their originally available chemical energy has been depleted. They are not designed to be recharged. Familiar examples of primary batteries are zinc-carbon dry cells, alkaline zinc-manganese dioxide flashlight batteries, zinc-mercuric oxide batteries used in early pacemakers (and still used in many other electronic devices), and lithium-iodine batteries used to power most modern cardiac pacemakers.

SECONDARY BATTERIES

Secondary batteries are designed to be repetitively discharged and recharged. The distinction between primary and secondary batteries is important, particularly because attempts to recharge a primary battery can be dangerous. Familiar examples of secondary batteries include the lead-acid batteries used to start automobiles and the cadmium-nickel oxide (nicad) batteries widely used in electronic devices and light power tools. Rechargeable cadmium-nickel oxide batteries were used to power some cardiac pacemakers built in the 1970s. However, cadmium-nickel oxide battery technology is being phased out of many applications because of its potential for environmental contamination with toxic cadmium-containing materials when the battery is thrown away. It appears that a direct technologic replacement will be the metal hydride-nickel oxide battery, which has voltage and current characteristics similar to those of nicad batteries, plus a significantly greater energy density and a greatly reduced environmental hazard.

Several newer rechargeable battery systems are being developed based on lithium as the negative electrode. Further discussion of secondary battery technology is omitted from this chapter because such cells are not being used in medical devices that are implanted today. The interested reader can find a good presentation of secondary battery technology in references 9 to 11.

AQUEOUS AND NONAQUEOUS BATTERIES

Another broad distinction between types of batteries is based on the choice of the electrolyte solvent. Batteries with aqueous electrolytes include many systems using zinc, lead, cadmium, aluminum, or magnesium anodes. Examples include zinc-mercuric oxide batteries, cadmium-nickel oxide rechargeable batteries, zinc-air batteries used in hearing aids, and alkaline zinc-manganese dioxide flashlight batteries. Water is an excellent solvent for salts and forms electrolyte solutions with excellent ionic conductivity. However, water cannot be used as a component for long-lived batteries employing alkaline metals, such as lithium or sodium, as anode materials because these metals undergo rapid reactions with water to form hydrogen gas and alkali hydroxides. Because of such reactions, alkaline metal anode batteries use nonaqueous electrolytes that react minimally with these materials. Most lithium-based batteries employ a mixture of organic ethers and esters as solvents for the electrolyte. For example, lithium-manganese dioxide batteries, widely used to power automatic cameras, use mixtures containing dimethoxyethane in which lithium trifluoromethane sulfonate or lithium perchlorate is dissolved to make the electrolyte. Some lithium batteries are designed with solid ceramic or polymeric electrolytes. The lithium-iodine battery, which is discussed in more detail later in this chapter, is one battery of this type. It does not contain any solvent, either aqueous or nonaqueous; its electrolyte is lithium iodide, the product of the discharge reaction.

Implantable Battery Design Requirements

Implantable medical devices must be thought of as a system. Longevity, end-of-service indications, and even basic reliability depend on optimal integration of the battery with the other components of the pulse generator. The type of battery selected for a particular application is determined by several critical requirements. Without question, the primary requirement in battery selection is high reliability. Other significant requirements include the longevity of the device and an appropriate indication of impending battery depletion (end-of-service warning). These are discussed in detail in this section.

The basic considerations when designing a battery for an implantable medical device include the electronic technology of the device that it will power and the voltage and current variations that will be required by the circuits and individual patients. The desired longevity of the device must also be established. Once these data are formulated, the current, voltage, and capacity requirements of the battery can be determined. An important limitation is the physical space, both of volume and shape, within the pulse generator that can be allotted to the battery. Once this is determined, the required energy density can be calculated, and various battery systems and designs can be considered and evaluated.

BATTERY CHEMISTRY

Different chemical systems have different battery characteristics. Voltage, energy density, and inherent current capability are all primary functions of the battery chemistry. The chemistry of the battery must be chosen to match the needs of the application. For example, the rate of energy delivery differs markedly for pacemakers and defibrillators. Pacemakers use very small amounts of energy when they stimulate the heart, on the order of 15 μJ. Defibrillators, on the other hand, require a much larger amount of energy when they discharge, as much as 35 J. Although the sizes of the batteries used in defibrillators and pacemakers are not greatly different, a pacemaker battery could never come close to supplying energy at the rate required for defibrillation. Likewise, the defibrillator battery would be a very poor choice to power a pacemaker, although it could easily supply the current needed. The high-power design of a defibrillator battery has a much lower energy density, perhaps by a factor of 3 lower than that of a pacemaker battery. Thus, if a defibrillator battery were used for pacing, it would need to be 3 times the volume of a pacemaker battery to obtain the same longevity. Additionally, a high-current cell poses more inherent safety risks (such as gross overheating from an internal short) than a low-current cell, so there are still other reasons for matching the battery to the application as closely as possible.

ELECTROLYTE AND ELECTRODE BALANCE

An ideal battery would contain the exact stoichiometric ratio of the active anodal and cathodal substances plus a very small amount of electrolyte. However, in practice batteries usually demand that one electrode be in excess of the other. For medical batteries this is nearly always the anode because the battery voltage would drop precipitously if the cell ever ran out of active anode material. The excess amount of anode (compared with the cathode) is often between 5% and 25%. The amount of electrolyte is also crucial to the long-term performance of batteries with liquid electrolyte. Minor parasitic or self-discharge reactions can consume significant amounts of the electrolyte over time. Thus, the battery must contain enough electrolyte so that it operates reliably over its entire intended service life.

POWER REQUIREMENTS

Another important consideration in designing an appropriate battery for a device is the peak power requirement. The battery must be capable of supplying the required power without a large drop in load voltage. The lithium-iodine battery, for example, has a high internal resistance, which increases as the battery is discharged. Its primary use is as a power source for implantable cardiac pacemakers, which typically have peak power demands on the order of 100 to 200 μW. Under these conditions, the lithium-iodine battery can maintain an adequate voltage even when its internal resistance is several thousand ohms. On the other hand, an implantable cardiac defibrillator may have peak power requirements approximately 10,000 times greater than those of a pacemaker, and a lithium-iodine battery would be incapable of meeting these requirements. This difference in peak power requirement may be made more obvious by realizing that if all of the lithium-iodine batteries ever produced were connected in an optimum series-parallel combination, they would operate fewer than five 100-W light bulbs. In contrast, every defibrillator battery must be capable of transiently supplying the current needed to light two 100-W bulbs.

AVERAGE VERSUS INSTANTANEOUS CURRENT DRAIN FROM THE BATTERY

A pacing circuit uses a capacitor to buffer the current drain on the battery. The battery charges the capacitor at a relatively low rate between pacing pulses. The pulse is delivered to the heart by discharging the capacitor through the pacing lead for a relatively short interval (i.e., the pacing pulse width). The use of a capacitor as a buffer allows the battery

to supply short bursts of power that may be more than two orders of magnitude higher than it could deliver directly. Thus, electronic buffering reduces the instantaneous power demands placed on the battery. It also allows the use of battery designs with reduced anode and cathode surface areas and improved volumetric efficiency.

SHAPE, SIZE, AND MASS CONSTRAINTS

Finally, all of these requirements (longevity, end-of-service indication, peak power, and so on) must be balanced against dimensional and mass constraints. The mass, dimensions, and shape of an implantable pulse generator are extremely important for safe implantation in children and for esthetic reasons in many adults. Because the battery is usually the largest component in an implantable pacemaker pulse generator, the battery design selected for a particular device must not only meet the electronic performance requirements but must also allow an acceptable longevity for the pulse generator, be small enough for long-term use, and have a good esthetic appearance.

The ratio of volume to surface area in the battery is an important factor. The performance of a battery of fixed volume can vary substantially depending on its electrode surface area-to-volume ratio. The operating current and longevity demanded from the battery determine both the minimum areas and the amounts of the anode and the cathode needed. Also, the area-volume ratio must not be made too large or the battery will be costly to make and will have a diminished energy density. Thus, these parameters can be changed only within certain ranges without jeopardizing either the long-term performance or the reliability of the battery.

RELATIONSHIP BETWEEN PACING CURRENT AND BATTERY SIZE

The relationship between average current and required battery size is not one of direct proportionality. For example, decreasing the average current by 50% will not permit a 50% reduction in battery size without compromising longevity. As battery size is decreased, the packaging efficiency of the battery also decreases because an increasing fraction of the battery weight and volume is composed of inactive materials (case, electrode separator material, current collectors, and so on). Also, the cell is balanced so there is an excess of lithium anode. In essence, this excess lithium is also an inactive material that reduces the packaging efficiency. This effect is most severe if the size reduction is accomplished by thinning the battery, which has been the trend in recent years. If battery size reduction is accomplished only by decreasing thickness, minimal change in the inactive material content inside the cell occurs because the mass and volume of the case, any separator material, and current collectors are largely unchanged. Thus, if a cell is made thinner, its capacity and energy density suffer far more than might be expected by the change in volume alone.

RELATIONSHIP BETWEEN ENERGY DENSITY AND CURRENT

Usable energy density is a function of the current demand on the cell. This is particularly true for a battery like the

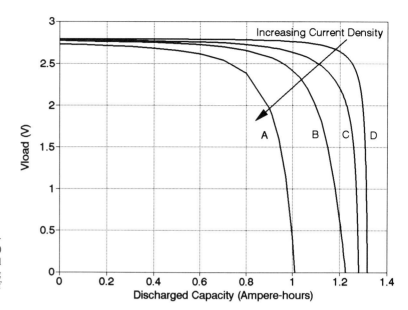

FIGURE 4–3. Load voltage–capacity plot for Li/I$_2$ battery discharged at four intensities of constant current. Curve A = 40 μA/cm^2, curve B = 20 μA/cm^2, curve C = 10 μA/cm^2, and curve D = 2 μA/cm^2. The capacity decreases with increasing current in this current range because of increasing effects of polarization.

lithium-iodine battery, which has an inherently high internal impedance. As the current from the cell is increased, the resulting voltage drop significantly reduces the period of time during which the cell can provide current at or above the specified minimum voltage level necessary to operate the pulse generator circuits (Fig. 4–3). Thus, the energy density, which is directly proportional to the area under the discharge curve (i.e., voltage vs. capacity), is also reduced.

EFFECT OF CLINICAL NEEDS AND PATIENT PREFERENCES ON BATTERY DESIGN

Marketing trends, which are intertwined with clinical needs, impose important limitations on the size and shape of batteries. For example, a thin, small pulse generator is a major clinical requirement for infants. For adults, a larger pulse generator with a greater battery capacity may be desirable for increased battery longevity. The major medical constraint is that the device must be designed so that side effects such as pocket and wound complication rates are not unacceptably higher in order to optimize other requirements such as longevity. Cosmetic appearance is also important for some patients.

Medical Battery Design Issues and the Management of the Patient

THE BATTERY AND LONGEVITY OF THE PULSE GENERATOR

Longevity is typically defined as the interval between implantation of the device and detection of the end-of-service indicator. Because longevity can vary dramatically with particular patients, the longevity requirement is typically linked to a specified set of nominal conditions and programmed parameters (i.e., pacing rate, pulse amplitude, pulse width, and lead impedance). The minimum battery capacity required to achieve the specified longevity can be calculated from the average current needed for this nominal set of conditions.

The following equation relates the deliverable capacity of the battery, Q, to the longevity of the pulse generator, L, and the average pacing current, I.

Eq 6 $Q = 8766 \times L \times I$

The units of Q are milliampere-hours (mAh), L is in years, and I is in milliamperes (mA). The conversion factor 8766 is needed because longevity is expressed in years, not hours.

PARASITIC AND OTHER NONUSEFUL BATTERY CAPACITY LOSSES

Other than pacing, there are numerous additional drains on battery capacity. First, self-discharge and possibly other parasitic losses of the anode or cathode begin from the date of battery manufacture and continue throughout use. Though small, these losses are not insignificant. Second, some current is required to power the circuit prior to implantation of the device. Thus, allowance must be made for capacity consumed during the expected period of shelf life between manufacture and implantation. Finally, substantial battery capacity must be kept in reserve to continue to power the device after the end-of-service indicator has been detected. For example, a device that requires a 72-month longevity and a 6-month end-of-service interval would need additional battery capacity of at least 8% (i.e., 6/72 × 100) more than the value calculated from equation 6.

FACTORS AFFECTING LONGEVITY OF PULSE GENERATORS

Two primary factors determine the longevity of an implanted pulse generator. The first factor is related to the size, design, and chemistry of the battery. The second factor is related to the rate at which the battery is discharged (i.e., the average current). The general relationships between battery size, average current, and longevity are obvious; larger batteries and lower current drains increase longevity. Because of better pacing electrodes and better electronic circuits, the average current drain has decreased substantially during the past decade. The trend throughout the evolution of cardiac pacemakers has been that reduced current demands lead to smaller batteries and pulse generators while maintaining relatively constant longevity.

OVERHEAD CURRENT

The battery must also supply the static (or overhead) current that is needed to power the electronic components even when no pacing pulses are being delivered. Advances in electronic technology have substantially reduced the static current drain in recent years. In most cases, the static current is a few microamperes. As a first approximation, static or overhead current can be considered to be independent of the programmed settings of the pulse generator.

EFFECT OF PULSE WIDTH ON PACING CURRENT DRAIN

Increasing the pacing rate, pulse width, or pulse amplitude increases the average pacing current. However, some of these relationships are highly nonlinear. For example, as shown later, doubling the pacing stimulus voltage quadruples the current drain on the battery.

The average pacing current (not including overhead current) is directly proportional to the pacing rate. However, the effect of pulse width on the average pacing current is not linear. Recall that the pacing pulse results from the discharge of a capacitor through a nominally resistive load (i.e., the electrode-heart interface). This produces a pacing pulse in which the current decays exponentially with time as shown for two pulse widths in Figure 4–4A and B. Thus, the time-dependent behavior of the delivered current during the pacing pulse is given by the following equation:

$$\text{Eq 7} \quad I = \frac{V_A}{R_H} e^{-\frac{t}{R_H C}}$$

where V_A is the amplitude at the beginning of the pacing pulse, R_H is the resistance of the heart, and lead C is the value of the capacitor that delivers the pacing pulse, and t is the time since the beginning of the pacing pulse. In Figure 4–4A and B the pulse width is given by t_w and $t_{w/2}$, respectively. The total charge delivered by each pulse is given by the area under its current-time curve. Although the width of the pulse in Figure 4–4B is half that of the pulse in Figure 4–4A, the charge delivered by this pulse is considerably more than half that of the longer pulse duration. It is not possible to calculate the exact ratio of the charge delivered in the two cases until the resistance and capacitance values are specified. Nevertheless, reducing the pulse width by a given fraction will always reduce the average pacing current by a substantially smaller fraction.

EFFECT OF PULSE AMPLITUDE ON PACING CURRENT DRAIN

The definition of pacing pulse amplitude may vary somewhat between manufacturers of implantable pulse generators. For our purposes, pulse amplitude is defined as the voltage delivered to the heart at the beginning of the pacing pulse (leading edge voltage). As stated earlier, the charge delivered

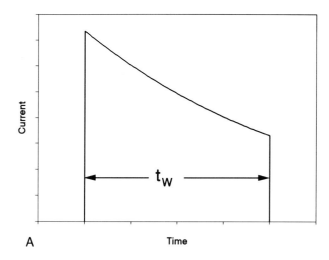

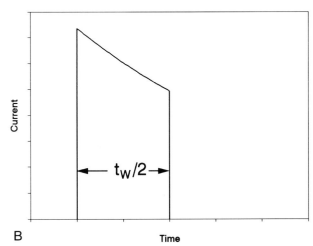

FIGURE 4–4. *A* and *B*, Comparison of charge delivered to the heart as the pacing pulse width is shortened. The two cases in *A* and *B* assume a discharge into the same patient. The pulse width, t_w, is typically between 0.2 and 1.5 msec, and the maximum current is between 2 and 15 mA, depending on the pulse generator output voltage and the lead-heart interface resistance.

per pulse is given by the area under the current-time curve. Thus, doubling the amplitude doubles the current and the total charge delivered to the heart. It might also appear that because the charge per pulse is doubled, the average pacing current drawn from the battery might also be doubled. However, the impact on the pacing current is much larger, as seen from the following argument. The energy per pacing pulse is defined by the equation:

$$\text{Eq 8} \quad E = V_A \times I_A \times t_w$$

where V_A is the average output voltage of the pulse generator, I_A is the average pacing current delivered to the heart, and t_w is the pulse width. If we consider the lead-electrode-heart interface to be mainly resistive, Ohm's law can be substituted in equation 8, i.e., $I = V/R$. When this is done, equation 8 becomes,

$$\text{Eq 9} \quad E = \frac{V_A^2}{R_H} \times t_w$$

where R_H is the effective ohmic load of the heart and lead. From this equation it is readily apparent that energy consumption increases with the square of the output voltage. Because all of the energy delivered to the heart is ultimately supplied by the battery at a relatively constant voltage, any increase in energy is accompanied by a proportional increase in current drawn from the battery. Thus, the average pacing current is proportional to the square of the pacing amplitude. In fact, this is the best situation; additional energy losses occur when the stimulus voltage is programmed to a higher level because the electronic processes for increasing the stimulus voltage are not 100% efficient.

EFFECT OF OHMIC LOAD ON PACING CURRENT

Finally, it is important to consider the effect of load of the lead and heart, R_H, on the average pacing current. In a sense, the term lead resistance is really a misnomer. The resistance of the lead itself is relatively small (in the range of 50 to 100 ohms), and most of the resistance actually arises at the electrode-tissue interface. The factors affecting the impedance of this interface are discussed in Chapter 1. In general, the average pacing current is approximately inversely proportional to lead resistance. Thus, there is a substantial interest in lead technologies that can increase the impedance of the electrode-tissue interface, thereby decreasing the pacing current, while maintaining a constant pacing threshold (voltage).

SUMMARY OF PROGRAMMING EFFECTS ON BATTERY LONGEVITY

In summary, the wide range of pacing parameters that can be selected can have a dramatic effect on the current drain from the battery in an implanted pulse generator. For example, in the same patient, a pulse generator with a 6-year longevity under nominal pacing parameters may reach its replacement time in 2 years at one extreme or more than 10 years at the other extreme. This is why the relationships between the programmed pacing parameters and the pacing threshold need to be quantitatively considered when the clinician is judging alternative programmable pulse generator settings or discussing predictions of future pulse generator replacement with the patient.

Battery End-of-Service Indication

End-of-service requirements result from the need to indicate impending battery depletion in a manner that allows the patient and physician adequate time to replace the device. In general, this requires a battery to have some measurable characteristic, such as voltage or impedance, that is related to its state of discharge. The pulse generator end-of-service indication must occur well before the battery loses so much voltage that it cannot sustain cardiac pacing or defibrillation. Again, this requirement is typically linked to a specific set of nominal pacing or defibrillation parameters. A detailed knowledge of the variations in battery performance, changes in load current with pulse generator settings, and the accuracy of the end-of-service measurement circuitry is necessary to ensure that these requirements will be met.

ELECTIVE REPLACEMENT INDICATOR

All modern implantable pulse generators have an elective replacement indicator (ERI) that alerts the clinician to im-

pending battery depletion and allows adequate time for replacement of the device. This point is also referred to as the recommended replacement time (RRT) or the end-of-service point (EOS). As a general rule, the ERI is designed to occur at least 3 months before the battery voltage drops to a level at which erratic pacing or loss of capture results.

METHODS FOR MONITORING STATE OF BATTERY DISCHARGE

Several means are used to monitor a battery's state of discharge.

BATTERY VOLTAGE

The most common method typically uses battery voltage. Historically, this was accomplished by comparing the battery voltage to a reference voltage in the pacemaker circuitry. The ERI was triggered when the battery voltage dropped below the reference level. Most modern pacemakers incorporate a voltage measurement circuit in the form of an analog-to-digital converter. The digitized battery voltage can be compared with a value stored in a nonvolatile memory to trigger the ERI, or it can be telemetered to the programmer where the comparison is made.

For most batteries, the battery voltage remains relatively constant throughout most of its discharge (Fig. 4–5). Because the battery voltage is relatively constant for much of the pulse generator's useful life, the telemetered voltage may not be particularly useful for estimating its remaining service life until the end-of-service time draws near. On the other hand, the measured voltage may be useful for determining the battery's ability to remain above the ERI voltage after reprogramming to a higher current condition has occurred or to indicate that the ERI is imminent.

BATTERY IMPEDANCE

Battery impedance is another parameter used to signal the elective replacement point. Battery impedance is generally much less dependent on current than is battery voltage and may convey more information about the battery's state of discharge. For example, although the voltage of a lithium-iodine battery remains relatively constant through most of its discharge, its impedance increases continuously. The increase in impedance is especially rapid as the battery approaches depletion (see Fig. 4–5). At this time, battery impedance is useful not only for signaling the elective replacement point but also for providing an estimate of remaining service life. This feature has been incorporated into some pacemaker designs.

CONSUMED CHARGE AS INDICATOR OF REMAINING BATTERY USE TIME

A final method used to indicate remaining battery life has been to measure the cumulative sum of the charge removed from the battery. This is accomplished by monitoring the current drawn from the battery or the current and voltage (i.e., energy) delivered to the heart. This method requires an accurate knowledge of the deliverable capacity of the battery because one is actually measuring capacity used, not what is left.

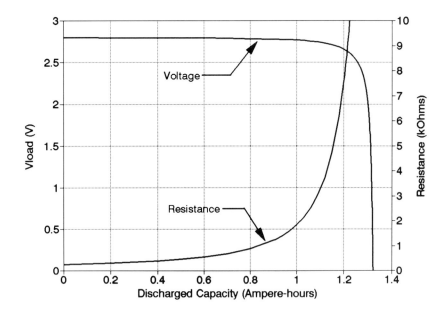

FIGURE 4–5. Relationship between voltage, resistance, and capacity of Li/I$_2$ battery showing rapid fall-off in voltage as resistance increases near time of end-of-service.

ERI TRIGGERING

The relatively high resistance of power sources like the lithium-iodine battery results in a battery voltage that is highly dependent on current. Thus, any large changes in average battery current in pulse generators that utilize battery voltage to indicate the elective replacement point (even if temporary) may drop the battery voltage below the ERI trigger value. Such changes in current can occur as a result of rate-responsive pacing, magnet-rate pacing, telemetry, and so on. This could also occur during electrophysiologic studies with noninvasive programmed stimulation (NIPS) in which the pacemaker is used to interrupt an episode of tachycardia by delivering short bursts of very high rate pacing. Because the ERI is usually latched (stored) when it is triggered, these temporary increases in current can cause a premature trigger of the ERI. The amount of service life lost to these premature triggers is typically relatively small (see the extreme example given later in this chapter). In most cases, devices are designed to make it possible to reset an ERI that has been prematurely triggered.

CLINICAL INDICATORS OF THE BATTERY REPLACEMENT TIME

The clinical indicators of battery depletion vary widely between manufacturers of pulse generators. In fact, there is often significant variation between various models provided by a single manufacturer. Some of the more common indicators are listed below.

1. Stepwise change in pacing rate. Elective replacement time is indicated by a change in the pacing rate to a predetermined fixed rate (such as 65 bpm) or a fractional change in rate (such as a 10% decrease from the programmed rate).
2. Stepwise change in magnet rate. The magnet pacing rate decreases in a stepwise fashion related to remaining battery life.

3. Pacing mode change. DDD and DDDR pulse generators may automatically revert to another mode such as VVI or VOO to reduce current drain and extend battery life.
4. Pulse width stretching. Some pulse generators increase the width of the pacing pulse to compensate for decreasing pulse amplitude associated with declining battery voltage. Pulse width stretching has also been used as an indicator of imminent ERI.
5. Telemetered battery voltage or impedance. In modern pacemakers the battery voltage or the battery impedance can be telemetered out to the programming device. This information can be useful in estimating remaining battery service life or in indicating an imminent ERI by algorithms performed outside the pulse generator.

All manufacturers provide technical manuals containing tables or graphs that indicate the relationship between battery voltage or impedance and the estimated remaining service life of the device. This time will differ for different loads on the battery as influenced by pacing rates and stimulus currents, as discussed previously.

The Elective Replacement Indicator in Practice

The ERI is both extremely useful and, if used uncritically, potentially misleading in some patients. The object of having an ERI is to allow the use of the pulse generator as long as safely possible. Several pertinent questions must be addressed by the clinician when considering elective pulse generator replacement based on the ERI: (1) how does the ERI for this particular pulse generator manifest itself; (2) if the goal is to replace the pulse generator before its continued use becomes unsafe, what is the definition of safe for the patient in question; and (3) how does one interpret the meaning of the appearance of the ERI in this patient (what other factors beside the nominal ERI must be considered for this patient)?

CONCERNS FOR THE PATIENT IF PACING STOPS

Having a probable expectation of the clinical consequences of loss of pacing in a particular patient is critically important. A small percentage of patients with pacemakers are extremely likely to develop asystole if pacing capture is lost. This group will die if pacing capture is lost outside a medical setting. Another fraction will be asystolic for a few seconds and then will develop an escape rhythm at very slow rates. This group will not die from asystole but may be injured during syncope. A third group will develop transient presyncope or lightheadedness but will then be able to function reasonably normally. A fourth, and probably the largest, group of patients will slowly develop symptoms such as reduced exercise tolerance but otherwise will be at least temporarily asymptomatic. The fifth and last group will not even know that the pacemaker has stopped working unless an Adams-Stokes attack occurs at some unpredictable time in the future. Thus, the consequences of loss of pacing vary tremendously, and for these reasons the time relationship between the appearance of the ERI and the loss of capture is much more important for some patients than for others.

EFFECTS OF HIGH CURRENT DRAINS IN OR NEAR ERI TIME

If the pacing threshold is very high, the output voltage of the pulse generator may decrease below the level necessary for capture before the ERI appears or reaches its nominal value. For example, the output voltage of some pulse generators starts to decrease when the magnet rate begins to decrease. If the normal magnet rate is 100 bpm and the ERI magnet rate is 85 bpm, capture in patients with very high thresholds may be lost when the magnet rate reaches 92 bpm rather than 85 bpm. Whether the potential loss of capture occurs or not depends on (1) the relationship between the magnet rate and the actual output voltage of the pulse generator at the programmed output voltage setting, and (2) the actual pacing threshold for the patient in question.

It is worth noting that reprogramming the pulse generator to a higher output voltage near its expected end-of-service life will have an especially large effect on reducing the remaining service life of the pulse generator. This is true because the current drain is increased when the battery's internal impedance is rising rapidly. The result is both an increase in current drain and a large increase in polarization voltage, which combine to shorten the remaining service life more than might be expected.

PACING OUTPUT VOLTAGE NEAR ERI

In most modern pulse generators the actual output voltage can be obtained by telemetry as discussed previously. With one otherwise excellent pulse generator that did not provide telemetry, we noticed that the measured output voltage at the time of replacement was consistently less than the graphs depicted in the technical manual. This information implies that it may be wise for the clinician who has patients requiring high-output pacing to be especially wary near the ERI time. The pulse generator output voltage decreases more rapidly when the cell is nearing or in the ERI phase than earlier

in its service period. When the magnet rate is changing because of ERI in pulse generators that feature a gradual rate change, the output voltage decreases faster at high-output voltages than it does for normal output settings. This should be expected because of the high current drain on the battery.

We also experienced an ERI anomaly in one series of modern rate-responsive pulse generators. In these devices the magnet rate indicated that the ERI time had come only a few days after implantation. This occurred during pacing at high voltage levels (7.5 V) into leads with normal impedance. Reprogramming of the pulse generator to 5.0 V restored the magnet rate to its beginning-of-life value. The explanation for this change in magnet rate is related to the fact that this series of pulse generators relates the magnet rate to the predicted time to end-of-service life at the programmed values regardless of battery impedance or voltage. This observation suggests that under some circumstances the clinician may wish to test such pulse generators at the time of implantation by temporarily pacing at the highest programmable voltage output. If the ERI magnet rate becomes manifest, the implanter may wish to confer with the manufacturer to be sure that the problem is not with the battery but rather with the ERI algorithm.

PULSE WIDTH STRETCHING EFFECTS ON SAFETY OF PACING DURING ERI TIME

A well-known but sometimes incompletely appreciated clinical point applicable to both low- and high-amplitude pacing is related to pulse width stretching. Certain pulse generators increase the pulse width as the cell output voltage decreases to maintain a nearly constant pulse energy. This feature is intended as both a marker of battery status and a threshold safety factor. The battery and stimulus output voltages decrease over time with cell use. Having the pulse generator automatically and gradually increase the stimulus duration does help to maintain the safety margin of the output pulse compared to the pacing threshold. However, it must be remembered that the strength-duration curve is curvilinear, and increases in pulse duration provide very little margin of safety if the pulse amplitude is near rheobase (see Chapter 1). Thus, when the voltage has decreased enough to reach or nearly reach the rheobase, further pulse width stretching provides little additional pacing threshold protection even though the pulse energy continues to increase.

COMMON SENSE CLINICAL GUIDELINES REGARDING ERI

The points discussed previously translate into two clinical guidelines that bear on the relationships between the status of the patient and the status of the pulse generator battery at ERI: (1) The physician should replace the pulse generator sooner than he or she otherwise would if the clinical history or present situation implies that something very serious may happen if pacing capture is lost; (2) the pulse generator (or the pulse generator and lead) should be changed even sooner if the pacing threshold is high. The time to change the pulse generator for life-preserving purposes cannot be decided on the basis of pulse generator and battery specifications alone.

Battery Reliability and Failure Modes

Battery reliability is the key concern for clinicians who implant pacing systems because these devices cannot operate without a battery.

METHODS OF ASSESSING BATTERY LONG-TERM RELIABILITY

The reliability of a long-term power source is difficult to assess except in retrospect after real-time experience. However, by then it may be too late to change anything if there is a problem. Therefore, battery and device designers attempt to make assessments of reliability based on accelerated and abuse tests along with quality tools such as fault tree analysis. Some potential failure mechanisms cannot be completely eliminated because they are also linked to characteristics that are required to meet the clinical needs of the application. The high-rate battery for the implantable defibrillator is a good example. High current capability means that the battery is vulnerable to failure from short circuits triggered either internally or externally. The high current capability could be eliminated, but then the battery would be incapable of performing its intended function. In this example the risk of battery failure is minimized by using external fuses, limiting the electrode areas within the battery, and using a fusible separator.

Battery reliability can be maximized by understanding all of the processes that occur in a battery and then supplementing this knowledge by careful, meticulous manufacturing and extensive testing for verification. Tables 4–2 and 4–3 list the impact of some major failure mechanisms on important battery characteristics and the principal methods that are used to eliminate them.

Battery Chemistries Used in Bradycardia Pacing

There have been many different battery chemistries used to power cardiac pacemakers over the years. This was particularly true 10 years ago. Table 4–4 compares the qualities of these various power sources. It also shows the power sources used for implantable defibrillators.

When implantable pacemakers were first developed in the late 1960s, lithium and other high-energy density batteries did not exist. The first implantable pacemaker used a nickel-

TABLE 4–2. **LIST OF BATTERY FAILURE MECHANISMS AND METHODS OF CONTROL**

FAILURE MECHANISM	METHODS OF CONTROL
High internal resistance	Choice of electrolyte
	Consistent manufacturing
Electrolyte loss and gas formation	Choice of electrolyte
	Dry electrolytes
	Enough electrolyte in cell
Internal short	Good manufacturing processes
	Good battery design
	Fusable separator
	Controlled contact area
External short	Fuse
	Care in handling
Manufacturing variations	Robust cell design
	Consistent manufacturing

cadmium oxide (nicad) battery, which was used as a primary battery. That implant only lasted a few hours. However, the concept of the battery-powered pacemaker was proved. The most practical power source for portable electronic devices at that time was the zinc-mercuric oxide battery that had been developed for military applications during World War II. It became the battery of choice by default and remained so until the mid-1970s.

MERCURY CELLS

The zinc-mercuric oxide (or mercury) battery has good energy density and high current capability but quite a low voltage (just over 1 V). Early pacemakers were designed to hold up to five or six mercury cells in series. The circuits and the pacing leads then in use put relatively high current and voltage demands on the cells within the pulse generator. In addition, this multiple-cell configuration allowed the pacemaker to continue to operate if one of the cells failed. Unfortunately, this happened unpredictably and frequently by today's standards. The longevity of pacemakers using mercury cells was typically between 1 and 3 years. These cells self-discharged and generated hydrogen gas. The pulse generators of that day were encapsulated in epoxy rather than being hermetically sealed, in part so that the small amounts of hydrogen gas produced could diffuse out of the pulse generator. Even more problematic was the propensity of this chemistry to develop a metal mercury short circuit through the separator. Such an event left that cell completely discharged and behaving very much like a wire. This is why the

TABLE 4–3. **EFFECT OF FAILURE MECHANISMS ON MEDICAL BATTERY PROPERTIES**

	CAPACITY LOSS	VOLTAGE DROP	HERMATICITY LOSS	SWELLING	UNPREDICTABLE END-OF-SERVICE
Water in cell	×	×			
Films on electrodes		×			×
Electrolyte loss				×	×
Feedthrough corrosion	×	×			
Gas formation				×	×
Internal short	×			×	
External short	×		×		×
Manufacturing variances		×			

TABLE 4–4. **COMPARISON OF CHARACTERISTICS FOR IMPLANTABLE MEDICAL BATTERY SYSTEMS**

SYSTEM	HIGH VOLTAGE	HIGH CURRENT	HIGH POWER	LOW SELF-DISCHARGE	HIGH ENERGY DENSITY	DEGREE OF RECHARGEABILITY	HIGHLY PREDICTABLE DISCHARGE	HIGHLY INHERENT RELIABILITY
Zn/HgO	1	4	4	2	2	0	2	2
Li/I$_2$	3	1	1	4	4	0	4	4
Li/MnO$_2$	3	3	4	3	3	0	4	3
Li/SOCl$_2$	4	3	4	2	4	0	3	3
Li/CuS	2	3	3	3	3	0	4	3
Li/SVO	3	4	4	3	3	0	3	3
Ni/CdO	1	4	4	1	2	4	3	2
Ni/H$_2$	1	4	4	2	2	5	3	2
Nuclear	0	1	1	5	5	0	5	5
Li/V$_2$O$_5$	3	4	3	2	3	0	2	3

For all parameters, 0, poor, 5, excellent.

strategy of the extra cell in series worked fairly well. This problem plagued the zinc-mercuric oxide battery chemistry for a long time. Just about the time a major improvement was made (by using multiple wraps of special separator material), the new lithium anode batteries had been sufficiently developed and tested for clinical use. In a very short time the lithium cells completely displaced the zinc-mercuric oxide batteries from implantable applications.

LITHIUM CELLS

The advent of lithium batteries in the early 1970s resulted in a dramatic revolution in cardiac pacing. Lithium was chosen as the anode material for several reasons. First, it has a very high capacity density (0.0768 equivalents/cm^3 or 2.06 Ah/cm^3). Lithium also forms many electrochemical couples that have appropriate stability, adequately fast discharge kinetics, and high energy density. The period from 1975 to 1980 could be characterized as "lithium mania." Lithium was the buzz word and physical chemists were on a bandwagon to develop new and exotic lithium batteries. Several lithium-based battery chemistries were developed for implantation during this period and were incorporated into cardiac pacemakers. These included three chemistries with liquid organic electrolytes: lithium-silver chromate, lithium-cupric sulfide, and lithium-manganese dioxide; one chemistry with a liquid cathode component, lithium-thionyl chloride; and one chemistry that behaved almost like a solid state battery, lithium-iodine. The chemistries of these battery systems are discussed in detail in reference 12.

TYPES OF LITHIUM CELLS

Although none of the several varieties of lithium batteries developed for implantable medical use proved to be inherently unreliable, only the lithium-iodine system remains in widespread use for cardiac pacing today. Device manufacturers, marketing and other business factors, and technical performance played roles in determining which battery chemistries became most widely used in cardiac pacemakers. In some cases not enough was known about the fundamental battery chemistry or critical design issues; these batteries did not always perform as expected and hence lost favor.

The lithium-cupric sulfide and lithium-silver chromate batteries had some very attractive features, although they are no longer used today. The type of lithium-manganese dioxide cells used in the late 1970s are also no longer made; however, newer versions of this system are beginning to be used again to power implantable cardiac pacemakers with higher power requirements such as optical sensors that measure mixed venous oxygen saturation. These sensors require battery currents in the range 0.1 to 1 mA at 2 V to power light-emitting diodes. Lithium-iodine batteries cannot provide this level of power without a significant loss of energy density. Thus, the longevity of a high current drain pulse generator using a low-current battery is significantly less than if a higher current battery such as lithium-manganese dioxide is used. For similar reasons, lithium-thionyl chloride batteries are still used in some implantable pulse generators for neurologic and drug delivery applications.

NUCLEAR BATTERIES

The evolutionary path to the lithium battery was not without it side branches. One of the most interesting of these was the development of nuclear batteries to power cardiac pacemakers. Approximately 3000 nuclear-powered pacemakers were implanted between 1970 and 1982.[13] Nuclear power sources harness the energy from radioactive decay as opposed to the chemical energy used in conventional batteries. Two types of nuclear batteries have been used in pacemakers. The first type works by the beta-voltaic effect. A beta emitter, such as promethium-147, gives off electrons that impinge on a semiconductor, producing an electric current. In the second type, the heat evolved during nuclear decay is converted to electric energy through a thermopile. Plutonium-238 is commonly used in this type of power source. Both power sources are described in detail in reference 13. The great advantage of nuclear power sources is their longevity and extreme reliability. The half-life of plutonium-238 is 88 years. In practical terms, a pulse generator powered by a nuclear source will last the life of the patient. Like many other power sources, nuclear batteries are no longer being used in implantable devices. Safety and regulatory requirements were the principal reasons for their demise. The absolute follow-up requirements were a major inconvenience for manufacturers, physicians, and patients, all of whom were held responsible for tracking the regulated power source and then returning it when it was no longer being used. In addition, the extreme longevity of nuclear power sources is in itself a problem. A patient with a functioning 20-year-old pacemaker does not benefit from any advances made in pacemaker technology, which typically changes substantially every 5 years. Also, nuclear batteries are relatively large and expensive. Their size was competitive with the zinc-mercuric oxide batteries of the 1960s, but they cannot compete with modern 1 Wh/cm³ primary lithium batteries.

RECHARGEABLE CELLS

The evolutionary tree of power sources for cardiac pacing also had one other interesting spur. The goals of small volume, low mass, and great longevity seem to be matched to rechargeable batteries. One device of this type was manufactured commercially. Approximately 5000 rechargeable nickel oxide-cadmium battery-powered pacemakers were implanted in the 1970s.[10] One coauthor of this chapter has had an ongoing, excellent clinical experience with patients who had rechargeable-cell pulse generators implanted between 1974 and 1978. These batteries functioned reliably, but most of them were eventually replaced by pulse generators powered by primary lithium batteries. However, even after more than 15 years, a few still remain implanted today.

There are two main reasons why rechargeable batteries did not continue to have commercial success. First, advances in electronics reduced the current drain of pacemakers so that designers could make an acceptably small pacemaker with a primary battery. The lower energy density of rechargeable batteries (0.2 Wh/cm³ compared with 1 Wh/cm³ for lithium-iodine batteries) combined with a high rate of self-discharge made rechargeable batteries less attractive. They no longer provided a volume savings when 1 Wh/cm³ lithium batteries became available. Another disadvantage was their need to be recharged about once a week. Some patients had psychological reactions to these devices because the need for regular recharging was a constant reminder of their cardiac problem. Reasons for removal of pulse generators powered by rechargeable cells in the author's experience ranged from a need for new pacing features (such as dual-chamber function or single chamber rate-response) to recurrent trouble with the recharging apparatus (which was subject to trauma or liquid spilling on it at home) to one patient's statement that he was simply too old to remember to recharge the device anymore. It seems unlikely that rechargeable batteries will replace lithium primary batteries to power bradycardia pulse generators in the foreseeable future.

The use of rechargeable cells in cardiac defibrillators is an attractive concept because it seems to allow a reduction in the defibrillator's volume or an increase in its service life. However, battery technology today is not sufficiently developed to ensure that the needed reliability can be designed into rechargeable high-current, high-energy density cells. Manufacturers probably will not incorporate such batteries into their implantable defibrillators until they have more confidence in the technology and in the clinical need for their use.

The Lithium-Iodine Battery

The lithium-iodine battery is the most important implantable battery because it has been used in the great majority of cardiac pacemakers manufactured during the past decade.[14] The first implant of a pacemaker powered by a lithium-iodine battery occurred in 1972.[15] About 3 million lithium-iodine-powered pacemakers have now been implanted. There are many factors favoring the use of this battery system. Lithium-iodine batteries have a high energy density (1 Wh/cm³) and low self-discharge (<1%/year), resulting in good longevity and small size. The inherent high impedance of the lithium-iodine battery is not a disadvantage because the current required by modern pacemaker circuits is so low, typically about 15 µA. (Note that the stimulus current is drawn from a capacitor, which can charge for a very long time compared to its discharge time.) The voltage and impedance characteristics of these lithium cells also allow the clinician to monitor the approaching end-of-service indication. This battery system is simple and elegant in concept and is inherently resistant to many common modes of failure, as will be discussed later. As a result, lithium-iodine batteries have attained a record of reliability unsurpassed among electrochemical power sources.[14]

LITHIUM-IODINE CELL COMPONENTS

Most lithium/iodine batteries consist of an anode of lithium coated with a thin film of poly-2-vinylpyridine (P2VP) and a cathode composed of a thermally reacted mixture of iodine and P2VP. Although lithium-iodine batteries are sensitive to moisture during manufacture, they can be safely and reliably manufactured in rooms maintained at low (1%) relative humidity.

Figure 4–6 shows a cutaway view of a typical lithium-iodine battery. Visible in the figure are the central anode with an embedded current collector grid and a surrounding piece of plastic to contain the lithium. The surrounding iodine-P2VP cathode mixture, which is in contact with both the anode and the inside of the battery container, is not visible but fills the remainder of the volume inside the battery. The figure also shows several other important structures. One of these is the electric feedthrough that connects the anode terminal to the outside of the cell. A second wire connector is shown on the top of the battery. This serves as the site of the electric connection to the battery cathode. The third is the fill port toward the top right side of the figure. The fill port is the means by which the cathode mixture is introduced into the cell.

ELECTROCHEMICAL PROPERTIES OF LITHIUM-IODINE CELLS

When lithium-iodine batteries are manufactured, the initial iodine reaching the surface of lithium reacts directly with the lithium, yielding lithium iodide. This reaction proceeds to only a small extent before the surface of the lithium is covered by lithium iodide, and the reaction rate slows greatly. The voltage of the cell quickly rises to 2.8 V, which is characteristic of the lithium-iodine couple, as this layer forms. The properties of the lithium iodide layer are responsible for most of the overt characteristics attributed to this system. Lithium iodide is an electronic insulator with enough lithium-ion conductivity to act as a solid electrolyte in the cell. The cell potential, 2.8 V, is not simply the difference in the two half-cell potentials for the lithium and iodine couples

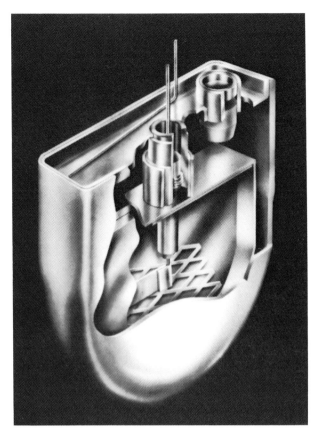

FIGURE 4–6. Cutaway view of a typical lithium-iodine battery showing its internal construction. Easily identifiable interior parts include the anode feedthrough, the anode current collector, a plastic band around the edge of the anode, and the port where the cathode material is poured into the cell.

given in Table 4–1. The values in Table 4–1 are calculated for the products in a standard state, in this case Li$^+$ and I$^-$, which are dissolved ions. In the lithium-iodine battery, which contains no solvent, the two ions combine to form the more stable, solid lithium iodide salt. This gives the cell a larger voltage than if the ions were dissolved in a solution. As the cell discharges, the lithium iodide produced is also the electrolyte. Lithium iodide accumulates near the surface of the anode because it is not soluble in the cathode mixture. Because the product of the direct reaction of the anode and cathode is also the electrolyte, a breach of the electrolyte layer in a cell simply results in the creation of more electrolyte. Thus, the electrolyte is said to be self-healing and contributes to the high reliability of this battery.

The iodine in the cathode is made conductive by reaction with P2VP. The reaction products are a viscous conductive liquid polyiodide material plus excess crystalline iodine.[16] Practical batteries are made with cathode compositions in the range of 20 to 50 parts of iodine per part of P2VP by weight. As the cell discharges, the crystalline iodine is consumed first, followed by iodine from the conductive liquid phase. As iodine is removed from the conductive liquid phase, the resistivity of the remaining material increases by several orders of magnitude before the cell is completely discharged.

LITHIUM CELL RESISTANCE

The resistivity of lithium iodide for lithium ion transport is significant; in practice, the measured resistance of the cell

is less than what would be expected from the buildup of a planar lithium iodide layer. This can be attributed to the P2VP coating originally on the anode. It reacts with lithium and iodine to produce a small amount of liquid electrolyte that enhances the conduction of the discharge product and also causes it to grow in a slightly irregular form.[17] The resistance of the electrolyte in a lithium-iodine cell increases during the course of discharge from a few hundred ohms to a few thousand ohms. This is a fundamental characteristic of this battery system and limits its application to uses that do not require very high or very frequent bursts of current.

ELECTROCHEMICAL PROCESSES IN THE LITHIUM-IODINE BATTERY

The electrochemistry of the lithium-iodine battery has been studied intensively. Several significant processes have been identified as contributing factors in the voltage loss seen under load.[18] They are (1) the bulk resistances of the electrolyte and cathode; (2) the charge-transfer resistance at the interface between the case and the cathode; (3) the concentration polarization in the cathode; and (4) the loss of open-circuit potential as the iodine becomes depleted.

Figures 4–7A and B show the characteristic shapes of the voltage and resistance curves as a function of discharge for a typical lithium-iodine battery. The most salient characteristic of these curves is the initial slow change of each parameter followed by a rapid change near the end of discharge. The point where the resistance curve becomes noticeably steeper corresponds to the point in the discharge where the crystalline iodine becomes depleted from the two-phase cathode mixture. Before this point, the resistance change is dominated by the growing electrolyte. Beyond it, the resistance rapidly becomes dominated by the cathode as iodine becomes depleted from the P2VP-rich liquid phase. The region of discharge dominated by cathode resistance is used to signal the approaching end-of-service for most pacemakers.

EFFECTS OF CURRENT DRAIN ON DELIVERABLE CAPACITY FROM LITHIUM-IODINE CELLS

The high energy density of the lithium-iodine battery may be negated if the application requires frequent periods of high current drain. This is because there is an optimum average current for the operation of this (or any) battery. Figure 4–8 shows a plot of the deliverable capacity versus the log average current drain for a typical lithium-iodine battery. The maximum in this curve is the optimum operating point for this battery. If higher currents are drawn from the battery, polarization lowers the deliverable capacity. If lower currents are required, self-discharge uses up capacity increasingly faster than the application current, resulting in a reduced deliverable capacity. For applications that require an average current drain that is significantly different from the maximum, a different battery system may result in a more favorable deliverable capacity and longevity, especially under high current conditions. For example, in the typical conditions encountered in an implanted cardiac pacemaker, a lithium-manganese dioxide battery has a volumetric efficiency of about 80% of that of a lithium-iodine battery. However, if the application requires frequent, intermittent current pulses at a 10-fold increase in magnitude, the overall deliverable

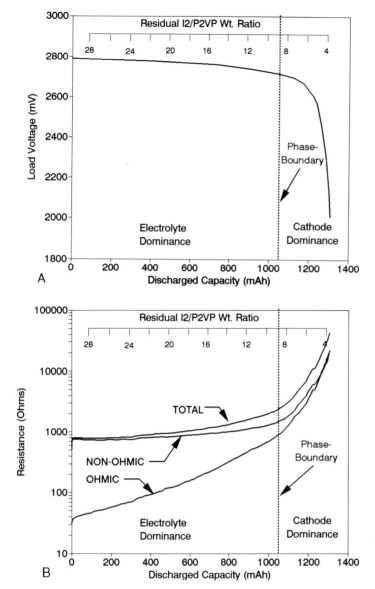

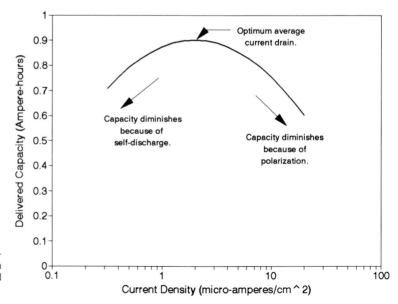

FIGURE 4–7. *A*, Voltage-capacity plot for Li/I$_2$ battery during discharge. The superimposed scale shows residual I$_2$/P2VP weight ratio (starting at 50). The vertical line defines the boundary between the two-phase and the single-phase cathode regions where the electrolyte and cathode, respectively, dominate the internal resistance. *B*, Resistance-capacity plot analogous to *A*. The ohmic and non-ohmic contributions to internal resistance are shown.

FIGURE 4–8. Capacity versus log current curve shows that deliverable battery capacity is a maximum between low and high average current drains due to the effects of self-discharge and polarization.

energy density of the lithium-manganese dioxide battery may become greater than that of the lithium-iodine battery. An example of a device requiring large intermittent current drains from the battery is a pulse generator that uses a light-emitting diode as part of a hemoglobin oxygen saturation measurement for pacemaker rate-response control.

Comparison of Implantable Cardiac Defibrillator and Pacemaker Batteries

Implantable defibrillators deliver up to 35 J to the heart in a few milliseconds. By contrast, the energy required to stimulate the heart in bradycardia pacing is on the order of 1 to 10 μJ. Clearly, the demands placed on the battery that powers an implantable defibrillator are much different from those of a battery that powers a bradycardia pacemaker. Implantable defibrillators are designed to deliver a shock within about 10 seconds (or less) after the fibrillation or tachycardia is detected. When the device determines that a shock will or may be required, it begins to charge a high-voltage capacitor. The time needed to charge the capacitor before the shock is delivered depends on the ability of the battery to sustain a very high current during this period. Thus, the implantable defibrillator requires a high peak-power battery. The energy delivered by the battery is the product of the battery voltage and the charge on the capacitor, or power times time. For example, the power required to charge the defibrillator for a 30-J shock in 10 seconds is 3 W, or 3 J/s. This assumes that all the energy in the capacitor is delivered to the heart. Actually, a substantial amount of the energy is left in the capacitor at the end of the defibrillator discharge pulse, so the actual power required from the battery is more than 3 W.

DEFIBRILLATOR BATTERIES MUST HAVE LOW INTERNAL IMPEDANCE

A further requirement is that the battery must deliver the high power level while maintaining a high voltage. In other words, the battery cannot polarize (a term that was discussed earlier) to a great extent. To accomplish this feat, the battery must have a low internal impedance. Two design features are the keys to attaining a low impedance. First, these batteries must contain a low-impedance liquid electrolyte in contrast to the solid electrolyte found in lithium-iodine batteries. The liquid electrolyte has no mechanical integrity, so a porous separator sheet is used to keep the anode and cathode apart as described before. Second, the anode and the cathode have high surface areas that lower the current density and also reduce impedance. Because of the high currents required to charge the capacitor, a substantial metallic current collector must be embedded in each active electrode to minimize voltage loss within the electrodes themselves. These features give the battery low impedance at the expense of increased volume.

DEFIBRILLATOR BATTERY CHEMISTRIES

Two different battery chemistries have been used in implantable defibrillators. Both chemistries contain lithium anodes and metal oxide cathodes. The first batteries to be implanted in defibrillators were lithium-vanadium oxide batteries.[19, 20] This chemistry was later supplanted by lithium-silver vanadium oxide.[21–23] The question is sometimes asked whether other battery chemistries could also be used. There is no reason why other battery systems could not be developed for this application. Other high current systems have been considered. One example is the lithium-thionyl chloride battery. This is a very high current battery that in principle could power a defibrillator very well. The problem with this battery is that when it is left inactive for long periods of time, as might happen with an implantable defibrillator, a film forms on the anode surface that inhibits immediate discharge of the battery when its service is again required. The film disappears after a few (about 5 to 30) seconds, but this delay is considered too long to wait for the battery to generate the high current needed to charge the capacitor in an emergency situation. This phenomenon is known as voltage delay and is much less important in the vanadium oxide and silver vanadium oxide cathode batteries. The deliverable capacity con-

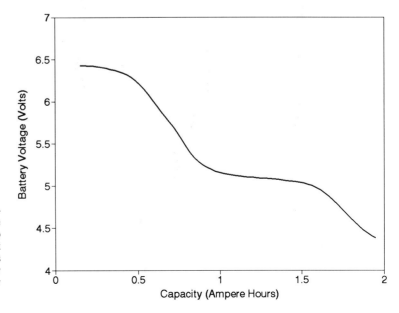

FIGURE 4–9. Typical voltage-capacity plot of a lithium silver–vanadium oxide battery, two cells connected in series, while under a low current drain. An implantable defibrillator reverts to a low current drain during monitoring and pacing activities. Most of its capacity is consumed under low current drain conditions because, although the defibrillation shocks draw an extremely high current from the battery, this happens infrequently and only for a very short period of time.

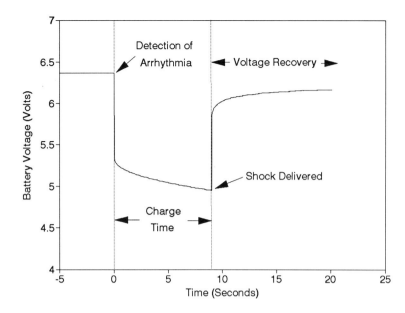

FIGURE 4–10. Typical voltage-time curve showing defibrillator battery load voltage before detection, during charging, and after delivery of the defibrillation shock.

tained in a defibrillator battery is typically 0.2 Ah/cm³, compared to 0.5 Ah/cm³ in lithium-iodine pacemaker batteries.

DEFIBRILLATOR BATTERIES USUALLY CONTAIN MORE THAN ONE CELL

Most implantable defibrillators contain two cells that are connected in series to form a battery with twice the voltage of an individual cell. This simplifies the task of electronically generating a high voltage charge on the capacitor. When the defibrillator is not charging the capacitor for a shock, it draws only a very small amount of current from the battery as overhead to run the sensing circuits (or in some tiered therapy devices, for antitachycardia pacing). As the battery is being depleted at low current, the voltage changes as shown in Figure 4–9. As the battery charges the capacitors to deliver a shock, the battery voltage changes, as shown in Figure 4–10.

DEFIBRILLATOR CAPACITOR CHARGE TIME AS INDICATOR OF BATTERY DEPLETION

The time required to charge the capacitor to the required energy level is known as the charge time. This is generally between 4 and 15 seconds. The charge time is longer for 30-J shocks than for 15-J shocks; it increases as the square of the delivered shock energy. The charge time also increases when the battery voltage during charging decreases, as happens when the battery capacity has been depleted through use. Thus, the time required to charge the capacitors is a useful measure of the battery's state of discharge and is used clinically as a replacement time indicator in some devices.

SAFETY

Safety is a concern with high-power batteries because they contain a large amount of energy and are designed to deliver it quickly. If an internal short circuit occurs, the power traveling through the short can heat the cell contents, and in some cases, initiate a violent chemical reaction. Batteries for implantable defibrillators are designed and constructed with great care to ensure that such a hazardous condition cannot occur. For example, a much thicker sheet of separator material is used in these batteries than in consumer lithium batteries of similar power capability. The polymeric separator materials chosen for this application are designed to melt at a relatively low temperature. This is very useful if either an external or an internal short develops in the battery. If a short occurs, the separator melts, and the porous structure of the separator is lost. The dense polymer sheet that results will not allow ions to pass through it, and the short circuit reaction is stopped. These batteries also undergo extensive testing under other abuse conditions to ensure that they are safe even if a hazardous condition should occur.

Summary

Cardiac pacemakers require batteries that are reliable, relatively compact, and have predictable indicators of cell depletion. A variety of battery chemistries are available, each with its own advantages and disadvantages. At present, lithium-iodine batteries are used for the great majority of pacemakers and have proved to be unsurpassed in long-term reliability.

REFERENCES

1. Brennen KR, Fester KE, Owens BB, Untereker DF: Pacemaker battery capacity: A consideration of the manufacturer's problem. Proceedings of the VIth World Symposium on Cardiac Pacing, Montreal, Pacesymp, 1979.
2. Brennen KR, Fester KE, Owens, BB, Untereker DF: A capacity rating system for cardiac pacemaker batteries. J Power Sources, 5:25, 1980.
3. Broadhead J: Electrochemical principles and reactions. In Linden D (ed): Handbook of Batteries and Fuel Cells. New York, McGraw Hill, 1983, pp 3(2–14).
4. Visbisky M, Stinebring RC, Holmes CF: An approach to the reliability of implantable lithium batteries. J Power Sources 26:185, 1989.
5. Schmidt CL, Skarstad PM: Impedance behavior in lithium-iodine batteries. In Abraham KM, Solomon M (eds): Proceedings of the Symposium on Primary and Secondary Lithium Batteries. The Electrochemical Society, PV91-3, pp 75–85, 1991.

6. Schmidt CL, Skarstad PM: Development of a physically based model for the lithium-iodine battery. *In* Keily T, Baxter BW (eds): Power Sources 13. Leatherhead, England, International Power Sources Committee, 1991, pp 347–361.

7. Untereker DF, Owens BB: Microcalorimetry: A tool for the assessment of self-discharge processes in batteries. Reliability Technology for Cardiac Pacemakers II. Gaithersburg, MD, National Bureau of Standards Workshop, October, 1977.

8. Untereker DF: The use of a microcalorimeter for analysis of load-dependent processes occurring in a primary battery. J Electrochem Soc 125:1907, 1978.

9. Abraham KM, Brummer SB: Secondary lithium cells. *In* Gabano JP (ed): Lithium Batteries. New York, Academic Press, 1983, pp 371–403.

10. Holleck GL: Rechargeable electrochemical cells as implantable power sources. *In* Owens BB (ed): Batteries for Implantable Biomedical Devices. New York, Plenum, 1986, pp 275–284.

11. Brummer SB: Ambient-temperature lithium batteries. *In* Ventatasetty HV (ed): Lithium Battery Technology. New York, John Wiley, 1984, pp 159–177.

12. Owens BB (ed): Batteries for Implantable Biomedical Devices. New York, Plenum, 1986.

13. Purdy DL: Nuclear batteries for implantable applications. *In* Owens BB (ed): Batteries for Implantable Biomedical Devices. New York, Plenum, 1986, pp 285–382.

14. Antonioli G, Baggioni F, Consiglio F, et al: Stimulatore cardiaco implantible con nuova battaria a sato solido al litio. Minerva Med 64:2298, 1973.

15. Greatbatch W, Holmes CF: The lithium/iodine battery: A historical perspective. PACE 15:2034, 1992.

16. Phillips GM, Untereker DF: Phase diagrams for poly-2-vinyl and 2-ethyl pyridene systems. Presented at the 156th National Electrochemical Society Meeting, Los Angeles, CA, October, 1979.

17. Phipps JB, Hayes TG, Skarstad PM, Untereker DF: In-situ formation of a solid/liquid composite electrolyte in Li/I_2 batteries. Solid State Ionics 18 & 19:1073, 1986.

18. Schmidt CL, Skarstad PM: Modeling the discharge behavior of the lithium-iodine battery. J Power Sources 43(1–3):111, 1993.

19. Walk CR: Lithium-vanadium pentoxide cells. *In* Gabano JP (ed): Lithium Batteries. London, Academic Press, 1983, pp 265–280.

20. Gabano JP, Broussely M, Grimm M: Lithium solid cathode batteries for biomedical implantable applications. *In* Owens BB (ed): Batteries for Implantable Biomedical Devices. New York, Plenum, 1986, pp 181–213.

21. Takeuchi ES, Quattrini JP: Batteries for implantable defibrillators. Med Electronics 119:114–117, 1989.

22. Liang CC, Bolster E, Murphy RM: Metal oxide cathode material for high energy density batteries. US Patents 4,310,609—1982 and 4,391,729—1983.

23. Holmes CF, Keister P, Takeuchi E: High rate lithium solid cathode battery for implantable medical devices. Prog Batteries & Solar Cells 6:64, 1987.

CHAPTER 5

PULSE GENERATOR CIRCUITRY

Jeffrey R. Ireland
G. Neal Kay

One of the most important technologies that has contributed to the development of modern pacing therapy is that of the electronic circuits used in implantable pulse generators. This technology is the backbone of pulse generators and has contributed greatly to improvements in the therapeutic and diagnostic features offered by modern pacemakers. These technologic improvements have allowed a rapid succession of increases in the new features offered by the pulse generator while simultaneously reducing their size. Despite these improvements in therapy and a reduction in the size of the battery, the longevity of these devices has generally been maintained by increased energy efficiency of the circuits. Most of the electronic technologies that are used in pulse generators today have been adapted from the commercial or consumer electronics industry. The most notable of these are integrated circuit technology, high-density packaging, and surface mounting of components. These engineering advances in the circuits of the pulse generator have had a dramatic impact on the clinical practice of pacing. The electronic circuits interact with the cellular biologic function of the myocardium, making decisions based on algorithms designed to mimic normal cardiovascular physiology. Thus, clinicians involved in the care of patients with permanent pacemakers must have an understanding of the implications of their programming decisions on the function and longevity of the pusle generator. The basic components of output and sensing circuits are emphasized in this chapter. First, an overview of the architecture of a typical pulse generator circuit is discussed. This is followed by a more detailed description of the circuits that have a direct interface with the myocardium. Next the ''brains'' of the pulse generator are discussed, including the diagnostic capabilities that are available. Finally, the clinical relevance of each of these circuits is reviewed in the context of managing patients with implanted pacemakers.

Pulse Generator Block Diagram

A typical pulse generator must perform many different functions. Of foremost importance, the pulse generator must provide pacing therapy by generating appropriately timed stimulation pulses that are synchronized to the intrinsic cardiac rhythm (the myocardial interface). For rate-adaptive pacemakers, the device must also interpret physiologic or biophysical parameters that are designed to indicate changes in metabolic demand. The pulse generator must allow its parameters to be modified by a programmer (the telemetry interface). In addition, most newer devices record the interactions of the pacemaker with the patient (the diagnostic system). An implantable pulse generator contains circuit blocks that control each of these functions. A typical block diagram of a pulse generator is shown in Figure 5–1.

THE PACING THERAPY CONTROLLER

The *pacing therapy controller* is the heart of any pulse generator. It provides the basic pacing therapy (stimulation and sensing) and contains the algorithms that implement the available pacing modalities (e.g., VVI, DDD). The pacing therapy controller may also modulate pacing rate in response to an artificial sensor or any other features that are related to the timing and sequencing of cardiac events. When timing parameters such as the lower rate interval, refractory intervals, or atrioventricular (AV) intervals are programmed, this information is stored in the pacing therapy controller. The interface between this block and the pacing lead(s) is provided by two sets of amplifiers: the output amplifiers and the sense amplifiers.

OUTPUT AMPLIFIERS

The *output amplifiers* accept commands (control signals) from the pacing therapy controller. These signals control

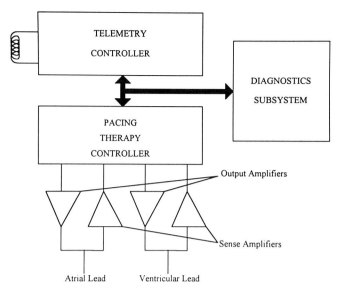

FIGURE 5–1. Diagram of the basic circuits in an implantable pulse generator. The pacing therapy controller (PTC) coordinates input from the telemetry controller and from the sense amplifiers. The logic in the PTC controls the appropriate timing of pacing stimulus delivery by the output amplifiers by determining which sensed events should be tracked, which should inhibit a pacing stimulus, and which should be ignored or trigger changes in pacing mode (refractory events). The PTC also sends data to be logged in the diagnostics subsystem. The contents of the diagnostic subsystem can be sent to the programmer through the telemetry controller.

when a pacing stimulus is to occur as well as the amplitude and duration of the stimulation pulse. The output amplifiers convert these control signals into an analog output voltage and apply that voltage to the lead system for a predetermined interval (the pulse width).

SENSE AMPLIFIERS

In contrast to the output amplifiers, the *sense amplifiers* send control signals *to* the pacing therapy controller. These signals indicate to the pacing therapy controller when an intrinsic cardiac event has occurred. The pacing therapy controller can use this information to inhibit the next pacing stimulus or to synchronize delivery of a pacing stimulus with the sensed atrial or ventricular electrogram.

DIAGNOSTICS SUBSYSTEM

Another block in this diagram is the *diagnostics subsystem*. This is typically the storage mechanism where detailed records of the interactions between the pacing therapy controller and the patient are kept. In addition, this block maintains records of a variety of other measurements and information about the pulse generator itself (such as the battery voltage, battery impedance, and so on).

TELEMETRY CONTROLLER

The *telemetry controller* provides the interface between the pulse generator and the pacemaker programmer. The telemetry controller provides bidirectional interaction between the pulse generator and the programmer. This is the portion of the pulse generator circuitry that allows program-

ming of parameters within the device. It also provides a means of exporting diagnostic information from the diagnostic subsystem, such as histograms, trends, and intracardiac electrograms to the programmer.

Output Amplifiers

The primary purpose of the output amplifiers is to deliver a pacing pulse to the myocardial tissue through the pacing lead. The pulse has a predetermined energy (pulse amplitude and pulse width) and is delivered at a time determined by the pacing therapy controller. The output amplifiers are programmable to allow selection of the pulse amplitude and duration. Once programmed, the circuitry in the output amplifiers of Figure 5–2 generates an analog voltage or current that represents the pulse amplitude. The pacing therapy controller then initiates a pacing stimulus by closing a switch that transmits the analog voltage or current pulse to the myocardial tissue through the tip electrode of the pacing lead. Pacemaker output amplifiers can be classified into two categories: constant-voltage and constant-current amplifiers. These are so named because of the characteristics of their respective output pulse waveforms (see later discussion).

OUTPUT PULSE WAVEFORMS

The constant-voltage output amplifier applies a voltage pulse to the tip electrode of the lead. A typical circuit diagram of a voltage output circuit is shown in Figure 5–3. This configuration contains a *pace amplitude generator* for generating an analog voltage. This analog voltage represents the stimulus amplitude and is stored on a holding capacitor, C_a. Two switches are used to deliver the pacing stimulus to the lead: (1) a PACE switch, and (2) a recharge switch (RCHG)

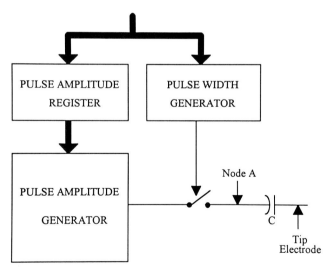

FIGURE 5–2. Schematic diagram of the manner in which the output circuit of a pulse generator is controlled by the pacing therapy controller. The output circuit receives instructions from the pacing therapy controller that regulate the timing of pacing stimuli and the amplitude and duration (pulse width) of the stimulus. The pulse amplitude generator determines the configuration of charging and output capacitors necessary to generate the programmed stimulus amplitude. The output switch is closed for a period of time that is controlled by the pulse width generator. When the output switch is closed, a pacing stimulus is delivered to the tip electrode of the pacing lead.

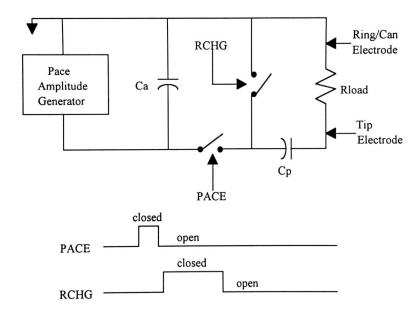

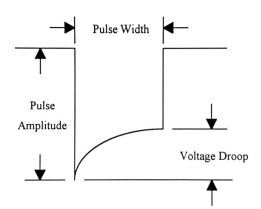

FIGURE 5–3. Schematic diagram of the output circuit. The pace amplitude generator generates the programmed stimulus amplitude (in volts) and stores the charge on an output holding capacitor (C_a). When the PACE switch is closed, the pacing stimulus is delivered to the tip electrode, and current flows across the lead and tissue (Rload) to the ring electrode (or pulse generator can). The PACE switch remains closed for the duration of the pulse (typically in the range of 0.5 msec). A direct current (DC) coupling capacitor (C_p) transfers the charge to the lead. Immediately following the pacing stimulus, the recharge (RCHG) switch is closed, allowing the residual charge on capacitor C_p to be dissipated. The sequence of opening and closing of the PACE and RCHG switches is shown in the lower portion of the figure.

that reestablishes the charge equilibrium after the pacing pulse has been delivered to the myocardium. However, these switches have leakage currents that can cause direct current (DC) currents to flow into the lead system. To prevent any possible corrosion that may result from the leakage of current in the lead, a DC blocking capacitor, C_p, is included. When the PACE switch is closed, the pulse amplitude analog voltage stored on the C_a holding capacitor is transferred to the tip electrode of the lead through the coupling capacitor, C_p. At the end of the pacing pulse, the PACE switch opens. Thus, the pulse duration is the interval from the closing of the PACE switch to its reopening. During the pacing stimulus, some of the charge stored on capacitor C_a has been transferred to capacitor C_p, and some has been delivered to the lead system to stimulate the myocardium (Rload). To reestablish equilibrium, the recharge switch (RCHG) is closed, and a rapid recharge pulse is delivered. This is intended to remove any residual charge remaining on the coupling capacitor (C_p) and the pacing electrodes on the lead (polarization). Thus, a pacing stimulus is delivered as the

result of the closing and opening of the PACE switch and the closing and opening of the RCHG switch. At this point, the charge on the holding capacitor (C_a) must be replenished by the pace amplitude generator before another pacing stimulus can be delivered.

A typical constant-voltage pulse waveform is shown in Figure 5–4. As can be seen from this diagram, the voltage is actually *not* constant during the pulse. Rather, the voltage on the tip electrode droops from the beginning of the pulse (leading edge) to the end of the pulse (trailing edge) by an amount that is dependent on the pulse amplitude, the pulse width, and the lead impedance. The voltage droop is given by the equation:

Eq 1 $\quad \Delta V = V_a \left(1 - e^{-\frac{PW}{R \times C}} \right)$

where V_a is the pulse amplitude in volts, PW is the pulse width, R is the lead impedance, and C is the effective output capacitance. It is in fact this voltage droop that is measured in many pacemakers to determine the lead impedance during real-time telemetry. Typically, the voltage droop is reported by the pulse generator to the programmer, the calculation of lead impedance being performed by the programmer. However, such calculations of lead impedance are only an approximation because the true lead impedance is not purely resistive but has capacitive and inductive components as well.

FIGURE 5–4. Typical constant-voltage (CV) pulse waveform. Note that the voltage is actually not constant with a CV pulse because there is a droop in voltage from the start to the end of the pulse. The lower the pacing impedance, the greater the current drained from the output capacitor and the greater the magnitude of the voltage droop. The voltage droop is used by some manufacturers to estimate pacing impedance.

ENERGY CONSUMPTION OF PACING STIMULI

It is important for clinicians to understand the amount of energy consumed by the output pulse because it determines in large part the battery longevity. Pulse energy is dependent upon three primary variables: (1) pulse amplitude, (2) pulse width, and (3) lead impedance. The amount of energy consumed by this pulse can be found by integrating the product of voltage and current over time, or, more explicitly:

Eq 2 $\quad E = \int_0^t V \times I$

where E is the pulse energy in joules, V is the pulse amplitude in volts, and I is the current in amperes. The limits of this integration range from zero to the pulse width (t) when zero is the start of the pulse and t is the end of the pulse. To simplify the calculation, if we assume that the lead impedance is a constant value (R) over this interval and that voltage and current follow Ohm's law:

Eq 3 $\quad I = \dfrac{V}{R}$

we can rewrite the equation for pulse energy as:

Eq 4 $\quad E = \dfrac{1}{R}\displaystyle\int_{o}^{t} V^2$

The output voltage can be expressed as:

Eq 5 $\quad V = V_a e^{-\frac{t}{R \times C}}$

where V_a is the peak stimulus amplitude (in volts), t is the pulse duration (in seconds), R is the lead impedance, and C is the output capacitance as shown in Figure 5–2. Substituting equation 5 into equation 4 yields:

Eq 6 $\quad E = V_a^2 \times \left(\dfrac{C}{2}\right) \times \left(1 - e^{-\frac{PW}{R \times C}}\right)$

where PW is the pulse width of the pace as shown in Figure 5–4. Keep in mind that this is only an approximation because the lead impedance, R, is not purely resistive as assumed here (see Chapter 1). Nor is lead impedance necessarily constant during the pacing stimulus because polarization increases during the pulse. However, the approximation is accurate enough for most pacing applications and serves to make understandable the clinical implications of programming the pulse amplitude and duration as they relate to pulse generator longevity. In fact, in many cases equation 6 can be simplified further by assuming that the pulse amplitude does not droop during the pacing stimulus as would be true if the pulse width were relatively short and the lead impedance were relatively large. In this case, equation 6 would reduce to:

Eq 7 $\quad E = \dfrac{V_a^2}{R} \times PW$

CONSTANT-CURRENT OUTPUT PULSE WAVEFORMS

In contrast to the constant-voltage output amplifier, a constant-current output amplifier applies a known amount of current to the tip electrode of the lead. The circuit diagram of a constant-current output circuit is very similar to that shown in Figure 5–3 except that an output current limiter is connected in series with the PACE switch. Thus, a constant-current generator discharges the pacing pulse through two resistors, including a high-resistance internal limiter and the impedance of the pacing lead. In comparison, a constant-voltage generator has only one resistor in the circuit (the lead). The internal resistance (current limiter) of a constant-current generator effectively limits the output current to a fixed (constant) value during the pulse, provided that the

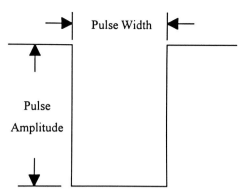

FIGURE 5–5. Typical constant-current (CI) pulse waveform. Note that within the range of expected pacing impedance, the pulse amplitude (mA) remains constant. CI pulses deliver current to the lead independent of load.

internal resistance is large compared with the lead impedance. A typical constant-current pulse waveform is shown in Figure 5–5. As can be seen from this diagram, the pulse has a constant amplitude that is measured in amperes. The amplitude of the constant-current pulse does not droop as does the amplitude of the voltage output pulse.

CONSTANT-CURRENT ENERGY CONSUMPTION

The amount of energy consumed by the constant-current output pulse is also dependent on the pulse amplitude, the pulse width, and the lead impedance. Just as for a constant-voltage stimulus, the amount of energy consumed by a constant-current pulse can be found by integrating the product of voltage and current over time (see equation 2). The current is constant during the pulse, and if we assume that the lead impedance is also constant, the integral of equation 2 reduces to:

Eq 8 $\quad E = I^2 \times R \times PW$

As discussed in Chapter 1, there are certain advantages and certain disadvantages to constant-current compared with constant-voltage output waveforms for implantable pacemakers. Basically, for a constant voltage generator, the *current* that is delivered during the pulse is determined by the pacing impedance. Thus, the flow of charge is load dependent. For a constant-current pulse generator, the *voltage* is determined by the pacing impedance. Therefore, flow of charge is load independent. Although many constant-current permanent pulse generators remain in service (manufactured by Cordis), only the constant-voltage type of pulse generator is marketed today. However, many temporary pacemakers use a constant-current output pulse because there can be marked variation in the impedance of temporary compared with permanent pacing leads. To minimize variations in pacing current as a result of the widely varying pacing impedances that are possible with the combinations of temporary pacing leads and cables that may be employed, the constant-current variety of pulse generator is probably preferable to the constant-voltage type for temporary pacing applications. However, because of the limited range of lead impedances available with permanent pacing leads, there is little practical importance to this distinction. One possible exception is the presence of lead insulation failure in which pacing impedance may fall drastically. In this situation, a constant-voltage pulse generator will deliver a marked increase in current with each pacing pulse, rapidly depleting the battery.

Voltage Dividers and Multipliers

In the preceding sections the basic structure of an output circuit was discussed. In addition, the energy required for a pacing stimulus was examined. This energy must, of necessity, be delivered from the internal power source or battery of the implantable pulse generator. The process of pacing results from the repeated charging of an output capacitor by charges drawn from the battery followed by discharge of the capacitor onto the pacing lead. Thus, the output capacitor is repeatedly charged and discharged. Because a battery contains a fixed amount of usable charge, to understand the impact of programming decisions about output pulse amplitude and duration on longevity of the implantable pulse generator, it is preferable to convert the expressions of stimulus energy into expressions of charge. Batteries are rated in units of charge known as ampere-hours (Ah—see Chapter 3). The chemical reactions in a battery generate a potential difference that is determined by its chemical constituents. For a lithium-iodine cell, the battery voltage is 2.8 V at the beginning of battery life. However, as all clinicians involved in programming permanent pacemakers know, the stimulus amplitude can be programmed to values as high as 8 V or as low as 0.5 V. How does a lithium-iodine battery with a potential of 2.8 V (at the beginning of life) generate a pacing stimulus that can be greater or less than the battery voltage? The answer lies in the use of voltage doublers, triplers, or dividers.

To explain the relationship between battery voltage and stimulus amplitude delivered to the lead more fully, it is important to understand the function of capacitors. A capacitor is used to store charge. It consists of two conductors isolated from each other and from their surroundings. The capacitance value of a capacitor (C) is measured in units of microfarads that express the magnitude of the charge on either conductor (Q) to the potential difference between them (V) as expressed by the equation:

Eq 9 $\quad C = \dfrac{Q}{V}$

Therefore, since the capacitance of a capacitor is constant, the amount of charge that is stored can only be increased by increasing the voltage. It can be shown that for a constant-voltage output pulse, the amount of charge (Q) *delivered to the lead* (and tissue) is given by:

Eq 10 $\quad Q = V_a \times C \times \left(1 - e^{-\frac{PW}{R \times C}}\right)$

However, as will be shown, this is not necessarily the same as the amount of charge taken from the battery to generate the output pulse. *Depending on the programmed stimulus amplitude, the battery charge required to deliver the pacing stimulus may be from one third to three times this amount.* In other words, the longevity of the pulse generator can be dramatically affected by the programmed output amplitude.

SINGLE OUTPUT (STIMULUS AMPLITUDE EQUAL TO THE BATTERY VOLTAGE)

Consider the simple case outlined in Figure 5–6 in which a pacing stimulus of 2.8 V is programmed. In this example, the pacing stimulus amplitude is equal to the battery potential of a lithium-iodine cell (2.8 V). Figure 5–6A represents the circuit diagram for recharging the output capacitor from the battery, whereas Figure 5–6B represents the circuit diagram during delivery of a 2.8 V (1×) pacing stimulus to the lead (represented by R). During the pace configuration, charge flows from the capacitor (C) to the lead system (R). Because charge is removed from the capacitor during the stimulus, the voltage on the capacitor at the end of the pulse is less than its initial value of 2.8 V. This final voltage (V_f) on the capacitor can be derived from equation 5 and is:

Eq 11 $\quad V_f = 2.8 \times e^{-\frac{PW}{R \times C}}$

Therefore, the amount of *charge* on the capacitor at the end of the pacing stimulus (Q_p) is:

Eq 12 $\quad Q_p = (C \times 2.8) \times e^{-\frac{PW}{R \times C}}$

When the capacitor is connected as shown in Figure 5–6A to recharge the capacitor after a pacing stimulus, charge flows from the battery and returns the voltage on the capacitor to 2.8 V. The amount of charge required from the battery to *recharge the capacitor* is given by its fully charged state minus the amount of charge on the capacitor after the pacing stimulus.

Eq 13 $\quad Q_p = (C \times 2.8) - \left[C \times 2.8 \times e^{-\frac{PW}{R \times C}}\right] =$

$$(C \times 2.8) \times \left(1 - e^{-\frac{PW}{R \times C}}\right)$$

From equation 10, the charge *delivered to the lead* is given by:

Eq 14 $\quad Q = (C \times 2.8) \times \left(1 - e^{-\frac{PW}{R \times C}}\right)$

Notice that the charge taken from the battery is exactly equal to that delivered to the lead system for a pacing stimulus of 2.8 V.

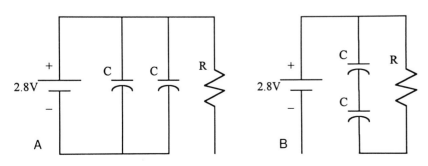

FIGURE 5–6. Charge *(A)* and pace *(B)* configurations of an output circuit programmed to deliver a pulse of 2.8 V. A lithium-iodine battery generates 2.8 V at the beginning of cell life. During charging of the holding capacitor, the charge is transferred from the battery to the capacitor. During delivery of a 2.8-V pacing stimulus to the lead (R), the capacitor discharges to the tip electrode. Thus, for delivery of a pacing stimulus equal in amplitude to the battery voltage (1×), the charge drawn from the battery is equal to the charge delivered to the lead.

VOLTAGE DOUBLERS (STIMULUS AMPLITUDE EQUAL TO TWICE THE BATTERY VOLTAGE)

As opposed to the simple single output situation just discussed, other capacitor switching configurations, such as doubling or tripling the battery voltage, do not yield the same result. A voltage doubler is required to generate pacing amplitudes that are larger than the battery voltage. Because the typical internal battery of an implantable pulse generator has a voltage of about 2.8 V, doublers are required to achieve 5.6-V pacing amplitudes. A diagram of the operation of a voltage doubler is shown in Figure 5–7. Operation is similar to that of the single output diagram of Figure 5–6 except that *two* capacitors are required to generate a leading-edge pacing voltage of 5.6 V. During the pacing stimulus (see Fig. 5–7B), the two capacitors are discharged in series, and charge flows from the capacitors onto the lead system, R. This results in a final voltage on the capacitors that is less than its initial value of 5.6 V. The final voltage on the capacitors can be derived from equation 5 and is equal to:

$$\textbf{Eq 15} \quad V_f = 5.6 \times e^{-\frac{PW}{R \times C_{eq}}}$$

where C_{eq} is the equivalent capacitance of the two capacitors connected in series. Because the capacitance of two capacitors in series is calculated as $\dfrac{1}{C_{eq}} = \dfrac{1}{C_1} + \dfrac{1}{C_2}$, then for two identical capacitors of capacitance C, $C_{eq} = \dfrac{C}{2}$. *Because the two capacitors are in series, an equal amount of charge must flow from each capacitor onto the lead system.* Therefore, the remaining voltage on each capacitor is $\dfrac{V_f}{2}$, and the charge on each capacitor is equal to:

$$\textbf{Eq 16} \quad Q_p = C \times \frac{V_f}{2} = (C \times 2.8) \times e^{-\frac{PW}{R \times C_{eq}}}$$

Figure 5–7A illustrates how the two capacitors of a voltage doubler are connected during the charge configuration. Note that although the capacitors are discharged in series, they are charged in parallel. During the charging configuration, charge flows from the battery onto both of the capacitors and returns the voltage on each to 2.8 V. When capacitors are connected in parallel, the equivalent capacitance is equal to $C_{eq} = C_1 + C_2$. Therefore, the equivalent capacitance of two identical capacitors connected in parallel is equal to $2 \times C$. The amount of charge *required from the battery* to perform this recharge operation is given by the fully charged value

minus the amount of charge on each capacitor after the pacing stimulus:

$$\textbf{Eq 17} \quad Q = 2 \times \left[(C \times 2.8) - \left(C \times 2.8 \times e^{-\frac{PW}{R \times C_{eq}}} \right) \right]$$

From equation 10, the charge *delivered to the lead system* is given by:

$$\textbf{Eq 18} \quad Q = C_{eq} \times 5.6 \times \left(1 - e^{-\frac{PW}{R \times C_{eq}}} \right)$$

$$\text{or } \frac{C}{2} \times 5.6 \times \left(1 - e^{-\frac{PW}{R \times C_{eq}}} \right)$$

Notice that for a voltage doubler, the charge taken from the battery is exactly equal to twice that delivered to the lead system. This may seem counterintuitive and may lead one to ask what happened to all the charge taken from the battery. The answer is that it was used to double the pacing voltage and is directly related to charging the two capacitors in parallel and discharging them in series. In fact, it can be shown that these equations observe the property of conservation of energy (i.e., energy is not generated by the process of transferring charge from the battery to the lead). The *energy* taken from the battery and that delivered to the lead are identical.

VOLTAGE TRIPLERS (STIMULUS AMPLITUDE EQUAL TO THREE TIMES THE BATTERY VOLTAGE)

These same derivations can easily be extended to the triple (3X) output. A tripler is required to generate 7.5- or 8.0-V pacing amplitudes. A diagram of the operation of a voltage tripler is shown in Figure 5–8. Again, during pacing, charge flows from the series connection of three capacitors onto the lead system, R. Recharging of the three capacitors is done in parallel. As with the voltage doubler, the charge taken from the battery by tripling the voltage is exactly equal to 3 times that delivered to the lead system because charge is used to triple the output voltage.

VOLTAGE DIVIDERS (STIMULUS VOLTAGE IS HALF THE BATTERY VOLTAGE)

This technique can also be extended to generate pacing amplitudes that are fractions of the battery voltage. Although a linear regulator can perform the same operation, it does not provide the same transformer operation that a voltage halver can. To understand this more fully, refer to the diagram shown in Figure 5–9. The operation is exactly the reverse of the voltage doubler in that two capacitors are charged in

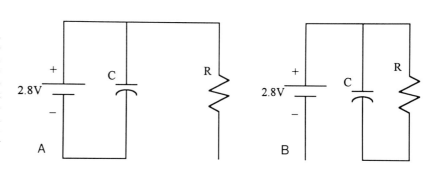

FIGURE 5–7. A voltage doubler. Charge and pace configurations of an output circuit programmed to deliver a pulse amplitude double that of the battery voltage (5.6 V). During charging, two capacitors (C_1 and C_2) are charged in parallel with the equivalent capacitance (C_{eq}) of $C_1 + C_2$. During the pace configuration, the two capacitors are connected in series, with the equivalent capacitance $1/C_{eq} = 1/C_1 + 1/C_2$. Because of the change in capacitor connections during charging and pacing, twice the charge is taken from the battery during charging as is delivered to the lead. See text for discussion.

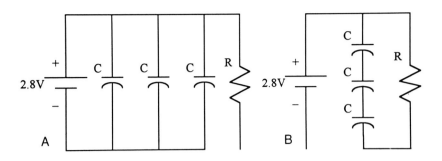

FIGURE 5–8. Capacitor configuration required to deliver a stimulus equal to three times the battery voltage. Note that during capacitor charging *(A)*, three capacitors are joined in parallel. During pacing *(B)*, the three capacitors are connected in series.

series but deliver the pacing stimulus in parallel. Because the capacitors are in series during the recharge phase, the equivalent capacitance is equal to $C_{eq} = \dfrac{1}{C_1} + \dfrac{1}{C_2}$, or $\dfrac{C}{2}$. This effectively divides the battery voltage in half, resulting in a stimulus voltage of 1.4 V. During delivery of the pacing stimulus, charge flows from the parallel connection of the capacitors onto the lead system (R). This results in a final voltage on the capacitors that is less than its initial value of 1.4 V. This final voltage is given by:

Eq 19 $\quad V_f = 1.4 \times e^{-\frac{PW}{R \times C_{eq}}}$

where the equivalent capacitance of the two capacitors connected in parallel is equal to $C_{eq} = C_1 + C_2$, or $C_{eq} = 2 \times C$. This is the final *voltage* on both capacitors. The *charge* on each capacitor at the end of a pacing stimulus (Q_p) is equal to:

Eq 20 $\quad Q_p = C \times V_f = C \times 1.4 \times e^{-\frac{PW}{R \times C_{eq}}}$

The amount of charge required from the battery to *recharge* the capacitors as shown in Figure 5–9A is equal to:

Eq 21 $\quad Q = (C \times 1.4) - \left(C \times 1.4 \times e^{-\frac{PW}{R \times C_{eq}}} \right) =$

$$C \times 1.4 \times \left(1 - e^{-\frac{PW}{R \times C_{eq}}} \right)$$

From equation 10, the charge delivered to the lead system is given by:

Eq 22 $\quad Q = C \times 2.8 \times \left(1 - e^{-\frac{PW}{R \times C_{eq}}} \right)$

Notice that the charge taken from the battery is exactly equal to *half* that delivered to the lead system. This should not be too surprising if it is noted that we have, in effect, swapped the battery and lead connections of the doubler output circuit. The same principles of energy conservation apply. This analysis of charge savings by programming the stimulus pulse as

low as possible can be extended to a one-third output charge multiplier. This can be useful in minimizing the effect of pacing current to maximize implantable pulse generator longevity.

CLINICAL IMPLICATIONS OF OUTPUT PULSE PROGRAMMING

The current drained from the battery of a modern pulse generator is influenced by several factors, including the static current requirements for operating the integrated circuits, the energy requirements of a rate adaptive sensor, and the energy required to operate diagnostic counters in the device. For example, the static current drain of recent pulse generators has been greatly improved compared with the older devices, with most newer models offering a static current drain of less than 5 uA. Because further improvements in static current drain of integrated circuits are likely to be rather small, it is critical to focus on the factors that can be controlled by the clinician. Although each of the factors mentioned earlier is important to the overall current drain, the current consumed in the delivery of pacing stimuli is the predominant determinant of how long a pulse generator will last. The effect of programming the stimulus voltage on the longevity of a pulse generator is shown in Tables 5–1 and 5–2. To illustrate this effect more dramatically, consider a typical case of a DDD pacemaker that paces both atrium and ventricle 100% of the time at a rate of 60 bpm. Table 5–1 lists the programmed parameters used for this illustration. Table 5–2 shows the impact on longevity that programming the output amplitude can have. The multiplier represents the pacing circuit configuration (halver, doubler, and so on), C_{eq} is the equivalent output capacitance, the pacing current column represents the current required for one chamber (atrial or ventricular), the total current represents the total current drain of a dual chamber device (including static current), and the longevity column is the estimated longevity of a device at these settings. As Table 5–2 illustrates, there is a *dramatic* difference in pacing current for the different output multiplier configurations. Notice that the pacing current for a 5.6-V pacing stimulus is 4 times that of a 2.8-V pacing stimulus. If the battery

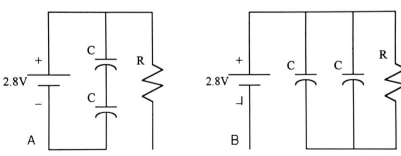

FIGURE 5–9. Capacitor configuration used to deliver a pacing stimulus equal to half the battery voltage. Note that two capacitors are charged in series *(A)* but are discharged during pacing in parallel *(B)*. See text for discussion.

TABLE 5–1. PROGRAMMED PARAMETERS

PARAMETER	VALUE	UNITS
Lead impedance (R)	500	ohms
Rate	60	bpm
Percent paced	100	%
Pulse width (PW)	0.5	msec
Output capacitance (C)	10	μF
Static current drain	10	μA
Battery capacity	1	Ah

TABLE 5–2. EFFECT OF STIMULUS AMPLITUDE ON PULSE GENERATOR LONGEVITY

STIMULUS AMPLITUDE (V)	MULTIPLIER (×)	C_{eq} (μF)	PACING CURRENT (μA)	TOTAL CURRENT (μA)	LONGEVITY (yr)
1.4	0.5	20	0.7	11.4	10.04
2.8	1	10	2.7	15.3	7.44
5.6	2	5	10.2	30.3	3.76
8.4	3	3.3	21.8	53.5	2.13

voltage is tripled, the pacing current would increase nine fold! Also note that as the stimulus amplitude is decreased below the battery voltage, the improvement in battery longevity continues to be significant. Because of the static current drain, there is a limit to battery longevity. Therefore, to achieve maximum longevity of a pulse generator, the long-term stimulation threshold of the pacing leads and the programmed parameters should be carefully evaluated (see Chapter 1).

Sense Amplifiers

A sense amplifier in an implantable pulse generator detects intrinsic cardiac electric signals and notifies the pacing therapy controller (see Fig. 5–1) that an electric event has occurred. In modern implantable pulse generators this is accomplished through the use of an electronic amplifier that filters and amplifies the intracardiac electrogram. Figure 5–10 is a block diagram of a multiprogrammable sense amplifier that can be programmed to either the unipolar (tip-to-can) or bipolar (tip-to-ring) sensing configuration. This amplifier also has sensitivity threshold settings that can be programmed by means of telemetry. These threshold values represent a minimum amplitude criterion that must be met by an electric signal to be sensed by the amplifier. Sensing amplifiers have at least four major components: (1) an input network connected to the sensing electrodes, (2) a front-end amplifier that increases the gain of the signal, (3) a bandpass filter that removes unwanted electric signals, and (4) a programmable sensitivity threshold and threshold comparator that compare the electrogram amplitude to a fixed reference voltage. Each of these components has an important function in the sensing amplifier and is discussed separately.

THE SENSE AMPLIFIER INPUT NETWORK

The sense amplifier depicted in Figure 5–10 is connected to the pacing lead through alternating current (AC) coupling capacitors, C. This is done to remove any DC or nonvarying electric potentials that may be present on the electrodes. The resistors shown in Figure 5–10 are used to establish a DC bias potential for the sense amplifier. Note that no AC coupling capacitor is shown connected to the implantable pulse generator can. The pulse generator can is typically used as a "ground" or return electrode (anode) in the implantable pulse generator pacing circuit, and thus DC blocking is not necessary (because it is already accomplished through the tip or ring electric connections). In addition, most modern sense amplifiers that can be programmed to either the unipolar or the bipolar sensing configurations include switches to control the connection of the amplifier to the electrodes on the pacing lead. For bipolar sensing operation, the sense amplifier input network is connected to the tip and ring electrodes. In this configuration the ring switch will be closed and the can switch will be open. Therefore, the pulse generator can is not

FIGURE 5–10. Diagram of a pulse generator sensing circuit (oriented from left to right in this figure). The tip and ring electrodes (bipolar configuration) or the tip electrode and pulse generator can (unipolar configuration) are connected by switches that are controlled by telemetry. The electrodes of the lead are connected to the input network of the sensing circuit with capacitors (C) that remove constant-voltage (DC) artifacts on the lead. The resistors (R) in the input network provide a DC bias potential for the sense amplifier. Note that there are switches at the junction of the input network with the "front-end" amplifier that can be opened to blank the amplifier at intervals fol-

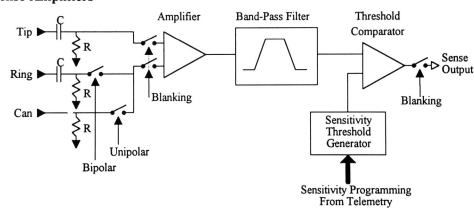

Sense Amplifiers

lowing a pacing stimulus. The amplifier increases the gain of the signal. The signal is then processed by a bandpass filter to attenuate signals outside the desired frequency range. The bandpass filter serves the purpose of distinguishing P waves and R waves from extracardiac signals. The output of the bandpass filter is then compared with a known reference voltage by the threshold comparator. If the signal exceeds a programmable sensitivity threshold, it will be registered as a sensed event and relayed to the pacing therapy controller. Also note that blanking switches may be present at the output of the threshold comparator to blank the sensing circuit following pacing stimuli. See text for discussion.

in electric contact with the sensing amplifier in the bipolar sensing configuration. For unipolar sensing, the sense amplifier input network is connected to the tip and can electrodes so that the can switch is closed and the ring switch is open. These switches are opened and closed by programmed instructions communicated between the programmer and the pulse generator by telemetry.

As discussed in Chapter 2, the intracardiac electrogram generated in the myocardium may not be the same signal seen by the sensing amplifier. In contrast to myocardial stimulation (in which the voltage source is the pulse generator), sensing involves recognition of a voltage source in the myocardium that must be transmitted to the pulse generator. Like pacing impedance, which opposes the flow of current between the pacing electrodes, the intracardiac electrogram voltage that originates in the myocardium is transmitted through the electrodes to the sensing amplifier input network. The impedance to current flow in the lead is determined by ohmic resistance of the lead conductors, resistance of the electrode-tissue interface, and capacitance of the electrode (see Chapter 2). The sense amplifier also offers impedance to the flow of current, known as input impedance. The input impedance of the sense amplifier is determined by its input network and is typically at least 20 kilo-ohms (kΩ) and occasionally as high as several hundred kΩ. The ratio of source impedance to input impedance is a critical determinant of the electrogram amplitude that will be sensed. To minimize attenuation of the electrogram from its source in the myocardium to its destination in the sense amplifer, the input impedance should greatly exceed the source impedance. If the input impedance offered by the input network is too low, or the source impedance offered by the lead is too high, the electrogram will be attenuated in amplitude and distorted. This phenomenon is known as *impedance mismatch.*

AMPLIFICATION

Amplification is used in modern sense amplifiers to transform a signal that may be less than 1 mV in amplitude to a signal that can be more easily detected by the integrated circuits in the pulse generator. Typical amplification levels afforded by sensing amplifiers are on the order of $100\times$. After input into the sensing amplifier through the input network, the electrogram undergoes initial amplification in a "front-end" amplifier. Although much of the amplification is performed in the first amplifier stage of the sense amplifier, the bandpass filter also performs some amplification. The front-end amplifier also performs the important function of converting a differential signal recorded between two electrodes (for example, the tip to ring electrodes in the bipolar configuration) into a single-ended or ground-referenced voltage waveform that can be more easily processed through the bandpass filter and threshold comparator. This conversion effectively subtracts the ring from the tip electrogram (i.e., output equals tip electrogram minus ring electrogram). It is, in fact, this subtraction operation that allows the improved signal-to-noise sensing performance of the bipolar sensing configuration. For example, an extracardiac interference signal (such as that originating from power lines or skeletal myopotentials) is likely to produce similar effects on both the tip and ring electrodes of a bipolar lead. By subtracting

the unipolar electrograms recorded from the tip and ring electrodes, most of the external interference is cancelled, leaving only the intracardiac signal at the output of the differencing amplifier. In clinical practice, externally induced signals are not identical as observed from the tip and ring electrodes. However, they are similar enough to afford significant improvements in sensing performance in the bipolar compared with the unipolar sensing configuration.

BANDPASS FILTERS

The ideal sense amplifier would detect only intracardiac depolarizations by excluding all extracardiac electric signals. In addition, an ideal atrial sense amplifier would detect only P waves and a ventricular amplifier would detect only R waves. However, sense amplifiers are not capable of such perfect signal discrimination. In reality, a sense amplifier records many different types of electric signals and must attempt to discriminate between the desired and the unwanted signals. Electric events that contribute to the intracardiac electrogram include intracardiac depolarizations, far-field signals originating in the opposite cardiac chamber, ectopic beats, power line signals, and electric noise from radar systems, electric appliances, theft detection systems, and so on. Sense amplifiers use electronic filtering techniques known as *bandpass filters* to aid in discriminating between intracardiac signals and this unwanted noise. A bandpass filter allows only signals within a certain frequency range (or band) to pass through it. It has a low-frequency cutoff point to exclude low-frequency signals and a high-frequency cutoff point to exclude high-frequency signals. Any signal in the frequency range below the low-frequency cutoff or above the high-frequency cutoff points is attenuated or diminished in amplitude relative to a signal whose frequency range is between these limits. The design of a sense amplifier requires careful choices for the low- and high-frequency cutoff points. Intrinsic intracardiac signals cannot be so neatly categorized into a sharply defined frequency band. The frequency content of an R wave or a P wave varies from patient to patient and is highly dependent on the intrinsic properties of the myocardium, the type of lead, its intracardiac location, and the maturity of the electrode-tissue interface. Therefore, the placement of the cutoff points of a bandpass filter is a compromise that attempts to maximize the intrinsic signal levels while minimizing unwanted signals.

SENSITIVITY THRESHOLDS

The output of the bandpass filter is continuously compared to a programmable sensitivity threshold to identify the electric signal as a sensed event. The signal that emerges from the bandpass filter is compared to a known reference voltage by the *threshold comparator.* The sensitivity threshold is generated by the *sensitivity threshold generator* according to the programmed sensitivity level. The sensitivity threshold is generated from a digital "code" received from the programmer when the sensitivity level is programmed. If the output of the bandpass filter exceeds the value of the threshold comparator, a voltage pulse is produced from the sense amplifier that is sent to the pacing therapy controller indicating a sensed event.

BLANKING AND REFRACTORY INTERVALS

Blanking and refractory intervals provide another method for distinguishing P waves and R waves from artifactual or otherwise unwanted signals. If the sense amplifier could reliably distinguish these electric signals, blanking and refractory intervals would not be required. However, because in practical applications a sense amplifier cannot reliably provide ideal signal-to-noise discrimination, these intervals are required for proper pacemaker operation. In general, blanking and refractory periods are time intervals during which the sense amplifiers do not respond to electric signals. Blanking intervals are somewhat different from refractory intervals. During *blanking*, the sense amplifier is completely disabled and cannot detect any electric signals. Blanking is used to reduce the amount of oversensing that can occur from detection of afterpotentials following pacing stimuli (see Chapter 2). In contrast, during a *refractory interval* the sensing amplifier can detect electric signals but responds to these signals differently than if the event had been detected outside the refractory interval. However, during a refractory interval a sensing amplifier output signal that is sent to the pacing therapy controller is interpreted or responded to in a manner that is different from that for a normal sensed event. For example, atrial signals that exceed the value of the threshold comparator during the postventricular atrial refractory period (PVARP) may be completely ignored by the pacing therapy controller or may trigger an automatic change in pacing mode depending on whether this feature is enabled. Because T waves may not be effectively attenuated by the lower frequency cutoff of the bandpass filter, a refractory period is designed into the ventricular sensing channel of all implantable pacemakers. If the T wave from the bandpass filter exceeds the threshold comparator value but falls within the refractory period, inhibition of ventricular output by T wave oversensing can be avoided. Similarly, refractory intervals are critical to the proper function of AAI pacemakers by masking far-field R waves in the atrial electrogram.

The techniques for implementing blanking and refractory intervals are different. For blanking, the sense amplifier is actually disconnected from the electrodes. Figure 5–10 shows how blanking switches can be used to perform this operation. The two switches at the input of the amplifier are opened to disconnect the electrodes, thereby completely preventing detection of any electric signals during this period regardless of amplitude. In addition, a switch (or logic gate) may be included at the output to prevent detection of any artifacts related to the opening or closing of the input switches as sensed events. Figure 5–11 shows the timing of sense amplifier blanking during dual-chamber operation. The ABLANK and VBLANK signals represent the blanking intervals for the atrial and ventricular sense amplifiers, respectively. In addition, the annotation on these signals represents the time during which the blanking switches shown in Figure 5–10 are opened or closed. When the switches are open the amplifier is blanked, and when they are closed the amplifier is not blanked.

Figure 5–11A shows how blanking is used to prevent detection of pacing stimuli or afterpotentials by the sensing amplifiers in the atrial and ventricular channels of a DDD pulse generator. Notice that both the atrial and ventricular sense amplifiers are blanked when either an atrial or a ven-

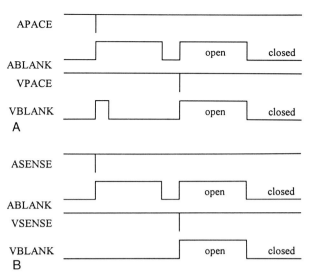

FIGURE 5–11. *A*, The sequence of opening and closing blanking switches in the atrial (ABLANK) and ventricular (VBLANK) sensing channels following pacing stimuli with a DDD pacemaker. Note that immediately following an atrial pacing stimulus (APACE), the blanking switches are opened in both the atrial and the ventricular sensing channels. The atrial blanking switches remain open longer in the atrial than in the ventricular channels following an atrial pacing stimulus. Following a ventricular pacing stimulus (VPACE), the blanking switches are opened in both the atrium and the ventricle. During blanking, no sensing is possible. *B*, The sequence of opening and closing blanking switches following sensed events in the atrium (ASENSE) and the ventricle (VSENSE). Note that the sequence is similar to that occurring after pacing except that cross-blanking does not occur in the ventricle following a sensed atrial event.

tricular pacing stimulus is delivered. These blanking intervals typically range from 100 to 125 msec in duration. An exception is the ventricular blanking period that follows an atrial pacing stimulus. This interval is sometimes referred to as cross-blanking and is intended to be as short as possible (typically 10 to 40 msec) to minimize the amount of time during which the ventricular amplifier is unable to detect intrinsic ventricular depolarizations resulting from normal AV conduction. Figure 5–11B shows that the blanking operation during sensed atrial and ventricular events is similar to that during pacing except that cross-blanking in the ventricle following atrial sensing is not used. The rationale for blanking for 100 to 125 msec after sensed events is that the biologic refractory period of the myocardium essentially excludes electric signals during this period from being desired signals. Blanking following sensing is used to prevent double counting of intracardiac electrograms of long duration. A practical complication of blanking is that it limits the detection of very rapid arrhythmias such as atrial fibrillation and may interfere with automatic mode conversion algorithms.

In contrast to blanking, refractory intervals are typically implemented in the pacing therapy controller rather than at the sense amplifier and are programmable by telemetry (Fig. 5–12). Refractory intervals usually start at the same time as blanking intervals but extend 50 to 300 msec past the completion of blanking. During the refractory period that follows blanking, the sense amplifier is reconnected to the electrodes and can detect any sensed events that may be present. Any sensed event that occurs during this interval is marked as a refractory sensed event (Fig. 5–13). Although the pacing therapy controller may not react to a refractory sensed event

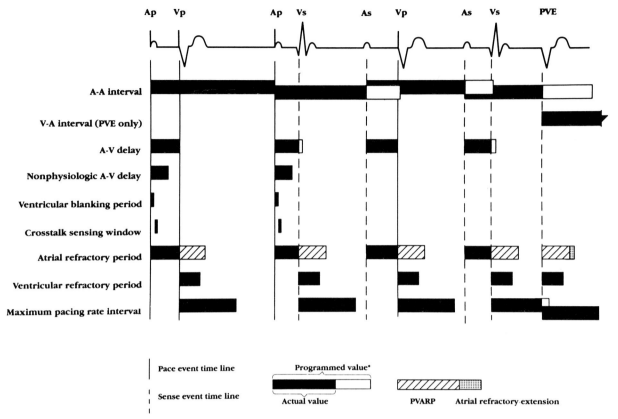

FIGURE 5–12. Diagram of the sequence of AV delay intervals, blanking periods, and refractory periods in a modern DDDR pulse generator (Intermedics 294-03, Intermedics Inc, Angleton, TX). PVARP, postventricular atrial refractory period. (Courtesy of Intermedics Inc.)

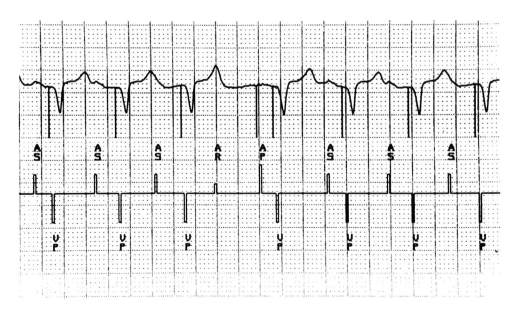

FIGURE 5–13. Atrial and ventricular sensing channel markers in a patient with a DDDR pacemaker (Medtronic 7074). Normal P waves are sensed by the pacemaker and denoted as AS (atrial sensed events). Premature atrial contractions that fall within the postventricular atrial refractory period (PVARP) are denoted by AR (atrial refractory events) and do not inhibit atrial pacing stimuli (AP). Ventricular pacing stimuli are denoted by VP.

in the same way as a normal sensed event, these events are annotated on the marker channel of the implantable pulse generator.

Protection of the Integrated Circuits

The circuitry of modern implantable pulse generators is susceptible to damage from external forces. Therefore, care must be taken in the design of the pulse generator to protect the circuitry from damage. Two of the sources from which the implantable pulse generator must be protected are defibrillation shocks and electrocautery. Damage to the pulse generator from a defibrillation shock can occur if the very high energies present during defibrillator discharge are transmitted to the pacemaker by the pacing leads. These high energies are present during the use of both implantable and external defibrillators. A typical technique for protecting an implantable pulse generator from very high energy levels is to divert the high currents away from the pulse generator's circuitry by using diodes. A diode conducts electric currents in one direction but not in the opposite direction. A Zener diode is capable of bidirectional conduction, conduction in one direction occurring only when the voltage exceeds a threshold value. These diodes are placed between the pulse generator's lead connections and the can. During normal operation the diodes have no effect because their activation voltage is higher than that of the implantable pulse generator's maximum pulse amplitudes. In the presence of very high voltages, the Zener diodes are capable of dissipating high currents, shunting the current away from the pulse generator. Although this technique works well in protecting the implantable pulse generator, it is not without limitations. A defibrillation pulse of sufficient energy may cause irreversible damage if it is discharged directly over an implantable pulse generator, necessitating replacement of the device. In addition, shunting of high-voltage shocks through the leads may result in effective ablation of the myocardium at the electrode-tissue interface.

Electrosurgical cautery can also affect pulse generator performance. Although it is possible for an implantable pulse generator to cease pacing permanently, it is more likely that the pulse generator will be temporarily inhibited during the use of electrocautery. The required level for such effects can vary greatly depending on the type of electrosurgical unit, its settings, and the distance of the current path from the implantable pulse generator and leads. Radiofrequency interference from transmitting devices can also cause temporary inhibition of an implantable pulse generator because the signals from these devices can be mistaken by the pulse generator for pulses that occur every second or half-second and can be interpreted as intrinsic cardiac events. Implantable pulse generators are typically protected from this type of interference by the use of filter capacitors placed between the lead connections on the inside of the pulse generator can.

Microprocessors

Although implantable pulse generators have been used clinically for many years, their construction and components have undergone steady evolution. Early pulse generators were constructed from an array of discrete components, including resistors, capacitors, and transistors. As integrated circuit technology became more reliable and readily available, these circuits were integrated into cardiac pacemakers. The use of integrated circuits in pulse generators has dramatically increased the complexity of these devices. Integrated circuit technology has provided the basis on which more sophisticated features are constructed. As these integrated circuits have become smaller, pacemaker manufacturers have been able to pack more features into the same space. This technologic evolution has now led to the incorporation of microprocessors into implantable pulse generators. This is the same technology that has made the personal computer popular and has brought us such devices as laptop computers, cellular phones, remote controlled TVs, and so on. Essentially, a microprocessor is a computer manufactured by using integrated circuit technology.

RAM VERSUS ROM

For a microprocessor to be programmed, it must have memory available to hold the operating instructions (software) and to store the data that it uses for calculations. In a microprocessor there are typically two types of memory— *random access memory* (RAM) and *read only memory* (ROM). The contents of RAM can be both changed (written) and read by the microprocessor. RAM is typically used to hold data used in calculations. Using RAM, data can be written or read from any memory location in any sequence. ROM is a form of memory in which the contents are unalterable and are determined at the time the ROM is manufactured. As its name implies, the microprocessor cannot write data into any ROM memory location but can only read the ROM memory contents. ROM is used to hold the software that determines what calculations are made and when. Another important distinction between RAM and ROM is that the contents of RAM can be lost if the voltage from the power source drops too low. In contrast, the contents of ROM cannot be lost by a fall in power supply. Because of this, ROM is used to store essential features of the pulse generator to ensure that the feature set will not change if the device is reset for any reason.

DATA STORAGE

One of the most prevalent uses for RAM is the storage of diagnostic data. Because the RAM contents can be written and read in any sequence, the RAM can be organized in ways that allow many different types of data to be stored simultaneously. The only limitation is in the size of the RAM. This size is usually measured in kilobytes (kbytes). One kbyte of RAM represents 1024 bytes. A byte is itself composed of 8 bits of data. Each bit can have a logic value of 0 or 1. Thus, a single byte has 2^8 possible combinations and can represent values from 0 to 256. Bits are grouped into bytes so that much larger numbers can be represented. Modern implantable pulse generators typically contain memories that range in size from 1 to 32 kbytes. It is anticipated that memories of 1 megabyte may soon be available in such devices as implantable cardioverter-defibrillators.

The types of data that are typically stored in RAM can be grouped into three major categories; histograms, trends, and

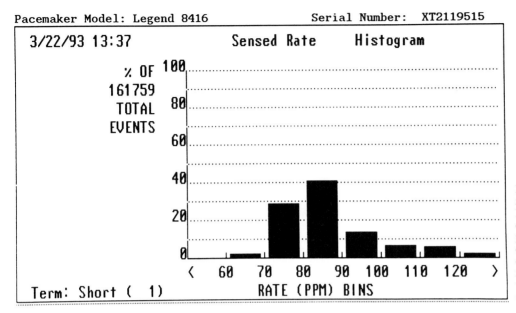

FIGURE 5–14. Typical short-term rate histogram in a patient with a DDDR pacemaker who had exercised prior to interrogation of the pulse generator. Note that the percentage of sensor rate events that occurred within the programmed ranges of rates (bins) are shown. Histograms require minimal memory for storage.

analog data. Histograms are common in many modern implantable pulse generators and provide a method of storing data in groups or bins over a long period of time. An example of a histogram is shown in Figure 5–14. Note that time information is not necessarily contained in the histograms but only the number of beats that occurred within a given range of heart rates. Histograms are a very efficient method of storing data because the count in the bin is updated with each occurrence of an event. For example, a histogram with 8 bins as shown in Figure 5–14 typically uses less than 50 bytes of RAM to log heart rate data over a period of up to several years, depending on the frequency of sampling. The less frequently data are sampled, the longer the duration of storage.

Another method for storing diagnostic data is the use of trends (Fig. 5–15). With a trend, each data point is time-stamped in some fashion. For example, if a heart rate trend is to be stored, the heart rate and the time at which the measurement was made are stored for each data point. Trend data consume considerably more memory than histograms because each data point itself must be stored instead of simply incrementing the count in a bin. For example, a 24 hour beat-by-beat trend can require over 100 kbytes of RAM at an average heart rate of 70 bpm. To reduce this memory requirement, the pulse generator can store a heart rate value every 10 seconds instead of every beat. This reduces the memory requirement to less than 9 kbytes. Because of these trade-offs, most clinicians use histograms to track long-term events. If the clinical need is to determine the pacing rate accurately during a period of known activity (such as treadmill exercise), a trend usually provides more useful information. Most modern pulse generators require the clinician to determine the type of data to be stored (whether the intrinsic heart rate, the sensor-indicated rate, the AV intervals, and so on), how it is to be stored (as a histogram or trend), the sampling frequency (every beat, every second, or less frequently), and whether the data are to be fixed or overwritten once the available memory has been exhausted. For example, if a heart rate trend with sampling every beat is chosen, the available RAM may be exhausted in as little as 15 minutes.

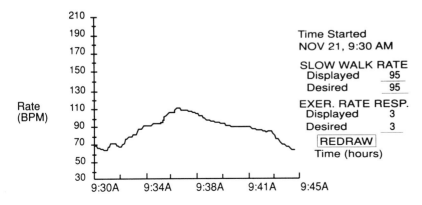

FIGURE 5–15. Diagnostic data stored as a trend of pacing rates versus time. Because each data point must be stored separately with the time of its occurrence, diagnostic trends require a far greater amount of memory than histograms do. (Courtesy of Intermedics Inc.)

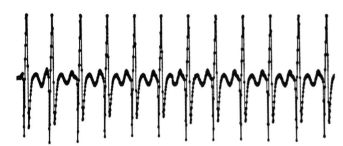

FIGURE 5–16. A stored intracardiac electrogram during an episode of ventricular tachycardia in a patient with an implantable cardioverter-defibrillator (Ventritex Cadence model V-100). Note that electrogram storage requires the recording of many data points, each with the electrogram amplitude (ordinate) and time (abscissa). Such stored electrograms require very large amounts of memory but provide clinically relevant information.

Therefore, most pulse generators offer the option of freezing the first 15 minutes of storage (a "frozen trend") or continually overwriting the memory (a "rolling trend"). In general, if the the clinician wants to know what the pulse generator was storing immediately prior to interrogation of the device, a rolling trend should be programmed. On the other hand, if the clinical need is to clear the diagnostic data and send the patient to perform a known physical activity with later interrogation of the pulse generator, a frozen trend should be used. Finally, if the clinical need is to store the long-term average performance of the device, a histogram is more useful.

The third method of storing diagnostic data is the use of analog signals such as those used in an intracardiac electrogram (EGM) (Fig. 5–16). This type of data can require huge amounts of RAM because many data points are required to represent the electrogram adequately over a very short period of time. Like trend data, an 8-bit data value (byte) is stored on every sample of the signal. The primary difference is that the sampling rate of an EGM signal is much higher than that used for trend data. To maintain the signal morphology and keep it visible, the EGM signal must be sampled at least 100 times per second. At this sampling rate, a 24-hour EGM recording would require over 8 million bytes of RAM. It is possible to use data compression techniques to reduce the memory storage requirements. However, the technology is not even close to achieving 24-hour EGM storage in the amount of RAM presently available in implantable pulse generators because most data compression techniques can achieve compression ratios ranging from only 2:1 to 10:1. Even at a 10:1 data compression ratio, over 800 kbytes of RAM would be required to store a 24-hour EGM. Nevertheless, in some clinical circumstances the intracardiac EGM provides critical information that cannot be adequately represented in any other way. For example, storage of the EGM prior to a mode switch allows accurate interpretation of the atrial EGM for diagnosis of an atrial arrhythmia. Intracardiac EGM storage is crucial for the management of patients with implantable cardioverter-defibrillators in whom the EGM can be used to distinguish ventricular from supraventricular arrhythmias or to sense lead malfunction. It is likely that as greater amounts of RAM become available in pulse generators, appropriate storage of EGM data will be made available for bradycardia pacemakers.

Summary

The modern implantable pulse generator offers greatly improved programmable features, automatic functions, and diagnostic storage capabilities. With further refinements in microprocessors, these capabilities can be expected to increase. It is critical for clinicians involved in the care of patients with pacemakers to understand the implications of their programming decisions on the performance of the pulse generator and to make optimum use of the capabilities of each device.

REFERENCES

1. DeCaprio V, Hurzeler P, Furman S: A comparison of unipolar and bipolar electrograms for cardiac pacemaker. Circulation 56:750, 1977.
2. Furman S, Hurzeler P, De Caprio V: Cardiac pacing and pacemakers III. Sensing the cardiac electrogram. Am Heart J 93:794, 1977.
3. Frohlig G, Schwendt H, Schieffer H, Bette L: Atrial signal variations and pacemaker malsensing during exercise: A study in the time and frequency domain. J Am Coll Cardiol 11:806, 1988.
4. Parsonnet V, Myers GH, Kresh YM: Characteristics of intracardiac electrograms II. Atrial endocardial electrograms. PACE 3:406, 1980.
5. Myers GH, Kresh YM, Parsonnett V: Characteristics of intracardiac electrograms. PACE 1:90, 1978.
6. Platia EV, Brinker JA: Time course of transvenous pacemaker stimulation impedance, capture thresholds, and intracardiac electrogram amplitude. PACE 9:620, 1986.
7. Mond HG, Stokes KB: The electrode-tissue interface: The revolutionary role of steroid elution. PACE 15:95, 1992.
8. Kleinert M, Elmqvist H, Strandberg H: Spectral properties of atrial and ventricular endocardial signals. PACE 2:11, 1979.
9. Klitzner TS, Stevenson WG: Effects of filtering on right ventricular electrograms recorded from endocardial catheters in humans. PACE 13:69, 1990.
10. Steinhaus DM, Foley L, Knoll K, Markowitz T: Atrial sensing revisited: Do bandpass filters matter? [Abstract]. PACE 16:946, 1993.
11. Medtronic Inc: Spectrax SX 5984, 5984 LP, 5985 Technical Manual. Minneapolis, Medtronic, Inc, 1984.
12. Barold SS, Kulkarni H, Thawani AJ, et al: Electrocardiographic manifestations of the rapid recharge function of pulse generators after sensing. PACE 11:1215, 1988.
13. Mond HG, Barold SS: Dual-chamber, rate-adaptive pacing in patients with paroxysmal supraventricular tachyarrhythmias: Protective measures for rate control. PACE 16:2168, 1993.
14. Lau CP, Tai YT, Fong PC, et al: Atrial arrhythmia management with sensor-controlled atrial refractory period and automatic mode switching in patients with minute ventilation–sensing, dual-chamber, rate-adaptive pacemakers. PACE 15:1504, 1992.
15. Ohm O-J: The interdependence between electrogram, total electrode impedance, and pacemaker input impedance necessary to obtain adequate functioning of demand pacemakers. PACE 2:465, 1979.
16. Fischler H: Polarization properties of small-surface-area pacemaker electrodes—implications on reliability of sensing and pacing. PACE 2:403, 1979.
17. Goldreyer BN, Olive AL, Leslie J, et al: A new orthogonal lead for P synchronous pacing. PACE 4:638, 1981.
18. Goldreyer BN, Knudson M, Cannom DS, Wyman MG: Orthogonal electrogram sensing. PACE 6:464, 1983.
19. Wainwright RJ, Crick JCP, Sowton E: Clinical evaluation of a single-pass electrode for all modes of pacing. PACE 6:210, 1983.
20. Antonioli GE, Ansani L, Barbieri D, et al: Single-lead VDD pacing. In Barold SS, Mugica J (eds): New Perspectives in Cardiac Pacing 3. Mt. Kisco, NY, Futura, 1993, pp 359–381.
21. Varriale P, Pilla AG, Tekriwal M: Single-lead VDD pacing system. PACE 13:757, 1990.
22. Curzio G and the Multicenter Study Group: A multicenter evaluation of a single-pass lead VDD pacing system. PACE 14:434, 1991.
23. Hurzeler P, Decaprio V, Furman S: Endocardial electrograms and pacemaker sensing. Med Inst 10(4):178, 1976.

24. Angello DA: Principles of electrical testing for analysis of ventricular endocardial pacing leads. Prog Cardiovasc Dis 27:57, 1984.

25. De Buitleir M, Kou WH, Schmaltz S, et al: Acute changes in pacing threshold and R- or P-wave amplitude during permanent pacemaker implantation. Am J Cardiol 65:999, 1990.

26. Nielsen AP, Cashion R, Spencer WH, et al: Long-term assessment of unipolar and bipolar stimulation and sensing thresholds using a lead configuration programmable pacemaker. J Am Coll Cardiol 5:1198, 1985.

27. Furman S: Bipolar pacing. PACE 9:619, 1986.

28. Scalhorn R, Markowitz T: Bipolar dual-chamber pacemakers: Is myopotential sensing still a problem? PACE 11:852, 1988.

29. Wirzfeld S, Lampadius M, Ruprecht EO: Unterdruckung von demand-Schrittmachern durch Muskelpotentials. Dtsch Med Wochenschr 97:61, 1972.

30. Levine PA, Klein MD: Myopotential inhibition of unipolar pacemakers: A disease of technologic progress. Ann Intern Med 98:101, 1983.

31. Watson WS: Myopotential sensing in cardiac pacemakers. In Barold SS, Mugica J (eds): Modern Cardiac Pacing. Mt Kisco, NY, Futura, 1985, pp 813–837.

32. Berger R, Warren J: Myopotential inhibition of demand pacemakers: Etiologic, diagnostic, and therapeutic considerations. PACE 2:596, 1979.

33. Fetter J, Hall DM, Hoff GL, Reeder JT: The effect of myopotential interference on unipolar and bipolar dual-chamber pacemakers in the DDD mode. Clin Prog Electrophysiol Pacing 3:368, 1985.

34. Brevik K, Ohm OJ: Myopotential inhibition of unipolar QRS-inhibited (VVI) pacemakers assessed by ambulatory Holter monitoring of the electrocardiogram. PACE 3:470, 1980.

35. Halpern JL, Camunas JL, Stern EH, et al: Myopotential interference with DDD pacemakers: Endocardial electrographic telemetry in the diagnosis of pacemaker-related arrhythmias. Am J Cardiol 54:97, 1984.

36. Secemsky SI, Hauser RG, Denes P, et al: Unipolar sensing abnormalities: Incidence and clinical significance of skeletal muscle interference and undersensing in 228 patients. PACE 5:10, 1982.

37. DeBoer H, Kofflard M, Scholtes T, et al: Differential bipolar sensing of a dual-chamber pacemaker. PACE 11:158, 1988.

38. Fetter J, Bobeldyk GL, Engman FJ: The clinical incidence and significance of myopotential sensing with unipolar pacemakers. PACE 7:871, 1984.

39. Brevik K, Ohm OJ, Engedal H: Long-term comparison of unipolar and bipolar pacing and sensing, using a new multiprogrammable system. PACE 6:592, 1983.

40. Barold SS, Ong LS, Falkoff MD: Inhibition of bipolar demand pacemaker by diaphragmatic myopotentials. Circulation 56:679, 1977.

41. El Gamal M, Van Gelder B: Suppression of an external demand pacemaker by diaphragmatic myopotentials: A sign of electrode perforation? PACE 2:191, 1979.

42. Barold SS, Falkoff MD, Ong LS, et al: Diaphragmatic myopotential inhibition in multiprogrammable unipolar and bipolar pulse generators. In Steinbach K (ed): Cardiac Pacing. Proceedings of the VIIIth World Symposium on Cardiac Pacing. Darmstadt, Germany, Steinkopff Verlag, 1983, p 537.

43. Rosenqvist M, Nordlander R, Andersson M, et al: Reduced incidence of myopotential pacemaker inhibition by abdominal generator implantation. PACE 9:417, 1986.

44. Gialafos J, Maillis A, Kalogeropoulos C, et al: Inhibition of demand pacemakers by myopotentials. Am Heart J 109:984, 1985.

45. Lau CP, Linker NJ, Butrous GS, et al: Myopotential interference in unipolar rate-responsive pacemakers. PACE 12:1324, 1989.

46. Volosin KJ, Rudderow R, Waxman HL: VOOR-nondemand rate-modulated pacing necessitated by myopotential inhibition. PACE 12:421, 1989.

47. Michalik RE, Williams WH, Hatcher CR Jr: Myopotential inhibition of unipolar pacing in children. PACE 8:25, 1985.

48. Griffin JC: Sensing characteristics of the right atrial appendage electrode. PACE 6:22, 1983.

49. Coombs WJ, Reynolds DW, Sharma AD, et al: Crosstalk in bipolar pacemakers. PACE 12:613, 1989.

50. Van Gelder LM, El Gamal MIH, Tielen CHJ: P-wave sensing in VVI pacemakers: Useful or a problem? PACE 11:1413, 1988.

51. Mond HG, Sloman JG: The malfunctioning pacemaker system. Part II. PACE 4:168, 1981.

52. Barold SS, Gaidula JJ: Evaluation of normal and abnormal sensing functions of demand pacemakers. Am J Cardiol 28:201, 1971.

53. Brandt J, Fahraeus T, Schuller H: Far-field QRS complex sensing via the atrial pace-maker lead. II. Prevalence, clinical significance, and possibility of intraoperative prediction in DDD pacing. PACE 11:1546, 1988.

54. Barold SS, Falkoff MD, Ong LS, et al: Double sensing by atrial automatic tachycardia-terminating pulse generator. PACE 10:58, 1987.

55. Warnowicz MA, Goldschlager N: Apparent failure to sense (undersensing) caused by oversensing: Diagnostic use of a noninvasively obtained intracardiac electrogram. PACE 6:1341, 1983.

56. Hauser RG, Susmano A: After-potential oversensing by a programmable pulse generator. PACE 4:391, 1981.

57. Shandling AH, Castellanet MJ, Messenger JC, et al: Utility of the atrial endocardial electrogram concurrent with dual-chamber pacing in the determination of a pacemaker-mediated arrhythmia. PACE 11:1419, 1988.

58. Shandling AH, Castellanet MJ, Thomas L, et al: Impaired activity rate responsiveness of an atrial activity triggered pacemaker. The role of differential atrial sensing in its prevention. PACE 12:1927, 1989.

59. Barold SS, Falkoff MD, Ong LS, et al: Interpretation of electrocardiograms produced by a new unipolar multiprogrammable ''committed'' AV sequential demand (DVI) pulse generator. PACE 4:692, 1981.

60. Levine PA, Brodsky SJ: Fusion, pseudofusion, pseudopseudofusion, and confusion. Clin Prog Pacing Electrophysiol 1:70, 1983.

61. Lindemans FW, Rankin IR, Murtaugh R, et al: Clinical experience with an activity-sensing pacemaker. PACE 9:978, 1986.

62. Waxman HL, Lazzara R, El-Sherif N: Apparent malfunction of demand pacemaker due to spurious potentials generated by contact between two endocardial electrodes. PACE 1:531, 1978.

63. Wilson JH, Lattner S: Apparent undersensing due to oversensing of low amplitude pulses in a thoracic impedance-sensing, rate-responsive pacemaker. PACE 11:1479, 1988.

64. Timmis GC, Westveer DC, Bakalyar DM, et al: Discrimination of anterograde from retrograde atrial electrograms for physiologic pacing. PACE 11:130, 1988.

65. Klementowicz PT, Furman S: Selective atrial sensing in dual-chamber pacemakers eliminates endless loop tachycardia. J Am Coll Cardiol 6:1338, 1986.

66. Leitch JW, Yee R, Klein GJ, et al: Correlation between the ventricular electrogram amplitude in sinus rhythm and ventricular fibrillation. PACE 13:1105, 1990.

67. Ellenbogen KA, Wood MA, Stambler BS, et al: Measurement of ventricular electrogram amplitude during intraoperative induction of ventricular tachyarrhythmias. Am J Cardiol 70:1017, 1992.

68. Sperry RE, Ellenbogen KA, Wood MA, et al: Failure of the second- and third-generation implantable cardioverter defibrillator to sense ventricular tachycardia: Implications for fixed-gain sensing devices. PACE 15:749, 1992.

69. Singer I, Adams L, Austin E: Potential hazards of fixed gain sensing and arrhythmia reconfirmation for implantable cardioverter defibrillators. PACE 16:1070, 1993.

70. Fontaine JM, Alma-Perri CA, El-Sherif N: DDD pacemaker pseudomalfunction during supraventricular tachycardia. PACE 11:1380, 1988.

71. Barold SS, Mond HG: Optimal antibradycardia pacing in patients with paroxysmal supraventricular tachyarrhythmias: Role of fallback and automatic mode-switching mechanisms. In Barold SS, Mugica J (eds): New Perspectives in Cardiac Pacing—3. Mt. Kisco, NY, Futura, 1993, pp 483–518.

72. Curry PVL, Raper DA: Single lead for permanent physiological cardiac pacing. Lancet 2:757, 1978.

73. Antonioli GE, Grass G, Baggioni FG, et al: New method for atrial triggered pacemaker. G Ital Cardiol 10:679, 1980.

74. Flammang DF, Renirie L, Begemann M, et al: Amplitude and direction of atrial depolarization using a multipolar floating catheter: Principles for a single-lead VDD pacing system. PACE 14:1040, 1991.

75. Ramsdale DR, Charles RG: Rate-responsive ventricular pacing: Clinical experience with the RS4-SRT pacing system. PACE 8:378, 1985.

CHAPTER 6

PROGRAMMERS FOR CARDIAC PACEMAKERS

Mark H. Schoenfeld
Luis E. Padula
J. Warren Harthorne

Programmability has been defined as a "noninvasive, reversible alteration of the electronic performance of an implanted pacemaker device."[1] The benefits of programmability have been discussed in detail with regard to both diagnostics and therapeutics.[2–4] The ability to adjust certain parameters to avoid second surgical interventions has received particular emphasis,[5] although attention has also been directed toward other goals such as optimizing cardiac output and reducing rate-related angina. Indeed, a policy conference of the North American Society of Pacing and Electrophysiology stated nearly a decade ago that "solely on the basis of patient safety, there is no indication for the implantation of a single- or dual-chamber pulse generator which is not programmable."[6]

Although the concept of programmability has been well established, there has been relatively little discussion in the medical literature about the particular devices that perform this function, namely, pacemaker programmers. Certainly, to the patient these devices appear to be "magical" wands that mysteriously and noninvasively adjust their pacemakers, but this "black box" impression also applies to most physicians involved in cardiac pacing. Furthermore, the vast array of programmers currently available through various manufacturers adds to the almost hopeless complexity faced by the physician (Fig. 6–1). It is the purpose of this chapter to trace the evolution of pacemaker programmers, examine their architecture, discuss certain idiosyncrasies of their function and dysfunction (without becoming too proprietary from the standpoint of manufacturers), address the concept of universal programming, and anticipate what lies ahead in programmer development.

A History of Programmers

The earliest technique for altering pacemaker function, albeit invasively, appeared in the early 1960s. This involved the use of two rate-controlling potentiometers manufactured by Medtronic Inc. (5870, 5842, 5900 series) that allowed percutaneous manipulation of the pulse generator by a triangular Keith needle;[7] another model allowed output voltage adjustment.[8] Other pacemakers permitted noninvasive adjustment of a bistable magnetic switch that selected one of two possible pacing rates.[9] The General Electric model A7020BA offered pacing rates of 70 or 85 bpm, which were programmed by temporary closure of a reed switch by the application of a pocket magnet.[1] In 1966 Tyers and colleagues reported on the first implant of a pacing system that allowed programmability of more than one parameter, including the stimulus voltage, pacing rate, and polarity.[10] This multiprogrammability was achieved by the external application of the appropriate pole of a bar magnet to one of five magnetically attuned reed switches in the pulse generator.[10] In 1970, Medtronic Inc. introduced a programming system (model 5531) with two external bar magnets rotated in an enclosed container, which was hand cranked over the pulse generator (model 5961). The pulse generator had two small bar magnets attached to a potentiometer, which was altered by the cranking process of the programmer (hence the term "coffee-grinder"), resulting in a change in the pulse duration.[11] At this time, temporary adjustments of stimulus intensity, pacing rate, sensitivity, and temporary facilitation of burst pacing or threshold testing were possible through the external application of a magnet that resulted in the closure of a reed switch

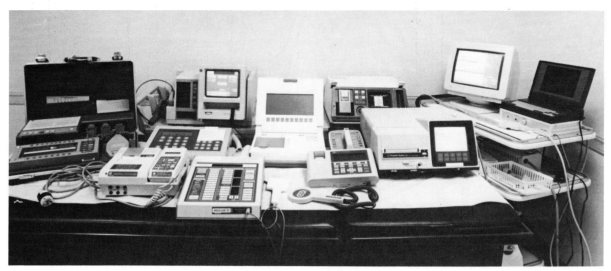

FIGURE 6–1. An array of programming devices typically required in a pacemaker center.

in the pulse generator.[12] In this case, the programmed change was transient, and the pulse generator subsequently returned to its original function when the magnet was removed. Introduction of the Cordis Omnicor series in 1973[13, 14] heralded the capability for *reversible* and *stable* noninvasive programming of changes in pulse generator function through the use of an external electromagnetic programmer that emitted a pulsed magnetic field to open and close a reed switch. This marked the age of true data transmission technology because magnetic signals were interpreted by the pulse generator as programming instructions. The ''dithering'' of the reed switch by pulsed magnetic fields resulted in voltage spikes that were detected by an 8-bit register encoded in a binary system (0 = reed switch open; 1 = reed switch closed). The smallest number of pulses required to alter the function of the pulse generator was 8, and there was a maximum of 73 pulses. In this device, the *number* of pulses encoded a specific combination of pacing rate, sensitivity, and stimulus intensity.

Along with the capability for programming came the need to confirm that a programming command had been successfully received by the pulse generator. This requirement for feedback from the pulse generator to the programmer, inherent in the concept of verification and bidirectional telemetry,[15] and the attendant desire for a fast and efficient method of transmission of information, ushered in the age of radio-frequency programming systems in the late 1970s. Early pacing systems that used radio-frequency signals to carry programming instructions included the Medtronic Xytron, Xyrel, and Byrel models. The radio-frequency modality also allowed greater security of the transmission code, minimizing pacemaker misprogramming and cross-programming (see later discussion).

Historically, the first parameters that could be programmed were the pacing rate (with a low rate for patients with angina, a standard rate, and a higher rate for pediatric patients), stimulus intensity (voltage and pulse duration), and sensitivity. These choices reflected the needs of patients in the early era of pacing and the limitations of battery and lead technology. *Programmer* development was essentially driven by the

evolution of technology of *pulse generators and leads* rather than the reverse. However, the advent of dual-chamber pacing technology required programmability for an ever-increasing array of parameters. Thus, the clinical requirement for multiprogrammability and the technologies of radio-frequency data transmission and microprocessors[16] were responsible for the development of modern pacemaker programmers.

Concepts in the Design of Pacemaker Programmers

Traditionally, programmers have been of either the hand-held or desk-top variety. The desk-top models generally allow a greater variety of functions, but the necessarily larger size limits their portability and increases their power consumption. It is anticipated that future refinements in microprocessor technology will allow reconciliation of these opposing goals of increased functionality and small size. An intermediate step in the evolution of pacemaker programmers may allow a portion of the desk-top unit to be removed for portable use as a hand-held module. The data telemetered from the pulse generator could then be stored in the hand-held module to be transported back to the desk-top workstation for printing or entry into a computerized data base.

CARRIERS FOR PROGRAMMING SIGNALS

The three forms of electromagnetic waves that have been used for communication between the programmer and the pulse generator are *magnetic coupling, inductive coupling,* and *radio-frequency energy.* A fourth modality, *ultrasound,* may be transmitted through a crystal oscillator but has not been generally employed for programming because it is critically dependent on a precise alignment between the transducer and receiver and on an intervening air-free medium.[8] *Magnetic coupling* occurs with application of a *continuous* magnet (such as that produced by a bar, toroidal, or horseshoe magnet) or through a *pulsed* magnetic field.[17] In both cases, the element used for detecting the magnetic field in the pulse generator is a reed switch. In the case of a pulsed magnetic field, the reed switch opens and closes with each pulse of the field (''dithering''). *Inductive coupling* occurs when pulsed magnetic fields are employed to transmit the programming instructions, which are detected by a receiving element that is an antenna coil. Essentially, these pulses of the magnetic field are transmitted in a coding scheme that induces current to flow in the antenna coil (Fig. 6–2). *Radio-frequency* (RF) waves are cycles of the electromagnetic field at frequencies typically ranging from 10 kHz to 175 kHz that allow rapid transmission of large amounts of information. Both the transmitter (in the programmer) and the receiver (in the pulse generator) have antennae for emitting and decoding RF signals. The selection of carrier frequencies for use in pacemaker programmers is quite variable and is manufacturer-specific. The RF frequency is varied with time (''modulated''), allowing the encoding of information during transmission by the programmer. The receiver coil is tuned through properly selected inductor-capacitor values to have unique sensitivity to the carrier frequency of the transmitted signals.

Certain programming systems employ both a radio-frequency field and a reed switch that must be magnetically dithered to allow detection of the radio-frequency waves by the pulse generator detector coil (antenna). In these systems, the requirement for a second electromagnetic field interaction (magnet-actuated reed switch closure) is viewed as a ''safety interlock'' or an environmental security measure against misprogramming or dysprogramming (see later discussion). The receiver circuit in this case does not remain constantly activated because of concern about current drain on the power cell of the pulse generator. The mechanical components tend to be the weakest link in any electromechanical system. Thus, a potential limitation of using a reed switch as the receiving element is the requirement for its mechanical motion, a factor that limits its speed. As a result, a relatively long transmission time is required for programming.[18] In one such system, 2.2 seconds was required to program one parameter.[19] The rates of opening and closure of the reed switch are several orders of magnitude slower than those obtained by electronic transistor switches.[17] Both reed switch–linked radio-frequency systems and the more traditional magnetic and inductive coupling schemes may malfunction in the event of a sticky or insensitive reed switch.[20] In addition, there are several theoretical and practical concerns about the extra current drain and the risk of asynchronous pacing that are associated with reed switch closure.[22] Furthermore, rather than serving as a security measure, the ubiquitous presence of magnetic fields in the environment[23] may inappropriately activate the reed switch mechanism.[17]

Signal attenuation is a potential concern in the interaction of the programmer with the pulse generator. Because the programming signal must pass from the programmer through the air intervening between the transmitter antenna and the skin, the subcutaneous tissues, and the pulse generator can, the signal that is received in the pulse generator may be of lower amplitude than the signal that was transmitted by the programmer. These same barriers serve to attenuate the signal emitted by the pulse generator during telemetry to the programmer. The extent to which these signals are attenuated is directly proportional to the distance between programmer and pulse generator. Attenuation by the pulse generator can is noted particularly at higher RF carrier frequencies.[17]

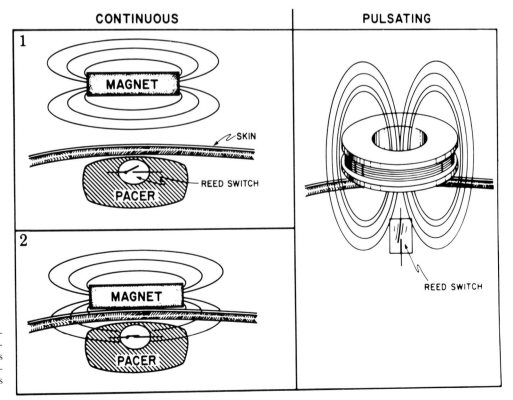

FIGURE 6–2. Examples of continuous and pulsed magnetic field applications. (From Parsonnet V, Rodgers T: The present status of programmable pacemakers. Prog Cardiovasc Dis 23:401, 1981.)

INTERFERENCE AND SIGNAL-TO-NOISE RATIOS

Other important concepts in the design of pacemaker programmers are those of electric interference and signal-to-noise ratios. Electric interference may be produced by a variety of sources but, for our purposes, can be conceptualized in the major categories of *radiation* (or "emissions") and *susceptibility*. Radiation is a measure of the interference given off by the programmer that may affect the operation of other electric equipment. Susceptibility is the sensitivity of the programmer to other sources of interference. For example, the programmer may be affected by electric interference that arises from a nearby electrocautery device. Because electric interference is ubiquitous in the medical environment, the pulse generator receiver coil must be able to discriminate between the appropriate signal from its corresponding programmer and electromagnetic noise emitted from other sources (including telemetry signals from the programmers of other manufacturers). Although the Food and Drug Administration (FDA) requires medical equipment manufacturers to test these aspects of interference, no precise U.S. standards exist (other than safety). In contrast, nonmedical devices such as computers must comply with FCC-generated emission standards. In contrast, medical devices must meet emission standards in Europe (the standard for emissions is German document VDE 0871, and for susceptibility the relevant document is IEC 850). Most pacemaker programmers do, however, meet at least one European standard (IEC 601-1) covering the safety of all medical instruments such as the risk of electric shock.[24] To discriminate between the appropriate programming instructions and electric interference, the signal-to-noise ratio should be as high as possible.

ENCODING SCHEMES FOR PROGRAMMING INSTRUCTIONS

The concept of *encoding* is critical to the function of pacemaker programmers. As mentioned earlier, the transmission of programming information involves manipulation of the carrier signal (continuous or pulsed magnetic fields, RF, or ultrasound) in a manner that is recognizable by the pulse generator as a valid set of instructions. This method of encoding information in the carrier input signals by the programmer is a process called modulation.[25] Thus, the process of modulation serves as a means of encoding the programming instructions in a language that is interpretable by the pulse generator. Modulation of signal amplitude (turning the carrier on and off between zero amplitude and a predefined value), pulse width, and time between pulses all have been employed in programming systems (Fig. 6–3). When modulation is accomplished by variations in pulse amplitude, encoding is based on the total number of pulses transmitted to the pulse generator. In such programming schemes, the time required for signal transmission is directly proportional to the number of pulses used for the code; furthermore, a minimum pulse count is required to identify the subsequent pulses as a valid code. Pulse width–modulated programming systems are ideally suited to binary coding, in which narrow and wide pulses may represent bit values of 0 and 1, respectively.[25] The information that can be encoded with X binary digits is 2^X. This allows more information to be conveyed in a smaller number of pulses. Thus, comparing the two coding schemes, a pacemaker with 4 programmable stimulus amplitudes, 8 programmable pacing rates, and 2 programmable sensitivities would have 64 potential combinations of parameters (4 × 8

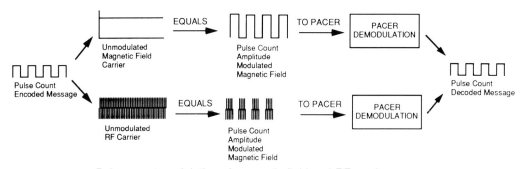

Pulse <u>count</u> modulation of magnetic field and RF carriers

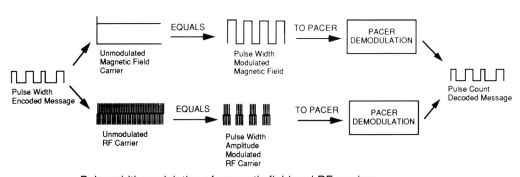

Pulse <u>width</u> modulation of magnetic field and RF carriers

FIGURE 6–3. Examples of modulation methods and carriers. (From Gold RD, Saulson SH, Macgregor DC: Programmable pacing systems: The medium and the message. PACE 5:776, 1982.)

× 2). An encoding scheme that transmitted this information as a series of pulses would require a minimum of 64 pulses (not including validation codes) to transmit the programming instructions. For example, 16 pulses might equal a pacing rate of 100 bpm, an amplitude of 5 V, and a sensitivity of 2 mV; similarly, 24 pulses might indicate a pacing rate of 90 bpm, an amplitude of 2.5 V, and a sensitivity of 4 mV. In contrast, only 6 pulses are required to encode all possible combinations with a binary pulse width–modulated scheme (i.e., $2^6 = 64$). The amount of information to be coded therefore depends not on the carrier type per se (i.e., RF, pulsed magnetic field) but on the coding scheme employed. The rate at which the information is transmitted may be influenced by the coding scheme as well as by the type of carrier used (faster transmission rates for high carrier frequencies, i.e., RF).

SECURITY OF THE PROGRAMMER CODE

The programming signal must be designed to be secure, both for proprietary reasons and to protect against misprogramming. Such programming security is of three types: message security, system security, and carrier security[25] (Fig. 6–4). *Carrier security* implies that a pulse generator will respond only to the carrier for which it has been designed to be sensitive. Magnetic pulses and low-frequency RF offer the greatest security from spurious environmental interference, whereas higher frequency RF systems may be "confused" by other signal sources such as radios, televisions, or even garage door openers. One form of *message security* has already been commented on, namely, using the first group of bits or pulses as an identification or access code. Restrictions

on pulse width and pulse rate are used as additional security measures. Thus, for example, in the case of the Pacesetter model 370 programmer:

. . . in the presence of a magnet-activated reed switch, a 14-bit pulsed, 37 KHz magnetic signal is transmitted to the pulse generator. The signal is analyzed by the pulse generator to insure that the correct timing, pulse shape, sequencing, and number of pulses are transmitted. It then executes the command and transmits a 5-bit confirmatory signal to the model 370 programmer. The received signal is compared with the expected response and only if there is a perfect match is the new parameter value or mode displayed on the CRT display. The command, INTERROGATE, initially produces a "search" signal which looks for the presence of the pulse generator and assists the operator in locating and properly aligning the programming/telemetry head . . .[26]

In another manufacturer's scheme (Intermedics), 80 impulses are organized into pairs to send a code message of 40 digital bits that allow four levels of "safety interlocks."[17–19] The first 16 bits allow the pulse generator to accept information only from an Intermedics programmer and contain the programming information (2^{16} or 65,536 programming commands possible), whereas the next 4 bits reflect the particular pulse generator model being programmed. The last 20 bits are in the binary code opposite to that of the first 20 bits (logical 1 becomes logical 0) and serve as a check against false signals (Fig. 6–5).

In the case of multiparameter programmability, the linkage of two or more parameters such as sensitivity and pacing rate may be used to verify that a change in one programmed value has occurred by verifying a change in another, more easily confirmed pacing parameter (*system security*; see Fig. 6–4). For example, the clinician may purposely change the

Example of Potential Elements in a Programming Security System

	Pulse Count Code (With No Telemetry)	Binary Code (With Telemetry)
Message Security (Modulation)	First Group of Bits as Identification Code	First N Bits as Unique Code Additional Model Specific Codes Fixed Length Message (i.e., 20 Bits)
	Checks on Pulse Width Checks on Time Between Pulses	Checks on Pulse Width of 0's and 1's Checks on Time Between Pulses Checks on Length of Delays Inserted within Code String Parity Check Internal Checks of Message Validity Transmission of Complement Others Possible
System Security (Modulation)	Linked Parameters	Linked Parameters Confirming Signal from Pacer Echoback of As-Received Signal for Comparison with As-Transmitted Signal Independently in Programmer Interrogation Automatic Reinterrogation

FIGURE 6–4. Examples of potential security elements in a programming system. (From Gold RD, Saulson SH, Macgregor DC: Programmable pacing systems: The medium and the message. PACE 5:776, 1982.)

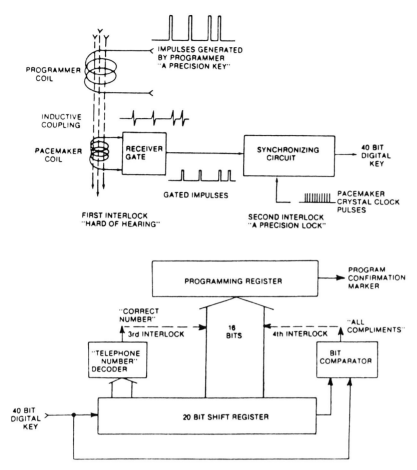

FIGURE 6–5. Multiple levels of "safety interlocks" in one manufacturer's security system. (From Gordon P, Calfee RV, Baker RG Jr: Multiprogrammable pacemaker technology. A tutorial review and prediction. *In* Barold SS, Mugica J [eds]: The Third Decade of Cardiac Pacing. Mt Kisco, NY, Futura, 1982, pp 127–143.)

programmed pacing rate simultaneously with a change in sensitivity. By confirming that a change in pacing rate has indeed occurred by physical or electrocardiographic (ECG) examination, the physician may be confident that the sensitivity was also programmed successfully. Although bidirectional telemetry is also used in most modern pacing systems to confirm that a programming sequence has been undertaken and completed successfully, it is incumbent on the physician to establish independently that appropriate programming has occurred by inspection of the electrocardiogram.

The Architecture of Pacemaker Programmers

All programming systems, independent of manufacturer, share certain fundamental features (Fig. 6–6). *Input* is the mechanism by which the user of the programmer sets up or enters the information that is to be conveyed from the programmer to the pulse generator. Typically, programming instructions are entered by means of a keyboard or a set of pushbuttons accompanied by a video display such as a light-emitting diode (LED) or liquid crystal display (LCD). Input of the programmed values may require interaction of the user and the programmer through a light pen or a touch-sensitive computer screen. These programming screens also provide a record of the programming session and are usually sent to an integrated printer. An invariable component of the input feature is a key for emergency programming to high-stimulus

output or rapid reprogramming to nominal or standard values.[27]

TELEMETRY

Telemetry involves the transmission of information from the pulse generator to an external programmer. As discussed previously, the telemetry interface is essential for modern programmers. The first telemetry systems used in implantable pacemakers were not associated with programmability. Rather, telemetry was used to assess the power source in pacemakers employing rechargeable batteries and served as a signal of when the batteries were fully recharged.[28] Telemetry was first applied to programmable pacemakers in 1978; transmission of information from the pulse generator was activated either by a bit controlled by the programmer or by reed switch closure in the pulse generator.[18] With telemetry, a coil in the pulse generator serves as the transmitting antenna, and the coil in the telemetry component of the programmer (usually in hand-held wand format) receives the telemetry signal[15] (Fig. 6–7). The telemetry circuit may be used to indicate the programmed values in the pulse generator or to confirm that a programming step has been successfully received and executed in the pulse generator. Real-time measurements of battery voltage and impedance, stimulus current, voltage and energy, and lead resistance may be conveyed from the pulse generator to the programmer. More recently, real-time intracardiac electrograms and marker channels as well as stored histograms of paced and sensed

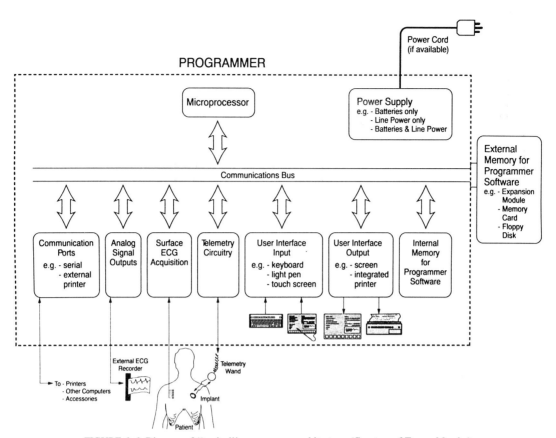

FIGURE 6–6. Diagram of "typical" programmer architecture. (Courtesy of Trevor Moody.)

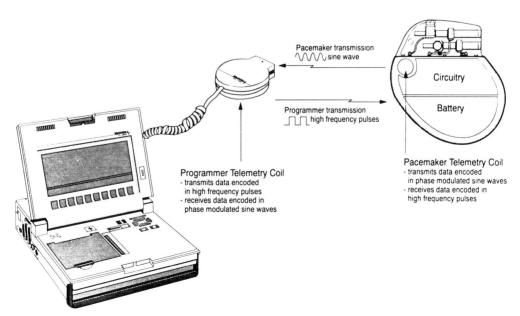

FIGURE 6–7. Example of bidirectional telemetry interaction. (Courtesy of Trevor Moody.)

events and rate-adaptive sensor data have been added to the features that may be telemetered from pacing systems.[3, 29–32]

The power supply for pacemaker programmers includes either DC batteries or a transformer for alternating line current. The power supply constitutes one of the "weightier" aspects of the programmer, and its size reflects the power requirements of the other components of the programming system. The most power-intensive component is typically the printer, particularly if it is high speed. Other, less apparent features that add to the power requirements include telemetry (especially real-time telemetry). Communication ports and outputs for analog signals allow connection to printers, external computers, and external ECG recorders. Many programmers are based on microcomputers and can be upgraded with new programmer software by use of a floppy disc or other software cartridges. These disc drives can also be used to copy data from the programmer when used with external computers.

Pacemaker and programmer technology has increasingly relied on advances made in the field of microprocessors and computers.[16] In the original hardware-organized design of pacemakers, memory registers (the inputs referred to earlier) were individually dedicated to storing specific parameters (such as rate, stimulus amplitude, and pulse duration) and were connected directly to hardware specifically designed to carry out the function. The programmer altered the content of the specific pacer register.[17] With the incorporation of software into pulse generators and programmer systems, microprocessors were interposed between hardware and register and could alter the contents of individual registers or determine what registers should be read and in what order (Figs. 6–8 and 6–9). Contents of registers were thereby interpreted as instructions and subsequently enacted. If the contents of these registers are completely alterable (by either the microprocessor or an external programmer), this form of memory is referred to as *random access memory* (RAM). Thus, RAM can be rewritten and is useful for storage of patient-specific data, paced and sensed events, electrograms, histograms, and other quantifiable information. For example, RAM allows the recording of information particular to a pulse generator such

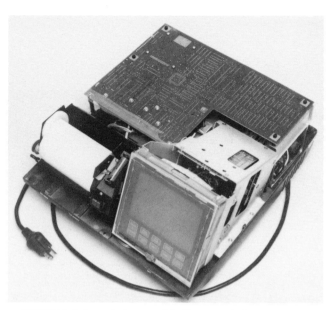

FIGURE 6–9. Internal circuitry of the Pacesetter desk-top programmer.

as implant values of lead type, threshold values, or serial numbers, as well as the storage of diagnostic information such as the number of paced events since the last interrogation. In the case of *read only memory* (ROM), processor instructions are stored in unchangeable fashion in specific registers, and a given location and type of register are associated with a unique bit pattern. Although the versatility of RAM is greater, ROM circuitry is simpler, uses less space, and is relatively immune to power interruption. Pacemaker model-specific ROM modules are commonly employed in programmer technology, taking the form of software cartridges, expansion modules, memory cards, and floppy discs. The modules enable the microprocessor to alter the numerical or qualitative pacing parameters (output, mode, and so on) for a given pacemaker model but not the contents of processor instructions contained in registers within the programmer's internal memory (Fig. 6–10). It is anticipated that the relative contributions of RAM and ROM in programmers and pacemakers will change as these devices become increasingly software-organized, particularly as the personal computer (PC) technology is incorporated (see later discussion).

THE RISKS OF PROGRAMMING: SPURIOUS PROGRAMMING AND DEVICE IDIOSYNCRASIES

Spurious programming has been categorized as *dysprogramming* (from an anomalous source of interference), *misprogramming* (the faulty transmission of programming instructions in which the pulse generator responds to the programmer in unanticipated fashion), *phantom programming* (by another "unknown" physician), and *cross-programming* (reprogramming of pulse generator from one manufacturer by the programmer of another manufacturer).[8, 17, 33–36] Early studies attributed dysprogramming to magnetically induced vibration of the programming reed switch.[34] Such early concerns led to the incorporation of security schemes such as the access codes and carrier frequencies discussed earlier. Of particular concern was the issue of cross-programming[5, 33, 37–39] (Fig. 6–11). Cross-programming can occur when a pro-

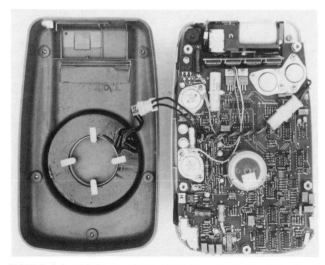

FIGURE 6–8. "Bird's eye view" of the internal circuitry of the Cordis hand-held programmer.

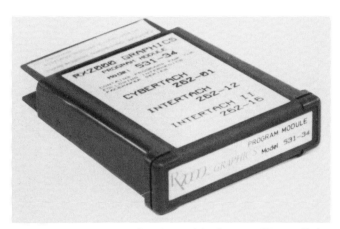

FIGURE 6–10. Example of a ROM module (Courtesy of Intermedics).

grammer satisfies the security code of another manufacturer's pulse generator. This can occur through an instability in the circuitry of the pulse generator that is created by transmission from the programmer, especially in systems utilizing a magnetic reed switch. Although the possibility of cross-programming is less likely with the increasing sophistication of coding and carrier schemes, manufacturers still appropriately warn of this phenomenon in their technical manuals. Another type of cross-programming is perhaps more correctly designated as nonprogramming. This is possible when the ROM memory module of one manufacturer's programmer is mechanically compatible with the programmer of another manufacturer, usually resulting in an inability to program the pulse generator.[40] We have also seen a patient with pacemaker undersensing who was carrying the identification card of the wrong manufacturer. The application of a programmer

over this patient's pulse generator resulted in a noninteraction (appropriately), producing the false impression of a malfunctioning pulse generator and (unnecessary) pulse generator replacement. These examples of cross-programming and nonprogramming have generated much interest in the pacing community in the concept of a universal programmer (see later discussion).

Environmental interference with both programmers and pulse generators has been discussed earlier. It is worthy of brief note that the pulse generator may be susceptible to reprogramming through exposure to electrocautery or defibrillatory shocks.[41] More recently, in a patient with both a Cardiac Pacemakers Inc. (CPI) implantable defibrillator and an Intermedics Intertach pacing system, an interaction between the Intermedics Rx 2000 programmer and a CPI model 2035 programmer was reported.[42] This interaction between programmers resulted in the inability of the CPI programmer to interact with the patient's implantable cardioverter-defibrillator (ICD) during noninvasive programmed stimulation performed through the Intermedics system. In another case, an ICD inappropriately discharged after responding to the high-frequency electromagnetic pulse signal generated during programming of his separate pacemaker.[43]

Malfunctions or idiosyncrasies of programming systems have long been appreciated, and some have even resulted in pulse generator or programmer recalls.[44–54] In perhaps one of the more well known reported series,[44] pacemaker inhibition occurred during programming to more rapid rates depending on when the programming command was received during the paced cycle. In most cases of idiosyncrasy, only isolated cases are reported, although the implications are potentially serious. In one report,[49] the pulse generator was either nonprogrammable or misprogrammed by the programmer, resulting in pacing at twice the selected rate. This anomalous

PACEMAKER MANUFACTURER	MODEL	ARCO	CPI	CORATOMIC	CORDIS	EDWARDS	INTERMEDICS	MEDCOR	MEDTRONIC 9701 (SPECTRAX)	MEDTRONIC 9600
ARCO	APP 153		I	I	I	*¹	I	O	*¹	*¹
CPI	MICROLITH 505	N		N	N,I	*	I	O	*,N	*,N
CORATOMIC	OVALITH P	I	I		I	*	I	O	*	*
CORDIS	OMNI STANICOR 206A	I	I	I		*	I	O	*	*
EDWARDS	23U	I	I	I	I		I²	O	*	*
INTERMEDICS	CYBERLITH 253-01	I	I	I	I	*		O	*	*
MEDCOR	LITHICRON 0511	I	I	I	I	*	I		*	*
MEDTRONIC	SPECTRAX 5984	O	O	I	O	*	O	O		*
MEDTRONIC	XYREL 5995VP	I	I	I	I	*	I	O	R³	

FIGURE 6–11. Table of effects on a pulse generator of programmers of other manufacturers. (N, noise mode; I, pacer inhibited for 1 to 2 beats; 0, no effect.) (From Parsonnet V, Rodgers T: The present status of programmable pacemakers. Prog Cardiovasc Dis 23:401, 1981.)

behavior was the result of programmer software problems. In a different case,[50] the ROM cartridge of a programmer incorrectly confirmed a programming transmission that was not received by the pulse generator, resulting in the pacemaker remaining in its previously programmed mode. In another report, persistent asynchronous pacing occurred after removal of the magnetic programming head during programming. This anomalous behavior was avoidable by pressing the interrogation button before removing the programmer head.[52] Conversely, pacemaker output inhibition has been reported during application of a programming head during interrogation.[53] This malfunction was attributed to the pulse generator sensing RF energy emitted from repetitive "interrogate" transmissions and may represent a form of "susceptibility." Familiarity with each device's real (or potential) idiosyncrasies is emphasized by another case report wherein a pulse generator reverted to a "stat set" mode and could not be reprogrammed by the programmer unless a new transmission "new patient–clear" command was used.[54] When in doubt about the adequacy of a programmer-pacemaker interaction, one should verify that errors in programming have not occurred, carefully scrutinize the appropriate technical manuals, and contact the manufacturer.

Universal, Emergency, and Multiprogrammers

Universal programming has been defined as "a system in which all, or at least a majority of programmable pacemaker systems would be programmable via the same hardware."[55] Arguments in favor of this concept have included the large number of programmers currently required to program all available pacemakers (see Fig. 6–1), the lack of general familiarity by physicians with all of these programmers, the lack of availability of all programmers in certain facilities (of great concern should emergent reprogramming be required), and the problems of cross-programming already discussed.[56, 57] The need for emergency reprogramming has led some clinicians to advocate fervently the introduction of a programmer that is capable, at a minimum, of reverting any pacemaker to the VOO mode at maximal stimulus output with a rate of 70 bpm.[58] Others, however, have suggested that the need for emergency reprogramming to such parameters is infrequent.[59] Implementation of an emergency programmer would necessitate the addition of unique circuitry and components to existing pacemakers to allow the appropriate response to the encoded carrier.

Still another concept is that of the *multiprogrammer*, which uses a common computer and control system with attachments that allow interaction with a variety of carrier types and modulation schemes.[60–64] In contrast, the universal programmer ideally would require a single carrier and encoding mechanism for all pacemakers.[25] Indeed, a multiprogrammer was actually used in the early 1980s and had the advantages of reliability, convenience, facilitation of interaction with an increasing array of pulse generators, and independence of pacing centers from manufacturers for programmer maintenance.[63] Its disadvantages at the time included slowness of the system, complexity of handling, cost, inability to update the software, and potential legal concerns.[63]

Against the concept of universal programming the following arguments have been made:

1. Pacemakers and their corresponding programmers are inextricably linked and are part of a unique pacing system. To standardize a programmer would entail standardizing all pacemakers similarly with regard to carrier type, encoding method, and actual codes used. The alternative would be to incorporate all carrier types, codes, and so on into a single programmer, which would result in a device prohibitive in both size and cost.
2. The cooperation that would be required among manufacturers to develop universal programming is problematic given the demands of free market competition. If one programmer existed, a company at the forefront of technology (requiring more from a programmer) would be the major driving force for upgrades or modifications of the programmer ("free rider" issue). Furthermore, programmers have never been profitable for manufacturers, who essentially provide these devices as a cost of supporting their customers; as such, programmers may be used to leverage competitive advantage as a "window" to the pacemaker. In addition, a universal programmer would require manufacturers to reveal technologic details, thereby inhibiting the development of novel pulse generators. (But note that cooperative interactions among manufacturers have led to significant improvements in pacemaker lead connectors and possibly the establishment of a national lead data base.[65, 66])
3. If one manufacturer (or even a manufacturer not presently involved in the pacing industry) makes the universal programmer but many manufacturers provide their own pulse generators, who is practically, medically, and legally responsible for ensuring the appropriate interactions between the programmer and the pulse generator?
4. Increased costs are inherent in the development of a universal programmer, including development time, technical complexity, and liability considerations.

Because of these concerns, at the time of this writing the universal programmer remains a concept rather than a reality.

The Future of Programmers: What Is the Ideal?

The ideal programmer must be easy to use ("user friendly"), safe and effective, and fast and efficient. Ease of use includes both the concept of portability and the provision of an intuitive user interface. The ideal interface is one that allows the user to perform the required actions intuitively, without the need for specialized training in the programmer operating system or the need to refer to a user's manual. A user-friendly interface is especially important for clinicians who use the programmer relatively infrequently. The user interface may be enhanced by a screen that is simple to understand and easy to read. Touch-sensitive screens provide an intuitive user interface that may enhance communication (Fig. 6–12). The use of graphics or icons (as in the graphical user interfaces employed in most personal computers) may facilitate the way in which information is presented to the user and, in turn, how the user may provide instructions to

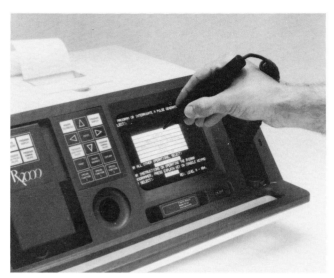

FIGURE 6–12. Example of touch-screen interface using light pen (Intermedics programmer).

the programmer. Designing a user-friendly interface entails guiding the user quickly and obviously (intuitively) to the required tasks; the most frequently used programming commands should be the most readily identified, and the least commonly used should have lower priority. The ability to turn on and access the programming system rapidly is another important feature of user friendliness. Ideally, this would include the ability to identify each model of pacemaker precisely without requiring the user to select a specific ROM module. Although many patients do not know the manufacturer or model of their pacing system, such a feature is rare in today's programmers. Batch programming (i.e., the ability to program multiple parameters simultaneously) is also essential and is not universal in present programmers. Backward compatibility of programmers with older pulse generator models that are no longer in production is also an important component of user friendliness. Portability implies not only that the programmer is lightweight but also that other accessories such as telemetry and ECG cables are easily stored and transported. The incorporation of an integrated, high-speed graphics printer provides an easily understood permanent record of the programmer-pacemaker interaction.

As the number of functions and programmable parameters of pacemakers expands, programmers will be increasingly asked to provide programming instructions to the pulse generator, gather and transmit data, analyze the data received from the pulse generator to provide useful information, and transmit this information to other computers for storage in a data base.[66, 67] The age of automaticity of pacemaker function is on us, and this too will require more from the programmer, namely, the ability to record data used to monitor automatic functions.[68] Artificial intelligence and rule-based logic will be needed to recommend pacing prescriptions of mode, rate, atrioventricular (AV) delay, and other parameters for individual patients. These recommendations from the programmer will also consider stored and real-time data regarding lead function, spontaneous arrhythmias, sensor information, and paced and sensed events. As the amount of RAM increases in pulse generators, more and more raw data can be stored. It will fall to the programmer to analyze these data so that clinically useful information is presented to the physician. Programmers must display the stored data in ways that are clinically meaningful, typically in a graphic format. The programmer must be capable of interpreting anomalies in the stored data, such as the implications of increasing or decreasing lead impedance, battery impedance, and the interaction between AV delay and intrinsic AV conduction in an individual patient. Although these innovations are likely to improve patient care, they clearly raise medicolegal and reimbursement issues. The ability of the programmer to capture and display both recorded and real-time data will also be essential to the operation of multisensor pacemakers. Incorporation of antibradycardia, antitachycardia, and cardiovertor-defibrillator programming schemes within the same programmer is also anticipated because the functions of pacemakers and implantable cardioverter-defibrillators are likely to be combined in single devices. The programmer must support other instrumentation used in the implantation and follow-up of pacing systems such as external cardioverter-defibrillator testing, pacing systems analyzers, and transmission of data to a computerized data base. It is also expected that programmers will provide other support such as generation of implantation procedure notes, reports from clinical follow-up sessions, and letters to referring physicians.

The move to a PC-based design for programmers has already been initiated. It reduces the manufacturers' investment in time, effort, and cost in making a programmer for several reasons: (1) the PC is already designed (the manufacturer buys a significant part of the programmer ''off the shelf''); (2) the writing of software for a PC has become standard, making the task relatively simple for software engineers; and (3) commercially available PC software with data base, word processing, and user-interface applications can be readily adapted to pacing applications. Compact, light-weight and smaller batteries have been employed increasingly as PC technology improves (e.g., notebook PCs), and this factor may contribute to the portability of future programmers. Enhancements in the area of user interfaces will also affect programmers favorably, making them easier to use. Ultimately, the programmer will no longer be viewed as a weighty and complex encumbrance to be overcome (or avoided by nonprogramming) but rather as a means of optimizing pacing function for the benefit of the patient and the education of the clinician.

Acknowledgments

The authors wish to acknowledge gratefully the tremendous help and insight provided by the following persons in the preparation of this work: S. Serge Barold, M.D., Trevor Moody (Telectronics Pacing Systems Inc.), Jonathan Lee (Telectronics Pacing Systems Inc.), Jeff Snell (Siemens-Pacesetter Inc.), Werner Hafelfinger (Siemens-Pacesetter Inc.), Marish Kothari (Cardiac Pacemakers Inc.), Alan Brewer and Michael Lee (Intermedics Inc.), and Terry Nadler (Medtronic Inc.).

REFERENCES

1. Harthorne JW: Programmable pacemakers: Technical features and clinical applications. *In* Dreifus L (ed): Pacemaker Therapy. Philadelphia, WB Saunders, 1983, pp 135–147.

2. Mugica J, Birkui P: Multiprogrammability of modern cardiac pacemakers. *In* El-Sherif N, Samet P (eds): Cardiac Pacing and Electrophysiology, 3rd ed. Philadelphia, WB Saunders, 1991, pp 504–523.

3. Schoenfeld MH: Follow-up of the pacemaker patient. *In* Ellenbogen K (ed): Cardiac Pacing. Cambridge, MA, Blackwell Scientific, 1992, pp 419–454.

4. Levine PA: Proceedings of the policy conference of the North American Society of Pacing and Electrophysiology on programmability and pacemaker follow-up programs. Clin Prog Pacing Electrophysiol 2:145, 1984.

5. Pannizzo F, Furman S: Clinical tests of the effects of simulated inadvertent "cross programming." *In* Meere C (ed): Cardiac Pacing. Proceedings of the VIth World Symposium on Cardiac Pacing. Montreal, Pacesymp, 1979, Chap 35-4.

6. Levine PA, Belott PH, Bilitch M, et al: Recommendations of the NASPE policy conference on pacemaker programmability and follow-up. PACE 6:1221, 1983.

7. Chardack WN, Gage AA, Federico AJ, et al: Five years' clinical experience with an implanted pacemaker: An appraisal. Surgery 58:915, 1965.

8. Mond H: Programmability. *In* Mond H (ed): The Cardiac Pacemaker: Function and Malfunction. New York, Grune & Stratton, 1983, pp 169–187.

9. Kantrowitz A: The treatment of Stokes-Adams syndrome in heart block. Prog Cardiovasc Dis 6:490, 1964.

10. Tyers G, Noto J, Danielson J: A new device for non-operative repair of internal cardiac pacemakers. Arch Surg 92:901, 1966.

11. Chardack WM, Baker EE, Bolduc L, et al: Magnetically activated pulse width control for implantable pacemakers. Ann Cardiol Angiol 20:345, 1971.

12. Grogler FM: Long-term experience with the EM 169 Vario pacemaker. Electromedica 4:135, 1975.

13. Harthorne JW: Preliminary experience with the Starr Edwards and Cordis Omnicor pacemaker systems. Proceedings of the IVth International Symposium on Cardiac Pacing. Amsterdam, Van Gorcum, 1973.

14. Parsonnet V, Cuddy T, Escher D, et al: A permanent pacemaker capable of external non-invasive programming. Trans Am Soc Artif Intern Organs 19:224, 1973.

15. Sholder J, Levine PA, Mann BM, et al: Bidirectional telemetry and interrogation. *In* Barold SS, Mugica J (eds): The Third Decade of Cardiac Pacing. Mt. Kisco, NY, Futura, 1982, pp 145–166.

16. Bernstein AD, Parsonnet V: Microcomputer and microprocessor applications in cardiac pacing. Med Instrumentation 17:329, 1983.

17. Hardage ML, Barold SS: Pacemaker programming techniques. *In* Barold SS, Mugica J (eds): The Third Decade of Cardiac Pacing. Mt Kisco, NY, Futura, 1982, pp 1–26.

18. Gordon PL, Calfee RV, Baker RG Jr: Multiprogrammable pacemaker technology: A tutorial review and prediction. *In* Barold SS, Mugica J (eds): The Third Decade of Cardiac Pacing. Mt Kisco, NY, Futura, 1982, pp 127–143.

19. Gordon P: The Intermedics Programming System. Technical Memo D4. Angleton, TX, Intermedics Inc., 1985.

20. Welti J: Reed switch anomalies. Stimarec Report. PACE 3:508, 1980.

21. Levine P, Klein M: Reed switch malfunction. PACE 2:377, 1979.

22. Bilitch M, Cosby RS, Cafferly EA: Ventricular fibrillation and competitive pacing. N Engl J Med 276:598, 1967.

23. Karson TH, Grace K, Denes P: Stereo speakers silence automatic implantable cardioverter-defibrillator. N Engl J Med 320:1628, 1989.

24. Trevor Moody: Personal communication, 1992.

25. Gold RD, Saulson SH, Macgregor DC: Programmable pacing systems: The medium and the message. PACE 5:776, 1982.

26. Physician's Technical Manual. Pacemaker model 370 AF and Genesis Series Analyzer Programmer System. Sylmar, CA, Pacesetter Systems Inc., 1985.

27. Sweesy MW, Batey RL, Forney RC: Activation times for "emergency back-up" programs. PACE 13:1224, 1990.

28. Tyers GFO, Brownlee RR, Hughes HC Jr, et al: Chronic testing of a pacemaker that needs recharging only once every four years. Arch Surg 111:1231, 1976.

29. Levine PA, Sholder J, Duncan JL: Clinical benefits of telemetered electrocardiograms in assessment of DDD function. PACE 7:1170, 1984.

30. Sanders R, Martin R, Fruman H, et al: Data storage and retrieval by implantable pacemakers for diagnostic purposes. PACE 7:1228, 1984.

31. Duffin EG Jr: The marker channel: A telemetric diagnostic aid. PACE 7:1165, 1984.

32. Levine PA, Vendetti FJ, Podrid PJ, et al: Telemetry of programmed and measured data, electrograms, event markers, and event counters: Luxury or necessity? *In* Barold SS, Mugica J (eds): New Perspectives in Cardiac Pacing. Mt Kisco, NY, Futura, 1988, pp 187–201.

33. Sinnaeve A, Piret J, Stroobandt R: Potential causes of spurious programming: Report of a case. PACE 3:541, 1980.

34. Fieldman A, Dobrow R: Phantom pacemaker programming. PACE 1:166, 1978.

35. Cameron J, Chisholm A, Froggatt G, et al: Phantom programming. *In* Meere C (ed): Cardiac Pacing. Proceedings of the VIth World Symposium on Cardiac Pacing. Montreal, Pacesymp, 1979.

36. Furman S: Spurious pacemaker programming. PACE 3:517, 1980.

37. Parsonnet V, Rodgers T: The present status of programmable pacemakers. Prog Cardiovasc Dis 23:401, 1981.

38. Response of AFP TM pacemakers to competitive programmers. Pacesetter Technical Memo M-8. Sylmar, CA, Siemens-Pacesetter Inc., 1985.

39. Fontaine G, Frank R, Petitot JC, et al: The risk of programmability. *In* Barold SS, Mugica J (eds): The Third Decade of Cardiac Pacing. Mt Kisco, NY, Futura, 1982, pp 77–103.

40. Intermedics Inc: Intermedics Technical Manual for RX 2000 Programmer. Angleton, TX, Intermedics Inc., 1988.

41. Barold S, Ong L, Scout J, et al: Reprogramming of implanted pacemaker following external defibrillation. PACE 1:514, 1978.

42. Rogers R, Ellenbogen KA, et al: Letter to the editor. PACE 13:1687, 1990.

43. Gottlieb C, Miller JM, Rosenthal ME, et al: Automatic implantable defibrillator discharge resulting from routine pacemaker programming. PACE 11:336, 1988.

44. Astrinsky EA, Furman S, Florio J: Asystolic episodes during pacemaker implantation. Circulation 63:1379, 1981.

45. Lindenberg BS, Hajan CA, Levine PA: Design-dependent loss of telemetry: Uplink telemetry hold. PACE 12:823, 1989.

46. Welti JJ, Godin JF: Stimarec report. PACE 6:668, 1983.

47. FDA Enforcement Rep Sept 25, 1991.

48. Lacombe MA: Letter to the editor. PACE 7:1087, 1984.

49. FDA Enforcement Rep Dec 11, 1985.

50. FDA Enforcement Rep Nov 19, 1986.

51. Welti JJ, Godin JF: Stimarec report. PACE 8:766, 1985.

52. Godin JF, Petitot JC, Pioger C: Stimarec report. PACE 14:1558, 1991.

53. Sweesy MW, Batey RI, Forney RC: Output inhibition upon application of programming head. PACE 11:1239, 1988.

54. Hayes DL, Holmes DR, Merideth J, et al: Apparent pacemaker failure due to reversion circuitry within the programming device. PACE 7:237, 1984.

55. Furman S: Universal programming. PACE 7:163, 1984.

56. Buffet J: The risk of the uncontrolled multiplication of programming systems for implantable cardiac pacemakers. Stimucoeur Med 11:37, 1983.

57. Gold D: Universal programmers for cardiac pacemakers and problems which may impede their development. Miami, FL, Cordis Corporation, Cordis Corporation Memo, 1982.

58. Boal BH: Emergency reprogramming of cardiac pacemakers. PACE 6:651, 1983.

59. Parsonnet V: Editorial. PACE 6:652, 1983.

60. Dodinot B: The universal programmer: Myth or reality? Stimucoeur Med 9:38, 1981.

61. Buffet J: The multi-programmer. Stimucoeur Med 9:48, 1981.

62. Buffet J, Gautier JP, Jacquet JP, et al: The universal programmer; feasibility and engineering consideration. *In* Barold SS, Mugica J (eds): Cardiac Pacing. The Third Decade of Cardiac Pacing. Mt Kisco, NY, Futura, 1982, pp 115–126.

63. Dodinot B, Kubler L, Buffet J, et al: Clinical investigation of a multiprogrammer. Proceedings of the VIIth World Symposium on Cardiac Pacing. Vienna, Springer-Verlag, 1983, pp 295–302.

64. Rottembourg JL, Stadler F, Fletcher E: A multifunction software based universal programmer. PACE 4:A-93, 1981.

65. Costeas XF, Schoenfeld MH: Undersensing as a consequence of lead incompatibility: Case report and a plea for universality. PACE 14:1681, 1991.

66. Schoenfeld MH, Benditt DG, Fletcher RD, et al: Recommendations for implementation of a North American multicenter arrhythmia device/lead database. NASPE policy statement. PACE 15:1632, 1992.

67. Byrd CL, Byrd CB, Tyler JE: Automatic transfer of information from pacemaker programmers to computers. PACE 10:148, 1987.

68. Hayes DL: Advances in pacing therapy for bradycardia. Int J Cardiol 32:183, 1991.

ARTIFICIAL RATE-ADAPTIVE SENSORS

CHAPTER 7

OVERVIEW OF IDEAL SENSOR CHARACTERISTICS

Chu-Pak Lau
A. John Camm

The cardiovascular system functions to ensure the optimal transport of oxygen to the tissues and the removal of the waste products of metabolism. The heart is intimately linked with the respiratory system, which adjusts the ventilatory response according to metabolic need. The availability of oxygen for aerobic metabolism in the tissues depends on the supply of oxygenated blood (cardiac output), the oxygen-carrying capacity of the blood (hemoglobin concentration), and the ability of the tissues to extract oxygen. During exercise a widening of the arteriovenous oxygen difference occurs as the extraction of oxygen by the metabolizing tissues increases. Cardiac output is increased during exercise by neurohumoral reflexes through a combination of an increase in both stroke volume and heart rate. This change in cardiac output is also modulated by the peripheral vascular system such that a local increase in acidosis results in arteriolar dilatation and a selective redistribution of the cardiac output to the various tissues.

In patients suffering from an inadequate heart rate, cardiac output can increase only as a consequence of increased stroke volume. Although relative bradycardia may result in a subtle reduction of cardiac output, a widening of the arteriovenous oxygen difference, and a redistribution of blood flow at rest, these abnormalities become more obvious during exercise when the compensatory mechanisms become overwhelmed. The aims of a physiologic pacemaker are to restore the rate and sequence of cardiac activation in the presence of abnormal cardiac automaticity and conduction. When sinoatrial function is adequate, the atrial electrogram can be used for rate control. Artificial implantable sensors are used primarily to overcome abnormal sinoatrial function ("chronotropic incompetence") or when the atrium is unreliable for sensing or pacing (such as during atrial fibrillation). Sensors must also be able to control atrioventricular (AV) conduction, adapting AV delay to changes in atrial rate. The future role of sensors will be expanded to include functions other than rate augmentation, as, for example, the detection of ventricular capture and the management of response to atrial arrhythmias.

Normal Heart Rate and Respiratory Responses to Exercise and Nonexercise Needs

Cardiac output is the product of heart rate and stroke volume. Stroke volume is enhanced during exercise when venous return, cardiac filling, and cardiac contractility increase in response to sympathetic stimulation and enhanced venous return from a more vigorous muscular pump. Because of the difference in venous return, the changes in heart rate and cardiac hemodynamics are highly influenced by whether the exercise was carried out in the upright or supine posture.

HEART RATE RESPONSE AT THE START AND END OF EXERCISE

An anticipatory response of the heart rate occurs in many individuals prior to exercise. With both supine and upright isotonic exercise, heart rate and cardiac output increase within 10 seconds of the onset of exercise.[1-3] The cardiac output may increase by as much as 40% within three heart beats following the onset of vigorous muscular exercise.

Both the cardiac output and the sinus rate increase exponentially, with a half-time that ranges from 10 to 45 seconds, the rate of rise being proportional to the intensity of work[1] (Fig. 7–1). At the termination of upright exercise there is a delay of approximately 5 to 10 seconds before cardiac output starts to decrease, followed by an exponential fall with a half-time of 25 to 60 seconds. The recovery time is related to age, work intensity, total work performed, and physical condition of the individual.[4] Although the optimal rate onset and decay kinetics for patients with pacemakers have not been firmly established, artificial sensors for rate-adaptive pacing should probably simulate the onset and recovery kinetics of the normal sinus node as the ideal physiologic standard.

HEART RATE AND RESPIRATORY CHANGES DURING EXERCISE

The change in heart rate during muscular exercise is linearly related to oxygen consumption and workload. The

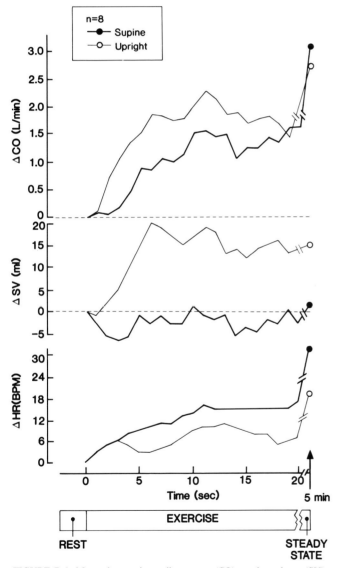

FIGURE 7–1. Mean changes in cardiac output (CO), stroke volume (SV), and heart rate (HR) during supine and upright exercise (cycle ergometry 300 kpm/min). Steady state hemodynamic response was achieved in 5 minutes. (Redrawn from Loeppky JA, Greene ER, Hoekenga DE, et al: Beat-by-beat stroke volume assessment by pulsed Doppler in upright and supine exercise. J Appl Physiol 50:1173, 1981.)

magnitude of the change in heart rate is a function of age, physical fitness, and the type of exercise used for testing (see Chapter 26). Because of the relationship between oxygen uptake and ventilatory volume during aerobic metabolism, minute ventilation is closely related to heart rate during exercise. At rest, the respiratory rate is typically between 10 and 20 breaths per minute. During low-intensity exercise an increase in tidal volume is the primary respiratory adaptation.[5] At higher work levels a further increase in tidal volume of up to 50% of the vital capacity occurs together with an increase in breathing frequency. The relationship between breathing rate and depth of respiration (tidal volume) varies considerably between individuals. In addition, the breathing rate is often synchronized with the work rhythm (the walking pace). However, because respiration is carefully controlled to maintain PCO_2 within a narrow physiologic range, compensatory adjustments in tidal volume ensure an appropriate minute ventilation.

Minute volume (the product of breathing rate and tidal volume) is linearly related to the rate of carbon dioxide production. At low- and medium-intensity workloads, minute ventilation is also linearly related to oxygen consumption. Resting values for minute ventilation are approximately 6 L/min and can increase to 100 L/min during exercise for normal men and up to 200 L/min for trained athletes. Tidal volume may rise from a resting value of 0.5 L/min to 3 L/min at maximal exercise in normal individuals. The breathing rate may increase from a resting value of 12 to 16 breaths/min to 40 to 50 breaths/min during peak exercise. In normal children and some adults with restrictive lung disease, the respiratory rate may exceed 60 breaths/min.

At about 70% of the maximum oxygen uptake, the rate of tissue metabolism outstrips the rate of tissue oxygen delivery, resulting in an accumulation of lactic acid, the so-called anaerobic threshold. Acidosis is initially prevented by plasma buffers, but continuous lactate production eventually leads to excess production of carbon dioxide from plasma bicarbonate. This excess carbon dioxide stimulates the respiratory center, leading to respiratory compensation (increased minute ventilation). The anaerobic threshold is defined more clearly using a protocol in which the work intensity is increased rapidly than with a more gradual exercise protocol. At an identical oxygen uptake, exercise involving small muscle groups, such as the arm muscles, results in a higher breathing rate than exercise performed with the muscles of the leg. At workloads that surpass the anaerobic threshold, carbon dioxide production and minute ventilation increase disproportionately to oxygen consumption.

HEART RATE MODULATION FOR NONEXERCISE NEEDS

Exercise is but one of the many physiologic requirements for variation in heart rate (Table 7–1). Emotions such as anxiety may trigger a substantial change in heart rate. Posture, for instance, has a significant effect on both the heart rate and the cardiac output. Thus, the sinus rate is higher when an individual moves from the supine to the upright posture. Isometric exercise also results in an increase in cardiac output and heart rate in most individuals.[6] The changes of heart rate that occur during various physiologic maneuvers (e.g., Valsalva maneuver), baroreceptor reflexes, and anxiety

TABLE 7–1. SOME RESPONSES OF THE SINUS NODE TO BODY REQUIREMENTS

1. Exercise—isotonic and isometric, during and after exercise
2. Postural changes
3. Anxiety and stress
4. Postprandial changes
5. Vagal maneuvers
6. Circadian changes
7. Fever

reaction may also be potentially important. Physiologic variations in heart rate are not confined to increases in response to increased metabolic demand. The lack of an ability to decrease the pacing rate in patients with VVI pacemakers during sleep may result in palpitations and sleep disturbances.[7] An appropriate compensatory heart rate response is especially important in pathophysiologic conditions such as anemia, acute blood loss, or other causes of hypovolemia.

Components of a Rate-Adaptive Pacing System

There are at least three aspects of a rate-adaptive pacing system that influence its rate-modulating characteristics. First, a sensor (or multiple sensors) must detect a physical or physiologic parameter that is related to metabolic demand either directly or indirectly. Each of the parameters used for control of pacing rate has its own intrinsic relation to exercise and emotion. Second, the rate-modulating circuit in the pulse generator must have an algorithm that relates changes in the sensed parameter to a change in pacing rate. The design of the rate-control algorithm may have a profound impact on the overall rate-response characteristics of a pacing system. Third, because the magnitude of the physical or physiologic changes that are monitored by the sensor differ between patients, physician input is usually necessary to adjust the algorithm (usually by programming one or more rate-responsive variables) to achieve the clinically desired rate response.[8]

CLASSIFICATION OF SENSORS

PHYSIOLOGIC CLASSIFICATION

Rickards and Donaldson classified sensors for rate-adaptive pacing according to the physiologic "level" they sense.[9] A *primary* sensor is defined as one that detects the *physiologic factors* that control the normal sinus node during varying metabolic needs. Primary sensed parameters include circulating catecholamines and autonomic nervous system activities. Although these parameters may be the most physiologically accurate indicators for use by a rate-adaptive pacing system, technical realization has yet to be achieved. The bulk of rate-adaptive sensors that have been proposed belong to the class of *secondary* sensors: those that detect physiologic parameters that are a *consequence* of exercise. Some of these parameters, such as the QT interval,[10] respiratory rate or minute ventilation,[11–15] average atrial rate,[16] central venous temperature,[17–19] venous blood pH,[20, 20a] right ventricular stroke volume,[21] preejection interval[22] or pressure,[23] and

mixed venous oxygen saturation ($S\bar{v}O_2$),[24] have been developed for either clinical or investigational pacing systems. Each of these physiologic variables responds to the onset of exercise with its own kinetics and has a different proportionality to exercise workload. A third group of sensors, the *tertiary* sensors, detects *external changes* that result from exercise. An example of a tertiary sensor is body movement.[25] As expected, the relationship between exercise workload and these sensed variables is less tightly linked, and there is often greater susceptibility to environmental influences such as vibration. Other measures, such as the use of the 24-hour clock to vary the lower pacing rate, can be considered tertiary sensors. Likewise, in one early rate-adaptive pacemaker, the pacing rate was changed by the patient using a hand-held programmer before exercise began.[26]

TECHNICAL CLASSIFICATION

Alternatively, sensors can be classified according to the technical methods that are used to measure the sensed parameter (Table 7–2). *Impedance* is a measure of all factors that oppose the flow of electric current and is derived by measuring resistivity to an injected electric current across a tissue. The impedance principle has been used extensively for measuring respiratory parameters[27–28] and relative stroke volume[29] in situations involving invasive monitoring. The elegant simplicity of impedance has enabled it to be used with implantable pacing leads, including both standard pacing leads and specialized multielectrode catheters. The pulse generator casing has been used as one electrode for the measurement of impedance in most of these pacing systems. Impedance can be used to detect changes in either ventilatory mechanics or right ventricular systolic function. In fact, a combination of cardiac and respiratory parameters can be derived from impedance measurements. Thus, measurements of impedance provide a convenient method for multisensor pacing. However, it should be remembered that neither minute ventilation nor right ventricular function is directly measured by impedance sensors and that these methods are susceptible to electrode motion artifacts. This propensity is inversely related to the number of electrodes used to measure impedance.[30] In rate-adaptive pacemakers, motion artifacts are usually the result of arm movement that causes the pulse generator to move within the prepectoral pocket,[31–32] thereby changing the relative electrode separation between the pacemaker and the intracardiac electrodes. Because arm movement accompanies normal walking, these artifacts in the impedance signal occur with both walking and upper limb exercises.

The *intracardiac ventricular electrogram* resulting from a pacing stimulus that captures the heart has been used to provide several parameters that can guide rate modulation. Following a suprathreshold pacing stimulus, a wavefront of depolarization propagates through the myocardium producing a characteristic intracardiac electrogram. The area under the curve inscribed by the depolarization phase of the electrogram (the intracardiac R wave) has been termed the ventricular depolarization gradient or paced depolarization integral (PDI).[33] In addition to depolarization, the total duration of depolarization and repolarization can be estimated by the interval from the pacing stimulus to the intracardiac T wave (the QT or stimulus-T interval). Both of these parameters are sensitive to changes in heart rate and circulating catechola-

TABLE 7–2. **MAJOR CLASSES OF SENSORS USED IN RATE-RESPONSIVE PACING, CLASSIFIED ACCORDING TO METHOD OF TECHNICAL REALIZATION**

		EXAMPLES	
METHODS	**PHYSIOLOGIC PARAMETERS**	MODELS	MANUFACTURERS
Impedance sensing	Respiratory rate Minute ventilation	Biorate Meta Chorus RM Legend plus	Biotec Telectronics Ela Medical Medtronic Inc.
	Stroke volume, preejection period, right ventricular ejection time	Precept	CPI
Ventricular evoked response and output pulse parameter sensing	Evoked QT interval Evoked R-wave area ("gradient") Trailing edge of output pulse	TX, Quintech, Rhythmx Prism CL	Vitatron Telectronics
Vibration sensing	Body movement	Activitrax, Legend Sensolog, Sensorhythm Relay, Dash Excel Ergos Swing	Medtronic Inc. Siemens Intermedics CPI Biotronik Sorin
Special sensors on pacing electrode	*Physical Parameters* 1. Central venous temperature 2. dP/dt 3. Average atrial rate 4. Right atrial pressure 5. Pulmonary arterial pressure *Chemical Parameters* 1. pH 2. Mixed venous oxygen saturation 3. Catecholamine levels	Kelvin 500 Nova MR Thermos Model 2503 RS4	Cook Pacemakers Intermedics Biotronic Medtronic Inc. CPI Medtronic Inc. Siemens

Manufacturers:
Biotec, S.P.A., Bologna, Italy
Biotronik, GmbH & Co., Berlin, Germany
Cardiac Pacemakers Inc., St. Paul, MN
Cook Pacemakers Corporation, Leechburg, PA
Ela Medical, Rougemont, France
Intermedics Inc., Angleton, TX
Medtronic Inc., Minneapolis, MN
Siemens Ltd., Solna, Sweden
Sorin Biomedica, Saluggia, Italy
Telectronics Pacing Systems, Englewood, CO
Vitatron Medical B.V., Dieren, The Netherlands

mines and can be derived from the paced intracardiac electrogram with conventional pacing electrodes. Since a large polarization effect occurs after a pacing stimulus (see Chapter 1), a modified waveform of the output pulse that compensates for afterpotentials is needed to eliminate this effect so that these parameters can be accurately measured. The interaction of the "square wave" output pulse with the endocardium of a ventricular pacemaker leads to a distortion of the pulse waveform,[34–35] and the "shape" of the resultant output pulse has been shown to be useful in estimating intracardiac volumes.

During isotonic exercise, body movements (especially those produced by heel strike during walking) result in changes in acceleration forces that act on the pacemaker. Sensors that are capable of measuring the acceleration or vibration forces in the pulse generator are broadly referred to as activity sensors. The sensing of *body vibrations* is therefore a simple way to indicate the onset of exercise. Technically, detection of body movement can be achieved using a piezoelectric crystal, an accelerometer, a tilt switch, or an inductive sensor. Each of these devices transduces motion of the sensor either directly into voltage or indirectly into measurable changes in the resistance of the crystal. Although a tertiary sensor, activity is the most widely used control parameter in rate-adaptive pacing because of its ease of implementation and its compatibility with standard unipolar and bipolar pacing leads.

The last group of sensors are those that are incorporated into the pacing lead. Examples of these specialized leads include thermistors (used to measure blood temperature), piezoelectric crystals (used to measure right ventricular pressure), and optical sensors (used to measure oxygen saturation in the venous blood). Some of these sensors are highly physiologic and can be used in closed-loop rate-adaptive pacing systems. On the other hand, because of the added technical complexity of incorporating a sensor into a conventional lead, they have not been widely used for rate-adaptive pacing and impose a number of potential technical problems. However, these sensors may be potentially useful for long-term hemodynamic monitoring in patients with other heart diseases, producing data that can be assessed through telemetry. Such an approach may be used to guide the effects of medical therapy in a variety of cardiac conditions.

CLOSED-LOOP VERSUS OPEN-LOOP SENSORS

A rate-adaptive pacing system can operate in either a *closed-loop* or an *open-loop* manner. In a completely closed-loop system (Fig. 7–2), the physiologic parameter that is monitored is used to effect a change in the pacing rate. In addition, changes in pacing rate in turn induce a physiologic change in the sensed parameter in the opposite direction. Thus, closed-loop pacing systems have *negative feedback* such that the sensed physiologic variable tends to return toward its baseline value in the presence of an appropriately modulated pacing rate. A partial degree of closed-loop negative feedback control is observed with pacemakers that use $S\bar{v}O_2$ as the rate-control parameter.[24] Exercise in the absence of adequate cardiac output (as in a patient with a fixed-rate pacemaker) increases tissue oxygen extraction from arterial blood, thereby decreasing the content of oxygen in the returning venous blood. This decrease in $S\bar{v}O_2$ can be measured and used to increase the pacing rate, thereby increasing the cardiac output to a value that is optimal for the level of exercise workload, resulting in improved oxygen delivery to the tissues. Under conditions of equilibrium, the pacing rate will be adjusted to maintain the maximum possible $S\bar{v}O_2$ for any level of metabolic demand. $S\bar{v}O_2$ is not a completely closed-loop system, however, because oxygen saturation declines during exercise even with a normal response of the cardiac output. Thus, even though there is a degree of closed-loop negative feedback with $S\bar{v}O_2$ pacemakers, the rate-control parameter ($S\bar{v}O_2$) cannot be strictly maintained at a constant value despite appropriate modulation of pacing rate. Another example of a closed-loop sensor is the PDI.[33] An increase in sympathetic activity decreases the PDI, whereas an increase in heart rate increases this parameter, thereby establishing a negative feedback loop that tends to maintain the sensed parameter at a relatively constant value during exercise. Theoretically, the physician input required for a closed-loop system should be minimal because the system is designed to be fully automatic. In practice, a rate-adaptive algorithm is still necessary because the available pacing systems provide only partial closed-loop negative feedback. In an ideal closed-loop system, the sensor automatically takes into account any changes in the patient's cardiovascular condition. Apart from setting the lower and upper rate limits, the physician can indirectly control the rate changes in a closed-loop system by determining the speed at which the pacing rate adjusts to return the sensed parameter to its baseline value.

Although a closed-loop sensor is theoretically attractive, the practical application of this concept has been less than ideal. Normal control of heart rate involves multiple parameters and feedbacks, and it is unlikely that a single sensor can accurately control heart rate in all clinical circumstances. In addition, a closed-loop sensor involved in rate control may be affected by factors other than metabolic demand. For example, adoption of an upright posture produces changes in ventricular size and geometry that increase the PDI. These factors can result in a paradoxical reduction in heart rate in a rate-adaptive pacing system controlled by this sensor. Thus, at present the potential of closed-loop sensors remains unrealized.

Open-loop logic is employed in most currently available sensors that measure either physiologic or biophysical parameters (see Fig. 7–2). In such open-loop systems a change in the heart rate does not result in a negative feedback effect on the physiologic or physical parameter used to modulate pacing rate. Thus, open-loop algorithms require the physician to prescribe the relationship between the parameter monitored by the sensor(s) and the desired change in pacing rate. An example of this is an activity-sensing pacing system that detects body movements. Physical exercise results in acceleration forces on the pulse generator that can be used to increase the pacing rate.[11-12] However, the resultant increases in pacing rate usually have minimal effects on body movement. An example of positive feedback of heart rate on the rate-control parameter is the QT interval. The QT interval shortens during exercise.[10] However, an increase in the pacing rate itself induces further shortening of the QT interval. For example, in the initial versions of QT-sensing pacemakers that used a linear slope to relate changes in the QT interval to changes in pacing rate, increases in pacing rate during exercise could shorten the QT interval excessively, leading to an excessive increase in rate.[36] This type of "sen-

FIGURE 7–2. Design of a rate-adaptive system. *Open loop*: The physiologic-physical change detected by the sensor is converted to a change in rate using an algorithm. The resultant rate change does not have a negative feedback effect on the physiologic-physical parameter. *Closed-loop*: The physiologic change detected by the sensor is converted to a change in rate using an algorithm. The resultant rate change induces a change in the physiologic parameter in the opposite direction, thus establishing a negative feedback loop. (From Lau CP: The range of sensors and algorithms used in rate-adaptive pacing [Review]. PACE 15:1177, 1992.)

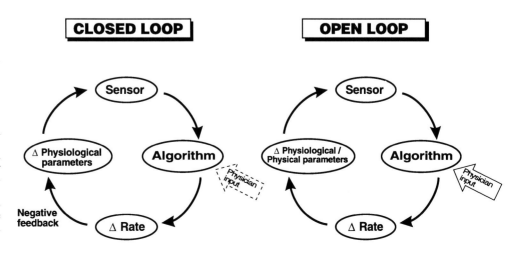

sor feedback tachycardia''[37] has also been described with rate-adaptive pacemakers that detect minute ventilation[38] and body activity.[39]

RATE-CONTROL ALGORITHMS AND RATE-RESPONSE CURVES

The term algorithm refers to the way in which the raw sensor data are converted to a change in pacing rate. Typically, sensor data are first filtered to exclude unwanted signals (e.g., signals outside the frequency range of the rate-control parameter) and then appropriately modified through rectification and gain control (Fig. 7–3). The processed signals are then used to modulate pacing rate through the use of a rate-control algorithm. The physician must determine the ultimate rate response that will be observed by choosing the lower pacing rate, the upper pacing rate, and a rate-response curve that determines the slope of the sensor-pacing rate relationship. In some pacemakers, the physician can also modify the rate response by changing the ''filter'' used to process the raw sensor signal. Examples of these filters include the threshold feature of activity-sensing pacemakers and the gain setting in the Sensolog activity-sensing pacemaker (Siemens Ltd., Solna, Sweden).

The relationship between the processed signals and pacing rate can be linear, curvilinear, or a more complex function

(see Fig. 7–3). A linear relationship was used to relate changes in minute ventilation to changes in pacing cycle length in the Meta MV pacemaker (Telectronics Pacing Systems Inc., Englewood, CO) (see Fig. 7–3A). Although this algorithm is linear, because the pacing *cycle length* is inversely related to *pacing rate,* the net result is an exponential relationship between changes in minute ventilation and heart rate. Newer generations of minute ventilation-sensing, rate-adaptive pacemakers provide a linear relationship between minute ventilation and pacing rate. A power or logarithmic function is often used in curvilinear rate-responsive curves. A curvilinear relation can be parabolic (e.g., in the Activitrax [Medtronic Inc., Minneapolis, MN]) or hyperbolic (Meta MV) (see Fig. 7–3B). A complex triphasic rate-response curve is used in an accelerometer-based, activity-sensing pacemaker (e.g., Dash or Relay [Intermedics Inc., Angleton, TX]) (see Fig. 7–3C). This allows a steep relationship between the sensor output and the pacing rate at low and high levels of exercise and a stable rate during ordinary levels of exertion. An example of an even more complex rate-response curve is the biphasic pattern of response of a more recent minute ventilation–sensing pacemaker, the Meta III (Telectronics Pacing Systems). This algorithm allows a steeper slope of the pacing rate–minute ventilation relationship at the beginning of exercise than at the end of the exercise. The initial aggressive slope is made possible by a separately pro-

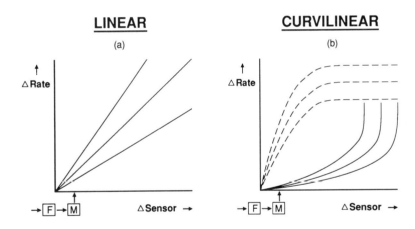

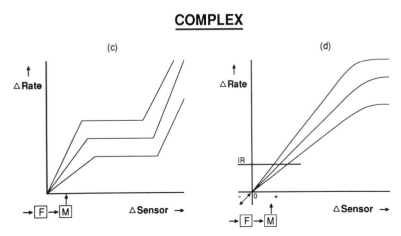

FIGURE 7–3. Types of rate-responsive curves currently used in rate-adaptive pacemakers employing a single sensor. An appropriate filter (F) eliminates unwanted raw signals (e.g., high- or low-pass frequency filters and thresholds). The filtered signals are then appropriately modified (M) (e.g., with gains and rectification) before being converted to a rate change. The curves can be linear, curvilinear, or complex. The physician can select an appropriate rate-responsive slope from a family of curves. (IR, interim rate). See text for further discussion. (From Lau CP: The range of sensors and algorithms used in rate-adaptive pacing [Review]. PACE 15:1177, 1992.)

grammable "rate augmentation factor," such that different slopes control the first and second halves of the pacing range. Perhaps the most sophisticated rate-response curves are those used for temperature sensing (see Fig. 7–2D). In one algorithm, a curvilinear relation is employed when the temperature increases. Because a temperature "dip" characteristically occurs at the beginning of exercise, this algorithm responds to a rapid decline in temperature with a rapid increase in the pacing rate to an interim value. Subsequent increases in temperature are used to modulate further increases in pacing rate. In addition to programming the rate-response curve, temperature-sensing pacing systems provide for a gradual decrease in the lower pacing rate in response to diurnal variation in blood temperature (bidirectional arrow in Fig. 7–3D). Thus, the rate of change in the rate-control parameter (in this case a slow fall in temperature during periods of rest) is used to vary the lower rate limit. Although the rate-response curves discussed previously define the relationship between the sensor output and increases in pacing rate during exercise, many rate-adaptive pacemakers use a different set of curves to control decreases in pacing rate during the recovery phase.

It should be recognized that the rate-response curves that have been discussed relate changes in the sensed parameter to changes in the *desired* pacing rate. In addition to these sensor-desired pacing rate–response curves, other factors control the speed (or time constant) with which the sensor-indicated *desired* pacing rate is translated into a change in the *actual* pacing rate. Obviously, an abrupt change in the sensed parameter must be translated into a gradual increase (or decrease) in the pacing rate. For example, if the activity signal of a pacemaker were to double abruptly, the rate-response curve might indicate that the pacing rate should be increased from 70 to 100 bpm. The interval required for the pacing rate to actually increase from 70 to 100 bpm is a programmable feature in some rate-adaptive pacing systems and has a fixed time constant in others. Similarly, if the sensor indicates that the pacing rate should be decreased from 100 bpm to 70 bpm, a time constant is required to translate this desired change into an actual decline in pacing rate. Thus, these "attack" and "decay" constants can have a major impact on the chronotropic response characteristics of different rate-adaptive pacemakers.

Characteristics of an Ideal Rate-Adaptive Pacing System

The normal human sinus node increases the rate of its spontaneous depolarization during exercise in a manner that is linearly related to oxygen consumption (VO_2). Because this response undoubtedly has evolutionary advantages, the goal of rate-adaptive pacemakers that modulate pacing rate by artificial sensors has been to simulate the chronotropic characteristics of the sinus node.[40] It should be plainly stated, however, that it is uncertain whether the sinus node provides the ideal rate response in patients who require permanent pacemakers. Nevertheless, until there is evidence indicating otherwise, rate-adaptive pacemakers will strive to reproduce this physiologic standard. Keeping these uncertainties in mind, the ideal rate-adaptive pacing system should provide

TABLE 7–3. CHARACTERISTICS OF AN IDEAL SENSOR FOR RATE-RESPONSIVE PACING

CONSIDERATIONS	EXAMPLES AND REMARKS
SENSOR CONSIDERATION	
Proportionality	Oxygen saturation sensing has good proportionality
Speed of response	Activity sensing has the best speed of response
Sensitivity	QT sensing can detect non–exercise-related changes such as anxiety reaction
Specificity	Activity sensing is affected by environmental vibration
	Respiratory sensing is affected by voluntary hyperventilation
TECHNICAL CONSIDERATION	
Stability	Stability of early pH sensor was a problem
Size	Large size or requirement for additional electrodes may be a problem
	Energy consumption must not harm pacemaker longevity unduly
Biocompatibility	Important for sensor in direct contact with the bloodstream
Ease of programming	Difficult programming in early QT sensing pacemakers

pacing rates that are *proportional* to the level of metabolic demand. In addition, the change in pacing rate should occur with kinetics (or *speed of response*) that are similar to those of the sinus node. The artificial sensor should be *sensitive* enough to detect both exercise and nonexercise need for changes in heart rate and yet be *specific* enough not to be affected by unrelated signals arising from both the internal and external environment. Although the ideal sensor should provide these functional characteristics, it must also be technically feasible to implement with a reliability that is acceptable with modern implantable pacemakers[41] (Table 7–3).

The overall chronotropic response obtained with a rate-adaptive pacing system is dependent on three major factors: (1) the intrinsic properties of the rate-control parameter, (2) the algorithm used to relate changes in the sensed parameter into changes in pacing rate, and (3) the way in which the pacing system is programmed. Each of these factors can dramatically change the rate modulation actually observed with a rate-adaptive pacing system. In addition, an appropriate rate-control algorithm or clever programming can overcome the intrinsic limitations of many sensors. In contrast, inappropriate programming of a pacing system can distort the chronotropic response of an otherwise ideal sensor so that a poor clinical result is observed. Thus, clinical skill is required to achieve optimal results with any rate-adaptive pacemaker.

Sensors for Purposes Other than Rate Modulation

Sensors may also be used for purposes other than modulation of pacing rate (Table 7–4). Several of the available sensors can be used to automate other diagnostic and therapeutic pacemaker functions. For example, the ability to detect the evoked intracardiac R wave may provide a means for capture detection and allow automatic regulation of the stim-

TABLE 7–4. **UTILITY OF SENSORS FOR PURPOSES OTHER THAN RATE AUGMENTATION**

FUNCTIONS	EXAMPLES
1. Pacing lead	Sensing and pacing in atrium and ventricle (may extend to the left heart) Automatic switchable polarity
2. Basic pacemaker parameters	Autosensing and capture Automatic AV interval and PVARP Interference protection Upper rate behavior
3. Mode variability	Spontaneous mode changes
4. Tachycardia management	Pacemaker-mediated tachycardias Diagnosis and action (in conjunction with antitachycardia devices) Ability to perform noninvasive electrophysiologic testing
5. Monitoring	Rate Hemodynamics Hormonal and metabolic profiles Myocardial function Myocardial ischemia

ulus amplitude based on threshold measurements. In a DDDR pacemaker, sensors such as minute ventilation have been used to control the AV interval and the postventricular atrial refractory period (PVARP).[42] In these devices, as the minute ventilation signal increases there is a concomitant decrease in both the AV delay and the PVARP. A sensor can be used to monitor the atrial rate, and a disproportionate increase in the atrial rate compared with the sensor-indicated rate is interpreted by the pacemaker as an atrial tachyarrhythmia, which triggers a change in the pacing mode from DDDR to VVIR. Thus, a rapid-paced ventricular response during atrial fibrillation can be avoided by an appropriate algorithm.[43] These uses of sensors may allow the use of automatic features in implantable devices other than pacemakers. For example, hemodynamic sensors can be incorporated into implantable cardioverter-defibrillators to monitor the hemodynamics of arrhythmias, allowing a tiered therapy such as pacing or cardioversion shocks to be administered more specifically.

Principles Used for Comparing and Evaluating Rate-Adaptive Systems

PROPORTIONALITY OF RATE RESPONSE

One of the best indicators of sensor proportionality is the correlation between the sensor-indicated pacing rate and the level of oxygen consumption during exercise.[44] In general, parameters such as minute ventilation are highly proportional to metabolic demand. The paced QT interval is also a proportional sensor during steady-state conditions. Some sensors using specialized pacing leads are also highly proportional. For example, $S\bar{v}O_2$ is closely related to oxygen consumption during exercise.

To assess the proportionality of chronotropic response during exertion, the exercise workload should be increased gradually. Traditional treadmill exercise protocols used to evalu-

ate coronary artery disease usually aim to reach maximum heart rate rapidly and tend to skip the lower workloads (3 to 5 Mets) that are performed normally by pacemaker recipients in their daily life. Thus, the use of exercise protocols with gradually increasing workloads such as the chronotropic assessment exercise protocol[45] are probably more appropriate for assessing the rate response of a pacemaker over the wider range of workloads (and oxygen consumption) that are relevant to these patients. Graded exercise testing to maximal tolerated workload may be impractical for some patients for assessing the function of a rate-adaptive pacemaker. Brief, submaximal ramp exercise tests are especially valuable for assessing the proportionality of current rate-adaptive pacing systems.[44] These tests can be "informal," for example, asking the patient to walk at different speeds or to ascend and descend stairs. In addition, monitoring of pacemaker function during activities of daily living may provide the most clinically relevant method of evaluating an elderly patient. Alternatively, submaximal exercises such as treadmill tests at a low speed and grade may be performed to assess the sensor response. These tests show that walking at a faster speed increases the pacing rate of most rate-adaptive pacemakers (Fig. 7–4). However, the rate is not necessarily increased by walking up a slope in patients with activity-sensing pacemakers, which respond according to the pattern of body motion or vibration associated with each type of activity. For example, ascending stairs is associated with a lower pacing rate than is descending stairs with many activity-sensing pacemakers. These findings suggest that there is only a moderate correlation between the rate achieved by activity-sensing pacemakers and exercise workload. These differences in chronotropic response may not be detected with graded treadmill exercise. Rather, incremental bicycle ergometry may provide a more relevant method for distinguishing the relative advantages of one sensor over another. Ambulatory electrocardiographic monitoring, rate histograms, or stored rate trends may provide useful methods of evaluating the chronotropic response of rate-adaptive pacing systems in patients who are less active or who cannot exercise. It should be kept in mind that very few patients with pacemakers (or, indeed the general population) exercise to maximal levels of workload on a regular basis. Thus, exercise testing may have little clinical relevance in these individuals.

SPEED OF ONSET OF RATE RESPONSE AND RECOVERY FROM EXERCISE

An appropriate speed of response of the pacing rate to the onset of and recovery from exercise is an essential feature of a rate-adaptive pacing system. The onset kinetics are best assessed during standard treadmill exercise, such as walking at a fixed speed on the treadmill. From continuous electrocardiographic (ECG) monitoring, the *delay time* for the onset of rate response, the time to reach half of the maximum change in pacing rate during exercise (half-time), and 90% of the maximum response can be derived and used as a basis for comparison. The exercise responses of six different types of rate-adaptive pacemakers (with sensors for activity, QT interval, respiratory rate, minute ventilation, and right ventricular dP/dt) were compared with normal sinus rate in one study.[44] The results of this study demonstrated that the activity-sensing pacemakers best simulated the normal speed of

Pacing rate (bpm)

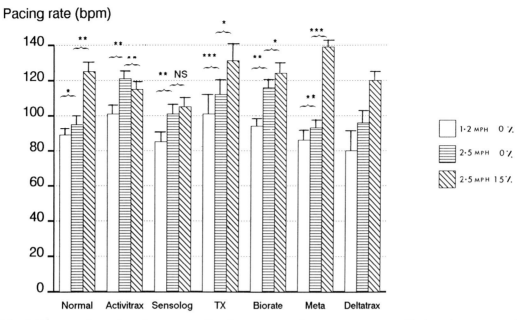

FIGURE 7–4. Brief activities are used to evaluate the proportionality of rate response of some common sensors. Maximum heart rate was derived from a 3-minute walking test done at different speeds (1.2 and 2.5 mph) and on different slopes (0 and 15%). There was no significant change in pacing rate when patients with the Sensolog pacemaker ascended an incline, whereas the pacing rate decreased significantly in patients with the Activitrax during the same activity. Bpm, beats/min; NS, not significant; * $p < .05$; ** $p < .01$; *** $p < .001$; Tx, QT sensing pacemaker. (From Lau CP, Butrous GS, Ward DE, Camm AJ: Comparison of exercise performance of six rate-adaptive right ventricular cardiac pacemakers. Am J Cardiol 63:833, 1989.)

rate response at the start of exercise. The rate response of activity sensors is usually immediate (no delay time), and the time needed to attain half of the maximum change in rate occurred within 45 seconds from the onset of exercise (Fig. 7–5). The maximum change in pacing rate is reached within 2 minutes of beginning an ordinary activity such as walking. The respiratory rate and the right ventricular dP/dt sensors had a longer delay time (about 30 seconds) and half-time (1 to 2 minutes), although the maximum change in rate was still attained within 2 to 3 minutes of exercise. The slowest sensor to respond to exercise was an early version of the QT-sensing pacemaker, which required up to 1 minute to initiate a rate response, and the maximum change in pacing rate was attained only in the recovery period following a short duration of exercise. The onset of rate responses and proportionality

to workload of the QT-sensing pacemaker were in sharp contrast to those of activity-sensing pacemakers. Other fast-reacting sensors include the PDI and the preejection interval (PEI).

The speed of onset of the QT-sensing pacemaker has been significantly improved by the use of a curvilinear rate-response slope that produces a larger change in pacing rate per unit change in QT interval at the onset of exercise than at higher workloads.[46] Similarly, the speed of rate response in an early minute ventilation–sensing pacemaker (Meta MV [Telectronics Pacing Systems]) was impeded by its curvilinear algorithm, which produced a lower slope at the lower range of minute ventilation (onset of exercise) than at higher ranges. This rate-response algorithm has been replaced by a linear slope, so that the rate of onset is significantly faster in

FIGURE 7–5. Speed of rate response of different pacemakers during walking at a nominal speed (2.5 mph at 0% gradient). The normal sinus rate responds almost immediately, half of the change being achieved in less than 30 seconds and most of the change within 1 minute. This speed of response was most closely simulated by the activity-sensing pacemakers. Significant differences were derived by comparing the response times of each pacemaker (T½ and T90) with those of the normal sinus response. Ninety percent of the maximum rate for this exercise was reached within the exercise period in all patients except those with the QT-sensing pacemaker (TX), who achieved this pacing rate only in the recovery phase. DT, delay time; T½ and T90, times needed to reach 50 and 90% of maximum heart rate. (From Lau CP, Butrous GS, Ward DE, Camm AJ: Comparison of exercise performance of six rate-adaptive right ventricular cardiac pacemakers. Am J Cardiol 63:833, 1989.)

Time (s)

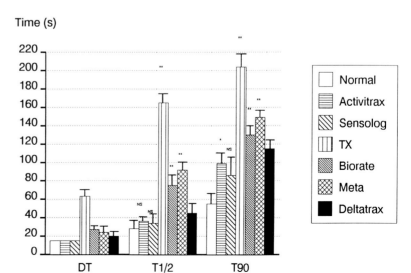

the more recent models (e.g., Meta II and Meta III [Telectronics Pacing Systems], Legend Plus [Medtronic Inc.], and Chorus RM [Ela Medical, Rougemont, France]). Thus, these minute ventilation–sensing pacemakers produce an increase in pacing rate that is linearly related to minute ventilation throughout exercise, providing the effect of shortening the rate-response half-time. Furthermore, the speed of onset of rate response is programmable in these newer generations of minute ventilation sensors.

Following termination of exercise, body movement decreases, and the pacing rate of an activity-sensing pacemaker returns toward the resting level based on an arbitrary rate decay curve.[47] If the rate decay is faster than is physiologically appropriate, adverse hemodynamic consequences may occur in the presence of a substantial drop in heart rate. In one study in which pacing rate was reduced either abruptly or gradually after identical exercise,[48] it was shown that an appropriately modulated rate recovery was associated with a higher cardiac output, lower sinus rate, and faster lactate clearance than with an unphysiologic rate recovery pattern (Fig. 7–6).[48] This complication can now be minimized in the newer generations of activity-sensing pacemakers, which have programmable rate-recovery curves.

SENSITIVITY OF A RATE-ADAPTIVE PACING SYSTEM TO CHANGES IN EXERCISE WORKLOAD AND OTHER PHYSIOLOGIC STRESSES

Table 7–5 shows the factors to which some rate-adaptive pacemakers are sensitive. Rate-adaptive pacemakers that are controlled by PDI and intracardiac hemodynamic parameters

are able to respond to emotional stresses. A reverse rate response has been observed during the Valsalva maneuver in patients with respiratory sensing pacing systems and some dP/dt sensing pacemakers. In these patients, the pacing rate is faster in the relaxation phase than in the strain phase (Fig. 7–7).[44] None of the currently available pacemakers reliably detects changes in posture, although several sensors may have the potential to do so.[49] A paradoxical decrease in heart rate may be observed during movement to the upright position with pacemakers that sense the PEI.[50] Although patients with rate-adaptive pacemakers that sense the PEI (Precept [Cardiac Pacemakers Inc., St. Paul, MN]) have had variable responses to posture, excessive tachycardia may occur with the adoption of upright posture. This response may require inactivation of the sensor in some patients.[51] A variable postural drop in heart rate has also been reported with a rate-adaptive pacemaker that detects the maximum first derivative of the right ventricular pressure (dP/dt) (Deltatrax [Medtronic Inc.]), although the changes were not clinically important.[52–53] A diurnal rate variation is possible with temperature-sensing and QT-sensing pacemakers. The clinical role of some of these rate changes to nonexercise stimuli remains to be determined, however.

SPECIFICITY OF RATE-ADAPTIVE PACING SYSTEMS

One of the main limitations of activity-sensing pacemakers is their susceptibility to extraneous vibrations. This typically occurs during various forms of transport. The degree of susceptibility to extraneous vibrations may vary with different types of activity sensors. For example, an accelerometer

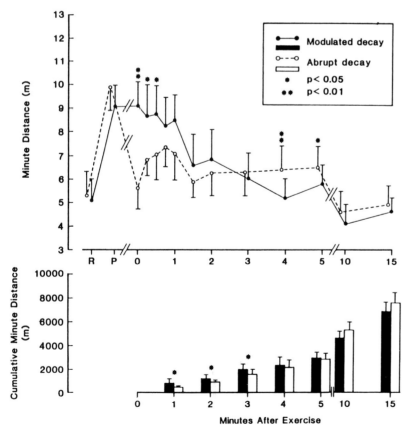

FIGURE 7–6. The change in instantaneous cardiac output (represented by Doppler-derived minute distance) at rest, at peak exercise, and during recovery *(upper graph)*. The lower panel shows the "cumulative cardiac output" during the 15-minute recovery period. The cumulative cardiac output during the two modes of recovery became identical at the fourth minute and thereafter remained similar. R, resting; P, peak exercise. (From Lau CP, Wong CK, Cheng CH, Leung WH: Importance of heart rate modulation on cardiac hemodynamics during post-exercise recovery. PACE 13:1277, 1990.)

TABLE 7–5. **PHYSIOLOGIC SENSITIVITY OF SOME CURRENTLY AVAILABLE RATE-ADAPTIVE PACEMAKERS**

| | EXERCISE | | EMOTION | VALSALVA | POSTURE | DIURNAL VARIATION |
	ISOTONIC	ISOMETRIC				
Sinus	+	+	+	+	+	+
Activity	+					
Respiration	+			R		
QT	+		+			+
Gradient	+	+	+		R	
Temperature	+		±			+
PEI	+	+	+		V	
dP/dt	+	+	+	V	V	
S$\bar{v}$O$_2$	+	+				

S$\bar{v}$O$_2$, Mixed venous oxygen saturation; dP/dt, maximum first derivation of right ventricular pressure; PEI, preejection interval; R, reversed response; V, variable.

using a tilt switch (Swing [Sorin Biomedica, Saluggia, Italy]) may be one of the least susceptible. The QT interval and the PDI may be significantly affected by such factors as cardioactive medications and myocardial ischemia. Ischemia may result in shortening of the QT interval, leading to an increase in pacing rate and further myocardial ischemia.[54] Sensors that use impedance to measure respiratory mechanics or the right ventricular PEI are susceptible to artifacts produced by arm movement, hyperventilation, and speech.[55–56] Electric diathermy is likely to cause inappropriate changes in pacing rate in pacemakers that measure impedance.[57] The same problem may be expected to occur during radio-frequency ablation in impedance-sensing pacemakers. In addition, external temperature change can significantly affect the pacing rate of temperature-sensing pacemakers.

CLINICAL CONTRAINDICATIONS TO SPECIFIC RATE-ADAPTIVE SENSORS

A number of clinical factors may preclude the use of some sensors for an individual patient (Table 7–6). When a param-

eter can be detected only at the ventricular level, the sensor cannot be used in an AAIR pacing system. The use of antiarrhythmic medications and the presence of myocardial ischemia may interfere with the detection of the PDI. Minute ventilation–sensing pacemakers are best avoided in young children, who may have very rapid respiratory rates during exercise that exceed the range detected by the pacemaker. Occupations associated with exposure to vibrations in the environment are a relative contraindication to the use of an activity sensor. In addition, replacing or upgrading a pulse generator requires that the sensor be compatible with the existing pacing lead.

Principles for Combining Rate-Adaptive Sensors and Algorithms

Regulation of the normal sinus node occurs through multiple physiologic inputs. Thus, theoretically a combination of sensors may best replicate the response of the sinus node during a variety of physiologic needs. However, the response of a sensor can be significantly enhanced by fine-tuning the characteristics of the sensor and the algorithms used to translate sensor output into modulation of pacing rate. On the other hand, the potential for combining sensors for purposes other than rate regulation during exercise is certainly a strong incentive for the development of multisensor pacemakers. Multisensor pacing may also offer the possibility of selecting an alternative sensor should one sensor fail or become inappropriate for an individual patient.

COMPONENTS OF A MULTISENSOR SYSTEM

There are five main components of sensor combinations (Table 7–7). Sensors for the purpose of rate modulation may be combined to improve the speed of rate response at the onset of exercise, proportionality of heart rate to workload, differential sensitivity to physiologic changes induced by exercise and nonexercise stresses, and rejection of unwanted environmental artifacts. These combinations aim to create a sensor system that best simulates the sinus node response in normal individuals. In addition, sensors may be implanted to control parameters other than pacing rate.

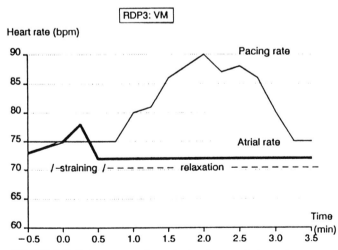

FIGURE 7–7. Rate response of a patient with a respiratory rate–sensing pacemaker (RDP3) during the Valsalva maneuver. The atrial rate increased during the straining phase and returned to baseline during the relaxation phase of this maneuver. The pacing rate, on the other hand, showed a paradoxical response as the patient hyperventilated after the strain phase, resulting in a postmaneuver tachycardia.

TABLE 7–6. CLINICAL FACTORS CONTRAINDICATING USE OF SOME CURRENTLY AVAILABLE RATE-ADAPTIVE PACEMAKERS

	ATRIAL PACING	ANTIARRHYTHMIC DRUGS	MYOCARDIAL ISCHEMIA	YOUNG CHILDREN OR RESPIRATORY DISEASE	STANDARD UNIPOLAR LEAD	EXPOSURE TO HIGH-VIBRATION ENVIRONMENT
Activity						−
Respiration				−	−	
QT interval	−	−	−			
Gradient	−	−	−		−	
Temperature	±				−	
PEI	−	−	−		−	
dP/dt	−	±	−		−	
S$\bar{v}$O$_2$	±			−	−	

PEI, Preejection interval; dP/dt, maximum first derivation of right ventricular pressure; S$\bar{v}$O$_2$, mixed venous oxygen saturation; −, unsuitable; ±, feasibility remains to be validated.

ALGORITHMS FOR COMBINING RATE-ADAPTIVE SENSORS

The algorithm for multisensor pacing serves not only to translate a change in each of the sensed parameters into a change in pacing rate but also combines the inputs from two or more sensors for rate optimization in individual patients (Fig. 7–8). The following categories of combination are possible:

ALGORITHMS FOR EXERCISE RESPONSE

Two basic methods for combining sensors to control chronotropic response have been used. The first of these methods is the use of one sensor to control a specific part of the rate response. For example, a fast-responding sensor (such as activity) can be used to modulate pacing rate at the onset of exercise, and a second sensor (such as minute ventilation) may modulate the pacing rate during more prolonged exercise. The pacing rate may increase to an "interim" or intermediate value when the faster sensor detects the onset of exercise, whereas a more proportional rate increase will occur when the slower, more proportional sensor "catches up." The other approach is simply to combine the rate response of both sensors, such that the pacing rate at any point during exercise reflects the output of the sensor with a higher rate. A variation of this approach is to calculate the output of each sensor in a relative proportion so that the ultimate rate profile is a blend of both (see later discussion).

ALGORITHMS FOR ENHANCING SENSITIVITY

The pacing rate can be controlled by two sensors that have different sensitivities to exercise and nonexercise physiologic stresses so that the system can respond to both exertional and emotional needs. It is conceivable that a separate rate-adaptive slope (or different upper and lower rates) can be programmed for modulation of rate in response to exertional and emotional needs. The algorithm can be designed to weigh the output of both sensors to diagnose a nonexercise physiologic stress and provide a different pattern of rate adaptation.

SENSOR CROSS-CHECKING

The response of one sensor can also be checked against the output from another sensor to improve the specificity of the chronotropic response. For example, the heart rate achieved in response to the output of a less specific sensor may be allowed to increase over a programmable range of pacing rates only for a limited time period (also programmable). In the absence of confirmation of exercise by the other sensor(s), the pacing rate returns to the baseline so that prolonged "false-positive" increases in pacing rate can be avoided. Sensor cross-checking can also be reciprocal, so that either sensor may limit the chronotropic response that results from the other. In contrast, cross-checking could be applied to limit only the less specific of the sensors.

POSSIBLE SENSOR COMBINATIONS

A number of sensor combinations have been suggested. These combinations are based on the chronotropic response characteristics of an ideal multisensor system as well as the convenience of having two or more sensors that are derived by similar technical methods. One of the simplest sensors is a 24-hour clock that can be used to vary the lower pacing rate. The normal diurnal variation in heart rate is well recognized, and an automatic decrease in the lower rate during

TABLE 7–7. COMPONENTS OF A MULTISENSOR SYSTEM FOR RATE-ADAPTIVE PACING (ONLY SENSORS USING STANDARD LEADS ARE USED FOR EXAMPLES)

	SPEED OF RESPONSE	PROPORTIONALITY	SENSITIVITY	SPECIFICITY	ENERGY SAVER
E	Activity	Minute ventilation	Diurnal variation: 24-hour clock	Minute ventilation	Detection of capture: Evoked QRS
X				QT	Stroke volume
A	Gradient	Preejection interval			
M			Emotional response:	Activity	
P		QT	QT		
L			Gradient		Rate reduction during sleep
E					Minimize myocardial oxygen
S					consumption

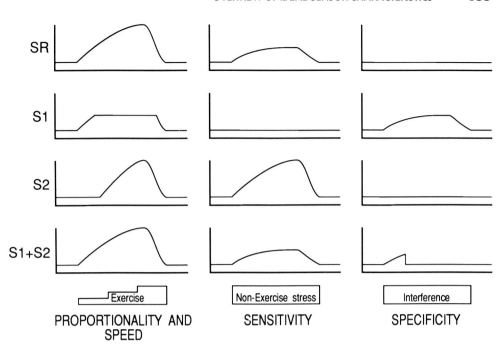

FIGURE 7–8. Different algorithms for sensor combinations needed to achieve better (1) proportionality and speed of response, (2) sensitivity, and (3) specificity. The graphs *(top to bottom)* depict the responses of the sinus node (SR), sensor 1 (S1), sensor 2 (S2), and the combined rate profile of S1 and S2. SR shows ideal proportionality, speed of rate response, and freedom from interference. S1 is a rapidly responding sensor, although it is neither proportional nor sensitive and is susceptible to interference. S2 is a proportional and sensitive sensor, although it has a slow response. It is also specific to exercise. Note the improved ability of the combined sensor approach in simulating the sinus rate under different conditions. (From Lau CP: Rate-Adaptive Cardiac Pacing: Single- and Dual-Chamber. Mt. Kisco, NY, Futura, 1994.)

the hours of sleep is physiologically appropriate. Battery consumption can also be reduced by this reduction in average pacing rate. A particularly attractive method of combining sensors is to incorporate an activity sensor (which has a fast response to exercise) and a sensor that provides a more proportional response to workload. An activity sensor can be easily added to the pulse generator without the need for a specialized lead. It also requires minimum energy consumption to operate and is compatible with most types of alternative sensors that are available. Activity has been combined with central venous temperature,[58] a parameter that is more proportional to metabolic need during prolonged exertion than is activity (Fig. 7–9). Similarly, the combination of the QT interval and activity enhances the speed of response compared with a QT sensor alone.[59–60] An activity sensor has been combined with a minute ventilation sensor in a single chamber pacemaker (Legend Plus, Medtronic Inc.). The sensing of intracardiac impedance is one of the simplest ways

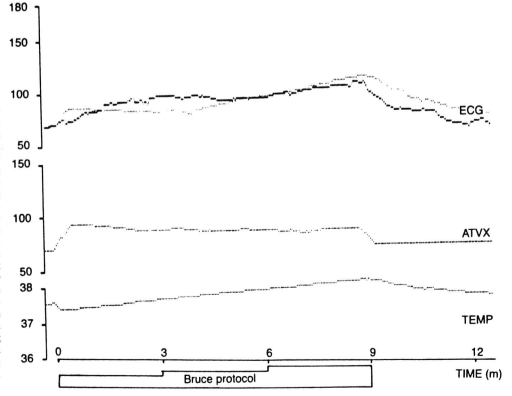

FIGURE 7–9. Combination of activity sensing and central venous temperature sensing. A simple algorithm for choosing the faster rate from either sensor is used. The activity sensor increases the rate rapidly with exercise, but thereafter the rate remains unchanged despite increases in workloads. Although temperature increase occurs late, it modulates the rate at higher workloads and in the recovery period. The overall rate response in the combined approach *(light line, top panel)* allows the best simulation of the intrinsic rate *(heavy line, top panel)*. ECG, intrinsic rate from surface lead II; TEMP, pulmonary arterial temperature in degrees Celsius; ATVX, pacing rate from an externally attached activity-sensing pacemaker (Activitrax). (From Lau CP: Rate-Adaptive Cardiac Pacing: Single- and Dual-Chamber. Mt. Kisco, NY, Futura, 1994.)

to combine sensors. Through the use of special filters, intra-cardiac impedance can be used to detect simultaneously low-frequency respiratory signals and higher frequency cardiac signals such as right ventricular stroke volume and the pre-ejection period (PEP). Most sensors are limited by their ina-bility to detect nonexercise needs, such as those occurring during changes in emotion. Among the commonly used sen-sors, a response to emotional stress can be achieved with the QT interval or the PDI. Because these parameters are easily measured using conventional pacing leads, their implemen-tation may enable a pacing system to detect non–exercise-related changes in catecholamine concentrations. Last but not least, because many sensors require the consumption of en-ergy to operate, it is desirable to minimize current drain by the use of steroid-eluting electrodes that produce a very low chronic stimulation threshold. Algorithms for the automatic detection of ventricular capture may be necessary to further minimize current drain so that multiple sensors can be used without reducing longevity of the pulse generator.

ADVANTAGES AND PROBLEMS OF COMBINING SENSORS

The use of multiple sensors to control pacing rate may theoretically improve the overall chronotropic response char-acteristics of pacing systems in terms of speed, proportional-ity, sensitivity, and specificity compared with a single sensor (Table 7–8). In addition, there is a clinical advantage in having an additional sensor for rate-adaptive pacing should one sensor fail to provide adequate rate modulation in an individual. In addition, the clinical status of patients may vary in ways that may preclude the use of one sensor. For example, the addition of antiarrhythmic medications to a patient's therapy may change the response characteristics of a QT sensor. Sensor combination may also allow a rate-adaptive system to be used during different periods of a patient's life. For example, the current minute ventilation sensors may not be appropriate for some pediatric patients. The addition of an activity sensor in a combined system may enable such a pacemaker to be used in this patient group during growth and maturity. Finally, multiple sensors may be required to assess the clinical status of a patient rather than providing rate augmentation. These functions may in-clude the measurement of right ventricular or pulmonary artery pressure and $S\bar{v}o_2$.

Despite these theoretical advantages of multisensor pace-makers, it should be emphasized that the clinical utility of such devices remains unproved. In addition, there are several potential disadvantages to combining sensors. Because of increased battery consumption, the pulse generator may need to be larger to provide comparable longevity. Furthermore, a second sensor may potentially adulterate the otherwise ideal rate-response characteristics of the first sensor. Because sen-sors may respond differently to different physiologic and environmental factors, the rate-control algorithm must assign a priority to each sensor, especially if the two sensors indi-cate that the pacing rate should change in opposite directions. Programming of a multisensor pacemaker is likely to be more complex than that for a single sensor alone. Apart from setting a priority to each sensor, certain combinations require programming of the relative contribution of each sensor to the overall chronotropic response. The time-related change in sensor response must also be considered, and repeated adjustment of rate-adaptive settings may be necessary. These programming decisions increase the complexity of multisen-sor pacing systems. Although the first generation of multi-sensor pacemakers is likely to increase the time required for follow-up clinic visits, it is anticipated that rate response may become fully automatic if each sensor is able to optimize the function of the other.

TABLE 7–8. **ADVANTAGES AND PROBLEMS WITH MULTISENSOR RATE-ADAPTIVE PACING**

	MULTISENSOR	**SINGLE SENSOR**
ADVANTAGES		
1. Combination of merits of different sensors	Improvement in speed, proportionality, and sensitivity	Better algorithm to improve sensor response
2. Improved specificity	Sensor cross-checking	Not possible
3. Sensor-controlled parameters other than rate	Multiple sensors may be needed to control other pacing parameters	
4. Sensor for back-up rate adaptation	One sensor may replace the other sensor if the latter fails, or a change in patient's condition precludes the use of one sensor	Not possible
5. Extended use for different populations of patients	Possible	Not possible
POTENTIAL PROBLEMS		
1. Increased cost	Multisensor devices may be more expensive	
2. Increased battery drain	Energy consumption is increased with two sensors. This may be reduced with the use of low-energy pacing electrodes or automatic pacing output control	Less energy expensive
3. Complexity in programming	a. A prioritization of multiple sensor inputs has to be made b. Sensors have to be individually programmed c. Automaticity may reduce the need for programming	
4. Clinical superiority	Clinical advantages of multisensor vs single-sensor pacing remain to be confirmed	Clinical superiority over fixed-rate devices demonstrated

Although the use of sensor combinations is technically interesting, the clinical benefit of sensor combinations compared with single sensors remains to be established. In terms of symptomatology, VVIR pacing is superior to VVI pacing. However, the overall contribution of improved control of symptoms to enhanced quality of life is probably small in the usual pacemaker recipient in whom quality of life is already close to that of age-matched normal individuals.[61] There is still no comparative study of different sensors in regard to their effect on symptomatology or quality of life. It is unlikely that studies comparing pacemakers with multiple sensors to those with a single sensor will show differences in objective measurements of functional responses such as exercise duration, maximal oxygen consumption, or anaerobic threshold. A very sensitive clinical indicator will probably be necessary to demonstrate any clinical benefits from multisensor pacing.

Programming Rate-Adaptive Pacing Systems

At the time of pacemaker implantation, most rate-adaptive pacemakers are programmed to the sensor-inactive mode. The activation of the rate-adaptive pacing mode involves matching the pacing rate provided by the sensor to the exercise workload. The factors that must be programmed include the upper and lower pacing rates, the speed of onset and recovery during exercise, and the rate-adaptive threshold and slope. By using submaximal exercise protocols, the rate-adaptive mode can be activated as soon as the patient begins to ambulate after pacemaker implantation. However, in our experience, reprogramming of initial sensor settings is often necessary during long-term follow-up as the condition of the patient and his or her physical activities change. Many rate-adaptive pacemakers are capable of monitoring the output of the sensor even when programmed to a sensor-passive mode. Thus, recording of sensor data can begin immediately after implantation to guide future programming decisions. A reassessment of the rate-adaptive function is usually carried out 6 to 8 weeks following implantation using standard methods of assessing sensing and pacing functions. A stored rate profile may also be used to adjust the sensor settings to obtain the desired response. For example, the choice of a rate-response slope may be narrowed to a small number of feasible alternatives so that programming can be simplified.

OPTIMAL TIME FOR PROGRAMMING RATE RESPONSE

As pointed out earlier, it is often prudent to be conservative with the programmed rate-response settings immediately following pacemaker implantation. Full activation of the sensor is often best delayed for at least several weeks because the patient's general condition is likely to fluctuate substantially in the early postoperative period. Factors such as postoperative pain, prolonged immobilization, anxiety, psychological acceptance of the permanent pacemaker,[62] physical rehabilitation, and reestablishment of daily routines are all important elements that vary during this period. There are additional reasons to delay programming of some sensors.

For example, in piezoelectric activity sensors, the nature of the rate response may be significantly affected by the maturation of the pacemaker pocket. In an early report[63] on the Activitrax pacemaker that involved weekly transtelephonic follow-up for 4 weeks and then every 3 months, 29 of 136 patients required reprogramming on clinical grounds. We observed that once these sensor variables stabilized, long-term reprogramming was seldom required.

A recent study[64] systematically evaluated the programming changes required for two activity-sensing, rate-adaptive pacemakers during clinical follow-up (Activitrax [Medtronic Inc.] and Synchrony [Siemens-Pacesetter, Sylmar, CA]). Most of the reprogramming of sensor variables occurred within the first month after implantation, and subsequent reprogramming became less frequent (Fig. 7–10). An objective assessment of sensor rate histograms was used for monitoring the rate-adaptive parameters of the Synchrony pulse generator, whereas the rate-adaptive parameters of the Activitrax were monitored clinically. There was no period that was associated with more frequent reprogramming of the Activitrax pulse generator during the first year. In patients receiving a Synchrony pulse generator, more reprogramming changes were noted during the first month than during later follow-up. When the full rate-adaptive settings were activated immediately after implantation, some patients with the Synchrony pacemaker developed rapid tachycardia and required reprogramming to a less sensitive setting. Based on these observations, it appears prudent to activate an activity sensor fully 6 to 8 weeks after implantation.

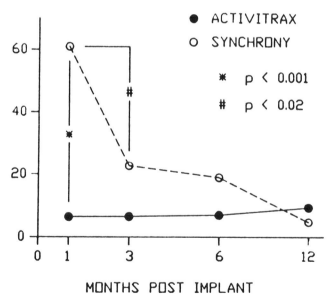

MONTHS POST IMPLANT

FIGURE 7–10. The incidence of activity parameter changes during 1-year follow-up for the Activitrax *(solid circle)* and Synchrony *(open circle)* devices. The incidence of changes noted in the Synchrony group (#) was significantly greater 1 month after implantation than at each subsequent period ($p < .02$). There was no significant difference in the incidence of activity parameter changes in the Activitrax group during the period of follow-up. Although the incidence of changes for the Synchrony and Activitrax groups (*) was markedly different at the 1-month interval ($p < .001$), there were no significant differences in the 3-, 6-, and 12-month intervals. (From Ahern T, Nydegger C, McCormick DJ, et al: Incidence and timing of activity parameter changes in activity responsive pacing systems. PACE 15:762, 1992.)

MATCHING SENSOR LEVEL TO WORKLOAD

Most rate-adaptive pacemakers use an open-loop logic, such that the physician must prescribe a clinically determined rate response–workload relationship, the so-called slope of rate response. A variety of exercise protocols and monitoring methods have been designed to standardize and simplify the choice of an appropriate rate-response slope.

EXERCISE METHODS

Treadmill exercise is one of the most widely employed methods for evaluating chronotropic response in patients with implanted pacing systems. Conventional exercise protocols are designed to quickly advance patients to their maximal exercise workload. As such, these exercise protocols are best suited for defining the presence of myocardial ischemia and for testing athletic individuals. However, because pacemaker recipients are often elderly, these maximal exercise protocols are often inadequate to define the chronotropic response of a pacing system. Treadmill exercise is useful for patients with implanted pacemakers provided that the exercise workload is increased in gradual increments that are relevant to the patient's normal activities. It is especially important to obtain heart rates during submaximal exercise intensities. Alt and Wilkoff and colleagues proposed the use of a more gradual exercise protocol to assess the degree of chronotropic incompetence in patients with pacemakers.[45, 65] The chronotropic assessment exercise protocol provides a very gradual increase in the treadmill speed and grade in 2-minute stages.[45] The predicted heart rate at any stage of exercise can be derived from the patient's age, resting heart rate, and functional capacity (maximal exercise capacity). Because a full treadmill protocol may be time consuming and cannot be performed by some patients, brief treadmill exercise lasting for 2 to 3 minutes at different speeds and grades may be used to assess the accuracy of programming.[44] Brief exercise tests can also be used to estimate the speed of rate response.

Bicycle ergometry has also been used to guide programming of rate-adaptive pacemakers. This obviates the influence of body weight on exercise workload so that the amount of exertion can be more accurately assessed. However, the rate response observed with some sensors is significantly less during cycle ergometry (e.g., activity and temperature sensing) than during treadmill exercise at comparable workloads.[44, 66]

The most common muscular exercise performed by pacemaker recipients is walking, and a walking test is both a convenient and a clinically relevant method for guiding the programming of rate-adaptive functions. Walking tests are inexpensive and can be performed by almost all patients with pacemakers. It has been previously demonstrated that a heart rate of approximately 90 to 100 bpm is usually achieved during a normal walking pace.[67] The clinical practice of evaluating patients during walking is supported by a previous study of the heart rates attained by 195 normal subjects during "casual" and "brisk" walking.[68] Despite variability in the resting heart rates, most normal subjects attained a rate of 85 to 100 bpm during casual walking and 100 to 110 bpm during brisk walking (Table 7–9).

Cardiopulmonary exercise testing with analysis of expired gases has been used increasingly to detect subtle differences in the physiologic consequences of different pacing modes. Although it is a highly sensitive and objective method, cardiopulmonary exercise testing cannot be performed by many pacemaker recipients because of the cost and complexity of the procedure. In the context of a minute ventilation sensor, the sensor slope determined during cardiopulmonary testing may be too sensitive for clinical use, and a submaximal step test may be more clinically relevant.[69] Whether these observations are equally applicable to other sensors is uncertain.

AUTOPROGRAMMABILITY

To simplify programming, some rate-adaptive pacemakers automatically determine the sensor output during a given workload and suggest sensor threshold or slope settings that will provide a prescribed pacing rate. In some activity-sensing pacemakers (Sensolog and Synchrony models [Siemens Ltd. and Siemens-Pacesetter Inc.]) sensor data are collected during casual and brisk walking, and the appropriate rate-adaptive parameters are then compared with published graphs to achieve the desired heart rate response.[70–72] The rate-response parameters determined by treadmill exercise tend to result in a higher than expected rate during ordinary walking and are highly dependent on the type of footwear worn.[70–71, 73] These facts should be considered during programming of this type of pacemaker.

Another approach to programming rate-adaptive parameters for ordinary exercise is that used in accelerometer-based pacemakers (Relay or Dash [Intermedics Inc.]).[74] Acceleration data are collected during a 3-minute exercise test (casual walking) and automatically coupled to a programmable rate response, a feature known as "tailor to patient." The rate-adaptive slope has a triphasic relation to workload (Fig. 7–3 C), a flat intermediate portion representing ordinary exer-

TABLE 7–9. **HEART RATE RESPONSE TO WALKING EXERCISE AS A FUNCTION OF AGE***

AGE GROUP (yr)	N (M/F)	RESTING HR	PEAK HR (CASUAL)	PEAK HR (BRISK)
20–34	74 (13/61)	79.5 (56–110)	90.5 (63–125)	109 (80–144)
35–49	32 (10/22)	81.5 (53–110)	92 (60–115)	102 (77–140)
50–69	42 (20/22)	75 (56–120)	89 (66–130)	104.5 (78–135)
70 +	27 (14/13)	77 (43–115)	90 (60–124)	100 (65–155)
Overall	175 (57/118)	79 (43–120)	91 (60–130)	107 (65–155)

*The "casual" and "brisk" walk are 94 and 132 steps/min respectively, as guided by a metronome. The number of volunteers in each age range are not equal, and there is a preponderance of younger volunteers.
HR, Heart rate.
From Hayes DL, Von Feldt L, Higano ST: Standardized informal exercise testing for programming rate-adaptive pacemakers. PACE 14:1772, 1991.

cise, and more aggressive curves indicating both lower and higher levels of exercise. The flat intermediate slope results in a relatively stable rate response during daily activities once the "tailor to patient" function is activated with ordinary walking. In addition, the rate response during ordinary workloads is only minimally affected by a change in slope because there is substantial overlap in the rate-response curves. Therefore, to ensure that the maximal pacing rate can be attained in the most active patients, a formal exercise test is still needed to assess the rate-response characteristics at higher workloads.

In a minute ventilation–sensing pacemaker (Meta MV [Telectronics]), the change in impedance associated with minute ventilation during exercise is reflected by the recommended rate response factor (RRF), which is telemetered by the programmer.[75] This parameter can be measured by performing an exercise test in either the VVI "adaptive" or VVIR pacing modes. The RRF value is determined at peak exercise. Using this RRF value to set the rate-responsive slope, the maximum pacing rate will occur when the impedance estimate of minute ventilation matches the impedance value determined during exercise testing. A more rapid adaptation to baseline minute ventilation is used in the newer versions of this sensor, and the rate-adaptive slope can be chosen using submaximal exercise tests. An automatic slope adaptation mechanism has been incorporated in the new version of the QT-sensing pacemaker (Rythmx [Vitatron Medical B.V., Dieren, The Netherlands]).[76] This algorithm involves two different rate-adaptive slopes, one slope designed for low exercise workloads and the other for higher workloads. The pacemaker automatically measures the QT–heart rate relationship at the lower rate when the patient is regularly at rest (usually during sleep). This value is used to determine the rate-response slope that is appropriate for the lower rate limit. Based on these measurements, the slope is automatically adjusted up or down one step. Similarly, if the QT interval continues to shorten when the maximum rate is reached, it is assumed that the slope at the upper rate is too aggressive, and this slope is reduced automatically so that the maximum rate is reached later during exercise. If the maximum rate is not reached after a certain number of days, this slope is automatically made more sensitive. Automaticity in rate-adaptive slope determination will be an important feature in future rate-adaptive pacemakers.

ONSET AND TERMINATION OF RATE RESPONSE

The normal sinus node increases its rate almost immediately at the onset of exercise. This prompt chronotropic response may be especially important for patients who normally exercise only for brief periods. Compared to the normal sinus node, activity-sensing pacemakers respond most rapidly to the onset of exercise.[44] It should be stressed that the normal response to exercise involves increased automaticity in the sinus node and conduction through the AV node. For patients with activity-sensing, rate-adaptive pacemakers in the AAIR mode, a sudden and inappropriately rapid increase in pacing rate may result in functional AV interval prolongation or AV Wenckebach block.[77–79] This is a special situation in which a programmable onset of rate response can be very useful in matching the atrial rate to the status of AV conduction.

The decay of pacing rate during recovery may also be clinically important. A physiologic rate decay[48] may contribute to improved hemodynamics and lower lactate accumulation after exercise than a rate decay that is too rapid. An appropriate pattern of pacing rate decrease is especially important for patients who have achieved a high rate at peak exercise. The rate-decay pattern is now programmable in a number of rate-adaptive pacemakers. In some pacemakers such as those sensing central venous temperature, oxygen saturation, and stroke volume, the decay of the sensor value after exercise is related to the previous workload and can be used to modulate the pacing rate decline after exercise.

MAXIMUM AND MINIMUM SENSOR-INDICATED RATES

Apart from rate-response slopes, a minimum and maximum pacing rate must also be programmed. In a VVI pacemaker, a lower rate must be programmed that is also the "average" pacing rate, which in most cases varies from 60 to 80 bpm. Some authors have suggested that the optimum lower pacing rate can be adjusted with the aim of achieving the minimum atrial rate in patients who have complete AV block.[80] However, it must be stressed that DDD is probably the appropriate pacing mode for these individuals. Unlike the VVI pacing mode in which a single, fixed pacing rate must be programmed to accommodate both rest and exercise, the lower rate limit becomes less critical in rate-adaptive pacemakers because higher rates can be achieved during exercise. It is clinically useful to program a lower pacing rate that is physiologically appropriate for the hours of sleep.[81] The lower resting heart rates also serve to improve the longevity of the pulse generator.[35] The patient's age and activity level and the presence of structural heart disease should be taken into account when choosing the maximum sensor-driven rate. In general, a higher upper rate may benefit young children. In a review of nine studies of physiologic pacemakers, Nordlander and colleagues found that the percentage of improvement in maximum exercise capacity was linearly related to the maximum heart rate achieved.[82] However, the proportion of time spent by these patients with heart rates near the upper rate limit must also be considered. A study using Holter recordings of 44 patients with complete heart block who were treated with VDD pacemakers showed that although the number of beats over a 24-hour period was similar for these patients in the VVI and VDD modes, the range of pacing rates was much wider in the VDD mode[83] (Fig. 7–11). However, only 5 of 39 patients with an upper rate of 150 bpm ever reached this limit during Holter recording. The typical pacemaker recipient in this study (mean age 68, range 18 to 84 years) achieved a rate of 150 bpm for less than 0.5% of the day[83] (Fig. 7–12). During 12-minute walking tests, there was no objective difference in the duration of exercise in patients with an upper rate limit of 125 and those with a limit of 150 bpm[67] (Fig. 7–13). Thus, it seems that an upper rate of between 125 and 150 bpm can be chosen for most patients. It has been convincingly demonstrated that rate-adaptive pacing may improve exercise tolerance in patients with angina pectoris, probably by decreasing ventricular volume and wall stress compared with VVI pacing.[84] Nevertheless, an aggressively programmed rate-adaptive pacemaker may induce angina in some individuals. Therefore, patients with

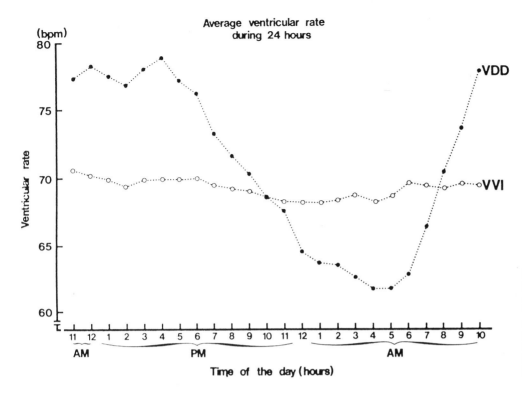

FIGURE 7–11. Ventricular rate with the Holter monitor in 43 patients with complete heart block in the VDD and VVI mode. (From Kristensson B, Karlson O, Rydén L: Holter-monitored heart rhythm during atrioventricular synchronous and fixed-rate ventricular pacing. PACE 9:511, 1986.)

angina pectoris may benefit from exercise testing to determine whether an appropriate chronotropic response can improve exercise capacity without exacerbating anginal symptoms.[84–86] A full clinical evaluation is required because myocardial ischemia is often subclinical. Provided that the upper rate is judiciously chosen, rate-adaptive pacing enhances cardiac efficiency compared with VVI pacing.

The values chosen for the lower and upper pacing rates can also affect submaximal rate response significantly. The "slopes" of rate response usually vary according to the lower and upper rates that have been programmed. Therefore, these lower and upper limits are as important to the overall chronotropic response as the rate-response threshold and slope parameters. This fact must be considered when programming a rate-adaptive pacing system[87] (Table 7–10).

SENSOR- AND RATE-MONITORING FUNCTIONS

The rate response during exercise can be monitored electrocardiographically during treadmill exercise and cycle er-

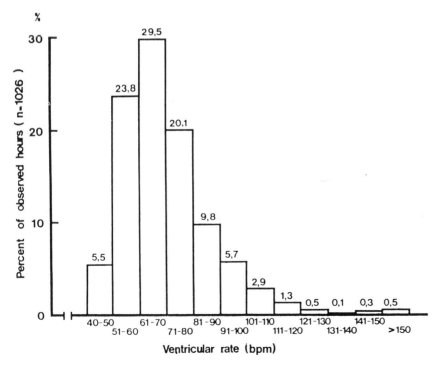

FIGURE 7–12. Proportion of time spent at various ventricular rates during 24 hours of Holter monitoring in 44 patients with a VDD pacemaker. (From Kristensson B, Karlson O, Rydén L: Holter-monitored heart rhythm during atrioventricular synchronous and fixed-rate ventricular pacing. PACE 9:511, 1986.)

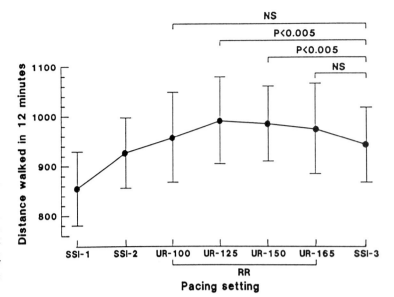

FIGURE 7–13. Distances covered in 12 minutes in patients with rate-adaptive pacemakers at different programmed settings. SSI-1 to SSI-3 represent repeated walking tests performed at a fixed rate, and SSI-3 is the distance covered after the "learning" effect resulting from SSI-1 and SSI-2. UR-100 to UR-165 represent the rate-adaptive pacing rates achieved during walking. The longest distance was covered with a maximum rate of 125 to 150 bpm. (From Lau CP, Butrous GS, Ward DE, Camm AJ: Comparison of exercise performance of six rate-adaptive right ventricular cardiac pacemakers. Am J Cardiol 63:833, 1989.)

gometry, or by ECG radiotelemetry if informal exercise is carried out. To simplify programming, most rate-adaptive pacemakers have the capability to monitor the heart rate of the patient, including the pacing rate that would have been observed had the sensor completely controlled the cardiac rhythm. In an activity-sensing pacemaker (Sensolog), the instantaneous pacing rate can be measured by telemetry with the programmer, using the so-called rate-read function.[70] The range of heart rates that occurs over a programmable time interval is stored in memory by the pulse generator. These data can be presented as percentages of the total beats that are within different ranges of heart rate (*rate histograms,* Fig. 7–14).[70, 72] The interval during which the data are collected may be programmed from minutes to many months. With longer intervals of time, the sampling frequency is typically longer. Rate histograms may be useful for evaluating the total rate response during the follow-up period between clinic visits or for a specific activity such as walking in the clinic or elsewhere. Rate histograms can also be used to collect the distribution of pacing rates during a 24-hour period, including the percentage of heart beats that are paced within each rate bin. For example, if the percentage of paced beats is high at the lower pacing limit but very low at the upper ranges of heart rates, the sensor may not have been programmed to provide an adequate chronotropic response. In

contrast, a 24-hour rate histogram that shows the majority of pacing rates above the lower limit may indicate that the pacemaker has been programmed too aggressively. In a study assessing time-related changes in 24-hour histograms,[88] a tendency was found for the higher rate ranges to be programmed during the follow-up, suggesting that patients might have increased their level of activities after permanent pacing.

The main limitation of rate histograms is that there is no information about *when* the recorded heart rates occurred. Thus, a rate acceleration (e.g., pacemaker-mediated tachycardia) may be overlooked as normal rate behavior in the histogram because there is no way to correlate the patient's activity with the recorded rate. In addition, the onset and recovery patterns of the chronotropic response cannot be directly assessed. An alternative diagnostic approach is to use built-in Holter functions or rate profiles as provided by the Rhythmx, Dash, and Relay pacemakers. In the Rhythmx pacemaker, the average pacing rate during a 20-second interval is sampled on a continuous basis and can be profiled during a 1-hour duration.[89] This has been shown to reflect accurately the recorded heart rate. When the automatic slope adaptation algorithm was activated, a spontaneous increase in the 24-hour rate-adaptive pattern was observed during follow-up.

A further refinement of this Holter monitor capability is that of the accelerometer-based pacemakers (Dash and Re-

TABLE 7–10. **EFFECT OF LOWER RATE PROGRAMMING IN 12 PATIENTS WITH DDDR PACEMAKERS***

	STAGES OF EXERCISE				
LOWER RATE	1	2	3	4	PEAK EXERCISE
80	102	106	112	110	137
70	96	103	110	101	130
60	87	97	103	113	127
50	86	91	110	111	125
p	<.01	<.05	NS	NS	NS

*Four patients had ventilation-sensing pacemakers; eight had activity-sensing devices. The pacing rate (bpm) attained during submaximal exercise stages was significantly affected by the programmed lower rate, although the maximum rate achieved at the end of exercise was not affected. The upper rate in all patients was 150 bpm.

Adapted from Leung SK, Choi YC, Lau CP, et al: Does the programmed low rate affect the rate response in rate-adaptive pacemakers [Abstract]? PACE 15:579, 1992.

HISTOGRAMS

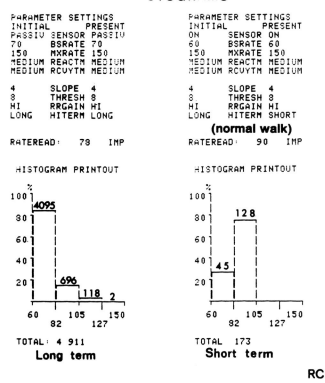

FIGURE 7–14. Rate histograms of a patient with an activity-sensing pacemaker (Sensolog). The number on top of each histogram bin (which was shown only on the programmer screen but is labeled here to give an idea of the size of each bin) represents the number of times that a pacing rate occurred within the bin range. The long-term histogram represents sampling over an 18- to 48-hour period, and the short-term histogram was made in this example during normal walking for 2 minutes. (From Lau CP, Tse WS, Camm AJ: Clinical experience with Sensolog 703: A new activity-sensing rate-responsive pacemaker. PACE 11:1444, 1988.)

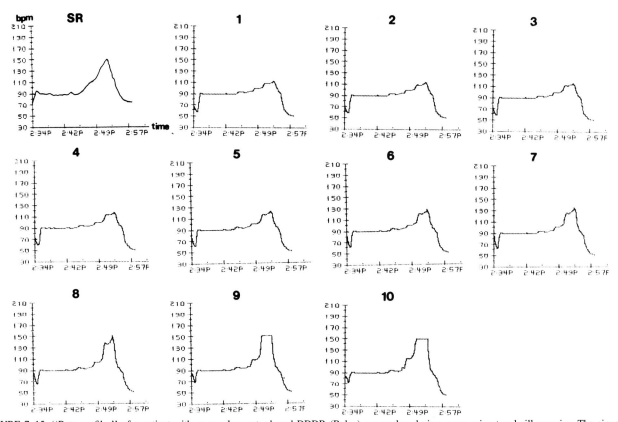

FIGURE 7–15. "Rate profiles" of a patient with an accelerometer-based DDDR (Relay) pacemaker during progressive treadmill exercise. The sinus rate (SR) is depicted in the upper left hand corner. Profiles 1 to 10 represent the calculated rate responses when the rate-adaptive slope is programmed as 1 to 10. Note that the main effect of increasing the rate-adaptive slope is on the rate response at the higher workload. A slope of 7 to 8 best simulates the SR during this exercise. (From Lau CP, Tai YT, Fong PC, et al: Clinical experience with an accelerometer-based activity-sensing dual-chamber rate-adaptive pacemaker. PACE 15:334, 1992.)

lay).[74] The duration of rate recording is programmable (15 minutes to 24 hours), and the recording can be continuous or frozen in memory once the programmed data collection period ends. Both the sensor-indicated pacing rate (calculated rate profile) and the actual heart rate can be obtained. It is also possible to display a simulation of the pacing rate profile that would have been produced with the same activity at different programmed rate-adaptive slopes, so that the optimum slope can be selected with a single exercise test (Fig. 7–15).

VALUE OF "CORRECT" RATE-ADAPTIVE PARAMETER PROGRAMMING

When programming in patients with rate-adaptive pacemakers is either above or below the "optimum" values, subjective well-being may be adversely affected.[90] Among 10 patients with activity-sensing, rate-adaptive pacemakers who were randomly programmed to the VVI mode, the VVIR mode with standard slope, or the VVIR mode with an excessively sensitive rate-adaptive slope, many requested early crossover from the VVI and the overprogrammed VVIR modes. Objective treadmill exercise tolerance was lowest in the VVI mode but no different between the two VVIR modes. A similar decrease in general well-being was observed with the dual chamber rate-adaptive modes, although objective differences in exercise tolerance were similar between DDD, DDDR, and an overprogrammed DDDR mode (Fig. 7–16). When a minute ventilation–sensing pacemaker was programmed to two different rate-response slopes (RRF equal to 23 and 25), it was shown that the anaerobic threshold was significantly enhanced by the higher slope (oxygen consumption at anaerobic threshold improved from 10.6 to 11.6 ml/kg per minute), with normalization of the minute ventilation–to–heart rate ratio compared with controls. Although both rate-adaptive settings were superior to fixed-rate pacing during exercise, the slight change in rate-response slope significantly improved anaerobic threshold and chronotropic competence during submaximal exercise.

How Often Is Rate Response Actually Required?

In the broadest sense, a rate-adaptive pacemaker should be considered for all patients who require pacing. For patients with complete AV block, the VDD and DDD pacing modes provide both rate modulation and AV synchrony in the presence of normal sinoatrial nodal function. Thus, an artificial sensor is not a requirement for rate-adaptive pacing. On the other hand, patients with chronic atrial fibrillation or flutter with AV block cannot be managed with these dual-chamber pacing modes and are ideal candidates for VVIR pacing, especially if the ventricular rate is inappropriately slow during exercise. For patients in whom sinoatrial disease is the primary indication for pacing, the need for rate-adaptive pacing is more variable. Some individuals with sinus node dysfunction may demonstrate normal chronotropic response to exercise and require AAI pacing only to prevent sinus pauses. In contrast, others with sinus node dysfunction may have little or no chronotropic response to exercise and are ideal candidates for AAIR or DDDR pacemakers, depending on the status of AV conduction. It should be recognized that the overall pattern of chronotropic response in an individual may evolve over time, making predictions regarding the ultimate need for rate-adaptive pacing unreliable. Furthermore, the frequency of chronotropic incompetence depends on the method of assessment and the definition that is chosen (see Chapter 26). In general, it is our practice to provide rate modulation and AV synchrony whenever possible to all patients who require permanent pacemakers. The sinus node is given priority as the primary modulator of heart rate when its function is unimpaired. For patients with paroxysmal or chronic atrial arrhythmias, a rate-adaptive pacing system that incorporates an artificial sensor is usually preferred, the choice of single- or dual-chamber pacing being dependent on the status of AV conduction and the frequency of atrial tachyarrhythmias.

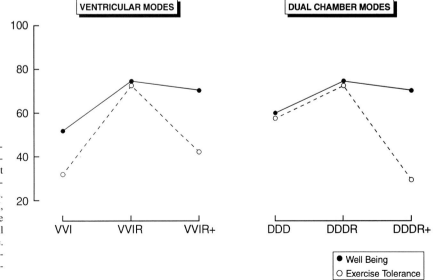

FIGURE 7–16. Subjective exercise tolerance and general well-being scores in 10 patients with activity-sensing DDDR pacemakers programmed at different modes. VVIR+ and DDDR+ represent overprogrammed rate-adaptive parameters in these modes. General well-being scores were lowest in the VVI, VVIR+, and DDDR+ modes. Subjective exercise tolerance (which correlates with objective treadmill exercise results) was decreased only in the VVI mode. (Redrawn from Sulke N, Dritsas A, Chambers J, Sowton E: Is accurate rate response programming necessary? PACE 13:1031, 1990.)

FORMAL EXERCISE TESTING

Most reported series have had a tendency to include pacemaker-dependent patients for assessment of the benefits of rate-adaptive pacing. Rickards and Donaldson estimated that about 55% of patients requiring permanent pacing may need additional chronotropic support for exercise.[91] In a recent review, Rosenqvist reported that an average of 40% (range, 28% to 50%) of patients with sinoatrial disease will need an artificial rate-adaptive sensor.[92] Chronotropic incompetence was found in 58% of patients (22 of 38) in another study that defined chronotropic incompetence as the inability to increase the heart rate above 80% of the age-predicted maximum.[93] Spontaneous variability of chronotropic incompetence over time is well recognized. Thus, a rate-adaptive sensor is likely to be required during exercise in nearly half of patients with pacemakers.

HOLTER RECORDING

Holter monitoring has not been widely used as a means of diagnosing chronotropic incompetence because of the lack of a consistent range of metabolic workloads performed during a 24-hour period. For example, in a study of 24 patients with sinoatrial disease who were referred for permanent pacing, the minimum, average, and maximum heart rates on Holter recordings were found to be 36, 51, and 100 bpm, respectively.[94] When these patients were exercised with the Bruce treadmill protocol, it was shown that they achieved 87% of their age-predicted maximum heart rate, and 49% of this increase occurred within the first stage of exercise. The normal sinus rate remained near the resting value most of the day, and the need for a rate response occurred during only a small proportion of the usual 24-hour period[83] (see Figs. 7–11 and 7–12).

One study attempted to quantify the rate responses observed with three different rate-adaptive pacemakers using full-disclosure Holter analysis.[95] Overall, rate response was active for less than 15% of the 24-hour study period. A moderate rate response (>100 bpm) was observed for 5% of the day, especially in the evening hours (4 to 8 PM). The magnitude of rate response otherwise was small (<100 bpm). In addition, the level of rate response was less for patients who were not pacemaker dependent. The percentage of the day showing a moderate rate response was higher for patients who had minute ventilation–sensing and activity-sensing pacemakers than for those with QT-sensing pacemakers.

STATISTICAL VERSUS FUNCTIONAL NEED FOR A RATE-ADAPTIVE SENSOR

Although chronotropic incompetence can be easily defined using statistical methods from a normal population, it does not necessarily follow that patients who fall outside the range of normal will derive benefit from rate-adaptive pacing. Perhaps the most clinically relevant definition of chronotropic incompetence is an abnormal response of the heart rate to changing metabolic demands that, when corrected, results in functional improvement.[96] In terms of maximal exercise capacity, reversal of chronotropic incompetence by pacing may improve exercise tolerance in only about 50% of patients. In one study, only 10 of 17 patients with severe chronotropic incompetence (maximum rate <100 bpm) derived clinical benefit from implantation of a rate-adaptive pacemaker.[97] In another study, 3 of 12 patients with chronotropic incompetence who were paced in the AAIR mode achieved no benefit compared with AAI pacing during exercise.[98] These observations may suggest that multiple compensatory mechanisms are operative during exercise, and exercise duration may not be the most sensitive indicator of chronotropic incompetence. Other methods such as the measurement of cardiac output and respiratory gas exchange during exercise may unmask more subtle benefits of rate-adaptive pacing.

Limitations and Adverse Effects of Rate-Adaptive Pacing

Rate-adaptive pacing is a rapidly developing field, in which many manufacturers are introducing new devices. It is therefore not surprising that a number of complications have been observed, especially with some of the early investigational models. The types of complications are summarized in Table 7–11. An overview is presented here because limitations of individual sensors will be separately detailed in succeeding chapters.

IMPLANTATION-RELATED COMPLICATIONS

In the early version of respiratory rate–sensing pacemakers (Biorate [Biotec, S.P.A., Bologna, Italy]), a subcutaneous auxiliary electrode was used to measure impedance to detect respiratory rate. This additional electrode could erode through the skin, requiring pacemaker replacement.[99] Early rate-adaptive pulse generators were bulky. For example, the mass of an early P-wave synchronous pulse generator (model RS4-SRT, Cardiac Pacemakers Inc.)[100] and the first DDDR pacemaker[101] were 82 g and 95 g, respectively. Although no specific complications during implantation and follow-up of these pacemakers were reported, the large size of these devices required a very large subcutaneous pocket. Size is no longer an important issue for rate-adaptive pacemakers because the newer devices are smaller and do not entail more difficult implantation.

SENSOR-RELATED COMPLICATIONS

It is useful to consider sensor-related complications in terms of the characteristics of an ideal sensor: speed, proportionality, sensitivity, and specificity. Any departure from these ideal characteristics may constitute a sensor-related complication in the broad sense. These limitations will be discussed in subsequent chapters.

TABLE 7–11. MAJOR CLASSES OF COMPLICATIONS AND INTERFERENCE ENCOUNTERED WITH RATE-ADAPTIVE PACING

1. Implantation-related
2. Sensor-related
3. Patient-related
4. Pacing mode– or programming-related
5. Technical problems
6. Pacemaker-mediated tachycardias

PATIENT-RELATED COMPLICATIONS

Certain clinical characteristics that are preexisting or develop after implantation may result in complications with rate-adaptive pacemakers. The QT interval is affected by myocardial ischemia and drugs. During myocardial infarction, QT-sensing pacemakers may either increase the pacing rate owing to increased sympathetic activity from congestive heart failure[102] or decrease the pacing rate owing to the effect of increased vagal tone on the QT interval.[103] Beta blockers can also cause a paradoxical increase in rate with pacemakers that sense the PDI.[104] These factors should always be considered in patients receiving pacemakers based on these principles.

During advanced heart failure, Cheyne-Stokes respirations may result in an unphysiologic tachycardia with minute ventilation–sensing pacemakers, resulting in a vicious circle that further aggravates heart failure.[38] The presence of chronic or acute lung problems may also cause undesirable rate acceleration with this type of sensor. A theoretical vicious cycle may also be established in a stroke volume sensor during heart failure. The increase in right ventricular volume resulting from myocardial failure would lead to an inappropriate rate increase, which might in turn aggravate the existing heart failure. The ability of rate-adaptive pacing to increase the heart rate has been shown to enhance cardiac output without increasing myocardial oxygen consumption compared to VVI pacing.[105] However, if the lower and upper rates and the rate-adaptive settings are not appropriately programmed, worsening of angina in patients with underlying heart disease may result.[85]

PACING MODE AND PROGRAMMING-RELATED COMPLICATIONS

A correct choice of pacing mode for different patient populations is crucial to optimize pacemaker function. An incorrect pacing mode prescription may result in complications. For example, if the status of AV conduction is not assessed prior to instituting AAIR pacing, advanced AV block may develop. Besides the possibility of AV block, the paced PR interval during AAIR pacing is also important. A markedly prolonged PR interval may cause the P wave to occur near the preceding R wave, resulting in a form of ''AAIR pacemaker syndrome.''[106–109] The influence of AV nodal blocking agents and class I antiarrhythmic agents should also be considered in this context.[109] This may be especially important for AAIR devices that are subject to false-positive increases in pacing rate (such as activity sensors).

Pacemaker syndrome is classically associated with VVI pacing, particularly in the presence of intact VA conduction. The VVIR pacing mode is also susceptible. This complication is avoided by the appropriate use of the DDDR mode. A number of sensor-based algorithms have been used to manage spontaneous atrial arrhythmias during DDDR pacing. In the presence of these arrhythmias, DDDR pacemakers may respond by automatically switching from the DDDR to the VVIR pacing mode (Telectronics Meta DDDR, model 1250). Mode switching may be effected either by an atrial ectopic beat that falls within the PVARP or by sinus tachycardia with a P wave that occurs during a long programmed PVARP.[110–111] Thus, AV dissociation and pacemaker syndrome may occur under either of these situations. A judiciously programmed PVARP is essential for this approach,[110] and the use of a more specific algorithm to detect pathologic tachycardia rather than relying on the occurrence of an atrial event in the PVARP is likely to improve the usefulness of the mode-switching feature.

TECHNICAL PROBLEMS

Technical problems with rate-adaptive pacemakers can arise from the leads, the pulse generator, or the sensor itself. The detection of the evoked QRS complex (QT interval and paced depolarization gradient) is significantly affected by electrode polarization. This resulted in failure of T-wave sensing in the early QT-sensing devices.[112–113] This problem is minimized with the use of low-polarization electrodes and specialized charge-balancing output pulses. Some sensors, such as the monitoring of pH, temperature, and the first derivative of right ventricular pressure (dP/dt), require special sensors that are incorporated into the pacing leads. Some of these investigational devices have been associated with a significant risk of lead failure. In an early report of seven patients with the pH-sensing pacemaker,[114] three devices were not functional because of lead failure. Early temperature-sensing pacing systems were also beset with lead complications.[115] Electrostatic discharges generated by opening the wrapping on the early dP/dt sensing leads could damage the sensor. This problem has been corrected by using different protective packaging in newer generations of these leads. Fibrin coating may affect the performance of the S$\bar{v}$O$_2$ sensor. This effect can be reduced by measuring the ratio of the reflectance of two wavelengths of light, thereby compensating for decreased light transmission.[116] Nevertheless, the long-term stability of these specialized sensors remains a persistent concern.

A number of sensor failures have been reported. In the early version of the PDI pacemaker (Prism-CL [Telectronics]), the range of the ''rate control factor'' (the target PDI to be achieved) was not optimally set, and this VVIR pacemaker often reverted to VVI pacing mode once the target rate-control factor was exceeded. Erratic pacing occurs in up to 10% of patients with a respiratory rate–sensing pacemaker (Biorate).[117] When the rate-response factor was assessed by telemetry during exercise in the DDDR mode, upper rate VVIR pacing developed, and the telemetry link was terminated. The sensor-mediated tachycardia of this device can be controlled with magnet application, which reverts the pulse generator to the VOO pacing at the magnet rate (99 bpm). These failures required pacemaker replacement, and the problem has been solved in the newer version of this device. A sensor problem resulting in inappropriate tachycardia was also reported in an early piezoelectric sensing device (Sensolog).[70] An error in rate-reprofiling software in the programmer occurred in an accelerometer-sensing pacemaker (Relay), allowing the calculated rate to be above the programmed upper rate. This error occurred only in the calculation but not in the actual pacemaker performance and has been corrected.

PACEMAKER-MEDIATED TACHYCARDIAS

Although pacemaker-mediated tachycardias are classically described with dual chamber pacemakers, rate-adaptive devices are not immune to this phenomenon.[118] In the broadest definition, sensor-mediated tachycardias occur when the sensor-determined rate is higher than the requirement dictated by the physiologic state. This may result from technical problems, inappropriate programming, or lack of specificity of the sensor. An example is the effect of interference on activity-sensing pacemakers by various forms of transport. These tachycardias terminate once the sources of interference are removed.

A special type of sensor-mediated tachycardia involves a "positive" feedback loop. In this tachycardia, sensor activation leads to an increase in pacing rate, which in turn further activates the sensor. Examples of this self-perpetuating tachycardia include the rate "oscillation" observed with the early generation QT pacemakers,[36] Cheyne-Stokes breathing with respiratory rate–sensing pacemakers,[38] and application of pressure over the pulse generator pocket of activity-sensing pacemakers.[39] Most cases of pacemaker-mediated tachycardia due to a rate-adaptive sensor can be corrected by making the appropriate adjustment of the rate-modulating parameters. The use of multisensor pacing may further reduce this problem.

Conclusion

Significant advances in rate-adaptive pacing have occurred since its inception, with respect both to the number of sensors available and the pacing modes that are offered. Technical innovations avoid many of the earlier sensor-related problems. Multisensor pacing may further enhance the properties of rate-adaptive pacing systems, including applications for purposes other than rate augmentation.

REFERENCES

1. Loeppky JA, Greene ER, Hoekenga DE, et al: Beat-by-beat stroke volume assessment by pulsed Doppler in upright and supine exercise. J Appl Physiol 50:1173, 1981.
2. Miyamoto Y: Transient changes in ventilation and cardiac output at the start and end of exercise. Jpn J Physiol 31:149, 1981.
3. Higginbotham MB, Morris KG, Williams RS, et al: Regulation of stroke volume during submaximal and maximal upright exercise in normal man. Circ Res 58:281, 1986.
4. Cardus D, Spenser WA: Recovery time of heart frequency in healthy men: Its relations to age and physical condition. Arch Phys Med 48:71, 1967.
5. Astrand P, Rodahl K: Textbook of Work Physiology: Physiological Basis of Exercise, 3rd ed. New York, McGraw-Hill, 1986, pp 260–261.
6. Longhurst JC, Kelley AR, Gonyea WJ, Michell JH: Cardiovascular responses to static exercise in distance runners and weight lifters. J Appl Physiol 49:676, 1980.
7. Neumann G, Grube E, Leschhorn JE, et al: Symptoms control and psychosocial rehabilitation of chronic pacemaker patients with different pacing modes. In Steinback K, Glogar D, Laczkovics A (eds): Cardiac Pacing, Proceedings of the VIIth World Symposium on Cardiac Pacing. Darmstadt, Steinkopff Verlag, 1983, pp 455–461.
8. Lau CP: The range of sensors and algorithms used in rate adaptive pacing [Review]. PACE 15:1177, 1992.
9. Rickards AF, Donaldson RM: Rate-responsive pacing. Clin Prog Pacing Electrophysiol 1:12, 1983.
10. Rickards AF, Norman J: Relation between QT interval and heart rate: New design of physiologically adaptive cardiac pacemaker. Br Heart J 45:56, 1981.
11. Rossi P, Plicchi G, Canducci G, et al: Respiratory rate as a determinant of optimal pacing rate. PACE 6:502, 1983.
12. Rossi P, Plicchi G, Canducci G, et al: Respiration as a reliable physiological sensor for the control of cardiac pacing rate. Br Heart J 51:7, 1984.
13. Nappholtz T, Valenta H, Maloney J, Simmons T: Electrode configurations for respiratory impedance measurement suitable for rate-responsive pacing. PACE 9:960, 1986.
14. Lau CP, Antoniou A, Ward DE, Camm AJ: Initial clinical experience with a minute ventilation–sensing rate modulated pacemaker: Improvements in exercise capacity and symptomatology. PACE 11:1815, 1988.
15. Mond H, Strathmore N, Kertes P, et al: Rate-responsive pacing using a minute ventilation sensor. PACE 11:1866, 1988.
16. Goldreyer BN, Olive AL, Leslie J, et al: A new orthogonal lead for P synchronous pacing. PACE 4:638, 1981.
17. Griffin JC, Jutzy KR, Claude JP, Knoutti JW: Central body temperature as a guide to optimal heart rate. PACE 6:498, 1983.
18. Alt E, Hirgstetter C, Heinz M, Blomer H: Rate control of physiologic pacemakers by central venous blood temperature. Circulation 73:1206, 1986.
19. Fearnot NE, Smith HJ, Sellers D, Boal B: Evaluation of the temperature response to exercise testing in patients with single-chamber, rate-adaptive pacemakers: A multicentre study. PACE 12:1806, 1989.
20. Cammilli L, Alcidi L, Papeschi G: A new pacemaker autoregulating the rate of pacing in relation to metabolic needs. In Watanabe Y (ed): Proceedings of the Vth International Symposium, Tokyo. Amsterdam, Excerpta Medica, 1976, pp 414–419.
20a. Cammilli L, Alcidi L, Papeschi G: Un huoro pacemaker sensible alle necessita metaboliche. Osped Ital Chir 28:85, 1975.
21. Salo RW, Pederson BD, Olive AL, et al: Continuous ventricular volume assessment for diagnosis and pacemaker control. PACE 7:1267, 1984.
22. Chirife R: Evaluation of systolic time interval as physiologic signals for rate-responsive pacing [Abstract]. PACE 10:1209, 1987.
23. Anderson KM, Moore AA: Sensors in pacing. PACE 9:954, 1986.
24. Wirtzfeld AL, Goedel-Meinen L, Bock T, et al: Central venous oxygen saturation for the control of automatic rate responsive pacing. PACE 5:829, 1982.
25. Humen DP, Kostuk WJ, Klein GJ: Activity-sensing, rate-responsive pacing: Improvement in myocardial performance with exercise. PACE 8:52, 1985.
26. Palmer G, de Bellis F, Solinas A, et al: Sensor-free physiological pacing. In Behrenbeck DW, Sowton E, Fontaine G, Winter UJ (eds): Cardiac Pacemakers. Darmstadt, Steinkopff Verlag, 1985, pp 781–785.
27. Pacela AF: Impedance pneumography—a survey of instrumentation technique. Med Biol Engin 4:1, 1965.
28. Van de Water JM, Mount B, Barela JR, et al: Monitoring the chest with impedance. Chest 64:597, 1973.
29. Rushmer RF, Crystal DK, Wagner C, Ellis RM: Intracardiac impedance plethysmography. Am J Physiol 174:171, 1953.
30. Sahakian AV, Tompkins WJ, Webster JG: Electrode motion artifacts in electrical impedance pneumography. IEEE Trans Bio Med Eng 32:448, 1985.
31. Lau CP, Ritchie D, Butrous GS, et al: Rate modulation by arm movements of the respiratory-dependent rate-responsive pacemaker. PACE 11:744, 1988.
32. Webb SC, Lewis LM, Morris-Thurgood JA, et al: Respiratory-dependent pacing: A dual response from a single sensor. PACE 11:730, 1988.
33. Callaghan F, Vollmann W, Livingston A, et al: The ventricular depolarization gradient: Effects of exercise, pacing rate, epinephrine, and intrinsic heart rate control on the right ventricular evoked response. PACE 12:1115, 1990.
34. Chirife R: Acquisition of hemodynamic data and sensor signals for rate control from standard pacing electrodes [Editorial]. PACE 14:1563, 1991.
35. Chirife R: Sensor for right ventricular volumes using the trailing edge voltage of a pulse generator output. PACE 14:1821, 1991.
36. Winter UJ, Behrenbeck DW, Candelon B, et al: Problems with the slope adjustment and rate adaptation in rate-responsive pacemakers: Oscillation phenomena and sudden rate jumps. In Behrenbeck DW, Sowton E, Fontaine G, Winter UJ (eds): Cardiac Pacemakers. Darmstadt, Steinkopff Verlag, 1985, pp 107–112.
37. Lau CP: Sensors and pacemaker mediated tachycardias [Editorial]. PACE 14:495, 1991.
38. Scanu P, Guilleman D, Grollier G, Potier JC: Inappropriate rate re-

sponse of the minute ventilation rate–responsive pacemaker in a patient with Cheyne-Stokes dyspnea [Letter to the editor]. PACE 12:1963, 1989.

39. Lau CP, Tai YT, Fong PC, et al: Pacemaker-mediated tachycardias in rate-responsive pacemaker. PACE 13:1575, 1990.
40. Gillette P: Critical analysis of sensors for physiological responsive pacing. PACE 7:1263, 1984.
41. Wen HK: A review of implantable sensors. PACE 6:482, 1983.
42. Lau CP, Tai YT, Fong PC, et al: The use of implantable sensors for the control of pacemaker-mediated tachycardias: A comparative evaluation between minute ventilation-sensing and acceleration-sensing dual-chamber rate-adaptive pacemakers. PACE 15:34, 1992.
43. Lau CP, Tai YT, Fong PC, et al: Atrial arrhythmia management with sensor controlled atrial refractory period and automatic mode switching in patients with minute ventilation-sensing, dual-chamber, rate-adaptive pacemakers. PACE 15:1504, 1992.
44. Lau CP, Butrous GS, Ward DE, Camm AJ: Comparison of exercise performance of six rate-adaptive right ventricular cardiac pacemakers. Am J Cardiol 63:833, 1989.
45. Wilkoff BL, Covey J, Blackburn G: A mathematical model of the cardiac chronotropic response to exercise. J Electrophysiol 3:176, 1989.
46. Baig MW, Wilson J, Boute W, et al: Improved pattern of rate responsiveness with dynamic slope setting for the QT sensing pacemaker. PACE 12:311, 1989.
47. Lau CP, Mehta D, Toff W, et al: Limitations of rate response of activity-sensing rate-responsive pacing to different forms of activity. PACE 11:141, 1988.
48. Lau CP, Wong CK, Cheng CH, Leung WH: Importance of heart rate modulation on cardiac hemodynamics during post-exercise recovery. PACE 13:1277, 1990.
49. Alt E, Matula M, Thilo R, et al: A new mechanical sensor for detecting body activity and posture, suitable for rate-responsive pacing. PACE 11:1875, 1988.
50. Paul V, Garrett C, Ward DE, Camm AJ: Closed-loop control of rate-adaptive pacing: Clinical assessment of a system analysing the ventricular depolarization gradient. PACE 12:1896, 1989.
51. Ruiter JH, Heemels JP, Kee D, et al: Adaptive rate pacing controlled by the right ventricular preejection interval: Clinical experience with a physiological pacing system. PACE 15:886, 1992.
52. Ovsyshcher I, Gutta V, Bondy C, et al: First derivative of right ventricular pressure, dP/dt, as a sensor for a rate-adaptive VVI pacemaker. PACE 15:211, 1992.
53. Bennett T, Sharma A, Sutton R, et al: Development of a rate-adaptive pacemaker based on the maximum rate-of-rise of right ventricular pressure (RV dP/dt max). PACE 15:219, 1992.
54. Edelstam C, Hedman A, Nordlander R, Pehrsson SK: QT-sensing rate-responsive pacing and myocardial infarction. PACE 12:502, 1989.
55. Lau CP, Ritchie D, Butrous GS, et al: Rate modulation by arm movements of the respiratory-dependent rate-responsive pacemaker. PACE 11:744, 1988.
56. Lau CP, Ward DE, Camm AJ: Single-chamber cardiac pacing with two forms of respiration-controlled rate-responsive pacemakers. Chest 95:352, 1989.
57. Von Hemel NM, Hamerlijnck RPHM, Pronk KJ, van der Veen EDP: Upper limit ventricular stimulation in respiratory rate responsive pacing due to electrocautery. PACE 12:1720, 1989.
58. Alt E, Theres H, Heinz M, et al: A new rate-modulated pacemaker system optimized by combination of two sensors. PACE 11:1119, 1988.
59. Landman MAJ, Senden PJ, van Pooijen, et al: Initial clinical experience with rate-adaptive cardiac pacing using two sensors simultaneously. PACE 13:1615, 1990.
60. Rickards AF: Initial experience with a new single-chamber dual-sensor rate-responsive pacemaker [Abstract]. Eur J Cardiovasc Electrophysiol 2:A23, 1992.
61. Lau CP, Rushby J, Leigh-Jones M, et al: Symptomatology and quality of life in patients with rate-responsive pacemakers: A double-blind crossover study. Clin Cardiol 12:505, 1989.
62. Romisowsky S: Psychological adaptation patterns in response to cardiac surgery. J Rehabil 46:50, 1980.
63. Hayes DL, Christiansen JR, Vlietstra RE, Osborn MJ: Follow-up of an activity-sensing, rate-modulated pacing device, including transtelephonic exercise assessment. Mayo Clin Proc 64:503, 1989.
64. Ahern T, Nydegger C, McCormick DJ, et al: Incidence and timing of activity parameter changes in activity-responsive pacing systems. PACE 15:762, 1992.

65. Alt E: A protocol for treadmill and bicycle stress testing designed for pacemaker patients. Stimucoeur 15:33, 1987.
66. Zegelman M, Winter UJ, Alt E, et al: Effect of different body-exercise modes on the rate response of the temperature-control pacemaker Nova MR. Thorac Cardiovasc Surg 38:181, 1990.
67. Lau CP, Leung WH, Wong CK, et al: Adaptive rate pacing at submaximal exercise: The importance of the programmed upper rate. J Electrophysiol 3:283, 1989.
68. Hayes DL, Von Feldt L, Higano ST: Standardized informal exercise testing for programming rate-adaptive pacemakers. PACE 14:1772, 1991.
69. Zegelman M, Sammer P, Treese N, et al: CPX versus step test—simple is better [Abstract]. PACE 15:576, 1992.
70. Lau CP, Tse WS, Camm AJ: Clinical experience with Sensolog 703: A new activity-sensing, rate-responsive pacemaker. PACE 11:1444, 1988.
71. Mahaux V, Waleffe A, Kulbertus HE: Clinical experience with a new activity-sensing, rate-modulated pacemaker using autoprogrammability. PACE 12:1362, 1989.
72. Hayes DL, Higano ST: Utility of rate histograms in programming and follow up of a DDDR pacemaker. Mayo Clin Proc 64:495, 1989.
73. Lau CP: Activity-sensing rate-responsive pacing [Letter to the editor]. PACE 13:819, 1990.
74. Lau CP, Tai YT, Fong PC, et al: Clinical experience with an accelerometer-based activity-sensing dual-chamber rate-adaptive pacemaker. PACE 15:334, 1992.
75. Lau CP, Antoniou A, Ward DE, Camm AJ: Initial clinical experience with a minute ventilation–sensing, rate-modulated pacemaker: Improvements in exercise capacity and symptomatology. PACE 11:1815, 1988.
76. Baig MW, Boute W, Begeman M, Perrins EJ: One-year follow-up of automatic adaptation of the rate response algorithm of the QT sensing, rate-adaptive pacemaker. PACE 14:1598, 1991.
77. Ruiter J, Burgersdij K, Zeeders M, Kee D: Atrial Activitrax pacing: The atrioventricular interval during exercise [Abstract]. PACE 10:1226, 1987.
78. Clarke M, Allan A: Rate-responsive atrial pacing resulting in pacemaker syndrome [Abstract]. PACE 10:1209, 1987.
79. Den Dulk K, Lindemens FW, Brugada P, et al: Pacemaker syndrome with AAI rate variable pacing: Importance of atrioventricular conduction properties, medication, and pacemaker programmability. PACE 11:1226, 1988.
80. Mitsui T, Hori M, Suma K, Saigusa M. Optimal heart rate in cardiac pacing in coronary sclerosis and non-sclerosis. Ann NY Acad Sci 167:745, 1969.
81. Swinehart JM, Recker RR: Tachycardia and nightmares. Nebr Med J 58:314, 1973.
82. Nordlander R, Hedman A, Pehrsson JK: Rate-responsive pacing and exercise capacity [Editorial]. PACE 12:749, 1989.
83. Kristensson B, Karlsson O, Rydén L: Holter-monitored heart rhythm during atrioventricular synchronous and fixed-rate ventricular pacing. PACE 9:511, 1986.
84. Kristensson BE, Arnman K, Ryden L: Atrial synchronous ventricular pacing in ischaemic heart disease. Eur Heart J 4:668, 1983.
85. De Cock CC, Panis JHC, Van Eenigl MJ, Roos JP: Efficacy and safety of rate-responsive pacing in patients with coronary artery disease and angina pectoris. PACE 12:1405, 1989.
86. Kenny RA, Ingram A, Mitsuoka T, et al: Optimum pacing mode for patients with angina. Br Heart J 56:463, 1986.
87. Leung SK, Choi YC, Lau CP, et al: Does the programmed low rate affect the rate response in rate-adaptive pacemakers [Abstract]? PACE 15:579, 1992.
88. Eisenger G, Hayes DL, Higano ST: Use of long-term and short-term histograms to optimize rate response parameters [Abstract]. Proceedings of Cardiostim 90. RBM 12:18, 1990.
89. Sermati S, Marconi M, Marzaloni M: Usefulness of 1-hour and 24-hour heart rate Holter inbuilt in new TX rate-adaptive pacemakers. PACE 13:1751, 1990.
90. Sulke N, Dritsas A, Chambers J, Sowton E: Is accurate rate response programming necessary? PACE 13:1031, 1990.
91. Rickards AF, Donaldson RM: Rate-responsive pacing. Clin Prog Pacing Electrophysiol 1:12, 1983.
92. Rosenqvist M: Atrial pacing for sick sinus syndrome. Clin Cardiol 13:43, 1990.
93. Gwinn N, Lemen R, Kratz J, et al: Chronotropic incompetence: A common and progressive finding in pacemaker patients. Am Heart J 123:1216, 1992.

94. Prior M, Masterson M, Morant VA, et al: Do patients with sinus node dysfunction and permanent pacemakers require an additional chronotropic sensor [Abstract]? PACE 10:418, 1987.
95. Sulke N, Pipilis A, Bucknall C, Sowton E: Quantitative analysis of contribution of rate response in three different ventricular rate-responsive pacemakers during out of hospital activity. PACE 13:37, 1990.
96. Holden W, McAnulty JH, Rahimtoola SH: Characteristics of heart rate response to exercise in sick sinus syndrome. Br Heart J 40:923, 1978.
97. Sutton R, Travill C, Fitzpatrick A: DDDR pacing in severe chronotropic incompetence [Abstract]. RBM 12:56, 1990.
98. Rosenqvist M, Aren C, Kristensson BE, et al: Atrial rate-responsive pacing in sinus node disease. Eur Heart J 11:537, 1990.
99. Lau CP, Ward DE, Camm AJ: Rate-responsive pacing with a pacemaker that detects the respiratory rate: Clinical advantages and complications. Clin Cardiol 11:318, 1988.
100. Ramsdale DR, Charles RG: Rate-responsive ventricular pacing: Clinical experience with the RS4-SRT pacing system. PACE 8:378, 1985.
101. Kappenberger LJ, Herpers L: Rate-responsive dual-chamber pacing. PACE 9:987, 1986.
102. Edelstam C, Hedman A, Nordlander R, Pehrsson SK: QT sensing rate-responsive pacing and myocardial infarction. PACE 12:502, 1989.
103. Robbens EJ, Clement DL, Jordaens LJ: QT-related rate-responsive pacing during acute myocardial infarction. PACE 11:339, 1988.
104. Lasaridis K, Paul VE, Katritsis D, et al: Influence of propranolol on the ventricular depolarization gradient. PACE 14:787, 1991.
105. Hedman A, Hjemdahl P, Nordlander R, et al: Effects of mental and physical stress on cardiac sympathetic nerve activity during QT-interval–sensing rate-responsive and fixed-rate ventricular inhibited pacing. Eur Heart J 11:903, 1990.
106. Clarke M, Allan A: Rate-responsive atrial pacing resulting in pacemaker syndrome [Abstract]. PACE 10:1209, 1987.
107. Ruiter J, Burgersdij K, Zeeders M, Kee D: Atrial Activitrax pacing: The atrioventricular interval during exercise [Abstract]. PACE 10:1226, 1987.
108. den Dulk K, Lindemens FW, Brugada P, et al: Pacemaker syndrome with AAI rate variable pacing: Importance of atrioventricular conduction properties, medication, and pacemaker programmability. PACE 11:1226, 1988.
109. Mabo P, Porillat C, Kermarrec A, et al: Lack of physiological adaptation of the atrioventricular interval to heart rate in patients chronically paced in the AAIR mode. PACE 14:2133, 1991.
110. Lau CP, Tai YT, Fong PC, et al: Atrial arrhythmia management with sensor-controlled atrial refractory period and automatic mode switching in patients with minute ventilation-sensing dual-chamber rate-adaptive pacemakers. PACE 15:1504, 1992.
111. Vanerio G, Patel S, Ching E, et al: Early clinical experience with a minute ventilation sensor DDDR pacemaker. PACE 14:1815, 1991.
112. Fananapazir L, Rodemaker M, Bennett DH: Reliability of the evoked response in determining the paced ventricular rate and performance of the QT or rate-responsive (TX) pacemaker. PACE 8:701, 1985.
113. Maisch B, Langenfeld H: Rate-adaptive pacing—clinical experience with three different pacing systems. PACE 9:997, 1986.
114. Cammilli L, Alcidi L, Shapland E, Obino S: Results, problems, and perspectives with the autoregulating pacemaker. PACE 6:488, 1983.
115. Laczkovics A, Laufer G, Ohner TH, Schlick W: First clinical results with a temperature-guided rate-responsive pacemaker [Abstract]. PACE 10:1216, 1987.
116. Wirtzfeld AL, Goedel-Meinen L, Bock T, et al: Central venous oxygen saturation for control of automatic rate-responsive pacing. PACE 5:829, 1985.
117. Rossi P, Prando MD, Magnani A, et al: Physiological sensitivity of respiratory-independent cardiac pacing: Four-year follow-up. PACE 11:1267, 1988.
118. Lau CP: The range of sensors and algorithms used in rate-adaptive cardiac pacing. PACE 15:1177, 1992.

CHAPTER 8

ACTIVITY-SENSING, RATE-ADAPTIVE PACEMAKERS

David G. Benditt
James L. Duncan

Among the most important functions of the cardiovascular system is the appropriate adjustment of cardiac output during rest, periods of increased physical exertion, and emotional or metabolic stress. Excluding the contributing peripheral vascular responses to exercise, modulation of cardiac output is achieved by a change in both heart rate (chronotropic response) and myocardial contractility (inotropic response). When greater cardiac output is needed, an increase in heart rate is the dominant contributor, providing approximately 66% to 80% of the total increase in cardiac output for the normal heart.[1–5]

Initially, cardiac pacemakers were incapable of providing the pacemaker-dependent patient with any increase in heart rate during periods of physiologic stress. The exclusive function of the first pacing modes (VOO/AOO, VVI/AAI, and VVT/AAT) was the prevention of bradycardia. These pacemakers provided a minimum pacing rate below which the heart rate was not permitted to fall. As technology advanced and the importance of rate augmentation for exercise tolerance became recognized, chronotropic responsiveness was provided by pacemakers that sensed the intrinsic atrial electrogram and synchronously paced the ventricle (VAT, VDD, and DDD modes).[6, 7] As long as the sinus node provided an appropriate chronotropic response, these "atrial-tracking" modes afforded an appropriate ventricular pacing response for patients with atrioventricular (AV) conduction system disease (within the programmed limitations of the pacemaker). However, atrial tracking does not furnish a normal chronotropic response for many patients with sinus node dysfunction.

The use of sensed parameters other than the intrinsic atrial rate (i.e., artificial sensors) to adjust the pacing rate of im-

plantable pulse generators was initially proposed by Krasner and colleagues[8] and later by Funke.[9] The specific use of an activity sensor for pacemaker rate augmentation was first described by Dahl[10] in 1979 (an accelerometer configuration) and later by Anderson and colleagues[11] in 1983 (a pressure-vibration configuration).

Initial Activity-Sensing, Rate-Adaptive Pacemakers

Although a variety of techniques can be used to estimate the magnitude of body activity, piezoelectric devices have been the most widely applied. These pacing systems have also been highly effective clinically.[3] Estimation of the intensity of physical activity by piezoelectric methods is an attractive concept for several reasons. First, because the concept of an activity sensor is easy to understand, it has been well accepted by physicians and patients alike. Second, the piezoelectric principle has been widespread in both medical and nonmedical applications (e.g., ultrasonic imaging and phonographs). Consequently, application of this concept to cardiac pacemakers did not raise concerns about the reliability of a "new" technologic development. Third, the approach is both inexpensive to implement and quite rugged (although bonding of the piezoceramic material to the pacemaker case has not been without potential pitfalls). Additionally, the piezoelectric method consumes very little energy from the battery, can be hermetically sealed within the pulse generator, and is compatible with conventional pacing leads in either the atrium or ventricle.

Activity sensors were first implemented clinically in an implantable pulse generator (Activitrax [Medtronic Inc., Minneapolis, MN]) by modifying an existing VDD pacemaker (Enertrax), which had been introduced in the early 1980s.[11-15] Because VDD pacemakers sense in both the atrium and the ventricle, the atrial channel was altered to respond to an electric signal from a piezoelectric element that was bonded to the inside of the pacemaker case rather than to the intrinsic atrial electrogram. Thus, this unique single-chamber pulse generator was controlled by the piezoelectric activity signal that was relayed to the atrial sensing amplifier. Instead of tracking the atrial electrogram, this device tracked the activity signal. Ten programmable slopes were available to control the sensor response. These so-called rate-response curves related electronically to the AV delay selections that had been present in the original VDD device. Additionally, three "activity thresholds" (low, medium, and high) could be programmed. These thresholds corresponded to the three original atrial sensitivity settings that had been present in the VDD pacemaker. These programmable activity thresholds provided flexibility for adjusting the sensitivity of the "activity" sense amplifier from patient to patient.[13-15] Numerous clinical reports attest to the reliability and appropriateness of the heart rate response of activity-based pacing systems.[13-22] However, *physical activity is not a direct indicator of metabolic demand.* The potential for false activation of the sensor by environmental stresses unrelated to physical activity[3, 22-24] and the inability of such systems to respond to metabolic stress not associated with physical movement are important limitations of these devices.[21-22, 24-26]

Almost 10 years have passed since activity sensors were introduced clinically for controlling the pacing rate of cardiac pacemakers. During this period, several other rate-adaptive sensors have been introduced as well. Nevertheless, on a worldwide basis the activity-based pacing systems have remained by far the most widely used. Furthermore, activity sensors not only have evolved in terms of clinical efficacy but also have been combined with other sensors in multisensor pacemaker applications.

Basic Concepts and Structure of Piezoelectric Activity Sensors

Piezoelectric elements may be natural materials (such as quartz) or can be produced synthetically as a ceramic (such as lead zirconate). For pacing applications, the piezoelectric element is typically a thin ceramic (approximate thickness 0.010 to 0.012 inch) that is bonded to the inside surface of the pacemaker case (Fig. 8–1). The ceramic material is metal-plated on both sides (nickel or gold) to provide a method for polarization of the crystal during manufacture and an electric connection to the monitoring electrodes. These electrodes are typically nickel wires that electrically connect the piezoelectric element to the circuitry of the pacemaker. The total surface area of the crystal is relatively large (in the range of 0.08 square inch) to provide a signal of sufficient strength to the activity-sensing circuit of the pulse generator.

Activity sensors using piezoelectric elements may be classified in a general sense as either the *accelerometer* or the

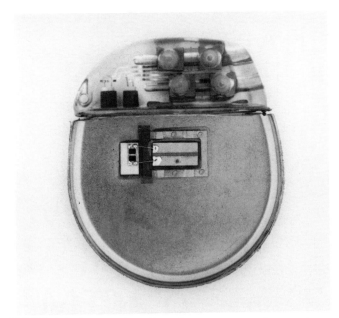

FIGURE 8–1. Cutaway view of a pulse generator case incorporating a piezoelectric activity sensor. The sensor is composed of a thin ceramic piezoelectric element that is bonded to the inside of the case. Two wires connect the sensor to the circuitry of the pulse generator.

pressure-vibration type. In both instances, physical movement elicits a small change in the structure of the piezoelectric element that changes its electric properties. The magnitude of the physical change in the piezoelectric element is usually related to the level of activity. Piezoelectric elements can be used in either of two ways as a physical activity detector. For example, deformation of the piezoelectric element may result in a change in the electric resistance of the piezoelectric material (*piezoresistance*) that can be identified by passing a low-level electric current through the material on a continuous or intermittent basis. However, piezoresistive sensors have the potential disadvantage of requiring a small amount of battery current to measure resistance. Therefore, an alternative property of piezoelectric materials is often used—the ability of the sensor itself to generate a small potential difference as a result of physical deformation. Because deformation of the piezoelectric sensor induces a voltage that is proportional to the degree of structural disturbance, measurement of these induced voltages permits estimation of the level of physical activity. This feature of piezoelectric ceramics, by virtue of their inherent energy conservation capabilities, has been the one favored for use in implanted rate-adaptive pacemakers.

In current clinical practice the pressure-vibration activity sensors have been by far the most commonly used (Fig. 8–2A). In this application, physical activity causes minute vibrations of the pacemaker case as pressure waves are transmitted to it from the body. The vibration results in a physical deformation of the piezoelectric element. An alternative approach has been to place the piezoelectric element on the circuit board in a cantilevered fashion to monitor accelerations in a single plane (see Fig. 8–2B), or, alternatively to use a conductive ball within an enclosure with multiple contact points.[27-28] In both of these configurations, the sensor functions as an accelerometer measuring the forces resulting from body movement.

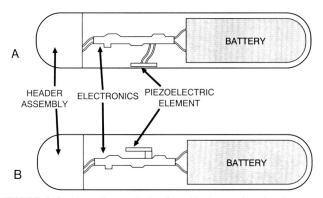

FIGURE 8–2. Alternative methods of positioning a piezoelectric sensor within a pulse generator. *A,* A traditional pressure-vibration sensor is bonded to the inside of the case. *B,* The piezoelectric element is bonded to the circuit board in a cantilevered fashion so that it is more sensitive to acceleration within a single plane.

In the usual application of activity-based sensor systems, pressure waves initiated in the skeleton and soft body tissues by physical activity result in a physical deformation of the piezoelectric element.[3, 11, 13–15, 27–29] The piezoelectric element is usually attached to the posterior surface of the pulse generator can during manufacturing so that it is positioned directly against the pectoralis major muscle to ensure good physical contact with the skeletal muscles. Although not advised, the pacemaker can be implanted with the sensor facing away from the muscle activity if the activity threshold can be programmed to compensate for the reduced signal amplitude with this orientation. Vibrations of the piezoelectric element induce electric potentials that are processed by the pacemaker to determine the appropriate pacing rate. As the level of physical activity increases, the amplitude of body vibrations also increases (Fig. 8–3). This results in greater deformation of the sensor element and production of a higher voltage. Generally, the piezoelectric element produces potentials in the range of 5 to 50 mV during rest and as much as 200 mV during vigorous activity.[12] The range of frequencies to which these systems are most sensitive is generally in the range of 10 Hz,[30] close to the typical resonant frequency of the human body.[31] Research using piezoelectric accelerometers suggests that physical activities produce pressure waves that are below 6 Hz, whereas most environmental interference occurs above 8 Hz for this sensor configuration.[32] Given

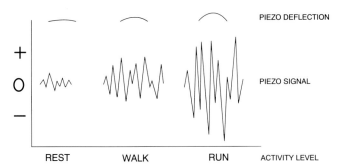

FIGURE 8–3. Electric signals generated by a piezoelectric sensor at rest, during walking, and during running. As the level of physical activity increases, the amplitude of body vibrations also increases. This results in greater flexion of the sensor element and production of a higher voltage. Potentials in the range of 5 to 50 mV may be recorded from an activity sensor during rest and may be as large as 200 mV during vigorous activity.

these signal characteristics, activity-based pacemakers using a piezoelectric element bonded to the inside of the pacemaker case appear to offer good correlation with upright physical movement involving walking or running.[14, 16, 18–20, 26, 33]

SIGNAL PROCESSING

Once the raw electric signal has been generated by the piezoelectric element, an algorithm must transduce the sensor output into clinically appropriate modulation of the pacing rate. Ultimately, the pacing rate should change in a manner that is proportional to the magnitude of the ''activity'' signal. Several options are available for accomplishing this goal. For example, the pacing rate could be made proportional to the peak amplitude of the piezoelectric signal. However, such a choice would leave the device susceptible to over-interpretation of large transient signals such as those produced by an abrupt slap on the back. Additionally, an algorithm that detected the peak sensor amplitude may be particularly susceptible to environmental factors such as the firmness of the ground on which the patient is walking or the material of the patient's shoes. Consequently, rather than simply assessing the amplitude of the induced signals, two separate processing methodologies have been developed. One group of devices counts the number of sensor signals that exceed a threshold amplitude per unit of time and provides an increase in the pacing rate that is proportional to the number of counts detected. This approach (which is discussed later under the section on the peak count system) allows two levels of flexibility. First, the minimum threshold amplitude for counted signals is a programmable setting, providing for patient-to-patient differences in the resonant characteristics of the body. The relationship between the number of counts detected per unit of time and the pacing rate can also be adjusted to provide further individualization of chronotropic response. An alternative strategy for activity sensors is to integrate the area under the activity signal derived from the sensor element (discussed later under the section on integration system). This approach also provides a threshold for instituting a change in pacing rate and a programmable slope of rate response according to the area under the activity curve. Because the integration method is also influenced by the number of counts detected, these two methods of processing the sensor signal tend to be similar in their effectiveness for many exercise workloads.

A critical element of signal processing with all rate-adaptive sensors is the ability of the sensor to distinguish those signals associated with physical exertion from those that are not. Discrimination of the desired signals from extraneous noise can be accomplished in two major ways. First, because the frequencies of signals related to physical exercise are often different from the frequencies of signals related to environmental interference, the sensor can be designed to respond to a desired frequency range. In the case of a rate-adaptive pacing system, the basic signal of interest is usually that associated with walking. However, the fundamental frequency of vibrations arising from walking (i.e., the walking rate) is itself an inadequate measure because of the somewhat higher frequency content associated with abrupt footfall. As a consequence, although slow to relatively fast walking may have a fundamental frequency of 1 to 4 Hz, the signal processing algorithm must be designed to encompass a wider range, usually up to 20 Hz or higher. In addition, the algorithm must exclude frequencies related to respiration (less than 1 Hz) and cardiac activity. The second method for improving signal-to-noise discrimination is to eliminate vibration signals below a threshold amplitude. As a rule, the amplitude of vibratory signals induced by walking or other comparable physical activities is greater than that associated with cardiac movement or other potentially confounding signals such as vehicular vibration or intention tremors. Consequently, establishing a threshold signal amplitude below which the device will not respond provides a relatively straightforward technique for separating signals associated with exercise from those that are not.

PEAK COUNT SYSTEM

The first rate-adaptive pulse generator to incorporate an activity sensor (Activitrax) used the peak counting method.[10, 13] Following initial filtering and amplification of the raw signal, the signal was passed through a threshold discriminator.[3, 15, 29, 32, 34, 35] Any energy deflections from the piezoelectric element that had an amplitude exceeding the programmed threshold were counted (Fig. 8–4). As described earlier, the three programmable activity thresholds in this device (low, medium, and high) were based on the three programmable atrial sensitivity thresholds of a VDD pacemaker. Later versions of this pacemaker increased the number of threshold selections to five. The peak counts could range from 0 to 15 per second, with 0 indicating a resting state and 15 reflecting a high level of activity.[34]

The processed count of the raw piezoelectric signal was passed through a programmable rate-modulation circuit that related the sensor output to a desired pacing rate. This circuit provided 10 separate "slope" or "rate-response" curves to control this sensor-pacing rate relationship (Fig. 8–5A). A rate-response curve of 1 provided the least change in pacing rate in response to an increase in the sensor output, whereas a rate-response curve of 10 resulted in the greatest increase in heart rate. Several of the lower programmed slopes provided an increase in heart rate with a curve that became relatively flat at higher activity levels. These rate-response curves resulted in the inability of the pacemaker to attain the programmed maximum sensor rate even with maximal exercise.[35] Later versions of this device provided a more linear

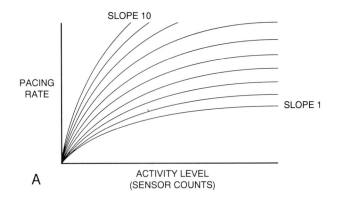

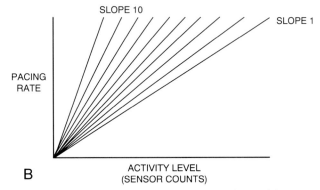

FIGURE 8–5. *A,* Original rate-adaptive algorithm of an activity sensor (Activitrax, [Medtronic]). This device provided 10 separate curves to relate output of the sensor (counts) to a change in pacing rate. A rate-response curve of 1 provided the least change in pacing rate in response to an increase in the sensor output, whereas a rate-response curve of 10 resulted in the greatest increase. Several of the lower programmed slopes provided an increase in heart rate with a curve that became relatively flat at higher activity levels. *B,* Later versions of activity sensors provided a more linear set of rate-response slopes.

set of rate-response slopes to correct this undesirable characteristic of rate modulation (see Fig. 8–5B).

The peak counting method is characterized by an algorithm that monitors the number of piezoelectric signals that exceed a programmable threshold (activity threshold). As the intensity of physical activity increases, further increases in the amplitude of the piezoelectric signal will not affect the rate response if the peak has already crossed the threshold (Fig. 8–6). This results in a sensor that characteristically responds to exercise in a relatively On or Off fashion.[30, 35] When a patient exercises, no rate response occurs until the amplitude of the piezoelectric signals exceeds the threshold. However, once this threshold has been passed, only increases in the number of the signals that are counted will result in an increase in the paced rate. Stangl and colleagues[30] reported that variation in the vibrational force applied to a peak counting sensor at a fixed frequency of 10 Hz increased the pacing rate to its maximum over a small range of forces. In clinical studies with this sensor, treadmill exercise testing with increasing speed (increasing step frequency) resulted in an incremental increase in the pacing rate. On the other hand, tests of patients on a treadmill at a constant speed of 3.2 km/hr with a changing incline from 0 to 15% resulted in an initial increase in pacing rate that subsequently leveled off and did not increase with further increases in workload. This

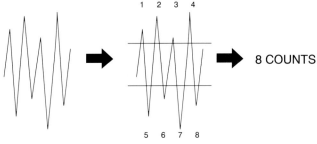

FIGURE 8–4. Effect of signal processing on sensor output. Note that in the peak counting method the number of deflections of the signal that exceed a programmable threshold value are counted. In this example, the raw signal exceeds the threshold eight times over the monitoring period, leading to a sensor output of eight counts.

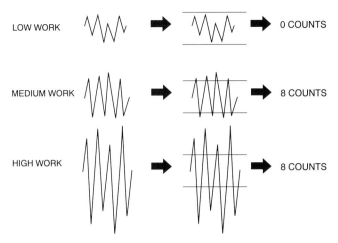

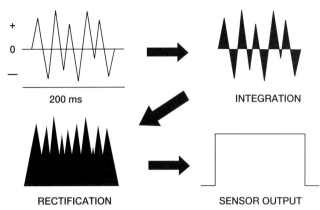

FIGURE 8–8. Integration method of signal processing. The raw activity signal *(upper left)* is processed by integrating the area under the curve inscribed by the sensor *(upper right)*. The integrated area is then rectified so that a uniform polarity is generated *(lower left)*. The rectified sensor signal is then converted into a square wave that is directly related in duration to the area under the curve.

FIGURE 8–6. Peak counting method of signal processing. Note that at low levels of exertion the amplitude of the sensor signals does not exceed the threshold amplitude, producing a sensor count of 0. At medium and high workloads the amplitude of the sensor signals increases. However, because this processing method counts only the number of threshold crossings, an identical sensor count is produced by medium and high workloads.

resulted in a weaker correlation between changes in pacing rate and changes in metabolic workload for this processing method (r = 0.2) compared with the integration method[30] (Fig. 8–7). On the other hand, Lau and associates[31] observed a more linear relation between oxygen consumption and pacing rate with the "peak count" method compared with the integration approach in patients who exercised using the Bruce protocol (r = 0.70 vs. r = 0.47).

INTEGRATION SYSTEM

The second technique for signal processing with a vibration activity sensor is the integration method[22, 28, 30, 35, 36] (Synchrony [Siemens-Pacesetter, Sylmar, CA]). The raw piezoelectric signal is integrated after initial filtering, amplification, and rectification (Fig. 8–8). All signals are used to determine the level of rate response because there is no amplitude

threshold that must be exceeded. The sensor is sampled for 200 msec after every sensed or paced ventricular complex. Following integration of the signal, the area under the curve of the piezoelectric signal is converted to a relative sensor number, which is directly related to the activity level of the patient (Fig. 8–9). As the activity level increases, the amplitude of the piezoelectric signals also increases, resulting in a greater area under the curve. By integrating the activity signals, the sensor output is influenced by increases in both signal frequency (step frequency) and amplitude.

The relative sensor number is then converted to a desired pacing rate by two programmable parameters, the threshold and the slope. In the integration method of signal processing, the threshold parameter is used in a different way from that used in the peak counting method. In the peak counting technique, the activity threshold is used as an integral part of the initial raw signal processing. In the integration technique, the threshold is used in the software algorithm to determine the desired pacing rate after initial signal processing has been

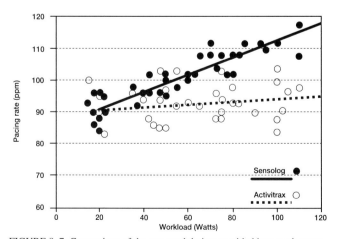

FIGURE 8–7. Comparison of the rate modulating provided by a peak counting algorithm (Activitrax) and an integration algorithm (Sensolog). Note that pacing rate is relatively independent of workload for the peak counting device, whereas the integration method provides a pacing rate that is related to workload.

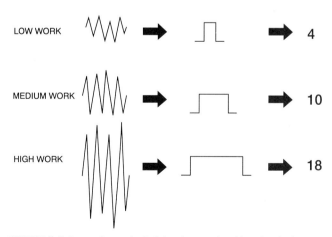

FIGURE 8–9. Integration method of signal processing. Note that the integration method is sensitive to both the frequency and amplitude of activity deflections. At low workloads a sensor count of 4 is generated. Note that the sensor output is related to workload, increasing to a count of 10 at medium workloads and 18 at high workloads.

completed. The selected threshold determines the minimum sensor area (sensor number) that is required before the device responds with a rate increase (Fig. 8–10). Once the sensor number exceeds this programmable threshold, the desired pacing rate is determined by the programmed slope. The devices currently available using the integration method provide 13 programmable threshold values. In addition, these devices also allow the pulse generator to automatically determine the activity threshold. The automatic threshold feature determines a running average sensor value over a period of 18 hours. This moving average is updated with each ventricular sensed or paced complex. There are four automatic threshold offset selections that can be programmed. These programmed automatic values add between 0 and 1.5 sensor units to the running average to determine the actual threshold used by the device for rate modulation. Because the average threshold approximates the resting activity level for most patients who are sedentary during most of the day, the offset values provide a means of reducing the responsiveness of the system. Sixteen slope settings that relate changes in the sensor output to changes in pacing rate are available, a value of 1 being the least responsive and 16 the most responsive (Fig. 8–11).

Prior research has confirmed the ability of the integration processing method to provide a linear response of pacing rate to exercise workload.[30, 36] However, the integration system also has the limitations inherent in all activity-based devices, such as false activation due to environmental vibrations[22] and diminished responsiveness to lower body exercise (i.e., bicycling) or nonactivity physiologic stress.[21, 22, 36]

RATE-ADAPTIVE ALGORITHMS

Perhaps the most useful and clinically important characteristic of an activity-based, rate-adaptive pacemaker is its ability to provide a prompt pacing response at the onset of physical activity. When physical activity begins, the device can identify the presence of the activity within one pacing cycle and determine the desired pacing rate according to the programmed threshold and slope settings. Although the *desired* pacing rate may change abruptly, there is a time delay between a change in the desired pacing rate and the change in the actual pacing rate. For example, if the onset of activity

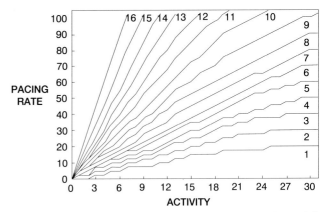

FIGURE 8–11. Relation of the sensor output to pacing rate of an activity sensor based on the integration method. A total of 16 slope curves relate the activity sensor output to a change in pacing rate.

results in the device calculating a desired pacing rate of 100 ppm, the pacemaker must use an algorithm to translate the change in desired pacing rate into a change in actual pacing rate. The rate-adaptive pacing algorithm incorporates an "acceleration" (also termed reaction) time that controls how fast the actual pacing rate can increase. In the currently available integration systems reaction times are programmable to 9, 18, 27, and 36 seconds, which correspond to the maximum time required to increase from a base rate of 60 ppm to a rate of 150 ppm. The peak count systems provide values of 15, 30, and 60 seconds, which correspond to the time required to achieve 90% of the difference between the programmed minimum and maximum rates. For the most part, these algorithms ensure development of an appropriately rapid heart rate response while preventing abrupt jumps in paced rate.

Following cessation of physical exertion, activity-based pulse generators are capable of promptly determining that no activity is present, thereby indicating that the device should return to its base rate. However, a dramatic drop in the paced rate would not be well tolerated by many patients. Therefore, these devices also incorporate "deceleration" (also termed recovery) times to smooth the return to the lower pacing rate. The integration devices provide recovery times of 2, 3.5, and 5 minutes, which correspond to the maximum time needed to decelerate from 150 ppm to 60 ppm. The most recent versions of the peak count pacing systems provide programmable deceleration constants of 2.5, 5, and 10 minutes, which control the time required for the pacing rate to decrease by 90% of the difference from the maximum to the minimum programmed rates. In both systems, the acceleration and deceleration constants provide a smooth transition of the paced rate even in the presence of abrupt changes in the sensor-indicated rate (Fig. 8–12).

When programmed to the VVIR or AAIR mode, the rate algorithm for activity-based pacemakers is very simple. As shown in Figure 8–12, the pacing rate increases and decreases according to the output of the activity sensor and the acceleration and deceleration constants. The rate-adaptive performance of these pacemakers is analogous to continual reprogramming of the lower pacing rate up or down, depending on the activity level of the patient. The pacemaker continues to sense the intrinsic ventricular (or atrial) electrogram

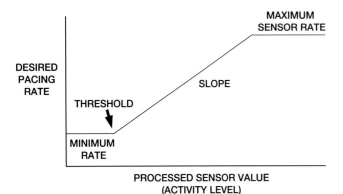

FIGURE 8–10. In the integration technique, the threshold is used in the software algorithm to determine the minimum processed sensor output that will produce an increase in pacing rate. Once the sensor number exceeds this programmable threshold, the sensor output is converted to a desired pacing rate by a programmable slope.

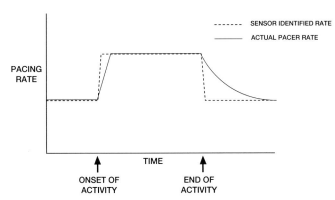

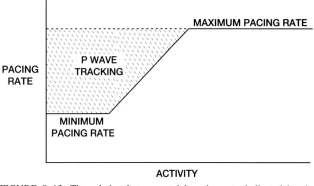

FIGURE 8–12. The relation between an instantaneously determined sensor rate *(dashed line)* and the actual pacing rate *(solid line)* of an activity sensor. Note that there is a lag between a change in the desired pacing rate and the achievement of an actual change in rate. Acceleration and deceleration (also termed ''recovery'') time constants smooth the increase and decrease in sensor-indicated pacing rate.

FIGURE 8–13. The relation between atrial pacing rate indicated by the activity sensor and normal P-wave tracking in a DDDR pacemaker. The lower pacing rate is effectively increased by the sensor up to the programmed maximum sensor-indicated rate. If the P-wave rate exceeds the lower pacing rate indicated by the sensor, normal tracking will occur.

and is inhibited by the presence of an intrinsic beat that occurs at a rate faster than the sensor-indicated pacing rate. The minimum and maximum limits of the pacing rate are programmable. When programmed to the DDDR mode, the rate-adaptive algorithm becomes more complicated (Fig. 8–13). Function in the DDDR mode is similar to that in the AAIR mode in regard to the lower pacing rate, which is continually adjusted by the activity sensor. As with the AAIR mode, sinus rates greater than the sensor-indicated lower rate

inhibit the atrial pacing stimulus. As with the normal DDD pacing mode, the device can also pace the ventricle faster than the sensor-indicated lower rate (Fig. 8–14) by tracking intrinsic P waves (atrial synchronous operation). Whether or not the ventricular pacing stimulus is delivered is determined by the presence or absence of intrinsic AV conduction within the programmed AV delay. Currently available DDDR devices can also be programmed to pace at different maximum P-wave tracking and sensor-indicated rates. When the pro-

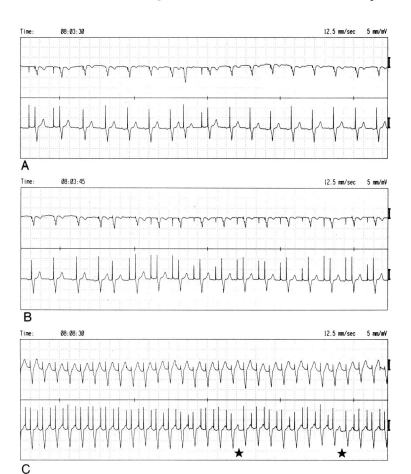

FIGURE 8–14. Normal DDDR pacemaker function over a range of atrial rates. As with a normal AAIR pacemaker, sinus rates greater than the sensor-indicated lower rate will inhibit the atrial pacing stimulus. However, a DDD pacing system will also pace the ventricle faster than the sensor-indicated lower rate *(A)* by tracking intrinsic P waves. Whether or not the ventricular pacing stimulus is delivered is determined by the presence or absence of intrinsic AV conduction within the programmed AV delay. Once the activity sensor indicates that the lower pacing rate should be increased above the intrinsic atrial rate *(B)*, atrial pacing stimuli are delivered. At rates above the upper atrial tracking limit, the device functions in the DDIR mode up to the maximum sensor-indicated rate *(stars)*.

grammed maximum sensor-indicated rate differs from the programmed maximum tracking rate, the device functions in the DDDR mode at rates below the upper tracking limit. At rates above the upper atrial tracking limit, the device functions in the DDIR mode up to the maximum sensor-indicated rate. Programming the sensor maximum rate higher than the P-wave tracking rate (Fig. 8–15A) has been found to be useful for patients with intermittent atrial fibrillation or flutter to avoid tracking of these arrhythmias while still allowing an appropriately high maximum sensor rate.[37] Alternatively, the maximum sensor rate can be set below the maximum P-wave tracking rate (see Fig. 8–15B), which may be helpful for patients who typically have normal chronotropic response during exercise to avoid pacemaker Wenckebach or 2:1 block upper rate behavior. With this combination of settings, the upper sensor-indicated rate is limited, although the sensor can provide back-up rate support should pacemaker Wenckebach or 2:1 block occur. The benefits of a DDDR pacemaker that provides this back-up support at the upper P-wave tracking limit have been termed sensor-driven rate smoothing.[38, 39]

The initial dual-chamber peak count pacemakers, when programmed to the DDDR mode, used one maximum upper rate for tracking both intrinsic P waves and output of the sensor. The upper rate was programmable from 80 to 180 ppm. Newer versions of these devices provide separately programmable maximum rates for atrial tracking and for sensor-driven pacing. DDDR pacemakers that use the inte-

gration system have always offered separately programmable maximum P-wave tracking and sensor rates. The maximum P-wave tracking rate can be adjusted from 90 to 175 ppm, and the maximum sensor rate from 90 to 150 ppm.

The algorithms of the current generation of activity-based devices that integrate the sensor output also include a rate-responsive AV delay. As the sensor-indicated rate increases, the paced AV delay shortens. Shortening of the AV delay is intended to approximate the response of the normal PR interval during exercise.[40] Because the total atrial refractory period is reduced as the AV delay is shortened, a rate-responsive AV delay allows a higher rate for tracking intrinsic atrial activity than would a fixed AV delay.[41] A drawback of this feature is that in patients with intact AV conduction automatic shortening of the AV interval may increase the likelihood of ventricular pacing (i.e., preempting conducted impulses), thereby increasing current drain from the battery. A paced ventricular complex may also reduce the stroke volume compared with an intrinsic QRS complex.

Clinical Experience with Activity-Based Sensors for Rate-Adaptive Pacing

PHYSIOLOGIC CORRELATION

Several important clinical advantages of activity-based, rate-adaptive pacemakers were enumerated earlier. From a physiologic perspective, however, their principal strength lies in the fact that they are inherently capable of providing a prompt response to activity signals of relatively low amplitude over a wide range of frequencies. On the other hand, activity-based pacemakers may be more susceptible to nonphysiologic vibrations such as those accompanying riding in a motor vehicle or using heavy machinery. Additionally, these sensors may vary considerably in the chronotropic response observed with different types of physical activity despite comparable metabolic workloads.[31, 42] For example, walking on a soft surface may induce a lower increase in heart rate than would be observed with the same rate of walking on a hard surface. Furthermore, activity-based pacemakers do not offer "closed-loop" operating characteristics. Thus, as the pacing rate rises in response to increasing physical activity, there is no inherent tendency of the sensed parameter (body motion) to return toward baseline. Finally, activity-based pacemakers are not capable of physiologic rate adaptation in the presence of emotional upset or fever (in the absence of shivering) or in anticipation of physical exercise. On balance, however, clinical studies have convincingly demonstrated that activity-based pacing systems offer the potential for greater exercise capacity and fewer exertionally related symptoms than fixed-rate (VVI) pacemakers. The clearest evidence of this benefit has been provided by exercise laboratory studies measuring both cardiopulmonary indices and the perception of exertion.

In an early clinical study of an activity-based, rate-adaptive pacemaker Benditt and colleagues[43] compared exercise tolerance during fixed-rate VVI pacing with that in VVIR pacing using cardiopulmonary treadmill exercise. Rate-adaptive pacing prolonged exercise duration by 35% and led to similar improvements in peak observed oxygen consumption

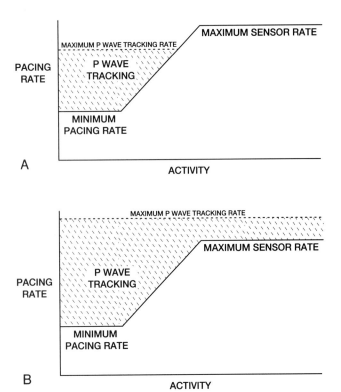

FIGURE 8–15. Separation of maximum sensor rate and maximum P-wave tracking rates. In A, the maximum sensor rate may exceed the maximum P-wave tracking rate. Such a programming scheme may prevent tracking of paroxysmal atrial tachyarrhythmias without limiting the maximum pacing rate that can be achieved with exercise. In B, the maximum P-wave tracking rate is programmed to a greater value than the maximum sensor rate. Such a programmed combination may be useful to avoid inappropriate sensor-indicated rates in patients with relatively intact sinus node function.

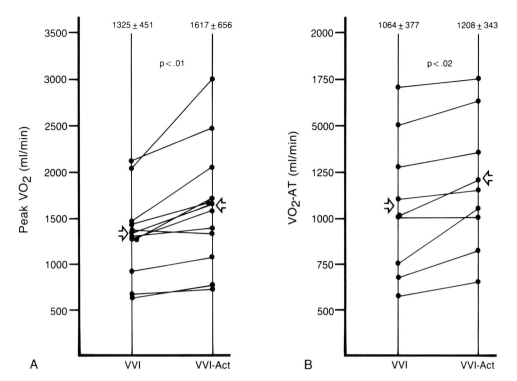

FIGURE 8–16. Effect of the VVIR pacing mode (labeled VVI-Act) on peak oxygen consumption (VO_2) and oxygen consumption at anaerobic threshold (VO_2-AT) with an activity-controlled pacing system. Note improvements in oxygen consumption with the VVIR pacing mode compared with the VVI mode. (Reproduced with permission from Benditt DG, et al: Single-chamber cardiac pacing with activity-initiated chronotropic response: Evaluation by cardiopulmonary exercise testing. Circulation 75:184, 1987. Copyright 1987 American Heart Association.)

and oxygen consumption at anaerobic threshold (Fig. 8–16). Rate-adaptive pacing also reduced the patient's perception of exertion at comparable exercise levels[44] (Fig. 8–17). In a subset of the same patients, it was demonstrated that the improved performance with VVIR pacing was sustained when exercise testing was repeated after an average of 5 months follow-up (Fig. 8–18).[45] Furthermore, at the time of follow-up exercise testing, reversion of the pacing system to a fixed rate (VVI) mode resulted in prompt deterioration of both observed oxygen consumption and exercise duration. Thus, the ability of a single-chamber activity-based pacing system to provide immediate and long-term improvements in exercise tolerance was clearly demonstrated.

Others have also reported improved exercise capacity with rate-adaptive pacemakers based on activity sensors, although the results from studies using bicycle exercise have been less dramatic than those observed with treadmill exercise.[20, 46–48] For example, Smedgard and coworkers[20] reported a 10% improvement and Alt and associates[47] a 6% improvement in exercise capacity with activity-based VVIR pacemakers compared with VVI pacing with bicycle exercise testing.

Buckingham and colleagues[48] used treadmill exercise testing to examine the impact of ventricular function on exercise responses of 16 patients with activity-based, rate-adaptive pacemakers in the VVI and the VVIR modes. The findings clearly indicated that provision of appropriate heart rate responsiveness by this technique resulted in a substantial increase in cardiac index that was independent of left ventricular systolic function (i.e., baseline ejection fraction). Whether diastolic function is helpful in predicting which patients might be more likely to benefit from chronotropic responsiveness was not examined. However, Lau and Camm[49] were unable to predict the potential hemodynamic benefits of rate-adaptive pacing in 22 patients using echocardiographic techniques to estimate left ventricular systolic and diastolic function.

Although the benefits of activity-based VVIR pacing are well established compared with those of fixed-rate ventricular pacing, the VVIR pacing mode has also been compared with atrial-tracking, dual-chamber pacing modes (VDD, DDD). Menozzi and colleagues[50] compared the DDD and VVIR pacing modes in a crossover study using a dual-chamber, activity-based pacemaker that offered selection of both

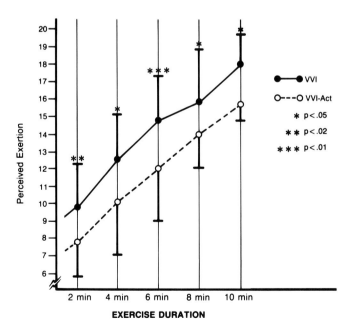

FIGURE 8–17. Effect of rate modulation provided by an activity-sensing VVIR pacing system on the perception of effort during exercise. Note that the perceived level of exertion was lower in the VVIR (VVI-Act) pacing mode than in the VVI mode at all stages of exercise. (Reproduced with permission from Benditt DG, et al: Sensor-triggered rate-variable cardiac pacing: Current technologies and clinical implications. Ann Intern Med 1987; 107:714–724.)

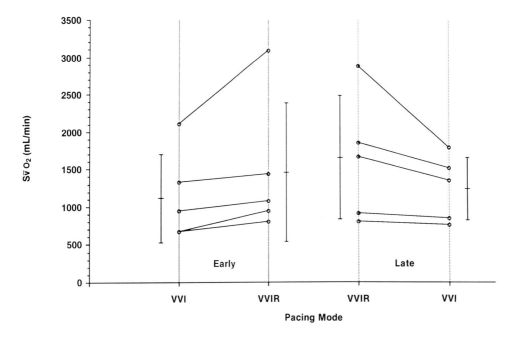

FIGURE 8–18. In a subset of the same patients shown in Figure 8–17 at the time of follow-up exercise testing, reversion of the pacing system to the VVI mode resulted in prompt deterioration of observed oxygen consumption ($S\bar{v}O_2$) compared with VVIR pacing. (From Buetikofer J, et al: Sustained improvement in exercise duration, rate pressure product and peak oxygen consumption with activity-initiated rate-variable pacing. *In* Belhassen B, et al (eds): Cardiac Pacing and Electrophysiology: Proceedings of the VIIIth World Symposium on Cardiac Pacing and Electrophysiology, Tel Aviv, R & L Creative Communications, 1987, pp 53–59.)

pacing modes. The pacemakers were programmed alternatively to VVIR or DDD for 6-week periods. Qualitative measures of symptomatic status, noninvasive estimates of cardiac output, and exercise capacity were evaluated. Not surprisingly, exercise tolerance was similar with the two modes (VVIR 68 ± 15W/min vs. DDD 70 ± 18 W/min). However, in this study the DDD mode was clearly preferred from a symptom perspective, suggesting the importance of AV synchrony from a quality-of-life viewpoint. In contrast to these results, Oldroyd and colleagues[51] found no significant difference between the DDD and VVIR modes with respect to symptom scores, maximal exercise performance (treadmill), or plasma concentrations of epinephrine, norepinephrine, and atrial natriuretic peptide (a finding disputed by Blanc and associates[52]). Furthermore, only one patient requested early reversion to the DDD mode from VVIR pacing, the only patient with intact retrograde conduction. Surprisingly, venous epinephrine and norepinephrine levels were not reported to be higher during exercise in the VVIR mode, as might have been expected given comparable exercise levels. The findings of Oldroyd and colleagues[51] have been more recently echoed by those of Linde-Edelstam and associates.[53] In their study, two activity-based VVIR and DDDR pacemakers were used to compare the DDD and VVIR pacing modes. Cardiac output at rest tended to be higher with DDD than with VVIR pacing. However, right atrial and pulmonary capillary wedge pressures, coronary sinus blood flow, coronary sinus arteriovenous O_2 difference, and myocardial oxygen consumption did not differ between these pacing modes.

In summary, activity-based VVIR pacemakers provide significant improvement in exercise capacity compared with fixed-rate VVI pacing. Additionally, exercise tolerance with the VVIR mode is essentially equivalent to that with DDD pacing in many patients. However, in certain cases (particularly patients susceptible to "pacemaker syndrome"), dual-chamber, rate-adaptive devices are clearly better tolerated. Additionally, dual-chamber pacing may offer other potential advantages including preservation of atrial electric stability

(i.e., a lower incidence of atrial fibrillation) and a lower incidence of congestive heart failure. Although the VVIR pacing mode offers similar exercise capacity compared with DDD pacing, the DDDR or AAIR pacing mode may be preferable for most patients with chronotropic incompetence who require a permanent pacemaker because of the inherent advantages of AV synchrony. Nevertheless, individuals with chronic atrial fibrillation and impaired AV conduction remain excellent candidates for activity-based VVIR pacemakers.

POTENTIAL FOR ATYPICAL OR UNDESIRED RESPONSES

In general, both the peak counting and integration piezoelectric configurations behave similarly in terms of their response to movement or vibration.[42] As a result, both may provide inappropriate heart rate responses when subjected to environmental vibrations such as those induced by the movement of a motor vehicle over rough terrain, or those resulting from air travel or the use of appliances or machinery. These pacemakers also respond to the application of static pressure on the pulse generator, as when the patient happens to lie on the pacemaker while sleeping in bed. Because static focal pressure on the posterior surface of the pacemaker case produces sensor deformation, an inappropriate pacing rate increase can occur in this situation. This can happen when a patient is sleeping or when the pulse generator is implanted directly over a rib. Respiratory movement of the rib cage can result in periodic pressure on the posterior surface of the pacemaker case, particularly in thin patients or when the device is implanted in a subpectoral location. This false-positive response to pressure is less of a problem with pacemakers that incorporate an accelerometer.[23]

Pacemaker-induced tachycardias caused by position are clearly undesirable in sleeping patients. On the other hand, in certain cases the heart rate increase associated with vehicular movement, rough air travel, or use of heavy machinery may in fact prove to be appropriate despite the fact that it is induced by nonphysiologic physical movement rather than by emotional stress. For instance, in a recent report by Matula and colleagues[54] the effects of various means of locomotion on pacing rate were assessed for different activity-based pacemakers. Three different activity-based pacing systems (peak detector, integration type, and accelerometer) were strapped to the chests of volunteers. Bicycling on the street resulted in higher pacing rates than did stationary bicycling for each type of pacemaker, although none of the pacemakers reached the heart rate achieved by the normal sinus node. During driving, the pacemakers increased the pacing rate, although the intrinsic sinus rate continued to be higher. In passively riding passengers, the pacemakers tended to produce a higher pacing rate than that of the normal sinus node. Of interest, the accelerometer-based system responded mainly to acceleration and curves, whereas vibration sensors responded primarily to vibrations and rough roads.

An additional category of potentially undesirable heart rate responses associated with activity-based pacing systems may be the responses resulting from the particular characteristics of an exercise or the manner in which physical exertion is performed. As noted earlier, the responsiveness of the devices may be affected by factors such as the softness of the patient's shoes or the nature of the terrain. Additionally, activity-based pacemakers have been shown to manifest paradoxically slower heart rates during walking uphill compared with walking downhill. This appears to be related to the fact that activity sensors respond to heel strike frequency. Although the workload is higher walking uphill, the incline results in a slower walking rate and a lower heel strike frequency than walking downhill. On the other hand, the apparently "poor" performance of activity-based systems during stationary bicycle exercise may be less important because when actual street bicycling is undertaken additional vibrations associated with movement occur.[54] Despite the potential for undesirable or nonphysiologic pacing responses, the great majority of patients are very well served by activity-based, rate-adaptive pacemakers. For example, in a recent study involving everyday activities (such as walking, climbing stairs, and mental stress), activity-based, rate-adaptive pacemakers proved quite sensitive during light physical exertion and compared favorably with respiratory-based and QT-based pacemakers.[55] When false-positive responses are detected, simple noninvasive programming steps usually alleviate the problem.[31]

POTENTIAL FOR COMBINATION WITH OTHER SENSORS

Despite the widespread popularity of activity sensors, there has been considerable interest in devising a more physiologic pacing system by combining two or more sensors. This strategy may balance the advantages and disadvantages of various technologies to optimize overall performance. In this regard, the sensitivity of activity sensors in detecting the onset of physical exertion and responding rapidly is unsurpassed. On the other hand, activity sensors are relatively unresponsive to many other conditions that call for increased heart rate, such as emotional stress, and may not be optimal for sustained physical activity. Consequently, the use of activity sensors in combination with more slowly responsive sensors has become the subject of both investigational interest and clinical application.

ACTIVITY AND TEMPERATURE SENSORS

The first study to combine an activity sensor with a second artificial sensor was reported by Heuer and associates in 1986.[56] In that report, central venous temperature was combined with activity to modulate pacing rate. If the temperature sensor confirmed that exercise was indeed in progress, central venous temperature would become the primary determinant of pacing rate. Until now, the combined use of an activity-based sensor with a temperature sensor has only been undertaken in an experimental setting. A conventional activity-based pulse generator was strapped to the chest wall of the patient, along with a temperature-sensing electrode located within the right atrium. The results of this combination indicated that treadmill exercise of short duration (<2 minutes) resulted in pacing that was predominantly controlled by the activity sensor. In addition, exposure of patients to passive vehicular vibrations demonstrated that the temperature sensor had essentially no impact on pacing rate. However, with extended periods of exercise the temperature sensor became the predominant controller of pacing rate. During recovery from extended exercise, the temperature sensor also maintained principal control, indicating the importance of thermoregulatory effects in determining the heart rate in the postexercise period. When the temperature sensor failed to confirm an increase in output of the activity sensor, the algorithm was designed to permit the pacing rate to gradually return to the baseline value. Consequently, passive vehicular vibrations resulted in only short periods of increased heart rate, which were subsequently countermanded by the absence of temperature confirmation.

The combination of an accelerometer and a temperature sensor has been reported by Alt and associates.[57] In this study, the accelerometer output was restricted to provide stepwise changes in pacing rate instead of the continuous adaptation possible in the Heuer model.[56] The contribution of the activity sensor to the algorithm was intended to confirm whether temperature recordings were indicative of continuing exercise. By testing the algorithm in healthy volunteers under a variety of exercise conditions, the investigators demonstrated a close correlation between the normal intrinsic sinus rate and the pacing rate proposed by the algorithm.

ACTIVITY AND QT INTERVAL SENSORS

A number of investigators have examined the combination of activity and the QT interval as the basis for a dual-sensor, rate-adaptive pacing system.[58–60] For the most part, the role of the activity sensor has been to detect the onset of physical activity, the QT interval being used to control the pacing rate during sustained exertion. An investigational dual-sensor pacing system incorporating activity and QT sensors was first implanted in 1990.[61, 62] This pacing system has evolved into the Topaz (Vitatron, The Netherlands). This pacemaker has been on the market in Europe since January 1992. In the Topaz and its recent dual-chamber version (Diamond), rate response is determined by two primary features: blending of sensors and cross-checking of each sensor against the other.[63, 64] With sensor blending, the pacemaker may be programmed to respond to the activity sensor alone, the QT sensor alone, or a combination of the sensors. In addition, the device can be programmed to give priority to one or the other sensor. Any of five combinations may be selected: QT only, activity only, QT less than activity, QT equal to activity, and QT more than activity. The cross-checking feature is designed to increase the specificity of the pacemaker for exercise and to reduce false-positive responses.[64] Thus, if the activity sensor indicates a need to increase the heart rate that is not soon confirmed by changes in the QT interval, a false-positive activity response is diagnosed by the algorithm, and the pacing rate returns to baseline. If exercise is indeed occurring, the pacing rate ultimately becomes dependent on changes in the QT interval. In an alternative circumstance, if the QT detector suggests the need for an increased pacing rate that is not confirmed by the activity sensor (such as may occur with an emotional upset or isometric exercise), the pacemaker limits the increase in heart rate to a value less than would have been the case had both sensors been concordant. The Topaz also features simplified programming and a considerable degree of automatic self adjustment.[64, 65] With automatic self adjustment of rate response, the device exhibits only a limited rate-response capability at implant and gradually adjusts over several weeks to optimize the rate-adaptive response.

ACTIVITY AND MINUTE VENTILATION

The combination of an activity sensor with a minute ventilation sensor is still another example of how the sensitivity and rapid responsiveness of activity are matched with a sensor that is perceived to be more ''physiologic'' in nature. One such pacemaker using this combination began clinical trials in Europe and North America in late 1992 (Legend Plus [Medtronic Inc.]). This pacemaker uses a piezoceramic sensor bonded to the inner aspect of the pulse generator case in conjunction with measurement of respiratory variation by transthoracic impedance. As discussed in Chapter 12, changes in transthoracic impedance correlate relatively well with actual minute ventilation, although the measurement is not without susceptibility for error (especially from nonres-

piratory chest or arm movements). In its current configuration, each of the sensors in this device is separately programmable, including independent upper rate limits and sensor slopes. Preliminary findings from clinical studies with this pacing system suggest that initial heart rate response is primarily driven by the activity sensor, with the minute ventilation sensor predominating during sustained levels of physical activity (Fig. 8–19).

ACTIVITY AND OXYGEN SATURATION

The combination of an activity sensor and a mixed venous oxygen saturation sensor is currently in the early stages of clinical investigation (OxyElite [Medtronic Inc.]). Other preliminary studies suggest that multisensor pacemakers incorporating mixed venous oxygen sensing may prove to be very effective.[66] Although the combination of activity with oxygen saturation has theoretical appeal, considerable technical development and clinical study are needed.

Practical Pearls for Activity Sensor Systems

Appropriate adjustment of the programmable rate-modulating parameters is crucial for maximizing the benefit attainable with activity-based pacemakers. Until fully automatic pacing systems are available, some form of exercise study will be needed to achieve optimal clinical results. Relying on the manufacturer's ''nominal'' values is usually inadequate.

INFORMAL TESTING FOR ESTABLISHING OPTIMAL PROGRAMMING

Clinical experience with exercise testing for adjusting the rate-modulating parameters of activity-based pacemakers is

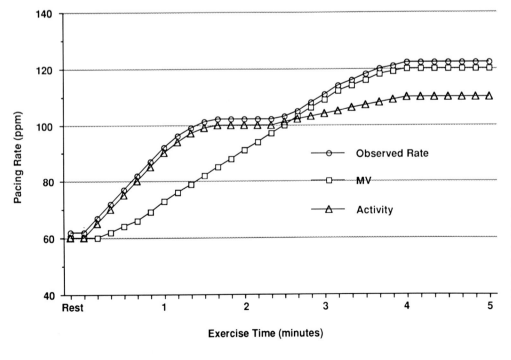

FIGURE 8–19. A dual-sensor pacing system using activity and minute ventilation sensors. In this algorithm, the pacing rate is determined by the faster of the two sensors. Note that an abrupt increase in pacing rate is provided by the activity sensor at the onset of exercise followed by a more linear increase in pacing rate provided by the minute ventilation (MV) sensor at higher workloads.

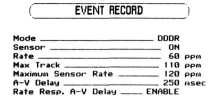

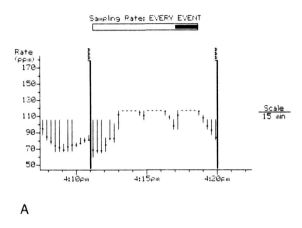

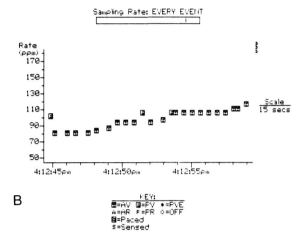

FIGURE 8–20. Examples of a rate trend *(A)* with a DDDR pacing system. Note that this device is programmed to log every pacing event, allowing the clinician to determine the pacing rate during a known period of time. In *B* the pulse generator stores and displays the sequence of pacing and sensing over a brief period. (AV, atrial pacing followed by ventricular pacing; PV, intrinsic P wave followed by ventricular pacing; AR, atrial pacing followed by intrinsic AV conduction; PR, intrinsic P wave followed by intrinsic AV conduction.)

extensive. In many cases an informal approach is quite adequate. This may entail briefly walking the patient at various rates on a flat surface and then proceeding up and down several flights of stairs. During this evaluation, the pacing rate should be monitored by an attendant or through the diagnostics of the device. Following appropriate reprogramming, informal exercise can be repeated. The attendant can also assess the patient's level of fatigue and other symptoms. For patients with newer versions of activity-based pacemakers, rate histograms can be used effectively for the purpose of assessing rate response.[67] Specifically, the rate histogram is adjusted to "short-term" monitoring. At the completion of walking, the pacemaker is interrogated. If the pacing rates achieved are not appropriate for the level of exertion or if excessive fatigue is reported, a programming adjustment can be made and the exercise repeated. Again the rate histograms are checked to validate the programmed changes.[67] The "event recorder" feature, which is available in some activity-based devices, can also be used to monitor the rate response of the device during exercise testing (Fig. 8–20). With this feature, a beat-for-beat record of the pacing rate is documented through the programmer to assess sensor response during activity. Finally, activity-based, rate-adaptive pulse generators can be strapped to the chest and used to "trigger" older implanted VVI or AAI pacemakers.[68] This technique permits assessment of the potential benefits of rate-adaptive pacing prior to surgery.

As an alternative to walking and stair climbing a series of stationary exercises that are more suitable to the clinic environment can be used. Benditt and associates[69] compared the

pacing rates of "strapped-on" and implanted rate-adaptive pacemakers during arm movement, walk-in-place exercise, and treadmill exercise. The findings indicated that the stationary exercise procedures could provide a useful assessment of rate response without resorting to formal exercise testing. Moura and colleagues[70] also found such an approach useful in comparing the rate response of an activity-based pacemaker with the response of the sinus node in control subjects.

A critical factor in selecting the appropriate programmed settings of a rate-adaptive pacemaker is an understanding of the range of heart rates that should be expected for a given form of exercise. Hayes and colleagues[71] provided these data for normal subjects during casual or brisk walking. Our own laboratory has similarly examined the heart rate responses of normal subjects across a broad range of ages, based on ambulatory monitoring data during activities of daily living.[72] As a result, the basic information with which to adjust pacemakers is now available in the clinic.[72, 73]

FORMAL TESTING FOR OPTIMIZING DEVICE PROGRAMMING

Formal treadmill exercise protocols have been developed for the purpose of assessing chronotropic competence that are applicable to patients with rate-adaptive pacemakers.[74] The most well known of these is the Chronotropic Assessment Exercise Protocol (CAEP).[75] We have developed an alternative protocol (Minnesota Pacemaker Response Exercise Protocol [M-PREP]) that is well tolerated and has pro-

TABLE 8–1. MINNESOTA PACEMAKER RESPONSE EXERCISE PROTOCOL (M-PREP)

STAGE	SPEED* (mph)	GRADE (%)	DURATION (min:sec)	METS
1	1.5	0.0	2:00	2.0
2	2.0	2.0	2:00	3.0
3	2.5	3.0	2:00	4.0
4	3.0	4.0	2:00	5.0
5	3.5	5.0	2:00	6.0
6	4.0	5.0	2:00	7.0
7	4.5	3.5	2:00	8.0
8	5.0	2.0	2:00	9.0
9	5.5	1.5	2:00	10.0
10	6.0	2.5	2:00	11.0
11	6.5	2.5	2:00	12.0
12	7.0	3.0	2:00	13.0
13	7.0	5.0	2:00	14.0
14	7.0	7.0	2:00	15.0
15	7.0	9.0	2:00	16.0
16	7.0	11.0	2:00	17.0

*The speed advances by 0.5 mph each stage to a maximum of 7.0 mph with grade adjustments to achieve a linear increase of 1 Met per stage.

vided a means for establishing appropriate programmed settings for activity-based, rate-adaptive pacemakers (Table 8–1). Unlike the CAEP protocol, the M-PREP increases workload on a linear basis starting at 2 Mets and increasing by one Met per stage. This protocol has been useful for evaluating a broad spectrum of patients with pacemaker and sinus node dysfunction, particularly those with activity-based, rate-adaptive pulse generators. The M-PREP nicely discerns the pacemaker response during lighter workloads that are representative of the activities of daily life. The variable speeds possible with this protocol are beneficial for assessing activity sensors because most patients do not maintain a constant gait as the treadmill grade increases. More typically, the gait is varied. Whichever protocol is used, the objective is to analyze the pacing rate at rest and during low and moderate levels of activity because these are the ranges utilized by most patients with pacemakers. As pointed out by

Wilkoff and associates,[74] conventional exercise protocols (e.g., Bruce protocol) tend to bypass these levels too quickly in an attempt to assess maximum tolerable workloads. The chronotropic protocols (i.e., CAEP, M-PREP) are more suitable for the older patient or the individual with orthopedic limitations and those who cannot tolerate more aggressive forms of exercise.

Treadmill exercise has proved quite effective for accurately programming activity-based pacemakers. Although formal exercise testing was routinely employed during initial clinical trials of pacemakers with activity sensors, treadmill exercise is usually reserved for patients in whom informal procedures do not provide an adequate rate response. Because commercially available pulse generators include greater data storage capacity, it is anticipated that automatic set-up and adjustment of the sensor will become an intrinsic feature of these pacemakers. Today, some levels of automaticity already exist, such as the autothreshold feature of the integration systems. This feature continually adjusts the activity threshold of the sensor based on the average activity level of the patient. An "autoset" feature is also available in some systems that offers enhanced selection of the proper rate-adaptive slope. The autoset feature allows the physician to select a desired pacing rate to be achieved during a brief walk and automatically determines the appropriate slope that will provide the selected pacing rate. As these automatic features become more sophisticated, the need for formal exercise testing will continue to diminish.

USE OF DIAGNOSTIC DATA TO EVALUATE DEVICE PERFORMANCE

Several rate-adaptive pulse generators incorporate advanced diagnostic features that can be telemetered from the device. The stored diagnostic data can be very helpful in the evaluation of pacemaker performance and can provide a guide for appropriate programming. For example, Figure 8–21 illustrates typical real-time telemetry information about battery and lead function that is obtainable with several rate-

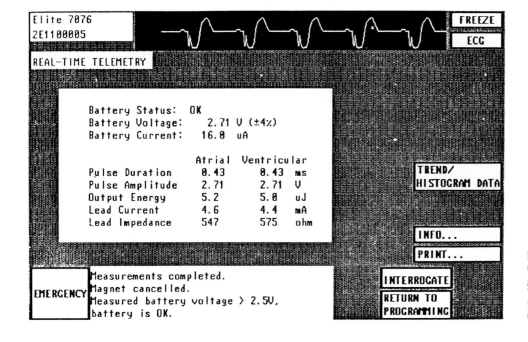

FIGURE 8–21. Example of real-time telemetry data provided by the programmer of a Medtronic Elite model 7076 pacing system. This system offers DDDR pacing using a well-established "activity" sensor.

adaptive pacemakers. The diagnostic data about sensor performance that are available include sensor-indicated histograms, event histograms, and event records. The event record provides a logged summary of the intrinsic and paced heart rates over a monitoring interval. The Synchrony II pulse generator (Siemens-Pacesetter) records the last 4096 events in a continuous loop fashion, which can be displayed through the programmer (see Fig. 8–20). When expanded to a detailed resolution, each recorded event is identified by the heart rate and whether the beats were paced or intrinsic (PR = sensed P wave, sensed R wave; PV = sensed P wave, paced ventricular stimulus; AR = paced atrial stimulus, sensed R wave; AV = paced atrial stimulus, paced ventricular stimulus; V* = premature ventricular event). This feature allows assessment of the chronotropic response characteristics of the sinus node, the activity sensor, and the status of intrinsic AV conduction. The collected data can be displayed by the programmer in several graphic formats.

The event histogram provides numerical data about pacemaker function. The number of events for the five pacing states listed in the preceding paragraph is recorded in separate rate bins (range of heart rates) (Fig. 8–22). Approximately 17 million events can be recorded within each of the 40 rate bins, providing data collection over 1 year. The sensor-indicated histogram can be used to record the sensor response during acute testing or chronic verification of the programmed settings (Fig. 8–23). The data can be collected with the sensor programmed to the active (On) or passive modes. In the sensor-passive mode, the activity sensor will not modulate pacing rate, although the pacing rate that would have been observed had the sensor been active can be stored. This allows the sensor to be adjusted without exposing the patient to potentially inappropriate pacing rates.

COMPARISON OF ACTIVITY SENSOR RESPONSES WITH OTHER RATE-ADAPTIVE PACING SYSTEM SENSORS

The basic goal of an optimal rate-adaptive pacing system is to provide a normal heart rate during a wide range of activities, from sleep to vigorous physical exercise. In this regard, the optimal rate-adaptive sensor should provide (1) a heart rate that is proportional to metabolic workload; (2) an appropriately rapid change in heart rate in response to a variable workload; (3) a high degree of sensitivity and specificity for exercise; and (4) an appropriate slowing of heart rate following exercise. McElroy and colleagues[75] have demonstrated a linear relationship between heart rate and oxygen consumption during exercise in normal volunteers and patients with varying degrees of cardiac impairment.[75]

Lau and associates[31] examined the heart rate–oxygen consumption relationship for six rate-adaptive pacing systems, including two with activity sensors. They observed reasonable correlations between pacing rate and oxygen consumption for both activity-based pacing systems (Fig. 8–24). Thus, it can be concluded that these devices appear to perform quite well despite the reported perception of them as "nonphysiologic." It is true that activity-based pacemakers appear to lack ideal proportionality with metabolic workload during treadmill exercise. Thus, as pointed out by Lau and associates,[31] both the Activitrax and the Sensolog failed to increase heart rate appropriately as treadmill *grade* was increased from 0% to 15% when the speed of walking remained constant (2.5 miles/hr). In contrast, Stangl and colleagues[30] observed a better correlation between pacing rate and metabolic workload for the Sensolog. Whereas increments in treadmill speed (heel strike frequency) routinely increase the pacing rate in both activity-based systems, a steeper grade does not necessarily result in an appropriate chronotropic response. Attention to device programming can largely obviate this limitation of activity-based sensors.

In addition to a proportional relationship between workload and heart rate, the speed of onset of a sensor may be important for maximizing exercise tolerance in patients. Lau and colleagues[31] examined exercise responses during walking and found that activity-based pacemakers best corresponded with the rate of the sinus node in normal subjects (Fig. 8–25). Not unexpectedly, the onset of an increased pacing rate was almost immediate in patients with activity-based systems and was considerably faster than that observed with rate-adaptive pacemakers based on minute ventilation, right ventricular pressure, or the QT interval.

In early activity-based, rate-adaptive pacing systems, the heart rate decay following termination of exercise occurred

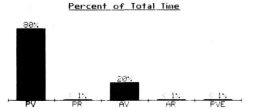

EVENT HISTOGRAM

Total Time Sampled: 29d 21h 20m 2s
Sampling Rate: EVERY EVENT

Mode	DDDR
Sensor	ON
Rate	60 ppm
Max Track	110 ppm
Maximum Sensor Rate	110 ppm
A-V Delay	175 msec
Rate Resp. A-V Delay	DISABLE

Note: The above values were obtained when the histogram was interrogated.

Rate ppm	PV	PR	AV	AR	PVE
0-60	13,534	0	340,666	5	0
61-67	447,645	34	18,436	16	0
68-75	707,956	108	28,620	5	44
76-85	596,406	15	53,823	0	59
86-100	886,231	21	38,450	0	13
101-119	12,070	16	29,705	2	3
120-149	0	14	0	0	6
> 149	0	7	0	0	10
Total:	2,663,842	215	509,750	28	135

Total Event Count: 3,173,970

Percent Paced in Atrium	16%
Percent Paced in Ventricle	> 99%
Total Time at Max Track Rate	4d 22h 49m 2s

Percent of Total Time

80% PV   1% PR   20% AV   1% AR   1% PVE

FIGURE 8–22. Event histogram provided by a Siemens-Pacesetter 2022 pulse generator indicating the sequence of paced and sensed events as a function of heart rate (see abbreviations given in Figure 8–20).

A

SENSOR INDICATED RATE HISTOGRAM

Total Time Sampled: 262d 21h 38m 13s
Sampling Rate: 1.6 seconds

Sensor _____	**ON**
Rate _____	**60 ppm**
Maximum Sensor Rate _____	**130 ppm**
Slope _____	**9**
Threshold _____	**2.0**
Reaction Time _____	**FAST**
Recovery Time _____	**MEDIUM**
Measured Average Sensor _____	**2.9**

Note: The above values were obtained
when the histogram was interrogated.

Bin Number	Range (ppm)	Time				Sample Counts
1	60 – 69	240d	1h	10m	31s	12,763,219
2	69 – 78	8d	17h	25m	14s	463,947
3	78 – 87	10d	17h	40m	18s	570,842
4	87 – 97	2d	0h	30m	6s	107,450
5	97 – 106	0d	19h	18m	44s	42,784
6	106 – 115	0d	7h	36m	34s	16,858
7	115 – 124	0d	3h	14m	8s	7,168
8	124 – 133	0d	2h	42m	38s	6,005
					Total:	13,978,273

Percent of Total Time

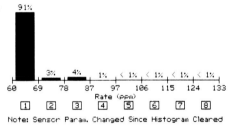

Note: Sensor Param. Changed Since Histogram Cleared

B

SENSOR INDICATED RATE HISTOGRAM

Total Time Sampled: 0d 0h 11m 27s
Sampling Rate: 1.6 seconds

Sensor _____	**ON**
Rate _____	**60 ppm**
Maximum Sensor Rate _____	**130 ppm**
Slope _____	**9**
Threshold _____	**2.0**
Reaction Time _____	**FAST**
Recovery Time _____	**MEDIUM**
Measured Average Sensor _____	**2.9**

Note: The above values were obtained
when the histogram was interrogated.

Bin Number	Range (ppm)	Time				Sample Counts
1	60 – 69	0d	0h	7m	33s	279
2	69 – 78	0d	0h	1m	33s	57
3	78 – 86	0d	0h	1m	36s	59
4	86 – 95	0d	0h	0m	46s	28
5	95 – 104	0d	0h	0m	0s	0
6	104 – 113	0d	0h	0m	0s	0
7	113 – 121	0d	0h	0m	0s	0
8	121 – 130	0d	0h	0m	0s	0
					Total:	423

Percent of Total Time

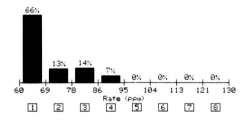

FIGURE 8–23. *A,* Sensor-indicated rate histogram of a Siemens-Pacesetter 2022 DDDR pacemaker with a sampling frequency of 1.6 seconds. Note that most of the sensor-indicated rates are near the lower programmed pacing rate, the usual finding with an appropriately programmed device. *B,* Sensor-indicated rate histogram determined during short-term clinical evaluation after a relatively slow walk.

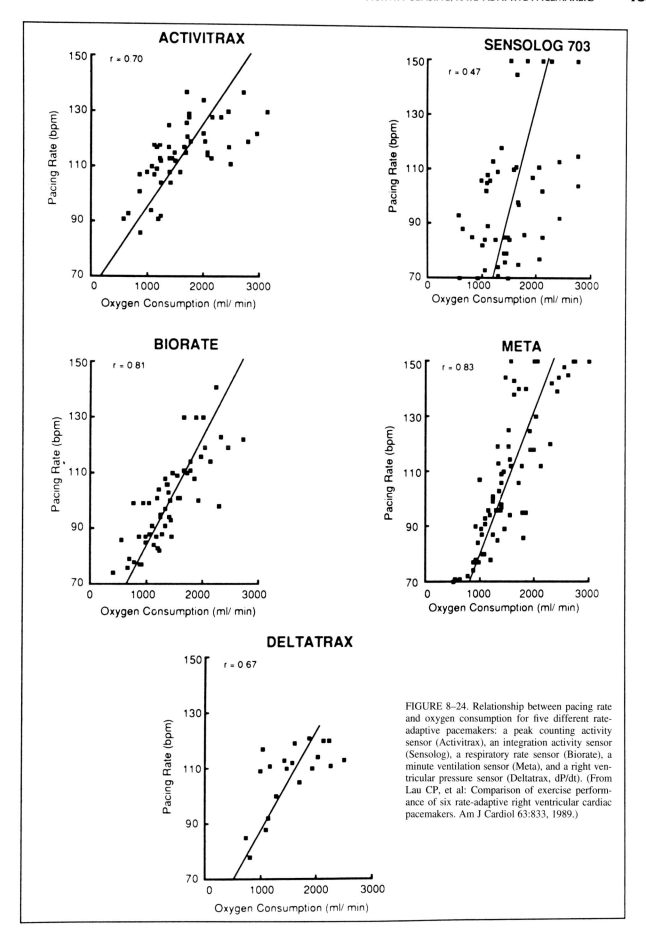

FIGURE 8–24. Relationship between pacing rate and oxygen consumption for five different rate-adaptive pacemakers: a peak counting activity sensor (Activitrax), an integration activity sensor (Sensolog), a respiratory rate sensor (Biorate), a minute ventilation sensor (Meta), and a right ventricular pressure sensor (Deltatrax, dP/dt). (From Lau CP, et al: Comparison of exercise performance of six rate-adaptive right ventricular cardiac pacemakers. Am J Cardiol 63:833, 1989.)

Time (s)

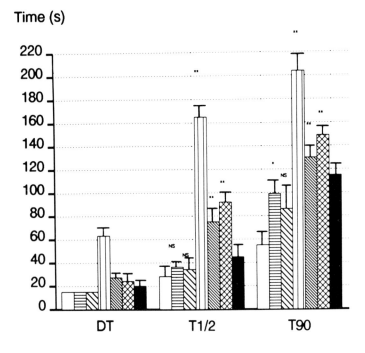

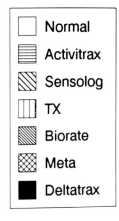

FIGURE 8–25. The time required to detect the onset of exercise as evidenced by an increase in pacing rate (DT), the time required for half the maximal rate response (T½), and the time required for 90% of the change in pacing rate for the normal sinus node (Normal) and six different rate-adaptive pacemakers. (From Lau, CP, et al: Comparison of exercise performance of six rate-adaptive right ventricular cardiac pacemakers. Am J Cardiol 63:833, 1989.)

more quickly than that observed with other sensors. However, this problem has been essentially eliminated in the newer generations of these devices with the development of programmable rate decay curves (see previous discussion). As a rule, physically active patients should have their pacemakers programmed to relatively long decay times. These values permit the heart rate to remain elevated for an extended time during recovery, thereby accounting for needs associated with reequilibration of thermoregulatory status after vigorous exercise.

The specificity and sensitivity of rate-adaptive pacing systems for detection of various physical or emotional maneuvers is quite variable. Activity-based sensors are probably best for rapid detection of physical activity. However, these sensors are incapable of detecting emotional stress such as that induced by mental arithmetic. In a direct comparison of an implanted minute ventilation sensor with an externally strapped-on, activity-based pacemaker, Lau and associates[76] found that for relatively low levels of physical exercise, both pacemakers resulted in adequate heart rate responses. However, for more strenuous activities, the activity-based pacemaker seemed to be less adequate with respect to maximum pacing rate, although the onset of response with the activity sensor was clearly faster. These findings support the potential utility of combining activity-based systems with minute ventilation sensing as is currently under evaluation (see previous discussion).

Conclusion

Activity sensors were used in the first clinically successful rate-adaptive pacemakers and have been the most thoroughly evaluated sensors in terms of patient benefit. These types of sensors have opened the door to a whole new aspect of "physiologic" cardiac pacing and remain the most widely used of all artificial sensors. They have the tremendous advantages of simplicity, reliability, and compatibility with all standard pacing leads. Given these facts, activity-based, rate-adaptive pacemakers are likely to retain their position as important clinical tools in both a "stand-alone" configuration and as part of more advanced multiple-sensor pacing systems.

Acknowledgments

We would like to thank Marcus Mianulli, Senior Scientist, University of Minnesota, Department of Medicine (Cardiovascular Division) for development of the M-PREP protocol, and both Stephanie Wiebke and Wendy Braatz for their valuable assistance in preparation of the manuscript.

REFERENCES

1. Rushmer RF: Cardiovascular Dynamics, 4th ed. Philadelphia, WB Saunders, 1976, pp 246–280.
2. Rickards AF, Donaldson RM: Rate-responsive pacing. Clin Prog Pacing Electrophysiol 1:12, 1983.
3. Benditt DG, Milstein S, Buetikofer J, et al: Sensor-triggered, rate-variable cardiac pacing: Current technologies and clinical implications. Ann Intern Med 107:714, 1987.
4. Gillette P: Critical analysis of sensors for physiological responsive pacing. PACE 7:1263, 1984.
5. Fananapazir L, Bennett DH, Monks P: Atrial synchronized ventricular pacing: Contribution of the chronotropic response to improved exercise performance. PACE 6:601, 1983.
6. Samet P, Castillo C, Bernstein WH: Hemodynamic sequelae of ventricular and atrioventricular sequential pacing in cardiac patients. Am Heart J 72:725, 1967.
7. Kruse I, Ryden L, Duffin E: Clinical evaluation of atrial synchronous ventricular inhibited pacemakers. PACE 3:641, 1980.
8. Krasner JL, Voukidis PC, Nardella PC: A physiologically controlled cardiac pacemaker. J Assoc Advanced Med Instrument 1:14, 1966.
9. Funke HD: Ein Herzschrittmacher mit Belastunsabhangiger Frequenzregulation. Biomed Technik 20:225, 1975.
10. Dahl JD: Variable rate timer for a cardiac pacemaker. US Patent 4,140,132, Feb 20, 1979.
11. Anderson K, Humen D, Klein GJ, et al: A rate variable pacemaker which automatically adjusts for physical activity [Abstract]. PACE 6:12, 1983.

12. Furman S: Rate-modulated pacing. Circulation 82:1081, 1990.
13. Humen DP, Kostuk WJ, Klein GJ: Activity-sensing, rate-responsive pacing: Improvement in myocardial performance with exercise. PACE 8:52, 1985.
14. Lindemans FW, Rankin IR, Murtaugh R, et al: Clinical experience with an activity-sensing pacemaker. PACE 9:978, 1986.
15. Benditt DG, Mianulli M, Fetter J, et al: Single-chamber cardiac pacing with activity-initiated chronotropic response: Evaluation by cardiopulmonary exercise testing. Circulation 75:184, 1987.
16. Perrins EJ, Morley CA, Chan SL, et al: Randomized controlled trial of physiological and ventricular pacing. Br Heart J 50:112, 1983.
17. Zeigler VL, Gillette PC, Kratz J: Is activity sensored pacing in children and young adults a feasible option? PACE 13:2104, 1990.
18. Zegelman M, Cieslinski G, Kreuzer J: Rate response during submaximal exercise: Comparison of three different sensors. PACE 11:1888, 1988.
19. Lau CP, Rushby J, Leigh-Jones M, et al: Symptomatology and quality of life in patients with rate-responsive pacemakers: A double-blind cross-over study. Clin Cardiol 12:505, 1989.
20. Smedgard P, Kristensson BE, Kruse I, et al: Rate-responsive pacing by means of activity sensing versus single rate ventricular pacing: A double-blind cross-over study. PACE 10:902, 1987.
21. Sulke AN, Pipilis A, Henderson RA, et al: Comparison of the normal sinus node with seven types of rate-responsive pacemaker during everyday activity. Br Heart J 64:525, 1990.
22. Kubisch K, Peters W, Chiladakis I, et al: Clinical experience with the rate-responsive pacemaker Sensolog 703. PACE 11:1829, 1988.
23. Wilkoff BL, Shimokochi DD, Schaal SF: Pacing rate increase due to application of steady external pressure on an activity-sensing pacemaker [Abstract]. PACE 10:423, 1987.
24. Lau CP, Mehta D, Toff W, et al: Limitations of rate response of activity-sensing rate-responsive pacing to different forms of activity. PACE 11:141, 1988.
25. Mehta D, Lau CP, Ward DE, et al: Comparative evaluation of chronotropic response of activity-sensing and QT-sensing rate-responsive pacemakers to different activities. PACE 11:1405, 1988.
26. Zegelman M, Beyersdorf F, Kreuzer J, et al: Rate-responsive pacemakers: Assessment after two years. PACE 9:1005, 1986.
27. Alt E, Matula M, Thilo R, et al: A new mechanical sensor for detecting body activity and posture, suitable for rate-responsive pacing. PACE 11:1875, 1988.
28. Alt E, Heinz M, Theres H, et al: Function and selection of sensors for optimum rate-modulated pacing. In Barold S, Mugica J (eds): New Perspectives in Cardiac Pacing 2. Mt Kisco, NY, Futura, 1991, pp 163–202.
29. Benditt DG, Buetikofer J, Milstein S: Physiologic cardiac pacing: Impact of ''on-line'' sensor technology. Can J Cardiol 4:1, 1988.
30. Stangl K, Wirtzfeld A, Lochschmidt O, et al: Physical movement-sensitive pacing: Comparison of two ''activity''-triggered pacing systems. PACE 12:102, 1989.
31. Lau CP, Butrous GS, Ward DE, et al: Comparison of exercise performance of six rate-adaptive right ventricular cardiac pacemakers. Am J Cardiol 63:833, 1989.
32. Alt E, Matula M, Theres H, et al: The basis for activity controlled rate variable cardiac pacemakers: An analysis of mechanical forces on the human body induced by exercise and environment. PACE 12:1667, 1989.
33. Faerestrand S, Breivik K, Ohm O: Assessment of the work capacity and relationship between rate response and exercise tolerance associated with activity-sensing rate-responsive ventricular pacing. PACE 10:1277, 1987.
34. Anderson KM, Moore AA: Sensors in pacing. PACE 9:954, 1986.
35. Lau CP: The range of sensors and algorithms used in rate-adaptive cardiac pacing. PACE 15:1177, 1992.
36. Lau CP, Tse WS, Camm AJ: Clinical experience with Sensolog 703: A new activity-sensing rate-responsive pacemaker. PACE 11:1444, 1988.
37. Higano ST, Hayes DL: Advantage of discrepant upper rate limits in a DDDR pacemaker. Mayo Clin Proc 64:932, 1989.
38. Hanich RF, Midei MG, McElroy BP, et al: Circumvention of maximum tracking limitations with a rate-modulated dual-chamber pacemaker. PACE 12:392, 1989.
39. Higano ST, Hayes DL, Eisinger G: Sensor-driven rate smoothing in a DDDR pacemaker. PACE 12:922, 1989.
40. Barbieri D, Percoco GF, Toselli G, et al: AV delay and exercise stress tests: Behavior in normal subjects. PACE 13:1724, 1990.
41. Hayes DL, Higano ST, Eisinger G: Electrocardiographic manifestations of a dual-chamber, rate-modulated (DDDR) pacemaker. PACE 12:555, 1989.
42. Lau CP: Clinical comparison of currently available sensor-based rate-adaptive pacing systems. In Benditt DG (ed): Rate-Adaptive Pacing. Boston, Blackwell Scientific Publications, 1993, pp 199–214.
43. Benditt DG, Mianulli M, Fetter J, et al: Single-chamber cardiac pacing with activity-initiated chronotropic response: Evaluation by cardiopulmonary exercise testing. Circulation 75:183, 1987.
44. Borg G: Perceived exertion as indicator of somatic stress. Scand J Rehab Med 2:92, 1970.
45. Buetikofer J, Milstein S, Mianulli M, et al: Sustained improvement in exercise duration, rate-pressure product and peak oxygen consumption with activity-initiated rate-variable pacing. In Belhassen B, Feldman S, Copperman Y (eds): Cardiac Pacing and Electrophysiology: Proceedings of the VIIIth World Symposium on Cardiac Pacing and Electrophysiology. Tel Aviv, R & L Creative Communications, 1987, pp 53–59.
46. Lau CP, Wong C-K, Leung W-H, et al: Superior cardiac hemodynamics of atrioventricular synchrony over rate-responsive pacing at submaximal exercise: Observations in activity-sensing DDDR pacemakers. PACE 13:1832, 1990.
47. Alt E, Theres H, Heinz M: Evaluation of temperature- and activity-controlled rate-adaptive cardiac pacemakers by spiroergometry. In Winter UJ, Wassermann K, Treese N, et al (eds): Computerized Cardiopulmonary Exercise Testing. Darmstadt, Steinkopff Verlag, 1991, pp 159–170.
48. Buckingham TA, Wodruf RC, Pennington G, et al: Effect of ventricular function on the exercise hemodynamics of variable rate pacing. J Am Coll Cardiol 11:169, 1988.
49. Lau CP, Camm AJ: Role of left ventricular function and Doppler derived variables in predicting hemodynamic benefits of rate-responsive pacing. Am J Cardiol 62:906, 1988.
50. Menozzi C, Brignole M, Moracchini PV, et al: Intrapatient comparison between chronic VVIR and DDD pacing in patients affected by high-degree AV block without heart failure. PACE 13:1816, 1990.
51. Oldroyd KG, Rae AP, Carter R, et al: Double-blind crossover comparison of the effects of dual-chamber pacing (DDD) and ventricular rate-adaptive (VVIR) pacing on neuroendocrine variables, exercise performance, and symptoms in complete heart block. Br Heart J 65:188, 1991.
52. Blanc JJ, Mansourati J, Ritter P, et al: Atrial natriuretic factor release during exercise in patients successively paced in DDD and rate-matched ventricular pacing. PACE 15:397, 1992.
53. Linde-Edelstam C, Hjemdahl P, Pehrsson SK, et al: Is DDD pacing superior to VVIR? A study on cardiac sympathetic nerve activity and myocardial oxygen consumption at rest and during exercise. PACE 15:425, 1992.
54. Matula M, Alt E, Fotuhi P, et al: Rate adaptation of activity pacemakers under various types of means of locomotion [Abstract]. Eur J Cardiac Pacing Electrophysiol 2:49, 1992.
55. Hamon D, Clementy J, Dulhoste MN, et al: Evaluation of four VVIR pacing systems using standardized usual everyday activities [Abstract]. Eur J Cardiac Pacing Electrophysiol 2:50, 1992.
56. Heuer H, Coch TH, Frenking B: Erfahrungen mit einem Zweisensorgesteuerten frequenzadattierenden Schrittmachersystem. Herzschrittmacher 2:64, 1986.
57. Alt E, Theres H, Heinz M, et al: A new rate-modulated pacemaker system optimized by combination of two sensors. PACE 11:1119, 1988.
58. Heuer H, Coch TH, Isbruch F, et al: Pacemaker stimulation by a two sensor regulation [Abstract]. PACE 10:688, 1987.
59. Senden PJ, Landman MAJ, vanRooijen H, et al: Clinical study of a dual sensor rate adaptive pacemaker using Activitrax and paced QT-interval mode [Abstract]. PACE 12:1574, 1989.
60. Velimirovic D, Cocovic D, Djordjevic M, et al: Clinical investigation using dual sensor (activity + QT) rate adaptive software [Abstract]. PACE 12:1574, 1989.
61. Boute W, Landman MAJ, Senden PJ, et al: Clinical studies for a dual-sensor rate-adaptive pacemaker [Abstract]. Eur Heart J 10:137, 1989.
62. Landman MAJ, Senden PJ, vanRooijen H, et al: Initial clinical experience with rate-adaptive cardiac pacing using two sensors simultaneously. PACE 13:1615, 1990.
63. DenDulk K, Landmann M, Senden PJ, et al: Initial experience with sensor blending in a dual sensor pacemaker [Abstract]. PACE 14:660, 1991.
64. Senden PJ, Landman MAJ, vanRooijen H, et al: Sensor cross checking in a dual sensor pacemaker during exercise and activity sensing artefacts [Abstract]. PACE 13:1209, 1990.
65. Daig NW, Boute W, Begemann MJS, et al: One-year follow-up of automatic adaptation of the rate response algorithm of the QT sensing rate adaptive pacemaker. PACE 14:1598, 1991.

66. Stangl K, Wirtzfeld A, Heinze R, et al: A new multisensor pacing system using stroke volume, respiratory rate, mixed venous oxygen saturation and temperature, right atrial pressure, right ventricular pressure and dP/dt. PACE 11:712, 1988.

67. Hayes DL, Higano ST, et al: Utility of rate histograms in programming and follow-up of a DDDR pacemaker. Mayo Clin Proc 64:495, 1989.

68. Fetter J, Benditt DG, Mianulli M: Usefulness of transcutaneous triggering of conventional implanted pulse generators by an activity-sensing pacemaker for predicting effectiveness of rate-response pacing. Am J Cardiol 62:901, 1988.

69. Benditt DG, Mianolli M, Fetter J, et al: An office-based exercise protocol for predicting chronotropic response of activity-triggered, rate-variable pacemakers. Am J Cardiol 64:27, 1989.

70. Moura PJ, Gessman LJ, Lai T, et al: Chronotropic response of an activity-detecting pacemaker compared with the normal sinus node. PACE 10:78, 1987.

71. Hayes DL, Von Feldt L, Higano ST: Standardized informal exercise testing for programming rate-adaptive pacemakers. PACE 14:1772, 1991.

72. Mianulli M, Lundstrom R, Birchfield D, et al: A standardized activities of daily living protocol for assessment of chronotropic incompetence [Abstract]. PACE 16:926, 1993.

73. Mianulli M, Lundstrom R, Birchfield D, et al: Pacemaker rate response optimization using a standardized activities of daily living protocol [Abstract]. PACE 16:873, 1993.

74. Wilkoff BL, Corey J, Blackburn G: A mathematical model of cardiac chronotropic response to exercise. J Electrophysiol 3:176, 1989.

75. McElroy TA, Janicki JS, Weber KT: Physiologic correlates of the heart rate response to upright isotonic exercise: Relevance to rate-responsive pacemakers. J Am Coll Cardiol 11:94, 1988.

76. Lau CP, Wong CK, Leung WH, et al: A comparative evaluation of minute ventilation–sensing and activity-sensing adaptive-rate pacemakers during daily activities. PACE 12:1514, 1989.

CHAPTER 9

Rate-Modulated Pacing Controlled by Mixed Venous Oxygen Saturation

G. Neal Kay
Gene A. Bornzin

The importance of chronotropic response for exercise tolerance is widely recognized and clinically applied in permanent pacing. Although the normal human sinus node is the ideal rate-modulating sensor for patients with impaired atrioventricular conduction, sinus node function may be unreliable in many patients requiring permanent pacemakers because of intrinsic disease, drug effects, or concomitant atrial arrhythmias. Thus, artificial sensors that measure a variety of biophysical parameters have been developed to modulate pacing rate in response to changing metabolic demands. In 1980, Wirtzfeld and Bock[1] described the use of mixed venous oxygen saturation as a rate-control parameter for permanent pacemakers. Wirtzfeld and colleagues[2, 3] later reported that mixed venous oxygen saturation could also be used to determine the optimal heart rate at any level of metabolic demand. Bornzin[4] described a pacing catheter employing dual wavelengths of light to measure the mixed venous oxygen saturation that could be used with an oxygen-controlled, rate-adaptive pacemaker. Since their initial descriptions, these ideas have been developed into implantable rate-adaptive pacing systems that modulate pacing rate in response to changes in mixed venous oxygen saturation.[5–9] Despite important technologic issues that have had to be addressed during the development of implantable oxygen sensors, these devices are now being frequently implanted in patients during clinical trials.[10–13] The widespread enthusiasm in the pacing community for this ''physiologic'' sensor is based on the perception that changes in mixed venous oxygen saturation accurately correlate with changes in the level

of metabolic demand. This chapter reviews the effects of exercise on mixed venous oxygen saturation, the influence of cardiac disease on this parameter, the considerable technical issues involved in the measurement of oxyhemoglobin saturation in vivo, and the clinical results with permanent pacemakers using this concept.

Relationship Between Oxygen Consumption, Mixed Venous Oxyhemoglobin Saturation, and Cardiac Output

Exercise, whether isometric or isotonic, is accomplished by the generation of force in skeletal muscles. This increase in muscular tension requires the consumption of energy in the form of high-energy phosphates, principally creatine phosphate, ATP, and ADP. With increased workload, there is an increase in the rate of oxidative metabolism within the skeletal muscles including the generation of ATP by the conversion of glucose and fatty acids to carbon dioxide and water via the glycolytic and tricarboxylic acid cycles. The increased use of oxygen by skeletal muscle is the result of two factors: (1) an increase in the flow of arterial blood into the exercising muscle as a result of local vasodilatation, and (2) an increase in the extraction of oxygen bound to hemoglobin in the arterial blood perfusing the muscle. The increase in exercise workload is associated with an increase in

187

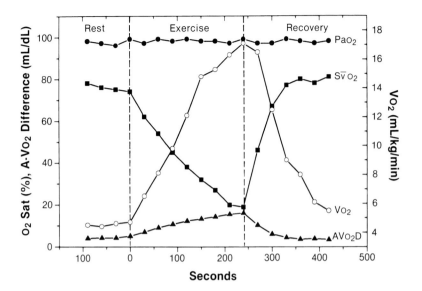

FIGURE 9–1. Treadmill exercise data from a patient with congestive heart failure and atrioventricular (AV) block in whom a rate-adaptive pacemaker was implanted. The onset and end of exercise are marked by vertical lines at 0 and 240 seconds. Note that aerobic exercise is associated with an increase in oxygen consumption *(open circles)*, and a decline in mixed venous oxygen saturation is measured in the pulmonary artery *(solid squares)*. Because the arterial oxygen saturation *(closed circles)* remains constant during exercise in the presence of a decreasing mixed venous oxygen saturation, the arterial-venous oxygen difference (A-Vo₂ difference, *triangles*) increases with increasing oxygen consumption.

the rate of oxygen consumption by the individual (increased Vo₂) and a decrease in the oxygen saturation of hemoglobin in the venous blood (Fig. 9–1). Because the great majority of the oxygen transported in arterial blood is bound to hemoglobin rather than dissolved in plasma, the oxyhemoglobin saturation in the venous blood serves as an indicator of the balance of oxygen supply (arterial blood flow) and oxygen demand (Vo₂) in a particular tissue. Exercise usually involves the generation of greater muscular tension in some muscle groups than in others so that the oxyhemoglobin saturation in the venous blood draining each muscle group varies inversely with the rate of oxidative metabolism. Therefore, the oxyhemoglobin saturation in a completely mixed sample of venous blood from all tissues such as that in the pulmonary artery reflects the total level of metabolic demand.

In individuals with adequate pulmonary function, the arterial oxyhemoglobin saturation remains constant or increases slightly from rest to exercise. Thus, the difference in content of oxygen between the arterial and mixed venous blood increases during exercise. The arterial-venous oxygen (A-Vo₂) difference is calculated from the formula:

$$\text{A-Vo}_2 \text{ difference} = (\text{Cao}_2 - \text{C}\bar{\text{v}}\text{o}_2)$$

where Cao₂ is the content of oxygen in arterial blood and C$\bar{\text{v}}$o₂ is the content of oxygen in mixed venous blood. If the small amount of oxygen that is dissolved in plasma is ignored, the content of oxygen in the arterial and venous blood can be calculated from the formulas:

$$\text{Cao}_2 = (\text{Sao}_2) \times (\text{g Hb}/100 \text{ mL}) \times (1.34 \text{ cc O}_2/\text{g Hb})$$

where Sao₂ is the saturation of hemoglobin with oxygen in the arterial blood; and

$$\text{C}\bar{\text{v}}\text{o}_2 = (\text{S}\bar{\text{v}}\text{o}_2) \times (\text{g Hb}/100 \text{ mL}) \times (1.34 \text{ cc O}_2/\text{g Hb})$$

where S$\bar{\text{v}}$o₂ is the saturation of hemoglobin with oxygen in the mixed venous blood.

It should be emphasized that the A-Vo₂ difference is also dependent on the adequacy of cardiac output for the level of metabolic demand. The percentage of oxygen that is extracted from arterial blood under resting conditions varies widely between organs, ranging from an A-Vo₂ difference of

1.0 mL/dL in skin to 11.4 mL/dL in the heart.[14] At resting levels of metabolic demand, the A-Vo₂ difference in individuals with normal cardiac output ranges from 3.5 to 5.5 cc O₂/dL. The mixed venous oxygen saturation decreases promptly with the onset of exercise in most individuals.[15] The concept of arterial-venous oxygen difference serves as the basis for the Fick equation[16] that is used to calculate cardiac output (CO).

$$\text{CO} = \frac{\text{Vo}_2}{\text{A-Vo}_2 \text{ difference}}$$

Since cardiac output is the product of heart rate and stroke volume:

$$\text{Vo}_2 = (\text{HR} \times \text{SV}) \times (\text{A-Vo}_2 \text{ difference})$$

where Vo₂ is the oxygen consumption measured in milliliters of oxygen per minute, A-Vo₂ difference is the arterial venous oxygen difference (mL O₂/dL), HR is the heart rate in beats per minute, and SV is the stroke volume in milliliters per beat. If the cardiac output at rest is insufficient to meet the resting level of oxygen consumption, the mixed venous oxyhemoglobin saturation declines and the A-Vo₂ difference increases. In contrast, if the cardiac output is inappropriately high for the level of metabolic demand (as with an arterial-venous shunt), the mixed venous oxyhemoglobin saturation increases and the A-Vo₂ difference decreases.

The normal mixed venous oxyhemoglobin saturation averages approximately 75% at rest, with an arterial oxygen saturation that usually exceeds 95%.[17] Assuming a hemoglobin concentration of 15 g/100 mL of blood, the arterial blood transports approximately 190 mL of oxygen per liter and the mixed venous blood contains approximately 150 mL of oxygen per liter. Thus, the normal arteriovenous oxygen extraction is approximately 40 mL of oxygen per liter. Because the normal resting oxygen consumption averages 3.5 mL/min/kg,[18] a 70-kg individual consumes approximately 245 mL of oxygen per minute and has a cardiac output of approximately 6 L/min.

$$\frac{245 \text{ mL/min}}{40 \text{ mL/L}}$$

The cardiac output increases 3- to 3.5-fold in response to maximum treadmill exercise in patients with little or no functional cardiac impairment.[18] This is associated with an increase in A-V_{O_2} difference to approximately 12 to 15 vol% and a minimum mixed venous oxyhemoglobin saturation of approximately 20% (see Fig. 9–1).[19] Thus, the extraction of oxygen from venous blood may exceed 80%, especially in venous blood from heavily exercising muscles.[20, 21] The normal maximal V_{O_2} (V_{O_2}max) is at least 20 mL/min/kg in patients without significant cardiac impairment[17–19] and decreases with age.[22] Assuming that the normal cardiac output triples with maximal exercise (from 6 to 18 L/min), an increase in the A-V_{O_2} difference to 15 vol% would allow at least a 10-fold increase in V_{O_2} (from 3.5 to 38.5 mL/min/kg) in a young, healthy individual. Thus, both an improvement in cardiac output and an increase in peripheral extraction of oxygen are important for exercise performance. In patients with impaired cardiac function, the V_{O_2}max declines in proportion to the degree of functional impairment.[17, 18]

The relationship between oxygen demand, cardiac output, and peripheral extraction of oxygen from arterial blood is complex. For example, a decline in mixed venous oxyhemoglobin saturation may reflect the normal response to exercise, an inappropriately low cardiac output, or a combination of these factors. Thus, for a given V_{O_2}, the greater the cardiac output, the higher would be the expected mixed venous oxygen saturation. This relation has been confirmed in patients with congestive heart failure in whom greater degrees of functional impairment are associated with a lower mixed venous oxyhemoglobin saturation for any V_{O_2}.[17–19, 23] Although increasing functional impairment in patients with congestive heart failure is associated with a lower V_{O_2}max, the mixed venous oxyhemoglobin saturation at peak exercise is similar across all functional classes.[17, 19] In addition, anaerobic threshold occurs at a similar mixed venous oxygen saturation ($32.9 \pm 7.8\%$) regardless of functional class.[23] Thus, in the presence of impaired cardiac output reserve, peripheral extraction of oxygen becomes the predominant means of increasing oxygen consumption. Increasing severity of congestive heart failure has also been associated with a higher ratio of change in heart rate to change in V_{O_2} during exercise.[23]

There is an inverse linear relationship between heart rate and mixed venous oxygen saturation during exercise that is independent of the degree of hemodynamic impairment in a variety of cardiac disorders.[19, 23, 24] For example, McElroy and colleagues[23] noted that the increase in heart rate during exercise was highly correlated with the decrease in mixed venous oxygen saturation in both normal individuals and patients with congestive heart failure.[23] For a decrease in mixed venous oxygen saturation of 1%, the average increase in heart rate was 1.8 ± 0.7 bpm in normals and ranged from 0.8 to 2.2 bpm per 1% decrease in oxygen saturation in patients with cardiac impairment.[23] Because of these relationships, a permanent pacemaker that increases the pacing rate in response to a decline in mixed venous oxyhemoglobin saturation should provide an appropriately greater pacing rate for any increment of exercise workload in a patient with impaired cardiac output than for an individual with normal cardiac function. Furthermore, mixed venous oxyhemoglobin saturation can also be used to ''optimize'' the cardiac output of patients requiring permanent pacing, so that the lowest

heart rate is provided to maintain the highest level of mixed venous oxyhemoglobin saturation at any level of exercise workload.[25, 26]

Rationale for Mixed Venous Oxygen Saturation as a Rate-Control Parameter

The preceding discussion of the response of mixed venous oxygen saturation to exercise suggests that this parameter may be ideal for modulating pacing rate. The theoretical advantages of mixed venous oxygen saturation as a physiologic sensor include proportionality to the level of metabolic demand, prompt response to the onset and termination of exercise, and predictable behavior (both qualitatively and quantitatively) over a wide range of functional cardiac impairment. In addition, because improvement in cardiac output at any level of metabolic demand is associated with an increase in mixed venous oxygen saturation, this parameter may provide a means of optimizing the pacing rate at all exercise workloads. The mixed venous oxygen saturation may also provide valuable diagnostic information about the adequacy of cardiac output in patients with structural heart disease. Despite these potential advantages, several technical challenges involving the chronic measurement of oxygen saturation in the heart had to be solved before this sensor could be implemented for permanent cardiac pacing.

Measurement of Oxygen Saturation In Vivo

To allow mixed venous oxygen saturation to become a reliable rate-control parameter for cardiac pacing, the saturation of hemoglobin in the right heart must be measured frequently and accurately. In addition, the accuracy of the sensor must be ensured under a variety of physiologic conditions such as variations in hematocrit, temperature, valvular and cardiac chamber motion, blood flow, and changes in the absolute level of oxyhemoglobin saturation itself. The sensor should remain accurate despite the pathologic changes associated with chronically implanted pacing leads, including fibrin coating, thrombosis, and encapsulation by a fibrous sheath.

The measurement of oxyhemoglobin saturation in blood is based on the principle of hemoreflectance—that is, oxygenated blood reflects light to a greater extent than does deoxygenated blood.[27] By using techniques first developed to measure oxygen saturation accurately in vitro that were based on the simple observation that arterial blood is brighter (more ''red'') than venous blood (which is darker or more ''blue''), Polanyi and Hehir used fiberoptics to measure the oxygen saturation of blood.[28, 29] The technique of fiberoptic oximetry was extensively refined by several investigators, including Mook and colleagues,[30, 31] Johnson and colleagues,[32] Kapany and Silbertrust,[33] and Shaw and Sperinde,[34] who used fiberoptic monofilaments to carry light from an external source into the bloodstream and to transport the light reflected from erythrocytes back to an external photosensor. Because oxygenated blood is more reflective than deoxygenated blood, the amount of light that is reflected is directly related to the oxyhemoglobin saturation.[35] Because catheters with polymer fiberoptics are relatively inexpensive and provide highly accurate measurements of oxyhemoglobin saturation, this technique has been widely accepted in critical care medicine.[36–40] However, because only a small fraction of the light emitted from the light source actually reaches the bloodstream in a fiberoptic catheter, this technique is energy inefficient. This is of little practical concern when using benchtop instruments coupling light to fiberoptic catheters powered by an alternating current power source. However, energy efficiency is highly relevant to the design of permanent pacemakers. Because permanent pacing systems are powered by a battery with limited charge capacity, fiberoptics are not practical for this application.

Solid-state electronics have allowed the development of an optical sensor that is suitable for a chronically implanted permanent pacing system. Implantable hemoreflectance oximeters using light-emitting diodes (LED) and a silicon photodetector were described by several teams including Yee and associates,[41] Schmitt and colleagues,[42] and Takatani and colleagues.[43] These solid-state devices placed the light source and the photodetector within the vasculature and proved that the entire sensor could be placed on a catheter. Solid-state sensors intended for incorporation into permanent pacing leads were proposed by Wirtzfeld and colleagues[25] and Baudino and associates.[44]

Hemoreflectance Oximetry

Although the amount of light reflected from blood is related to the percentage of hemoglobin that is bound to oxygen, this observation is highly dependent on the wavelength of light used to illuminate the blood. As shown in Figure 9–2, the reflectance of light from blood is most influenced by the extent of oxygen saturation when a wavelength of 660 nm (in the visible red range) is used. Thus, the 660-nm wavelength provides the highest level of discrimination of oxygenated from deoxygenated blood. In contrast, wavelengths of light in the 800- to 900-nm (infrared) range are reflected from blood nearly independently of the percentage of oxygen saturation.

The reflectance of light in both the red and the infrared ranges is also related to the number of erythrocytes that are present within a given volume of blood (the structures from which light is actually reflected). Studies by Mook and colleagues,[31] Renolds and coworkers,[45] Schmitt and associates,[42] and Bornzin and colleagues[46] have shown that the intensity of reflected light increases as the hematocrit increases (until a plateau is reached). Thus, the hematocrit has a marked influence on the reflectance of blood. In addition, other factors such as the orientation, size, and shape of erythrocytes have important effects on the back-scattering of light. Takatani and colleagues[43] demonstrated that the mean corpuscular volume (MCV) of red blood cells affects the intensity of photons reflected during illumination of the bloodstream with either the red or infrared wavelengths.[43] The orientation of disc-shaped erythrocytes is influenced by blood flow. Low-flow states lead to stacking of erythrocytes (rouleaux formation) and a change in light reflectivity.[31] In addition, osmolality and pH have been shown to affect the size and shape of erythrocytes and alter the light-scattering properties of blood.[47, 48] To compensate for these nonspecific effects, oxygen saturation is commonly measured with two wavelengths of light (red and infrared) that have different reflective properties with respect to the proportion of hemoglobin in a sample of blood that is bound to oxygen.

Because both red and infrared wavelengths are influenced by the nonspecific effects of hematocrit, red cell orientation, size, and shape on light reflectance, the ratio of light reflectance from these two wavelengths tends to cancel out these factors (leaving oxygen saturation as the major factor determining the reflectance of light). If the reflectance for both the red (660-nm) and the infrared (880-nm) wavelengths of light is known, an accurate estimate of the percentage of hemoglobin bound to oxygen can be calculated. The ratio of infrared to red light reflectance is used to measure oxyhemoglobin saturation by use of the formula:

$$R = I_{IR}/I_R$$

where R is the ratio of infrared (I_{IR}) to red (I_R) light reflectance. Although early studies assumed that oxygen saturation was linearly related to this ratio, this assumption is true only for a narrow range of oxygen saturations, for instance, 40% to 85%. This formula is most accurate at an oxygen saturation of approximately 80% because the red (660-nm) and infrared (880-nm) light scatter and decay are almost identical at this level. At oxygen saturations of less than 40%, the effects of red cell size, shape, and hematocrit become more significant than at higher saturation, leading to inaccuracies in the measurement. Figure 9–3 demonstrates the effect of hematocrit on the reflectance of red (660-nm) and infrared (880-nm) wavelengths of light. Note that at a saturation of 75%, the effect of hematocrit on reflectance is minimal, but greater sensitivity to this variable occurs at lower saturations in which the decay in red and infrared light intensities with reflection are most different. Figure 9–4 illustrates how the precision and linearity of this formula can be improved if constants are added to infrared and red intensity.[44, 49] Further improvements in the accuracy of oxyhemoglobin saturation

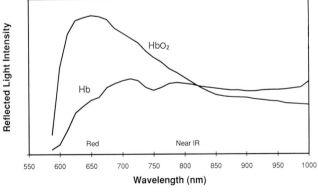

FIGURE 9–2. Reflectance of light by hemoglobin in blood that is oxygenated (HbO$_2$) and deoxygenated (Hb). Note that wavelengths of light in the red range (660 nm) are reflected with much greater intensity from oxygenated blood than from deoxygenated blood. In contrast, at wavelengths in the near-infrared region (805 nm), there is very little difference in the reflectance of light from oxygenated or deoxygenated blood. By constructing a ratio of the reflectance of light from red and infrared wavelengths, an absolute oxygen saturation can be calculated (see text for discussion).

FIGURE 9–3. The effect of hematocrit on the reflectance of light from blood is demonstrated for a pacing system with an oxygen saturation sensor using red and infrared wavelengths of light. Note that the slope of the relationship between the ratio of light reflectance with red and infrared wavelengths and the oxygen saturation changes with changes in hematocrit. In the oxygen saturation range of approximately 78%, the ratio of light reflectance is independent of the hematocrit. At this saturation level, the infrared and red wavelengths of light decay at nearly identical rates following illumination of blood, so changes in scattering due to hematocrit do not affect the ratio of light reflectance. At lower saturations the decay of red light is more sensitive to hematocrit than for infrared wavelengths. Thus, the ratio of red to infrared reflectance increases as the hematocrit increases. (Data from Seifert GP, Moore AA, Graves KL, Lahtinen SP: In vivo and in vitro studies of a chronic oxygen saturation sensor. PACE 14:514, 1991.)

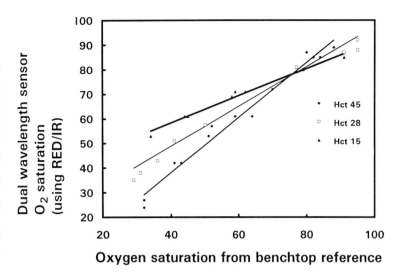

Oxygen saturation from benchtop reference

measurements are afforded by the use of three wavelengths of light and the calculation of two reflectance ratios; one ratio is most accurate at an oxygen saturation of 80% and the other at a saturation of 40%.[34]

Design of Pacing Leads and Pulse Generators That Measure Oxygen Saturation

Chronically implantable oxygen saturation sensors must meet several stringent performance criteria. First, the sensors must operate while drawing only small amounts of current (in the microampere range). Second, the optical and electronic components must be protected from the harsh environment of the bloodstream. Third, the lead must be capable of withstanding the flexion stress of hundreds of millions of heart beats. Fourth, another challenge relates to variations in the adequacy of mixing of venous blood within the right ventricle. At present, two manufacturers have developed and

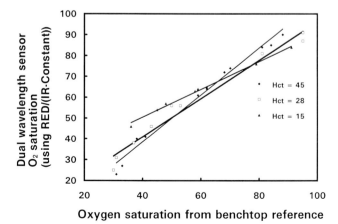

Oxygen saturation from benchtop reference

FIGURE 9–4. The results from Figure 9–3 were recalculated by subtracting a constant from the infrared light reflectance. This approach increases the accuracy of the ratio of infrared to red light reflectance despite changes in hematocrit. (Data from Seifert GP, Moore AA, Graves KL, Lahtinen SP: In vivo and in vitro studies of a chronic oxygen saturation sensor. PACE 14:514, 1991.)

investigated oxygen saturation-controlled pacemakers (Medtronic Inc., Minneapolis, MN and Siemens-Pacesetter, Sylmar, CA). These devices differ somewhat in the method of oxygen saturation measurement, the Siemens-Pacesetter device using a single red wavelength of light and the Medtronic device using two wavelengths. There are several trade-offs between these approaches to the measurement of oxygen saturation that will be discussed later.

The Siemens-Pacesetter model 1104C oxygen saturation pacing catheter is an 8 F bipolar lead that is insulated with silicone rubber. An oxygen saturation sensor is located proximal to the tip of the lead and is deployed in the right ventricular cavity. A close-up photograph of the sensor capsule is shown in Figure 9–5. A transparent glass capsule with platinum end-caps is used to protect the optical sensor electronics mounted on a hybrid ceramic circuit from the bloodstream. When driven by a nominal current in the 200-μA range, an LED illuminates the blood with a relatively constant intensity at a wavelength of 660 nm. Light passes through the transparent capsule and polymer coating into the bloodstream. The red light is reflected from erythrocytes and is detected by a photodetector. The LED remains "on" until enough reflected light has been detected by the solid-state photodetector to charge a capacitor to a reference voltage. The interval required to charge the capacitance is dependent on the intensity of reflected light. Under high oxygen saturation conditions (about 75%), the blood is highly reflective, and the interval required to charge the capacitor is short (about 1 msec). When the saturation drops during exercise, the blood is less reflective, and the charging times increase to the 2- to 3-msec range (Fig. 9–6). Considering that measurements are made every cardiac cycle with a nominal LED current requirement of 200 μA for a charging time of 1 msec, the sensor drains only a fraction of a microampere from the battery. This is only a small fraction of the current required for the pacing pulse (approximately 6 μA with nominal settings).

This single-wavelength design provides for a small size of the sensor capsule and lead (8 F) and relatively high energy efficiency. Optimizing the design of a single-wavelength sensor requires selection of the optimal spacing between the light source (LED) and the photodetector. As the hematocrit increases, the intensity of reflected light increases to a plateau

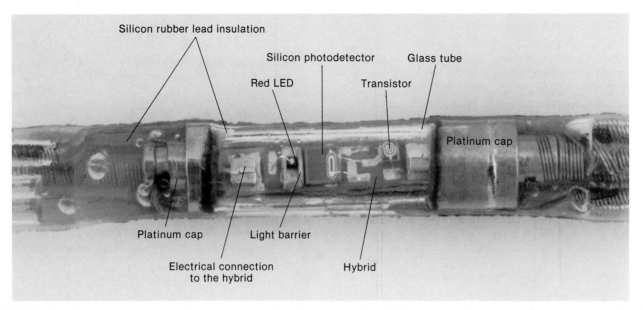

FIGURE 9–5. Magnified photograph of the optical sensor capsule of the Siemens-Pacesetter 1104C pacing lead. The optical sensor is composed of solid state elements located on a hybrid circuit that is sealed in a glass tube with platinum caps at each end. The photodetector is the large circular element located on the hybrid circuit to the right of a light barrier. The red light–emitting diode (LED) is shown opposite the detector to the left of the barrier. A transistor *(extreme right)* converts the reflectance of red light into a time interval. The platinum caps are welded to provide a hermetic seal and an electric connection to the conductor coils in the lead.

before decreasing at very high values. Figure 9–7 illustrates how the plateau varies with the distance between the light source and the photodetector. The single-wavelength sensor uses a spacing on the order of 1 mm. Consequently, the intensity of reflected light is directly proportional to both the hematocrit and the oxygen saturation. Since both of these variables influence the oxygen-carrying capacity of blood, this single-wavelength sensor has the potential advantage of tracking the mixed venous oxygen content.

The Siemens-Pacesetter 1104C lead was designed to be connected to either the model 2070 dual-chamber or the model 2080 single-chamber rate-adaptive pulse generator

(Fig. 9–8). These devices are powered by a 1.8-Ah lithium-iodide battery and weigh 41 and 38 g, respectively. The rate-adaptive algorithm provides for automatically setting the sensitivity of the sensor based on typical day-to-day variations in oxygen saturation. Maximal oxygen-controlled heart rate occurs at the typical minimum achieved oxyhemoglobin saturation. Tissue overgrowth, which may be expected to reduce the amount of light detected by the sensor, is compensated for by automatically increasing the sensitivity of the sensor. A piezoelectric activity sensor is located in the pulse generator and allows the pacing rate to be controlled by either oxygen saturation or activity alone or by a combination of the two sensors. The activity and oxygen saturation sensors can be programmed to prevent changes in pacing rate occurring without confirmation by the alternate sensor, minimizing the potential for ''false-positive'' responses. The activity sen-

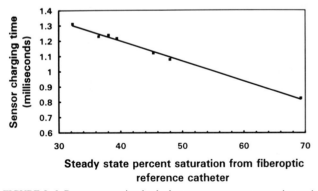

FIGURE 9–6. Permanent pacing leads that measure oxygen saturation emit a known quantity of light into the bloodstream and quantitate the intensity of light reflected from red blood cells with a photodetector. The photons received by the photodetector charge a capacitor to a reference voltage. The charging time required to charge the capacitor is plotted as a function of the steady state percentage of oxygen saturation measured with a fiberoptic reference catheter. Note that as the oxygen saturation increases, the charging time decreases because more light is reflected from the brighter oxygenated blood and received by the photodetector. At low oxygen saturations, the intensity of reflected light decreases, thus requiring a greater interval for the photodetector to charge the capacitor to the same charge.

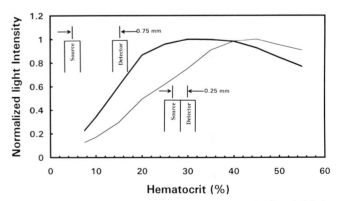

FIGURE 9–7. The effect of hematocrit on the intensity of reflected light is shown for two optical sensors with different distances between the light source and the photodetector (0.25 mm and 0.75 mm). Note that a distance of 0.75 mm between the source and the detector provides a relatively stable intensity of reflected light over the physiologic range of hematocrits (18–50%).

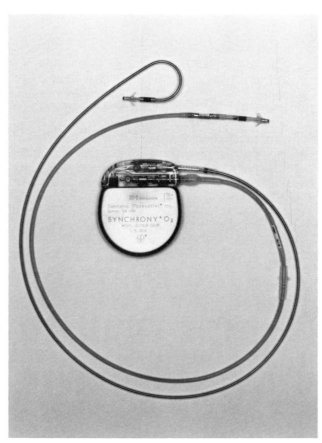

FIGURE 9–8. Photograph of the Siemens-Pacesetter model 2070 oxygen saturation–controlled pulse generator and atrial and ventricular leads. The 41-g pulse generator is connected to a tined, 8 F bipolar lead (model 1104C) that emits light with a wavelength of 660 nm and registers the quantity of light that is reflected from the bloodstream. The optic sensor is located 4 cm from the tip of the ventricular lead. This pacing system also has the capability of controlling pacing rate by a piezoelectric activity sensor.

sor provides for a rapid response to the onset of exercise when the mixed venous oxygen saturation may tend to lag in the presence of impaired venous return. If activity levels are inappropriately high with respect to venous oxygen saturation, the activity-driven rate increase is limited to prevent an excessive rate response. Conversely, marked declines in mixed venous oxygen saturation that are not accompanied by an increase in the activity signal are also prevented from modulating pacing rate excessively.

Following the alternative approach of using both red and infrared wavelengths of light to measure absolute oxygen saturation, an 11 F lead has been developed by Medtronic Inc. (Fig. 9–9). Two LEDs and other electronic components, including a photodiode detector, are hermetically sealed in an optically pure sapphire and titanium capsule.[44] Like the single-wavelength system described earlier, a charged capacitor scheme inside the sensor transduces reflected light intensity into time intervals. The Medtronic model 2505A and 8007 oxygen saturation pacing systems use both red and infrared wavelengths of light to determine oxygen saturation. For these dual-wavelength sensors, the red LED (660 nm) is first activated to illuminate the bloodstream. The light continues to be transmitted until the photodetector has detected sufficient photons to charge a capacitor to a reference level.

Once the photodetector is charged to a predetermined level, the red LED is turned off. Then the infrared LED is turned on, and the photodetector is again used to charge a capacitor to a reference level at this wavelength. The red LED is then activated again. It is this second red-cycle interval that is used for measurement of the light reflectance ratio (the first red interval is used to stabilize the circuitry and is discarded). The interval required for charging of the photodiode by the red wavelength depends on the oxygen saturation, hematocrit, temperature, and flow pattern of the venous blood as well as on any surface deposits that are located on the sensor. The red interval is typically 1.5 to 2.0 msec at a resting mixed venous saturation of 75% and increases to 4 to 5 msec during exercise. A current of approximately 3 mA is required to illuminate the red LED. The infrared LED emits a wavelength of 880 nm and consumes approximately 1 mA of current. The infrared activation interval (typically 2 to 3 msec) is relatively independent of oxygen saturation but is influenced by hematocrit, temperature, flow pattern, and surface deposits on the sensor. By using the ratio of red to infrared wavelengths, these variables can be minimized in the calculation of oxyhemoglobin saturation. Although use of a single red wavelength of light (660 nm) allows detection of relative changes in oxyhemoglobin saturation, quantitation of the ratio of reflectance from the red (sensitive to oxyhemoglobin saturation) and the infrared (insensitive to oxyhemoglobin saturation) wavelengths allows an absolute value of oxygen saturation to be determined.

The battery used for the Medtronic 2505A (VVIR) and 8007 (DDDR) pulse generators is based on lithium-manganese dioxide. This battery chemistry was chosen because of its low internal resistance, which allows current to be delivered to the sensor without a decline in voltage that would interfere with the pacing pulse. The beginning of life (BOL) battery voltage of this cell is 3.1 V (compared with 2.8 V for lithium iodide), and it has an elective replacement indicator (ERI) voltage of 2.5 V.

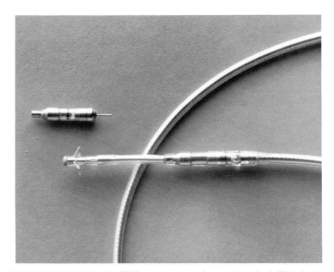

FIGURE 9–9. Medtronic 6227 oxygen saturation–sensing lead. This device uses two LEDs emitting light at wavelengths of 660 and 805 nm with a single photodetector. The optic components are incorporated into a hermetically sealed sapphire and titanium capsule.

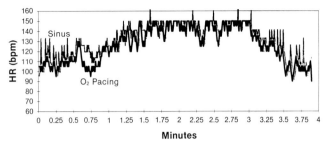

FIGURE 9–10. Effect of treadmill exercise in a dog on the rate of the normal sinus node and an oxygen saturation–controlled VVIR pacing system using a single wavelength of light. Note that there is a close correlation between the sinus rate and the pacing rate, suggesting that mixed venous oxygen saturation provides a suitable sensor for chronotropic modulation of the heart.

Animal Experiments with Implanted Oxygen-Controlled Pacing Systems

ACUTE STUDIES

Oxygen saturation–controlled pacing was compared to atrioventricular (AV) synchronous (VDD) pacing and pacing modulated by right ventricular dP/dt and stroke volume in dogs with complete AV block during treadmill exercise.[50, 51] These animals were implanted with atrial and ventricular leads, right atrial dP/dt pressure sensors, electromagnetic flow probes for measurement of cardiac output, and cannulas for measurement of arterial pressure. Fiberoptic catheters were placed in the right ventricle for measurement of mixed venous oxygen saturation. External pacing was used as the canines exercised on a treadmill at a speed of 6.6 mph and grades of 6%, 12%, and 18%. There was no difference in the hemodynamics with sensor-controlled VVIR pacing compared with VDD pacing. The chronotropic response times (the interval required for the heart rate to increase from the resting value to 90% of the steady-state value) were 15, 20, 33, and 35 seconds for VDD pacing, and VVIR pacing controlled by dP/dt, mixed venous oxygen saturation, and stroke volume, respectively.[52]

Animal experiments with pacing systems controlled by mixed venous oxygen saturation have generally shown a very close correlation between the oxyhemoglobin saturation measured from single- or dual-wavelength sensors and a reference three-wavelength fiberoptic catheter. Figure 9–10 demonstrates the rate response of the normal sinus node and the pacing rate provided by a permanent pacing system using a single red wavelength sensor during exercise in a canine. The permanent oxygen saturation sensor had been implanted 2 days previously into the right ventricle. Note that the sinus rate and the pacing rate controlled by oxygen saturation in the right ventricle are closely matched. The effect of exercise on mixed venous oxygen saturation as determined by a fiberoptic reference catheter using three wavelengths of light is shown in Figure 9–11 for a dog at three workloads (variable treadmill grade with constant speed). Note that the mixed venous oxygen saturation falls promptly at the onset of exercise and reaches a steady state that is proportional to the workload. Figure 9–12 demonstrates the response of a single-wavelength pacing system during treadmill exercise in a dog at three workloads. The charging time required for reflected light detected by the photodetector to charge a capacitor is inversely related to the mixed venous oxygen saturation. Note that the charging time increases to a plateau value that is proportional to the treadmill grade. At high workloads this device responds with a brisk onset. There is a smooth and gradual increase in oxygen saturation with a constant slope during the recovery phase at each workload. From these acute animal experiments the accuracy, feasibility, and physiologic correlation of right ventricular oxygen saturation has been demonstrated.

CHRONIC STUDIES

Although the acute studies of oxygen-controlled pacing systems have suggested that this device has very desirable properties, there has been considerable concern about the long-term stability of an optical sensor positioned within the heart. Because transvenous pacing leads frequently become encased with a fibrous sheath and thrombi,[53] the effect of these pathologic changes on the function of an optical sensor that must illuminate the bloodstream and measure the quantity of light that is reflected has been proposed as a potential clinical problem with a chronically implanted device. Limited data exist about the long-term fate of optical sensors on permanent pacing leads in the right ventricle. The available data suggest, at least in canines, that an opaque fibrotic

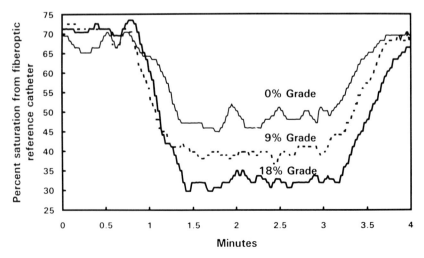

FIGURE 9–11. Effect of treadmill exercise on mixed venous oxygen saturation measured with a fiberoptic reference catheter in the right ventricle in a dog. Exercise was performed at three workloads using a variable treadmill grade and constant treadmill speed. Note that the oxygen saturation decreases promptly following the onset of exercise to a relatively constant value that is proportional to the workload. After 30 seconds of standing on the treadmill, exercise was performed by ramping the treadmill to a speed of 6.5 km/hr. The treadmill was stopped after approximately 3 minutes of exercise.

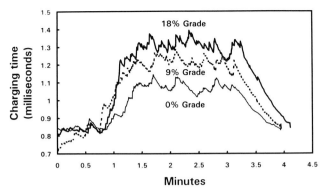

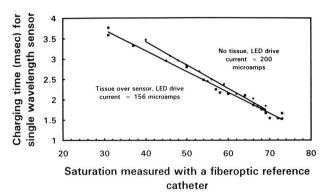

FIGURE 9–12. The effect of treadmill exercise on an implanted right ventricular oxygen sensor in a dog at three workloads. Exercise was performed with the pacing system programmed to the DDDR mode with sensor measurements recorded in the memory of the pulse generator. The charging time is inversely related to the mixed venous oxygen saturation. As the oxygen saturation declines, the intensity of light reflected from the bloodstream decreases. Thus, at lower saturations a longer interval is required for the photodetector to charge the capacitor to a reference value.

FIGURE 9–14. The results of a study of the effects of simulated tissue overgrowth on a single wavelength sensor are shown in this figure. A control study was performed in a canine in which the sensor was placed in the right ventricle. The mixed venous oxygen saturation was then varied. Tissue overgrowth was simulated by covering the sensor with a portion of excised jugular vein. This device used an algorithm that adjusts the current delivered to the sensor to maintain a consistent range of light reflectance. Although the overall light intensity was reduced by tissue overgrowth, the adjustment in current to the sensor reestablished the recorded oxygen saturation toward the control value. This algorithm is designed to compensate for changes in sensor sensitivity that may be caused by factors such as tissue overgrowth.

sheath may cover the sensor capsule in some animals. The clinical data accumulated during extraction of transvenous leads suggests that fibrotic attachments to permanent pacing leads may develop at almost any point in the central veins, right atrium, or right ventricle.

Studies have been performed on both the single- and dual-wavelength systems to approximate the effects of tissue overgrowth on the optical sensor. The dual-wavelength sensor was studied with freshly excised pericardial tissue that was wrapped around the sensor in vitro. The results of these experiments are shown in Figure 9–13 and demonstrate that this simulated tissue overgrowth tended to cause the sensor measurements of oxygen saturation to read higher than the control lead. In a study performed with a single-wavelength oxygen saturation system, tissue overgrowth was simulated by covering the optical sensor with a section of excised jugular vein (Fig. 9–14). To compensate for the reduction in the intensity of reflected light, the current delivered to the sensor was reduced from 200 to 156 μA. This reestablished an oxygen saturation sensitivity similar to the control conditions. It remains to be demonstrated how often such fibrotic encapsulation will interfere with the accuracy of a mixed venous oxygen sensor in the right ventricle and whether or

not self-calibrating algorithms can be designed to effectively deal with this possibility.

Clinical Experience with Rate-Modulated, Oxygen-Controlled Pacing Systems

ACUTE STUDIES

Wirtzfeld and colleagues[54] demonstrated the feasibility of controlling pacing rate based on central venous oxyhemoglobin saturation in 10 human volunteers with VVI pacemakers previously implanted for complete AV block. In this initial report, a fiberoptic pulmonary artery catheter was used for measurement of oxyhemoglobin saturation during supine bicycle exercise at a constant workload of 25 W. The oxyhemoglobin saturation was used to modulate the pacing rate of a temporary transvenous pacing system. Compared with VVI pacing, oxygen-controlled temporary pacing resulted in an

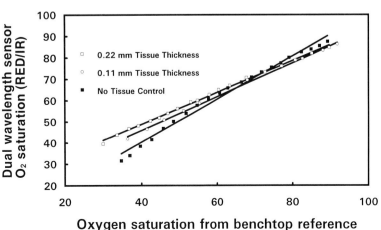

FIGURE 9–13. The effect of simulated tissue overgrowth on an optical sensor in the right ventricle that uses both red and infrared (RED/IR) wavelengths of light. Tissue overgrowth was simulated by wrapping pericardial tissue around the sensor with an extracorporeal oxygenator. Tissue overgrowth causes the sensor to register somewhat higher than the actual value (referenced to a benchtop oximeter).

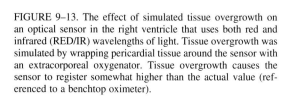

increase in maximum heart rate during exercise (106 bpm VVIR vs. 70.5 bpm VVI), cardiac output (8.4 L/min VVIR vs. 7.14 L/min VVI), and minimum mixed venous oxyhemoglobin saturation (46% VVIR vs. 44% VVI).

Based on these encouraging results, Wirtzfeld and colleagues developed an optical sensor integrating the light-emitting and light-receiving elements of a hemoreflectorimetry system within a hermetically sealed capsule that was suitable for use with a permanent pacing lead. This lead used a single wavelength of light (660 nm) and was demonstrated to provide oxyhemoglobin saturation measurements that were reliable and reproducible. Studies of right ventricular oxyhemoglobin saturation measured by this permanent pacing lead using a single transmitted wavelength of light have generally demonstrated a close correlation with the results of fiberoptic catheters using three wavelengths (660 nm, 700 nm, and 805 nm) in humans at the time of cardiac catheterization. The raw signal from a light-reflective sensor positioned in the right ventricle demonstrates marked fluctuations with each cardiac cycle.[55] These dynamic fluctuations reflect movement of the right ventricular walls, the tricuspid valve and subvalvular apparatus, and the sensor itself within the right ventricle. Therefore, the sensor output must be processed to attenuate these motion artifacts.[55] The artifact-rejection filter for a single-wavelength (660 nm) oxyhemoglobin saturation signal is used to reject high-intensity peaks and defines the oxygen saturation as the minimum value during the cardiac cycle.

In healthy volunteers there is a slight fall in right ventricular oxyhemoglobin saturation with a change from the supine to the upright position, corresponding to the expected postural decrease in venous return and cardiac output. Figure 9–15 demonstrates the effect of posture on mixed venous oxygen saturation in a normal volunteer. Note that the oxyhemoglobin saturation in the right ventricle decreased from 68% to 63% with a change from the supine to the sitting position. In patients with impaired cardiac output the decline in oxyhemoglobin saturation may be more marked. These data suggest that, in contrast to other sensors (such as right ventricular dP/dt or stroke volume), the oxygen sensor may provide an effective means of detecting (and treating) posturally induced decreases in cardiac output in patients with impaired autonomic reflexes.

Acute studies of the oxygen sensor in human subjects during exercise have also demonstrated a generally close correlation with the results obtained with a fiberoptic catheter using three wavelengths of transmitted light. Figure 9–16 was taken from a 63-year-old man with normal exercise tolerance and no structural heart disease during upright bicycle exercise. There is a sharp fall in right ventricular oxyhemoglobin saturation following the onset of exercise at a workload of 30 W. Note that the oxyhemoglobin saturation from the pacing lead closely tracks the output from the fiberoptic catheter from a baseline value of 73% to a value of 44% at this workload. After increase in the exercise workload to 45 W, there is a further decline in the oxyhemoglobin saturation to a nadir value of 38%. Following a decrease in the exercise workload, the oxyhemoglobin saturation increases to 56%. Also note that there is a phase lag between the oxyhemoglobin saturation recorded by the pacing lead and that of the fiberoptic catheter. This is likely an artifact of the signal processing algorithm used for this study. Figure 9–17 demonstrates similar findings in a 57-year-old man during upright bicycle exercise. Note that the oxyhemoglobin sensor from the pacing lead closely tracked the output of the fiberoptic catheter during exercise with a slight lag in the recorded saturation during recovery.

Further studies by Stangl and associates[12] in human volunteers have demonstrated that a closed-loop pacing system with modulation of pacing rate controlled by this oxyhemoglobin saturation sensor was both feasible and provided heart rates that were very similar to those of the normal sinus node. The mixed venous oxyhemoglobin saturation has an exponential relationship to exercise workload, with the highest sensitivity for changes in mixed venous oxyhemoglobin saturation occurring at low levels of metabolic demand. As the exercise workload increases, changes in workload result in smaller changes in oxyhemoglobin saturation. Thus, these acute studies suggest that mixed venous oxyhemoglobin saturation is likely to be an especially useful discriminator of exercise workload for patients with relatively limited exercise tolerance. Figure 9–18 demonstrates the effect of a supraventricular tachycardia on right ventricular oxyhemoglobin saturation in a patient with an acutely implanted oxygen saturation catheter at the time of electrophysiologic study. In this individual, an abrupt increase in the tachycardia rate from

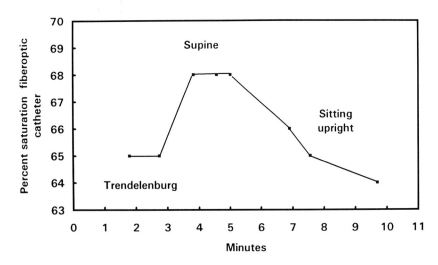

FIGURE 9–15. Effect of posture on mixed venous oxygen saturation. Right ventricular oxygen saturation was measured at rest in the Trendelenburg, supine, and sitting positions. Note that the supine position is associated with a higher oxygen saturation than the sitting position. This effect has been quite consistent in patients studied acutely with fiberoptic reference catheters and with implanted oxygen saturation pacing systems.

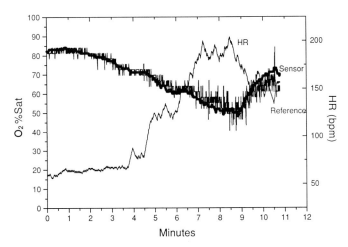

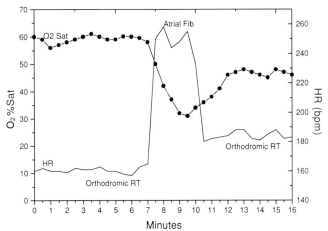

FIGURE 9–16. Effect of upright bicycle exercise on heart rate (HR) and right ventricular oxygen saturation measured with a fiberoptic reference catheter (Reference) and a single wavelength, implantable, oxygen saturation–sensing pacing lead (Sensor) in a healthy volunteer. Note that oxygen saturation measured with both devices is similar and promptly decreases at the start of exercise (3 minutes). The oxygen saturation measured by the implantable lead is lower than that measured by the reference catheter during recovery. This is an artifact of the averaging technique used during this study.

FIGURE 9–18. Effect of supraventricular tachycardia on mixed venous oxygen saturation in a patient with the Wolff-Parkinson-White syndrome. Note that the right ventricular oxygen saturation is relatively decreased (to approximately 60%) during supraventricular tachycardia at a rate of 165 bpm. With a transient increase in heart rate due to the development of atrial fibrillation to 250 bpm at approximately 7 minutes, there is an abrupt decline in oxygen saturation to 35%. With a decrease in heart rate (termination of atrial fibrillation and recurrence of AV reciprocating tachycardia), the oxygen saturation increases to approximately 43%.

160 to 250 bpm resulted in a decline in right ventricular oxygen saturation from 60% to 35% in a patient with reduced cardiac output (during supraventricular tachycardia). Note that with a decrease in the heart rate the oxyhemoglobin saturation gradually increased in this patient to approximately 43%. It is likely that the mixed venous oxygen saturation may provide a means of detecting an inappropriately rapid heart rate. These observations also raise the possibility of a closed-loop, positive feedback amplification of the pacing rate. If the pacing rate is excessively rapid, resulting in ischemia or hemodynamic compromise, the mixed venous oxygen saturation may decline, inducing further increases in pacing rate and further worsening of the hemodynamics.

Faerestrand and colleagues have reported their experience with a right ventricular oxyhemoglobin saturation sensor that

uses two wavelengths of light (660 nm and 805 nm).[56] The ratio of reflectance from the red and infrared wavelengths measured after every fourth QRS complex was used as the rate-control parameter. During supine arm exercise (25 W for 3 minutes), the oxyhemoglobin saturation measured by the pacing lead in the right ventricle correlated closely with that measured with right ventricular blood samples in six subjects with AV block at the time of cardiac catheterization. With rate-modulated pacing based on the oxyhemoglobin saturation, the heart rate increased from a mean of 96 bpm at rest to 127 bpm after 3 minutes of exercise. The oxyhemoglobin saturation was greater during rate-modulated pacing than during spontaneous AV block at rest and exercise.

Chronic Studies with Permanent Pacing Systems

Clinical data with oxyhemoglobin-controlled permanent pacing systems are quite limited. Stangl and colleagues were the first to report the clinical experience in two patients implanted with an oxygen-controlled, rate-adaptive permanent pacing system.[12] This VVIR device used an oxyhemoglobin saturation sensor that was located 9 cm proximal to the tip of a standard bipolar pacing lead. This sensor was hermetically sealed with a LED (660 nm) and a phototransistor that converts the light reflectance into an analog electric signal that is processed by the pulse generator. As the oxyhemoglobin saturation declines, the time required for the reflected light to charge a capacitor in the sensor capsule increases. Thus, the oxyhemoglobin saturation is inversely related to the charging time. The pacing rate is modulated between programmed minimum and maximum values in response to the sensor signal. The time required to achieve a 10% change in pacing rate in response to treadmill exercise ranged from 6 to 17 seconds. The time constant to achieve 67% of the observed increase in pacing rate at a given exer-

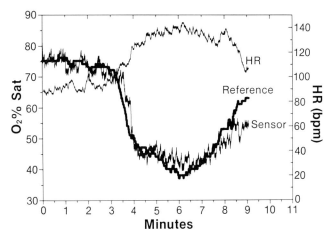

FIGURE 9–17. Effect of upright bicycle exercise on heart rate (HR) and right ventricular oxygen saturation measured with a fiberoptic reference catheter and a single wavelength implantable sensor in a 57-year-old man. Note that there is a smooth decline in oxygen saturation following the start of exercise (2 minutes), and similar values are recorded by both devices.

cise workload ranged between 38 and 44 seconds in these patients and was independent of workload. The decay constant (the time required for a 67% fall in pacing rate at the termination of exercise) was directly related to the intensity of exercise (47.5 seconds after a 25-W workload and 115 seconds after a 75-W workload). These investigators also determined whether an ''optimal'' pacing rate at any level of metabolic demand could be determined by measuring the oxyhemoglobin saturation over a range of rates. The optimal pacing rate was defined as the lowest pacing rate at any metabolic demand that does not result in a decline in right ventricular oxyhemoglobin saturation. Although no deterioration of the sensor signal was observed in this study, the follow-up time was only 5 months, which is inadequate to draw conclusions about long-term stability of the sensor.

Faerestrand and colleagues have reported their initial clinical results in four patients with VVIR pacing systems in which heart rate was controlled by right ventricular oxyhemoglobin saturation.[13] This device used a hemoreflectance sensor emitting both red and infrared wavelengths located in the right ventricle. The right ventricular oxyhemoglobin saturation decreased from a mean of 65% at rest to 36% during exercise (bicycle and treadmill) with an increase in heart rate to a mean of 110 bpm. Ambulatory electrocardiographic monitoring demonstrated appropriate variation in pacing rate during a follow-up period ranging from 1 to 6 months. Although long-term data have not yet been published, the initial experience with this pacing system has been characterized by an excellent rate response in 12 patients, marked variability in the resting heart rate in 1 patient, and an inadequate response to exercise in 1 patient. Despite a follow-up period extending beyond 4 years from the date of the initial implants, the limited number of study patients does not allow firm conclusions to be drawn about the long-term stability of the sensor.

The Medtronic model 2505A VVIR pacing system allows separately programmable upper and lower pacing rates as well as two rate-modulating parameters, the rate response slope and the rate offset. There are 10 values for the rate response slope and 2 rate-offset choices. These variables define a family of rate-modulation curves that determine the relationship between oxygen saturation and pacing rate. Thus, at each value of mixed venous oxygen saturation the pacing rate can be predicted. The results of exercise testing with a dual wavelength oxygen saturation pacing system (Medtronic model 2505A) are shown in Figure 9–19. Note that the mixed venous oxygen saturation declines rapidly following the onset of exercise from approximately 60% to a telemetered nadir of less than 10% at peak exercise. The actual minimum oxygen saturation is probably somewhat higher (approximately 20%) because the assumption of a linear relationship between the reflectance of red and infrared light and the oxygen saturation does not hold at very low oxygen saturations. Nevertheless, the decrease in oxygen saturation is associated with a smooth increase in pacing rate from approximately 90 bpm at rest to a maximum value of 140 bpm in this individual. Following the termination of exercise there is a sharp increase in mixed venous oxygen saturation to resting values of approximately 65%. Figure 9–20 illustrates how this device can be used to measure the cardiac output by the Fick method. Although precise Fick cardiac output calculations should be made under steady-

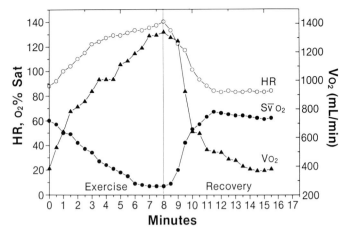

FIGURE 9–19. Effect of treadmill exercise on right ventricular oxygen saturation in a patient with an implanted Medtronic 2505A VVIR pacing system. This patient had severe left ventricular dysfunction and chronic atrial fibrillation with complete AV block following AV nodal catheter ablation. Note that oxygen saturation decreases from a resting value of 60% to a telemetered value of 8% at peak exercise. The nadir value is actually higher than that recorded in this individual by telemetry because the red-infrared ratio at low oxygen saturations is nonlinear. The heart rate (HR) increases with a slope that is slightly less than that of the measured oxygen consumption (Vo_2) in this patient. The slope is a programmable function with this pacing system and was increased from a programmed value of 1 to a setting of 5 following this exercise test.

state conditions, measurement of the mixed venous and the arterial oxygen saturation as well as collection of expired gases allows calculation of the cardiac output. Note that the cardiac output increases in this individual with poor left ventricular function during exercise and declines to resting values during recovery. Figure 9–21 shows the telemetered mixed venous oxygen saturation and pacing rate during low- and medium-intensity walks in a patient with severe congestive heart failure who has a Medtronic 2505A pacing system. Note that minimal exertion produced an abrupt decline in oxygen saturation from a resting value of 58% to 42%. With a medium-level walk there was a decrease in oxygen saturation from 58% to 22%. The initial experience with this pacing system has shown it to provide predictable rate modulation and valuable diagnostic information that can be used to assess the hemodynamic status of the patient.

Potential Clinical Problems

There are several theoretical limitations to the oxyhemoglobin saturation sensor. First, and perhaps most important, the long-term reliability of the sensor remains to be established. Because permanent pacing leads often become coated by a sheath of opaque fibrous tissue, the intensity of the light emitted by the sensor capsule may decline over time. It is likely that this obstacle can be overcome with algorithms that adjust the gain of the pacing system over time. Second, the optimal location of the sensor within the heart has not been firmly established. Although positioning of the sensor in the right atrium may decrease the likelihood of fibrous encapsulation, valvular interference, and wall motion artifact, the venous blood is not as well mixed in the right atrium as it is more distally in the venous circulation. In addition, a catheter

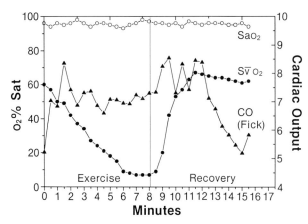

FIGURE 9–20. Effect of exercise on cardiac output measured with the Fick technique in a patient with an implanted Medtronic 2505A VVIR pacing system (same patient as shown in Figure 9–19). The arterial oxygen saturation was measured with a transcutaneous saturation monitor. Although precise application of the Fick technique requires a steady-state oxygen consumption, the Fick equation was used to estimate cardiac output during exercise. Note that the cardiac output increased from a resting value of 5.3 L/min to 8.5 L/min during peak exercise, with a decrease to resting values during recovery. The potential diagnostic value of an absolute mixed venous oxygen saturation pacing system is demonstrated by this example.

in the right atrium may be likely to become more heavily influenced by the markedly deoxygenated blood returning from the coronary sinus, further enhancing the potential for inaccuracy.

Third, a closed-loop pacing system controlled by mixed venous oxyhemoglobin saturation has the potential for positive feedback. For example, in the presence of myocardial ischemia, inappropriately high pacing rates have the theoretical potential to worsen the degree of ischemia, thereby decreasing ventricular performance and decreasing mixed venous oxyhemoglobin saturation. Such a scenario could lead to further increases in pacing rate and more ischemia. It should be recognized that such a situation for positive feedback may also exist for other sensors such as minute ventilation, evoked ventricular response, and right ventricular dP/dt. It should be stressed that, as with all rate-adaptive pacing

systems, clinical judgment is required for programming of the minimum and maximum pacing rates.

Fourth, the characteristics of the venous circulation on the performance of the oxyhemoglobin saturation sensor must be considered. As with pacing systems that monitor right ventricular temperature, the capacitance of the venous circulation is likely to influence the time delay between the onset of exercise and the fall in right ventricular oxyhemoglobin saturation. Because most acute studies of this sensor have involved volunteers in the catheterization laboratory, the spectrum of exercise response times encountered in elderly patients with varying degrees of venous incompetence is likely to differ from the results of initial studies.

Summary

Mixed venous oxygen saturation is a physiologic indicator of metabolic demand with characteristics that are ideally suited to control heart rate. This parameter can be measured reliably using the hemoreflectance technique with catheters suitable for an implantable pacing system. Initial studies in humans and animals have demonstrated that chronic measurement of oxygen saturation in the right ventricle is feasible. Despite these initially encouraging results, the long-term stability of this sensor remains to be demonstrated. Because of the physiologic characteristics of oxygen saturation during exercise, it is likely that this sensor will become widely accepted in the pacing community if the chronic reliability of the sensor can be ensured.

REFERENCES

1. Wirtzfeld A, Bock T: Cardiac Pacemaker. US Patent No. 4,202,339, 1980.
2. Wirtzfeld A, Goedel-Meinen L, Bock T, et al: Central venous oxygen saturation for the control of automatic rate-responsive pacing. PACE 5:829, 1982.
3. Wirtzfeld A, Heinze R, Liess HD, et al: An active optical sensor for monitoring mixed venous oxygen saturation for an implantable rate-regulating pacing system. PACE 6:494, 1983.
4. Bornzin GA: Rate-adaptive demand pacemaker. US Patent No. 4,467,807, 1984.
5. Anderson KM, Moore AA: Sensors in pacing. PACE 9:953, 1986.
6. Stangl K, Wirtzfeld A, Heinze R, et al: A new multisensor pacing system using stroke volume, respiratory rate, mixed venous oxygen saturation, and temperature, right atrial pressure, right ventricular pressure, and dP/dt. PACE 11:712, 1988.
7. Faerestrand S, Skadberg BT, Ohm O-J: Acute hemodynamic evaluation of a new pacemaker responding to central venous oxygen saturation [Abstract]. PACE 12:1158, 1989.
8. Faerestrand S, Skadberg BT, Anderson K, Ohm O-J: Acute clinical testing and follow-up of a new rate-variable pacemaker controlled by central venous oxygen saturation [Abstract]. J Am Coll Cardiol 13:112A, 1989.
9. Bennett T, Bornzin G, Baudino M, Olson W: Rate-responsive pacing using mixed venous oxygen saturation in heart blocked dogs [Abstract]. Circulation 70:II-246, 1984.
10. Faerestrand S, Skadberg BT, Ohm O-J: Follow-up of a new rate-responsive pacemaker controlled by central venous oxygen saturation [Abstract]. PACE 12:1231, 1989.
11. Faerestrand S, Ohm O-J: Central venous oxygen saturation at rest and exercise during bradycardia and rate-responsive pacing [Abstract]. PACE 13:529, 1990.
12. Stangl K, Wirtzfeld A, Heinze R, et al: First clinical experience with an oxygen saturation controlled pacemaker in man. PACE 11:1882, 1988.
13. Faerestrand S, Skadberg BT, Ohm O-J: Long-term rate responsive pacing controlled by central venous oxygen saturation [Abstract]. PACE 12:671, 1989.

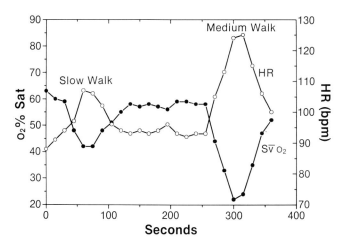

FIGURE 9–21. Effect of slow- and medium-intensity walking on telemetered mixed venous oxygen saturation and pacing rate in a patient in whom a Medtronic 2505A pacing system was implanted (see text for discussion).

14. Wade OL, Bishop JM: Cardiac Output and Regional Blood Flow. Philadelphia, FA Davis, 1962.

15. Casaburi R, Daly J, Hansen J, et al: Abrupt changes in mixed venous blood gas compositions after the onset of exercise. J Appl Physiol 67:1106, 1989.

16. Fick A: Über die Messung des Blutquantums in den Herzventikeln. Sitz der Physik-Med ges Wurtzberg. 1870, p 16.

17. Weber KT, Kinasewitz GT, Janicki JS, Fishman AP: Oxygen utilization and ventilation during exercise in patients with chronic cardiac failure. Circulation 65:1213, 1982.

18. Weber KT, Janicki JS: Cardiopulmonary exercise (CPX) testing. In Leff AR (ed): Cardiopulmonary Exercise Testing: Physiologic Principles and Clinical Applications. Philadelphia, WB Saunders, 1986.

19. Weber KT, Janicki JS: Cardiopulmonary exercise testing for evaluation of chronic cardiac failure. Am J Cardiol 55:22A, 1985.

20. Wilson JR, Martin JL, Schwartz D, Ferraro N: Exercise intolerance in patients with chronic heart failure: Role of impaired nutritive flow to skeletal muscle. Circulation 69:1079, 1984.

21. Kugler J, Maskin C, Frishman WH, et al: Regional and systemic metabolic effects of angiotensin converting enzyme inhibition during exercise in patients with severe heart failure. Circulation 66:1256, 1982.

22. Astrand I, Astrand P-O, Hallback I, Kilbom A: Reduction in maximum oxygen uptake with age. J Appl Physiol 35:649, 1973.

23. McElroy PA, Janicki JS, Weber KT: Physiologic correlates of the heart rate response to upright isotonic exercise: relevance to rate-responsive pacemakers. J Am Coll Cardiol 11:94, 1988.

24. French W, Casaburi R, Lewis D, et al: Relationship between mixed venous oxygen saturation and heart rate during exercise in normal subjects and patients with cardiac disease [Abstract]. PACE 13:515, 1990.

25. Wirtzfeld A, Heinze R, Bock T, Liess HD: Process and device for regulating the stimulation frequency of heart pacemakers. US Patent No. 4,399,820, 1984.

26. Inbar GF, Heinze R, Hoekstein KN, et al: Development of a closed loop controller regulating mixed venous oxygen saturation level. IEEE Trans Biomed Eng 35:679, 1988.

27. Horecker B: The absorption spectra of hemoglobin and its derivatives in the visible and near infra-red regions. J Biol Chem 148:173, 1943.

28. Polanyi ML, Hehir RM: New reflection oximeter. Rev Sci Instrum 31:401, 1960.

29. Polanyi ML, Hehir RM: In vivo oximeter with fast dynamic response. Rev Sci Instrum 33:1040, 1962.

30. Mook GA, Zijlstra WG: Direct measurement of the oxygen saturation of human blood during cardiac catheterization. Proc Kon Nederl Akad Wet, Series C 60:158, 1957.

31. Mook GA, Osypka P, Sturm RE, Wood EH: Fibre optic reflection photometry on blood. Cardiovasc Res 2:199, 1968.

32. Johnson CC, Palm RD, Stewart DC, et al: A solid state fiberoptic oximeter. J Assoc Adv Med Instrum 5:77, 1971.

33. Kapany NS, Silbertrust N: Fibre optics spectrophotometer for in vivo oximetry. Nature 204:138, 1964.

34. Shaw RF, Sperinde JM: Catheter oximeter apparatus and method. US Patent No. 4,114,604, 1978.

35. Nahas GG: Spectrophotometric determination of hemoglobin and oxyhemoglobin in whole hemolyzed blood. Science 113:723, 1951.

36. Groom D, Wood EH, Burchell HB, Parker RL: The application of an oximeter for whole blood to diagnostic cardiac catheterization. Mayo Clin Proc Staff Meet 23:601, 1948.

37. Cole JS, Martin WE, Cheung PW, Johnson CC: Clinical studies with a solid state fiberoptic oximeter. Am J Cardiol 29:383, 1972.

38. Bossina KK, Mook GA, Zijlstra WG: Direct-reflection oximetry in routine cardiac catheterization. Circulation 22:908, 1960.

39. Enson Y, Briscoe WA, Polanyi ML, Cournand A: In vivo studies with an intravascular and intracardiac reflection oximeter. J Appl Physiol 17:552, 1962.

40. Harrison DC, Kapany NS, Miller HA, et al: Fiber optics for continuous in vivo monitoring of oxygen saturation. Am Heart J 71:766, 1966.

41. Yee S, Schibli E, Krishman V: Proposed miniature red/infrared oximeter suitable for mounting on a catheter tip. IEEE Trans Biomed Eng 18:27, 1977.

42. Schmitt JM, Mihm FG, Meindel JD: New methods for whole blood oximetry. Ann Biomed Eng 14:35, 1986.

43. Takatani S, Noda H, Takano H, et al: A miniature hybrid reflection type optical sensor for measurement of hemoglobin content and oxygen saturation of whole blood. IEEE Trans Biomed Eng 45:187, 1988.

44. Baudino MD, de Franco MD, Lessar JF, et al: Oxygen sensing pacemaker. US Patent Nos. 4,791,935, 4,804,629, 4,813,421, 1988.

45. Renolds L, Johnson C, Ishiaru A: Diffuse reflectance from a finite blood medium. Appl Optics 15:2059, 1976.

46. Bornzin GA, Mendelson Y, Moran B, et al: Proceedings of the IEEE 9th Annual Conference of Eng Med Biol Soc, 1987, pp 807–809.

47. Mendelson Y, Galvin JJ, Wang Y: In-vitro evaluation of a dual oxygen saturation/hematocrit intravascular fiberoptic catheter. Biomed Instrum Technol 24:199, 1990.

48. Tremolieres F, Lecompte F, Sinet M, et al: In vivo measurements of oxy-hemoglobin saturation by a fiberoptic catheter. Eur J Intens Care Med 2:177, 1976.

49. Seifert GP, Moore AA, Graves KL, Lahtinen SP: In vivo and in vitro studies of a chronic oxygen saturation sensor. PACE 14:1514, 1991.

50. Bennett T, Bornzin G, Baudino M, Olson W: Rate-responsive pacing using mixed venous oxygen saturation in heart blocked dogs [Abstract]. Circulation 70(II):246, 1985.

51. Bennett T, Olson W, Bornzin G, Baudino M: Alternative modes for physiological pacing. In Gomez FP (ed): Cardiac Pacing and Electrophysiology: Tachyarrhythmias. Mt. Kisco, NY, Futura, 1985.

52. Bennett TD, Olson WH, Bornzin GA, Baudino MD: Rate-responsive pacing: Alternative modes for physiological cardiac pacing. Proceedings of the AAMI Annual Meeting, 1985, p 12.

53. Becker A, Becker M, Claudon D, Edwards JE: Surface thrombosis and fibrous encapsulation of intravenous pacemaker catheter electrode. Circulation 46:409, 1972.

54. Wirtzfeld A, Heinze R, Stangl K, et al: Regulation of pacing rate by variations of mixed venous oxygen saturation. PACE 7:1257, 1984.

55. Stangl K, Wirtzfeld A, Gobl G, et al: Rate control with an external SO_2 closed loop system. PACE 9:992, 1986.

56. Faerestrand S, Skadberg B, Anderson K, et al: Bradycardia and rate-responsive pacing: comparison of central venous oxygen saturation at rest and during exercise [Abstract]. PACE 12:1187, 1989.

CHAPTER 10

TEMPERATURE-CONTROLLED RATE-ADAPTIVE PACING

T. Duncan Sellers
Neal E. Fearnot
Heidi J. Smith

Basic Concept of Sensor

HISTORY OF DEVELOPMENT

Because of its physiologic link to metabolism, body temperature was thought by several investigators to be a potential metabolic sensor for rate-adaptive pacing. Encouraged by early animal experiments that showed that blood temperature is elevated during increasing exercise workloads and returns to baseline during recovery,[1, 2] the relationship between blood temperature and heart rate was extensively investigated.[3–7] These studies indicated that the measurement of blood temperature in the right ventricle provided an ideal sensor location for rate modulation. The results of preclinical studies were confirmed in humans using external pacemaker prototypes that implemented a variety of algorithms for modulating pacing rate based on right ventricular blood temperature.[8–10] Blood temperature was shown to be a metabolic indicator that was highly correlated with the rate of the normal sinus node, thus demonstrating its potential for use in rate-adaptive pacing.[9, 11–13] One aspect of the effect of exercise on this parameter was discovered in early *clinical* studies that was not appreciated in animal studies: A transient decrease in right ventricular blood temperature was often found to occur at the onset of exercise.[7] Therefore, rather than simply increasing the pacing rate as a direct function of blood temperature, more complex processing of the temperature signal was required to provide for appropriate rate modulation in patients. These observations led to the development of algorithms that increased the pacing rate in response to a decrease in the temperature of the right ventricular blood at the onset of exercise as well as providing an increase in pacing rate in response to increasing blood temperature, which typically occurs during later stages of exercise. Several manufacturers have developed implantable pacing systems that modulate heart rate based on the temperature of the right ventricular blood. For each of these pacing systems, temperature was measured by a thermistor located near the tip of the pacing lead in the right ventricle.[14–16] Various algorithms have been implemented in permanently implantable devices, each of which provides a somewhat different rate response. In this chapter we discuss the factors that influence the temperature of blood in the right ventricle, the kinetics of temperature change, the important considerations in the design of temperature-controlled pacing systems, the rate-modulating algorithms that have been developed, and the clinical results of trials evaluating temperature-controlled, rate-adaptive pacing.

PHYSIOLOGIC FACTORS AFFECTING TEMPERATURE

Right ventricular blood temperature differs significantly from oral, rectal, and skin temperature. Blood returning from all parts of the body mixes in the right heart. Therefore, right ventricular blood temperature provides an average temperature of the entire venous return. At least nine physiologic factors are known to affect the temperature of the right ventricular blood, including the amount of heat produced during muscular exercise, changes in peripheral circulation in the extremities, vasodilation associated with anticipation of exercise, emotional stress, the temperature of the environment, ingestion of hot or cold foods and liquids, fever, diurnal metabolism, and sleep.

HEAT PRODUCTION DURING EXERCISE

Because skeletal muscles are only about 20% efficient, they produce heat during work. The contribution of the skeletal muscles to total body heat production increases from approximately 18% at rest to approximately 73% during peak exercise.[17] The heat generated by exercising muscles is carried by the venous blood that returns to the right heart before reaching the organs of heat dissipation, principally the skin and lungs. The increase in right ventricular blood temperature (Fig. 10–1) is dependent on the intensity and duration of exercise, especially at higher workloads.[3, 9, 11–13] During exercise, heat loss is regulated to maintain a temperature equilibrium.[18] Approximately 20% of body heat is lost by evaporation, 25% by conduction, 45% by radiation, and 8% by ventilation.[17]

INCREASED CIRCULATION IN THE EXTREMITIES AT ONSET OF EXERCISE

During exercise, much of the cardiac output is redirected to perfuse the skin and extremities.[19, 20] Because the skin and extremities are cooler than the core body temperature at the beginning of exercise, the increased blood flow to the extremities results initially in the return of cooler blood to the heart, causing a decrease in right ventricular blood temperature. Following this initial dip in temperature, the increased heat production in the exercising muscles begins to warm the venous return, resulting in a steady rise in right ventricular blood temperature (Fig. 10–2). The transient decrease in blood temperature at the onset of exercise is more prolonged in patients with congestive heart failure, in whom a greater quantity of blood is pooled in the extremities.[21]

VASOACTIVITY ASSOCIATED WITH ANTICIPATION

The transient decrease in temperature occurs not only at the beginning of exercise but also in anticipation of exercise (Fig. 10–3), indicating that this response is independent of muscle work or body movement.[9] Transient decreases in right ventricular blood temperature have also been observed when patients are startled. Because of the speed of this response, a neurogenic mechanism has been postulated. This is further supported by observations of right ventricular blood

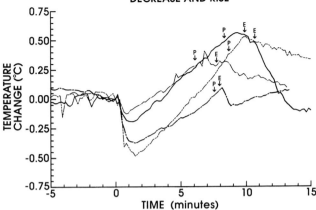

FIGURE 10–2. Right ventricular blood temperature change in four patients during Bruce protocol treadmill exercise. When patients were at rest prior to exercise (time −5 to 0), temperature fluctuated 0.1°C. During the first 1 to 2 minutes of exercise, temperature decreased 0.13° to 0.48°C. Following the temperature dip at the onset of exercise, temperature rose steadily to the end of peak exercise (P). Temperature decreased following the end of exercise (E). (From Sellers TD, Fearnot NE, Smith HJ, et al: Right ventricular blood temperature profiles for rate-responsive pacing. PACE 10:467, 1987.)

temperature in patients with autonomically mediated syncope during tilt table testing. It has been reported that the right ventricular blood temperature actually increases in response to venous pooling in these individuals at the onset of syncope as the amount of cooler venous blood returning to the heart suddenly decreases.

EMOTIONAL STRESS

Right ventricular temperature has been shown to increase significantly in response to emotional stress (Fig. 10–4).[22] This phenomenon has been observed in a variety of conditions such as anxiety during office visits or while awaiting

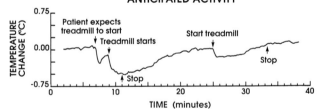

FIGURE 10–3. Vasodilation associated with anticipation. The patient was told that the treadmill would start. The switch was thrown but the treadmill itself did not turn on. There was a prompt drop in the right ventricular blood temperature of 0.34°C in the absence of physical exercise and a slow return toward baseline as the patient waited for the treadmill to be reset and turned on. When the warm-up exercise began, there was a further abrupt drop of 0.4°C, followed by a slow rise as exercise continued. The exercise was stopped at the end of the warm-up period, and temperature returned to baseline over 10 minutes. After temperature returned to baseline, the patient underwent exercise, during which there was a smaller, 0.16°C drop in the right ventricular blood temperature and an increase from there of 0.28°C at peak exercise. (From Sellers TD, Fearnot NE, Smith HJ, et al: Right ventricular blood temperature profiles for rate-responsive pacing. PACE 10:467, 1987.)

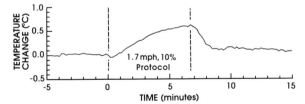

FIGURE 10–1. Blood temperature rise during exercise. Temperature rose shortly after the beginning of exercise (time 0) and continued to rise throughout the treadmill exercise period. After exercise ended, temperature returned to baseline. (From Fearnot NE, Smith HJ, Sellers TD, et al: Evaluation of the temperature response to exercise testing in patients with single-chamber, rate-adaptive pacemakers: A multicenter study. PACE 12:1806, 1989.)

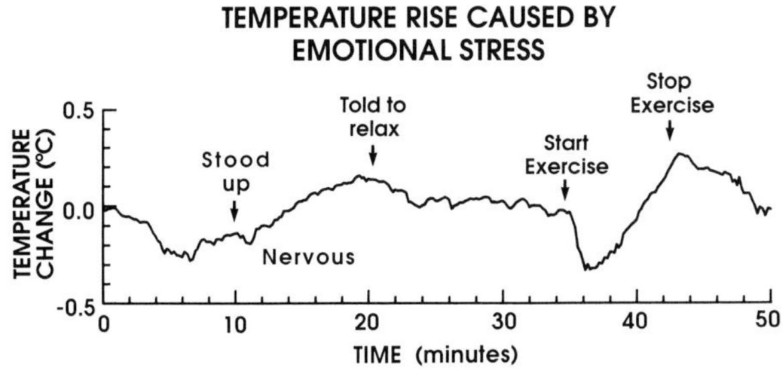

TEMPERATURE RISE CAUSED BY EMOTIONAL STRESS

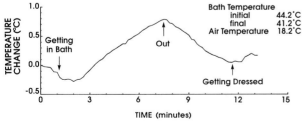

FIGURE 10–4. Temperature response to anxiety. Throughout the period of anxiety, between the time the patient stood up and was told to relax, temperature rose. Temperature returned to baseline after the patient was told to relax. Later, the patient underwent treadmill exercise, which caused a transient decrease followed by a subsequent rise through peak exercise. (From Fearnot NE, Kitoh O. Fujita T, et al: Case studies on the effect of exercise and hot water submersion on intracardiac temperature and the performance of a pacemaker that varies pacing rate based on temperature. Jpn Heart J 30:353, 1989.)

exercise tests. In some cases, emotion can cause the right ventricular blood temperature to decrease owing to the vasoactivity discussed earlier. Significant temperature changes have been reported during emotional stress, such as occurs with mental arithmetic testing and mirror-drawing tests.[23, 24]

ENVIRONMENTAL HEAT STRESS

Under normal conditions, the body temperature of warm-blooded animals is closely regulated within a physiologic range. However, under some severe conditions of environmental and exercise stress, the heating and cooling capabilities may be exceeded. These conditions have been studied by controlling outer body surface temperature with perfusion suits or submersion (Fig. 10–5).[13, 19, 22] Under severe heat stress, blood temperature changes linearly until the animal becomes unconscious. The temperature rise is dependent on the environmental temperature and the duration of exposure. In a hot environment with increasing blood temperature, resting heart rate is also significantly elevated.[13, 22] Normal hot or cold showers and baths have insignificant effects on right ventricular blood temperature, even though large effects on skin temperature may be observed.[13]

INGESTION

There may be a transient response of the right ventricular blood temperature to the ingestion of hot or cold foods or liquids. The change in right ventricular blood temperature is dependent on the difference between the temperature of the ingestant and the body, the volume consumed, and the rate of consumption. Although normal eating has little effect on right ventricular temperature, transient changes of -0.2 to $+0.2°C$ have been observed when very hot or very cold liquids are consumed quickly.[9, 13] Temperature increases of 0.07° to 0.36°C have been observed during eating; however, most of this change may be related to the general activity of eating and not specifically to the ingestion of heated substances.[9]

FEVER

Infection, inflammation, or allergic reactions may cause a febrile response of variable magnitude and character. Important to pacing is the difference between a sustained fever and an oscillating or spiking fever. Typically, the physiologic response to fever is an increase in heart rate.

DIURNAL VARIATION IN RIGHT VENTRICULAR BLOOD TEMPERATURE

The right ventricular blood temperature normally demonstrates a diurnal variation that parallels the overall rate of metabolism and the heart rate. Each of these parameters increases during waking hours and decreases during sleep (Fig. 10–6).[9] Superimposed on the diurnal variation of core temperature are the effects of exercise, emotion, and other factors. The magnitude of the diurnal variation has been reported to be as high as $1.95 \pm 0.98°C$.[25]

CYCLIC VARIATION DURING SLEEP

Minor cyclical variations in right ventricular blood temperature have been noted during deep sleep (Fig. 10–7). Al-

ENVIRONMENTAL HEAT STRESS (HOT BATH)

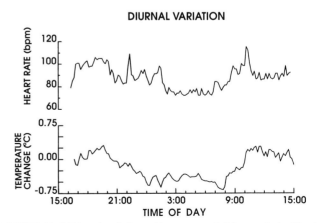

FIGURE 10–5. Effect of extreme skin temperature. During submersion in a 44.2°C bath, right ventricular temperature rose at the rate of 0.2°C/min. This temperature increase is associated with increased heart rate in normal subjects. (From Fearnot NE, Kitoh O, Fujita T, et al: Case studies on the effect of exercise and hot water submersion on intracardiac temperature and the performance of a pacemaker that varies pacing rate based on temperature. Jpn Heart J 30:353, 1989.)

FIGURE 10–6. Diurnal variations of heart rate and right ventricular blood temperature, averaged over 10-minute intervals, show corresponding increases during the day, when the subject is generally more active, and decreases at night when the subject is sleeping or resting. (From Sellers TD, Fearnot NE, Smith HJ, et al: Right ventricular blood temperature profiles for rate-responsive pacing. PACE 10:467, 1987.)

CYCLIC VARIATION DURING DEEP SLEEP

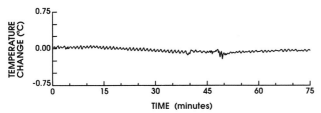

FIGURE 10–7. Temperature variation during deep sleep. This record shows a 1-minute cycle length variation in temperature of up to 0.15°C.

though the mechanism is not known, this may be due to slowing of the body's temperature control process causing oscillations.

The Kinetics of Right Ventricular Blood Temperature

EXERCISE AND EMOTION

Since rate modulation is possible only in response to a *change* in temperature, the timing between the onset of activity and the subsequent change in right ventricular blood temperature is critically important. Although in most patients temperature begins to change within a few seconds of the onset of exercise, changes in right ventricular blood temperature often slightly *precede* the onset of exercise owing to the anticipatory response. During a study of patients undergoing 68 exercise tests in which right ventricular blood temperature was measured every 10 seconds, a change in right ventricular temperature was detected an average of 10 seconds after the onset of exercise, with a standard deviation of 16 seconds.

In a cohort of 25 patients performing treadmill exercise, a change in right ventricular blood temperature preceded the onset of exercise by as much as 36 seconds in a few patients owing to the anticipatory response. The decrease in right ventricular temperature at exercise onset averaged 0.26° ± 0.14°C (range, 0.07° to 0.54°C). In this study, the rate of temperature decrease averaged 0.24° ± 13°C/min (0.06°/min to 0.58°C/min). Following the transient initial decrease, right ventricular blood temperature rose throughout exercise, with an average increase of 0.41° ± 0.28°C (range, 0.03° to 1.11°C) and an average rate of rise of 0.08° ± 0.05°C/min (0.03°/min to 0.26°C/min).[10] The rate of temperature rise is related to the difference between heat production and heat dissipation. The temperature rise is highly correlated with both the exercise workload over a given period of time and the duration of exercise at a fixed workload.

BLUNTING OF TEMPERATURE DECREASE

The presence of the initial decrease in right ventricular blood temperature is variable among individuals because of their varied physiologic responses. The decrease is related to cardiac condition, body build, and fitness as well as other possible factors. With repeated exercise sessions, the transient decrease in temperature is blunted when there is insufficient time to cool the extremities between periods of exer-

BLUNTING OF TEMPERATURE DECREASE WITH REPEATED EXERCISE

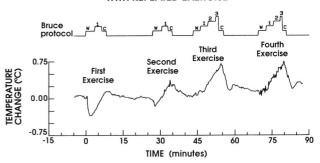

FIGURE 10–8. Blunting of temperature decrease during four successive Bruce treadmill exercise periods. Treadmill protocol is indicated (W, warm-up; 1–3, Bruce protocol stages 1–3; C, cool-down). During the first exercise period, there was an initial decrease in right ventricular blood temperature, followed by a rise. After a period of rest, a smaller, blunted decrease in the right ventricular blood temperature accompanied onset of the second exercise. During the third and fourth exercise periods, no temperature decrease was seen owing to equilibration of the right ventricular blood temperature and the peripheral circulation. (From Sellers TD, Fearnot NE, Smith HJ, et al: Right ventricular blood temperature profiles for rate-responsive pacing. PACE 10:467, 1987.)

cise (Fig. 10–8).[9] In a series of 31 patients undergoing treadmill exercise tests, a temperature decrease of greater than 0.1°C at onset of exercise was observed in 91% of patients.[26] In another group of treadmill and bicycle exercise tests among 21 patients, the initial temperature decrease was observed in 57% of patients. The duration of the temperature decrease averaged 3.5 ± 1.9 minutes.[27]

DECAY CHARACTERISTICS

The time period over which temperature returns to baseline after exercise depends on multiple factors, including patient condition and the absolute temperature increase (or decrease) from baseline that occurs during exercise. In general, however, temperature and heart rate follow a parallel course, returning toward baseline over a few minutes after exercise ends (Fig. 10–9).[9, 11, 12]

HEART RATE AND TEMPERATURE DURING EXERCISE AND RECOVERY

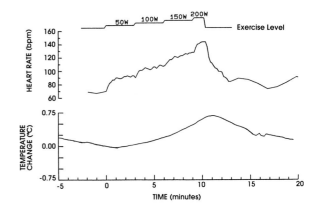

FIGURE 10–9. Right ventricular blood temperature and heart rate during and following supine ergometry at 50 to 200 W in a healthy volunteer. During exercise, temperature rose steadily (0.71°C in 10 minutes), paralleling the heart rate increase. Following exercise, heart rate and temperature showed similar declines toward baseline. (From Sellers TD, Fearnot NE, Smith HJ, et al: Right ventricular blood temperature profiles for rate-responsive pacing. PACE 10:467, 1987.)

Measurement of Temperature in the Right Ventricle

Temperature-sensing pacing systems require a special pacing lead that incorporates a temperature sensor near its tip. For reliable temperature measurement during long-term implantation, the design of the lead is critical. Several important design features have been identified.

LEAD REQUIREMENTS, MATERIALS, AND MANUFACTURING

Although temperature can be sensed by thermocouples, thermotransistors, and optics, all temperature-sensing pacing systems to date have used a thermistor near the tip of the pacing lead. Thermistors have been available for decades, are extremely stable, and can be made very small. Thermistors are formed of a semiconductive material that changes resistance inversely with changes in temperature. The temperature range that is necessary for rate-adaptive pacing must be at least 34° to 40°C with a resolution of at least 0.01°C. The type and resistance of the thermistor are also important design criteria. To withstand the rigors of lead implantation without semiconductor failure, only thermistors that are hermetically sealed in a fluid-impenetrable material such as glass are suitable. The nominal resistance of the thermistor affects the current drain of the pulse generator battery and the degree to which modest lead damage can compromise rate-adaptive behavior. High thermistor resistance lowers current drain, whereas low thermistor resistance decreases the measurement error caused by body fluid between the conductor coils in a damaged pacing lead. Thermistor resistances of clinical pacing leads range from 5000 ohms to 100,000 ohms. The temperature-sensing circuit must minimize battery current drain by energizing the thermistor for measurement of temperature only intermittently. The frequency of measurements must be at least once every 10 seconds to adequately detect the temperature drop at the beginning of exercise. The promptness of the heart rate response to exercise is dependent on both the frequency with which measurements are made and how quickly body activity results in an actual change in right ventricular temperature.

Temperature-sensing leads require at least three conductors (two for the thermistor, one for sensing and pacing). A bipolar temperature-sensing lead is possible with three conductors if the thermistor and the bipolar ring electrode share one conductor coil. The configuration of the conductor coils in the lead has proved to be an important design consideration. The conductor wires connecting the thermistor to the pulse generator may be configured either as two separate and parallel insulated coils[28] or as a coaxial design, with one coil wound around the other.[15] The ground wire may be either the outer or inner coil. Unfortunately, the coaxial design with the common wire as the outer coil has been shown to be subject to fractures, insulation breaks, and sensing failures.[15]

SENSOR ACCURACY

The accuracy and precision of temperature measurement are dependent on the drift characteristics of the sensor as well as the measurement circuitry within the pulse generator. The pacemaker models that have relied on absolute rather than relative temperature measurement have experienced drift problems in some cases.[25, 29] The resolution of temperature measurement was 0.025°C, 0.021°C, and 0.004°C for the Biotronik, Intermedics, and Cook pacemakers, respectively.[15, 28, 30]

DURABILITY AND RELIABILITY

Because of the high reliability of the thermistor as a sensor, the durability of the pacing system is most often dependent on the lead design and its handling during implantation. The lead must be impervious to body fluids. Damage to the terminal block grommet or seal of the pulse generator during lead attachment allows fluid to enter and may cause a conductive bridge between terminals, affecting the temperature measurements. Therefore, proper sealing at the time of implantation is important to ensure sensor accuracy. Like all pacing leads, the conductor coils and insulation must withstand the trauma of implantation. The critical areas that have been associated with lead damage are the areas lying between the first rib and the clavicle (where the lead may become compressed between these bones),[31, 32] at the points of suture (where sutures may cut through the insulation), and within the pocket (where surgical instruments may inadvertently pierce the insulation). Therefore, use of the cephalic vein or more lateral entry into the subclavian vein, use of suture collars for all ligatures around the pacing lead, and protection of the lead during pocket closure are essential to ensure proper sensor function. The incidence of these problems is low when systems are properly implanted.

Susceptibility to lead damage is not unique to temperature-sensing leads; in fact, these failure mechanisms have been reported for all lead types. What is unique for a temperature-sensing pacemaker is that when these conditions occur, the temperature measurement is often affected before pacing and sensing are lost. Even less likely than lead damage is failure of the connection between the conductor coil and thermistor, failure of the temperature-sensing circuit in the pulse generator, or failure of the thermistor. Because of the added complexity of a specialized lead, there has been a concern about its long-term reliability. However, 5-year follow-up of the Cook Pacemaker temperature-sensing leads showed that their reliability with regard to pacing function was $99.8 \pm 1.1\%$, and reliability with regard to temperature-sensing function was $97.3 \pm 1.4\%$, exceeding the reliability of some well-known standard leads.[33, 34]

ENERGY CONSUMPTION

Energy consumption is dependent not only on the nominal resistance of the thermistor but also on how often temperature is measured and how long the thermistor must be energized for each measurement. As with all rate-responsive pacemakers, current drain and energy consumption are affected by the pacing rate during periods of activity. In the Kelvin pulse generators, the current needed to energize the thermistor is about 0.1 mA and has a duty cycle of 3%.[28] This causes minimal battery drain to sample the temperature. The battery life has not been significantly decreased by this, with some pacemakers now functioning 8 years after implantation.

ARTIFACTS OF TEMPERATURE MEASUREMENT

Unlike some physiologic sensors, temperature measurement is not affected by cardiac arrhythmias or abnormalities, medications, or environmental noise. However, temperature measured in the right ventricle may have unwanted components related to mixing, respiration, and heart rate. To suppress these temperature variations, the temperature signal is typically filtered by designing the thermomechanical properties of the lead to have a 5-second time constant.[28]

EFFECT OF RIGHT VENTRICLE ANATOMY AND BLOOD MIXING ON TEMPERATURE MEASUREMENTS

Central blood temperature may be measured in the right atrium, the right ventricle, or the trunk of the pulmonary artery (Fig. 10–10).[35] It has been demonstrated that mixing of blood is inadequate in the inferior and superior venae cavae, and respiratory artifacts are more prominent in the branches of the pulmonary arteries.[36] The temperature response is not known to be affected by anatomic anomalies, conduction patterns, valve function, or other anomalies.

Rate-Adaptive Algorithms

The relationship between heart rate and core temperature is both workload dependent and time dependent. It is inadequate to consider the relationship between heart rate and temperature as a simple linear function. The complexity of this relationship demands a sophisticated algorithm. Because heart rate does not simply parallel the temperature response, the pacing rate during activity can vary widely, depending on the design of the rate-adaptive algorithm. Important design factors include: (1) a prompt response to the onset of exercise, (2) proportionality to exercise workload, (3) short-term heart rate response to emotion, and (4) response to diurnal variation in metabolism. To address these factors, the

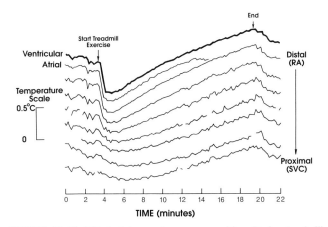

LOCATIONS FOR TEMPERATURE SENSING

FIGURE 10–10. Effect of temperature sensor position. During treadmill exercise, temperature response was measured simultaneously by a thermistor in the ventricle and by eight thermistors spaced 1 cm apart on an atrial J lead. Temperature recordings in the right atrial appendage or middle right atrium paralleled the ventricular temperature changes. However, temperature changes became less pronounced nearer to the superior vena cava.

TEMPERATURE-BASED PACEMAKER ALGORITHMS

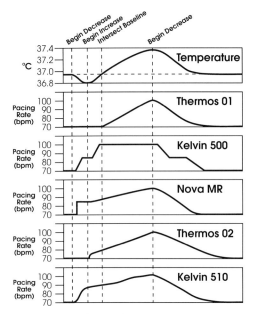

FIGURE 10–11. Generalized pacing rate responses to temperature during exercise for five algorithms. For this diagram, the lower rate was set at 70 and the upper rate at 100 for each model. The figures are arranged in order of sophistication, not chronologically.

temperature-based pacemaker must separately process diurnal, emotional, and exercise responses. A rate increase of 80 to 100 bpm per degree Celsius is appropriate for exercise, whereas a 5- to 15-bpm rate increase per degree Celsius is more appropriate for diurnal temperature variation. Responsiveness to the initial temperature decrease, when present, is also necessary to provide a reasonably prompt response to the onset of exercise. In the absence of such an algorithm for detecting the dip in right ventricular blood temperature, the onset of rate response can be delayed by as much as several minutes, which is clinically unacceptable. Initially, many investigators viewed the decrease in right ventricular blood temperature at the beginning of exercise as an insurmountable barrier to a prompt chronotropic response. However, with the development of algorithms that respond to the initial temperature decrease, reasonably prompt pacing rate responses have been achieved. Many algorithms have been proposed, and at least five pacing systems for single-chamber temperature-based rate response have been implanted in humans. These are described in Figure 10–11. At least two dual-chamber temperature-based pacing algorithms have also been designed.

DESCRIPTION OF SPECIFIC ALGORITHMS

THERMOS 01. In the simplest algorithm, based on the early work of Csapo,[37] the programmer pre-assigns a specific pacing rate to each possible temperature value in 0.1°C increments (Biotronik, Berlin, Germany).[37, 38] The temperature-rate relationship for temperature increase and for temperature decrease after exercise can be programmed separately. Nine standard temperature-rate relationships are available. When right ventricular blood reaches a specific temperature, the assigned pacing rate is produced (see Fig. 10–11A). In this early algorithm, no rate increase occurred during the initial temperature decrease. Instead, the rate increase was delayed and the heart rate maintained at a lower pacing rate until temperature exceeded the baseline value.[39]

KELVIN 500 SERIES. The Kelvin 500 series pacemakers (Cook Pacemaker, Leechburg, PA) do not assign specific pacing rates to specific temperatures but instead use temperature change and the rate of temperature change to detect the beginning and ending of exertion.[40, 41] Pacing rate is determined using a somewhat mechanistic approach. The algorithm recognizes the temperature decrease at exercise onset and elevates the pacing rate to an interim rate, programmed to a level appropriate for light exercise. If sufficient exercise continues, producing an appropriate temperature rise, the pacing rate is increased from the interim rate to the programmed upper rate (see Fig. 10–11B). If a rise in temperature does not occur following the dip, the pacing rate begins to slowly decrease to the lower pacing rate after a programmed "interim time" (2 to 12 minutes). The sensitivity of the pacemaker to temperature changes (Kelvin Set 1 to 8) and rate smoothing ("rate ramp," 20 to 80 msec) is programmable. With appropriate adjustments of temperature sensitivity, interim time, pacing rates, and rate smoothing, it is possible to produce a smooth or step-wise increase and decrease in heart rate with exercise.[9, 26]

NOVA MR. In response to an initial temperature decrease, the Nova MR (Intermedics, Angleton, TX) algorithm increases the pacing rate to an intermediate value. As temperature begins to rise following the initial dip, the pacing rate is further increased in a manner that is proportional to the temperature change (see Fig. 10–11C).[11, 42] Since the relationship between changes in heart rate and right ventricular temperature is not linear, this algorithm uses a variable heart rate–temperature slope over the physiologic range of core temperatures. Therefore, as the temperature increase becomes greater, the slope of the change in rate to the change in temperature decreases. The gain of the rate response to temperature is programmable with 10 possible steps (1 to 10). Because of the relationship between temperature and exercise workload, the pacing rate was found to be proportional to workload in most cases, especially for higher workloads.[27] A separate diurnal rate component of 15 bpm per degree Celsius is dependent on baseline temperature.[42] The temperature measurement is calibrated with oral temperature, although blood temperature and oral temperature often differ.

THERMOS 02. The second-generation Thermos pacemaker calculates the exercise pacing rate based on the temperature increase above a baseline temperature (see Fig. 10–11D), like the Kelvin 500 and the Nova MR. Thus, this pacing system responds to changes in temperature rather than fixing the pacing rate to an absolute temperature as in the Thermos 01.[16] This allows the algorithm to discriminate between baseline temperature and rate increase due to exercise. The baseline temperature is calculated as the average temperature over a few minutes prior to temperature rise. As temperature begins to increase, an augmentation based on the increase is added to the pacing rate. Thus, large diurnal temperature increases and sustained higher temperatures no longer result in sustained high pacing rates. The relationship between temperature change (instead of absolute temperature) is programmable in 0.1°C increments; 10 standard temperature-rate curves are available. In addition, the temperature-rate values

can be individually programmed. The pacemaker averages temperature over several days to produce autocalibration to compensate for temperature measurement drift.[16] This pacemaker also responds to the fall in right ventricular blood temperature with an increase in pacing rate.

KELVIN 510 SERIES. The Kelvin 510 series combines a proportional response to the initial temperature decrease with a proportional response during temperature rise (see Fig. 10–11E). Pacing rates are based on the magnitude of temperature change and rate of change with respect to various baseline temperatures.[10] In response to the initial temperature decrease at the beginning of exercise, the algorithm produces a prompt increase in pacing rate that is proportional to the magnitude of change and rate of temperature change during the temperature decrease. As temperature begins to increase during further exertion, additional rate augmentation is based on the rise and rate of rise in blood temperature. This results in a pacing rate increase that is proportional to workload throughout exercise. Programmable parameters include the lower and upper rate limits, the gain of the rate response to temperature (Kelvin Set 1 to 10), and rate smoothing (rate ramp, 12 to 60 bpm per minute limit for increasing pacing rate, 6 to 30 bpm per minute limit for decreasing pacing rate). In addition to exercise rate augmentation, there is also a diurnal rate augmentation. Diurnal variation is related to the averaged temperature increase above minimal temperature during the previous 24 hours.

With this algorithm, a correlation coefficient between intrinsic heart rate and pacemaker rate of 0.92 (Fig. 10–12) has been reported.[10] The mean time to a change in pacing rate at the onset of exercise was 16 ± 21 seconds. No significant difference was found between the mean pacing response times of patients who had or had not been engaged in prior physical activity (a factor that reduces or eliminates the initial temperature decrease at exercise onset).[10] The response to repetitive exercise is illustrated in Figure 10–13.

CIRCADIA. The Nova MR temperature algorithm has been combined with a dual-chamber algorithm in a DDDR pacemaker.[43] The pacemaker tracks atrial rate until the tempera-

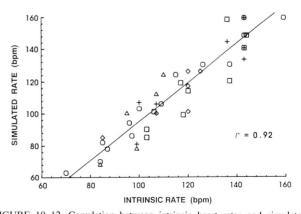

CORRELATION BETWEEN INTRINSIC RATES AND SIMULATED RATES FOR KELVIN 510 SERIES

FIGURE 10–12. Correlation between intrinsic heart rates and simulated rates during treadmill exercise during five exercise periods using the Kelvin 510 series algorithm. (From Fearnot NE, Evans ML: Heart rate correlation, response time, and effect of previous exercise using advanced pacing rate algorithm for temperature-based rate modulation. PACE 11:1846, 1988.)

RESPONSE TO REPEATED EXERCISE
(KELVIN 510 SERIES)

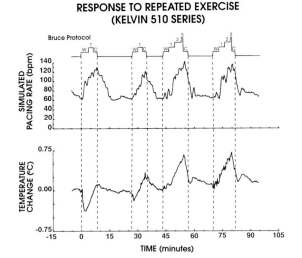

FIGURE 10–13. Response of the Kelvin 510 series algorithm to repeated exercise. Pacing rate responded promptly to all exercise tests regardless of the presence or absence of temperature decrease at exercise onset.

ture-based pacing rate exceeds the atrial sensed rate, then switches to pacing at the temperature-based rate. The programmed responsiveness to temperature determines the degree of impact of temperature sensing on pacing rate.

KELVIN 700 SERIES. The Kelvin 510 series algorithm has been incorporated in a dual-chamber (DDDR) device. Unique to the dual-chamber version is the pacemaker's coordination of atrial rate tracking and sensor-based rate. With separately programmable upper rates for tracking the atrial rate and that of the temperature sensor, sensor-based pacing above the maximum atrial tracking rate is possible. Likewise, the upper atrial tracking rate is automatically adjusted based on the sensor (dynamic tracking rate), allowing diurnal variation of upper and lower atrial tracking rates.[44] Both the sensor response and the atrial sensed event timing are used for advanced mode switching. Rate histograms and extensive telemetry assist in understanding these features.

SUMMARY OF ALGORITHMS. The evolution of algorithms has led to increased sophistication, faster responses, and better proportionality of pacing rate to exercise workload. Factors found to be important in the design of temperature algorithms include measuring relative temperature (to avoid problems with drift), discriminating between diurnal changes and those related to exercise, properly responding during the initial temperature decrease, and offering multiple slopes for the relationship between changes in temperature and changes in heart rate. With these factors, appropriate physiologic response to a variety of daily activities has become possible. In terms of dual-chamber pacing, the appropriate combination of the sensor-indicated rate and the sensed atrial rate offers potentially improved pacing therapy for patients with intermittent atrial arrhythmias.

Clinical Experience with Implantable Temperature-Controlled Pacemakers

Temperature-based pacemakers from Biotronik (Thermos 01, Thermos 02), Intermedics (Nova MR, Circadia), and Cook Pacemaker (Kelvin 500 series, Kelvin 510 series) have been implanted in a large number of patients.[22–27, 29, 32, 38, 39, 43, 45–50]

The specific pacing rate observed in response to exercise and emotion depends on the pacing algorithm, the programmed parameters controlling rate response (such as sensitivity to temperature, lower and upper rate limits, and speed of rate increase and decrease), and on the integrity of the thermistor-pacing lead. Most single-chamber pulse generators were VVIR, although AAIR pacing was reported in a few patients.[48]

Because of variations in the temperature response between patients, the ability to adjust the rate response to temperature proved to be important. With some of these systems, the effect of changing the parameters, given individual temperature curves, could be graphically shown on a computer display, allowing the physician to rapidly optimize the programmed parameters. This process was labor intensive but was quite easily learned.

PHYSIOLOGIC CORRELATION WITH EXERCISE

Increased exercise duration has been shown in several studies that have compared temperature-based rate-responsive pacing using various algorithms to fixed-rate pacing.[25, 26, 39, 48] The pacing rate has been correlated with exercise workload with both treadmill and bicycle exercise tests.[27] In addition, the temperature-based pacing rate has been shown to be favorably related to oxygen uptake (Fig. 10–14).[48] A decrease in perceived exertion has also been observed.[48] With optimal programming, rate increase during exercise was reliably achieved for most patients, although the response time varied with different pacemaker models and was slower for those that lacked adequate detection of or response to the temperature decrease at exercise onset.[27, 39] For the Kelvin 500 and the Nova MR, average response times of less than 25 seconds from exercise onset to beginning of a rate increase were reported.[26, 49] Elevated pacing rates during normal daily activities such as gardening, housework, and meal preparation have also been demonstrated.[38] In general, the algorithms that produced rates related to workload and had adequate detection and response to temperature decrease at

RELATION OF PACING RATE TO OXYGEN UPTAKE

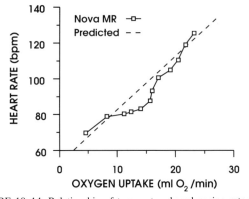

FIGURE 10–14. Relationship of temperature-based pacing rate to oxygen uptake during bicycle ergometry using the Nova MR. The dotted line shows the predicted normal heart rate at a given oxygen uptake, calculated according to age, sex, weight, and size. (Redrawn and reproduced with permission from Alt E, Volker R, Hogl B, et al: First clinical results with a new temperature-controlled rate-responsive pacemaker. Circulation 78(Suppl III):111-116, 1988. Copyright 1988 American Heart Association.)

exercise onset provided more prompt and appropriate responses.

CORRELATION OF PACING RATE WITH EMOTION

Psychological factors affecting temperature and pacing rate have been reported in several studies. Because of anxiety, pacing rate can increase while the patient is still "at rest" during an office visit or while awaiting an exercise test.[22, 27] This correlates with the normal response to anxiety often demonstrated by increased blood pressure and pulse rate during office visits. Pacing rate increases have also been reported with mental stress testing such as mental arithmetic tests or mirror-drawing tests.[23, 24] Because of the temperature change that occurs in response to changes in posture, temperature-based pacemakers have been proposed as ideal for patients with chronotropic incompetence and postural syncope.[43]

POTENTIAL FOR ATYPICAL OR UNDESIRED RESPONSES

One major difference between successful and unsuccessful pacemakers is whether the algorithm relies on absolute temperature. Early pacing systems that used absolute temperature were troubled by a drift in temperature measurement with time.[25, 29] In some patients, this resulted in sustained high rates and the eventual switching of the pulse generator to a non–rate-adaptive mode, leading to clinical abandonment of some of these models. Pacing systems based on relative temperature are not as susceptible to undesired responses caused by temperature drifts over time. In some Nova MR patients, a decrease in pacing rate was observed owing to a constant or slightly decreasing venous blood temperature, and changing the rate and duration of the response to temperature decrease was proposed.[27] Temperature rise was not always seen with low workloads, especially if the duration of the workload was short. For example, workloads of 10 to 30 W over 2 to 4 minutes did not increase absolute temperature;[27, 46] however, algorithms with an adequate response to the temperature decrease at exercise onset could still provide increased pacing rate under these conditions.

Pacemaker-mediated tachycardia was reported for one patient with a single-chamber Kelvin 500 pacemaker.[50] This patient experienced diaphragmatic pacing that caused an increase in right ventricular blood temperature, leading to sustained pacing at the upper rate limit. The problem was resolved by decreasing the output to prevent diaphragmatic capture.

Potential for Combination with Other Sensors

The use of temperature in combination with other sensors, including activity or acceleration, oxygen saturation, and respiration, has been investigated.[51–53] The combination most likely to be introduced clinically is that of temperature and activity. A piezoelectric crystal or an accelerometer offers nearly instantaneous response to abrupt activity, whereas temperature offers a more physiologic and workload-related response. Therefore, this combination could provide the advantage of each sensor while minimizing the disadvantages of both. Other studies are ongoing to determine the feasibility of correlating changes in temperature sensed in the pacemaker pocket (using thermistors in the pulse generator or in the muscle) with exercise. At present, the most difficult problem is related to the environmental effects at the pocket site.

Practical Aspects of Using a Temperature-Based Sensor

PROGRAMMING AND PACEMAKER FOLLOW-UP

As with other rate-responsive pacemakers, temperature-based pacing systems offer programmable sensor responsiveness (gain) and other parameters. Telemetry of temperature, either during real-time or as stored histograms, is available with some models and has proved valuable for understanding the physiology of blood temperature and the reason for individual rate responses. It has also been helpful for optimizing the rate relationship (gain) and demonstrating appropriate operation.

Because of variations in temperature response between patients, individualized programming is often required to yield optimal rate modulation. Although not always practical, an exercise treadmill test may provide the best data for optimal programming of the exercise response. However, these parameters have been adequately programmed using a variety of simple office procedures such as step tests or walking in the hallway. Temperature data that are telemetered during a single exercise test can be "replayed" to demonstrate the pacing rate that would have occurred with different programmed rate-response settings, facilitating optimal programming without requiring repeat exercise testing. Proper programming of these features is enhanced by programmer-based diagnostics in many models. More sophisticated programmer models provide autoprogramming of some rate-response parameters based on the stored temperature history.

There has been a misconception that temperature-based pacing provides rate increases only during physical activity. Because of changes in right ventricular blood temperature in response to changes in emotional activity, the pacing rate may be increased above the programmed lower rate in many patients during office visits because of associated anxiety. Because blood temperature reflects anticipation, increases in pacing rate have frequently been observed just prior to beginning a treadmill or bicycle exercise test. These rate increases have often been misconstrued as inappropriate due to failure to recognize the connections between a patient's emotional state, metabolism, and blood temperature. The physiologic nature of temperature must be understood to properly interpret anomalous behavior and to optimally program the rate response parameters.

Augmentation of pacing rate by diurnal variation in temperature, emotionally induced variations, and those related to physical activity make this sensor highly physiologic. However, because temperature responds to many different factors, follow-up of these pacing systems can be more challenging because the pacing rate often exceeds the programmed lower rate. Pacemaker follow-up services should be aware of the metabolic nature of the pacemaker, since rates higher than the programmed lower pacing rate are often observed. Pacemaker evaluation may be more dependent on the programmer diagnostics, such as rate histograms from treadmill exercise tests or from longer periods of activity between office visits, and on selective programming of specific rate-response features. Delineation of the respective contributions to rate augmentation provided by the programmer may be helpful in explaining the origin of any unexpected responses.

If abnormal temperature patterns are sensed by the pacemaker, most pacemakers alert the physician by altering the magnet rate. In some models, abnormal temperatures result in magnet rates similar to the end-of-service magnet rate. Other models provide magnet rates between the normal magnet rate and the end-of-service magnet rate. These alternative magnet rates due to the sensor circuit should provoke further pacemaker evaluation. Careful investigation may indicate that (1) the cause was temporary and no longer exists, (2) reprogramming of rate-response parameters is needed, or (3) rate-responsive pacing is no longer available unless the lead or pulse generator is replaced. Impending lead failure may be indicated by the temperature-sensing circuitry prior to total failure of pacing and myocardial sensing, giving cause for more frequent follow-up or lead replacement. If temperature sensing is lost owing to lead failure, lead replacement is necessary to restore rate response.

REVISIONS, UPGRADES, AND GENERATOR REPLACEMENT

The major disadvantage of temperature-based rate-responsive pacemakers is common to all lead-based sensors—that is, a special lead is required. This raises potential concerns about lead longevity and sensor vulnerability. If the sensor fails, restoration of rate response requires implantation of a new lead. When replacing a pulse generator in a patient with a standard pacing lead, upgrading to a temperature-based pacemaker is difficult to justify because a specialized lead with a thermistor must be placed. When replacing the pulse generator of a system that has a special sensor lead with another pulse generator, the new pulse generator must be compatible with the sensor lead. It should be emphasized that temperature sensing leads from different manufacturers are not interchangeable.

In temperature-responsive pacing systems using VS-1 or IS-1 standard leads, pulse generator replacement with a non–temperature-responsive pulse generator is often straightforward, although the thermistor connection must be capped. This is especially important with a bipolar version because the thermistor has a direct connection to the bipolar ring. Because a standard for sensor-based leads is nonexistent, the configuration of pins varies between models and manufacturers. The manufacturer's specifications and recommendations should be checked.

Perspectives on Temperature-Based Pacing

Right ventricular blood temperature has been successfully used as a metabolic sensor for rate-responsive pacing. The sensor, a thermistor, has been proved reliable. Temperature-based pacing systems provide a prompt rate response to the onset of exercise and a proportional increase in heart rate with increasing exercise workload, especially at higher levels. However, despite the advantages of this simple sensor, it has not become the primary sensor for rate-responsive pacing, primarily due to the requirement for a special lead. Although the physiology of temperature may be superior to that of some of the more popular rate-responsive sensors (e.g., vibration), a question that remains to be answered is how much practical patient benefit results from a more physiologic sensor.

REFERENCES

1. Bazett HC: Theory of reflex controls to explain regulation of body temperature at rest and during exercise. J Appl Physiol 4:245, 1951.
2. Brundin T: Temperature of mixed venous blood during exercise. Scand J Clin Lab Invest 35:539, 1975.
3. Weisswange A, Csapo G, Perach W, et al: Frequenzsteuerung von Schrittmachern durch Bluttemperatur. Dtsch Ges Kreislaufforsch 44:152, 1978.
4. Griffin JG, Jutzy KR, Claude JP, et al: Central body temperatures as a guide to optimal heart rate. PACE 6:498, 1983.
5. Jolgren D, Fearnot N, Geddes L: A rate-responsive pacemaker controlled by right ventricular blood temperature. PACE 7:794, 1984.
6. Fearnot NE, Jolgren DL, Tacker WA, et al: Increasing cardiac rate by measurement of right ventricular temperature. PACE 7:1240, 1984.
7. Sellers TD, Fearnot N, Johnson W, et al: Central venous temperature profiles for a pacemaker algorithm [Abstract]. PACE 8:294, 1985.
8. Laczkovics A: The central venous blood temperature as a guide for rate control in pacemaker therapy. PACE 7:822, 1984.
9. Sellers TD, Fearnot NE, Smith HJ, et al: Right ventricular blood temperature profiles for rate-responsive pacing. PACE 10:467, 1987.
10. Fearnot NE, Evans ML: Heart rate correlation, response time, and effect of previous exercise using advanced pacing rate algorithm for temperature-based rate modulation. PACE 11:1846, 1988.
11. Alt E, Hirgstetter C, Heinz M, et al: Rate control of physiologic pacemakers by central venous blood temperature. Circulation 73:1206, 1986.
12. Alt E, Hirgstetter C, Heinz M, et al: Measurement of right ventricular blood temperature during exercise as a means of rate control in physiological pacemakers. PACE 9:970, 1986.
13. Alt E, Hirgstetter C, Heinz M, et al: Central venous blood temperature for rate control of physiological pacemakers. J Cardiovasc Surg 29:80, 1988.
14. Cook WA, Fearnot NE, Geddes LA: Exercise-responsive cardiac pacemaker lead. U.S. Patent 4,726,383, February 23, 1988.
15. Baker RG, Phillips RE, Frey ML, et al: A central venous temperature-sensing lead. PACE 9:965, 1986.
16. Schaldach M: Compensation of chronotropic incompetence with temperature-controlled rate-adaptive pacing. Biomed Technik 33:286, 1988.
17. Aschoff J, Guenther B, Kramer K: Energiehaushalt und Temperatur Regulation. Münich, Urban & Schwarzenberg, 1971.
18. Nielsen M: Die Regulation der Korper temperatur bei Muskelarbeit. Skand Arch Physiol 79:193, 1938.
19. Rowell LB, Murray JA, Brengelmann GL, et al: Human cardiovascular adjustment to rapid changes in skin temperature during exercise. Circ Res 24:711, 1969.
20. Rowell LB: Circulatory adjustments to dynamic exercise. *In* Human Circulation Regulation During Physical Stress. New York, Oxford University Press, 1986, pp 213–256.
21. Shellock FG, Swan HJC, Rubin SA: Muscle and femoral vein temperatures during short-term maximal exercise in heart failure. J Appl Physiol 58:400, 1985.
22. Fearnot NE, Kitoh O, Fujita T, et al: Case studies on the effect of exercise and hot water submersion on intracardiac temperature and the performance of a pacemaker which varies pacing rate based on temperature. Jpn Heart J 30:353, 1989.
23. Maddalena G, Santomauro M, Fazio S, et al: Initial clinical experience with a temperature-controlled rate-modulated pacemaker [Abstract]. Rev Eur Technol Biomed 12:53, 1990.
24. Umemura J, Kasanuki H, Ohnishi S, et al: The influence of emotional stress in rate-responsive pacemaker [Abstract]. PACE 10:1231, 1987.
25. Winter UJ, Alt E, Zegelman M, et al: Clinical experience with 65 temperature-guided (TP) pacemakers Nova MR in Europe [Abstract]. PACE 12:1567, 1989.

26. Fearnot NE, Smith HJ, Sellers TD, et al: Evaluation of the temperature response to exercise testing in patients with single-chamber, rate-adaptive pacemakers: A multicenter study. PACE 12:1806, 1989.

27. Zegelman M, Winter UJ, Alt E, et al: Effect of different body-exercise modes on the rate response of the temperature-controlled pacemaker Nova MR. Thorac Cardiovasc Surg 38:181, 1990.

28. Shirey R, Johnson W, Bowser D, et al: The Kelvin central venous temperature sensing/pacing lead. PACE 10:742, 1987.

29. Zegelman M, Kreuzer J, Beyersdorf F, et al: Temperature-guided pacemaker Nova MR—problems due to temperature shift [Abstract]. Rev Eur Technol Biomed 12:99, 1990.

30. Schaldach M: Current status of pacemaker technology. *In* Atlee JL, Gombotz H, Tscheliessnigg KH (eds): Perioperative Management of Pacemaker Patients. Berlin, Springer-Verlag, 1992, pp 1–26.

31. Arakawa M, Kambara K, Ito H, et al: Intermittent oversensing due to internal insulation damage of temperature-sensing rate-responsive pacemaker lead in subclavian venipuncture method. PACE 12:1312, 1989.

32. Magney JE, Flynn DM, Parsons AJ, et al: Anatomical mechanisms explaining damage to pacemaker leads, defibrillator leads, and failure of central venous catheters adjacent to the sternoclavicular joint. PACE 16:445, 1993.

33. Sellers TD, Smith HJ: Specialized pacing leads for rate-adaptive pacing systems: Implications for lead implantation, longevity, and removal. *In* Benditt DG (ed): Rate-Adaptive Cardiac Pacing: Current Technologies and Clinical Applications. Cambridge, Blackwell Scientific Publications, 1993.

34. Furman S, Benedek ZM: Implantable Lead Registry: Survival of implantable pacemaker leads. PACE 13:1910, 1990.

35. Sellers TD, Fearnot N, Smith H, et al: Differential temperature measurements in the atrium and ventricle: Implications for chronic AAI temperature-controlled rate-adaptive pacing [Abstract]. PACE 11:794, 1988.

36. Afonso S, Rowe GG, Castillo CA, et al: Intravascular and intracardiac blood temperatures in man. J Appl Physiol 17:706, 1962.

37. Csapo G: Katheter für Herzschrittmacher. European Patent GM 7606824, August 25, 1977.

38. d'Alnoncourt CN, Schnabel P, Baumanns B, et al: Temperaturgesteuerter Herzschrittmacher Thermos 01 nach Hisbundel-ablation. Herzschrittmacher 7:168, 1987.

39. Crussard BFG: Experience with temperature-controlled pacemakers [Abstract]. PACE 13:1191, 1990.

40. Cook W, Fearnot NE, Geddes LA: Exercise-responsive cardiac pacemaker. US Patent 4,436,092, March 13, 1984.

41. Fearnot NE: The pacing rate algorithm of the temperature-controlled Kelvin 500 rate-modulated pacemaker [Abstract]. PACE 11:807, 1988.

42. Theres H, Alt E, Atkins A, et al: Temperature-controlled pacing: Benefits of a new optimized algorithm [Abstract]. Clin Prog Electrophysiol Pacing 4 (Suppl):8, 1986.

43. Singer I, Peavler P, Johnson B, et al: Temperature may be an ideal sensor for rate modulation in patients with posture-related syncope and chronotropic incompetence [Abstract]. J Am Coll Cardiol 21:426A, 1993.

44. Fearnot NE, Heggs KS, Johnson WL, et al: Pacemaker with activity-dependent rate limiting. U.S. Patent 4,945,909, August 7, 1990.

45. Anelli-Monti M, Machler H, Iberer F, et al: Problems in programming different rate-responsive (RR) pacemaker (PM) systems [Abstract]. PACE 12:1577, 1989.

46. Koch T, Isbruch FM, Frenking B, et al: Long-term results with the temperature-controlled pacemaker Thermos 01 [Abstract]. PACE 11:807, 1988.

47. Schroder E, Klein H, Siclari F, et al: Erste Erfahrungen mit einem Temperaturgesteuerten frequenzadaptierenden Schrittmachersystem. Herzschrittmacher 7:22, 1987.

48. Alt E, Volker R, Hogl B, et al: First clinical results with a new temperature-controlled rate-responsive pacemaker. Circulation 78 (Suppl III):III-116, 1988.

49. Alt E, Theres H, Hogl B, et al: Function of the temperature-controlled Nova MR pacemaker in patient's everyday life: Preliminary clinical results [Abstract]. PACE 12:1158, 1989.

50. Volosin KJ, O'Connor WH, Fabiszewski R, et al: Pacemaker-mediated tachycardia from a single-chamber temperature-sensitive pacemaker. PACE 12:1596, 1989.

51. Alt E, Theres H, Heinz M, et al: A new rate-modulated pacemaker system optimized by combination of two sensors. PACE 11:1119, 1988.

52. Sigiura T, Kimura M, Mizushina S, et al: Cardiac pacemaker regulated by respiratory rate and blood temperature. PACE 11:1077, 1988.

53. Stangl K, Wirtzfeld A, Heinz R, et al: A new multisensor pacing system using stroke volume, respiratory rate, mixed venous oxygen saturation, and temperature, right atrial pressure, right ventricular pressure, and dP/dt. PACE 11:712, 1988.

CHAPTER 11

RATE-ADAPTIVE PACING CONTROLLED BY DYNAMIC RIGHT VENTRICULAR PRESSURE (dP/dtmax)

Raymond Yee
Thomas D. Bennett

Physiologic Basis for RV dP/dtmax Pacing

The maximum rate of pressure development in the right ventricle (RV dP/dtmax) is one of several parameters that reflect the contractile state of the right ventricle. Right ventricular contractility, like that of the left ventricle, is modulated by both hemodynamic and autonomic factors and is susceptible to exogenous influences such as a variety of drugs.[1–8] Any physical or emotional stress that increases circulating or endogenous catecholamines may potentially augment contractility of the ventricles and increase the dP/dtmax that is recorded within these chambers[2] (Fig. 11–1). The increased sympathetic tone and vagal withdrawal that occur with physical or emotional stress normally increase the intrinsic heart rate concomitant with the changes in ventricular contractility. Although the rate of pressure rise in either the right or the left ventricle could be used as an index of these changes in autonomic tone, only the right ventricle is suitable for long-term implantation of a pressure transducer located on a permanent pacing lead. Thus, RV dP/dtmax has been developed as an indirect measure of sympathetic tone that can be used as a physiologic variable for controlling the pacing rate of a permanent pacing system.[9–30]

Potentially Confounding Physiologic Effects

Although RV dP/dtmax is a directly measureable physiologic variable, it responds to a complex set of inputs that could potentially complicate its application as a rate-controlling parameter in a rate-adaptive pacemaker. For example, changes in RV preload such as those induced by changes in posture, venous pooling, or fluid loading will alter the RV dP/dtmax by the Frank-Starling mechanism.[1, 3] Since decreased venous return to the heart results in a reduced intraventricular end-diastolic pressure and volume, the RV dP/dtmax may decline with a change from the supine to the upright posture.[18, 31] The normal sinus node compensates for a transient decline in right ventricular filling pressure (and left ventricular stroke volume) with an increase in heart rate that is mediated by the carotid body baroreceptors. The increase in sinus rate tends to limit the postural changes in cardiac output (the product of stroke volume and heart rate). However, for patients with a rate-adaptive pacemaker that is controlled by RV dP/dtmax, these hemodynamic effects could produce an inappropriate decrease in pacing rate.[18, 31] The respiratory cycle also causes cyclic variation in ventricular loading that may result in oscillating RV contractility.[1, 7, 8]

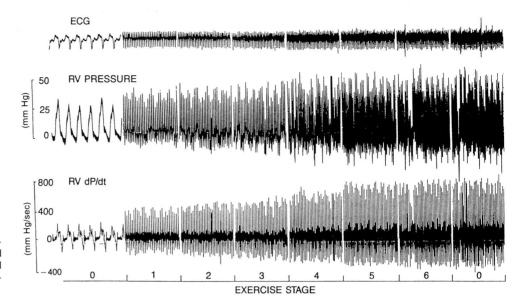

FIGURE 11–1. Illustration of electrocardiogram (ECG), telemetered right ventricular (RV) pressure, and RV dP/dt signals from a patient during graded treadmill exercise.

Such cycles of right ventricular volume and pressure could potentially result in an oscillating pacing rate. In addition to these effects of changes in venous return and intraventricular volume, the contractile state of the myocardium is positively related to heart rate.[5] Increases in heart rate result in an increase in ventricular contractility that is independent of any autonomic influences. Thus, simple increases in the intrinsic or paced cardiac rate will increase dP/dtmax, a phenomenon termed the Treppe effect, which is modulated by changes in intracellular calcium concentration. Such positive feedback could potentially result in an inappropriate increase in pacing rate. Although it is a potential limitation to the use of dP/dtmax pacing, the magnitude of the Treppe effect has been found to be quite small and has not been identified as a clinical problem in clinical studies of this sensor.

In addition to these known physiologic factors that could complicate a rate-adaptive pacemaker controlled by RV dP/dtmax, there are additional pathologic factors that need to be considered. For example, the intrinsic contractility of the right ventricular myocardium is likely to influence the manner in which RV dP/dtmax responds to physiologic stress. Any acute or chronic cardiac or pulmonary disease state that depresses RV function could potentially limit the usefulness of RV dP/dtmax as a rate-controlling parameter. Right ventricular infarction or ischemia would be expected to impair the normal contractile response to exercise. Similarly, long-standing pulmonary disease or intrinsic vascular disease in the pulmonary circulation may chronically increase resistance to blood flow, thereby increasing afterload on the right ventricle. Changes in afterload have an important influence on ventricular contractility. The effects of such changes in right ventricular afterload on systolic performance are related to the chronicity with which they develop and the compensatory mechanism of ventricular hypertrophy. For example, acute increases in pulmonary vascular resistance (e.g., following thromboembolism) are likely to have a much greater impact on right ventricular function than are more gradual increases. Thus, the magnitude of right ventricular dP/dtmax and its response to stress may be altered by these pathologic conditions in unpredictable ways.

A variety of cardioactive drugs may also significantly alter the RV dP/dtmax.[3] Drugs such as digoxin or dobutamine increase ventricular contractility. In patients with a pacemaker controlled by dP/dtmax, unwanted increases in pacing rate related to these drug effects may occur. The net effect of drugs that decrease pulmonary artery and right ventricular pressure may be especially complex. For example, diuretics or vasodilators can be expected to decrease dP/dtmax if the decline in right ventricular preload is greater than the decrease in afterload. If the effect of these agents is to decrease right ventricular afterload to a greater extent than preload, an increase in RV dP/dtmax may result. Thus, the effect on pacing rate may be either a decrease or an increase. It should also be recognized that interventions directed at the hemodynamic status may be either offset or accentuated by reflex changes in the autonomic nervous system. Thus, in the case of diuretics or vasodilators, if there is a decrease in left ventricular stroke volume, an increase in sympathetic tone may be evoked that reflexively enhances contractility. If the cardiac output is increased by these drugs, the sympathetic tone and heart rate might be expected to decrease.

On balance, the complexity of these interrelating factors that modulate RV dP/dtmax constitutes a desirable feature for a physiologic pacing sensor, since the cardiac output is usually modified within the physiologic range. However, complexity also represents clinical and technical challenges. Therefore, pacemakers using RV dP/dtmax for rate control must provide adequate programmability to compensate for pathologic conditions and to limit any undesired behavior.

Lead and Sensor Technology for Measurement of RV dP/dtmax

The clinical acceptance of any sensor-based pacemaker system is directly linked to the reliability of the sensor technology. The right ventricular pressure sensor used to determine dP/dtmax is based on a piezoelectric crystal that transduces small deflections of an intravascular sensor diaphragm into an electric signal. The diaphragm is coupled to the piezoelectric crystal.[29] As the pressure in the right ventricle changes, movement of the diaphragm results in distortion of the crystal. An intrinsic property of piezoelectric crystals is that a change in their shape produces a voltage difference across the crystal. The voltage that is produced is proportional to the degree of mechanical deformation and can be calibrated to represent known pressures causing the diaphragm distortion. Differentiation of the voltage signal provides a dV/dt signal that is representative of the instantaneous rate of change in pressure (dP/dt). Following each pacing stimulus or sensed QRS, the peak positive value of right ventricular dP/dt (dP/dtmax) that is recorded during a 200-msec window spanning the initial portion of mechanical ventricular systole is used for input into the rate response algorithm of the pacemaker. Operation of the pressure sensor in pacemakers based on RV dP/dtmax requires power. During *continuous operation,* the current drain of the sensor is approximately 20 μA. However, the sensor operates only for a brief period following the QRS, so the average current drain by the sensor is much smaller and has only a small impact on overall pulse generator longevity.

A key requirement for long-term function of indwelling physiologic sensors is that the electric components are isolated from the harsh environment of the body. The right ventricular pressure sensor used with the RV dP/dtmax pacemaker is hermetically sealed, protecting it from chemical degradation. Long-term performance of the sensor has been demonstrated with no reported sensor failures with implants for as long as 5 years.[17, 29] Another requirement for sensors in continuous use for applications such as the control of pacing rate is stability of the sensed parameter over time. Drift in a sensor signal can result in unacceptable shifts in pacing rate over time. The piezoelectric sensor found in the dP/dtmax pacemakers has inherent baseline values of 0 volts (AC coupled). Thus, the sensor responds only to *changes in pressure,* rather than to gradual drift in baseline right ventricular pressure. This also means that the pressure transducer cannot measure *absolute pressure values* (right ventricular systolic or diastolic pressure). Although knowledge of the patient's right ventricular systolic and diastolic pressures would provide potentially useful diagnostic information for the clinician, the only parameters that the dP/dt pacemaker

can reliably measure are changes in pressure over the cardiac cycle (e.g., right ventricular pulse pressure) and the rate of change of pressure (dP/dt) (Fig. 11–2). While the lack of absolute pressures imposes certain limitations, it simultaneously provides for very high inherent stability.

Physiologic sensors that are incorporated on a pacing lead in the right ventricle are likely to become encapsulated by tissue as part of the normal foreign body reaction. Normal tissue encapsulation has not proved to compromise the right ventricular pressure transducers that have been used, to date, in RV dP/dtmax–based pacemakers because the tissue covering the sensing ports is highly compliant compared with the sensor diaphragm. However, entrapment or ingrowth of the sensor into muscular trabeculae can isolate the transducer from the true hydraulic pressures of the ventricular cavity and result in an erroneous dynamic pressure waveform and dP/dtmax measurement. While this has been noted to occur in chronic animal studies,[33] this complication has not been observed in patient studies to date.

Operation of a rate-adaptive sensor that is incorporated on a pacing lead also requires a minimum of one additional electric conductor in the lead to operate the sensor. This means that, for unipolar pacing and sensing, two conductor coils are required for the right ventricular pressure sensor lead that has been used in the dP/dtmax–based pacemakers. Thus, all dP/dt leads that have been implanted in clinical trials provide only unipolar pacing and sensing operation. To date, the lead function and longevity of the pressure-based leads used (Models 6220, 6220S, and 2431, Medtronic Inc., Minneapolis, MN) have been comparable to those of standard coaxial bipolar leads. One negative aspect of all right ventricular pressure-sensing leads that have been studied, to date, is the size of the introducer that is required for implantation. While the lead bodies of these leads are of standard dimension for a coaxial bipolar lead, the sensor capsule is approximately 10 F in diameter. Therefore, unless the lead is introduced directly into the vein by the cutdown technique, a 10.5 to 11.0 F introducer is required for lead implantation. Perhaps a more significant factor for lead implantation is that the stylet cannot be passed beyond the sensor to the tip of the lead. Since the stylet ends at the sensor, the distal 2.8 cm of the lead is without stylet control. Although this limitation

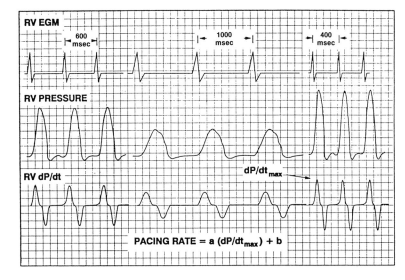

FIGURE 11–2. Illustration of electrogram (EGM), telemetered right ventricular pressure, and RV dP/dt signals showing the RV dP/dtmax pacing concept in which pacing cycle length increases (pacing rate decreases) as RV dP/dtmax decreases, and pacing cycle length decreases (pacing rate increases) as RV dP/dtmax increases. The linear relation between pacing rate and RV dP/dtmax is shown in the equation at the bottom of the figure.

has proved an inconvenience in some cases and requires some adjustment in lead handling technique, it has not been reported to be a serious drawback.

Pacemaker Technology Review

Three rate-adaptive pulse generators based on RV dP/dtmax have been implanted in human subjects. These are the Medtronic models 2451, 2503, 8225, and 8227. None of these pacemakers has yet gained universal market approval throughout the world; they are limited to investigational use in some countries, including the United States. The initial model 2451 pacemaker was a VVI pacemaker capable of right ventricular pressure telemetry only. This device served to provide limited, early evidence of the feasibility of the sensor lead and dP/dtmax concept (see following section on clinical studies). The model 2503 pulse generator was the first VVIR pacemaker that used RV dP/dtmax to control pacing rate and was coupled with the original model 6220 lead. This pulse generator and lead required a bifurcated lead connector configuration. The model 2503 pacemaker had 20 programmable, curvilinear rate-response curves with selectable upper and lower rate limits (Fig. 11–3). The model 8225 pulse generator was designed to function with the model 6220S pressure lead. This system had several improvements over its predecessor, including a steroid-eluting electrode at the tip of the lead and an in-line bipolar connector. The pulse generator had a new, smaller profile. It contained 16 programmable, linear rate-response curves and 16 rate-offset curves to allow more flexibility for matching the sensor response to the patient's right ventricular pressure profile. The model 8227 pulse generator is similar to the model 8225 except that it shifted the rate-response curves into a range that was found to be more appropriate for the expected range of RV dP/dtmax values that are encountered in typical patients (Fig. 11–4). In addition, this device is connected to an

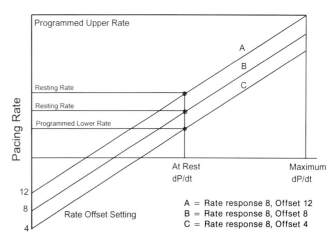

FIGURE 11–4. Effect of programming rate offset on pacing rate. Three curves (A, B, and C) are demonstrated with offsets of 4, 8, and 12. Note that the rate-response setting is constant (8) for each of these curves. A higher rate offset increases the pacing rate at any dP/dt value, thus shifting the curve upward. Also note that the choice of rate offset influences the heart rate that will be observed at rest for any resting dP/dt (although the pacing rate will never be less than the programmed lower pacing rate).

upgraded model 4321 lead that utilizes a standard IS-1 in-line connector.

Several limitations in these pacemakers are notable. First, the dP/dtmax devices described to date have been only single-chamber, VVIR pacing systems. Although dual-chamber pacemakers based on this sensor have been planned, none have yet been introduced. The pulse generators are larger than many VVIR pacemakers currently in use that are based on other sensors. The devices are programmed by older, less convenient programmers than those of newer pacing systems. Finally, because there is considerable variability between patients with respect to their right ventricular pulse pressures and dP/dtmax, the lack of features to aid in the optimal programming of the rate-response features may lead to a prolonged patient follow-up session. However, it must be pointed out that none of these limitations is an integral part of the dP/dtmax sensor. Rather, these relate to the fact that these pacing systems have not been developed for commercially released products.

Clinical Studies

Following earlier animal studies[9, 17, 33] and temporary pacing studies in patients,[12, 26] Heynen and colleagues[21] conducted initial trials of the first implantable unipolar, tined pressure-sensing lead (model 6220, Medtronic Inc.) in a small number of patients requiring permanent pacemaker implantation. At the time, a fully rate-responsive pacemaker device based on RV dP/dtmax was not available. Instead, the lead was implanted with a VVI pulse generator (model 2451, Medtronic Inc.) that was capable of telemetering dynamic right ventricular pressure via a radio-frequency programming head to a computer with an algorithm for determining the appropriate pacing rate. The computer determined the rate of chest wall stimulation that would drive the implanted pulse generator, which had been programmed to the VVT mode. Thus, this research system emulated a rate-responsive pacemaker with the rate determined by the RV dP/dtmax. A

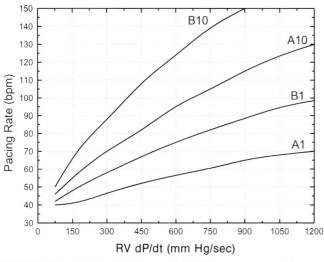

FIGURE 11–3. Relationship between RV dP/dtmax expressed in mm Hg/sec and pacing rate at various combinations of offset and slope. At an identical right ventricular dP/dt, note that at the highest combination of offset (B) and slope (10), the pacing rate is faster than at the least sensitive setting (A1). Also note that offset and slope are not independent of each another.

pacing rate of 70 bpm was assigned to the resting RV dP/dtmax value, and the RV dP/dtmax value at a submaximal exercise workload during a treadmill exercise test was arbitrarily associated with a pacing rate of 130 bpm. A linear relationship between RV dP/dtmax and pacing rate was assumed. A total of nine patients (mean age 54 years) with complete heart block received the dP/dt lead. Evaluation of the lead during exercise was limited to six patients. In the VVIR pacing mode, the RV dP/dtmax averaged 223 ± 55 mm Hg/sec at a resting heart rate of 82 ± 13 bpm and increased to a maximum level of 405 ± 181 mm Hg/sec with a corresponding heart rate of 119 ± 13 bpm during exercise. The interval from the onset of the intracardiac R wave to the RV dP/dtmax increased from 106 ± 30 to 119 ± 12 msec during exercise. The paced rate approximated the sinus rate during exercise, indicating that the closed loop external pacing mode emulated function of the normal sinus node quite well. Other relevant right ventricular pressure parameters are listed in Table 11–1.

Subsequently, a fully rate-responsive pacemaker (model 2503, Medtronic Inc.) capable of interfacing to the same model 6220 pressure-sensing lead was developed. This pacing system offered two selectable families of rate-response curves that were curvilinear, converging at the lower levels of RV dP/dtmax while becoming shallower at the high end. Bennett and associates[29] reported on the experience in 12 patients (mean age 65 years), the majority of whom had complete atrioventricular (AV) block and all of whom had chronotropic incompetence. Pacing responses to exercise, normal daily activity (Holter recording), respiratory stress, and posture were evaluated. During formal exercise testing in the VVIR mode, the heart rate increased from 67 ± 5 to 114 ± 27 bpm. This increase in rate of 47 ± 26 bpm was highly significant statistically ($p < 0.05$), whereas the change in heart rate in the VVI mode was not. However, since the VVI exercise test was conducted first to determine the appropriate rate-response setting, these were not randomized comparisons. A subset of five patients underwent an additional crossover comparison of the VVI and VVIR pacing modalities. In these patients, the lower rate of the device was set at 50 bpm, with an upper rate setting of 130 bpm. Because of the small number of subjects and the presence of some intrinsic chronotropic competence during VVI pacing, the increase in exercise duration (from 12.9 to 14.5 minutes) and exercise stage reached (6.0 to 6.9) with VVIR mode was not statistically significant. Holter recordings performed 1 to 3 months after implantation confirmed the continued reliable function of the device, with heart rates averaging a minimum of 51 ± 6 bpm and reaching a maximum of 110 ± 22 bpm. As in the previous study of the model 2451 pulse generator, postural changes (headup tilt test) and respiratory cycle changes including Valsalva maneuver evoked only minimal changes in RV dP/dtmax. Interestingly, three patients exhibited paradox-

ical decreases in pacing rate with upright tilt, although none experienced symptoms related to hypotension. It was concluded that chronic rate-responsive pacing based on RV dP/dtmax was possible and does respond physiologically to stresses such as exercise and respiratory cycle variation.

The next development in the RV dP/dtmax pacing system was the model 8225 pulse generator and the model 6220S steroid-eluting version of the pressure-sensing polyurethane lead. Between 1988 and 1990, a total of 36 devices were implanted in 13 women and 23 men with a mean age of 69 ± 13 years. The dP/dtmax system constituted a replacement of a preexisting pacing system in 11 patients. Eleven patients had left ventricular dysfunction of varying etiology. At implantation, the resting dP/dtmax averaged 332 ± 101 mm Hg/sec with a mean RV pulse pressure of 25 ± 8 mm Hg. Over the ensuing 3-month follow-up, the telemetered pulse pressure value did not diminish appreciably. All patients were chronically programmed to VVIR pacing mode, with the exception of a single patient whose device manifested aberrant rate-responsive behavior. During follow-up, the telemetered right ventricular pressure values remained stable. Holter recordings documented appropriate increases in pacing rate related to physical and emotional stresses. There were no adverse effects or inappropriate rate increases related to environmental factors or evidence of significant positive feedback rate behavior (Treppe effect). There have been no device-related deaths during long-term follow-up. On formal exercise testing in 22 patients with an implanted dP/dtmax pacing system, the peak heart rate was a mean of 132 bpm with a 90% decay time during a postexercise recovery period of 5 to 6 minutes. This rate recovery characteristic, in addition to the rate increase at the onset of exercise, reflected appropriate physiologic modulation.

The most recent version of the RV dP/dtmax–based rate-responsive pacemaker utilizes the model 8227 pulse generator with a new steroid-eluting, tined, unipolar polyurethane lead with an IS-1 connector (model 4321, Medtronic Inc.). To date, there have been more than 115 of these devices implanted in patients with a mean age of 69 ± 11 years. Fifty-five percent of those receiving the device were men. The indication for pacemaker implantation was complete AV block created by catheter ablation of the AV node because of refractory atrial fibrillation in almost all patients. Recruitment for the clinical trial has been completed, but limited information has been published. One preliminary report by Bailin and coworkers[15] in 10 patients with the model 8227 pacemaker showed significantly improved heart rate, maximal workload, and Vo₂max in the VVIR mode compared with the VVI mode during paired treadmill testing. These investigators also reported a similar pattern of rate-responsive VVIR pacing when the patients participated in paired tests with either treadmill or bicycle exercise. These important findings led the investigators to conclude that the rate response was related to workload but was independent of the type of exercise.

In another series of 13 patients, Kay[18] reported the results of rate-responsive pacing based on RV dP/dtmax with the model 8227. The VVIR mode was associated with an exercise duration of 511 ± 220 seconds, which was significantly greater than that during exercise in the VVI mode (418 ± 233 seconds, $p = 0.006$). The Vo₂max increased from 12.6 ± 4 mL/kg per minute (VVI) to 15.9 ± 6 mL/kg per minute

TABLE 11–1. RV PRESSURE PARAMETERS WITH EXERCISE TESTING IN VVIR MODE

	HEART RATE	POS dP/dtmax	NEG dP/dtmax	RV PULSE PRESSURE
Rest	82 ± 13	223 ± 55	222 ± 66	13.6 ± 4.8
Exercise	119 ± 13	405 ± 181	335 ± 180	17.6 ± 6.5

(VVIR) ($p = 0.02$) and was associated with a maximal heart rate of 72 ± 6 bpm (VVI) versus 124 ± 18 bpm (VVIR). Using a newly developed scheme for evaluating overall chronotropic performance based on dividing exercise into 25% phases for each patient, Kay[32] found that the dP/dtmax–based pacemaker provided an increase in pacing rate during exercise that closely paralleled the expected heart rate based on Vo_2. When the rate-response curve was plotted and expressed as a percentage of the area under the expected heart rate curve, the dP/dtmax pacing system provided a mean rate response that was $96.7\% \pm 45.7\%$ of that expected during increasing exercise workloads. During recovery, the mean area under the heart rate curve was $100.1\% \pm 43\%$ of that expected. When the exercise tests were analyzed by each quartile of workload, the heart rate response tended to be somewhat greater than that expected during low levels of exercise and most closely reflected the expected rate during higher levels. These investigators also reported that the heart rate fell during a change from the supine to the upright posture in 3 of 13 patients, with a maximum decline of 7 bpm (from 77 to 70 bpm). In one patient, a reproducible increase in pacing rate to the maximal programmed rate occurred when she turned onto her left side.

In summary, clinical experience indicates that RV dP/dtmax–based pacing systems provide excellent long-term rate-responsive pacing behavior in response to changes in both physical and emotional physiologic conditions. Growing experience with this pacing sensor over several years suggests that the technical pathophysiologic complications of this sensor are minimal, although larger clinical trials remain to be fully reported.

Future Developments

The potential clinical utility of pacemakers that are capable of beat-by-beat measurement of right ventricular pressure are intriguing. Since this sensor allows measurement of mechanical function of the right ventricle, it may have utility as a method for verifying ventricular capture. Patients with high pacing thresholds or for whom use of low stimulation energy is desired to prolong battery longevity could potentially benefit from automatic capture detection or threshold tracking. Reports indicate beat-by-beat ventricular capture detection can be accomplished by checking after each pacing stimulus for appropriate pressure development by the right ventricular pressure sensor. Except in cases of electromechanical dissociation, right ventricular pressure provided a reliable signal for identifying loss of capture and automatically adjusting the pacing stimulus to immediately regain capture.

While the prior experiences with the VVIR version of this pacing system have shown merit in patients with persistent atrial arrhythmias, a dual-chamber, rate-adaptive pacemaker using RV dP/dtmax could be beneficial in certain other patient groups. Patients with a particularly strong dependence on appropriately timed atrial synchrony could have AV interval dynamically adjusted to provide optimized ventricular contractions, rather than a fixed AV interval or a simple rate-dependent AV interval.

Rate-adaptive pacing based on cardiac parameters such as dP/dtmax may, in the future, benefit still other patient groups, such as those with heart failure. Reynolds and associates[4] conducted a retrospective analysis of right ventricular pressures in 100 patients having right heart catheterizations with recordings of right ventricular pressures. Reports from this analysis confirmed the baseline values of right ventricular pulse pressures and dP/dtmax reported from the dP/dtmax pacing studies. Also, the investigators confirmed that patients with low left ventricular ejection fractions (LVEF <50%) associated with elevated pulmonary artery pressures (PA systolic pressure >50 mm Hg) had significantly elevated right ventricular pulse pressure (35%) and dP/dtmax (37%). The authors speculated on the potential diagnostic merit of telemetered right ventricular pressures, although their retrospective

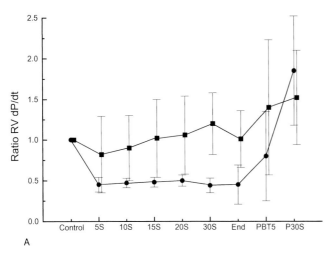

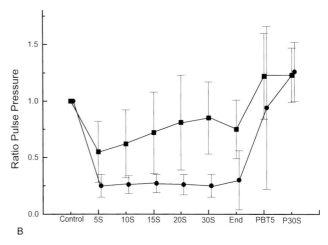

A

B

FIGURE 11–5. Illustration of changes in right ventricular pulse pressure and RV dP/dtmax from a group of patients during hemodynamically stable and unstable ventricular tachyarrhythmias. *A*, The ratio of RV dP/dt during sinus rhythm (control) and during ventricular tachycardia (VT) is demonstrated. The squares represent the ratio of RV dP/dt during hemodynamically stable VT to the control value. Note that there is a slight but abrupt decrease in RV dP/dt within 5 seconds of the onset of VT, which quickly returns toward baseline values. Within 5 seconds of the termination of VT (PBT5), the RV dP/dt exceeds the baseline value. The same measurements were made during hemodynamically unstable VT *(circles)*. Note that the right ventricular dP/dt falls below the control value throughout VT, with a somewhat greater overshoot in right ventricular contractility following VT termination. *B*, The ratio of the right ventricular pulse pressure to the control value is shown for hemodynamically stable *(squares)* and unstable *(circles)* VT. Note that the findings are similar to these observed for RV dP/dt.

study did not identify specific right ventricular pressure parameters that were indicative of the level or degree of left ventricular dysfunction in their patients. A limitation of this study was that there were no serial data within any patient subgroup for analysis.

Right ventricular pressure has been reported by several investigators as having potential value as a hemodynamic discriminator in implantable cardioverter defibrillator (ICD) devices as well. Sharma and colleagues,[35] Reynolds and associates,[4] and Ellenbogen and coworkers[34] have identified that right ventricular pressure parameters can help differentiate hemodynamically tolerated ventricular tachyarrhythmias from hemodynamically unstable rhythms[36, 37] (Fig. 11–5). Sharma and colleagues conducted their studies using a temporarily placed pressure sensing lead (model 6220, Medtronic Inc.) and reported sustained decreases in right ventricular pulse pressure and RV dP/dtmax by 10 seconds into ventricular tachycardia–ventricular fibrillation episodes. Reynolds and associates[4] used micromanometer catheters (Millar Instruments, Houston, TX) and Ellenbogen and coworkers[34] used fluid-filled catheters with external transducers in their studies. Despite these pilot studies, pressure sensor incorporation into ICD lead system architectures has not yet been reported. In addition, there is considerable concern regarding the sensitivity and specificity of right ventricular pressure recordings to accurately reflect the hemodynamic status of the systemic circulation. In summary, the RV dP/dtmax–based pacemakers described to date represent only the early stages of the potential value such technology may hold for future devices.

REFERENCES

1. Morris J, Wechsler A: Right ventricular function: The assessment of contractile performance. *In* Fisk R (ed): The Right Heart. Philadelphia, FA Davis, 1987, pp 3–18.
2. Korner PI: Central nervous control of autonomic cardiovascular function. *In* Berne RM, Sperelakis N, Geiger SR (eds): Handbook of Physiology, Sec. 2, Vol. 1. Bethesda, MD, American Physiological Society, 1979, pp 691–739.
3. Quinones M, Gaasch W, Alexander J: Influences of acute changes in preload, afterload, contractile state, and heart rate on ejection and isovolumic indices of myocardial contractility in man. Circulation 53:293, 1976.
4. Reynolds D, Turner S, Bridges S, et al: Right ventricular pressure parameters in patients with normal and reduced cardiac function [abstract]. PACE 10:436, 1987.
5. Schmidt H, Hoppe H, Muller K: The effect of changes in cardiac frequency on left and right ventricular dP/dtmax at different contractile states of the myocardium. Eur J Appl Physiol 42:183, 1979.
6. Schmidt H, Hoppe H: Maximal rate of pressure rise and time parameters in the right ventricle under isovolumic conditions. Basic Res Cardiol 71:521, 1976.
7. Cody R, Kubo S: Assessment of right and left heart interactions: Application of the resistance ratio in congestive heart failure. *In* Fisk R (ed): The Right Heart. Philadelphia, FA Davis, 1987, pp 133–144.
8. Baker B, Franciosa J: Effect of left ventricle on the right ventricle. *In* Fisk R (ed): The Right Heart. Philadelphia, FA Davis, 1987, pp 145–155.
9. Sharma A, Sutton R, Bennett T, et al: Physiologic pacing based on beat-to-beat measurement of right ventricular dP/dtmax: Initial feasibility studies in man [abstract]. J Am Coll Cardiol 7:3A, 1986.
10. Bennett TD, Baudino M, Bornzin G, et al: Rate-responsive pacing using dynamic right ventricular pressure in heart-blocked dogs [abstract]. J Am Coll Cardiol 5:393, 1985.
11. Bennett TD, Olson WH, Bornzin GA, et al: Alternative modes for physiologic pacing. *In* Perez-Gomez F (ed): Cardiac Pacing. Mt Kisco, NY, Futura Pub., 1985, pp 577–587.
12. Sharma A, Bennett T, Erickson M, et al: Rate-responsive pacing based on maximum positive right ventricular dP/dt: Effects of respiratory

maneuvers. *In* Belhassen B, Feldman S, Cooperman S (eds): Cardiac Pacing and Electrophysiology: Proceedings of the VIIIth Symposium on Cardiac Pacing and Electrophysiology. Jerusalem, Israel, Keterpress Enterprises, 1987, pp 67–76.
13. Bennett T, Beck R, Erickson M: Right ventricular pressure parameters for differentiation of supraventricular and ventricular rhythms [abstract]. PACE 10:415, 1987.
14. Bennett T, Erickson M: Telemetered right ventricular pressure from an implanted pacemaker: One-year follow-up in dogs [abstract]. Rev Eur Technol Biomed 12:48, 1990.
15. Bailin SJ, Fetter J, Johnson B, et al: Clinical effectiveness with a dP/dt VVIR pacemaker utilizing a right ventricular pressure sensor during treadmill and bicycle exercise testing [abstract]. PACE 16:895, 1993.
16. Lau CP, Butrous GS, Ward DE, et al: Comparison of exercise performance of six rate-adaptive right ventricular cardiac pacemakers. Am J Cardiol 63:833, 1989.
17. Erickson M, Bennett T: Pacing rate responses with the dP/dt VVIR pacemaker: One-year follow-up in heart blocked dogs [abstract]. PACE 13:529, 1990.
18. Kay GN: Rate-modulated pacing based on right ventricular pressure (dP/dt): Quantitative analysis of chronotropic response. PACE (in press).
19. Paul V, Farrell T, Ward D, Camm J: Long-term reliability of the dP/dt sensor. Rev Eur Technol Biomed 12:47, 1990.
20. Ohlsson A, Astrom H, Beck B, et al: Monitoring of right ventricular pressure and mixed venous oxygen saturation with a multisensor lead [abstract]. PACE 16:885, 1993.
21. Heynen H, Sharma A, Sutton R, et al: Clinical experience with VVIR pacing based on right ventricular dP/dt. Eur J Pacing Electrophysiol 1:138, 1991.
22. Stangl K, Wirtzfield A, Heinze R, et al: A new multisensor pacing system using stroke volume, respiratory rate, mixed venous oxygen saturation, and temperature, right atrial pressure, right ventricular pressure, and dP/dt. PACE 11:712, 1988.
23. Stangl K, Munteanu J, Wirtzfield A: Right atrial pressure, right ventricular pressure, and dP/dt: New parameters for regulating rate response in pacemakers [abstract]. PACE 10:1230, 1987.
24. Sutton R, Sharma A, Ingram A: Ventricular rate-responsive pacing using first derivative of right ventricular pressure as a sensor [abstract]. J Am Coll Cardiol 11:167A, 1988.
25. Sharma AD, Bennett TD, Erickson M, et al: Randomized single-blind assessment of rate-responsive pacing based upon maximum positive right ventricular dP/dt during treadmill exercise. PACE 11:487, 1988.
26. Sharma A, Yee R, Bennett T, et al: The effects of ventricular pacing on right ventricular maximum positive dP/dt: Implications for a rate-responsive pacing system based on this parameter [abstract]. PACE 10:1228, 1987.
27. Sutton R, Sharma A, Ingram A, et al: First derivative of right ventricular pressure as a sensor for an implantable rate-responsive VVI pacemaker [abstract]. PACE 11:487, 1988.
28. Anderson K, Moore A: Sensors in pacing. PACE 9:954, 1986.
29. Bennett T, Sharma A, Sutton R: Development of a rate-adaptive pacemaker based on the maximum rate-of-rise of right ventricular pressure (RV dP/dtmax). PACE 15:219, 1992.
30. Cohen TJ, Liem LB: Biosensor applications to antitachycardia devices. PACE 14:322, 1991.
31. Bennett TD, Olson WH: Effects of postural stress on several rate-responsive pacing modes in conscious dogs [abstract]. PACE 10:645, 1987.
32. Kay GN: Quantitation of chronotropic response: Comparison of methods for rate-modulating permanent pacemakers. J Am Coll Cardiol 20:1533, 1992.
33. Bennett T, Erickson M: Telemetered right ventricular pressure from an implanted pacemaker: One-year follow-up in dogs [abstract]. Rev Biol Med 12:48, 1990.
34. Ellenbogen KA, Lu B, Kapadia K, et al: Usefulness of right ventricular pulse pressure as a potential sensor for hemodynamically unstable tachycardia. Am J Cardiol 65:1105, 1990.
35. Sharma A, Bennett T, Erickson K, et al: Right ventricular pressure during ventricular arrhythmias in humans: Potential implications for implantable antitachycardia devices. J Am Coll Cardiol 15:648, 1990.
36. Wood M, Ellenbogen KA, Lu B, Valenta H: A prospective study of right ventricular pulse pressure and dP/dt to discriminant-induced ventricular tachycardia from supraventricular and sinus tachycardia in man. PACE 13:1148, 1990.
37. Olson WH, Bennett TD, Huberty KP, et al: Automatic detection of ventricular fibrillation with chronically implanted pressure sensors [abstract]. J Am Coll Cardiol 7:182A, 1986.

CHAPTER 12

RATE-ADAPTIVE PACING BASED ON IMPEDANCE-DERIVED MINUTE VENTILATION

Tibor Nappholz
James D. Maloney
G. Neal Kay

The concept of ''rate-responsive'' pacing is viewed by many as a revolutionary trend, born from the rapid advances in pacing therapy. A different perspective may be obtained if we realize that the concept of using respiration as a rate-responsive parameter was being extensively discussed by Krasner and Voukydis as early as 1966.[1] In fact, Krasner and Nardella patented the concept in 1967.[2] Many potential rate-control parameters have been visited and abandoned since then, but the simplicity and high specificity of respiration as an indicator of metabolic demand has earned its preeminence in the small and select rank of metabolic sensors for rate-responsive pacing. The following discussion focuses on the utility of respiration as a rate-responsive parameter in current pacing therapy and includes some historical perspective.

Biomedical Impedance

The mechanics of respiration involve the cyclic expansion and contraction of the thoracic cavity. It should be emphasized that ''minute ventilation'' pacemakers do not actually measure air flow through the lungs. Rather, associated with the mechanical movements of ventilation is a change in the electric impedance across the human torso. It is the measurement of these changes in impedance that enables the respiratory process to be monitored by relatively simple means that are adaptable to an implantable pacemaker. The measurement of impedance in biomedical applications is commonly referred to as plethysmography and has its basis in Ohm's law. This law states that the ratio of the applied voltage (V) to the current (I) flowing is:

$$R = \frac{V}{I}$$

where R is the impedance. If the current (I) is kept constant, then the voltage (V) that is measured will reflect the changes in resistance. The value of R is related to the resistivity (ρ) of the medium (blood, tissue, etc.), the length of the path (L), and inversely by the cross-sectional area ($A + \Delta A$) of the conducting medium as indicated by the following equation:

$$R = \rho \frac{L}{A + \Delta A}$$

Note that the cross-sectional area is displayed as having two components, a constant component (A) and a dynamic component (ΔA) that changes with respiration (and other factors).

Placing any two electrodes subcutaneously across the human torso will result in the impedances shown in Figure 12–1. A measurement of this type is termed a *bipolar* measurement. The resistances R_1 and R_2 and the capacitances C_1 and C_2 are due to the effects of polarization at the electrode-electrolyte interface. The values of these parameters are dependent on the frequency of the measurement current. At

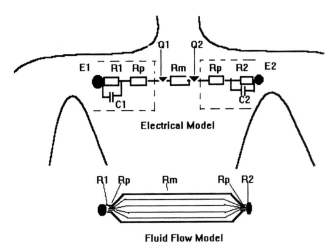

Electrical Model

Fluid Flow Model

FIGURE 12–1. Constituents of impedance measurement across the human torso. When voltage is applied between electrodes E1 and E2, separate measurement points Q1 and Q2 give respiration changes independent of contact resistances. R_1, C_1, R_2, C_2, polarization elements; RP, contact resistance; RM, torso resistance containing respiration signal.

frequencies above a few thousand cycles per second (Hz) their contribution becomes negligible. For this reason, as well as for the purposes of minimizing battery drain and maintaining patient safety, the measurements in implantable devices are performed with high frequencies or very narrow pulse widths. As an example, a current pulse used in one of the minute-ventilation pacing systems is 15 μsec wide, roughly equivalent to a frequency of 33 kHz. This frequency eliminates all polarization effects.

We can use a "fluid flow" analogy to further understand the bipolar impedance measurement. Using this model, we see that impedance consists of three "conduits" that impede the flow of electric current. The narrow conduits (R_p) are related to contact resistance at the electrode-tissue interfaces and have a considerably larger impedance than the wider conduit R_m, which is related to resistance across the torso (both R_p values are shown as equal for convenience). The impedance R_m contains the respiration signal that we want to measure to control the pacing rate of a rate-adaptive pacemaker. As a rule, the values of R_p are greater than those of R_m, especially for electrodes with a small surface area. This makes the regions around the electrodes prone to artifacts related to movement of the skin and underlying tissues. To eliminate this source of inaccuracy, normally either a four-electrode (quadripolar) system, as shown by the measurement points Q1 and Q2 in Fig. 12–1, is used, or the electrodes are made large, thereby minimizing this funneling. It is important at the outset to understand these simple concepts as they relate to implanted pacemakers, because the electrodes available are generally small and very limited in number.

MAGNITUDE OF IMPEDANCE SIGNALS

When considering how a minute-ventilation pacemaker operates it is instructive to look at the size of the signals that such an impedance measurement system must detect. The usual tip electrode-tissue impedance of a pacing lead is on the order of 400 ohms (the value of R_p in Fig. 12–1). For a larger electrode, such as those used subcutaneously, the im-

pedance is about 200 ohms. The impedance around a pacemaker case depends on its size but is usually less than 20 ohms. The impedance across the torso (R_m in Fig. 12–1) is on the order of 50 ohms. The change in R_m that is related to respiration (the value that we want to measure) is in the vicinity of 1 ohm. To detect small changes in minute ventilation, we have to be able to distinguish changes of 0.06 ohm. This gives some indication of how sensitive the measurement system has to be.

History of Development

As mentioned previously, respiration was recognized very early in the history of pacing as the most likely candidate for monitoring metabolic demand by an implanted pacemaker. After the work of Krasner and his associates, work further on this theme was done by Funke, who used an intrapleural pressure sensor,[3] and by Ionescu.[4] The early work of Krasner and associates, however, formed the basis for the first production of a rate-responsive device by Rossi and colleagues in collaboration with Biotec, S.P.A., Bologna, Italy, in April 1982.[5–7] This device, as prescribed by Krasner and associates, used a subcutaneous lead for sensing the respiratory rate. The measurement was made in a bipolar mode between the pulse generator case and an additional subcutaneous lead that had to be tunneled into the chest wall, usually across the sternum. Around the same time (1983), Medtronic, Inc. (Minneapolis, MN) introduced a rate-responsive pacer based on activity, the Activitrax.[8] In a way, this device was also a byproduct of the respiration approach, because it was during the search for a simple sensor to detect respiration by the measurement of chest wall movement that it was realized that the artifacts of motion were a clearer signal than the artifacts of respiration.

TRANSVENOUS APPROACH TO MEASUREMENT OF MINUTE VENTILATION

Krasner and associates, and subsequently Rossi and his colleagues, measured respiration with the use of an auxiliary lead across the chest, as shown in Figure 12–2. In both of these configurations the test current was delivered between the same electrodes (E1 and E2) that were used to measure the resultant voltage. Krasner's work never became a reality, and it was really Rossi and his colleagues who made it into a practical concept. There were a couple of disadvantages even to Rossi's implementation from the perspective of con-

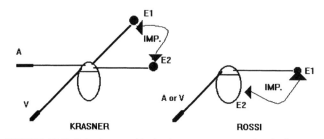

FIGURE 12–2. Subcutaneous bipolar transvenous approaches to the measurement of minute ventilation according to Krasner and Rossi. A and V, atrial and ventricular electrodes; E1 and E2, electrodes applying current and measuring impedance.

ventional pacing therapy. First, the use of subcutaneous leads involved tunneling procedures during pacemaker implantation that are laborious and time consuming and are an acquired skill. In addition, subcutaneous leads are prone to erosion and are generally an additional component that can fail. This was borne out by the experience with the Biotec devices,[7] which had a complication rate of 2%. Second, bipolar measurements that are done subcutaneously are more prone to motion artifacts because of continued movement during normal activity, making accurate quantitative measurements of respiration more difficult. Third, respiratory rate is only one component of ventilation, the other being the depth of breathing (tidal volume).

With these disadvantages in mind, Nappholz, in collaboration with J. Maloney and A. Simmons of the Cleveland Clinic, carried out a series of studies to explore the use of transvenous electrodes to measure minute ventilation in exercising patients.[9–14] Minute ventilation (MV), the product of respiratory rate and tidal volume, was chosen because it was known to have excellent correlation with the rate of the normal sinus node and had a good dynamic range. These qualities had been demonstrated previously by Pearce and colleagues,[15, 17] and Whipp and Wasserman,[16] and more recently by the work of Weber and associates[18] and McElroy and colleagues,[19, 20] who emphasized studies in patients with cardiac disease. The other reason for selecting MV was the belief, on theoretical grounds, that the transvenous approach would be less prone to motion artifacts than the subcutaneous approach. Initial work on the transvenous system focused on plethysmographic measurements in the superior vena cava (SVC) because it was known from general clinical observation that this large vessel changed dimensions dramatically in response to changes in intrapleural pressure.

Figure 12–3 illustrates the relationship between intrapleural pressure and tidal volume, based on the work of Weber and Janicki.[26] Changes in intrapleural pressure are related in a monotonic manner to tidal volume. It is also apparent that the pressure range in the pleural cavity is comparable to pressures in the SVC, thus leading to dramatic changes in SVC volume during respiration. The impedance measurements at first were done using a quadripolar system in the SVC of dogs and subsequently in patients. The correlation of changes in impedance with actual changes in MV was excellent (r > 0.9).[9] It was noted in some of the subse-

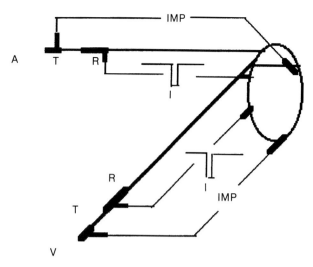

FIGURE 12–4. Measurements explored for conventional configurations. Measurements in both chambers of the heart are shown. A, V, atrium, ventricle; T, R, tip, ring; I, constant-current pulse; IMP, impedance measured.

quent experiments, however, that when the impedance measurements were extended through the innominate and subclavian veins to encompass some of the pectoral region, certain anomalies appeared. These anomalies could have been due to the nature of respiration, in that during inspiration the thoracic cavity increases in volume during filling of the lungs, the greater volume of air leading to a higher impedance, while at the same time the SVC is also increasing in blood volume, leading to a decrease in impedance. These observations encouraged a departure from a pure venous approach and promoted a slightly modified configuration that was also more suitable for pacemaker implants. A cutaneous defibrillation pad was placed over the prepectoral region (the site of the pacemaker case), and the measurement current was generated between the right ventricle and the cutaneous pad. The resultant voltage was sensed in the SVC.[10] The results confirmed that the use of a common electrode for both generating the current pulses and measuring the impedance was appropriate and that the impedance of a cutaneous pad was about the same as that for a pulse generator case (<20 ohms). At the same time, with this approach and with all subsequent ones, the highest impedance was through the thoracic cavity, which dominated the measurement. This work was followed by a series of studies, first with dogs and then with patients, by Valenta and colleagues[11] and Fischer and associates[12] using the configurations shown in Fig. 12–4, which encompassed all the possibilities with standard pacemakers.

The results, specific to five exercising patients, are shown in Table 12–1. These experiments clearly show the good correlation between heart rate and MV that is obtained in the ventricle and the atrium.[21] Using these raw data the algorithm for an implantable system was developed. A configuration in which the current pulse was generated between the pulse generator case and the ring electrode (A or V), and the measurement was taken between the tip electrode (A or V) and the case was found to be the most suitable compromise. These measurements validated the application of this sensor for either atrial or ventricular pacemakers. It is important to

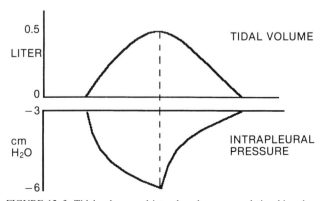

FIGURE 12–3. Tidal volume and intrapleural pressure relationships showing close relation and pressures similar to venous pressures. Six cm of H_2O translates roughly to 5 mm Hg.

TABLE 12–1. **RESPIRATION–HEART RATE CORRELATION**

PATIENT	LEAD	RESPIRATION PARAMETER	CORRELATION
AO1	SVC	Minute ventilation	0.681
		Respiration rate	0.861
AO3	AB	Minute ventilation	0.908
		Respiration rate	0.896
		Tidal volume	0.867
AO5	AB	Minute ventilation	0.959
		Respiration rate	0.867
		Tidal volume	0.347
	VE	Minute ventilation	0.956
		Respiration rate	0.852
		Tidal volume	0.309
A13	AB	Minute ventilation	0.921
		Respiration rate	0.621
		Tidal volume	0.761
	VE	Minute ventilation	0.898
		Respiration rate	0.609
		Tidal volume	0.736
A27	AB	Minute ventilation	0.965
		Respiration rate	0.670
		Tidal volume	0.904
	VE	Minute ventilation	0.767
		Respiration rate	0.585
		Tidal volume	0.547

Abbreviations: For atrium, AB = current from ring to case, measurement tip to case. For ventricle, VE = current from ring to case, measurement tip to case. For superior vena cava, current from ventricular ring to case, measurement in SVC.

note that this configuration is very close to a quadripolar configuration, as shown in Figure 12–1, because the size of the pacemaker case overcomes the main disadvantages of this configuration, namely, that the pacemaker case is both the source of the measurement current and the reference for its measurement. The encouraging results from this work led to the use of right ventricular impedance for the measurement of stroke volume during arrhythmias by two biomedical engineers, Yeh[42] and Khoury.[43]

Appropriateness of Respiratory Parameters as Indicators of Metabolic Demand

RELATIONSHIP BETWEEN HEART RATE AND RESPIRATORY PARAMETERS DURING EXERCISE

The process of aerobic metabolism requires the consumption of oxygen that is transported to the tissues by the heart. In fact, changes in heart rate during exercise are closely related to changes in Vo_2 at all levels of exertion. At metabolic workloads of less than anaerobic threshold, oxygen consumption (Vo_2) and heart rate are also directly proportional to MV. This is borne out by the work performed by several investigators.[18, 19, 22] The correlation coefficient for heart rate to MV has been found to be greater than 0.9 in most investigational work.[12, 21, 22]

The seminal work on rate response done by McElroy and associates[19, 20] and later confirmed by Vai and colleagues[22] showed that the correlation between respiratory rate and oxygen uptake during submaximal exercise was not particularly good, with both studies demonstrating correlation coefficients of less than 0.54. It is important to note that McElroy's

study consisted of 81 patients with heart failure or hypertension and 27 normal subjects. This study, more than any other, resolved the question of the impact of heart disease on the relationship between heart rate and respiratory parameters. Rossi and his colleagues[5–7] reported a correlation coefficient of 0.7 for respiratory rate with heart rate. Although this was slightly better, it is still not ideal. The early work of Beaver and Wasserman,[23] Pearce and associates,[15, 17] and the more recent work of Alt and colleagues[24] clearly indicated that the ventilatory response at the onset of exercise is predominantly a reflection of a more pronounced change in tidal volume (V_T) than in respiratory rate. In a number of studies it was noted that the tidal volume increased to a plateau within 2 minutes after the onset of exercise. The relative speed of changes in respiratory rate and MV (the product of tidal volume and respiratory rate) during exertion is best illustrated by the study of Alt and colleagues[24] (Fig. 12–5). It is instructive to note from this study that the respiratory rate not only rises slowly during exercise but also declines faster than tidal volume at the cessation of exercise.

ANAEROBIC THRESHOLD

In all patients there comes a point during exercise when continued increases in oxygen demand cannot be matched by increases in oxygen delivery to the tissues by the cardiovascular system. When the heart is unable to meet the increased oxygen demand of the working muscles, anaerobic metabolism is initiated, resulting in an increased production of lactic acid. Lactic acid dissociates into lactate and H^+, which is buffered by bicarbonate, resulting in an abrupt increase in carbon dioxide production. Because MV is largely controlled by carbon dioxide production and blood pH rather than Vo_2, this increase in carbon dioxide increases MV out of proportion to oxygen consumption and heart rate. In a rate-responsive pacemaker that uses MV as the controller of pacing rate, the onset of anaerobic metabolism may lead to an increase in the pacing rate in excess of true demand. The onset of anaerobic metabolism in patients with New York Heart Association (NYHA) class III and IV heart disease can become manifest by a drop in respiratory rate, but in all classes MV increases disproportionately to oxygen demand.[18] This implies that in an MV-controlled pacer the switch to anaerobic metabolism will lead to a drop in the correlation coefficient for Vo_2 and heart rate. In contrast to this MV response, a fall in respiratory rate at workloads exceeding anaerobic threshold could lead to a decrease in pacing rate in some patients in a pacemaker that responds only to respiratory rate. Rossi[7] noted that up to 20% of patients with respiratory-rate pacemakers had erratic responses at workloads above anaerobic threshold.

SENSITIVITY AND SPECIFICITY OF MINUTE VENTILATION AS A METABOLIC SENSOR

For a parameter to be appropriate for the control of heart rate, it must have good correlation with metabolic demand (i.e., oxygen consumption). In addition, it must have a dynamic range that allows reliable sensing of changes in the signal (sensitivity) and should not be prone to interference from various nonspecific sources (specificity). Based on the work of Pearce and Milhorn[17] and others, the increase in the

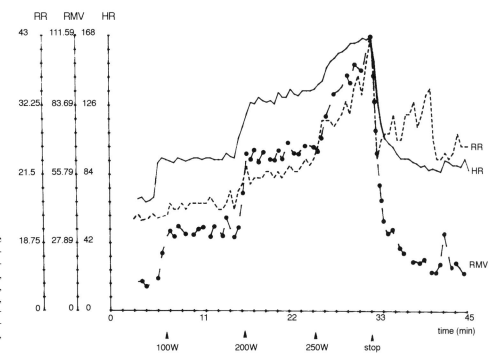

FIGURE 12–5. Study emphasizing the slower response of respiratory rate compared with minute ventilation. RR, respiratory rate (breaths per minute); RMV, minute ventilation (L per minute); HR, heart rate (bpm). (From Alt A, Heinz M, Hirgestetter C, et al: Control of pacemaker rate by impedance-based respiratory minute ventilation. Chest 92:247, 1987.)

respiration rate from rest to the anaerobic threshold is influenced by learned responses of the individual. The change in respiratory rate over this range tends to be on the order of 100% or less (e.g., 15 bpm to 30 bpm). In the case of MV, typically about a 600% change occurs from rest to anaerobic threshold (e.g., 10 L/min to 60 L/min). As a simple comparison, when temperature is monitored for the same range of metabolism, it often results in a change of about 3% from the baseline value.[20]

However, MV is not directly measured to control the pacing rate. Rather, it is the byproduct of ventilatory mechanics that must be sensed, that is, changes in thoracic impedance.

In the subcutaneous respiratory-rate pacemaker RDP3 (Biotec), Rossi and colleagues[7] observed problems in sensing the respiration signal in about 10% of 143 implanted devices. The exact cause of this problem was not clear, but it implies insufficient size of the impedance signal. In the transvenous MV system, early indications were that the changes in impedance signal during respiration were very small. Figure 12–6 shows the values of the programmed rate-response factor (RRF) in the clinical study summary of the Meta MV (Telectronics Pacing Systems, Englewood, CO).[25] This presentation highlights the relationship between RRF values and the actual impedance changes that were measured.

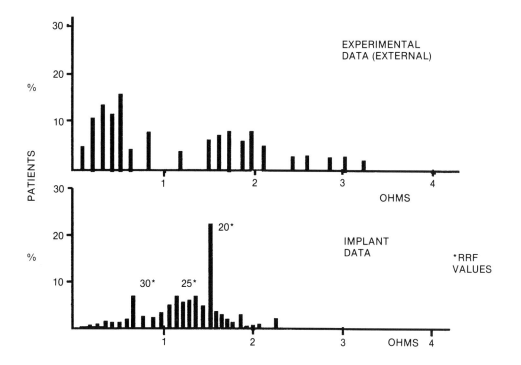

FIGURE 12–6. Early externally obtained experimental results and results of implanted device. RRF, rate response factor; Ohms, dynamic change of impedance due to minute ventilation.

The RRF is the relationship between the change in MV and the corresponding change in pacing rate. The larger this value, the smaller the change in MV that is required to produce a desired change in heart rate. In the implantable device, the RRF is the programmable parameter used by the physician to control the change in pacing rate for observed changes in MV. Among patients within any NYHA heart failure class, the relationship between heart rate and MV is reasonably constant, about 1.5 bpm per/L.[20] In patients with chronotropic incompetence, this value is different; hence, the need for the programmable RRF. The reason why the RRF is not identical for all patients is because the transformation from the tidal volume in the lungs to a change in the measured impedance is different for each patient. The results from the clinical study of the Meta MV indicated that there was a tight distribution for the RRF (and impedance). These results were certainly better than those obtained during the early external experimental work. The reason for this difference can be attributed to two factors. First, the use of external cutaneous electrode pads is notoriously prone to artifacts of motion. Second, the measurements of impedance during the external studies were based on maximum voluntary ventilation (MVV), a value that bears a loose relationship to the maximum attainable MV during peak exercise. In the large population of patients with permanent implants of the Meta MV, sensitivity to changes in respiration has not been a clinical problem. The peak RRF of 20 that is shown (see Fig. 12–6) is due to excessive use of a recommended setting and is not related to any physiologic phenomenon.

The specificity of the MV-sensing pacemaker for changes in metabolic workload may be reduced by mechanical movement of the implanted pulse generator, changes in right ventricular stroke volume (for the transvenous system), talking, coughing, voluntary hyperventilation, and anaerobic threshold. The influence of mechanical manipulation of the pulse generator case is minimized by its large surface area as well as by certain considerations in the design of the algorithm. With the use of a small area auxiliary subcutaneous lead, as in the respiratory-rate device, mechanical movement tends to be more of a clinical problem.[34]

Stroke volume is an inherent problem in transvenous pacing systems that sense MV. An example of an early recording is shown in Fig. 12–7. As shown by the telemetered data (on an expanded time scale), the stroke volume component is very effectively controlled by the design of the algorithm. Kay and associates[39] carried out studies to validate the ability of the system to reject stroke volume interference. These were accomplished by the use of isoproterenol to increase stroke volume but not respiration and resulted in the finding that the algorithm of the implanted device effectively rejected the change in stroke volume and produced no statistical effect on the paced rate. The other possible sources of interference (talking, coughing, hyperventilation) all generate changes in intrapleural pressure and tend to be transient events. It was decided during early external experimental work that their contribution could be ascertained only with implanted devices. Numerous studies have since been carried out by Lau and associates[33, 34] and others and have indicated that these factors are of minor practical relevance. Dr. Lau's extensive work in this field also encompassed a comparison of the respiratory-rate pacing system using a subcutaneous lead with the totally transvenous MV system.[34] The trans-

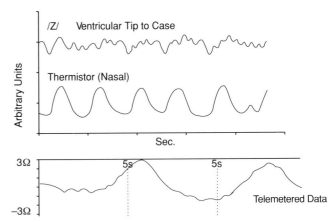

FIGURE 12–7. Comparison of stroke volume on unprocessed and processed ventilation signals. Telemetered data are made on a different time scale and are shown only to illustrate results of processing of signal.

venous MV pacing system showed less sensitivity to arm movement than the respiratory-rate pacemaker. Mechanical ventilators create an artificially large variation in intrapleural pressure. All MV-based pacemakers sense these changes in transthoracic impedance, resulting in a large change in pacing rate. Consequently, when patients require mechanical ventilation the rate-response function should always be turned off.

CHANGES IN MINUTE VENTILATION AT THE ONSET AND CESSATION OF EXERCISE

As discussed, the cardiac and pulmonary systems are closely integrated, their interdependency being modified only under conditions of anaerobic metabolism. Several careful studies[15–17] have shown that there is no loss in the coupling of MV to heart rate either at the onset of exercise or at its cessation. Despite the known transient anaerobic metabolism (oxygen deficit) that occurs at the start of exercise, Pearce and Milhorn[17] found that the correlation coefficient between heart rate and MV was not significantly affected at the start or termination of exercise. Mond and Kertes,[40] working with the Meta MV pacing system, observed that the correlation coefficient between the actual MV and the pacing rate was more than 0.9 following the end of exercise. Hence, the linking of MV (as measured by thoracic impedance) is very effective during this transition stage.

EFFECT OF PULMONARY DISEASE ON MINUTE VENTILATION SENSORS

The true impact of various pulmonary diseases on the relationship between heart rate and respiratory parameters as measured by thoracic impedance was unknown during the early development stage of an implantable rate-response pacing device. We know that for patients with emphysema, chronic bronchitis, and restrictive lung disease it is the pulmonary system that usually limits exercise, not the cardiovascular system. In a normal patient at the end of exercise MV is about 50% of MVV. In the patient with pulmonary disease this reserve is less and in many cases disappears prior to initiation of the anaerobic threshold, indicating that the patient will not reach this condition. The transthoracic estimate of MV is very often higher for the same oxygen consumption in patients with pulmonary disease, providing a strong signal for the implantable device to control heart rate, though often with a more limited range. To complicate matters, many patients requiring pacemakers have both cardiac and pulmonary disorders. This complex medical subject has been thoughtfully addressed by Weber and Janicki.[26] How these issues affect the use of respiration as a rate-control parameter is best seen in reports of the results of implants of the Meta MV.[25, 27] The clinical study summary[25] included 35 patients with chronic lung disease who received this pacing system without reported complications. In addition, Kay and associates[27] reported on two patients with advanced pulmonary disease who demonstrated excellent rate response with this pacemaker during cardiopulmonary exercise testing. One study result is shown in Figure 12–8. The conclusion is that pulmonary disease does not present a problem in specificity and sensitivity of MV-sensing pacemakers. Unfortunately, the conclusions about the use of respiratory rate as a control parameter in patients with pulmonary disease are not as well defined.

CHRONIC STABILITY OF IMPEDANCE MEASUREMENTS

The measurement of impedance to estimate MV is done with conventional pacing catheters. Although generally stable, these leads show some degree of evolution following implantation when used for the measurement of electric potentials in the heart. The process of fibrosis around the electrodes leads to a small change in pacing impedance but does not affect the dynamic component, which represents changes in respiration. This dynamic component is further helped by generating the test current at the ring electrode while measuring the voltage at the tip. As long as the value of the current and the measurement electronics are stable, the impedance value will depend only on the physiologic influences

of the respiratory process (and the possible confounding factors discussed previously). However, it is possible that a variety of pulmonary parameters can change in an individual over time, altering the relationship between MV and heart rate. Studies of this possibility in patients with implanted devices have indicated that it is of little or no practical consequence.[30]

UNIPOLAR AND EPICARDIAL IMPLANTS

In the very early stages of development of an MV pacemaker, implementation for a unipolar pacing system using a bipolar impedance measurement from the pulse generator case to the tip electrode was rejected because of very large stroke volume components, a tendency toward erratic behavior,[13] and instabilities with intermittent pacing and sensing (Fig. 12–9). Since then, Luttikhuis and Tuinstra[28] and others have shown that replacement of the ring electrode of a standard bipolar lead with a subcutaneous plate electrode in the prepectoral region allows accurate measurements of respiration using a transvenous unipolar pacing lead. The subcutaneous plate used in the study by Luttikhuis and Tuinstra was about 2 cm² and displaced about 15 cm from the pulse generator.

With totally epicardial implants, the specificity of the MV system has not been proved to date. From the early developmental work, the stroke volume component of the impedance signal was found to be considerably greater with this approach. This problem can be alleviated to some extent by separating the two epicardial electrodes as much as possible. However, to date the clinical results from epicardial implants of MV pacing systems have been mixed.

Implantable Minute Ventilation Pacing Systems

At present several manufacturers have products on the market that control rate response using respiration parameters. These include Biotec S.P.A. (Bologna, Italy) with the Biorate (RDP and MB series), which uses respiratory rate as the rate-control parameter. Telectronics Pacing Systems, Inc. (Englewood, CO) was the first manufacturer to use MV to modulate pacing rate. The Meta series includes both single- and dual-chamber pacemakers using MV. In addition, the Legend Plus pacing system (Medtronic Inc., Minneapolis, MN) combines MV and activity as possible rate-control parameters with the option to use either sensor alone or in combination with the other. The Telectronics and Medtronic devices use almost identical transvenous approaches to measure MV. In this section the key considerations in the design of an implantable respiration-controlled device are described, so that the reader may gain a better appreciation of the issues that are relevant to such an implementation. It is not meant to be a design lesson or an exhaustive coverage of the technical considerations.

MEASUREMENT PULSES

As discussed previously, the measurement of impedance can be accomplished by using either constant-current or constant-voltage pulses. Constant-current pulses are the most

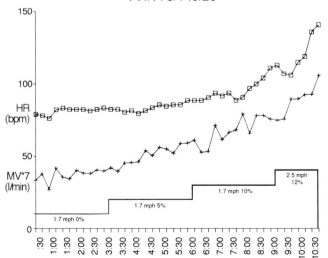

FIGURE 12–8. Patient with chronic obstructive pulmonary disease. Note small range of minute ventilation (MV) from about 5 L/min to 13 L/min. HR, heart rate.

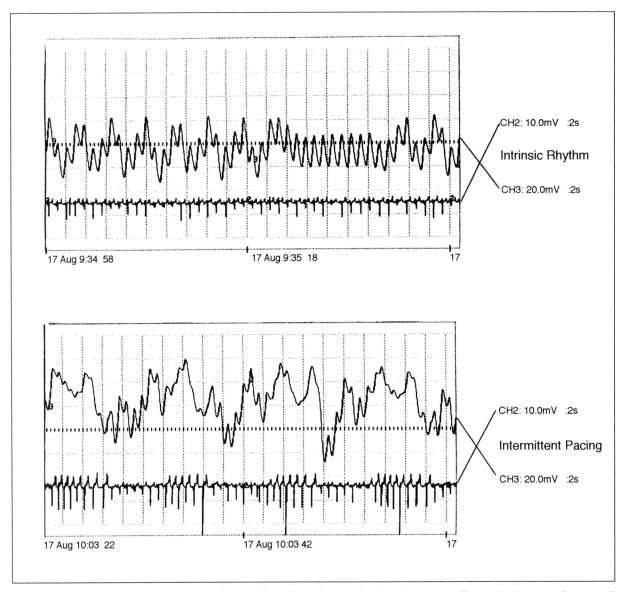

FIGURE 12–9. Unipolar impedance measurement showing the effect of intermittent pacing from the same tip. Top tracing shows ventilator turned off at about 9:35 for 8 seconds. Lower tracing shows pacing turned on and off with dramatic results.

commonly used, and the main considerations regarding their intensity are the signal-to-noise ratio and patient safety (avoidance of myocardial capture by the impedance pulses). If too small a pulse amplitude is used, the noise in the sensing electronics tends to mask the signal to be measured. The lower limit of the impedance pulse is probably around 100 μA. The pulse width is not relevant as long as it is stable and is wide enough to be generated conveniently with the electronics in the pulse generator but not so wide that it captures the myocardium in a transvenous system. An optimum value is usually from 7 to 30 μsec, because this value can be derived from the clock cycle of conventional pacemakers. If we consider 10 mA (average) as a safe current in the heart (the international standard for devices), then the average current of a 1-mA, 15-μsec pulse occurring 20 times per second would be equivalent to about 0.3 μA. This would be very safe in itself. In addition, because the pulses are delivered at very high frequency, they are far less likely to

capture cardiac cells, providing an added order of magnitude of safety. In the Biotec pacing system a current pulse of 125 μsec and 200 μA is used. Because this current pulse is delivered subcutaneously, its width is not critical. The Meta MV systems use 15- and 7-μsec pulses, and the Legend Plus uses a 30-μsec pulse. In all these devices, the current is 1 mA in amplitude.

INTERFERENCE WITH SENSING

It is quite possible for some sense amplifiers to sense these small impedance pulses unless some preventive steps are taken. In some products, a blanking of about 1 μsec is applied to the amplifiers to ''blind'' them to these pulses. In other cases, special balancing of the pulse is carried out, achieving the same objective. Wilson and Lattner[29] reported an incident in which the sense amplifier did see the measurement pulse. This occurred in a patient with one of the early

Meta MV pacemakers who was one of four patients noted to have this problem in the Meta MV clinical study summary.[25] The problem was traced to a residue of medical epoxy on the ring electrode of some Cordis-Telectronics pacing leads. This thin layer affected the impedance of the electrode during delivery of the 1-mA current pulses. Because the ring is a common electrode with the electrocardiographic (ECG) sense amplifier, this increase in impedance resulted in a sizable increase in the signal seen by the amplifier, enough to inhibit the pacing pulse under certain circumstances. In addition, the polarization of the ring also increased, thereby accentuating the problem during the blanking of the 15-μsec impedance pulse. A multitude of leads have been used since then with no reported problem.[25]

INTERFERENCE WITH THE SURFACE ELECTROCARDIOGRAM

Sensing of the impedance pulses by a surface ECG monitor is always a possibility and depends on the sensitivity of the ECG machine. The pulse width and the balancing of the impedance pulse influence this possibility. The clinical study summary for the Meta MV reported this phenomenon with some of the monitors and transtelephonic systems (those with pulse stretch capabilities). This irritating occurrence could be minimized by repositioning the surface electrodes. In subsequent models of the Meta series, this problem has been almost eliminated, as shown in Figure 12–10. The problem was due to a balanced current pulse that was 7 μsec in duration instead of 15 μsec. The effect of decreasing the pulse width was not as noticeable as balancing it.

INTERFERENCE FROM ELECTRIC SIGNALS

As discussed earlier, the monitoring of impedance involves the conversion of an impedance measurement into a voltage signal. This implies that other voltage signals can be mistaken for changes in impedance. The impedance is measured only for the duration of the narrow, 7-μsec pulse. As long as the electric signal does not change during this short interval, interference from underlying electric signals is rejected. This problem can be visualized by noting that a signal with a frequency of 60 Hz takes about 7000 μsec to change from its minimum to its maximum value. In the 15 μsec required to make the impedance measurement, an intracardiac signal will obviously change very little. Hence, the ef-

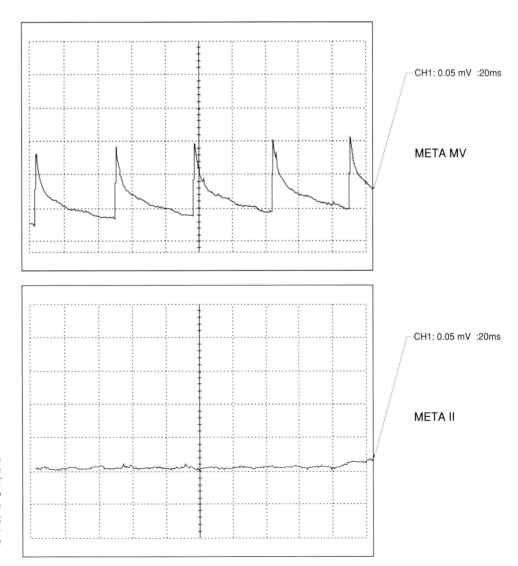

FIGURE 12–10. Improvement in surface ECG display of artifact size due to balancing and narrowing of measurement pulse in META II. Top tracing was made with 15 μsec pulse, no balancing. Bottom tracing was made with 7 μsec pulse followed by 60 μsec lower amplitude balance pulse in reverse direction.

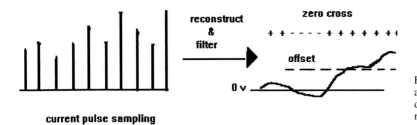

current pulse sampling

FIGURE 12–11. Signal sampling with current pulse filtering and processing. Reconstructed signal on right shows polarity decisions. The offset would be a threshold set only in rate-respiration–based devices.

fect of an intracardiac electrogram on the impedance pulse will be negligible. This type of filtering ensures that most common power frequencies, myopotentials, and endocardial signals do not affect the rate-response parameter measurement. Frequencies above about a few kHz could have some effect on the rate responsiveness of the device but become manifest only when the frequency is in very specific ranges (at an exact multiple of the sampling frequency). The chances of this happening must be very rare because there have been no reported instances with any of the thousands of devices implanted to date. Electrocautery and electrosurgery generate very high energy, broad-band frequency interference. Because of their intensity and wide range of frequencies, these signals could be picked up by the rate-response circuitry and could drive the pacemaker to its maximum rate. In fact, this was reported by Van Hemel and colleagues[32] and must be avoided at all times by turning the rate-response function off whenever electrosurgery is to be used.

PARAMETER MEASUREMENT

As discussed in the section on impedance measurement, respiration is sampled with constant-current pulses. These pulses are then reconstructed into the original respiration signal and processed (Fig. 12–11). The respiration signal contains all its relevant information under 1 Hz (under 60 breaths/min). Thus, after reconstruction from the impedance pulses, the signal is generally filtered for information between 0.1 Hz and 1 Hz. In pacemakers controlled by respiratory rate, the physician must program the "offset" of the signal (as shown in Fig. 12–11) to allow adequate sensing of crossovers of the offset line from rest to heavy exercise. In a transvenous system, in which the objective is to measure the product of the respiratory rate and the tidal volume, accurate measurement of the waveform is mandatory. In Figure 12–11 we can see that to obtain the MV value we have to measure the tidal volume and the number of these cycles per minute. Each sample shown in the figure is checked for the polarity of the signal. If 7 samples of 10 are of one polarity, the signal is considered to be of that polarity. Each time this polarity changes it is registered and used to compute the respiratory rate. This mode of measurement makes allowances for considerable noise in the respiratory signal and allows accurate measurement of rate independent of wave-

form distortions. In the Meta MV pacing system, for example, the signal is digitized and filtered, allowing establishment of the baseline as shown in Figure 12–12.

In addition to analog filtering, digital filtering is used to eliminate as much of the stroke volume as possible as well as any signal in excess of 60 breaths per minute (Telectronics Meta MV). The Medtronic Legend Plus pacemaker filters impedance signals that occur faster than 48 per minute. The filtered respiration component is rectified, averaged, and then multiplied by the respiratory rate to give the MV value (called the delta MV), which controls pacing rate. As explained earlier, the respiratory rate is obtained by noting the number of times each minute that the impedance signal crosses the baseline. Conversion of the delta MV to pacing rate is done by the rate-response factor (RRF), also discussed previously. The MV at rest is the baseline information that defines the lower pacing rate, corresponding to the "rest MV" shown in Figure 12–12. In the first Meta MV pacemaker, this is the value that was determined with the patient resting for 1 hour. This processing sequence is shown in Figure 12–12.

The purpose of filtering the signal is to ensure, among other things, that the effect of random fluctuations is minimized. As a result, a step change in MV will not be manifest as a step change in heart rate. Rather, the pacing rate will gradually rise from the present pacing rate to a new level that is determined by the sensor. The time required for this change in pacing rate is dependent on the time constant of the filter (Fig. 12–13). In the original Meta MV, the time constant needed for the pacing rate to change from baseline to 66% of the target pacing was about 30 seconds. In addition to this time constant, the RRF controls the relationship between changes in MV and changes in heart rate and can consequently be seen as a "sensitivity" control for MV. Figure 12–13 shows the trade-off between time constants and RRF adjustment. It can be seen that if the RRF had been set to achieve target 2, the time constant would still be the same, but the heart rate would have risen faster. Changing the RRF at any time will generate an immediate response in heart rate.

OTHER RATE-RESPONSE FACTORS

The relationship between the MV signal and the desired heart rate is the RRF. In the original Meta MV, because of

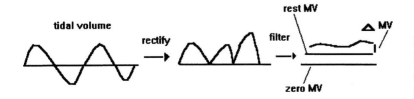

FIGURE 12–12. Processing of respiratory signal to obtain pacemaker rate driver (ΔMV). Tidal volume is as processed in Figure 12–11. ΔMV is change in minute ventilation and is converted to heart rate response factor. Filter step involves filtering and multiplication by respiration rate.

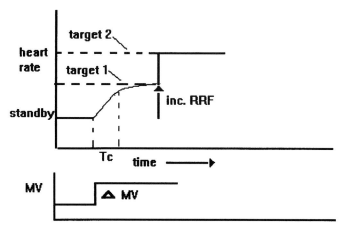

FIGURE 12–13. Diagram showing that changing RRF changes only the target heart rate, not the time needed to reach target. RRF, sensitivity controller needed to convert ΔMV to heart rate; RRF, rate response factor; TC, time constant of heart rate change to step change in minute ventilation; MV, minute ventilation.

the need to simplify the computations, *the MV signal was made proportional to pacing interval*. This resulted in a slower chronotropic response because identical changes in *pacing cycle length* at *slow rates* result in far smaller changes in pacing rate than identical changes in cycle length at *fast rates*. Thus, this initial device suffered from a relatively slow onset of rate response at the onset of exercise and brisk increases in pacing rate near the end of exercise (Fig. 12–14). This design anomaly has been corrected in later versions of these pacing systems by making the *MV signal linear to pacing rate*. Typically, a step increase in MV (marked by the dotted line) from rest resulted in a heart rate increase (for the original curve, target 1) of about 20 ppm compared to 35 ppm (for the linear response, target 2). In the currently available devices this shortcoming has been corrected, and additional augmentation has been added as shown in Figure 12–14. This augmentation is used mainly to overcome the delays generated by the filtering, at the onset of exercise. In the previous discussion it was pointed out that augmentation of RRF increases response time without affecting the filtering of random respiratory changes.

The Medtronic Legend Plus SSIR pacemaker incorporates

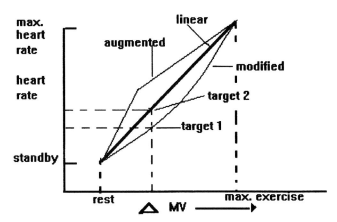

FIGURE 12–14. Various relationships between heart rate and minute ventilation change (ΔMV). The same change in minute ventilation (MV) can produce dramatically different heart rates.

both a piezoelectric crystal for sensing activity and MV as dual rate-adaptive sensors. The sensors can be combined, with the fastest sensor controlling the pacing rate. The maximum pacing rate for each sensor is separately programmable. Thus, the maximum activity rate is often programmed to a lower level than the maximum MV rate. In this way the activity sensor can be programmed with an aggressive slope to provide a very rapid response to the onset of exercise while the more proportional MV sensor provides for pacing rates during prolonged exercise at higher workloads. This separation of the upper rates for each sensor also limits false-positive responses with activity. In addition to allowing the combination of two sensors, the Legend Plus also allows either activity or MV alone to control the pacing rate.

The Legend Plus pacemaker provides a programmable feature known as the *MV range* that is designed to limit the influence of upper body motion and other artifacts on the MV impedance signal. These values clip the peak MV signal by a programmable percentage of the transthoracic impedance range. Four MV range settings, allowing a maximal change in impedance of 12.5%, 25%, 50%, and 100% of the MV signal range, are available.

PROGRAMMING THE RATE-RESPONSE SLOPE

Programming of most MV-sensing, rate-adaptive pacemakers requires selection of a lower pacing rate, an upper pacing rate, and a slope that relates changes in MV to changes in pacing rate. For the Meta MV series of pacemakers this slope parameter is known as the RRF. The RRF value is directly related to the slope of the rate-response curve. Thus, high RRF values provide very steep rate-response curves, whereas low values provide a more gradual rate response.

Programming the RRF is usually accomplished by asking the patient to exercise to his or her symptomatic limit (usually past the anaerobic threshold). The programmer automatically uses the measured maximum value of MV that is stored in the pulse generator to calculate the RRF value that will give the maximum pacing rate for this level of MV. This method of determining the clinically optimal RRF has several limitations. First, patients may not exercise to a workload that approaches their symptomatic limit. In this instance, the RRF suggested by the programmer may be inappropriately high, providing a chronotropic response that is overly aggressive. Second, other patients may exercise well beyond their anaerobic threshold. Because MV increases rapidly and out of proportion to oxygen consumption at workloads past anaerobic threshold, the RRF value suggested by the programmer may be lower than is appropriate, providing a very low level of chronotropic response. A refinement in the method of defining the RRF has been discussed by Brachmann and colleagues.[31] This revised method involves averaging the suggested RRF values at anaerobic threshold and at peak exercise to calculate the correct RRF. This revised method is the direct result of the break in the relationship between heart rate and MV that occurs beyond the anaerobic threshold. Future MV pacing systems will account for this factor as well as providing automatic regulation of the RRF.

The Legend Plus pacemaker provides a programmable *MV rate response* that controls the relationship between changes in impedance and changes in pacing rate. There are 16 settings, with a value of 1 providing the smallest change in pacing rate in response to an increase in MV signal and a value of 16 providing the greatest change. All of these settings are linear and allow the pacing rate to increase to the maximum MV rate for most values. The programmer recommends a specific MV rate response setting based on a low-level exercise protocol that involves exercising the patient for 2 minutes. The physician selects a target heart rate for the level of exercise. The programmer analyzes the MV signal to determine the appropriate MV rate-response curve that will provide the target heart rate. In addition to this programmable setting, acceleration and deceleration times can also be programmed. These values control the interval required for a change in the MV-indicated pacing rate to be converted into a change in the actual pacing rate. The possible acceleration times are 0.25, 0.5, and 1 minute. The settings for deceleration times are 2.5, 5.0, and 10 minutes.

POWER CONSUMPTION OF MINUTE VENTILATION SENSORS

As discussed, the current pulses used for measurement of transthoracic impedance in an MV pacing system are of extremely low amplitude and duration (1 mA and 0.015 msec, respectively). The amount of current needed to power the rest of the rate-response algorithm is a function of its implementation. If the MV sensor is totally controlled with a microprocessor, the current drain is generally about 3 to 5 µA. If analog circuitry and special digital circuits are used, the current drain can be kept below 1 µA. The use of MV as the rate-control parameter, when processed using the optimum methods available in modern pacemakers, is no more expensive in terms of longevity than the addition of any other simple sensor. For example, the projected longevity of the Legend Plus pacemaker with both the activity and MV sensors active is approximately 8.6 years at a pacing amplitude of 5 V and 0.48 msec pulse duration (500 ohm load, 100% pacing). This compares to a projected longevity of approximately 9.8 years for the pacemaker using the activity sensor alone.

DDDR Pacemakers Controlled by Minute Ventilation

In the early development work on transvenous MV pacing systems (see Table 9–1), the correlation coefficients for the relationship between heart rate and transthoracic impedance estimates of MV are comparable in the atrium and ventricle. These observations suggest that MV is feasible for AAIR and DDDR pacing and provides considerable flexibility. Thus, the same configuration for impedance measurement has been used in both the atrium and ventricle. At present there are two DDDR pacemakers based on MV, the Telectronics Meta DDDR and the Ela Chorus RM (Ela Medical, Montrouge, France).

The Meta DDDR pacing system processes the impedance signal in a manner similar to that used in the Meta MV model 1202. In the model 1250 DDDR device, the MV signal is linearly related to the paced cycle length (curvilinear with respect to pacing rate). The acceleration and deceleration

constants were decreased from 30 seconds to 18 seconds. This allows a somewhat faster response time than with the Meta MV 1202 pacing system. The deceleration time is also faster with the Meta DDDR pacemaker. The same upper rate applies to both atrial tracking and sensor-driven pacing. This device requires a bipolar ventricular lead for measurement of the MV signal but allows either unipolar or bipolar pacing and sensing to be programmed independently in the atrium and ventricle.

The Chorus RM DDDR pacemaker measures MV with a bipolar atrial pacing lead. This device provides rate response that is linear with the MV signal. The Chorus RM uses a programmable rate-response slope that can be selected from one of 15 settings (a value of 1 providing the least and a value of 15 the greatest rate-response slope). The acceleration and deceleration constants are programmable with two possible values (fast or slow). The fast acceleration constant corresponds to a 31-msec change in the pacing interval every fourth cardiac cycle, whereas the slow constant is associated with a 16-msec change. The Chorus RM also allows the rate response to be calibrated automatically by the pulse generator. The pacemaker determines the resting and maximum MV values on a daily basis and stores the mean values over the last 30 days. The MV signal is determined every 32nd respiratory cycle. The resting MV value is decreased by 6% if the mean value of MV calculated for the last 64 respiratory cycles is 6% or more below the present value. The resting MV is increased by 6% if more than 8 mean values for the MV signal (calculated every 64 respiratory cycles) are at least 6% above the present value. The maximal increase in the resting MV value is limited to 20% of the mean resting value the day before. The device calculates the exercise MV signal by looking for the maximal MV signal and recalculates this value every eighth cycle during which a change has occurred. The exercise MV value is increased or decreased in 6% intervals. The mean resting and exercise MV values are used to adjust the rate-response slope automatically over the range of values from 1 to 15 in steps of 0.1. By automatically adjusting the rate-response slope in this manner, the Chorus RM may be able to provide rate response that is individualized for each patient and can vary this as physiologic conditions evolve.

AUTOMATIC MODE SWITCHING

Telectronics made the important decision to use MV as the means of distinguishing pathologically high rates in the atrium from physiologically appropriate sinus tachycardia. This could only be done if there was strong confidence that the sensor would always respond to metabolic demand. Based on the extensive work in physiology and the establishment of impedance as a reliable indicator of respiration, the specificity of the transvenous MV sensor was thought to be very high. Thus, the Meta DDDR pacemaker was designed to track high atrial rates if the MV sensor indicated a high level of respiration but to revert to the VVIR pacing mode at the rate indicated by the sensor if the MV signal was not increased.

The *automatic mode switching* (AMS) operation of the Telectronics model 1250 DDDR pacemaker is explained in Figure 12–15. On the X-axis is plotted an increasing level of metabolic demand as indicated by the MV impedance sensor.

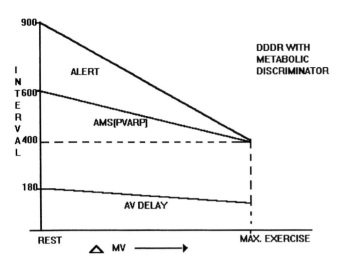

FIGURE 12–15. Response of DDDR timing parameters to metabolic demand. AMS, Automatic mode switch zone in which atrial events contribute to decision to switch to ventricular control; Alert, atrial events in this zone trigger ventricular pacing after corresponding AV delay; PVARP, postventricular.

On the Y-axis are the atrial pacing rates that the device is allowed to track, corresponding to the level of the MV signal. If the atrial rhythm is faster than the bounds set for it, the rhythm is judged to be inappropriately rapid, and AMS to the VVIR mode occurs. The device will then continue in the VVIR mode until the atrial rate moves back into the "legal" limits indicated by the MV sensor, when reassociation will occur. One of the main objectives of this approach was protection against pacemaker-mediated tachycardias (PMT). In this device the MV signal defined the length of the AV delay as well as the postventricular atrial refractory period (PVARP). The greater the metabolic demand indicated by the MV sensor, the shorter the AV delay and PVARP. Atrial electrograms that occurred within the PVARP were sensed by the atrial sense amplifier and interpreted as physiologically inappropriate. The initial implementation of AMS in the Meta DDDR pacing system needed three premature atrial events in the PVARP (the AMS zone) for it to switch to VVIR. If only a single premature event occurred in this zone no atrial pacing pulse was delivered to protect the atrium from pacing in the vulnerable zone. This partial mode change was sensed by some patients as frequent atrial ectopic beats due to the transient loss of AV synchrony. This was an infrequent occurrence, reported by less than 1% of patients,[35] although some individuals were extremely symptomatic from inappropriate mode switching. More rigorous studies of AMS have demonstrated that inappropriate VVIR pacing may occur in up to 50% of individuals. In addition to these limitations, the Telectronics model 1250 did not allow inactivation of the AMS feature in the DDDR mode.

Clinical experience with the initial implementation of AMS in the Meta DDDR device indicated that this concept has very high sensitivity for detecting atrial fibrillation and flutter but suffers from relatively low specificity. These findings have been subsequently corrected in a newer model, the Telectronics 1254. In this new model a greater number of events must occur within the AMS zone to trigger for a mode switch and to inhibit atrial pacing. The problem of protecting the atrium from being paced with a very short interval be-

tween the last sensed complex within the vulnerable zone is solved by introducing an *atrial protection interval* (API), which is always timed from a preceding atrial event. If the minimum rate is to be violated by the API, AV interval prolongation takes place instead.

The Chorus RM DDDR pacemaker offers the option of programming the device to a fallback mode with rate-adaptive pacing. This operation can be programmed to occur with the device in either the DDD or DDDR modes. When programmed in this manner, normal DDD or DDDR atrial tracking occurs at rates between the lower and upper rate limits. At rates above the upper rate limit, Wenckebach behavior occurs. The MV sensor is activated as soon as the pacemaker detects an atrial rate above the upper tracking rate. The Wenckebach upper rate behavior is allowed to function for a programmable number of cycles before the device changes modes to the VDIR mode (VVIR pacing with continued atrial sensing) with fallback to the sensor-indicated rate. As soon as the atrial rate decreases below the upper tracking limit there is reassociation of the atria and ventricles with return to the DDD(R) mode. The Chorus RM also offers the option of programming rate smoothing, a function that prevents abrupt changes in ventricular rate. Shortening of the AV delay also occurs with changes in the MV-indicated or intrinsic sinus rate with this device.

CLINICAL FINDINGS FOR USE OF MV IN A DDDR DEVICE

A good summary of the performance of MV in a dual-chamber device is available in the Clinical Study Summary[35] of the Meta DDDR, the first device to make use of this sensor. The study included 782 patients, 63% of whom were male. Atrial or ventricular arrhythmias were reported in 43% of the patients. The most relevant findings of the study were:

- Seventy percent of the patients had an RRF setting of between 20 and 24.
- Ninety percent of the patients were in DDDR mode after 1 month.
- Eighty percent of the patients had a PVARP setting of 360 msec or 400 msec, the lowest values that were programmable.
- Seventy percent of the patients were programmed to maximum rates between 120 ppm and 140 ppm (55% at 120 ppm).

Of the patient group discussed, 13 were selected to undergo cardiopulmonary exercise testing. These patients were judged to be chronotropically incompetent owing to a maximum attainable heart rate of less than 100 bpm or a maximum increase in heart rate that was less than 50% of their heart rate reserve. Each patient was exercised in the dual-chamber rate-responsive mode and the non–rate-responsive dual-chamber mode utilizing the Chronotropic Assessment Exercise Protocol (CAEP).[41] The pacing modes were randomized, and the patients were blinded to the mode. Expired respiratory gases were analyzed continuously. The key results of this study are shown in Figures 12–16 and 12–17. When programmed to the DDDR mode, these patients had a workload that increased by 85.2%, from 26 W to 50 W. Comparing the DDD with the DDDR modes, a statistically significant increase in oxygen uptake at an anaerobic thresh-

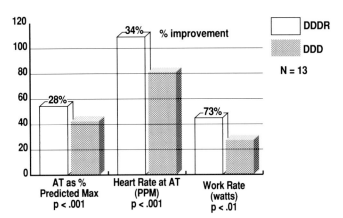

FIGURE 12–16. Improvements in DDDR versus DDD mode. Refer to text for discussion.

- The transvenous measurement of MV has a high level of accuracy and high specificity.
- The use of MV as a metabolic sensor is highly effective for rate-responsive pacemakers.
- The intentional limitation of the MV measurement to respiratory rates below 45 to 60 breaths per minute necessitates caution when this device is used in children or in those with breathing rates in excess of 45 to 60 breaths per minute.
- The calibration of the rate-responsive device to individual patients using the maximal exercise method remains chronically stable.
- Few external sources of interference have been noted, although arm movement may produce false-positive increases in the MV signal.

old of 27% was observed in the DDDR mode (9.7 vs. 12.1 mL/kg per minute). The anaerobic threshold occurred at 43.2% compared with 54.6% of the predicted Vo_2max in the DDD and DDDR modes, respectively. The time to anaerobic threshold (indicated by maximum Vo_2 consumption) increased by 50% with DDDR pacing. The heart rate-oxygen consumption slope improvement indicates that there was a more prompt heart rate response in the DDDR mode with an increase in slope from 1.1 to 4.5. The heart rate slope increased to 1.9, (Ve) which is the average as predicted by McElroy and associates.[20] This pacing system has now been extensively reviewed in several publications.[36–38]

Summary

At present, a number of single-chamber and dual-chamber rate-responsive pacemakers based on respiration are approved for general use or are in clinical trials. The considerable number of publications available on this subject stand as proof of the extensive scrutiny received by this sensor. From clinical observations of these pacing systems we can draw a number of conclusions:

- Respiratory *rate* alone has limitations in terms of speed of response at the onset of exercise and specificity above the anaerobic threshold.

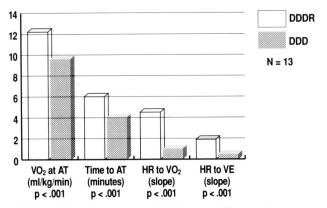

FIGURE 12–17. Improvements in DDDR versus DDD mode. Refer to text for discussion.

REFERENCES

1. Krasner JL, Voukydis PC, Nardella PC: A physiologically controlled cardiac pacemaker. J Assoc Adv Med Instrum 1:14, 1966.
2. Krasner JL, Nardella PC: US Patent No. 3,593,718. Filed 1967.
3. Funke HD: Ein Herzschrittmacher mit belastung abhanginger Frequenzregulation. Biomed Tech 20:225, 1975.
4. Ionescu VL: An on-demand pacemaker responsive to respiration rate [Abstract]. PACE 3:375, 1980.
5. Rossi P, Plicchi G, Canducci G, et al: Respiratory rate as a determinant of optimal pacing rate. PACE 6:502, 1983.
6. Rossi P, Plicchi G, et al: Respiration as a reliable physiological sensor for the control of cardiac pacing rate. Br Heart J 51:7, 1984.
7. Rossi P, Rognoni G, Occhetta E, et al: Respiration-dependent ventricular pacing compared with ventricular and atrial-ventricular synchronous pacing: Aerobic and hemodynamic variables. J Am Coll Cardiol 6:646, 1985.
8. Humen PP, Anderson K, Brunwell D, et al: A pacemaker which automatically increases its rate with physical activity. In Cardiac Pacing: Proceedings of the VIIth World Symposium on Cardiac Pacing, Vienna 1983.
9. Nappholz TA, Lubin M, Maloney J, Simmons A: Measuring minute ventilation with a pacing catheter [Abstract]. Third Asian Symposium on Cardiac Pacing and Electrophysiology, Melbourne, Australia, October 1985.
10. Simmons A, Maloney J, et al: Exercise-responsive intravascular impedance changes as a rate controller for cardiac pacing [Abstract]. PACE 9:285, 1986.
11. Valenta H, Maloney J, McElroy P: Correlation of heart rate with an intravenous impedance respiratory sensor. Instrumen Soc of America, No. 86-0002, 1986.
12. Fischer S, Nappholz TA, et al: Optimizing respiration as a parameter for rate-responsive pacing [Abstract]. Internal Document.
13. Nappholz TA, Valenta H, Maloney J, Simmons A: Electrode configurations for a respiratory impedance measurement suitable for rate-responsive pacing. PACE 9 pt. II:960, 1986.
14. Simmons A, Valenta H, et al: Verification of a minute ventilation rate-responsive algorithm with a computer-based external pacing system. PACE 11:505, 1988.
15. Pearce DH, Milhorn HT, et al: Computer-based system for analysis of respiratory responses to exercise. J Appl Physiol 42(6):968, 1977.
16. Whipp BJ, Wasserman K: Oxygen uptake kinetics for various intensities of constant-load work. J Appl Physiol 33(3):351, 1972.
17. Pearce DH, Milhorn HT: Dynamic and steady-state respiratory responses to bicycle exercise. J Appl Physiol 42(6):959, 1976.
18. Weber KT, Kinasewitz GT, Janicki JS, Fishmann AP: Oxygen utilization and ventilation during exercise in patients with chronic cardiac failure. Circulation 65(6):1213, 1982.
19. McElroy P, Weber KT, Nappholz TA: Heart rate, ventilation, mixed venous temperature, pH, and oxygen saturation during incremental upright exercise. Third Asian Pacific Symposium on Cardiac Pacing and Electrophysiology, Melbourne, Australia, October, 1985.
20. McElroy P, Janicki JS, Weber KT: Physiologic correlates of the heart rate response to upright isotonic exercise: Relevance to rate-responsive pacemakers. J Am Coll Cardiol 11(1):94, 1988.

21. Fischer S: Internal document, Telectronics Pacing Systems, Inc.
22. Vai F, Bonnet JL, Ritter PH, Pioger G: Relationship between heart rate and minute ventilation, tidal volume and respiratory rate during brief and low level exercise. PACE 11 (pt II):1860, 1988.
23. Beaver WL, Wasserman K: Tidal volume and respiratory rate change at start and end of exercise. J Appl Physiol 29(6):872, 1970.
24. Alt E, Heinz M. Hirgestetter C, et al: Control of pacemaker rate by impedance-based respiratory minute ventilation. Chest 92:247, 1987.
25. Telectronics Pacing Systems: Meta MV, Clinical Study Summary. Document No. 130-2531, Rev 1, April 1989.
26. Weber KT, Janicki JS: Cardiopulmonary Exercise Testing. Philadelphia, WB Saunders, 1986.
27. Kay GN, Bubien SR, Epstein AE, Plumb VJ: Rate-modulated pacing based on transthoracic impedance measurements of minute ventilation: Correlation with exercise gas exchange. J Am Coll Cardiol 15:1283, 1989.
28. Luttikhuis HA, Tuinstra E: Unipolar pacemaker replacement—the option for minute ventilation rate response [Abstract]. Eur J Cardiac Pacing Electrophysiol Cardiostim 2:729, 1992.
29. Wilson J, Lattner S: Apparent undersensing due to oversensing of low amplitude pulses in a thoracic impedance-sensing rate-responsive pacemaker. PACE 11:1479, 1988.
30. Li H, Neubauer SA, Hays DL: Follow-up of a minute ventilation rate-adaptive pacemaker. PACE 15:1826, 1992.
31. Brachmann J, MacCarter DJ, Frees U, et al: Minimal algorithm changes in the rate-adaptive pacemaker slope cause significant differences in patient exercise capacity [Abstract]. ACC, March, 1991.
32. Van Hemel N, Hamerlijnck RP, Pronk KJ, Van Der Veen EP: Upper limit ventricular stimulation in respiratory rate-responsive pacing due to electrocautery. PACE 12:1720, 1989.
33. Lau CP, Antoniou A, Ward DE, Camm AJ: Reliability of minute ventilation as a parameter for rate-responsive pacing. PACE 12:321, 1989.
34. Lau CP, Ward DE, Camm AJ: Single-chamber cardiac pacing with two forms of respiration-controlled rate-responsive pacemaker. Chest 95:352, 1989.
35. Telectronics Pacing Systems: Meta DDDR, Clinical Study Summary. Document No. 130-3081, Rev 1, April 1992.
36. Brinker J, MacCarter D, Shewmaker S, et al: Improved functional capacity with DDDR pacing in patients with chronotropic incompetence. PACE 14:684, 1991.
37. Lau CP, Fong PC, et al: Atrial arrhythmia management with sensor-controlled atrial refractory period and automatic mode switching in patients with minute ventilation sensing dual chamber rate-adaptive pacemakers. PACE 15:1504, 1992.
38. Lemke B, Dryander B, Jager D, et al: Aerobic capacity in rate-modulated pacing. PACE 15:1914, 1992.
39. Kay GN, Bubien R, et al: Transthoracic impedance measurement with minute ventilation-sensing pacemakers. Discrimination of respiratory and stroke volume components. PACE 12:671, 1989.
40. Mond HG, Kertes PJ: Rate-Responsive Cardiac Pacing. Englewood, CO, Telectronics Pacing Systems, 1990.
41. Wilkoff B, et al: Mathematical model of the cardiac chronotropic response to exercise. J Electrophysiol 3:176, 1989.
42. Yeh E: The hemodynamic importance of atrio-ventricular synchrony during ventricular tachycardia in man. Thesis, Case Western Reserve University, Cleveland, OH, 1988.
43. Khoury DS: Continuous right ventricular volume assessment by catheter measurement of impedance for antitachycardia system control. Thesis, Case Western Reserve University, Cleveland, OH, 1989.

CHAPTER 13

THE USE OF INTRACARDIAC IMPEDANCE-BASED INDICATORS TO OPTIMIZE PACING RATE

Rodney Salo
Susan O'Donoghue
Edward V. Platia

The goal of rate-adaptive pacing is to mimic the "natural" response of an intact system of impulse formation and conduction to variations in metabolic demand. To that end, an "autonomic nervous system sensor" would seem to be the ideal. Such a sensor is not available per se, but the sensors discussed in this chapter may come close to achieving this goal. Two pacing systems currently undergoing evaluation use impedance-based measurements to track parameters that correlate closely with the inotropic state of the myocardium. This chapter reviews the background work leading to the development of these sensors, the physiologic basis for their validity, the engineering aspects of the pacing systems, and the clinical data available from patients in whom such systems have been implanted.

History of Intracardiac Impedance

The measurement of intracardiac impedance may be tracked back to studies by Rappoport and Ray.[1] In 1927 they reported a 10% change in impedance observed during contraction of an isolated tortoise heart placed in a beaker of saline. The impedance signal as a function of time was suggestive of ventricular volume, but no attempt was made to relate measured impedance to actual ventricular volume.

In the early 1950s Rushmer and colleagues[2] extended these measurements to a canine heart. They monitored impedance between pairs of electrodes sutured onto the surface of the heart and found that the relationship between volume and impedance was quite complex and difficult to predict. This complexity was partially explained by the fact that the epicardial electrode system was sensitive to wall thickness as well as chamber volume, as pointed out by Geddes and associates.[3]

In 1966 Geddes and associates[3] published the results of a series of studies using an improved electrode system comprising electrodes that pierced the heart, allowing the electrode tips to directly contact the ventricular blood volume. Tracings from this electrode system exhibited the expected characteristics of a ventricular volume waveform. Geddes' group also attempted to calibrate the measured impedance by filling the left ventricle with known blood volumes. The results were not particularly satisfactory because they were highly nonlinear with calibration constants that varied from 0.6 to 2.6 mL/ohm in vitro and 4.2 to 10.0 mL/ohm in vivo. In 1970 Palmer[4] submitted a thesis that included the first measurements of intracardiac impedance with a multielectrode cardiac catheter. However, calibration of the catheter-based system also proved to be difficult.

The first major improvement in catheter-based impedance

measurement was introduced by Baan and colleagues[5] in the early 1980s. They developed an eight-electrode catheter system that permitted simultaneous monitoring of five longitudinal volume segments[5] and simplified the measurement of total ventricular volume.[6]

Two pacemaker manufacturers have developed impedance-based sensors for rate-adaptive pacing. In 1980 Salo and colleagues[7] began exploring the use of intracardiac impedance-derived parameters to control the stimulation rate of implantable cardiac pacemakers. The results of the initial human studies were published in 1984 and demonstrated the feasibility of controlling heart rate based on changes in right ventricular stroke volume. This work led to the development of a first-generation implantable device, the Precept pacemaker (Cardiac Pacemakers, Inc., St. Paul, MN), which was under clinical investigation from 1989 to 1992. The second manufacturer, Biotronik (Berlin, Germany), developed a pacing system based on measurement of localized cardiac motion from unipolar pacing leads. This device, the Neos-PEP, is currently undergoing clinical trials.

Technical Details of Intracardiac Impedance Measurements

The measurement of intracardiac impedance involves injection of a known current (usually a constant sinusoidal current, although current pulses are sometimes used to reduce current drain) between a pair of catheter (drive) electrodes within the blood volume of the chamber of interest. Two or more additional (sense) electrodes, spaced between the drive electrodes, sense the electric potential generated by passage of the current. The voltage difference between the sense electrodes, when divided by the current, yields an impedance (or, in this case, since the reactance is very small, a resistance), which is related to the volume of blood between the sense electrodes. Equation 1 is most commonly used to relate resistance (R), chamber volume (V), blood resistivity (ρ), and distance between sense electrodes (L), although it was derived for an insulated cylindrical volume with a uniform current density. A typical impedance waveform, shown in Figure 13–1, exhibits the characteristics of a volume waveform but is inverted owing to the reciprocal relationship between volume and impedance.

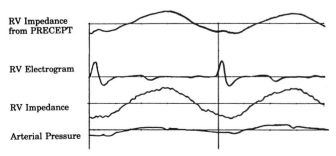

FIGURE 13–1. Typical canine waveforms during sinus rhythm from tripolar lead 1 month after implantation. The waveforms, from top to bottom, are right ventricular impedance signal from implanted Precept pacemaker, right ventricular electrogram from the tripolar lead, right ventricular impedance from external impedance circuitry directly connected to the tripolar lead, arterial pressure.

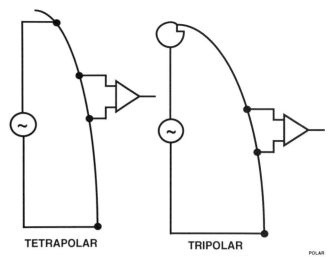

TETRAPOLAR   **TRIPOLAR**

POLAR

FIGURE 13–2. Tetrapolar. Diagram of a typical tetrapolar impedance measurement system. A sinusoidal constant current is driven between a distal and a proximal pair of electrodes, and the electric potential generated by this current is measured at two points between the current sources. The difference between the two measured potentials (in volts) is divided by the current (in amperes) to compute the impedance (in ohms) between the measuring electrodes. Tripolar. Diagram of a tripolar impedance measurement system. This system is identical to the tetrapolar system except that the proximal current source is located remotely from the other three electrodes. In the case of the Precept device, this remote electrode is the pacemaker can. With this approach, the pacing lead contains only three electrodes and conductors, thus reducing the complexity of the lead and the chance of lead failure.

Eq 1 $\quad R = \rho \cdot \dfrac{L^2}{V}$

Typical arrangements for the measurement of intracardiac impedance are shown in Figure 13–2. Although the actual volume-impedance relationship is quite complex,[6, 8] if the change in resistance measured during a cardiac cycle (the peak-to-peak resistance change, ΔR), is small

Eq 2 $\quad SV = -\rho \cdot L^2 \dfrac{\Delta R}{R_{EDV} \cdot (R_{EDV} + \Delta R)}$

compared to the end-diastolic resistance (R_{EDV}), it is generally possible to relate the change in resistance to the actual volume change (or stroke volume, SV) during the cycle by a simple equation, equation 2, which is derived from equation 1.[8] If the total resistance remains relatively constant over time, the denominator is fixed, and a simple proportionality exists between stroke volume and resistance change. A linear correlation between stroke volume and right ventricular ΔR with r^2 values of between 0.82 and 0.98 in individual animals has been reported.[9] This simplified model, which assumes that stroke volume is directly proportional to the change in impedance during a cardiac cycle, has been the basis for all rate-control studies done to date.

The resistivity of human blood is approximately 150 ohm-cm at the low frequencies (1 to 10 kHz) used for intracardiac impedance measurements. At these frequencies, surrounding structures such as the ventricular wall and lungs exhibit resistivities that are 3 to 10 times that of blood.[10] Thus, these structures are also conductors, and a portion of the drive current passes through them. The effect of these parallel current paths is to reduce the overall measured resistance and, by equation 1, increase the computed blood volume.[6, 8] This additional measured volume, or volume offset, must be independently determined if an accurate computed volume is required. If the resistance of the parallel structures remains constant, the effect on equation 2 is to change the proportionality constant between SV and ΔR. However, the resistance of the lungs changes during a respiratory cycle, and this is reflected in a periodic variation in the measured intracardiac impedance. This variation is difficult to separate from actual chamber volume variation owing to changes in preload and afterload as a result of respiration.

Device Design Considerations

One of the major advantages of the impedance sensor is its use of standard pacing electrodes and lead construction. The advantage of the use of standard electrode (e.g., platinum-iridium) and lead materials (e.g., silicone) cannot be overestimated. These materials have proven reliability and biocompatibility, and the manufacture of leads containing these materials is well understood. In addition, the functional lifetime of such leads has been well established and meets implant requirements.

Total current required for the impedance sensor includes the sum of the current driven between the lead electrodes (the current that appears in the computation of intracardiac impedance) and the current required to power the internal amplifiers, filters, demodulators, and logic associated with processing the impedance signal. For example, the drive current used with the Precept was programmable anywhere from 2 to 12 μA but was almost universally programmed to the default value of 6 μA. The current required to power impedance-related electronics was approximately 20 μA at 2.5 V. Total current related to the impedance measurement was, therefore, 25 to 30 μA at the battery voltage. The drive current necessary to measure impedance with a desired signal-to-noise ratio is largely a function of the sophistication of the sensing electronics. Excellent signals have been obtained with a sinusoidal drive current of less than 1.0 μA, but the additional circuitry required to work with such small signals may consume most or all of the apparent current savings. Sense amplifiers are generally high-input impedance devices that draw minimal current from the sense electrodes, reducing electrode polarization effects to essentially zero and permitting very small electrode surface areas.

Lead and Electrode Characteristics

Four different electrode configurations have been proposed or are routinely used to measure intracardiac impedance. These configurations are tetrapolar, tripolar, bipolar, and unipolar, based on the number of electrodes (four, three, two, and one, respectively) positioned in the chamber volume. Each of these configurations displays a characteristic volume, shape, and position dependence, which determine its accuracy. The four-electrode, or tetrapolar, system shown in Figure 13–2, has long been considered the standard for impedance measurements because the drive and sense electrodes are spatially separated. This minimizes the current that passes through the sense electrode–blood interface, thereby reducing the electrode polarization voltage. The tripolar electrode system, also displayed in Figure 13–2, has similar characteristics and is identical to a tetrapolar system except that one of the drive electrodes (the pacemaker can) is distant from the other electrodes.

The signal-to-noise ratio for a tripolar lead, considering the signal to be the volume dependence and the noise to be the position dependence of the patch (or pacemaker can), is comparable to that seen with the tetrapolar system. Overall, the tripolar system is comparable to the standard tetrapolar system except that it displays increased sensitivity to the shape of the ventricle.

The problem of lead motion is greatest at the time of implant when the electrodes are most loosely fixed in position. During subsequent weeks, as the lead is stabilized by normal tissue growth, the amplitude of motion-related artifacts decreases, reaching a minimum 7 to 28 days after implantation.[12] The impedance signal remains stable and relatively constant from this time on.

Definition and Characteristics of Physiologic Parameters

Two factors govern the utility of a potential physiologic indicator: (1) the appropriateness of the indicator in describing metabolic demand and the hemodynamic state of the patient, and (2) the accuracy with which the indicator can be measured. To determine the appropriateness of an indicator, it is necessary to assess its response to workload, heart rate, emotion, posture, and body motion. Assessing accuracy requires a comparison of measured values with those derived from "standard" techniques under all conditions that may influence the results. Thus, measurements must be made at rest (supine, sitting, and standing), during various forms of exercise, and in the presence of environmental noise and vibration.

Three intracardiac impedance-derived indicators, operationally defined in Figure 13–3, have been incorporated into

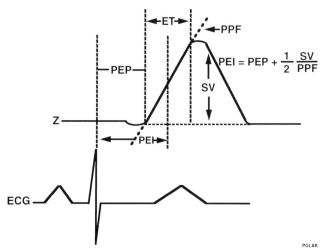

FIGURE 13–3. The definition of stroke volume (SV) and preejection interval (PEI) as used by Precept. PEI may be computed from other parameters: SV, preejection period (PEP), and peak pulmonary flow (PPF) as indicated.

implantable devices to control pacing rate: (1) relative stroke volume or cardiac output (CO),[7] (2) preejection period (PEP), which is determined from localized cardiac motion,[13] and (3) preejection interval (PEI),[14, 15] a right heart analog of PEP, which also includes a portion of the ejection time (ET). A fourth indicator, the peak time derivative of intracardiac impedance (dZ/dt), either during ejection or during filling of the ventricle, has been studied[16] but has not yet been incorporated into a pacemaker algorithm.

Stroke Volume as a Sensor

RESPONSE TO EXERCISE

Ventricular stroke volume, the amount of blood ejected with each contraction, is calculated as the difference between end-diastolic (EDV) and end-systolic volumes (ESV). Stroke volume is dependent on preload, afterload, and contractility, which are themselves interdependent to some extent. During exercise or stress, cardiac output increases owing to both a rise in heart rate and an increase in stroke volume. The augmentation of stroke volume is the result of the Starling mechanism, meaning that increased volume results in greater force of contraction. Increased contractility mediated by the sympathetic nervous system also occurs, lowering ESV and thus increasing stroke volume independent of the Starling mechanism.

In anticipation of exercise, centrally mediated vagal withdrawal and increased adrenergic drive lead to vasoconstriction, which augments venous return, thus raising stroke volume. During supine exercise in normal individuals stroke volume increases, and parallel increases occur in left ventricular EDV throughout light and moderate exercise.[17] EDV and stroke volume are nearly maximal at rest in a supine position and do not, therefore, increase during supine exercise. In the upright position at rest, stroke volume and EDV are initially lower than they are in the supine position. During upright exercise, stroke volume and EDV increase exponentially, reaching maximum values comparable to resting supine values[18, 19] at a workload corresponding to 50% of maximal oxygen uptake.[20] Interestingly, a study using radionuclide angiography found that trained athletes increase their ejection fraction by decreasing ESV, whereas normal subjects attain a similar increase in ejection fraction by increasing EDV.[21] Continued augmentation of cardiac output at higher workloads is due entirely to a progressive increase in heart rate. Overall, increased heart rate is the major contributor to cardiac output, especially at high levels or prolonged duration of exercise.[22, 23] The increases in heart rate and stroke volume that occur in normal subjects permit cardiac output to attain a value of 18 to 30 L per minute. This, combined with normal oxygen extraction by the tissue, produces a maximal oxygen uptake (Vo₂ max) of 3 to 5 L of oxygen per minute. Since the resting metabolism is 0.2 to 0.3 L per minute, the average subject can increase his rate of metabolism 15- to 20-fold over the resting value.

In sharp contrast, patients at a fixed pacing rate can respond to increased metabolic demand only by increasing stroke volume.[7, 24] These patients exhibit a nearly linear relationship between workload and stroke volume (Fig. 13–4) up to their maximum stroke volume, which is determined by

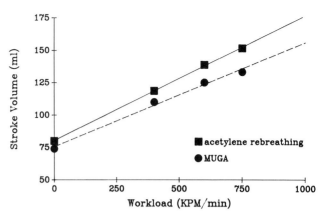

FIGURE 13–4. The stroke volume measured by acetylene rebreathing or radioisotope imaging during bicycle exercise as a function of workload during fixed-rate pacing at 70 ppm in a healthy 45-year-old subject.

filling pressures, ventricular distensibility, and contractility. These factors ultimately limit the stroke volume (and, in this case, cardiac output) increase to 50% to 100%. For example, a healthy person at a fixed rate of 70 ppm may achieve a stroke volume of 150 mL during exercise, which corresponds to a cardiac output of 10.5 L per minute. With a maximal oxygen extraction of 170 mL, this would result in a Vo₂max of about 1.8 L per minute. Such an individual would be severely limited in his ability to exercise at high workloads and would benefit significantly from increased pacing rate.

At a fixed workload in a healthy heart, cardiac output is maintained at a reasonably constant level over a wide range of heart rates because stroke volume decreases proportionately with increased rate, as shown in Figure 13–5 for six patients with chronic tripolar leads. Under these conditions, stroke volume[25] and EDV[26] are approximately inversely related to heart rate. Generally, a three-phase relationship exists between cardiac output and pacing rate, as depicted in Figure

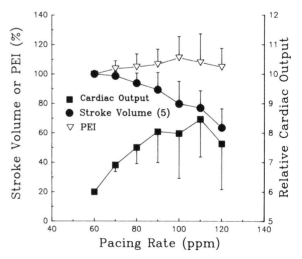

FIGURE 13–5. Mean relative stroke volume, relative cardiac output, and preejection interval (PEI) measured as a function of pacing rate at rest in six Precept patients with chronic tripolar pacing leads. Three values of SV and PEI were recorded for each patient at each pacing rate. Each of these values was the mean of 16 heartbeats. The error bars indicate standard deviation. Stroke volume and PEI values are normalized, in percentages, against the values at a rate of 60 ppm. Cardiac output is computed as the product of relative stroke volume and heart rate.

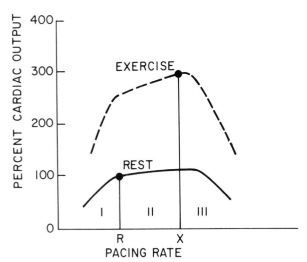

FIGURE 13–6. Conceptual representation of the relationship between cardiac output and pacing rate at rest and during exercise at a fixed workload. These schematic representations are derived from the experimental canine model. (From Wessale JL, Geddes LA, Fearnot NE, et al: Cardiac output vs pacing rate at rest and with exercise in dogs with AV block. PACE 11:575, 1988.)

13–6.[27] At a fixed workload, as pacing rate is increased, cardiac output initially increases, then reaches a plateau, and finally falls. During the initial phase at low heart rates, stroke volume is at a maximal value, and cardiac output increases directly with rate. In the middle phase, maximal stroke volume is not required to generate sufficient cardiac output, and stroke volume decreases inversely with rate to maintain a constant cardiac output. In the final phase, filling of the ventricle is compromised by excessive heart rate, resulting in increased right atrial pressure and decreased venous return and thus decreased cardiac output.[28]

STROKE VOLUME AND AGING

It is well known that the maximum expected exercise heart rate declines with age. Many early studies had suggested that there was also a decline in cardiac output and cardiovascular performance during exercise with advancing age.[29–31] However, it is likely that these study populations included elderly patients with occult coronary artery disease. A radionuclide angiographic study of subjects aged 25 to 79 years who were rigorously screened to exclude heart disease found no age-related changes in cardiac output, left ventricular EDV (LVEDV), left ventricular ESV (LVESV), or ejection fraction at rest.[32] During exercise there was no decline in cardiac output related to age. However, the mechanism by which cardiac output increased was different in older people than in younger patients. With advancing age, exercise heart rate was lower, whereas EDV and stroke volume were higher for a given cardiac output, as shown in Figure 13–7. Thus, older patients, in whom heart rate response is limited by decreased catecholamine sensitivity, are more dependent on the Starling mechanism to augment cardiac output during exercise.

STROKE VOLUME AND HEART DISEASE

Given the complexity of the circulatory response, it is not surprising that heart disease alters cardiovascular perform-

ance. There is a substantial body of data on exercise performance in patients with coronary artery disease, most derived from groups with stable angina pectoris or healed myocardial infarctions. Although there is a broad spectrum of individual responses, in general the presence of coronary disease results in reduced exercise capacity, marked by failure to increase stroke volume or an actual fall in stroke volume.[33] However, there is wide disparity between the performances of different individuals with seemingly similar baseline hemodynamics and left ventricular ejection fraction. Some data suggest that

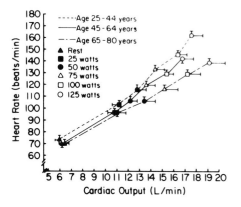

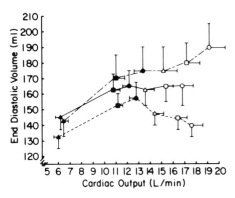

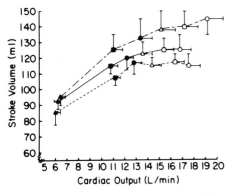

FIGURE 13–7. Relationship between heart rate (top), end-diastolic volume (EDV, middle), and stroke volume (bottom) versus cardiac output across a range of workloads for various age groups. In the older age group, the same higher cardiac output during exercise is attained with a lower heart rate, higher EDV, and higher stroke volume. The effect of age was significant by analysis of covariance for heart rate ($p = .001$), end-diastolic volume ($p = .04$), and stroke volume ($p = .002$). (Reproduced with permission from Rodeheffer RJ, Gerstenblith G, Becker LC, et al: Exercise cardiac output is maintained with advancing age in healthy human subjects: Cardiac dilatation and increased stroke volume compensate for a diminished heart rate. Circulation 69:203, 1984. Copyright 1984, American Heart Association.)

right ventricular performance may be a key to understanding this disparity. A decline in right ventricular stroke volume during exercise has been shown in patients with coronary artery disease, coupled with an increase in pulmonary vascular resistance.[34] In patients with congestive heart failure, right ventricular ejection fraction but not left ventricular ejection fraction correlates with maximal oxygen consumption.[35] The most cogent explanation is that high left ventricular end-diastolic pressure (LVEDP) during exercise results in pulmonary hypertension, thereby increasing right ventricular afterload and reducing the output of the right heart. Right ventricular ischemia may also play a role, but these findings are present even in patients without disease of the right coronary artery.

Patients with chronic obstructive pulmonary disease have also been found to have abnormal right ventricular function with impaired stroke volume response, probably due in part to increased total pulmonary resistance.[36] Similarly, patients with isolated mitral valve stenosis demonstrate a fall in right ventricular ejection fraction with exercise, and return to a normal exercise response postoperatively.[37] In a group of patients with symptomatic aortic or mitral valve disease, predominantly of the regurgitant variety, no clear conclusions could be drawn about the role and pathophysiology of right ventricular dysfunction.[38]

The goal of a rate-adaptive pacing system is to control heart rate in a manner consistent with the needs and capabilities of the patient. Most indicators of metabolic demand, whether loosely (e.g., body activity or core temperature) or more closely (e.g., minute ventilation) related to workload, do not actually monitor the patient's hemodynamic condition. If the rate is driven by these indicators without regard to the underlying hemodynamic state, it is possible to push the heart outside of its normal operating range and into failure or at least into less efficient operation. This occurs in pacing-induced angina. A patient with coronary artery disease who is paced at a high rate may develop ischemia and reduced systolic function, shown by an increase in LVEDP, accompanied by a decrease in left ventricular distensibility, as indicated by an upward shift in the diastolic function curve. In contrast, a patient with normal coronary arteries in the same situation demonstrates an increase in systolic function and distensibility.[39] Thus, whereas an inappropriate rate may inconvenience a patient with a healthy heart, it could severely compromise a patient with coronary artery disease or a failing heart.

Current rate-adaptive pacemakers adequately increase pacing rate in response to workload to improve exercise tolerance in patients with good cardiac function. Patients with good systolic and diastolic function can maintain cardiac output despite inappropriately high pacing rates providing they do not have substantial coronary artery disease. However, patients with slow filling rates, due either to valvular disease or compromised relaxation, those who are unable to increase contractility to shorten ejection time, and those with angina demonstrate decreased cardiac output at inappropriately high pacing rates. Maintenance of cardiac output is critical in diseased hearts. Unfortunately, cardiac output measures are not generally useful for rate control because the typical patient population can maintain a nearly constant cardiac output over a wide range of rates.[28] Cardiac output is, however, the product of stroke volume and heart rate, and the stroke volume factor is sensitive to cardiac function. For example, under stroke volume rate control, if pacing rate increases inappropriately, stroke volume decreases below its baseline value, which results in a decreased (and therefore more appropriate) rate. Thus, any stroke volume–based pacemaker already contains elements of rate optimization, and this function could be improved by using a negative feedback algorithm to minimize stroke volume variation.

STROKE VOLUME AND MENTAL STRESS

In daily life, the human cardiovascular system must respond not only to exercise but also to emotional duress, pain, fear, and intense mental concentration. These conditions activate the sympathetic nervous system, with the expected increases in heart rate, contractility, and cardiac output. Available data suggest that stroke volume remains unchanged or falls during experimental stress testing in the laboratory[40, 41] in normal individuals, suggesting that the required augmentation in cardiac output is met entirely by an increase in heart rate. This may be caused by an absolute or relative increase in afterload due to alpha-adrenergic vasoconstriction, or, alternatively, a disproportionate heart rate response might result in relative deficiency in preload.[58] The response of peripheral vascular resistance to mental stress is highly variable, falling in some subjects and rising in others.[41] Thus, there is no uniform pattern of hemodynamic response to stress. However, any increase in metabolic demand, whether related to exercise or emotion, must result in increased stroke volume if the patient has a fixed heart rate or is chronotropically incompetent but requires increased cardiac output. In these patients, increased sympathetic drive results in increased contractility, increased ejection fraction, increased stroke volume, and increased cardiac output. The lack of stroke volume response in the normal population indicates that the most appropriate rate algorithm is one that maintains stroke volume at an approximately constant level during emotional stress. In this algorithm, the rate increase must counterbalance the stroke volume increase to maintain a fixed stroke volume value. An example of such an algorithm can be seen in Figure 13–8.

POSTURE DEPENDENCE

Unlike impedance parameters, which are derived from whole torso measurements (e.g., currently available units based on minute ventilation) and are, therefore, sensitive to movements of the torso and limbs,[42] stroke volume and PEI, measured by intracardiac electrode systems such as the tripolar lead, are not sensitive to external motion. However, posture does have a well-known effect on stroke volume, which is reflected in measurements of stroke volume made with implanted sensor systems.[43] Interestingly, in some patients there are large differences between measurements made on the left and right sides despite the lack of major shifts in blood pools during this maneuver. However, the heart as it hangs from the great vessels is oriented differently with respect to the lungs and other surrounding organs, and current densities through these tissues are modified. Also, the lead may be oriented somewhat differently within the heart, resulting in altered sensitivity to heart motion. In either case, most of the apparent stroke volume difference is almost cer-

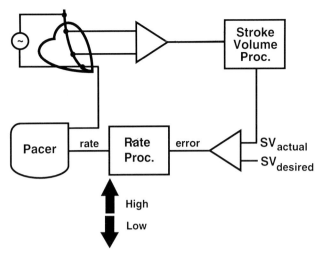

FIGURE 13–8. Simplified diagram of a closed-loop, rate-adaptive pacing system based on relative stroke volume measurements. $SV_{DESIRED}$ is initially acquired with the patient at rest and represents the desired stroke volume value. If the measured SV is greater than $SV_{DESIRED}$, a positive error signal $(SV_{ACTUAL} - SV_{DESIRED})$ is generated, and the heart rate is increased. The increase in heart rate (at a fixed workload) decreases the measured stroke volume until it approaches $SV_{DESIRED}$ and the error signal is minimized. The heart rate is maintained until the level of exercise (or emotional stress) is decreased, resulting in a decrease in stroke volume, a negative error signal, and a decrease in pacing rate. The rate continues to decrease until SV_{ACTUAL} equals $SV_{DESIRED}$. Thus, by modulating the heart rate the stroke volume is maintained at a nearly constant value during increases and decreases in workload.

tainly due to artifact. In contrast, the stroke volume difference between the upright and supine measurements, as evident in Figure 13–9, is probably a real effect resulting from the increased venous return in the supine position. If, however, the stroke volume increase results in excessive cardiac output, the patient who is kept at a fixed heart rate modulates the peripheral resistance to reduce cardiac output (i.e., stroke volume) to a more reasonable value. Thus, these stroke volume changes are generally transitory.

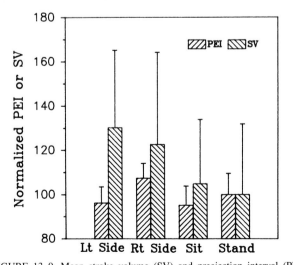

FIGURE 13–9. Mean stroke volume (SV) and preejection interval (PEI) responses to posture in six Precept patients. Three values of SV and PEI were measured at each postural position for each patient. Each value was a mean over 16 heartbeats. The error bars indicate standard deviation.

SUMMARY

Stroke volume seems to have many of the features needed for an ideal sensor for rate-adaptive pacing. It is part of the primary response to increased metabolic demand and in fact is the primary response (except for increased oxygen extraction) for pacemaker-dependent or chronotropically incompetent patients. It changes quickly, is proportional to workload, and exhibits negative feedback with respect to changes in heart rate. Thus, it may be used in a negative feedback control loop.

The stroke volume response to changes in metabolic demand in pacemaker-dependent or chronotropically incompetent patients with coronary disease or congestive heart failure, whether demand is due to exercise or mental stress, has not been well characterized. However, an increase in sympathetic drive should result in increased cardiac output, which in these patients can only arise from increased stroke volume.

Systolic Time Intervals as Sensors

Systolic time intervals have long been used to provide noninvasive information about the circulation and cardiovascular performance. The technique of simultaneously recording the electrocardiogram, phonocardiogram, and central arterial pressure was introduced in 1923.[44] The preejection period is classically defined as the interval from the beginning of the QRS complex to the onset of the carotid upstroke, as illustrated in Figure 13–10. It is calculated by subtracting

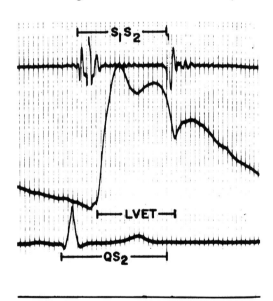

PEP = QS₂ − LVET

ICT = S₁S₂ − LVET

Q–1 = QS₂ − S₁S₂

FIGURE 13–10. Simultaneous recording of the phonocardiogram, carotid arterial pulse tracing, and electrocardiogram in a normal subject. QS_2, total electromechanical systole; S_1S_2, heart sounds interval; LVET, left ventricular ejection time; PEP, preejection period; Q-1, interval from onset of QRS to first heart sounds; ICT, isovolumic contraction time. (Reproduced with permission from Weissler AM, Harris WS, Schoenfeld CD: Systolic time intervals in heart failure in man. Circulation 37:149–159, 1968. Copyright 1968, American Heart Association.)

the left ventricular ejection time from the duration of electromechanical systole, the QS_2 interval.[45] The PEP, which includes the isovolumetric contraction period and the electromechanical interval, averages 0.08 to 0.11 seconds in normal individuals. Using right ventricular impedance measurements, a closely related interval can be derived. The preejection interval (PEI) is measured from the onset of the sensed or paced intracardiac electrogram to the onset of right ventricular ejection. Relative changes in PEP (and PEI) appear to reflect sympathetic drive closely,[46] and thus they may be applicable to rate-adaptive pacing.

PEP AND EXERCISE

The relationship between PEP and heart rate has been the subject of some controversy, most likely related to choice of subjects and measurement technique. Early data suggested an inverse correlation, that is, a slightly shorter PEP at higher resting heart rates.[45] Subsequent studies refuted this conclusion, finding no effect of PEP on heart rate[47, 48] in normal individuals. In pacemaker-dependent patients, PEP increases nearly linearly with increased pacing rate at rest if PEP is defined as the interval between the ventricular pacing pulse and the opening of the aortic valve. As the pacing rate is increased at rest, arterial diastolic pressure increases (because isovolumetric contraction begins earlier in diastolic filling), and the beginning of ejection is delayed until the greater arterial pressure is overcome, allowing the aortic valve to open. Because ejection time decreases and PEP increases with increased rate, PEI, which is a linear combination of PEP and approximately half of the right ventricular ejection time, can show either behavior.

PEP does shorten markedly during epinephrine infusion in normal individuals.[48] Shortening of the PEP also occurs in response to exercise.[49, 50] Shortening of the PEI during bicy-

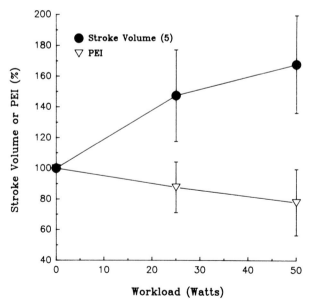

FIGURE 13–11. Mean stroke volume (SV) and preejection interval (PEI) as a function of workload at a fixed pacing rate of 80 ppm during upright bicycle exercise for six Precept patients with chronic tripolar pacing leads. Three values of SV and PEI were recorded for each patient at each workload. Each of these values was the mean over 16 heartbeats. The error bars indicate standard deviation.

TABLE 13–1. FACTORS INFLUENCING PREEJECTION PERIOD (PEP)

CAUSES OF PROLONGED PEP
Bradycardia
Reduced left ventricular preload
Negative inotropic agents (beta-adrenergic blockade, etc.)
Decreased myocardial function
Systemic hypertension
Left ventricular conduction delay (left bundle branch block, left anterior hemiblock)
Hypothyroidism

CAUSES OF SHORTENED PEP
Tachycardia
Increased stroke volume
Positive inotropic agents (digitalis glycosides, etc.)
Beta-adrenergic stimulation (anxiety, exercise, drugs)
Decreased afterload (left ventricle)
Aortic stenosis
Aortic insufficiency
Hyperthyroidism

Modified with permission from Weissler AM, Harris WS, Schoenfeld CD: Systolic time intervals in heart failure in man. Circulation 37:149, 1968. Copyright 1968, American Heart Association.

cle exercise in six patients who were paced at a fixed rate is demonstrated in Figure 13–11. Taken together, the data consistently demonstrate that PEP and PEI shorten as sympathetic drive increases.

PEP AND HEART DISEASE

Systolic time intervals have been used extensively as a sensitive noninvasive measure of cardiac function. Nonvalvular heart disease produces a lengthening of the PEP and a shortening of the ejection time.[51] The left ventricular ejection time (LVET)/PEP ratio is reported to be a predictor of ejection fraction. For PEP to be useful as a sensor, the direction of change in PEP with varying metabolic demand must be consistent. The magnitude of the baseline PEP is less important because a pacemaker may be designed to respond only to relative changes in PEP. The effect of exercise on systolic time intervals has been compared in healthy subjects and patients who have recovered from myocardial infarction.[48] Shortening of the PEP in response to exercise occurred in both groups, whether the subjects were generally sedentary or active. Unfortunately, the technique involved in measurement of the carotid pulse tracing and phonocardiogram limited the measurements to those made before and immediately after exercise. Thus, the PEP response at different times during exercise could not be plotted in this type of study.

Patients with more significant impairment of cardiac function can have a different pattern of response to exercise. Compensated congestive heart failure is associated with a prolonged PEP, which may further lengthen rather than shorten with exercise.[52] This finding may limit the utility of PEP as a sensor. However, it must be remembered that impedance-based pacing systems derive the PEI from the right ventricle. The data are not clear about whether right-sided systolic time intervals show the same changes as left-sided intervals in the presence of heart failure.

A variety of other factors influence the PEP, as indicated in Table 13–1. Left ventricular conduction delay lengthens the PEP.[53] Positive inotropic agents shorten the PEP, whereas beta-adrenergic blockade lengthens it, although not significantly at clinically meaningful doses. Again, however, as long as the PEP shortens from baseline in response to exercise or stress, these factors do not affect its use for rate control.

Right ventricular failure is of interest with regard to its effect on PEI. Significant chronic obstructive pulmonary disease has been associated with a prolonged PEP, as have mitral stenosis and pulmonary emboli.[54, 55] If right-sided PEI lengthens further with exercise in such patients, analogous to the left-sided PEP that occurs in patients with congestive heart failure, the value of PEI as a sensor would be limited in some patients. There are at present insufficient data that address this issue.

PEP AND POSTURE

The effect of posture on PEP is unclear. One study examining this relationship reported a lengthening of PEP with passive head-up tilt.[56] However, PEP was "corrected" for heart rate, thereby obscuring any catecholamine-mediated shortening of PEP that may have occurred. PEP measurements, as shown in Figure 13–9, appear to be relatively unaffected by posture. Any actual change is probably due to modification of peripheral pressure, which would affect the timing of the opening of the aortic and pulmonic valves as discussed earlier.

SUMMARY

There are many features of the PEP which make it attractive as a potential sensor for rate-adaptive pacing. PEP is sensitive to sympathetic drive and responds rapidly and proportionally to exercise. PEP is also expected to respond to emotional stress in the same way it responds to exercise. Although it has not been observed in clinical trials, in the presence of cardiac decompensation, PEP could conceivably change in the opposite direction during exercise compared to the response seen in normal subjects. Whether this potential behavior represents a limitation or a safeguard to patients remains to be seen.

Contractility Sensors

dZ/dt AS A SENSOR

It is possible to compute peak positive dZ/dt from an impedance signal in a manner analogous to that used for ventricular dP/dt assessments of contractility. This corresponds roughly to the peak rate of ejection of blood from the ventricle and may be related to contractility, although it is obviously load dependent. Only preliminary studies have been conducted with this sensor so far,[13, 16, 62] and no current device uses this measure for rate-responsive pacing.

LOCALIZED MOTION SENSING—VENTRICULAR INOTROPIC PARAMETER

The region immediately adjacent to a drive electrode in an impedance-based system is the region of highest current density (which decreases as $1/r^2$ with distance from the source).

This current density may be modified by local factors such as motion of the electrode relative to the tissue interface or localized changes in tissue impedance. These factors are not related to the volume of the chamber, and their influence on intracardiac impedance measurements is normally considered an undesirable artifact. The influence of localized changes in the region of the drive electrode is usually reduced by using a tetrapolar electrode system to separate the impedance-sensing electrodes from the drive electrodes. This positions the sensing electrodes in regions of decreased current density, where the current density is also more homogeneous and dependent on chamber volume and is less influenced by local environment. However, the impedance between drive electrodes may be monitored directly to monitor the current source "microenvironment." Because this immediate environment includes cardiac tissue, the timing of cardiac events, specifically the beginning of ejection in the right and left ventricles, could conceivably be monitored by this approach.

A major advantage of this impedance system is that it could use a standard unipolar or bipolar pacing lead. However, because the physical properties of the electrode (surface area, material, and so on) influence its interface characteristics, the same results would not be obtained from different leads, and a system based on this approach might only function with a subset of all available pacing leads.

A disadvantage of a system based on changes in the electrode-tissue interface is an inability to relate these changes to the commonly measured parameters. Because there are no clinical data on the topic, studies must be conducted in a large number of patients under a variety of conditions to prove clinical viability. A second disadvantage of such a system is its extreme sensitivity to lead motion. Patient activity generates lead motion, which is sensed at the electrode-tissue interface. Thus, it is almost certainly necessary to use a filtering technique such as ensemble averaging to remove random uncorrelated noise due to patient activity.

The average slope (dZ/dt) over a particular interval (or region of interest) of an averaged impedance (or conductance) waveform from a unipolar lead system has been reported to be related to the beginning of left ventricular ejection and therefore to the inotropic state of the heart.[13] An essential feature of this measurement is the determination of the interval over which the relationship is valid, and it is not clear whether this interval must be independently determined for each patient. The value of the ventricular inotropic parameter (VIP), which is the rate-control parameter, varies between 0 at rest and 1.0 during maximal exercise and is derived from the measured slope value, RQ, as shown in equation 3. RQ_{rest} and $RQ_{exercise}$ are the slope values at rest and during maximal exercise, respectively.

$$\textbf{Eq 3} \quad VIP = \frac{RQ - RQ_{rest}}{RQ_{exercise} - RQ_{rest}}$$

CPI Precept Pacing System

Based on promising data on the use of stroke volume and PEI as sensors, Cardiac Pacemakers Inc., St. Paul, MN (CPI) developed the Precept pacing system, which entered clinical trials in 1989. These trials were completed in 1992. The pacing system consists of a pulse generator and a special tripolar ventricular lead. Due to the small drive currents used (2 to 12 μA), the surface of the drive electrodes is not a critical factor. Also, because a symmetrical sinusoidal alternating current (AC) drive signal is used, few irreversible electrochemical reactions occur at the electrodes, and there is minimal electrode erosion. The dual-chamber version of Precept employs a standard atrial lead. The only novel aspect of the tripolar impedance lead is the addition of one electrode to the standard bipolar lead system. The tripolar lead for the Precept system is a 9-French lead containing two ring (sense) electrodes. The distal ring electrode is located 14.7 mm from the distal tip, and the proximal ring electrode is 23 mm from the distal ring electrode. This spacing is sufficient to obtain an impedance signal representative of the entire right ventricle while ensuring that the proximal electrode will remain in the ventricle on small human hearts.

Impedance measurements are made between the proximal and distal ring electrodes of the tripolar lead. A 6-μA, 2700-Hz constant current maintained between the tip electrode and the pacemaker generator is used to measure impedance. Impedance varies with right ventricular volume throughout the cardiac cycle. From these changes, the pacemaker derives a "sensorgram," which allows measurement of relative changes in stroke volume and PEI. An actual patient sensorgram with a simultaneously recorded electrocardiogram is shown in Figure 13-12.

The mean stroke volume and PEI relationship to workload at a fixed pacing rate derived from the Precept intracardiac impedance measurements is shown in Figure 13-11 for six patients with chronic tripolar leads. This figure shows the increase in relative stroke volume and decrease in PEI expected during exercise.

The Precept rate-adaptive pacemaker uses a simple linear algorithm (the algorithm is linear for cycle length vs. sensor change from baseline) to generate pacing rates from sensor measurements. With this simple algorithm it is only necessary to program the lower rate limit (corresponding to the resting heart rate), the sensor upper rate limit (i.e., maximum sensor rate or MSR), and the response slope (the increase in pacing rate per unit change in sensor value). In practice, the algorithm works adequately as demonstrated in the rate-adaptive exercise responses shown in Figures 13-13 and 13-14. The response slope was not optimally programmed for each patient, but it is apparent that appropriate reprogramming would have resulted in a virtually identical response in each patient.

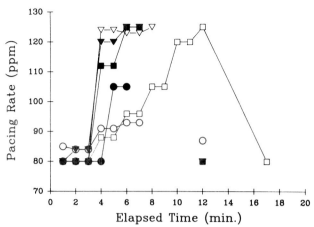

FIGURE 13-13. Pacing rate as a function of workload in six Precept patients during bicycle ergometry. Each patient was in the rate-adaptive mode with the pacing rate controlled by preejection interval (PEI). The protocol included 2 minutes of rest, 2 minutes of exercise at 25 W, 2 minutes of exercise at 50 W, and recovery beginning at an elapsed time of 6 minutes. One patient (indicated by open squares) exercised for 2 minutes each at 25 W, 50 W, 75 W, 100 W, and 125 W. He began recovery at 12 minutes total elapsed time. Because the slope of the rate versus PEI relationship was not reprogrammed for each patient to optimize the rate response, the rate increase occurred overly rapidly in several patients. Each point is a mean value over 16 heartbeats. The error bars indicate standard deviation. Each symbol represents data derived from an individual patient.

An alternative algorithm, a simple closed-loop control system, is shown in Figure 13-8. This system attempts to maintain a constant stroke volume by modulating the heart rate.[7] An increase in stroke volume generates an increase in heart rate sufficient to reduce the stroke volume to the reference value. Likewise, a decrease in stroke volume generates a heart rate decrease. The major advantage of closed-loop con-

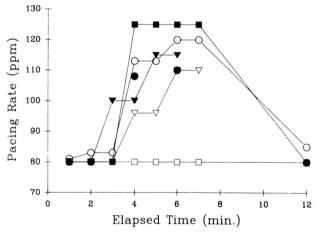

FIGURE 13-14. Pacing rate as a function of workload in six Precept patients during bicycle ergometry. Each patient was in the rate-adaptive mode with the pacing rate controlled by stroke volume. The exercise protocol was the same as that described for Figure 13-13. Because the slope of the rate versus stroke volume relationship was not reprogrammed for each patient to optimize the rate response, the rate increase occurred rapidly in several patients. Each point is a mean value over 16 heartbeats. The error bars indicate standard deviation. One patient *(open squares)*, had an impedance waveform that was unusable for stroke volume–based rate control and showed no rate increase. Fortunately, this same patient demonstrated an excellent PEI increase (see Figure 13-13).

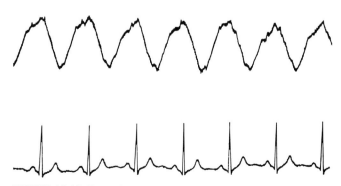

FIGURE 13-12. Pacemaker-generated "sensorgram" demonstrating relative changes in right ventricular volume and simultaneous electrocardiogram from a patient with an implanted Precept pacemaker.

trol is that reprogramming for individual patients is not generally required.

IMPLANTATION AND PROGRAMMING

A critical step in the clinical application of intracardiac impedance is the positioning of the impedance lead. The volume that most directly influences the measured impedance is that bounded by planar surfaces perpendicular to the lead at the positions of the sense electrodes and circumferentially by the walls of the chamber. Ideally, the impedance lead should be positioned with the tip at the apex of the right ventricle and the catheter body coincident with the longitudinal axis of the right ventricle. The proximal sense electrode should be below the tricuspid valve to minimize contamination by valvular or atrial motion. Because, by equation 1, the impedance varies directly as the square of the distance between the sense electrodes, this distance should remain fixed during ventricular contraction. Thus, the catheter should show limited motion under fluoroscopy, and motion of the sense electrodes toward or away from each other should be minimized. As discussed earlier, signals at implant are not necessarily representative of chronic signals and may not be useful during positioning. Fortunately, lead positions that look appropriate under fluoroscopy almost always result in usable chronic impedance signals.

Placement of the Precept system is carried out using standard permanent pacemaker implantation techniques. The tripolar lead requires an 11.5- or 12-French introducer. To select the most appropriate sensor settings, the patient performs an exercise test in the non–rate-adaptive mode. The pacemaker acquires stroke volume and PEI measurements during this test. The physician can then review these data on the programmer screen and select the sensor that demonstrates the best response. The pacemaker employs a linear algorithm by which the pacing rate increases in response to an increase in relative stroke volume or a decrease in relative PEI. The response slope can be chosen by monitoring the patient during a period of steady moderate activity and choosing the slope that yields the desired heart rate response.

The pacemaker acquires baseline values for stroke volume and PEI at the time of sensor programming. These serve as reference points for the sensor. The patient should be inactive for this 30-second acquisition period. A baseline tracking feature can also be used, which allows the pacemaker to modify baseline values according to ongoing average sensor values. This feature is designed to prevent long-term changes in stroke volume or PEI measurements from adversely affecting sensor function.

Precept uses a simple linear algorithm to generate pacing rates from sensor measurements. In this simple algorithm it is only necessary to program the lower rate, the sensor upper rate limit, and the response slope (the increase in pacing rate per unit change in sensor value). The algorithm is most appropriate for sensors that are independent of rate (e.g., body activity) but not optimal for stroke volume or PEI. In practice, the algorithm works adequately, as demonstrated by the mean rate-adaptive exercise response of six patients shown in Figure 13–15.

The raw values for stroke volume and PEI may differ for a paced ventricular complex compared with an intrinsic QRS complex. PEI is generally longer following a paced complex

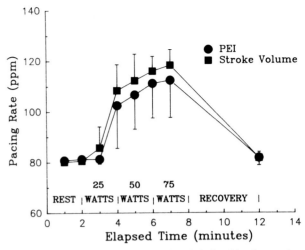

FIGURE 13–15. Mean pacing rates achieved during bicycle exercise at various workloads in rate-adaptive pacing models controlled by either stroke volume (SV) or preejection interval (PEI) for six Precept patients with chronic tripolar leads. Error bars indicate standard deviation.

compared with an intrinsic complex. The stroke volume response is less uniform. Therefore, in patients who are not fully paced in the ventricle, sensor values should be acquired during both paced and intrinsic ventricular rhythm. Review of these values may demonstrate a greater consistency of one sensor compared with the other. If a significant but fairly constant difference in values is present, the pacemaker's "pace-sense offset" feature can be utilized. This allows automatic compensation for paced versus sensed complexes by adding a correction factor to the raw values. Through this programming detail and the use of average rather than individual sensor values, the pacemaker can avoid large beat-to-beat variations in pacing rate.

Burns and colleagues[57] attempted to validate the accuracy of the impedance signal for determining stroke volume by simultaneously measuring right and left ventricular stroke volume using echocardiographic and Doppler techniques and comparing those values to those interrogated from the pacemaker. Comparisons of stroke volume were made during pacing at different heart rates and atrioventricular (AV) intervals and during handgrip and lower body negative pressure. There was a close correlation between changes in pacemaker-derived stroke volume and the Doppler time velocity integral measurements. Both techniques detected a decrease in stroke volume with lower body negative pressure. The pacemaker was able to determine optimal stroke volume in about 70% of the interventions.[57] This work was extended by Sperry and associates[58] in this group of patients by measuring PEI during pacing at different heart rates, AV intervals, handgrip, and lower body negative pressure. PEI as determined by telemetry from the pacemaker was compared with an echocardiographically derived right and left ventricular preejection period. The direction and magnitude of change were roughly proportional in the pacemaker and the echocardiographically derived measurements.[58]

RESULTS FROM CLINICAL TRIALS

Approximately 300 patients have received Precept pacemakers during phase I and phase II clinical trials; two thirds of these were dual-chamber pacemakers. Resting sensor values were obtained at all follow-up visits, and periodic exercise tests were carried out in the rate-adaptive and non–rate-adaptive pacing modes during the first year after implantation. Figure 13–16 shows the change in PEI and stroke volume during exercise testing from a subset of the Precept population.[33] Data from the initial exercise test done 2 days following pacemaker implantation are shown, along with data obtained from a second exercise test 2 weeks later. The close correlation between data from the two tests suggests that sensor stability is achieved very early after implantation. The stroke volume values decline during a shift from the supine to the upright posture, consistent with the known effects of posture on stroke volume. Therefore, patients with stroke volume as the selected sensor may experience a transient increase in pacing rate when assuming a supine position and, conversely, a decrease in pacing rate when assuming an upright posture. On the other hand, PEI values shorten with the upright position, consistent with the expected increase in sympathetic tone. The shortening of the PEI translates to an increased pacing rate when the patient changes from a supine

to an upright position. In this regard, PEI may provide a more physiologic response to postural changes.

A comparison of paired exercise data from patients with chronotropic incompetence in both rate-adaptive and non–rate-adaptive modes is shown in Figure 13–17 and Table 13–2. A clear increase in exercise heart rate and duration of exercise is evident in the rate-adaptive compared with the non–rate-adaptive pacing modes.

Ruiter and coworkers[60] reported their experience in 10 patients with Precept impedance-based pacemakers. Nine patients received a DDDR pacemaker, and 1 had a VVIR pacemaker programmed to PEI as the sensor. Each patient underwent symptom-limited maximal bicycle exercise testing, Holter monitoring, and measurement of sensor values and heart rates during postural changes. After 1 year of follow-up, the PEI values were adequate for reliable rate-modulated pacing. PEI continued to demonstrate a rapid and proportional decrease at all levels of exercise. In two patients, uncomfortable and symptomatic palpitations occurred with postural changes.[60] This increased heart rate on changing from a supine to a standing position may be beneficial in patients with refractory orthostatic hypotension. Grubb and colleagues[61] described a patient whose pacemaker showed ventricular rate acceleration with standing when it was programmed to the PEI sensor. It was reasoned that the sudden drop in venous return and right ventricular filling would result in shortening of the PEI and accelerated pacing when it was needed during sitting or standing, with return to a lower rate while lying supine.[61]

The results of clinical trials suggest that the Precept pacing system provides appropriate rate-adaptive pacing. Further, analysis of the clinical data will address issues of long-term sensor performance and generator longevity. It may also be possible to gain more information about the use of stroke volume and PEI as sensors in patients with congestive heart failure and in other groups by examining data from the appropriate subgroups in the Precept clinical trials.

PRE-EJECTION INTERVAL

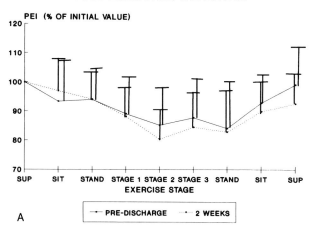

A

STROKE VOLUME

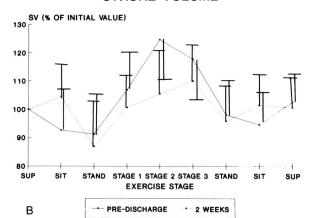

B

FIGURE 13–16. Changes in preejection interval (PEI [*A*]) and stroke volume (SV [*B*]) sensor values from patients with Precept pacemakers during exercise testing. Data from predischarge and 2-week follow-up studies are shown. (Reprinted from Burns CA, Sperry RE, Arrowood JA, et al. Doppler echocardiographic assessment of an impedance-based and dual-chamber rate-responsive pacemaker. American Journal of Cardiology, Vol 71, sect 7, 1993, pp 569–574.)

Biotronik Neos-PEP Pacing System

Biotronik has also developed a pacing system that uses impedance-based measurements of local cardiac motion as the sensor for rate adaptation. The Biotronik Neos-PEP is presently being evaluated in clinical trials in Europe and Australia. This VVI pacemaker employs a standard unipolar pacing lead and thus can be used at initial implantation or as a replacement generator with a previously implanted lead. A 4097-Hz continuous square wave current of 40 μA is injected through the pacing tip for a short period following a paced or sensed complex. By monitoring the resulting voltage between the lead tip and the generator, an impedance or conductance signal is obtained. Signal filtering and processing are necessary to diminish the contribution from ventilation, motion, and other influences. Because the pacing electrode area is so much smaller than that of the generator, the current density is highest near the electrode tip. Therefore, the conductance signal is purported to represent primarily local intracardiac rather than distant phenomena.[13] In the initial phase of clinical evaluation, a measurement related to PEP was used in the pacing algorithm. Subsequently, a new algorithm was developed based on clinical data, which are

Rate Response in DDD vs. DDDR - Incompetent Patients

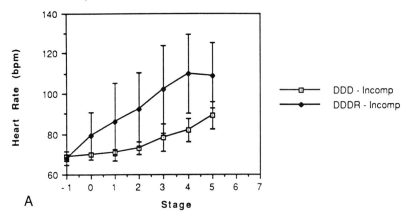

A

Rate Response in VVI vs. VVIR Mode - Incompetent Patients

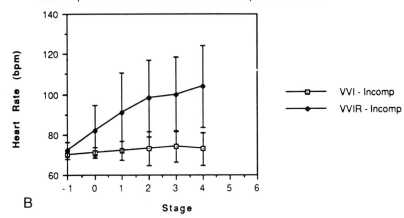

B

FIGURE 13–17. Comparison of heart rate response with exercise in patients with chronotropic incompetence who underwent treadmill testing in both the rate-adaptive and non–rate-adaptive pacing modes. Paired exercise data are shown for DDD versus DDDR *(A)* and VVI versus VVIR *(B)* pacing modes.

thought to provide a more accurate and predictable heart rate response. This method uses shifts in the conductance waveform during early systole to gauge metabolic demand. Figure 13–18 shows an example of conductance (the reciprocal of impedance) waveforms during rest and exercise for an individual patient.[13] The time window in early systole demonstrating the greatest change in conductance compared to baseline (RQ) is the designated region of interest. By limiting measurements to the region of interest, power consumption can be reduced. The gradual shift in the cardiac conductance waveform during exercise is shown in Figure 13–19. From conductance measurements in the region of interest, the VIP is calculated.[62]

The VIP, which is considered a measure of sympathetic tone by virtue of its relationship to ventricular motion and its time course during exercise, is used to adjust pacing rate. Data from individual patients show a favorable heart rate response. Figure 13–20 compares the sensor-controlled pac-

TABLE 13–2. **EXERCISE DATA FROM PATIENTS WITH SINGLE- AND DUAL-CHAMBER PRECEPT PACEMAKERS**

	MAXIMUM HEART RATE (BPM)			EXERCISE TIME (MIN)		
	NONADAPTIVE RATE MODE	ADAPTIVE RATE MODE	DIFFERENCE (*P* VALUE)	NONADAPTIVE RATE MODE	ADAPTIVE RATE MODE	DIFFERENCE (*P* VALUE)
VVI/VVIR (NL = 38)						
Competent (18)	122 ± 15	125 ± 14	.22	9.6 ± 3.4	10.2 ± 3.1	.56
Incompetent (20)	75 + 9	111 ± 16	.001	7.9 ± 3.4	9.2 ± 3.9	.005
PEI (22)	92 ± 24	113 ± 17	.005	8.8 ± 3.7	9.8 ± 3.7	.002
SV (16)	104 ± 29	123 ± 14	.005	8.6 ± 3.3	9.5 ± 3.4	.035
DDD/DDDR (N = 65)						
Competent (51)	123 ± 17	125 ± 18	.33	10.29 ± 3.54	10.45 ± 3.39	.208
Incompetent (14)	90 ± 6	115 ± 16	.0007	8.73 ± 2.59	9.81 ± 2.72	.068
PEI (39)	118 ± 21	125 ± 19	.05	9.97 ± 3.58	10.68 ± 3.35	.0003
SV (26)	112 ± 18	121 ± 17	.04	9.93 ± 3.19	9.83 ± 3.08	.746

Competent, patients with chronotropic competence; Incompetent, patients with chronotropic incompetence; PEI, patients with preejection interval selected as sensor; SV, patients with stroke volume selected as sensor.

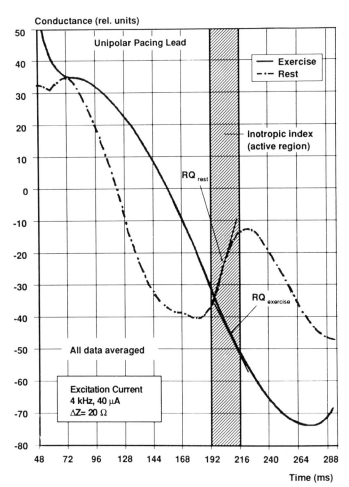

FIGURE 13–18. Conductance waveforms during rest and exercise from the Biotronik Neos-PEP pacing system. (From Schaldach M: Electrotherapy of the Heart. New York, Springer-Verlag, 1992. Copyright 1992 by Springer-Verlag.)

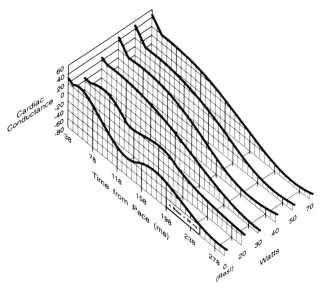

FIGURE 13–19. Conductance waveforms at various levels of exercise from the Biotronik Neos-PEP pacing system. (From Schaldach M: Electrotherapy of the Heart. New York, Springer-Verlag, 1992. Copyright 1992 by Springer-Verlag.)

ing rate to the sinus rate in a patient with AV block during exercise. A response slope, or "individual adaptation characteristic," is achieved by the inotropic index, a variable that normalizes the change in VIP by comparing the conductance measurements during exercise, at maximal performance, and at rest. Data from the overall clinical experience are not yet available for review, but preliminary clinical data from acute exercise testing show good correlation between the spontaneous sinus rhythm and the stimulation rate predicted by the VIP algorithm. Ongoing studies are examining the long-term stability and the effect of medication on this algorithm.

Summary

The pacemakers discussed in this chapter are the first clinically viable systems with sensors that measure the primary indicators of metabolic demand. The data available to date suggest that in terms of the appropriateness and proportionality of pacing rate in a wide variety of circumstances the results are impressive. These results have been achieved using relatively simple linear pacing algorithms. Closed-loop control systems may also prove useful and may simplify

programming. The relationship between heart rate and sensor response at a fixed workload is important in determining the stability of a pacing system. A sensor parameter, such as stroke volume, which exhibits negative feedback (i.e., the response to increased rate is opposite to the response to increased workload) tends to be stable and can be used safely in a feedback system. A parameter that is essentially independent of pacing rate, such as body motion (activity) and minute ventilation, is also stable but cannot be used in a feedback system (because there is no feedback). Instead, a mapping between sensor value and desired pacing rate must be determined experimentally and programmed into the device. Finally, a sensor that exhibits positive feedback (i.e., the response to increased rate occurs in the same direction as the response to increased workload) is inherently unstable and requires sophisticated algorithms and careful programming. An example of this latter class of sensor is the QT interval.

Another intriguing aspect of these impedance-based pa-

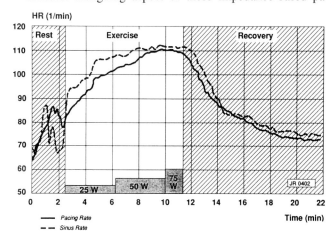

FIGURE 13–20. Comparison between sinus rate and pacing rate in a patient with complete atrioventricular (AV) block with a Biotronik Neos-PEP pacing system. (From Schaldach M: Electrotherapy of the Heart. New York, Springer-Verlag, 1992. Copyright 1992 by Springer-Verlag.)

rameters is that they permit monitoring of cardiac performance. This has two important implications. The first is the potential to optimize performance in impaired hearts by avoiding inappropriate rapid pacing. This can occur automatically when, for example, an increase in pacing rate causes ischemia leading to a decrease in stroke volume, which in turn decreases pacing rate to a more appropriate level. The second important implication is the possibility of using impedance-based measurements to confirm capture. Ongoing capture verification would be a valuable safety feature and could be used to automatically adjust pacing output to ensure capture while minimizing wasted energy.

In the coming years, further refinements in impedance-based sensors can be expected to enlarge and redefine our definition of physiologic pacing.

REFERENCES

1. Rappoport D, Ray GB: Changes in electrical conductivity in the beating tortoise ventricle. Am J Physiol 80:126, 1927.
2. Rushmer RF, Crystal TK, Wagner C, et al: Intracardiac plethysmography. Am J Physiol 174:171, 1953.
3. Geddes LA, Hoff HE, Mello A, et al: Continuous measurement of ventricular volume by electrical impedance. Cardiac Res Cen Bull 4:118, 1966.
4. Palmer CL: Continuous measurement of stroke volume by electrical impedance in the unanesthetized animal. Thesis (Ph.D.), Baylor University, 1970.
5. Baan J, Aouw Jong TT, Kerkhof PLM, et al: Continuous stroke volume and cardiac output from intraventricular dimensions obtained with impedance catheter. Cardiovasc Res 15:328, 1981.
6. Salo R, Wallner TG, Pederson BD: Measurement of ventricular volume by intracardiac impedance: Theoretical and empirical approaches. IEEE Trans Biomed Eng BME-33:189, 1986.
7. Salo RW, Pederson BD, Olive AL: Continuous ventricular volume assessment for diagnosis and pacemaker control. PACE 7:1267, 1984.
8. Salo RW, Pederson BD, Hauck JA: The measurement of ventricular volume by intracardiac impedance. In Wise DL (ed): Bioinstrumentation: Research, Developments and Applications. Boston, Butterworths, 1990, pp 853–891.
9. Woodward JC, Bertram CD, Gow SB: Right ventricular volumetry by catheter measurement of conductance. PACE 10:862, 1987.
10. Geddes LA, Baker LE: The specific resistance of biological material—a compendium of data for the biomedical engineer and physiologist. Med & Biol Eng 5:271, 1967.
11. Salo RW: The theoretical basis of a computational model for the determination of volume by impedance. Automedica 11(4):299, 1989.
12. Chastain S: Personal communication, 1988.
13. Schaldach M: Electrotherapy of the Heart. New York, Springer-Verlag, 1992, pp 105–143.
14. Chirife R: Physiological principles of a new method for rate-responsive pacing using the pre-ejection interval. PACE 11:1545, 1988.
15. McGoon MD, Shapland JE, Salo RW, et al: The feasibility of utilizing the systolic preejection interval as a determinant of pacing rate. J Am Coll Cardiol 14(7):1753, 1989.
16. Salo RW, Pederson BD, Chirife R: Exercise studies in animals of three chronic sensors for rate-responsive pacing. PACE 11:511, 1988.
17. Polinar LR, Dehmer GJ, Lewis SE, et al: Left ventricular performance in normal subjects. A comparison of response to exercise in upright and supine positions. Circulation 62:528, 1980.
18. Gauer OH, Thron HL: Postural changes in the circulation. In Hamilton WF, Dow F (eds): Handbook of Physiology: Circulation. Washington, DC, American Physiological Society, 1965, pp 2409–2439.
19. Stenberg J, Astrand PO, Ekblom B, et al: Hemodynamic response to work with different muscle groups, sitting and supine. J Appl Physiol 22:61, 1967.
20. Honig CR: Modern Cardiovascular Physiology. Boston, Little, Brown, 1981, p 150.
21. Bar-Shlomo B-Z, Druck MN, Morch JE, et al: Left ventricular function in trained and untrained subjects. Circulation 65:484, 1982.
22. Iskandrian AS, Hakki A-H, DePace NL, et al: Evaluation of left ventric-

23. Kitamura K, Jorgensen CR, Gobel FL, et al: Hemodynamic correlates of myocardial O_2 consumption during upright exercise. J Appl Physiol 32:516, 1972.
24. Benchimol A, Yeou-bing L, Dimond EG: Cardiovascular dynamics in complete heart block at various heart rates. Circulation 30:542, 1964.
25. Samet P, Bernstein WH, Medow A, Nathan DA: Effect of alterations in ventricular rate on cardiac output in complete heart block. Am J Cardiol 14:477, 1964.
26. van der Werf T: Interdependence of left ventricular end-diastolic volume and heart rate. Chest 73:683, 1978.
27. Wessale JL, Geddes LA, Fearnot NE, et al: Cardiac output vs pacing rate at rest and with exercise in dogs with AV block. PACE 11:575, 1988.
28. Katz AM: The working heart. In Physiology of the Heart, 2nd ed. New York, Raven Press, 1992, p 378.
29. Gerstenblith G, Lakatta EG, Weisfeldt ML: Age changes in myocardial function and exercise response. Prog Cardiovasc Dis 19:1, 1976.
30. Julius S, Antoon A, Whitlock LS, Conway J: Influence of age on the hemodynamic response to exercise. Circulation 36:222, 1967.
31. Granath A, Jonsson B, Strandell T: Circulation in healthy old men studied by right heart catheterization and rest and during exercise in supine and sitting position. Acta Med Scand 176:425, 1964.
32. Rodeheffer RJ, Gerstenblith G, Becker LC, et al: Exercise cardiac output is maintained with advancing age in healthy human subjects: Cardiac dilatation and increased stroke volume compensate for a diminished heart rate. Circulation 69:203, 1984.
33. Clausen JP: Circulatory adjustments in dynamic exercise and effect of physical training in normal subjects and in patients with coronary artery disease. Prog Cardiovasc Dis 18:459, 1976.
34. Heywood JT, Grimm J, Hess OM, et al: Right ventricular systolic function during exercise with and without significant coronary artery disease. Am J Cardiol 67:681, 1991.
35. Baker BJ, Wilen MM, Boyd CM, et al: Relation of right ventricular ejection fraction to exercise capacity in chronic left ventricular failure. Am J Cardiol 54:596, 1984.
36. Morrison DA, Adcock K, Collins CM, et al: Right ventricular dysfunction and the exercise limitation of chronic obstructive pulmonary disease. J Am Coll Cardiol 9:1219, 1987.
37. Cohen M, Horowitz SF, Madrac J, et al: Response of the right ventricle to exercise in isolated mitral stenosis. Am J Cardiol 55:1054, 1985.
38. Morrison DA, Lancaster L, Henry R, Goldman S: Right ventricular function at rest and during exercise in aortic and mitral disease. J Am Coll Cardiol 5:21, 1985.
39. Aroesty JM, McKay RG, Heller GV, et al: Simultaneous assessment of left ventricular systolic and diastolic dysfunction during pacing-induced ischemia. Circulation 71:889, 1985.
40. Schulte W, Neus H: Hemodynamics during emotional stress in borderline and mild hypertension. Eur Heart J 4:803, 1983.
41. Rudel H, Langewitz W, Schachinger H, et al: Hemodynamic response patterns to mental stress: Diagnostic and therapeutic implications. Am Heart J 116:617, 1988.
42. Alt E, Theres H, Heinz M, et al: Does transthoracic impedance reflect ventilation or body activity? PACE 13(9):1189, 1990.
43. van Mechelen R, Wortel HJJ, de Boer JGA: Impedance measurements in the human right ventricle. PACE 13(9):1203, 1990.
44. Katz LN, Feil HS: Clinical observations on the dynamics of ventricular systole. I. Auricular fibrillation. Arch Intern Med 32:672, 1923.
45. Weissler AM, Harris WS, Schoenfeld CD: Systolic time intervals in heart failure in man. Circulation 37:149, 1968.
46. Ahmed SS, Levinson GE, Schartz DJ, et al. Systolic time intervals as measures of the contractile state of the left ventricular myocardium in man. Circulation 46:559, 1972.
47. Spodick DH, Doi YL, Bishop RL, Hashimoto T: Systolic time intervals reconsidered. Reevaluation of the preejection period: Absence of relation to heart rate. Am J Cardiol 53:1667, 1984.
48. Salzman SH, Wolfson S, Jackson B, Schecter E: Epinephrine infusion in man. Standardization, normal response, and abnormal response in idiopathic hypertrophic subaortic stenosis. Circulation 43:137, 1971.
49. Whitsett TL, Naughton J: The effect of exercise on systolic time intervals in sedentary and active individuals and rehabilitated patients with heart disease. Am J Cardiol 27:352, 1971.
50. Spodick DH, Quarry-Pigott VM: Effects of posture on exercise per-

formance: Measurement by systolic time intervals. Circulation 48:74, 1973.

51. Weissler AM, Harris WS, Schoenfeld CD: Bedside techniques for the evaluation of ventricular function in man. Am J Cardiol 23:577, 1969.

52. Sugimoto T, Inasaka T, Basta LL, Takeuchi J: Relationships of left-ventricular systolic time intervals with hemodynamic variables in intact and failing hearts. Jpn Heart J 16:433, 1975.

53. Tavel ME: Systolic and diastolic time intervals. *In* Clinical Phonocardiography and External Pulse Recording, 4th ed. Chicago, Year Book, 1985, pp 279–299.

54. Hooper RG, Whitcomb ME: Systolic time intervals in chronic obstructive pulmonary disease. Circulation 50:1205, 1979.

55. Alpert JS, Rickman FD, Howe JP: Alteration of systolic time intervals in right ventricular failure. Circulation 50:317, 1974.

56. Stafford RW, Harris WS, Weissler AM: Left ventricular systolic time intervals as indices of postural circulatory stress in man. Circulation 41:485, 1970.

57. Burns CA, Sperry RE, Arrowood JA, et al: Doppler echocardiographic assessment of an impedance-based dual-chamber rate-responsive pacemaker. Am J Cardiol 71:569, 1993.

58. Sperry RE, Burns CA, Wood MA, et al: Validation of pre-ejection interval as a sensor for a dual-chamber, rate-responsive pacemaker. J Am Coll Cardiol 19(3):65A, 1992.

59. Platia EV, O'Donoghue S, Waclawski SH: Stroke volume and pre-ejection interval as sensors in a dual-chamber rate-modulated pacemaker [Abstract]. PACE 14:659, 1991.

60. Ruiter JH, Heemels JP, Kee D, et al: Adaptive rate pacing controlled by the right ventricular preejection interval: Clinical experience with a physiological pacing system. PACE 15:886, 1992.

61. Grubb BP, Wolfe DA, Samoil D, et al: Adaptive rate pacing controlled by right ventricular preejection interval for severe refractory orthostatic hypotension. PACE 16:801, 1993.

62. Schaldach M, Hutten H: Intracardiac impedance to determine sympathetic activity in rate-responsive pacing. PACE 15:1778, 1992.

CHAPTER 14

THE EVOKED QT INTERVAL

Derek T. Connelly
Anthony F. Rickards

It has long been known that the evoked potential recorded from a unipolar endocardial ventricular lead consists of depolarization and repolarization components, analogous to the QRS complex and the T wave, respectively, on the surface electrocardiogram (ECG). In 1981 a microprocessor-based pacemaker was developed that was capable of recording and measuring the interval from the pacing stimulus to the maximum gradient of the repolarization component of the evoked potential (''stimulus-to-T'' or ''evoked QT'' interval), and could vary the pacing rate in accordance with the value of this parameter. This chapter describes the rationale behind the use of the paced QT interval as a biosensor, the development of a ventricular pacing system that uses this sensor for rate-responsive ventricular pacing, the clinical efficacy of this pacing system, and its recent combination with other sensors and incorporation into rate-responsive, dual-chamber (DDDR) systems.

QT Interval Variability and Its Use as a Biosensor

The observation that the QT interval on the surface ECG tends to decrease with increasing heart rate was first made in the early years of this century. Several investigators have attempted to quantify the variation in QT interval with heart rate, and the most enduring estimate of the QT-RR relationship is that of Bazett.[1] Bazett's formula for correcting the QT interval for heart rate (dividing the QT interval by the square root of the RR interval in seconds) is still widely quoted[2] and has been incorporated into computerized algorithms for ECG interpretation. Other authors have suggested a cube root relationship,[3, 4] a logarithmic relationship,[5] an exponential relationship,[6, 7] and a straight line relationship.[8] Some recent studies have suggested that the QT interval varies in direct proportion to the heart rate (i.e., in inverse proportion to the RR interval),[9–12] and a theoretical derivation based on cardiac thermodynamics has suggested that such a relationship accords with the principle of conservation of energy as applied to the duration of systole as a function of the RR interval.[13]

Several factors other than the instantaneous heart rate influence the QT interval at any given time. There is a diurnal variation that produces small changes in the QT interval, so that for a given heart rate the QT interval will tend to be longer during the night.[14–16] More important is the nonlinear adaptation of QT interval with changes in heart rate during and after exercise:[17] at a given heart rate, the QT interval is usually longer during exercise than during recovery because it takes a finite amount of time for the action potential duration (and hence the QT interval) to adapt to a change in heart rate.[18, 19] There is some evidence that beta-adrenergic blocking agents alter the slope of the relationship between QT interval and heart rate, so that the corrected QT interval tends to be longer at rest and shorter at peak exercise.[20, 21] Furthermore, stimuli such as breath holding, hyperventilation, the Valsalva maneuver, and the cold-pressor test produce marked changes in heart rate but very small changes in QT interval.[22] All these studies suggest that the QT interval does not vary simply in relation to the heart rate but may be affected by other factors such as sympathetic tone.

The first suggestion that variation in the QT interval may be a useful biosensor for rate-modulated pacing was made by Rickards and Norman.[11] They studied the relation between QT interval and heart rate in patients undergoing exercise, in a group of patients undergoing atrial pacing without exercise, and in a group of patients with complete heart block and fixed-rate ventricular pacing undergoing exercise. In the first group, a linear relation between QT interval and heart rate was observed, so that the QT interval fell by 187 msec for an increase in heart rate of 100 bpm; in the atrially paced group, the decrease in QT interval observed with increasing heart rates was considerably less marked (66 msec decrease in QT interval, for an increase in heart rate of 100 bpm). Interestingly, in the group with complete heart block, there was a pronounced reduction in stimulus-to-T interval on exercise despite the fact that the ventricular rate remained constant; when the stimulus-to-T interval was plotted against the *atrial* rate during exercise, a linear relationship was observed, so that for a 100-bpm rise in atrial rate the stimulus-to-T interval decreased by 95 msec. The authors concluded that the changes in QT interval observed during exercise were strongly influenced by the effect of circulating catecholamines and less influenced by the intrinsic alteration in heart rate. Similar results were obtained by Fananapazir and colleagues.[23] Rickards and Norman[11] also described a system by which the endocardial paced evoked response could be sensed from a unipolar lead within 5 msec of delivery of the stimulus; the system depended on a modified pulse waveform and automatic postpulse compensation to eliminate the effect of polarization at the electrode-myocardium interface.

The first implantation of a prototype rate-adaptive cardiac pacemaker using the stimulus-to-T wave as sensor (TX [Vitatron Medical B.V., Dieren, The Netherlands]) was performed in 1981. In addition to standard programmable variables, this device permitted analysis of the amplitude of the evoked T wave and the duration of the stimulus-to-T interval. Following delivery of a pacing pulse, the pacemaker was refractory to all input for 200 msec. There then followed a window (programmable out to 450 msec after the stimulus) during which a signal corresponding to the frequency content of an endocardial T wave could be sensed and timed (Fig. 14–1). The subsequent stimulus was delivered as a function of the preceding stimulus–to–T wave interval (measured from the pacing stimulus to the point of maximal negative slope of the evoked T wave), so that a decreasing stimulus-to-T interval resulted in a faster heart rate and vice versa. The pacemaker's programmable parameters included the sensitivity of the heart rate–QT interval relation, defined in terms of bpm/msec, the maximal pacing rate, the maximal rate of change of pacing rate, and the rate of slow drift back to the minimal programmed rate.[24]

PHYSIOLOGIC FACTORS AFFECTING THE STIMULUS-TO-T INTERVAL

Initial studies with the QT-sensing pacemaker demonstrated satisfactory increases in pacing rate and cardiac output on exertion.[24, 25] Subsequent studies have shown appropriate increases in pacing rate on exertion in more than 90% of patients.[26, 27] The pacing rate during exercise has been shown to correlate with plasma noradrenaline levels in patients with QT-sensing pacemakers,[28] and, as stated earlier, the QT interval appears to be influenced by circulating catecholamine levels rather than by heart rate alone. A number of investigators have shown that stimuli other than exercise that are associated with catecholamine release can increase the pacing rate of QT-sensing pacemakers. The pyrexia associated with bacterial endocarditis,[29] the pain of acute myocardial infarction,[30, 31] and psychological stress[32, 33] have been shown to result in an appropriate increase in pacing rate in patients with implanted QT-sensing pacing systems.

KINETICS OF PACED QT INTERVAL VARIATION

A significant limitation of rate-modulated pacing systems using "physiologic" sensors is that many of them respond rather slowly to rapid changes in physiologic demand. Lau and associates studied the rate of change of stimulus-to-T adaptation to abrupt changes (increase and decrease) in pacing rate in seven patients with newly diagnosed complete atrioventricular (AV) block. The time course of stimulus-to-T adaptation was shown to be exponential, with a time constant of 49 seconds when the rate was increasing and 60 seconds when it was decreasing. The practical implication of this delay in stimulus-to-T shortening or lengthening is that, after a short burst of exercise (such as ascending a staircase), the maximum heart rate may not be achieved until after the exercise has been completed. In addition, the heart rate may remain elevated for 2 to 3 minutes after the end of exercise. In recent years some improvements have been made in the rate-response algorithm to improve the pacing response at the onset of exercise (see later section; Rate-Adaptive Algorithms).

MEASUREMENT OF THE PACED QT INTERVAL

For the stimulus-to-T wave interval to be measured, the sensing circuit of the pulse generator must be capable of discriminating the T wave from artifactual signals. A conventional pacing stimulus typically delivers a pulse of about 5 V for 0.5 msec into a load of approximately 500 ohms. This results in polarization at the electrode-myocardium interface in such a way that after the end of the pulse a voltage exists

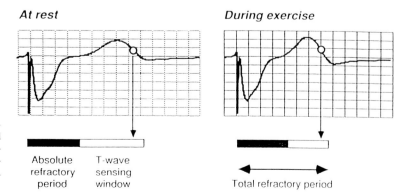

FIGURE 14–1. Evoked endocardial T-wave sensing. The T-wave sensing window begins 200 msec after the window and has a duration (programmable) of up to 250 msec. The maximum slope of the evoked T wave is sensed, and T-wave sensing ends (and QRS sensing is enabled) 25 msec after this. During exercise the stimulus–T interval shortens.

between the cathode and anode of opposite polarity to the pacing stimulus. The time course of decay of this potential may be several hundred milliseconds, causing difficulties in sensing small amplitude potentials during that period. Rickards and Norman[11] described the development of a pacing input-output circuit that, by delivering charge-balanced pulses, was capable of eliminating this polarization effect. This system was shown to be capable of sensing the evoked response within 5 msec of the pacing pulse delivered across a conventional unipolar lead system. Recordings of the evoked response using this system showed a negative depolarization component (''QRS complex''), which reached a maximum amplitude 45 msec after the stimulus and was followed by a clearly defined positive repolarization component (''T wave'') (see Fig. 14–1). The evoked T-wave amplitude was 3 to 12 mV, approximately half the amplitude of the evoked QRS complex and considerably larger than the T wave of spontaneous (nonpaced) complexes.

A major advantage of the paced QT interval as a biosensor is that it can be sensed from a standard unipolar pacing lead. There is no need for additional or specially constructed sensing leads, and the QT-sensing pacemaker can be connected to a chronically implanted lead when the pulse generator is replaced if desired. A study of T-wave sensing in 1500 pacemaker patients[34] showed satisfactory T-wave amplitudes in 94.1% of patients. Among these patients, 81% had an acutely implanted lead and 19% had a chronic lead. There was no evidence of long-term deterioration of T-wave sensing in the patients with chronically implanted leads. Thus, it seems that T-wave sensing is feasible in the great majority of pacemaker patients, and the T-wave amplitude appears to be stable with the passage of time. In one small study of the long-term efficacy of the QT-sensing pacemaker, the rate-response parameters remained satisfactory 5 years after implantation in the majority of patients.[27]

Rate-Adaptive Algorithms

NONLINEAR SLOPE OF THE HEART RATE–QT INTERVAL RELATIONSHIP

The relationship between heart rate and QT interval, which was initially implemented as a linear function,[11] was recently reevaluated by Baig and colleagues.[35] They showed that the relationship was nonlinear, the degree of QT shortening being least at low heart rates. Therefore, a linear algorithm would provide very small increases in pacing rate at the onset of exercise and excessively rapid increases at high workloads. To overcome this undesirable property of the QT interval, a new algorithm for determination of the pacing rate was developed and was first evaluated clinically in 1988 (TX919 and Rhythmyx [Vitatron Medical]) (Fig. 14–2). This new algorithm provided a higher heart rate–QT slope at slow pacing rates than at faster rates. The net result was a more natural increase in pacing rates at all workloads. Subsequently, the old and new algorithms were compared in an open study in 10 patients[36] and in a double-blind crossover study[37] in 11 patients. The new algorithm did not produce a significant increase in peak pacing rate, exercise capacity, or oxygen consumption, but did produce a faster initial acceleration in heart rate at the onset of exercise. The nonlinear

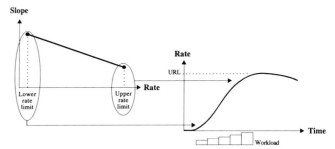

FIGURE 14–2. Nonlinear relationship between heart rate and QT interval. At rest, the slope of the rate response is high (i.e., a small decrease in QT interval produces a relatively large increase in heart rate). This produces a more brisk increase in pacing rate at the onset of exercise. At peak exercise the slope of the rate response is low, resulting in a smooth approach to the upper rate limit (URL).

algorithm was also associated with fewer cases of rate instability (oscillation) during exercise.

AUTOMATIC SLOPE ADAPTATION

A potential problem with rate-responsive pacemakers of all types is the number of parameters that must be programmed and the amount of time and effort required to optimally program the pacemaker for an individual patient. With the QT-sensing pacemaker, the programmable parameters include the pacing mode, output and pulse width, lower and upper rate limits, QRS and T wave sensitivity, and the slope of the rate response at the lower and upper rate limits. Recent modifications in the software of QT-sensing pacemakers have allowed some of these functions to be performed automatically by the pulse generator.[38, 39] At the time of implantation, the slope is set to relatively low values. The slope at the lower rate limit is automatically adjusted every night (when the pacemaker's 24-hour clock signals that it is night-time and the pacing rate is at the lower rate limit) by temporarily disabling the rate response and increasing the pacing rate by 10 bpm, thereby assessing the difference in stimulus-to-T interval between these two rates. The slope of the QT-pacing rate relationship is then adjusted accordingly. The slope at the upper rate limit is adjusted whenever the patient exercises strenuously enough to drive the pacing rate to the upper rate limit. If at that time the stimulus-to-T interval shortens further, this is taken as an indication that the patient has not reached his maximum workload and the upper rate limit has been reached too early in exercise. The slope is therefore decreased, so that a higher level of exercise is required to reach the upper pacing rate. By contrast, if the upper rate limit is not reached over a period of 8 days, the slope at the upper rate limit is automatically increased, making it easier to reach the upper pacing rate. Recently, Baig and colleagues[40] reviewed their experience with automatic slope adaptation in 17 patients in the first year after implantation of a QT-sensing pacing system. They showed that most of the changes in slope at the lower rate limit occurred within the first 2 to 4 weeks after its enablement, whereas little change occurred in the slope at the upper rate limit. They concluded that this self-calibrating rate-adaptive system functioned successfully and that this system ought to simplify follow-up of these patients. They also found the pacemaker's built-in Holter monitoring facility useful in evaluating their patients, as did Murdock and coworkers.[41]

AUTOMATIC ADJUSTMENT OF REFRACTORY PERIOD

When the pacemaker is programmed to the rate-adaptive mode the refractory period is automatically adjusted after every stimulus. After an absolute refractory period of 200 msec, T-wave sensing is enabled. The T-wave sensing window ends 25 msec after the T wave has been sensed, after which QRS sensing is enabled immediately. Thus, the refractory period adapts automatically to the stimulus-to-T interval and the pacing rate, mimicking the normal behavior of cardiac cells.

Clinical Experience

Initial experience with the earliest models of the QT-sensing pacemaker was generally encouraging, with appropriate increases in pacing rate and cardiac output occurring on exertion in most patients.[24, 25] Subsequent studies have shown satisfactory increases in pacing rate in more than 90% of patients during exercise.[26, 27] Hedman and Nordlander[42] performed a double-blind crossover comparison of rate-modulated pacing versus fixed-rate VVI pacing in 18 patients with QT-sensing pacemakers and showed that rate-modulated pacing resulted in a 9% increase in exercise tolerance, with significantly less dyspnea and fatigue at comparable workloads. Eleven of the 18 patients preferred the rate-modulated pacing mode, 5 could not distinguish between the two modes, and 2 preferred fixed-rate VVI pacing because their angina pectoris became worse at high heart rates during rate-modulated pacing.

Several investigators have compared the rate-response characteristics of QT-sensing pacemakers with those of other sensors. Maisch and colleagues[43, 44] reported their experience with eight patients with QT-sensing pacing systems, six with respiratory rate-sensing devices, and eight with activity-sensing pacemakers. These authors also surveyed 11 other centers to obtain data on a further 132 patients with rate-responsive pacemakers. They reported that the early QT-sensing pacemakers had more problems than pacemakers using other sensors because of voltage polarization at the electrode tip that limited accurate T-wave sensing in the early models. Zegelman and associates[45] performed submaximal exercise testing (Kaltenbach's step test) in 19 patients with QT-sensing pacemakers, 12 patients with respiratory-sensing pacemakers, and 45 patients with activity-sensing pacemakers, and compared the results with those obtained by 52 patients with dual-chamber pacemakers. They found that the rate-response characteristics of the QT-sensing pacemakers were less reproducible than those of the other sensors; however, the patient groups were not necessarily well matched with regard to age, cardiac diagnoses, and duration of pacing.

Mehta and associates[46] performed treadmill exercise testing in nine patients with activity-sensing pacemakers and five patients with QT-sensing pacemakers. They found that the maximum pacing rates in each group were not significantly different. Patients with activity-sensing pacemakers showed

an increase in pacing rate in response to each increase in speed but not in response to increases in gradient. Patients with QT-sensing pacemakers responded to increases in both treadmill speed and gradient, although there was a delay in achieving the maximum rate at each stage and a longer delay in returning to the baseline pacing rate at the end of exercise. Thus, there appeared to be advantages and disadvantages with each type of sensor. Further studies from the same group[47] compared six different rate-responsive pacemakers (two activity-sensing, one QT-sensing, two respiratory rate-sensing, and one that sensed right ventricular dP/dt) in 46 patients. Activity-sensing pacemakers responded most rapidly, but their rate responses were not related to workload, whereas the QT-sensing pacemaker's output was proportional to exercise workload. Similar findings were reported by Sulke and colleagues,[48] who studied 59 patients in whom seven different types of rate-responsive pacemakers were implanted. As well as performing graded exercise testing, this group studied the effect of everyday activities such as ascending and descending stairs, lifting a suitcase with a pacemaker arm, and mental stress. Activity-sensing pacemakers overresponded to staircase descent, changes in walking speed, and lifting a suitcase, and these devices did not respond to mental stress. The QT-sensing pacemaker responded satisfactorily to mental stress, but "physiologic" sensors (QT and minute ventilation) responded slowly to rapid changes in physical demand. More recently, Bellamy and coworkers[49] compared the latest version of the QT-sensing pacemaker (which has a nonlinear relationship between QT interval and heart rate) with a second-generation activity-sensing pacemaker (Legend, [Medtronic Inc., Minneapolis, MN]). They found that both pacemakers showed improvements compared with their previous counterparts, but the QT-sensing pacemaker was still relatively slow to respond to changes in metabolic demand, showing an "overshoot" of pacing rate on cessation of exercise. The activity-sensing device was quick to adapt at the onset of exercise, but its pacing rate did not change significantly with different levels of exercise.

LIMITATIONS OF QT-SENSING PACEMAKERS

Twelve years of experience with QT-sensing pacemakers have produced a substantial amount of data on the problems and limitations of the stimulus-to-T wave interval as a biosensor. Obviously, patients with repolarization abnormalities such as the long QT syndrome are not suitable candidates for this type of pacemaker because the window for T-wave sensing cannot be prolonged beyond 450 msec. Similarly, patients who are receiving drugs with class III antiarrhythmic activity may not benefit from this type of pacemaker if their resting QT interval is grossly prolonged. Class Ia antiarrhythmic drugs also prolong the QT interval and impair the QT shortening that normally occurs with increasing heart rate.[50] Beta-blockers attenuate the QT interval shortening that occurs with increasing catecholamine levels.[23] This is a physiologic effect and might be viewed as an advantage of this type of pacemaker because patients requiring beta blockade will not develop unduly fast heart rates with this pacemaker; a similar effect is seen in patients with dual-chamber pacemakers who are taking beta-blockers. In contrast, patients who have undergone adrenalectomy or who have severe autonomic neuropathy may not be suitable candidates for this type of pacemaker because the QT interval may not vary physiologically in these patients. Finally, in patients with myocardial ischemia, it is theoretically possible that ischemia can induce changes in the QT interval, although this has not presented problems in clinical practice.

Occasionally a positive feedback loop was triggered in the first-generation QT-sensing pacemakers in which a reduction in the QT interval produced an increase in pacing rate, which itself led to a further reduction in the QT interval; in some patients this resulted in nocturnal episodes of tachycardia,[33] which may have precipitated myocardial ischemia in susceptible patients. Another problem that occurred in the early devices was rate instability or oscillation, particularly during exercise. If the gain of the rate-response parameter was high, small changes in stimulus-to-T interval could induce changes in the pacing rate despite a constant workload; the result of this instability was that, when the patient was exercising and the pacing rate was close to the upper rate limit, the pacing rate varied spontaneously. This problem has been largely overcome[37] by changes made in the rate-response algorithm that produce a lower slope in the QT interval–heart rate relationship near the upper rate limit, as described earlier.

Combination of the QT Interval with Other Rate-Adaptive Sensors

In view of its delayed response at the onset of exercise, the paced QT interval must be considered less than ideal as a single sensor for rate-responsive pacing. The possibility of combining the paced QT interval with another sensor that responds rapidly to changes in physiologic demand has therefore aroused interest. The combination of two sensors (QT interval and activity) was explored by Landman and colleagues,[51] who studied nine patients with implanted QT-sensing pacemakers. By strapping an activity-sensing pacemaker to the chest wall and analyzing the rate-response data generated by both pacemakers with a computer, they were able to develop a rate-adaptive algorithm using information derived from both the activity signal and the stimulus-to-T interval. Exercise testing using the combination of sensors (Fig. 14–3) resulted in a more rapid increase in pacing rate at the onset of exercise (triggered by the activity sensor) and a proportional increase in pacing rate with increasing workload (triggered by shortening the stimulus-to-T interval).

An algorithm incorporating data from both activity and stimulus-to-T sensors has now been incorporated in a single-chamber, rate-responsive pacemaker (Topaz [Vitatron Medical]).[52] This pacemaker incorporates all the features of the most recent models of the QT-sensing pacemakers and, in addition, has a piezoelectric crystal in the pulse generator similar to that in use in other activity-sensing pacemakers. Because activity sensors provide a prompt increase in pacing rate at the onset of exercise and QT sensors produce a pacing rate that is proportional to workload during exercise, the combination of the two sensors is expected to combine the positive attributes of each sensor (Fig. 14–4). From a practical viewpoint, the fact that the QT interval is sensed from a unipolar lead and activity is sensed from movement of the

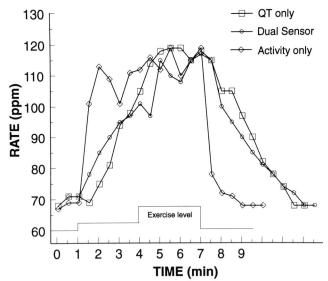

FIGURE 14–3. Rate response of QT, activity, and dual sensor modes during three successive exercise tests in one patient.

generator means that implantation of this rate-responsive pacemaker does not require insertion of extra leads (as would be required with most other ''physiologic'' sensors). The sensitivity of the QT slope and the activity slope are independently programmable, and the pacemaker can be programmed for automatic adjustment of both slope parameters.[53] In addition, the relative contribution of each sensor to the overall rate response can be programmed for each patient individually (Fig. 14–5). If problems occur with T-wave sensing, the activity mode alone can be programmed; if there are too many activity artifacts, the QT sensor alone can be used. Using both sensors, the relative weight given to the QT interval or activity (ACT) may be varied (QT > ACT, QT = ACT, or QT < ACT). In addition, either sensor may be used to cross check the other. This sensor cross-checking should help to minimize inappropriate changes in heart rate (Fig. 14–6). For example, if the activity sensor is activated without initiating a concomitant change in the QT interval, the increase in pacing rate can be limited, the assumption being that such a scenario is most likely due to motion artifact. The first prototypes of this device were implanted in the Netherlands in 1990, and the first commercially available units were implanted in patients in September 1991 in the

	QT	ACT	QT+ACT
Onset of rate response	Gradual	Fast	Fast
Proportional to workload	Yes	Partial	Yes
Rate decay	Physiologic	Preset	Physiologic
Specificity	High	Medium	High
Standard implantation	Yes	Yes	Yes

FIGURE 14–4. Theoretical advantages of a combination of QT and activity sensing.

SENSOR	INDICATION
QT	QT satisfies; many activity artifacts
QT > Act	Standard sensor selection
QT = Act	Standard sensor selection
QT < Act	Low QT response (diabetic, etc.)
Act	AAIR; QT related difficulties

FIGURE 14–5. Factors influencing choice of sensors in a patient with a dual sensor VVIR pacemaker.

Netherlands and in London. Initial assessment of this pacemaker was promising,[52, 54] and treadmill exercise testing and other studies have demonstrated that the device may have advantages over single-sensor pacemakers using either the QT interval or an activity sensor alone. Furthermore, tests of the sensor cross-checking function appear to demonstrate that inappropriate activity sensing can be effectively "ignored" by the dual-sensor pacemaker after a few minutes because the QT interval does not adapt. Nevertheless, some authors have cast doubt on the utility of the sensor cross-checking function,[55] suggesting that its full implementation leads to an inadequate rate response at the onset of exercise, and it may be that further refining of the algorithm may be required in future.

DUAL-CHAMBER, DUAL-SENSOR PACING

The algorithm described earlier that combines the paced QT interval and activity sensing has been implemented in a new series of dual-chamber pacemakers that became available in Europe in 1992. The Vitatron Ruby is a dual-chamber (DDD) pacemaker that is capable of mode switching to VVIR behavior in the presence of atrial tachycardia or atrial fibrillation. The Vitatron Saphir is a VDD pacemaker that uses a single-pass lead with a proximal pair of electrodes for atrial sensing. The Vitatron Diamond is a DDDR pacemaker capable of sensor-driven (QT and activity) increases in atrial pacing rate in the presence of chronotropic incompetence. Rather than implementing a mode switch to VVIR in the event of atrial arrhythmia, the Diamond continually uses sensor information to determine on a beat-to-beat basis

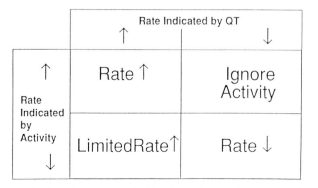

FIGURE 14–6. Sensor cross-checking in dual sensor VVIR pacemakers should help minimize heart rate changes induced by activity artifacts.

whether or not to track the atrial rate. All three of these pacemakers employ unipolar ventricular sensing to detect the evoked T wave but can be programmed to either the unipolar or bipolar ventricular pacing configuration. The Ruby and the Diamond can be programmed for either unipolar or bipolar atrial pacing or sensing, and the Saphir employs bipolar atrial sensing through the proximal electrodes of the single-pass lead. Early clinical trials of these three novel devices have recently been completed in Europe, and their long-term efficacy is currently being evaluated.

Future Developments

OTHER SENSOR COMBINATIONS

The use of sensor combinations for rate-responsive pacing is being evaluated by several investigators and manufacturers.[56] Res and Boute[57] studied the combination of two components of the evoked potential (the T-wave amplitude and the QT interval) and concluded from a small study that the combination of these parameters was superior to the QT interval alone. This combination of parameters has not subsequently been adopted for implantable devices. However, it is feasible that combinations of QT interval and other sensors may become available in the future.

BIPOLAR ENDOCARDIAL T-WAVE SENSING

Currently available QT-sensing pacemakers employ unipolar ventricular sensing for detection and analysis of the evoked T wave. Unipolar leads are more susceptible to external interference than bipolar systems, and QT-sensing pacemakers have been shown to be susceptible to extraneous electric interference.[58] Furthermore, myopotentials can interfere with the rate response of these devices.[59] The feasibility of recording endocardial T waves using a bipolar lead has recently been studied by Snoeck and associates,[60] who showed that problems of electrode polarization can be overcome and satisfactory evoked T-wave sensing obtained. Bipolar T-wave sensing has not yet been incorporated into currently available QT-sensing rate-responsive pacemakers.

ANTITACHYCARDIA PACING

Antitachycardia pacing involves the delivery of pacing stimuli, either singly or in rapid trains, in electric diastole during a reentrant tachycardia to attempt to terminate the tachycardia. The timing of the delivered stimuli is often critically important in determining the outcome of a termination attempt—stimuli that are too late may fail to penetrate the tachycardia circuit, and stimuli that are too premature may fall within the refractory period and be ineffective. It has been suggested that T-wave sensing may help to identify the end of the absolute refractory period and hence guide the appropriate timing of antitachycardia pacing stimuli.[61] Recently, den Dulk and colleagues[62] have shown that the use of the stimulus-to-T interval can be helpful in defining the refractory period on a beat-to-beat basis when the heart rate is changing rapidly and have suggested that this interval may be useful in determining appropriate antitachycardia pacing algorithms.

Puddu and Torresani[63] have pointed out that QT interval prolongation may be a harbinger of ventricular arrhythmias and sudden death in certain patients. They suggested that QT-sensing pacemakers may be useful in such patients to predict the occurrence of arrhythmic events and that these devices may prevent ventricular arrhythmias by increasing the heart rate in response to an abnormally prolonged QT interval (thereby shortening this parameter). Although of theoretical interest, this idea has not yet been put into practice, and the problem of sensing spontaneous (rather than paced) T waves has not been fully addressed.

Conclusions

The evoked QT interval was the first practical sensor to be developed for rate-adaptive pacing, and 12 years of development have resulted in several improvements and refinements in the algorithm relating the evoked QT interval to the pacing rate. The most recent major development has been the combination of evoked QT interval and activity sensing in a family of dual-sensor pacemakers for both single- and dual-chamber pacing. Whether these new technologic developments will result in a more physiologic rate response during everyday activities and will lead to a better quality of life for patients who require pacemakers in the long term remains to be determined, and the results of further studies utilizing these novel devices are eagerly awaited.

REFERENCES

1. Bazett HC: An analysis of the time-relations of electrocardiograms. Heart 7:353, 1920.
2. Ahnve S: Correction of the QT interval for heart rate: Review of different formulas and the use of Bazett's formula in myocardial infarction. Am Heart J 109:568, 1985.
3. Fridericia LS: Die Systolendauer im Elektrokardiogram bei normalen Menschen und bei Herzkranken. Acta Med Scand 53:489, 1920.
4. Puddu PE, Jouve R, Mariotti S, et al: Evaluation of 10 QT prediction formulas in 881 middle-aged men from the seven countries study: Emphasis on the cubic root Fridericia's equation. J Electrocardiol 21:219, 1988.
5. Ashman R: The normal duration of the QT interval. Am Heart J 23:522, 1942.
6. Sarma JS, Sarma RJ, Bilitch M, et al: An exponential formula for heart rate dependence of QT interval during exercise and cardiac pacing in humans: Reevaluation of Bazett's formula. Am J Cardiol 54:103, 1984.
7. Lecocq B, Lecocq V, Jaillon P: Physiologic relation between cardiac cycle and QT duration in healthy volunteers. Am J Cardiol 64:481, 1989.
8. Simonson E, Cady LD Jr, Woodbury M: The normal QT interval. Am Heart J 63:747, 1962.
9. Akhras F, Rickards AF: The relationship between QT interval and heart rate during physiological exercise and pacing. Jpn Heart J 22:345, 1981.
10. Boudoulas H, Geleris P, Lewis RP, Rittgens SE: Linear relationship between electrical systole, mechanical systole, and heart rate. Chest 80:613, 1981.
11. Rickards AF, Norman J: Relation between QT interval and heart rate. New design of physically adaptive cardiac pacemaker. Br Heart J 45:56, 1981.
12. Romano M, di Maro T, Carella G, et al: Relation between heart rate and QT interval in exercise-induced myocardial ischemia. Am J Cardiol 56:861, 1985.
13. Kovacs SJ: The duration of the QT interval as a function of heart rate: A derivation based on physical principles and a comparison to measured values. Am Heart J 110:872, 1985.
14. Bexton RS, Vallin HO, Camm AJ: Diurnal variation of the QT interval—influence of the autonomic nervous system. Br Heart J 55:253, 1986.
15. de Leonardis V, de Scalzi M, Fabiano FS, Cinelli P: A chronobiologic study on some cardiovascular parameters. J Electrocardiol 18:385, 1985.
16. Djordjevic M, Kocovic D, Pavlovic S, et al: Circadian variations of heart rate and stim-T interval: Adaptation for nighttime pacing. PACE 12:1757, 1989.
17. Sarma JS, Venkataraman Sk, Samant DR, Gadgil U: Hysteresis in the human RR-QT relationship during exercise and recovery. PACE 10:485, 1987.
18. Seed WA, Noble MIM, Oldershaw P, et al: Relation of human cardiac action potential to the interval between beats: Implications for the validity of rate corrected QT interval (QT_c). Br Heart J 57:32, 1987.
19. Lau CP, Freedman AR, Fleming S, et al: Hysteresis of the ventricular paced QT interval in response to abrupt changes in pacing rate. Cardiovasc Res 22:67, 1988.
20. Algra A, Roelandt JR, Tijssen JG, et al: Effect of beta-blockers on the relation between QT-interval and heart rate in exercise ECG. Eur Heart J 8(Suppl D):71, 1987.
21. Sarma JS, Venkataraman K, Samant DR, Gadgil UG: Effect of propranolol on the QT intervals of normal individuals during exercise: A new method for studying interventions. Br Heart J 60:434, 1988.
22. Davidowski TA, Wolf S: The QT interval during reflex cardiovascular adaptation. Circulation 69:22, 1984.
23. Fananapazir L, Bennett DH, Faragher EB: Contribution of heart rate to QT interval shortening during exercise. Eur Heart J 4:265, 1983.
24. Rickards AF, Donaldson RM, Thalen HJT: The use of QT interval to determine pacing rate: Early clinical experience. PACE 6:346, 1983.
25. Donaldson RM, Fox K, Richards AF: Initial experience with a physiological, rate responsive pacemaker. Br Med J 286:667, 1983.
26. Fananapazir L, Rademaker M, Bennett DH: Reliability of the evoked response in determining the paced ventricular rate and performance of the QT or rate-responsive (TX) pacemaker. PACE 8:701, 1985.
27. Bloomfield P, MacAreavy D, Kerr F, Fananapazir L: Long-term follow-up of patients with the QT rate adaptive pacemaker. PACE 12:111, 1989.
28. Jordaens L, Backers J, Moerman E, Clement DL: Catecholamine levels and pacing behavior of QT-driven pacemakers during exercise. PACE 13:603, 1990.
29. Kaye GC, Baig W, Mackintosh AF: QT sensing rate responsive pacing during subacute bacterial endocarditis: A case report. PACE 13:1089, 1990.
30. Robbens EJ, Clement DL, Jordaens L: QT-related rate-responsive pacing during acute myocardial infarction. PACE 11:339, 1988.
31. Edelstam C, Hedman A, Nordlander R, Pehrsson SK: QT-sensing rate-responsive pacing and acute myocardial infarction: A case report. PACE 12:502, 1989.
32. Hedman A, Nordlander R: Changes in QT and Q-aT intervals induced by mental and physical stress with fixed rate and atrial triggered ventricular-inhibited cardiac pacing. PACE 11:1426, 1988.
33. Hedman A, Hjemdahl P, Nordlander R, Astrom H: Effects of mental and physical stress on central haemodynamics and cardiac sympathetic nerve activity during QT interval-sensing rate-responsive and fixed rate ventricular-inhibited pacing. Eur Heart J 11:903, 1990.
34. Boute W, Derrien Y, Wittkampf FHM: Reliability of evoked endocardial T-wave sensing in 1,500 pacemaker patients. PACE 9:948, 1986.
35. Baig MW, Boute W, Begemann M, Perrins EJ: Non-linear relation between pacing and evoked QT interval. PACE 11:753, 1988.
36. Baig MW, Wilson J, Boute W, et al: Improved pattern of rate responsiveness with dynamic slope setting for the QT-sensing pacemaker. PACE 12:311, 1989.
37. Baig MW, Green A, Wade G, et al: A randomized double-blind, crossover study of the linear and nonlinear algorithms for the QT sensing rate adaptive pacemaker. PACE 13:1802, 1990.
38. Baig W, Begemann M, Rickards A, Perrins EJ: Automatically adjusting slope setting for the QT-sensing pacemaker—initial clinical evaluation [Abstract]. PACE 10:1207, 1987.
39. Boute W, Gebhardt U, Begemann MJS: Introduction of a new generation of QT-driven rate responsive pacemakers [Abstract]. PACE 10:1208, 1987.
40. Baig MW, Boute W, Begemann M, Perrins EJ: One-year follow-up of automatic adaptation of the rate response algorithm of the QT sensing, rate adaptive pacemaker. PACE 14:1598, 1991.
41. Murdock CJ, Kelin GJ, Yee R, et al: Feasibility of long-term electrocardiographic monitoring with an implanted device for syncope diagnosis. PACE 13:1374, 1990.
42. Hedman A, Nordlander R: QT sensing rate responsive pacing compared

to fixed rate ventricular inhibited pacing: A controlled clinical study. PACE 12:374, 1989.

43. Maisch B, Langenfeld H: Rate adaptive pacing—clinical experience with three different pacing systems. PACE 9:997, 1986.

44. Maisch B, Langenfeld H, Steilner H: Clinical experiences with three different rate-adaptive pacemaker systems. Z Kardiol 75:480, 1986.

45. Zegelman M, Cieslinski G, Kreuzer J: Rate response during submaximal exercise: Comparison of three different sensors. PACE 11:1888, 1988.

46. Mehta D, Lau CP, Ward DE, Camm AJ: Comparative evaluation of chronotropic responses of QT sensing and activity sensing rate-responsive pacemakers. PACE 11:1405, 1988.

47. Lau CP, Butrous GS, Ward DE, Camm AJ: Comparison of exercise performance of six rate-adaptive right ventricular cardiac pacemakers. Am J Cardiol 63:833, 1989.

48. Sulke AN, Pipilis A, Henderson RA, et al: Comparison of the normal sinus node with seven types of rate responsive pacemaker during everyday activity. Br Heart J 64:25, 1990.

49. Bellamy CM, Roberts DH, Hughes S, Charles RG: Comparative evaluation of rate modulation in new generation evoked Q and activity sensing pacemakers. PACE 15:993, 1992.

50. Kadish AH, Weisman HF, Veltri EP, et al: Paradoxical effects of exercise on the QT interval in patients with polymorphic ventricular tachycardia receiving type Ia antiarrhythmic agents. Circulation 81:14, 1990.

51. Landman MAJ, Senden PJ, van Rooijen H, van Hemel NM: Initial clinical experience with rate adaptive cardiac pacing using two sensors simultaneously. PACE 13:1615, 1990.

52. Connelly DT, The Topaz Study Group: Initial experience with a new single chamber, dual sensor rate responsive pacemaker. PACE 16:1833, 1993.

53. van Krieken F, Perrins J, Sigmund M: Clinical results of automatic slope adaptation in a dual sensor rate responsive pacemaker. PACE 15:1815, 1992.

54. Provenier F, van Acker R, Backers J, et al: Clinical observations with a dual sensor rate-adaptive single-chamber pacemaker. PACE 15:1821, 1992.

55. Cowell R, Morris-Thurgood J, Paul V, et al: Are we being driven to two sensors? Clinical benefits of sensor cross-checking. PACE 16:1441, 1993.

56. Connelly DT, Rickards AF: Sensor combinations—which, how and why? *In* Barold SS, Mujica J (eds): New Perspectives in Cardiac Pacing 3. New York, Futura, 1993, pp 325–335.

57. Res JCJ, Boute W: A dual sensor in a rate-responsive pacemaker: The QT interval and the T wave amplitude [Abstract]. Eur Heart J 11:199, 1990.

58. Butrous GS, Lau CP, Ward DE, Camm AJ: Interference of 50-Hz alternating current on implanted rate responsive pacemakers [Abstract]. PACE 11:513, 1988.

59. Lau CP, Linker NJ, Butrous GS, et al: Myopotential interference in unipolar rate responsive pacemakers. PACE 12:1324, 1989.

60. Snoeck J, Berkhof M, Vrints C: Simultaneous bipolar pacing and sensing during EPs. J Electrocardiol 22(Suppl):224, 1989.

61. Begemann M, Boute W, Wittkampf FH. Evoked endocardial potentials in tachycardia management [Abstract]. PACE 10:608, 1987.

62. den Dulk K, Leerssen H, Vos M, et al: Applicability of the stimulus-T interval for antitachycardia pacing. PACE 14:1757, 1991.

63. Puddu PE, Torresani J: The QT-sensitive cybernetic pacemaker: A new role for an old parameter? PACE 9:108, 1986.

CHAPTER 15

EVOKED POTENTIALS AS A SENSOR FOR RATE-ADAPTIVE PACING

Igor Singer
Frank J. Callaghan

An electric stimulus of an intensity that exceeds the threshold value results in initiation of a self-propagating wave of depolarization in the myocardium. The cardiac action potentials that combine to produce this wave of myocardial activation are characterized by an initial phase of rapid depolarization, followed by a plateau phase in which the cell membrane remains in a depolarized state, and finally a phase of repolarization to the resting membrane potential. The combined electric currents generated by myocardial depolarization and repolarization in the ventricle are manifest in the surface electrocardiogram as the QRS and T waves, respectively. Wilson and colleagues[1] reported that the sum of all the vectors resulting from ventricular depolarization and repolarization were represented by the QRST integral. The amplitude and duration of the T wave (the period of repolarization) are influenced by heart rate and autonomic tone, factors that change in response to exercise.[2–6] These observations on ventricular repolarization have formed the fundamental basis for the development of rate-adaptive pacemakers that modulate pacing rate in response to changes in the QT interval.[7, 8] In addition to the influencing ventricular repolarization, exercise produces changes in myocardial depolarization that are manifest in the QRS complex of the surface electrocardiogram. The *intracardiac* ventricular electrogram during depolarization (termed the evoked response or the ventricular depolarization integral) also responds to changes in heart rate, exercise, and autonomic tone in characteristic and measurable ways.[9, 10] Because implantable pacemakers are capable of recording these electric signals using standard pacing leads, the evoked response to an artificial pacing stimulus has been developed as a rate-modulating parameter for rate-adaptive pacing. This chapter reviews the technical challenges involved in measuring the evoked response, the factors that affect this parameter, its potential diagnostic uses, and the results of clinical trials with implantable pacemakers based on this concept.

Rationale for the Use of the Evoked Response as a Rate-Modulating Parameter

The ventricular depolarization gradient has been shown to be inversely dependent on sympathetically mediated stress and directly dependent on pacing rate.[9–11] With increased sympathetic stimulation, the area under the curve inscribed by the ventricular electrogram during depolarization *decreases*.[9] Thus, a pacing system that monitored the ventricular depolarization integral should be designed to increase the pacing rate in response to a decrease in this parameter. In contrast, in the absence of sympathetic stimulation, increasing the heart rate *increases* the area under the ventricular depolarization integral. Because exercise is associated with both an increase in sympathetic stimulation (which decreases the ventricular depolarization integral) and an increase in the heart rate (which increases the ventricular depolarization integral), the net result of these offsetting effects is to maintain the ventricular depolarization integral nearly constant.[9] The contrasting effects of heart rate and sympathetic stimulation have the advantage of negative feedback, preventing an increase in heart rate from augmenting the parameter used to control the pacing rate.

More recent studies have demonstrated that the paced depolarization integral (PDI), as the ventricular depolarization integral is now called by the principal manufacturer of pacemakers using this concept, is inversely related to intraventricular conduction velocity and directly related to ventricular mass.[12, 13] Exercise results in increased sympathetic tone due to circulating and locally released catecholamines. The effect of the catecholamines is to increase myocardial contractility and sinus rate in hearts with an intact sinus mechanism and autonomic control.[14] Increases in venous return and augmentation of diastolic dimensions are also observed.[15] Increased contractility results in a more complete ventricular emptying in systole, resulting in a decreased end-systolic ventricular dimension with a consequent decrease in end-diastolic myocardial wall thickness. A decrease in wall thickness and an increase in conduction velocity may explain the observed decrease in PDI measured during exercise and during epinephrine infusion.[16, 17] Increases in pacing rate at rest result in decreases in ventricular filling time, stroke volume, and diastolic dimensions.[17–19] The resulting increase in ventricular wall thickness and decrease in conduction velocity[20] may explain the increase in PDI that is measured during pacing.[13]

THE CHALLENGE OF DETECTING THE EVOKED RESPONSE

The cardiac evoked response to a suprathreshold stimulus in the atrium or ventricle is easily recognized on the surface electrocardiogram, although it is recognized more readily with ventricular than with atrial stimulation. If *intracardiac* electrodes are used, the task of detecting and measuring the evoked response presents significant technical challenges, particularly when the stimulation electrodes are also used for sensing. These challenges are directly related to the electrochemical behavior of electrodes placed in a complex electrolyte solution such as blood, and the effect of polarization when it is used to deliver an electric current from a pacemaker output circuit. To understand how the evoked response is measured, the events that follow delivery of a pacing stimulus to the myocardium must be considered.

The interface between an electrode and the underlying myocardium can be modeled, in its simplest form, by a parallel combination of a resistor and a capacitor. The resistor is known as the Faradaic resistance, and it is dependent largely on the electrode material, surface area, and composition of the aqueous media. The capacitor is the double-layer capacitance, and it is inversely related to the effective surface area of the electrode in contact with the solution. In a practical sense, these interfacing elements represent electrode system inefficiencies in that electric energy is wasted as a consequence of these factors when the tissue is stimulated by the pacemaker.

The Faradaic resistance and the double-layer capacitance comprise a simple parallel resistor-capacitor (RC) energy storage network that is actively charged during stimulation and passively discharges during the subsequent pacemaker cycle. During stimulation, the electrically driven interface presents a temporally increasing resistance to the pacemaker. This is known as the polarization impedance, and it increases over time as the double-layer capacitance is charged by the pacemaker stimulus (see Chapter 1). Following stimulation, the electric energy stored within the double-layer capacitance must passively discharge through its parallel Faradaic resistance; this energy dissipates at a rate determined by the time

constant of the RC network, creating an exponentially decaying polarization voltage. It is this poststimulus polarization voltage that creates the challenge for detecting the cardiac evoked response.

A hypothetical ideal electrode would have zero Faradaic resistance and infinite double-layer capacitance. Such an idealized electrode would not provide electric inefficiency to the pacemaker system by the electrode interface. Since such a hypothetical electrode would store no charge at the interface with the myocardium following stimulation, there would be no poststimulus polarization voltage to obscure detection of the cardiac evoked potential. In practice, however, ideal electrodes do not exist, although there has been considerable progress in the design of pacing leads through the advent of specialized coatings and manufacturing processes employing platinum-black, carbon, iridium oxide, titanium nitride, and "Ottenization." These new electrode materials are likely to decrease polarization and enhance the ability to detect the paced depolarization integral for automatic control of pacing rate, stimulus intensity, and other programmable parameters. However, pulse generators that use PDI as a rate-modulating control parameter, when intended as replacements, must also be designed to function appropriately with leads made with older technology. Thus, pulse generators have been developed that circumvent the need for special electrode materials by using special stimulus waveforms and new methods of pacing.

Methods for Detecting PDI

To use stimulating electrodes to detect cardiac evoked responses, one must be able to stimulate the tissue and detect the resultant electric response within an interval of 200 msec or less. If measurement of atrial or ventricular *depolarization* is required, one must overcome the effects of electrode polarization within the first 10 to 20 msec following the pacing pulse. The exponentially decaying polarization voltage is often hundreds or thousands of millivolts in amplitude, and it is not possible to reliably filter these large potentials because their frequency spectra significantly overlap those of cardiac electric activity. This polarization "noise" is often three or more orders of magnitude larger than a 1-mV cardiac evoked response. Therefore, the polarization artifact must be minimized so that the signal of interest (the PDI) is not obscured. To assist in detection of the evoked response, two different electric techniques have been developed that operate to reduce polarization to amplitudes below that of the cardiac PDI.

The first technique developed to detect PDI employed special output circuitry to reduce poststimulus polarization. With this "active postcharge" technique, an initial cathodal stimulus is followed immediately by an anodal pulse. The polarity of the pulse is abruptly reversed, the integral of the current delivered in this manner is theoretically zero. Because no net charge has been delivered, there is little or no poststimulus polarization at the electrode-tissue interface. The cardiac evoked depolarization integral can, therefore, be distinguished from the noise of polarization.

The first implantable device capable of evoked response detection was designed to detect the T wave and was primarily intended to measure the QT interval as the rate-control parameter.[5] Although this method successfully detected the T wave, its polarization recovery was not sufficient to permit reliable measurement of the paced intracardiac R wave. Recent advances in the active-recharge technique[21–24] have made it possible to decrease the poststimulus polarization enough to reliably detect paced ventricular depolarizations. Accurate electronic balancing of the recharge circuitry is critical for successful detection of R waves with this technique because the circuit needs to recover from polarization almost instantaneously, and variations in electrode materials between lead manufacturers may render the system effective for one lead system but ineffective for others. One recent development[23, 24] provides for automatic adjustment of the output circuit's recharge balance by triggered stimulation into refractory tissue while adjusting the recharge until no polarization is present. Hence, rapid detection of ventricular depolarization has become possible and reliable using this active-recharge technique.

A second technique used for detection of evoked depolarization integrals in the Prism-CL pacing system (Telectronics Pacing Systems, Inc., Englewood, CO) has addressed the problem of poststimulus polarization by divorcing the stimulation electrode from the evoked response-sensing electrode and by creating an evoked response amplifier and measurement circuit that is separate from that used for normal alert-period sensing.[9, 10, 11, 25, 26] This technique is passive in that additional energy is not consumed in the act of generating a recharge pulse, and the only requirement imposed by the technique is that a bipolar lead must be used with the pacing system.[9] Considering that the pacemaker case provides an additional electrode, a three-electrode system is used to combine the features of unipolar and bipolar configurations. As shown in Figure 15–1, alert-period sensing is differential bipolar, using the remote pacemaker case as the reference electrode to a common dual-input difference amplifier. During stimulation, a unipolar cathodal stimulus is emitted between the tip electrode of the lead and the pulse generator case, and this is immediately followed by a temporary 10-msec short circuit of the pacemaker's output circuit. This "charge dump" operation permits rapid, passive discharge of the pulse generator's coupling capacitor and creates anodic currents at the stimulating electrode that serve to reduce the electrode polarization afterpotential. This reduction in polarization is sufficient to permit high-fidelity evoked response recordings, including depolarization of the atrium and the ventricle, from the proximal ring electrode of the bipolar lead using a unipolar single-ended amplifier referenced to the pacemaker case.[9, 26] This technique has been effective with stimulus intensities of up to 5 mA and 1 msec (Fig. 15–2).

Immediately following charge dump, an evoked response window (lasting up to 125 msec) occurs during which the paced cardiac depolarization is measured. Since the ring electrode is not used for stimulation, it is not polarized by the stimulus, and cathodal polarization potentials occurring at the tip electrode appear as far-field signals and are dramatically reduced in amplitude. Also, the spatial separation between the stimulating and recording electrodes creates a physiologic propagation delay between the initial site of stimulation in the myocardium and the arrival of the excitation wavefront at the ring electrode; this delay creates additional time during which the electrodes may dissipate the afterpotential. When electronically integrated (Fig. 15–3) the ventricular gradient

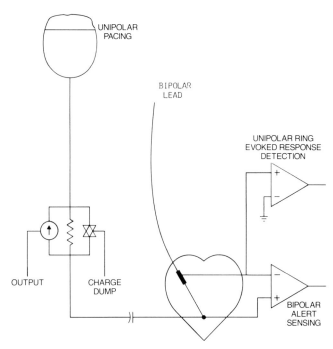

FIGURE 15–1. Schematic diagram of the evoked response detection method. Pacing is unipolar with charge dump, and alert period sensing is bipolar. Following charge dump, the unipolar ventricular evoked response is amplified and electronically integrated from the ring electrode. (From Callaghan FJ, Vollmann W, Livingston AR, et al: The ventricular depolarization gradient: Effects of exercise, pacing rate, epinephrine, and intrinsic heart rate control on the right ventricular evoked response. PACE 12[1]: 1115, 1989.)

is obtained, the peak negative value of which provides a measure of activation time dispersion known as the depolarization gradient.[1, 9]

Clinical Implementation of the PDI Concept for Rate-Adaptive Pacing

Prism-CL model 450A ventricular pacemaker (Telectronics Pacing Systems) was designed to provide rate-adaptive pacing based on the PDI concept.[27] A schematic for the implementation of this pacemaker is shown in Figure 15–1. The Prism-CL 450A pacemaker incorporated two innovative concepts: (1) closed-loop rate-adaptive pacing based on continuous analysis of PDI, and (2) automatic output regulation.[27]

Rate response is based on the PDI measurement. Because the effects of exercise on PDI are opposite those that occur with an increase in pacing rate, a physiologic negative feedback mechanism is established, and the heart rate is adjusted continuously to maintain a constant value of the PDI. The PDI was also synonymously termed the rate-control parameter (RCP) in this pacemaker. A constant target value of RCP is maintained that is analogous to the set point of any control system. Target RCP is initially established by acquiring and averaging 20 paced beat measurements when the pacemaker is implanted and the system has been turned on. Subsequently, the RCP measurement is obtained every fourth beat and compared with the target RCP. If the measured RCP is less than the target RCP, the pacing rate is increased. If

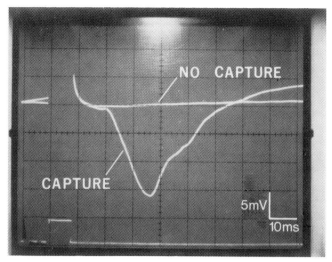

FIGURE 15–2. Fidelity of the evoked response detection method. The ability to quickly recover from poststimulus electrode polarization is illustrated in this dual-sweep oscilloscope record. The "capture" tracing shows the entire paced ventricular depolarization evoked with a 5 mA/1 msec stimulus. The "no capture" tracing demonstrates system recovery (at the same output intensity) without an evoked R wave, obtained by pacing into refractory tissue. The lower channel is a charge dump marker.

measured RCP is greater than the target RCP, the pacing rate is decreased (Fig. 15–4).

RCP drifts are possible over time owing to physiologic changes such as lead maturation and the influence of antiarrhythmic drugs. The algorithm is designed to respond to these changes by compensating for gradual drifts, producing minimal effects on the exercise response. This compensation is achieved by adjusting the target RCP in the direction of the long-term drifts in the measured RCP values.

The calibration algorithm involves two parameters: (1) the calibration register, and (2) the target RCP. After each meas-

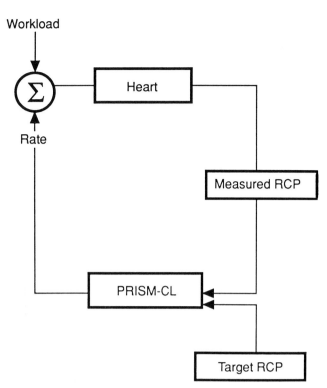

FIGURE 15–4. Closed-loop rate modulation is based on the opposing effects of workload and heart rate on the rate control parameter (RCP), so that measured RCP is more continuously compared to the *target* RCP, and heart rate is adjusted until the measured RCP is equal to the target RCP.

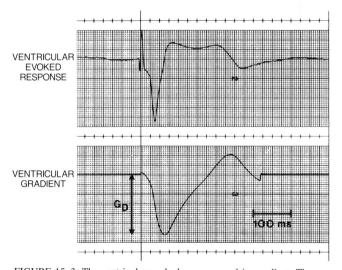

FIGURE 15–3. The ventricular evoked response and its gradient. The gradient is generated with an electronic integrator. The ventricular depolarization gradient (GD) is the peak negative amplitude of the integral and represents the area under the evoked R wave. (From Callaghan FJ, Vollmann W, Livingston AR, et al: The ventricular depolarization gradient: Effects of exercise, pacing rate, epinephrine, and intrinsic heart rate control on the right ventricular evoked response. PACE 12[1]: 1115, 1989.)

ured value of the RCP (every fourth beat) the calibration register is adjusted either upward or downward by a small numerical value, which is determined by the programmable calibration speed (slow, medium, or fast). When the calibration register exceeds the target RCP, the target RCP is increased by approximately 3%. Conversely, when the calibration register is less than the target RCP, the target RCP is decreased by approximately 3%. Because the calibration register is adjusted in small increments after each RCP measurement, many adjustments in the same direction are required to change the target RCP. Transient changes in the measured RCP have little effect on the target RCP, although they cause immediate changes in pacing rate, resulting in chronotropic response. The fast calibration speed can accommodate drifts as fast as 20% per hour by allowing adjustments in the target RCP as frequently as every 8.5 minutes. Medium and slow speeds can track drifts of 15% or 10%, with target RCP changes allowed every 11.5 or 17 minutes, respectively.

During periods of prolonged continuous exercise, the target RCP adjusts to a lower value. This feature was designed to prevent prolonged periods of elevated pacing rate. When the patient rests, the rate returns to the minimum rate. To reestablish the baseline target RCP the minimum rate of calibration is much faster than that occurring during rate response for all calibration speeds. Therefore, a brief rest period adjusts the target RCP so that the high rates can be achieved again with repeat exercise effort.

AUTOMATIC OUTPUT REGULATION

Automatic output regulation consists of automatic capture verification and threshold search, which together provide au-

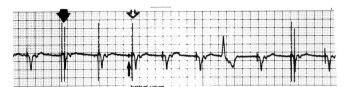

FIGURE 15–5. An example of a threshold test. A noncaptured second and third beat *(small black arrow)* is followed by a backup pulse *(white open arrow)* until the output is augmented sufficiently to regain capture. Double vertical lines represent a "signature" marking the beginning and end of the test *(large black arrow)*. (From Singer I: Paced depolarization integral. *In* Ryden L, Sutton R, Bourgeois I, [eds]: Individual Clinical Descriptions of Different Sensor-Driven Systems. Mt Kisco; Futura, NY, 1993.)

tomatic regulation of the output pulse from the pulse generator. The purpose of the capture verification algorithm is to check for ventricular capture automatically following a paced beat. If loss of capture is detected, the pacemaker output is automatically adjusted on a beat-by-beat basis until capture is regained. The safety margin is then added to the measured threshold. To ensure capture, particularly in a pacemaker-dependent patient, a back-up pulse of 10 mA and 1 msec in duration is issued by the pacemaker when a loss of capture is detected. In addition, an automatic threshold search occurs approximately every 12 hours (Fig. 15–5). If the capture threshold plus the pacing safety output exceed the maximum output for PDI detection (5 mA and 1 msec), stat-set pacing is initiated (10 mA and 1 msec), and the pacemaker reverts to VVI pacing. This backup function was provided as a safety mechanism to ensure myocardial capture for pacemaker-dependent patients.

Clinical Experience with Prism-CL Model 450A Pacemaker

Clinical trials of the Prism-CL 450A pacemaker began in August, 1988 in Europe and were extended to the United States and Canada subsequently. A total of 152 patients were enrolled in phases I and II of the clinical trial. The initial experience with the ventricular rate-modulated pacemaker has already been reported.[27–30] Patient characteristics are summarized in Table 15–1. The primary indication for pacemaker implantation in these 152 patients was sick sinus syndrome, which was associated with symptomatic bradyar-

rhythmias in 66% of patients and atrioventricular block in 34%. The mean implant duration was 23 months at the time of the published reports. However, in 83% of the patients the implant duration had been longer than 1 year when the clinical trial ended (October, 1990). Ninety-two percent of the patients were alive as of June 15, 1991, the date of the last compiled clinical report, 12 patients having died during the course of the study. The causes of death were congestive heart failure (three patients), pulmonary emboli unrelated to the pacemaker lead (one patient), myocardial infarction (one patient), noncardiac causes (three patients), and unwitnessed death (four patients). None of these unwitnessed deaths were judged by the investigators to be related to the function of the pacemaker.

The pacemaker was explanted in five patients. The reasons for explantation were pocket erosion (one patient), oversensing that could not be corrected by reprogramming (one patient), pacemaker syndrome (one patient), inappropriately high pacing rates in recumbent position (one patient), and repeated stat-set behavior that could not be corrected by reprogramming in one patient.

CHRONOTROPIC RESPONSE TO EXERCISE

All phase I patients receiving the Telectronics 450A pacing system underwent treadmill testing within 1 month of the implant (36 patients). Physiologic rate response was observed in all patients. The paced heart rate increased from 75 ± 9 ppm at the baseline to 127 ± 14 ppm at peak exercise ($p < .0001$). Maximum achievable heart rate was limited by the programmed upper rate limit. An anticipatory rate increase prior to the onset of exercise (defined as an initial rate response due to anticipation of exercise) was noted in 61% of patients. This resulted in a mean paced heart rate increase of 14 ppm prior to the onset of exercise.

RESPONSE TO STRESS AND MENTAL ACTIVITY

PDI response to epinephrine and anticipation of exercise in dogs with Prism-CL pacemaker implants was noted by Callaghan and colleagues.[9] These investigators postulated that the PDI response was modulated by circulatory epinephrine. Based on this initial observation, Singer and associates[27–30] postulated that similar effects may occur in response to mental stress in human subjects with Prism-CL pacemaker implants. Eight patients with Prism-CL pacemakers were tested using a mental stress protocol.[29, 30] Heart rate and blood pressure were continuously recorded during the test. All patients were studied while in the supine position, in a quiet environment in the electrophysiology laboratory. The protocol consisted of 10 stages: baseline recording (stage 1), difficult arithmetic tasks (stages 2 to 6), verbalization of a stressful event (stage 7), talking about a positive life event (stage 8), thinking only about a positive life event without talking (stage 9), and reassurance (stage 10). Stages 8 and 9 were designed to exclude motor activity (talking) from mental stress as a causative factor of heart rate response. The results are shown in Figure 15–6. Mental stress was associated with an increase in paced heart rate. In response to "positive thinking" and reassurance, the paced heart rate returned to the baseline values.

Similar results have also been reported by Paul and col-

TABLE 15–1. **PATIENT CHARACTERISTICS (N = 152)**

Age	70 + 10 years (47–91 years)
Sex	94 M, 58 F
LVEF*	0.54 + 0.17 (0.12–0.80)
Follow-up (mean)	23 months
NYHA Class†	
Class I	27%
Class II	49%
Class III	20%
Class IV	4%

*Left ventricular ejection fraction, reported in 22 patients.
†NYHA = New York Heart Association functional class for heart failure.
From Singer I: Evoked potentials for rate-adaptive pacing. *In* Benditt DG (ed): Rate-Adaptive Cardiac Pacing: Current Technologies and Clinical Applications. Cambridge, MA, Blackwell Scientific Publications, 1992. Reprinted by permission of Blackwell Scientific Publications, Inc.

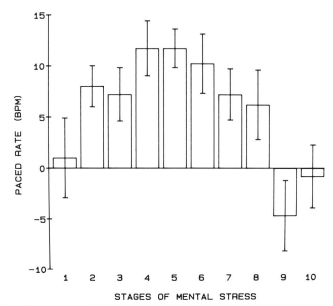

FIGURE 15–6. Heart rate response to mental stress. Stages of mental stress protocol 1–10 (abscissa) and paced heart rate, adjusted to baseline pacing rate (ordinate). Changes in peak heart rate are significant ($p < .05$, ANOVA). Refer to text for details. (From Singer I, Brennan AF, Steinhaus B, et al: Effects of stress and beta₁ blockade on the ventricular depolarization gradient of the rate modulating pacemaker. PACE 14:460, 1991.)

leagues[28] using a different mental stress protocol. The results of these two studies suggest that circulating catecholamines, which are presumably increased during mental stress, modulate PDI either directly or indirectly.

Effect of Postural Changes on Heart Rate

Paul and colleagues[28] studied paced heart rate responses to head-up tilt.[28] When patients were tilted from the standing to the supine position, the paced heart rate increased. However, when the baseline pacing rate was increased, prompt deceleration in heart rate occurred when patients were tilted from the supine to the standing position. The mechanism underlying these physiologically paradoxical effects has not been fully elucidated. However, it is likely that alteration in the right ventricular preload and wall stress have a direct effect on PDI. These effects may be clinically undesirable, particularly in patients with postural syncope.

Effect of Beta-1 Selective Antagonist (Esmolol) on PDI

The foregoing discussion has suggested that PDI may be directly modulated by circulating or locally released catecholamines. It would be anticipated, therefore, that beta-1 selective blockade would reverse or prevent catecholamine-induced changes on PDI and in paced heart rate response. With this hypothesis in mind, we set out to demonstrate that mental stress effects on paced heart rate, and by implication on PDI, could be blocked by a beta-1 selective blocker (esmolol).[30] Six patients were studied using the previously de-

scribed mental stress protocol.[30] Esmolol was administered as an intravenous bolus (15 μg/kg) given over 1 minute. This resulted in an increase in paced heart rate from 70 ± 7 to 80 ± 6 ppm ($p < .05$) with no significant alteration in diastolic or systolic blood pressure. During esmolol infusion (75 to 125 μg/kg/min) the paced heart rate increased from 69 ± 5 to 84 ± 11 ppm ($p < .05$). Systolic and diastolic blood pressures did not change significantly during the continuous infusion of esmolol. The mental stress test was administered to three patients prior to the esmolol infusion, and subsequently the protocol was repeated during the infusion. A reverse sequence was followed in three other patients. This design was used to eliminate a potential bias due to the learning process. The heart rate response was blunted in the presence of esmolol. However, an unexpected increase in heart rate was observed in response to the esmolol bolus and infusion, which could not be predicted from the original hypothesis that epinephrine alone was responsible for PDI modulation. These data suggested that esmolol may have a direct effect on PDI (i.e., that it causes a decrease in PDI independent of its beta₁-blocking properties and, further, that the direct effect blunts the heart rate response to mental stress.[30]

This hypothesis was further tested in the animal laboratory.[30] Paced depolarization gradient waveforms were studied at fixed pacing rates during a control saline infusion and during bolus infusion of esmolol in dogs. Figure 15–7 shows

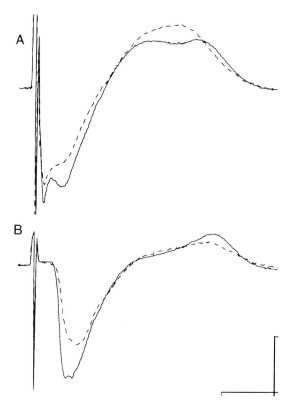

FIGURE 15–7. Evoked potential recording during control *(solid lines)* and during infusion of esmolol *(broken lines)* from the catheter tip *(A)* and catheter ring *(B)*. Pacing stimulus can be seen as the first fast deflection from the baseline. Calibration bars of 50 msec and 15 mV. Note a decrease in paced depolarization integral (PDI) in response to esmolol infusion. (From Singer I, Brennan AF, Steinhaus B, et al. Effects of stress and beta₁ blockade on the ventricular depolarization gradient of the rate modulating pacemaker. PACE 14:460, 1991.)

the unipolar waveform from the tip electrode (*A*) and from the ring electrode (*B*) of a bipolar pacing catheter in the right ventricular apex of the dog. Esmolol infusion reduced the PDI recorded from the tip and ring electrodes, confirming a direct effect of esmolol on PDI. It is interesting to note, however, that propranolol (a nonselective beta-adrenergic antagonist) did not affect PDI in a similar manner. It is hypothesized that myocardial contractility or alteration in right ventricular preload may be the mechanism producing the esmolol effect. The reasons for differences in effect of esmolol and propanolol are not understood at present.

Effects of Antiarrhythmic Drugs on Paced Depolarization Integral

Because PDI is dependent on conduction velocity, antiarrhythmic drugs may be expected to influence PDI. For example, it may be anticipated that class 1 or class 3 drugs will decrease conduction velocity, thereby increasing PDI and causing a decrease in the pacing rate of a device controlled by this parameter. However, since the calibration mechanism is designed to adjust the target RCP in the direction of the drift in RCP, it is likely that drugs administered by the enteral route will result in a gradual increase in serum concentrations. In contrast, rapid infusions of antiarrhythmic drugs may have an effect that overwhelms the calibration adaptation algorithm.

Antiarrhythmic drugs may affect PDI by altering conduction velocity or by directly affecting the right ventricular preload in a manner analogous to that seen with esmolol or tilt table testing. Since the effect of antiarrhythmic drugs on PDI has not been systematically studied, these remarks are based on theoretical considerations only. It is possible, then, that PDI may be potentially useful for continuous measurement of drug concentrations in patients with implanted pacemakers or antiarrhythmic drug infusion systems.

Limitations of the Prism-Cl 450A Pacemaker

Although the Prism-CL 450A pacemaker performed generally as anticipated during the clinical trial, some limitations were recognized. These were related to hardware constraints and to biologic variability that was unanticipated from the initial and preliminary animal data. An intrinsic limitation of PDI as a sensor is the requirement for delivery of a pacing pulse to measure the evoked response. Because many patients require pacing only intermittently, delivery of a VVI pacing pulse at a rate slightly faster than the intrinsic heart rate may be associated with uncomfortable sensations related to the transient loss of AV synchrony. The most troubling problems encountered in the clinical trial of the Prism-CL pacing system were related to automatic output regulation. In the initial software design (software 20.5) a 60-msec window was available for capture recognition. In some patients this window was too short for the software to recognize the paced depolarization. Inappropriate output augmentation occurred occasionally owing to pseudofusion beats, which was followed by an inappropriate increase in the intensity of the

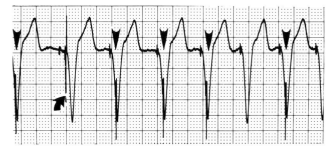

FIGURE 15–8. An example of an appropriate classification of a noncaptured beat (second beat) followed by appropriate output augmentation *(curved arrow)* and a false-negative classification resulting in inappropriate output augmentation (first, third, fourth, fifth, seventh beats). Note that despite ventricular capture the beats were classified as noncaptured beats, and backup pulses were issued *(arrowheads)*. Augmentation of output eventually results in a *stat-set*. (From Singer I: Evoked potentials for rate-adaptive pacing. *In* Benditt DG (ed): Rate-Adaptive Cardiac Pacing: Current Technologies and Clinical Application. Cambridge, MA, Blackwell Scientific Publications, 1993. Reprinted by permission of Blackwell Scientific Publications, Inc.)

output pulse. When the upper safety limit was reached (5 mA and 1 msec), stat-set occurred with automatic reprogramming to the VVI mode (disabling rate-adaptive pacing) at the maximum stimulus output (10 mA and 1 msec) (Fig. 15–8). This problem was partially eliminated by extending the time window for capture verification to 75 msec (software version 20.6). This software modification helped to decrease the number of patients with false-negative capture verifications but did not completely eliminate the problem (Table 15–2). In most patients, the automatic capture verification threshold-tracking algorithm functioned appropriately (see Fig. 15–5).

Yet another cause of stat-set behavior resulted from low measured RCP values. Because of the limitation of the hardware design, RCP values below 160 μV-seconds could not be reliably measured. Because the pacemaker was designed to be "safe," if the RCP value could not be measured consistently, stat-set at the maximum output was instituted to protect the patient from loss of capture. In other words, rate response and automatic output regulation were sacrificed in the interest of preserving myocardial capture. These limitations notwithstanding, in the majority of patients, the algorithm performed reliably, and physiologic rate response was satisfactory. Based on the most recent review of the clinical data, in the majority of patients both rate response and automatic threshold function were turned on (see Table 15–2).

TABLE 15–2. **PERCENTAGE OF PRISM-CL PATIENTS WITH RATE RESPONSE AND AUTO THRESHOLD ALGORITHMS ENABLED**

Software version	20.5	20.6
Rate response (RR)	82%	86%
Auto threshold (AT)	77%	93%
RR and AT	55%	70%
Stat-Set* (% of patient visits)	25%	14%

*See text for discussion.
From Singer I: Evoked potentials for rate-adaptive pacing. *In* Benditt DG (ed): Rate-Adaptive Cardiac Pacing: Current Technologies and Clinical Applications. Cambridge, MA, Blackwell Scientific Publications, 1992. Reprinted by permission of Blackwell Scientific Publications, Inc.

Future Applications of PDI Technology

Based on the clinical experience gathered during the Prism-CL 450A clinical trial, a number of improvements were implemented in the next generation of VVIR pacemakers based on the PDI concept. The first of these was an extension of the time window required to verify capture. Based on the available data, it appears that this window may need to be extended in some patients to as long as 125 msec, or possibly longer, following delivery of the pacing pulse. The second requirement may be to extend the range for paced depolarization gradient measurement below 160 μV-seconds.

Future developments may allow unipolar pacing leads to be used for PDI-controlled rate-adaptive pacing. In this application, polarization artifact due to the pacing stimulus must be minimized to allow accurate PDI recording from the same electrode used for stimulation. A triphasic stimulus pulse and an automatic balancing algorithm, which uses a test stimulus in the refractory period to balance the polarization artifact, has been described.[24, 31] This type of system may also be used for automatic threshold verification and tracking. It is expected that with this detection algorithm patient-to-patient variability in the capture time window, which was seen in the Prism-CL pacemaker trial, may not be an issue. New hardware designs combined with this development may allow a greater range of measurements for RCP values. A dual-chamber rate-adaptive pacemaker based on the PDI concept has also been considered. Atrial capture detection has been examined by Livingston and colleagues.[26] The early data suggest that a similar concept may be applicable in the atrium, although the data are so far only preliminary.

The PDI sensor and the minute-volume ventilation sensor have been combined in another VVIR pacemaker (Sentri [Telectronics Pacing Systems]) that is undergoing phase I clinical trials in Europe. The rationale for combining the two sensors is to maximize the benefits of each sensor while minimizing the disadvantages of both. For example, an early rapid response of the PDI sensor in anticipation of exercise or emotional stress may have an advantage over the minute-volume ventilation sensor in these situations. On the other hand, the minute ventilation sensor (estimated by transthoracic impedance) responds more slowly and may be used to modulate the paced response during continuous exercise. The problem of deciding which of the two competing sensors should prevail at any one time is a formidable one. Mediation between the two competing sensor inputs is somewhat empiric. The use of two sensors, therefore, may provide some theoretical benefits but still must be proved in the clinical environment. The differences between the newest generation of pacemaker (Sentri) and the Prism-CL 450A are detailed in Table 15–3.

Future research studies may identify additional factors that affect PDI. Further studies should focus on elucidating the effects on PDI of lead maturation, cardioactive drugs, hemodynamic perturbations, changes in autonomic tone, antiarrhythmic drugs, and ischemia. PDI may also find additional clinical applications. Because PDI is influenced by conduction velocity, it may also prove useful in noninvasive antiarrhythmic drug monitoring or in detection of ischemia. Be-

TABLE 15–3. COMPARISON OF PDI SENTRI MODEL 1210 AND PRISM-CL 450A PULSE GENERATORS

SENTRI	PRISM-CL
Unipolar pacing pulse delivered through the tip and PDI sensed from the tip (overcomes latency time and variability due to ring motion)	Unipolar pacing pulse delivered to the tip electrode and PDI sensed from the ring
Bandpass filter starts at 16-Hz (eliminates the effect of the T-wave)	Bandpass starting at 1.5 Hz for measurement of PDI
Dynamic range is greatly expanded for measurement of PDI	Limited dynamic range for measurement of PDI
Integrator is continued to the zero-crossing point	Integrator of the negative portion of the PDI is continued for a preset period, independent of the zero-crossing point
Overdrive after a sensed intrinsic QRS is 10 ppm	Overdrive after a sensed intrinsic is 50 ms
Overdrive after non-capture is 25 ppm, then 40 ppm, then 50 ppm	Overdrive after non-capture: the cycle shortens by 50 msec, then 70 msec, then 125 msec
Capture threshold is checked every 36 hours	Capture threshold is checked every 12 hours
Capture verification is every fourth paced beat	Capture verification is continuous
The second and third pulses with loss of capture have back-up pulses	Every pulse with loss of capture has a back-up pulse

From Singer I: Evoked potentials for rate-adaptive pacing. *In* Benditt DG (ed): Rate-Adaptive Cardiac Pacing: Current Technologies and Clinical Applications. Cambridge, MA, Blackwell Scientific Publications, 1992. Reprinted by permission of Blackwell Scientific Publications, Inc.

cause myocardial ischemia profoundly influences conduction velocity and repolarization, it may have a significant and readily detectable effect on PDI. One limitation of this application is that measurement of the right ventricular PDI during ischemia may not reflect alterations in PDI due to left ventricular myocardial ischemia. This application clearly needs further clinical study. Anecdotal observations also suggest that profound alterations in PDI may occur with the onset of ventricular tachycardia or ventricular fibrillation. These observations merit further study, because if confirmed, this application may be useful in future implantable cardioverter defibrillator (ICD) devices to provide hemodynamic monitoring.

Overview

PDI is a parameter that is suitable for automatic rate modulation and automatic threshold tracking. This rate-modulating sensor uses standard pacing leads but requires low-polarization electrodes. Despite the potential advantages of this rate-control parameter, the technical challenges encountered during early clinical trials of pacemakers based on PDI have suggested that these devices may not provide predictable rate modulation in all individuals. In addition, the clinical trials of these devices have suggested that automatic output regulation is a complex technologic challenge. Whether this parameter will be developed and marketed in the United States remains to be determined. Further research should focus on the use of PDI for automatic dual-chamber rate-adaptive pacemakers and other potential applications.

REFERENCES

1. Wilson F, Macleod AG, Barker P, et al: The determination and the significance of the areas of the ventricular deflections of the electrocardiogram. Am Heart J 10:46, 1934.
2. Rickards AT, Norman J: Relation between QT interval and heart rate: New design of a physiologically-adaptive cardiac pacemaker. Br Heart J 45:56, 1981.
3. Oda E: Changes in QT interval during exercise testing in patients with VVI pacemakers. PACE 9:36, 1986.
4. Milne JR, Ward DE, Spurrell RAJ, Camm AJ: The ventricular paced QT interval—the effects of rate and exercise. PACE 5:352, 1982.
5. Donaldson PM, Rickards AT: The ventricular endocardial paced evoked response. PACE 6(2):253, 1983.
6. Boute W, Wittkampf FHM: Evoked intracardiac signals: Detection morphology and their use in pacemakers. PACE 10:650, 1987.
7. Fananapazir L, Rademaker M, Bennett DH: Reliability of the evoked response in determining the paced ventricular rate and performance of the QT or rate responsive (TX) pacemaker. PACE 8:701, 1985.
8. Baig MW, Perrins EJ: A reappraisal of the relationship between the evoked QT-interval and ventricular pacing rate. PACE 10:1029, 1987.
9. Callaghan FJ, Vollmann W, Livingston AR, et al: The ventricular depolarization gradient: Effects of exercise, pacing rate, epinephrine, and intrinsic heart rate control on the right ventricular evoked response. PACE 12(1):1115, 1989.
10. Callaghan FJ, Livingston AR, Camerlo J, et al: Ventricular activation as the basis for closed-loop rate adaptive pacing. Proceedings of the Association for the Advancement of Medical Instrumentation, 23rd Annual Scientific Sessions, Washington, DC, 1988.
11. Callaghan FJ: Automatic functions in cardiac pacing: Optimization of device and pacing therapy. IEEE Eng Biol Magazine 9(2):28, 1990.
12. Plosney RA: A contemporary view of the ventricular gradient of Wilson. J Electrophysiol 12:337, 1979.
13. Steinhaus BM, Nappholz TA: The information content of the cardiac electrogram at the stimulus site. Proceedings of the 12th Annual Conference of the IEEE Engineering in Medicine Biology Society, 1990, pp 607–609.
14. Rushmer RF, Smith OA KR, Lasher EP: Neural mechanisms of cardiac control during exertion. Physiol Rev 40:27, 1990.
15. Sedney MI, Weyers E, Van Der Wall E, et al: Short-term and long-term changes of left ventricular volumes during rate adaptive and single-rate pacing. PACE 12:1863, 1989.
16. Seibens AA, Hoffman BF, Enson Y, et al: Effects of 1-epinephrine and 1-norepinephrine on cardiac excitability. Am J Physiol 175:1, 1953.
17. Wallace AG, Sarnoff SJ: Effects of cardiac sympathetic nerve stimulation on conduction in the heart. Circ Res 14:86, 1964.
18. Ross J Jr, Linhart JW, Braunwald E: Effects of changing heart rate in man by electrical stimulation of the right atrium. Circulation 32:549, 1965.
19. Benchimol A, Li Y, Diamond EG: Cardiovascular dynamics in complete heart block at various heart rates. Circulation 30:542, 1964.
20. Viersma JW, Bouman LN, Mater M: Frequency, conduction velocity, and rate of depolarization in rabbit auricles. Nature 217:1176, 1968.
21. Boute W, Candelon B, Wittkampf FHM: Characterization of the endocardial evoked potentials. Clin Prog Electrophysiol Pacing 4:47, 1986.
22. Baig W, Boute W, Wilson J, et al: Use of the paced evoked response in the determination of pacing threshold. PACE 11:822, 1988.
23. Nappholz TA, Whigham R, Hansen J, et al: Automatic detection of atrial and ventricular capture. Clin Prog Electrophysiol Pacing 4:46, 1986.
24. Curtis AB, Vance F, Shifrin K: Diminution of the stimulated bipolar electrogram at stimulus amplitudes above threshold. PACE 12:683, 1989.
25. Byrd CL, Livingston AR, Callaghan FJ, et al: A special circuit designed for high fidelity ventricular evoked response measurement using a standard bipolar lead. PACE 11(4):505, 1988.
26. Livingston AR, Callaghan FJ, Byrd CL, et al: Atrial capture detection with endocardial electrodes. PACE 11(11):1770, 1988.
27. Singer I, Olash J, Brennan A, et al: Initial clinical experience with a rate-responsive pacemaker. PACE 12:1458, 1989.
28. Paul V, Garratt C, Ward DE, Camm AJ: Closed loop control of rate adaptive pacing: Clinical assessment of a system analyzing the ventricular depolarization gradient. PACE 12:1896, 1989.
29. Singer I, Camm J, Brown R, et al: Results with Prism-CL rate modulating pacemaker [Abstract]. RMB 12:17, 1990.
30. Singer I, Brennan AF, Steinhaus B, et al: Effects of stress and beta₁-blockade on the ventricular depolarization gradient of the rate modulating pacemaker. PACE 14:460, 1991.
31. Curtis AB, Vance F, Miller-Shifrin K: Characteristic variation in evoked potential amplitude with changes in pacing stimulus strength. Am J Cardiol 66:416, 1990.

CHAPTER 16

ACCELEROMETERS

Eckhard Alt
Jay O. Millerhagen
Jan-Pieter Heemels

An accelerometer is a sensor designed to measure acceleration, defined as the rate of change in velocity. Accelerometers have widespread applications when accuracy in motion detection is important. Extremely sensitive accelerometers are used for navigational equipment in the aerospace industry. Other applications include sensors in automotive active-suspension systems, antilocking braking systems, and airbag deployment mechanisms.[1]

Accelerometers are ideally suited for pacemakers because they are compact and highly reliable and produce a sensor signal capable of being matched to body motion. This chapter introduces the accelerometer concept and discusses the design of these sensors for application in rate-adaptive cardiac pacemakers. In addition, the performance of the sensor in its early clinical applications is discussed.

Basic Concept of Accelerometers

Activity has achieved wide clinical acceptance as the primary rate-controlling parameter. More than 300,000 rate-adaptive pacemakers controlled by body activity have been implanted since the first implant was performed in 1984. Although body activity constitutes a nonphysiologic parameter, activity-based pacemakers are theoretically and operationally simple and do not require a special sensor outside the pulse generator can. They work with virtually any type of pacing lead, have excellent long-term stability, and are highly reliable. Activity-guided pacemakers are easy to implant and, in general, react promptly to the start and end of physical exercise. The first activity sensors were piezoelectric crystals that responded mostly to the frequency of vibrations that were transmitted to the pulse generator.

In 1987 the possibility of using acceleration for pacing rate control was reported for the first time.[2, 3, 5] In an accelerometer-based pacemaker, the changes in movement of the body are detected by means of a miniature accelerometer situated on the hybrid electronic circuitry of the pulse generator. Physiologic studies have shown that rhythmic body motions, such as walking and riding a bicycle, fall within a narrow frequency range, typically 1 to 4 Hz,[5-8] in which accelerometers are most sensitive.

Measurement of Acceleration

Accelerometer technology makes use of either piezoelectric or piezoresistive material properties. The piezoelectric effect was discovered and researched using natural crystals, such as tourmalines and quartz, by the Curie brothers more than 100 years ago. Today piezoceramic materials with several characteristic properties are produced artificially. When a mechanical force is applied along the mechanical axis of a piezoelectric element, the shape of the element changes slightly, generating a voltage proportional to the force applied along the electric axis (Fig. 16–1). Similarly, application of a mechanical force on some materials with piezoresistive properties results in proportional changes in resistance of the material. These physical characteristics can be applied in the construction of mechanical-electric converters.

The main difference between an accelerometer and a piezoelectric crystal sensor that measures vibration is in the actual mass that, on activity, deforms the piezoelectric or piezoresistive material. This is referred to as the coupling mass. In the case of the vibration-measuring device, the crystal is bonded to the inside of the pulse generator can (Fig. 16–2). The coupling mass is the body tissue in close proximity to the sensor, which actually exerts a force on the pulse generator can during activity. This mass, consisting of the connective tissue and muscles surrounding the pacemaker, may vary considerably among patients. Therefore, variation in rate response from patient to patient for the same level of

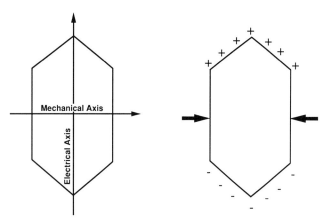

FIGURE 16–1. Piezoelectric effect. Pressure applied along the mechanical axis of materials with piezoelectric properties causes a voltage to be generated along the electric axis of the material.

activity can be expected from the vibrational piezoelectric crystal sensor.

GENERAL PRINCIPLES OF ACCELEROMETERS

In accelerometers the coupling mass is a small seismic mass, typically weighing less than 100 mg, suspended on one or more levers (Fig. 16–3). The structure is mechanically insulated from the pulse generator can. On acceleration, this mass deflects the lever by an amount that is proportional to the change in velocity and the direction of acceleration. In accelerometers this deflection can be translated into an electric signal by piezoelectric or piezoresistive material applied to the suspension levers. Because the pulse generator moves with the patient, the accelerometer detects acceleration or deceleration associated with body motion.

The main advantage can be found in the fact that the seismic mass of the accelerometer is constant. Equal acceleration forces induce equal sensor signals independent of the tissue mass surrounding the pacemaker or the physical properties of the individual, such as weight and height. This may be an improvement over the conventional piezoelectric crystal sensors because the constant coupling mass of the accelerometer provides a consistent and predictable rate response.

This concept can be rephrased using Newton's second law of motion:

$$F = m \cdot a$$

where m is the seismic (coupling) mass of the device and F is the force applied to the coupling mass as a result of body

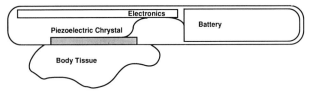

FIGURE 16–2. The piezoelectric sensor is bonded to the inside surface of the pacemaker case. Vibration is sensed through tissue contact. The mechanical forces are transmitted by the surrounding connective tissue, fatty tissue, and muscles. The extent of contact and the coupling mass of the mechanical forces can vary considerably.

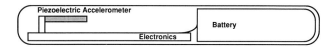

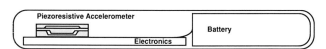

FIGURE 16–3. The accelerometer is mounted on the pacemaker's hybrid circuitry. The seismic mass of the accelerometer is fixed. Therefore, measured accelerations are independent of surrounding tissue and patient physical properties.

acceleration a. Thus, the force acting on the coupling mass and hence on the suspension system depends only on the coupling mass and the acceleration being applied to the pulse generator.

POTENTIAL CLINICAL BENEFITS

Although algorithms for a conventional piezoelectric crystal sensor bonded to the pacemaker housing can take into account both the frequency and the magnitude of the acceleration signal, they are not fully effective unless the coupling mass remains constant. As a result, nominal rate response parameters for conventional activity devices may not be appropriate for many patients. Since accelerometers have a constant coupling mass that is consistent for all devices, nominal parameter settings may provide appropriate rate response for many patients.[9] Studies some years ago showed that, regardless of age, weight, and physical condition, normal volunteers and pacemaker patients produced similar acceleration signals on performing the same kind of exercise.[5, 6]

In addition, the accelerometer sensor may be able to detect smaller changes in activity levels than a conventional vibration sensor. Thus, this improved resolution may provide a more gradual increase in pacing rate that is more proportional to the exercise workload.

Accelerometer-based pacing has currently been introduced by two manufacturers. Cardiac Pacemakers, Inc. (CPI; St. Paul, MN) uses a piezoresistive accelerometer in the Excel VR, Vigor DR, and Vigor SR pacemakers. Intermedics, Inc. (Freeport, TX) uses a piezoelectric type of accelerometer in the Dash and Relay devices.

PIEZOELECTRIC ACCELERATION SENSORS

In piezoelectric accelerometers, piezoelectric material is applied to the lever on which the seismic mass is suspended. On deflection, a voltage proportional to the amount of deflection is generated. This voltage is measured and used for rate modulation. This type of accelerometer does not require input current to generate a signal.

PIEZORESISTIVE ACCELERATION SENSORS

With advances in silicon micromachining technology, a new class of accelerometers is emerging: silicon-based piezoresistive accelerometers. This type of accelerometer is now

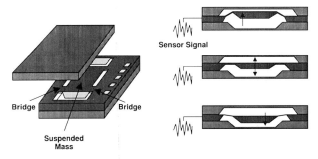

FIGURE 16–4. The silicon-based piezoresistive accelerometer consists of three layers of silicon bonded together to form a single integrated circuit chip.

small enough to be used in cardiac pacemakers. The piezoresistive accelerometer is contained entirely within a silicon chip. The silicon accelerometer consists of three layers of silicon wafers bonded together to form a sandwich. The center layer forms the mass and is suspended by silicon bridges within a cavity in the sandwich (Fig. 16–4). The silicon bridges suspending the mass act as springs. As the mass moves up and down or forward and backward in response to body motions, piezoresistors on each bridge are compressed or expanded. A constant current (3 to 4 μA) is applied to the resistors in the accelerometer. As the resistance changes with motion, the resultant voltage varies in direct proportion ($V = IR$). In the absence of acceleration, the mass moves back to its resting location. Protective stops limit movement of the mass and guard against excessive shock or forces. This type of piezoresistive accelerometer is very sensitive and specifically allows for detection of low-frequency, low-amplitude signals. Although a small current drain is required for operation of the piezoresistive sensor, this energy cost may be balanced by the ability of this sensor to detect small changes in body motion. Both types of accelerometers have constant coupling masses, exhibit a linear frequency response, and are most sensitive in the lower frequency range, below 8 Hz, which corresponds with typical body motions. The characteristic properties of the piezoelectric crystal, piezoelectric accelerometer, and the piezoresistive accelerometer are summarized in Table 16–1.

ACCELEROMETERS MONITOR THE ANTEROPOSTERIOR AXIS

The motion of the upper body in an anteroposterior direction mainly determines the energy expenditure.[10, 11] Figure 16–5 shows original recordings of acceleration signals in the three axes during treadmill exercise: vertical, lateral, and horizontal (anteroposterior). Note that treadmill exercise produces the most significant acceleration signals in the vertical and horizontal axes.

Figure 16–6 shows the orientation of the three axes. Although accelerations along the vertical axis generate a larger signal during walking or running, the anteroposterior axis generates signals that are more proportional to the exercise workload. In addition, other activities, such as cycling, gardening, and dishwashing, are best represented by acceleration signals in the horizontal plane. Because the orientation of a pulse generator in the pocket is likely to change somewhat following implantation, the vertical and lateral axes may change. For these reasons, accelerometer-based pacemakers are oriented along the horizontal axis.

SIGNAL PROCESSING

Several studies have shown that measurement of acceleration provides a better correlation with the level of exertion than measurement of the frequency of activity signals alone.[10, 11] Since the accelerometer measures acceleration continuously and instantaneously, there is no delay between the onset of acceleration and the moment at which sensor data are made available to the device's rate-adaptive algorithms. These rate-adaptive algorithms, controlled by programmable parameters, determine the actual speed of rate increase and decrease in response to exercise.

Figure 16–7 shows an example of the Vigor Sensorgram (raw accelerometer signal) recorded during the transition between light walking and heavy walking. Both the frequency and the amplitude of the accelerometer signal are evaluated during signal processing. The raw sensor signal is rectified and integrated by the pacemaker's analog circuits to yield the energy content of the motion associated with physical activity (Fig. 16–8). The integrated result is available instantaneously for further algorithmic processing.

FILTERING

Signal processing is important to sensor performance. A key advantage of accelerometer technology is the ability to limit the sensor signal to frequencies that are associated with true body motion. Studies[2, 3, 5, 8, 13, 14, 15] have shown that the frequency content as determined by Fourier analysis of accelerometer signals during physical stress is in the low-frequency range (Fig. 16–9), with signals of maximum ampli-

TABLE 16–1. **CHARACTERISTICS OF THREE TYPES OF ACTIVITY SENSORS USED FOR ADAPTIVE-RATE PACING**

	PIEZOELECTRIC	PIEZOELECTRIC	PIEZORESISTIVE
Activity sensor	Crystal bonded to can	Accelerometer	Accelerometer
Abbreviation	PZ	AC	AC
Indicator	Vibration	Body motion	Body motion
Mechanics	Bonded to pacemaker	Mounted on hybrid	Integrated chip
Coupling mass	Body tissue	85-mg seismic mass	12-mg seismic mass
Sensitivity	10–15 Hz	1–4 Hz	1–8 Hz
Current drain	0.0 μA	0.0 μA	3–4 μA
Signal analysis	Frequency dominant	Frequency and amplitude	Frequency and amplitude
Size	Approx. 4 mm × 20 mm	4.6 mm × 3.8 mm × 1.5 mm	6.0 mm × 6.0 mm × 1.5 mm

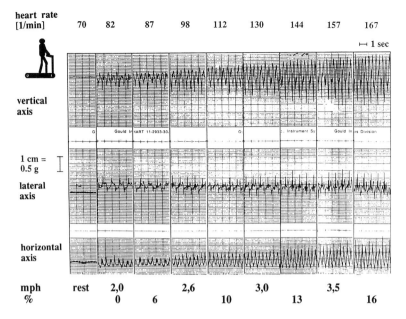

heart rate [1/min] 70 82 87 98 112 130 144 157 167

⊢⊣ 1 sec

vertical axis

1 cm = 0.5 g

lateral axis

horizontal axis

mph rest 2,0   2,6   3,0   3,5
%   0   6   10   13   16

FIGURE 16–5. Acceleration signals in the vertical, lateral, and horizontal (anteroposterior) directions recorded from a healthy volunteer undergoing treadmill exercise. The protocol increased speed, starting with 2 mph and a 0% grade and ending with a maximum of 3.5 mph and a 16% grade. The heart rate of the volunteer increased from 70 bpm to 167 bpm in a linear manner. The frequency and amplitude of the acceleration signals provide a rather linear increase with increase in speed and slope. (From Alt E, Matura M: Comparison of two activity-controlled, rate-adaptive pacing principles: Acceleration vs. vibration. Cardiol Clin 10 [4]:635, 1992.)

tude below 4 Hz. Signals originating from external noise sources such as electric drills reach a maximum amplitude in the 10- to 50-Hz frequency range (Fig. 16–10). Note that accelerometers respond to frequencies that are typical of body motion, whereas conventional piezoelectric crystals are associated with a wider range of frequencies. The accelerometers currently used in accelerometer-based pacemakers are designed to be highly sensitive in the low-frequency ranges associated with body movements. The Intermedics pacemakers employ a frequency range of from 0.5 to 4 Hz, and the CPI pacemakers use the signals between 1 and 8 Hz. This selective filtering effectively discriminates between wanted and unwanted signals. The result is a pacing system that is less susceptible to external noise and more appropriately responsive to true physiologic activities. Piezoelectric crystals are highly sensitive in the 10- to 50-Hz frequency range.[16] Therefore, it is clear that discrimination between noise signals from true physical signals is more difficult in vibrational pacemakers.

MECHANICAL CONSIDERATIONS

A second major advantage of accelerometer technology is that the sensor fits into the hybrid electronics of the pace-

maker circuitry. Both accelerometers currently used in clinical practice are very small. The piezoelectric version used in Intermedics pacemakers is 4.6 × 3.8 × 1.5 mm, and the piezoresistive accelerometer in CPI pacemakers is 6.0 × 6.0 × 1.5 mm. Because the accelerometer is mechanically insulated from the can, it shows no reaction to external pressure applied to the pacemaker implant site.

RELIABILITY

The excellent sensing properties of accelerometers have been proved in epidemiologic studies conducted to track the activity levels of patients. In one such study, a modified accelerometer and a signal recorder were worn by subjects during exercise testing.[17] Results confirmed that accelerometer measurements correlated more closely with oxygen consumption than did measurements taken with other types of activity sensors. In another study, continuous monitoring of subjects over several days showed that the accelerometer closely followed the motion of activities such as walking, running, climbing stairs, and washing windows.[18] Accelerometer output increased in intensity with increased activity and effectively paralleled physiologic increases in heart rate.

Adaptive-Rate Algorithms

Typically, the response to activity can be managed by changing the rate-response parameters to the patient's needs. In CPI devices there is a linear relation between the rectified integrated accelerometer signal and the pacing rate (Fig. 16–11A). Nominal slopes are provided, and optimal adjustments can be made easily. The Intermedics devices use a three-stage relation between the acceleration signal and the pacing rate (see Fig. 16–11B).

Clinical Results

Because accelerometer-based adaptive-rate pacing systems have been clinically introduced only recently, fewer studies

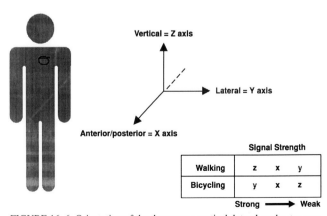

Vertical = Z axis

Lateral = Y axis

Anterior/posterior = X axis

	Signal Strength		
Walking	z	x	y
Bicycling	y	x	z

Strong ——➤ Weak

FIGURE 16–6. Orientation of the three axes: vertical, lateral, and anteroposterior. The accelerometer is oriented in the anteroposterior axis.

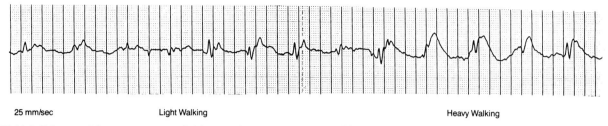

25 mm/sec   Light Walking   Heavy Walking

FIGURE 16–7. Telemetered Sensorgram as recorded from a Vigor DR during the transition between light and heavy walking at approximately one step per second.

have been performed with them than with vibrational devices. Lau and colleagues[19] compared the behavior of accelerometer-based devices with that of piezoelectric crystal devices and reported that the accelerometer showed a better response to walking, jogging, and standing. They also observed that the subject's footwear had no significant effect on the results seen with the accelerometer as opposed to the results obtained with vibrational piezoelectric devices. Increasing grade of the treadmill had a significant effect on pacing rate with the accelerometer device, whereas there was no change in pacing rate with the piezoelectric vibrational sensors. They concluded that, compared to the vibrational device, the accelerometer sensor-controlled devices showed a more adequate rate response and were less susceptible to direct pressure or to tapping on the pulse generator. From visual inspection of the linear behavior of the sensor during exercise (see Fig. 16–5), it is evident that rate adaptation based on the accelerometer's signals provides an excellent basis for mimicking the natural heart-rate response in many individuals.

Figure 16–12 shows the results of an elderly subject walking on a treadmill according to the Chronotropic Assessment Exercise Protocol (CAEP). The CAEP test was designed to provide small incremental work rates that approximate typical daily activities of pacemaker patients. The piezoresistive accelerometer-based pacemaker strapped to the chest generated a paced rate that compares favorably to the subject's intrinsic rate for various speeds and grades of the treadmill.[20] The piezoresistive accelerometer also showed proportionately small changes in pacing rate for small incremental levels of exercise. Bacharach and associates[9] (Fig. 16–13) found that the response of the accelerometer to graded treadmill testing was more strongly correlated with the patient's intrinsic heart rate (r = 0.80) than that of a vibrational

adaptive-rate device (r = 0.27). They also compared the response of walking up and down stairs using a piezoresistive accelerometer device and a vibrational piezoelectric pacemaker (Fig. 16–14) with the intrinsic sinus rate in 10 elderly subjects. The accelerometer responded appropriately when subjects walked upstairs (103 ppm) and walked downstairs (98 ppm). The response of the vibrational devices was paradoxical, with a slower pacing rate when subjects walked upstairs (83 ppm) than when they walked downstairs (89 ppm).

Recent studies[10, 11] compared the response of an acceler-

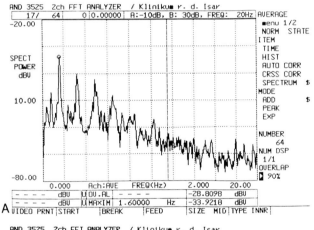

A

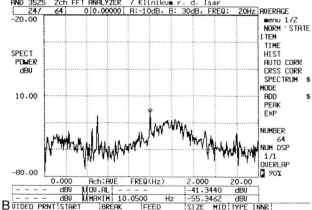

B

FIGURE 16–9. A, Fourier analysis of an accelerometer signal during walking (4.2 km/hr, 10% incline). The ordinate gives the power spectrum in a logarithmic manner, and the abscissa gives the frequency content from 0 to 20 Hz. The energy peak occurs at 1.6 Hz. B, Fourier analysis of signals from an accelerometer attached to a patient performing work with an electric drill. In the low-frequency range, very little signal amplitude is present, whereas in the 10- to 12-Hz range a signal of −55 dB can be detected.

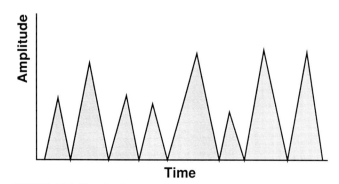

FIGURE 16–8. The signal processing of the accelerometer signal integrates the rectified signal to measure energy content.

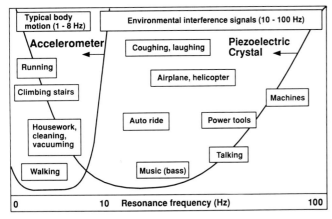

FIGURE 16–10. The low-filter bandpass of accelerometer technology detects mechanical resonance frequencies associated with typical body motion in the low-frequency range. Environmental signals greater than 8 Hz that can distort rate response are undetected.

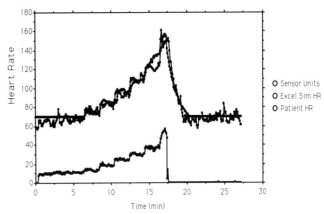

FIGURE 16–12. The results of an elderly subject walking on a treadmill according to the Chronotropic Assessment Exercise Protocol (CAEP). The piezoresistive accelerometer system strapped to the chest generated a paced rate that is comparable to the intrinsic rate for various speeds and elevations of the treadmill. The piezoresistive accelerometer shows a proportionately small rate response for small incremental levels of exercise.

ometer with a vibrational device during treadmill exercise involving increasing and decreasing speed and grade. To avoid biasing the results by using different settings, the researchers calibrated the strapped-on pacemakers for six patients and six healthy subjects using identical methods. The basic pacing rate in each subject and patient was set to 70 ppm, and the individual systems were tailored to a response of 95 ppm with a treadmill speed of 2 mph and 0% grade. The sinus rate of the six subjects was recorded continuously as a reference. The treadmill protocol[21] represented a smooth and constant increase and decrease in the workload (Fig. 16–15). The accelerometer pacing rate correlated well with the natural sinus rhythm, responding not only to an increase in speed but also to an increase in grade over the entire protocol. In a second test, the effect of increasing and decreasing grade was studied at a constant treadmill speed (Fig. 16–16). The accelerometer showed a more desirable behavior compared to vibrational devices. The correlation of sinus rate with treadmill grade was high (r = 0.97). The accelerometer device was close to this and produced a more appropriate response (r = 0.90) than the Activitrax (r = 0.52) or the Sensolog (r = 0.87).

Accelerometer systems typically demonstrate appropriate rate response with light changes in typical activities of daily living. In the European clinical evaluation of a piezoresistive accelerometer system (Excel VR [CPI]), small changes in paced rate response were noted with postural changes: supine (3 ± 2 ppm), sitting (7 ± 3 ppm), standing (10 ± 5 ppm), slow walk (29 ± 9 ppm), and brisk walk (44 ± 11 ppm)[22] (Fig. 16–17).

In another study, Erdelitsch-Reiser and associates[23] administered a clinical protocol to observe the adaptive-rate response of an implanted piezoresistive accelerometer in seven patients during typical daily activities and incremental exercise on a treadmill. Mean pacing rates (Fig. 16–18) were 50 ppm (supine), 56 ppm (standing), 77 ppm (descending stairs), 81 ppm (slow walk), 83 ppm (slow stair climb), 91 ppm (fast walk), and 92 ppm (fast stair climb). When the arm proximal to the pulse generator was used for window washing, the rate

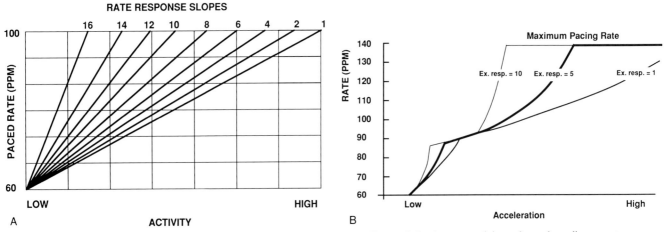

FIGURE 16–11. Different correlations between activity signals and pacing rate. A, A linear relation between activity and rate depending on rate-response slopes is established with CPI's Excel and Vigor accelerometers. B, Intermedics' exercise rate-response curves have three stages corresponding to different levels of physical activity used in a "tailor to patient" protocol. (From Alt E, Matura M: Comparison of two activity-controlled, rate-adaptive pacing principles: Acceleration vs. vibration. Cardiol Clin 10 [4]:635, 1992.)

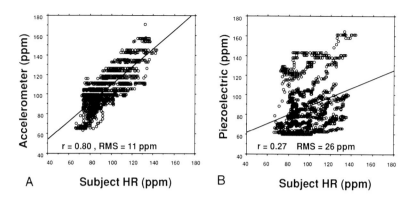

FIGURE 16–13. *A,* Clinical results obtained with CPI's Excel accelerometer-based rate-adaptive system. The heart rate of chronotropically competent patients was compared with the calculated pacing rate obtained from an externally strapped-on device. The correlation was found to be r = 0.80; the average rate variation noted by the root mean square (RMS) was 11 ppm. *B,* The performance of the vibrational device during treadmill testing was more variable. This variation depended on the individual subject. As a result, the correlation coefficient for the piezoelectric device rate and the intrinsic heart rate was 0.27; the average rate variation noted by the RMS was 26 bpm.

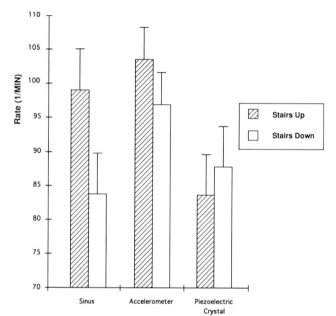

FIGURE 16–14. Strap-on accelerometer and piezoelectric crystal vibrational sensor response to stair climbing. The accelerometer's response parallels the subject's intrinsic response to stair climbing and descent, respectively. The piezoelectric crystal shows a paradoxical response to intrinsic rate, similar to clinical experience and published reports.

FIGURE 16–15. Comparison of a strap-on accelerometer (Relay) with vibrational devices (Sensolog and Activitrax). All three devices were individually calibrated to the same basic conditions. The pacing rate at rest was set to 70 ppm, and the individual rate response was tailored to obtain a rate of 95 ppm with an initial treadmill walking speed of 2.0 mph at a 0% grade. The paced response of the accelerometer with increasing and decreasing work rate closely follows the natural sinus rhythm. At rest, the sinus rate was about 20 beats above the pacemaker-indicated resting rate of 70 ppm. This difference in paced to natural heart rate continued throughout the trial. (From Alt E, Matura M: Comparison of two activity-controlled, rate-adaptive pacing principles: Acceleration vs. vibration. Cardiol Clin 10 [4]:635, 1992.)

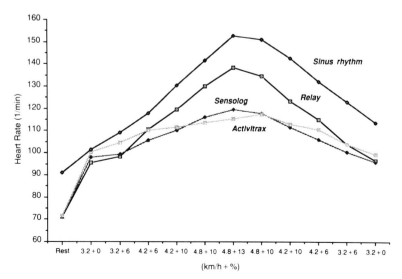

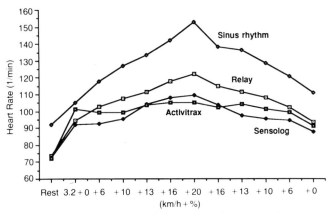

FIGURE 16–16. Response of accelerometer and vibrational devices to constant speed with increasing and decreasing slopes. The vibrational devices show little reaction to increasing workloads resulting from increasing slopes on a treadmill. The accelerometer corresponds more closely to the change in workload resulting from varied slopes. (From Alt E, Matura M: Comparison of two activity-controlled, rate-adaptive pacing principles: Acceleration vs. vibration. Cardiol Clin 10 [4]:635, 1992.)

rose to 87 ppm. When the opposite arm was used, the rate was 63 ppm. During treadmill testing, rates between 82 ppm (1.2 mph) and 104 ppm (3 mph) were observed. These investigators concluded that the device provided a proportional response to graded activities of treadmill exercise and daily living.

BICYCLE EXERCISE

Activity-controlled pacemakers typically are less responsive to bicycle exercise than to treadmill exercise due to the reduced upper body activity with bicycle ergometry, especially with stationary ergometers. Figure 16–19 shows the results with a strapped-on piezoelectric accelerometer-based pacemaker during stationary bicycle ergometry and compares the generated rate with the sinus rate seen in the same subjects with the same kind of activity. Bicycling on the street produced higher pacing rates than those observed on the stationary bicycle.

In a comparative evaluation of the piezoresistive acceler-

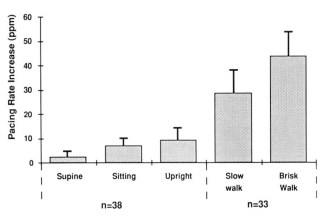

FIGURE 16–17. In the European clinical evaluation of patients with an implanted piezoresistive accelerometer system (CPI's Excel VR), appropriate changes in paced rate response were noted with postural changes and slow and brisk walks.

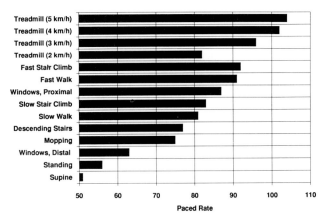

FIGURE 16–18. The rate-adaptive response of the piezoresistive accelerometer implanted in seven patients during typical daily activities and incremental exercise on a treadmill.

ometer system and a vibrational piezoelectric system during bicycle ergometry, rate responses of strapped-on devices were compared with the intrinsic response seen in 10 elderly subjects. The protocol consisted of two parts: (1) a progressively higher workload with constant revolutions per minute (rpm), and (2) a constant workload with progressively higher revolutions per minute. Although the accelerometer pacemaker did not achieve the intrinsic rate, it generated a significantly higher pacing rate than did the piezoelectric vibrational pacemaker during all stages of the cycling tasks (Fig. 16–20).

Practical Aspects

When implanting an accelerometer device, no special orientation of the pulse generator is needed. It may be flipped over or rotated in the pocket, and excess lead may be coiled beneath it. The physician can use the simplest and most convenient surgical procedure without risk of sacrificing sensor response.

Conclusion

The new generation of accelerometer-based devices overcomes some of the limitations of vibrational piezoelectric devices. Because of their sensitivity to body movements in the anteroposterior direction and their constant coupling mass, their response to graded treadmill exercise and walking up and down stairs is more reflective of the true energy expenditure of these activities. The filter characteristics that limit the sensitivity of the accelerometer to signals below 8 Hz enable the device to discriminate more accurately between true physical activity and noise stemming from machines or from other environmental sources.[2]

Because the accelerometer is incorporated into the hybrid circuit board rather than attached to the pacemaker housing, susceptibility to direct pressure and tapping on the pacemaker is reduced significantly compared to that of piezoelectric crystal devices (Fig. 16–21). This is of practical importance for patients who lie on their chest during sleep, compressing the pacemaker case.

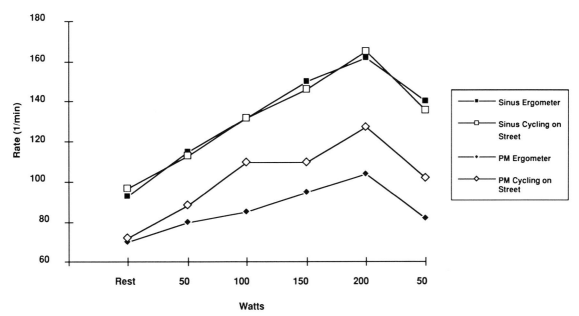

FIGURE 16–19. Comparison of pacing rate and intrinsic heart rate with bicycling on a stationary ergometer and on the street. Although the sinus rate of the subject with the strap-on device is the same with street cycling and bicycle ergometry, the accelerometer responds better to cycling on the street than to stationary ergometry; however, the paced rate is still below the sinus rate (PM, pacemaker). (From Alt E, Matura M: Comparison of two activity-controlled, rate-adaptive pacing principles: Acceleration vs. vibration. Cardiol Clin 10 [4]:635, 1992.)

Although the accelerometer is a nonmetabolic sensor and therefore cannot react to emotions, fever, and stages of increased overall metabolism, the accurate detection of movement and proportional response of the accelerometer form the basis for simple, reliable algorithms that result in excellent chronotropic response and ease of use.

Truly metabolic adaptive-rate pacemakers of the future might incorporate a combination of an accelerometer with another sensor such as minute ventilation, temperature, or QT interval, as suggested in earlier reports.[24–27] In addition, more sophisticated algorithms will help to create even better performance by activity-based pacemakers. With increased clinical use, the silicon chip accelerometer may become the standard sensor for pacemakers and defibrillators offering

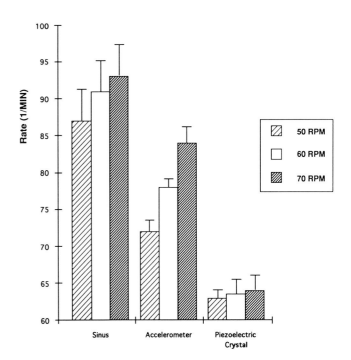

FIGURE 16–20. Comparison of pacing rate and intrinsic heart rate with bicycling on a stationary ergometer. Constant work rate with various pedaling speeds. In general, the piezoresistive accelerometer device generated approximately half the rate response of the intrinsic heart rate (HR), whereas the piezoelectric-based vibrational pacemaker provided only a moderate response in both cases.

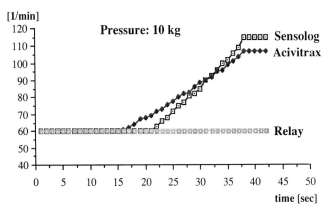

FIGURE 16–21. Application of 10-kg pressure results in an increase in pacing rate with Activitrax and Sensolog in an in vitro laboratory trial. The accelerometer-based pacemaker (Relay) shows no sensitivity to externally applied pressure. (From Alt E, Matura M: Comparison of two activity-controlled, rate-adaptive pacing principles: Acceleration vs. vibration. Cardiol Clin 10 [4]:635, 1992.)

accurate, reliable, and predictable rate adaptation as one of many programmable features within a multiprogrammable device.

Acknowledgments

The authors wish to give special thanks and credit to Markus Matula, M.D., and Kristi Fuller for their technical and editorial support.

REFERENCES

1. Howe RT, Muller RS, Gabriel KJ, Trimmer WSN: Silicon microme-chanics: Sensors and actuators on a chip. IEEE Spectrum 7:29–3S, 1990.
2. Alt E, Heinz M, Theres H, et al: A new body motion activity-based rate-responsive pacing system. PACE 10:422, 1987.
3. Lau CP, Stott JR, Toff WD, et al: Vibration sensing: New design of activity-sensing rate-responsive pacemaker. PACE 10:1217, 1987.
4. Mehta D, Lau CP, Ward DE, et al: Comparative evaluation of chrono-tropic response of QT-sensing and activity-sensing rate-responsive pacemakers. PACE 11:1405, 1988.
5. Alt E, Matula M, Theres H, et al: The basis for activity-controlled rate-variable cardiac pacemakers: An analysis of mechanical forces on the human body induced by exercise and environment. PACE 12:1667, 1989.
6. Alt E, Matula M, Theres H, et al: Grundlage Aktivitatsgesteuerter fre-quenzvariabler Herzschrittmacher: Analyse von belastungs- und um-weltbedingten mechanischen Einflussen am menschlichen Korper. Z Kardiol 78:587, 1989.
7. Anderson KM: An activity sensor to control heart rate. In Ko WH (ed): Implantable Sensor for Closed-Loop Prosthetic Systems. Mt. Kisco, NY, Futura Publishing, 1985.
8. Lau CP, Stott JR, Toff WD, et al: Selective vibration sensing: A new concept for activity-sensing rate-responsive pacing. PACE 11:1299, 1988.
9. Bacharach DW, Hilden RS, Millerhagen JO, et al: Activity-based pac-ing: Comparison of a device using an accelerometer versus a piezoelec-tric crystal. PACE 15:188, 1992.
10. Matula M, Alt E, Fotuhi P, et al: Influence of varied types of exercise to the rate adaption of activity pacemakers. PACE 15:578, 1992.
11. Matula M, Alt E, Schrepf R, et al: Response of activity pacemakers controlled by different motion sensors to treadmill testing with varied slopes. PACE 15:523, 1992.
12. Alt E, Volker R, Hogl B, et al: First clinical results with a new tem-perature-controlled rate-responsive pacemaker. Circulation 78(Suppl III):116, 1988.
13. Anderson KM: Sensor pacing: Research leads to major breakthrough in rate-responsive pacemaking. Med Electron 86:89, 1986.
14. Cardiac Pacemakers Inc: Recent Developments in Adaptive Rate Pacing Technology. St. Paul, MN, Cardiac Pacemakers Inc, 1991.
15. Matula M, Alt E, Theres H, et al: Rate-responsive pacing based on a new activity sensing principle. PACE 10:1220, 1987.
16. Stangl K, Wirtzfeld A, Lochschmidt O, et al: Moglichkeiten und Gren-zen eines ''aktivitatsgesteuerten'' Schrittmachersystems. Herz/Kreislauf 19:351, 1987.
17. Wong TC, Webster JG, Montoye HJ, et al: Portable accelerometer device for measuring human energy expenditure. Trans Biomed Eng 6:467, 1981.
18. Servais SB, Webster JG, Montoye HJ: Estimating human energy expen-diture using an accelerometer device. IEEE Frontiers of Engineering in Health. 1982, pp 309–312.
19. Lau CP, Tai YT, Fong PC, et al: Clinical experience with an activity-sensing DDDR pacemaker using an accelerometer sensor. PACE 15:334, 1992.
20. Millerhagen J, Bacharach D, Street G, et al: A comparison study of two activity pacemakers: An accelerometer versus piezoelectric crystal de-vice. PACE 14:665, 1991.
21. Alt E: A protocol for treadmill and bicycle stress testing designed for pacemaker patients. Stimucoeur 15:33, 1987.
22. Charles RG, Heemels JP, Westrum BL, et al: Accelerometer-based pacing: A multi-center study. PACE 16:418, 1993.
23. Erdelitsch-Reiser E, Langenfeld H, Millerhagen J, Kochsiek K: New concept in activity-controlled pacemakers: Clinical results with an ac-celerometer-based rate-adaptive pacing system. PACE 15:2245, 1992.
24. Alt E, Heinz M, Theres H, et al: Function and selection of sensors for optimum rate-modulated pacing. In Barold S, Mugica J (eds): New Perspectives in Cardiac Pacing. Mt Kisco, NY, Futura Publishing, 1991, p 163.
25. Alt E, Theres H, Heinz M, et al: A new rate-modulated pacemaker system optimized by combination of two sensors. PACE 11:1119, 1988.
26. Mugica J, Barold S, Ripart A: The smart pacemaker. In Barold S, Mugica J (eds): New Perspectives in Cardiac Pacing. Mt Kisco, NY, Futura Publishing, 1991, p 545.
27. Schroeppel EA: Current trends in cardiac pacing technology. I. Brady-cardia pacing. Biomed Sci Tech 3:90, 1992.

CLINICAL CONCEPTS

CHAPTER 17

PACEMAKER AND DEFIBRILLATOR CODES

Alan D. Bernstein
Victor Parsonnet

The need for specialized symbols to describe pacemaker function has evolved together with pacemaker technology itself. Most pacemakers of the 1960s presented no problem in this regard because they were all essentially the same: they paced a single cardiac chamber, had no sensing capability (and thus no response to sensing that needed to be identified), and had no adjustable characteristics whose settings had to be communicated readily. With the subsequent development of atrial and ventricular pacemakers whose output was triggered or inhibited by spontaneous cardiac activity, awareness of the pacemaker's configuration and functional design became indispensable to verifying its proper operation or identifying possible problems.

From the beginning it was evident that two quite separate tasks needed to be addressed in designing a code to be used in describing cardiac-pacemaker function: first, identifying the information that needs to be conveyed and in what circumstances; second, defining appropriate symbols and code structure to convey that information. These considerations are central to the design of each of the pacemaker codes described in this chapter.

The Generic Codes: Historical Perspective

THE THREE-POSITION ICHD CODE (1974)

In 1974 the Inter-Society Commission for Heart Disease Resources (ICHD) proposed a three-position "generic" or "conversational" pacemaker code to meet an increasingly apparent need for distinguishing different types of pacemakers according to three fundamental attributes: (1) the chamber or chambers paced, (2) the chamber or chambers in which native cardiac events were sensed, and (3) what the

pacemaker did when a spontaneous depolarization was sensed. The 1974 code, which was based on an initial structure suggested several years previously by Smyth, is summarized in Table 17–1,[1] and the existing pacing modes for which this code was formulated are listed in Table 17–2.

Position I represents the location of pacing (atrium, ventricle, or both), position II shows where spontaneous events are sensed (atrium, ventricle, or both), and position III denotes the pacemaker's response to sensing. Thus, a VVI pacemaker stimulates the ventricle (V), and whenever a spontaneous event is sensed in the ventricle (V) the pacemaker inhibits (I) a pending ventricular stimulus.

A certain degree of ambiguity is inherent in position III, although much of that ambiguity may be resolved by the context in which the code is used. For example, a VVT pacemaker is one that paces the ventricle, senses spontaneous ventricular depolarizations, and produces a triggered ventricular output immediately upon ventricular sensing. In VAT pacing, on the other hand, triggering means something else: the production of a triggered ventricular output in response to atrial sensing after a delay intended to simulate the normal temporal pattern of atrioventricular (AV) conduction. The

TABLE 17–1. **THE 1974 THREE-POSITION ICHD CODE OR THREE-LETTER IDENTIFICATION CODE**[a]

FIRST LETTER	SECOND LETTER	THIRD LETTER
Chamber paced	Chamber sensed	Mode of response

[a]Letters: V = ventricle I = inhibited
A = atrium T = triggered
D = double chamber O = not applicable

Adapted with permission from Parsonnet V, Furman S, Smyth NPD: Implantable cardiac pacemakers: Status report and resource guideline. Circulation 50:A-21, 1974. Copyright 1974 American Heart Association.

TABLE 17–2. PACING MODES DESCRIBED BY THE THREE-POSITION ICHD CODE

MODE	DESCRIPTION
VOO	Asynchronous ventricular pacing; no sensing function
AOO	Asynchronous atrial pacing; no sensing function
DOO	Dual-chamber (AV sequential) asynchronous pacing; no sensing function
VVI	Ventricular pacing inhibited by ventricular sensing
VVT	Ventricular pacing triggered instantaneously by ventricular sensing
AAI	Atrial pacing inhibited by atrial sensing
AAT	Atrial pacing triggered instantaneously by atrial sensing
VAT	Ventricular pacing triggered after a delay by atrial sensing
DVI	Dual-chamber (AV-sequential) pacing inhibited by ventricular sensing

Abbreviation: AV, atrioventricular.
Modified with permission from Parsonnet V, Furman S, Smyth NPD: Implantable cardiac pacemakers: Status report and resource guidelines. Pacemaker Study Group, Inter-Society Commission for Heart Disease Resources (ICHD). Circulation 50:A21, 1974. Copyright 1974 American Heart Association.

delay is assumed implicitly in this use of the code, as in other dual-chamber modes, such as DVI, DDD, and DDI.

This was the first of the recognized generic or conversational codes. Its designers' identification of information priorities (the first task referred to above) was so insightful and its design so convenient (the second task) that the code has been in continuous use worldwide since its publication and has served as the kernel of each of three successive generic codes that superseded it. Its forward compatibility stands as a tribute to its designers, particularly with respect to pacemakers that could sense in both chambers, which had not yet come into existence when the code was formulated.

THE FIVE-POSITION ICHD CODE (1981)

In 1981 a revised code was published by the same designers (Table 17–3).[2] Although it incorporated all of the features of the previous code, it was augmented by two additional positions to allow it to describe two major developments of the intervening 5 years: programmability and antitachyarrhythmia pacing.

With the advent of pacemakers some of whose operating parameters could be adjusted noninvasively by means of a programming device, if became important to know that the pacemaker's rate, output amplitude, mode, or timing characteristics could be changed at will so that the reflections of

such changes in the electrocardiogram would not be mistaken as evidence of a device malfunction. A fifth position was added to provide information about antitachyarrhythmia pacing functions and the means by which they were activated, whether automatically or by external command using a separate triggering device. The information about antibradycardia pacing modes represented by the five-position code remained in the first three positions and was expressed in the same fashion as before, so that compatibility with the previous code was retained. Table 17–4 lists examples of pacing modes described by the five-position ICHD code that did not exist at the time the original three-position code was designed.

In 1983 this code was amended once again, this time to include the option of the letter C (communicating) in position IV to denote any of three categories of pacemaker telemetry, defined as the ability of the implanted device to transmit (1) internally stored information such as a serial number, (2) device-status information such as the internal resistance of the battery, or (3) physiologic data such as an intracardiac-electrogram signal.[3] The presence of C in position IV of the revised ICHD code was hierarchical in the sense that it implied that either simple programmability (usually rate and output) or multiprogrammability was present as well. For example, a VVI,C pacemaker would perform ventricular antibradycardia pacing inhibited by ventricular sensing and would be capable of pacemaker telemetry and some degree of programmability.

The NASPE/BPEG Generic (NBG) Pacemaker Code

The pacemaker code in most common use at present was introduced in 1987 by the Mode Code Committee of the North American Society of Pacing and Electrophysiology (NASPE) together with the British Pacing and Electrophysiology Group (BPEG) in response to the continually growing need for a conversational code that could clearly signify the presence of device characteristics beyond basic antibradycardia-pacing capabilities.[4] This newest generic code is summarized in Table 17–5.

This code retains all of the characteristics of the 1974 ICHD Code and some of those of the later five-position codes. To deal with the increasing complexity of later devices, however, it was considered necessary to clarify several

TABLE 17–3. THE 1981 FIVE-POSITION ICHD CODE

POSITION	I	II	III	IV	V
Category	Chamber(s) paced	Chamber(s) sensed	Modes of response(s)	Programmable functions	Special antitachyarrhythmia functions
Letters used	V = ventricle A = atrium D = double	V = ventricle A = atrium D = double O = none	T = triggered I = inhibited D = double O = none R = reverse	P = programmable (rate and/or output) M = multiprogrammable C = communicating O = none	B = bursts N = normal rate competition S = scanning E = external
Manufacturer's designation only	S = single chamber	S = single chamber		Comma optional here	

[a]Triggered and inhibited response.
Adapted from Parsonnet V, Furman S, Smyth NPD: A revised code for pacemaker identification. PACE 4:400, 1981.

TABLE 17–4. **PACING MODES DESCRIBED BY THE FIVE-POSITION ICHD CODE**

MODE	DESCRIPTION
VDD,M (VDDM)	Ventricular antibradycardia pacing inhibited by ventricular sensing, triggered after a delay by atrial sensing. Multiprogrammable device. No antitachyarrhythmia function
DDD,M (DDDM)	Dual-chamber (AV-sequential) antibradycardia pacing inhibited by sensing in either chamber, with ventricular pacing triggered after a delay by sensing in the atrium following a ventricular event. Multiprogrammable device. No antitachyarrhythmia function.
VVI,MB (VVIMB)	Ventricular antibradycardia pacing inhibited by ventricular sensing. Multiprogrammable device. Pacing bursts for ventricular tachyarrhythmia, means of activation unspecified.
AAR,ON (AARON)	No antibradycardia function. Nonprogrammable device. Normal-rate competition for termination of atrial tachycardia, activated by atrial sensing.
AOO,OE (AOOOE)	Asynchronous atrial antibradycardia pacing. Nonprogrammable device. Externally activated atrial antitachycardia pacing, nature unspecified.

Modified from Parsonnet V, Furman S, Smyth NPD: Revised code for pacemaker identification. PACE 4:400, 1981.

features and to define more explicitly how the code was to be used.

The first three positions of the NBG Code are reserved exclusively for antibradycardia-pacing functions. As a result, the R in position III of the 1981 and 1983 ICHD Codes, which denoted reverse pacing, or pacing that was invoked only in the presence of a tachycardia, is absent. O may be used in all five positions, to accommodate either antibradycardia or antitachycardia pacing without the other, although antibradycardia pacing is the intended focus of the code.

Position IV serves a dual purpose, describing two distinctly different device characteristics: the degree of programmability (P, M, or C) as in the revised ICHD Code and the presence or absence of rate modulation (R). Like the C in the revised ICHD Code, the R is hierarchical in that it takes precedence over programmability; it is assumed that adaptive-rate pacemakers are multiprogrammable and usually

are capable of some degree of pacemaker telemetry. (All existing adaptive-rate pacemakers are multiprogrammable and incorporate telemetry capabilities.)

Position V indicates the presence of one or more *active* antitachyarrhythmia functions (i.e., excluding normal-rate competition or fixed-rate pacing to suppress a tachyarrhythmia), whether initiated automatically or by external command. A distinction is made between antitachycardia-pacing (P) and shock (S) interventions for cardioversion (low energy) or defibrillation (high energy) applied using cardiac electrodes. Position V is thus more general than the corresponding position of the 1981 and 1983 ICHD Codes. In designing the NBG Code, this modification was considered necessary, partly because of the increasing variety of anti-tachycardia-pacing patterns and partly because the B, S, N, E descriptors of the earlier codes were felt to be intrinsically restrictive, mixing function (B and N), timing (S), and means of activation (E) in a fashion that allowed only one of the three properties to be represented at a time.[4, 5]

To avoid possible confusion, it was also found necessary to identify the possible contexts in which the code could be used: to represent the maximal capabilities of a device (e.g., DDD), the mode to which the device is programmed (e.g., DVI), or the mode in which it is operating at a given moment (e.g., VAT).

The use of the NBG Code is illustrated in Table 17–6.

Specific Codes

Identifying high-priority information that needs to be conveyed quickly in clinical practice, although a prerequisite for designing a generic code, involves an inherent compromise because some information must be left out if the code is to be of practical value. Because this compromise inevitably generates ambiguity (as in the dual meaning of "triggered," a need was identified in some situations for summarizing more information than a generic code allows. One such situation is the task of determining whether an electrocardiographic rhythm strip reflects normal or abnormal operation of a complex dual-chamber pacemaker, particularly if instantaneous triggering is present in either chamber, a feature that cannot be conveyed by the NBG Code or its predecessors.

In 1981 a ratio-format code was described that provided separate descriptions of the pacing-mode elements operative in the atrial and ventricular channels of the pulse generator.[6]

TABLE 17–5. **THE NASPE/BPEG GENERIC (NBG) PACEMAKER CODE**

POSITION	I	II	III	IV	V
Category	Chamber(s) paced	Chamber(s) sensed	Response to sensing	Programmability, rate modulation	Antitachyarrhythmia function(s)
Letters:	O = none A = atrium V = ventricle D = dual (A + V)	O = none A = atrium V = ventricle D = dual (A+ V)	O = none T = triggered I = inhibited D = dual (T + I)	O = none P = simple programmable M = multiprogrammable C = communicating R = rate modulation	O = none P = pacing (anti-tachyarrhythmia) S = shock D = dual (P + S)
Manufacturers' designation only	S = Single (A or V)	S = Single (A or V)			

[a]Positions I through III are used exclusively for antibradyarrhythmia function.
Adapted from Bernstein AD, Camm AJ, Fletcher RD, et al: The NASPE/BPEG Generic Pacemaker Code for antibradyarrhythmia and adaptive-rate pacing and antitachyarrhythmia devices. PACE 10:794, 1987.

TABLE 17–6. **EXAMPLES OF THE NASPE/BPEG GENERIC (NBG) CODE**

CODE	MEANING
VOOO or VOOOO	Asynchronous ventricular pacing; no adaptive rate control or antitachyarrhythmia functions (also VOO in clinical use but not in device labeling)
DDDM or DDDMO	Multiprogrammable physiologic dual-chamber pacing, no adaptive rate control or antitachyarrhythmia functions
VVIPP	Simple programmable VVI pacemaker with antitachyarrhythmia-pacing capability
DDDCP	DDD pacemaker with telemetry and antitachyarrhythmia-pacing capability
OOOPS	Simple-programmable cardioverter, defibrillator, or cardioverter/defibrillator
OOOPD	Simple-programmable cardioverter, defibrillator, or cardioverter/defibrillator with antitachyarrhythmia-pacing capability
VVIMD	Multiprogrammable VVI pacemaker with defibrillation (or cardioversion) and antitachyarrhythmia-pacing capabilities
VVIR or VVIRO	VVI pacemaker with escape interval controlled adaptively by one or more unspecified variables
VVIRP	Programmable VVI pacemaker with escape interval controlled adaptively by one or more unspecified variables, also incorporating antitachyarrhythmia-pacing capability
DDDRD	Programmable DDD pacemaker with escape interval controlled adaptively by one or more unspecified variables, also incorporating antitachyarrhythmia-pacing capability and cardioversion (or defibrillation, or cardioversion and defibrillation) functions

Adapted from Bernstein AD, Brownlee RR, Fletcher RD, et al: Report of the NASPE Mode Code Committee. PACE 7:395, 1984.

This code, with relatively few modifications, was adopted by NASPE a few years later as the NASPE Specific Code, which is summarized in Table 17–7.[5, 7]

Although inappropriate for conversational use, this code provides a means of summarizing pacing-mode characteristics, including antitachyarrhythmia-pacing features, in a concise but accurate fashion that is, incidentally, convenient for computer processing. We have found it particularly useful in teaching and as a shorthand when notation for an unusual mode is desired. For example, it clarifies the basic difference between the DDD and DDI modes:

$$DDD = \frac{PSIaIv}{PSIvTa} \qquad DDI = \frac{PSIaIv}{PSIv}$$

The difference lies in the ventricular-channel function: it may be seen that Ta is missing from the ventricular-channel descriptor (the denominator) of the DDI code. In the DDI mode, ventricular pacing is not triggered by atrial sensing as in DDD, but the other functions remain the same. In DDI, therefore, fast atrial rates are not tracked by ventricular pacing but merely inhibit pending atrial outputs, so that AV synchrony is not maintained when the spontaneous atrial rate exceeds the basic pacing rate.

Without the strict constraints on complexity that affect generic codes, the NASPE Specific Code is more amenable to amendment. For example, it has been suggested that adaptive functions such as rate modulation and AV-interval hysteresis could be represented by additional symbols appended in square brackets.

The NASPE/BPEG Defibrillator (NBD) Code

On January 23, 1993, the NASPE Board of Trustees approved the adoption of the NASPE/BPEG Defibrillator Code (NBD Code), which is summarized in Table 17–8.[8] It was developed by the NASPE Mode Code Committee, comprising members of NASPE and BPEG, and is intended for describing cardiac-defibrillator capabilities and operation in conversation, record keeping, and device labeling. The NBD Code is patterned after the NBG Code and is compatible with it. Like the NBG Code, it is a generic code, but whereas the NBG Code describes antibradycardia-pacing functions in detail and indicates the presence of shock capability without

TABLE 17–7. **THE NASPE SPECIFIC CODE**[5, 7]

Basic structure	Atrial- and ventricular-channel functions are described in numerator and denominator, respectively, of a ratio-format code, or separated by a virgule (slash) or hyphen when restriction to a single line is unavoidable. Example: $$DDD = \frac{PSIaIv}{PSIvTa} = PSIaIv/PSIvTa$$		
Antibradycardia-pacing symbols	Function: O = none P = pace S = sense	Pacing type: T = triggered I = inhibited	Signal source a = atrium v = ventricle
	Function U = underdrive B = burst R = ramp	X = extrastimulus C = cardioversion D = defibrillation	Activation: a = atrial sensing v = ventricular sensing e = external
Antitachycardia-therapy symbols	Antitachycardia-therapy symbols are appended in parentheses as needed. Thus a multiprogrammable DDD pacemaker with atrial-burst capability, either automatically or externally activated, plus automatic defibrillation would be represented as $$DDDMD = \frac{PSIaIv(BaBe)}{PSIvTa(Dv)} = PSIaIv(BaBe)/PSIvTa(DV)$$		

TABLE 17–8. **THE NASPE/BPEG DEFIBRILLATOR CODE (NBD CODE)**[8]

I SHOCK CHAMBER	II ANTITACHYCARDIA- PACING CHAMBER	III TACHYCARDIA DETECTION	IV ANTIBRADYCARDIA- PACING CHAMBER
O = none A = atrium V = ventricle D = dual (A + V)	O = none A = atrium V = ventricle D = dual (A + V)	E = electrogram H = hemodynamic	O = none A = atrium V = ventricle D = dual (A + V)

Adapted from Bernstein AD, Camm AJ, Fisher JD, et al: The NASPE/BPEG defibrillator code. PACE 16:1776, 1993.

providing specific information, the NBD Code gives more information about cardioversion and defibrillation capabilities and indicates the presence of antibradycardia pacing without providing details.

The NBD Code does not indicate shock energy levels and thus does not distinguish between cardioversion and defibrillation. Positions I, II, and IV indicate only the location of shock, antitachycardia-pacing, and antibradycardia-pacing functions, respectively. Position III indicates the means of tachycardia detection and is hierarchical in the sense that a device that monitors hemodynamic variables is assumed to monitor the intracardiac-electrogram signal as well. In this sense, H implies E.

In conversation, at least the first two positions are used, with others added as needed for clarity. In device labeling and record keeping, the first three positions are used, followed by a hyphen and the first four positions of the NBG Code. For example, a ventricular defibrillator with adaptive-rate ventricular antibradycardia pacing would be labeled VOE-VVIR or VOH-VVIR, depending on its tachycardia-detection mechanism.

As an additional means of distinguishing concisely among devices limited to cardioversion or defibrillation and those that incorporate antitachycardia and antibradycardia pacing as well, a short-form code was defined, as summarized in Table 17–9. It is intended only for use in conversation.

Concluding Comments

In the context of clinical pacing, pacing education, and the development of pacing technology, additional symbolic rep-

TABLE 17–9. **THE NASPE/BPEG DEFIBRILLATOR CODE (NBD CODE), SHORT FORM**[8]

ICD-S	= ICD with **s**hock capability only
ICD-B	= ICD with **b**radycardia pacing as well as shock
ICD-T	= ICD with **t**achycardia (and bradycardia) pacing as well as shock

Abbreviation: ICD, implanted cardioverter/defibrillator.
Adapted from Bernstein AD, Camm AJ, Fisher JD, et al: The NASPE/ BPEG defibrillator code. PACE 16:1776, 1993.

resentations not discussed in this chapter have been developed. These potentially useful resources, primarily diagrammatic, include pictorial mode codes,[7, 9] mechanisms for annotating electrocardiograms and other records with concise summaries of pacing mode and programmable-parameter settings,[10] diagrammatic aids to interpreting paced electrocardiograms,[9] and state diagrams for illustrating pacemaker-timing design characteristics.[11]

Agreed-upon symbols are a basic requirement of successful communication. Not surprisingly, therefore, the search for practical symbols for describing the function of increasingly versatile devices is an ongoing task, which will continue as rhythm-management technology continues to evolve.

REFERENCES

1. Parsonnet V, Furman S, Smyth NPD: Implantable cardiac pacemakers: Status report and resource guidelines. Pacemaker Study Group, Inter-Society Commission for Heart Disease Resources (ICHD). Circulation 50:A21, 1974.
2. Parsonnet V, Furman S, Smyth NPD: Revised code for pacemaker identification. PACE 4:400, 1981.
3. Parsonnet V, Furman S, Smyth NPD, Bilitch M: Implantable cardiac pacemakers: Status report and resource guidelines, 1982. Pacemaker Study Group, Inter-Society Commission for Heart Disease Resources (ICHD). Circulation 68:227A, 1984.
4. Bernstein AD, Camm AJ, Fletcher RD, et al: The NASPE/BPEG Generic Pacemaker Code for antibradyarrhythmia and adaptive-rate pacing and antitachyarrhythmia devices. PACE 10:794, 1987.
5. Bernstein AD, Brownlee RR, Fletcher RD, et al: Report of the NASPE Mode Code Committee. PACE 7:395, 1984.
6. Brownlee RR, Shimmel JB, Del Marco CJ: A new code for pacemaker operating modes. PACE 4:396, 1981.
7. Bernstein AD, Brownlee RR, Fletcher RD, et al: Pacing Mode Codes. In Barold SS (ed.): Modern Cardiac Pacing. Mount Kisco, NY, Futura, 1985, pp 307–322.
8. Bernstein AD, Camm AJ, Fisher JD, et al: The NASPE/BPEG Defibrillator Code. PACE 16:1776, 1993.
9. Lindemans F: Diagrammatic representation of pacemaker function. In Barold SS (ed.): Modern Cardiac Pacing. Mount Kisco, NY, Futura, 1985, pp 323–353.
10. Parsonnet V, Bernstein AD: An annotation system for displaying operating-parameter values in dual-chamber pacing. Am Heart J 111:817, 1986.
11. Bernstein AD: Visualizing pacing modes. In course notebook, Cardiac Pacing 1988, Bethesda, MD, American College of Cardiology, 1988, pp C1–C24.

CHAPTER 18

SINUS NODE DISEASE

Richard Sutton

Definition

Sinus node disease has many names, all of which describe the same set of syndromes. Sinoatrial node disease is probably the most accurate, whereas sick sinus syndrome is possibly the most memorable. This name was coined by Lown[1] early in the appreciation of this clinical phenomenon. Sinus bradycardia, sinus arrest, sinoatrial exit block, and bradycardia-tachycardia syndrome are additional names used to describe different presentations of this disease.

This condition is defined as an affliction of the sinoatrial node that either prevents impulse generation or prevents or delays the conduction of sinoatrial impulses to the surrounding atrial tissue. This affliction may be a pathologic process in or around the sinoatrial node, or it may be a pathophysiologic phenomenon of abnormal function of the autonomic nervous system that adversely influences impulse generation within the node or conduction out of it. This implies at least two different types of pathologic processes, which have been termed intrinsic and extrinsic. Intrinsic sinus node disease is present when a histologically confirmable lesion can be demonstrated, and extrinsic sinus node disease exists when the abnormality appears to be solely in the autonomic nervous system. This can be confirmed by the achievement of normal sinus node function when the heart is separated, usually chemically, from the influence of the autonomic nervous system. These two entities overlap, as shown by recent data that suggest an increased incidence of autonomic abnormalities (e.g., as defined by tilt table testing and carotid sinus testing) in patients with intrinsic sinus node disease.

The identification of and later the understanding of the function of the sinoatrial node originated from the work of Keith and Flack,[2, 3] who demonstrated that this structure is the heart's pacemaker. The development of cellular electrophysiology culminated in the work of Hoffman,[4] who identified the characteristic phase 4 depolarization in pacemaker cells, and later by West,[5] who confirmed by intracellular recordings the exact role of the sinoatrial node as pacemaker in the rabbit.

The first reports of sinus node disease are credited to Laslett[6] in 1909, Schott[7] in 1912, and Levine[8] in 1916. Thereafter there were sporadic case reports until the 1960s, when Irene Ferrer focused on this condition at Columbia-Presbyterian Medical Center in New York. After her important scientific articles,[9, 10] she wrote a magnificent monograph on the subject.[11]

Anatomy and Pathophysiology

The pioneering work of Keith and Flack[2] showed that the sinoatrial node is situated in the upper anterolateral epicardial right atrium. Its shape is elliptical or crescentic at the junction of the superior vena cava and the root of the right atrial appendage. It is 5 to 8 mm long and 1.5 mm wide. On cross-section the sinus node cells surround its central structure, the sinus node artery. This artery is derived from the right coronary artery in 55% of individuals and from the circumflex branch of the left coronary artery in the other 45%.[12] Histologically, the sinoatrial node consists of three types of cells:

1. P cells, which are believed to be the principal pacemaker cells and contain a few myofilaments. They are seen only on electron microscopy. There are only a few thousand cells (about 5000), which are localized to a small area of the sinus node.
2. Transitional cells, which contain more myofilaments.
3. Myocytes, which are similar to atrial myocytes.

In addition, there is collagen and connective tissue, and there are ramifications of nerve tissue. P cells are interwoven with transitional cells and collagen. They are in contact with transitional cells but not with atrial myocytes. Transitional cells conduct the impulse from the P cells to the atrial myocytes, which are in turn in contact with the specialized atrial conduction pathways, the atrial myocardium, and the atrial perinodal fibers, which are slow conductors.[13] The collagen in the structure of the sinoatrial node increases with age until it is the dominant histologic finding in the elderly.[14] This aging change is independent of the degree of atherosclerosis present.[15]

The sinoatrial node is highly innervated by both the parasympathetic (vagal-cholinergic) and sympathetic (adrenergic) systems.[16, 17] These nerves exert their influence by means of the chemical transmitters acetylcholine and norepinephrine and by their interaction with phase 4 depolarization and the threshold voltage (point of onset of phase 0 depolarization) to modulate control of the heart rate.

Electrotonic conduction within the sinoatrial node is slow (1–8 cm/s^{-1}),[16] which is attributed to the paucity of desmosomes or areas of low resistance between P cells. The relative lack of ability of P cells to conduct impulses from one to another and then to transitional cells and the increasing collagen content in the node may account for intrinsic sinus node disease in some patients. Even in the normal sinoatrial node, different groups of P cells are dominant in driving the heart
at different rates and under different autonomic influences.[18–20] Classically, firing of a group of P cells depends on three factors:

1. The rate of diastolic depolarization.
2. The resting potential (at the start of phase 4).
3. The threshold potential.

Different groups of P cells may differ in these three respects, and these differences may be more marked in disease states of the sinoatrial node.

Pathophysiology

Probably the most common cause of sinus node disease is a loss of P cells to a greater extent than that expected with aging. The cause is uncertain but has been attributed to an autoimmune process, amyloid deposition, or collagen disease.[21–23] Sinus node disease has been associated with thyroid disease,[24] myocarditis, trauma secondary to recent or remote cardiac surgery, collagen vascular diseases, rheumatic heart disease, cardiomyopathy, neuromuscular diseases, and past diphtheria.[21, 25] Unfortunately, in many cases the cause is not readily apparent, and the structural changes in the sinoatrial region may be indistinguishable from those that occur with normal aging. The sinoatrial node has been found to be hypoplastic in sporadic cases of sinus node disease in children[26] and in familial cases.[27] Ischemic heart disease is rarely a cause of sinoatrial node disease,[21, 28, 29] although this was not the impression gained by some of the early clinical workers in the field.[30–33] As more cases have been recognized and more thorough investigation has been completed, the small role played by coronary artery disease has been brought into perspective. Transient sinus node dysfunction occurs frequently during myocardial infarction.[34, 35] This may be due to direct ischemia or to adenosine released from damaged tissues,[36] which antagonizes cholinesterase. Atropine is often effective in managing this condition. Permanent sick sinus syndrome due solely to ischemic heart disease is rare, as discussed earlier. Adenosine has also been claimed to play an etiologic role in nonischemic cases.[37, 38]

In some cases no histologic abnormality of the sinoatrial node or its surrounding tissue has been demonstrated.[39] Presumably, these are cases of extrinsic sinus node disease in which the sinus node functional abnormalities are imposed by the autonomic nervous system. The closeness of the relationship between extrinsic sinus node disease, carotid sinus syndrome,[40] and, more recently, vasovagal syndrome has been clearly shown by Brignole and colleagues[41] and suggests an intimate etiologic process among these three syndromes. The etiology is uncertain, but at present it is considered to lie chiefly at the vasomotor center level in the brainstem,[42] perhaps associated with some abnormalities of acetylcholine production or metabolism in the region of the sinoatrial node.[43] This possibility is highlighted by the recent report of Alboni and colleagues[44] comparing two groups of patients with sinus bradycardia (with heart rates as low as 50 bpm). Both groups had similar clinical characteristics, ambulatory electrocardiographic (ECG) monitoring data, and invasive electrophysiologic study measurements of sinus node function before and after autonomic blockade. The group of patients with sinus bradycardia and syncope differed from those with sinus bradycardia alone by a higher incidence of abnormal response (induction of syncope or presyncope with hypotension or bradycardia) to head-up tilt table testing or carotid sinus massage. Results of at least one test (head-up tilt table testing or carotid sinus massage or both) were positive in 76% of patients with sinus bradycardia and syncope but only in 36% of patients with sinus bradycardia alone.

ATRIAL PARALYSIS

Atrial paralysis is rare and involves severe damage to the atrial tissue with replacement by fibrosis. There is no electric or contractile activity of the atria. The condition is often familial and may also involve more extensive conduction system disease including the His-Purkinje system.[45, 46] Atrial paralysis is also seen as a cardiac manifestation of muscular dystrophy, after myocarditis, or associated with congenital heart disease such as Ebstein's anomaly. Transient atrial paralysis may occur after cardiac surgery and after intravenous flecainide administration.

Epidemiology

Sinus node disease occurs at any age, but its incidence increases with age. In the elderly, sinus node dysfunction has been shown to be very common,[47] although it is often not associated with symptoms and therefore it may not come to clinical attention. As described earlier, the etiology varies with the patient's age at presentation. In children, congenital causes are likely, and presentation often follows cardiac surgery for congenital heart disease. In middle age, systemic disease and coronary artery disease are important, but in the elderly degeneration of the sinus node and possibly also its nervous connections are the major causes. By virtue of the aging populations in developed countries, sinus node disease must be expected to increase, and demand for its treatment will increase in parallel with it. It is estimated that 150 to 200 new patients per million population per year will require pacing for symptoms due to sick sinus syndrome in the future.[48] In most Western countries, sinus node dysfunction accounts for 40% to 60% of patients undergoing new permanent pacemaker implantation. The coexistence of sinus node dysfunction in 25% to 50% of patients who have undergone permanent pacemaker implantation for complete or high-grade atrioventricular (AV) block has also been noted.

The role of sinus node disease in the huge numbers of patients with atrial fibrillation is still unclear, but it seems likely that many patients with this arrhythmia pass through a phase of sick sinus syndrome before atrial fibrillation becomes chronic.

Clinical Presentation

Symptoms of sinus node disease that can occur at any age[30, 49] and that draw prompt clinical attention are dizziness and syncope. These symptoms tend to be dramatic and demand effective therapy. However, there are many more subtle symptoms such as paroxysmal palpitations, tiredness, dyspnea on exertion, unrefreshing sleep, reduced powers of concentration, and poor memory. Sinus node disease is occasionally associated with frank congestive heart failure or pulmonary edema.

Any of these subtle symptoms should prompt the cardiologist to consider sinus node disease. If symptoms are intermittent they may be due to transient bradycardias or tachycardias that may not be present at the time of examination. If they are exercise related, again they may be due to arrhythmias or possibly to a failure of the sinus node to accelerate known as chronotropic incompetence.[50] Some symptoms such as memory loss, personality changes, and demented states are due to persistent severe arrhythmias, such as bradycardia or tachycardia, and these conditions must be present for these symptoms to be considered cardiac.

Dizziness and syncope in patients with sinus node disease can be caused by bradycardia, asystole, or tachycardia and may be indistinguishable from these symptoms in patients with AV block. But at times there are differences. Syncope may occur with a little more warning, such as preceding dizziness or palpitations in patients with sick sinus syndrome. It may also be more prolonged. It is possible for the cardiac rhythm to reestablish itself following a pause but still be insufficient to generate an adequate cardiac output; thus, life is preserved but unconsciousness persists. This may cause diagnostic difficulties because cardiac syncope is expected to be brief, and distinguishing it from epilepsy is more difficult. Syncope and dizziness in patients with sinus node disease are more often associated with neurologic sequelae due in part to the possibility of more prolonged depression of cardiac output and also to the possibility of cerebral embolism complicating the event. Once again, this may make diagnosis difficult, and patients are labeled with a diagnosis of a transient ischemic attack (TIA). Loss of consciousness, however, is rare with TIAs.

Physical examination in patients with sinus node disease may reveal nothing abnormal. The most likely finding, however, is sinus bradycardia. The presence of this rhythm in an elderly person should arouse suspicion immediately. Sinus pauses and atrial tachyarrythmias are not often seen in the clinic and usually require longer periods of monitoring to become evident. Signs of heart failure should not be expected unless there is also an arrhythmia, either slow or fast. Other, possibly causative, systemic diseases should be sought as well.

Because therapy for sinus node disease has been limited in

TABLE 18–1. SYMPTOMS OF SINUS NODE DISEASE

DRAMATIC	SUBTLE
Dizziness	Palpitations
Syncope	Tiredness
Heart failure	Unrefreshing sleep
	Memory loss
	Poor concentration
	Early dementia
	Dyspnea on exertion

its efficacy, it has been restricted to patients with dramatic symptoms (Table 18–1). Now that therapy of much broader scope is available, using pacing modes that include the atria and provide rate responsiveness that can overcome chronotropic incompetence, the cardiologist is obligated to seek the more subtle symptoms (see Table 18–1) and to consider what treatment can be used to ameliorate them.

Diagnosis

The standard diagnostic tools available to the cardiologist are 12-lead electrocardiography, ambulatory ECG (Holter), and invasive electrophysiologic studies. Despite the sophistication of these tools, the diagnosis of sinus node disease often remains elusive and is seldom absolutely established by one test. The diagnosis of sinus node disease is a clinical diagnosis that requires the presence of *both* symptoms and objective ECG findings in most cases.

Ferrer, in her book in 1974,[11] listed a group of what she called 'indirect diagnostic criteria' (Table 18–2). All of these criteria are still pertinent today, and all can be approached by ECG (routine or Holter) except criterion number 5, which requires cardioversion. Today we add to these criteria those acquired from invasive electrophysiologic studies, which include sinus node recovery time, sinoatrial conduction time (with and without autonomic blockade), and direct recordings from the sinoatrial node.

It is important to note that a substantial number of patients with sinus node disease also show features of AV block.[51–53] In their literature review in 1986 of published work on sinus node disease, Sutton and Kenny[54] found that 16.6% of patients with sick sinus syndrome showed evidence of clinically significant AV block at initial diagnosis.

TABLE 18–2. FERRER'S DIAGNOSTIC CRITERIA FOR SINUS NODE DISEASE

1. Persistent, severe and unexpected sinus bradycardia, including inappropriately slow sinus rate or relatively slow sinus rhythm
2. Sinus arrest
   a. Short-lived—with no escape rhythm
   b. Longer-lived—replacement by atrial or junctional escape rhythms
   c. Long periods of sinus arrest without a rescue rhythm producing cardiac arrest and often ventricular arrhythmias
3. Sinoatrial exit block not related to drug therapy
4. Chronic atrial fibrillation replaces sinus rhythm, which has ceased. Atrial fibrillation is often accompanied by a slow ventricular rate in the absence of digitalis (due to accompanying AV nodal disease)
5. No sinus rhythm after cardioversion

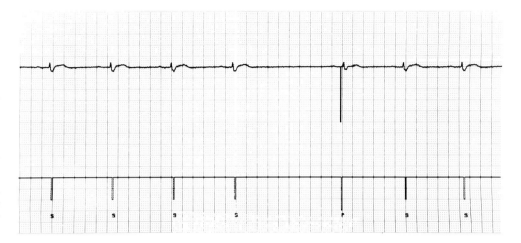

FIGURE 18–1. Single-channel electrocardiogram taken from a pacemaker programmer concurrent with a marker channel. The first four complexes are of sinus origin at 50 bpm. After the fourth complex, there is second-degree sinoatrial block. The next three complexes are again sinus bradycardia at 53 bpm. The pacemaker is ventricular demand (e.g., VVI) set at 30. A pacemaker stimulus is delivered in pseudofusion fashion in complex 5. All other ventricular complexes are correctly sensed.

Another factor that must be considered in the assessment of sinus node disease is the possible role of drugs. An accurate appraisal requires cessation of all antiarrhythmics, beta-blocking agents, vasodilators (e.g., certain calcium and alpha-blocking agents), digitalis preparations,[55] and other cardiovascular drugs[56] because many can create a clinical situation that mimics sinus node disease and a few can mask abnormal findings.

ECG documentation of sinoatrial block and sinus arrest is shown in Figures 18–1 and 18–2. In sinoatrial block there is a relationship between the pattern and the basic cycle length, and both Mobitz types I and II second-degree block are seen. With sinus arrest there is no relationship between the pause and the basic cycle length. Depressed AV nodal and atrial tachyarrhythmic escape mechanisms are shown in Figures 18–3 and 18–4. These rhythms plus atrial fibrillation, often with a slow ventricular response (which has not been illustrated), are the whole panoply of arrhythmias seen with sinus node disease. Approximately 50% of sinus node disease patients can be expected to show features of the bradycardia-tachycardia syndrome. First- and third-degree sinoatrial blocks are not detectable on the ECG. Patients with sinus node disease may also show atrial tachyarrhythmias that are not bradycardia dependent. This may be due to coincident atrial muscle disease.[57] A progression of arrhythmias over time is thought to occur beginning with sinus bradycardia and followed by sinoatrial block and sinus arrest, which are complicated by atrial tachyarrhythmias; the final rhythm is atrial fibrillation. This progression was recognized by Ferrer[11] and was certainly apparent in the clinical review by Sutton and Kenny.[54] It is important to bear in mind that sinus bradycardias, sinoatrial block, and sinus arrest can occur normally in young people and in atheletes.[58–60]

The duration of sinus pause or sinus arrest resulting in symptoms is variable. Asymptomatic pauses of up to 3 seconds in duration are relatively common and may be even more common in the elderly. Pauses of up to 3 seconds are not associated with adverse clinical consequences. Sinus pauses longer than 3 seconds are rare during ambulatory monitoring (<5% of patients) and are often associated with symptoms. Pauses longer than 3 seconds warrant careful clinical assessment, and attempts should be made to *correlate* clinical symptoms with ECG abnormalities.

INVASIVE ELECTROPHYSIOLOGY STUDIES

Electrophysiology studies may be indicated (1) in patients in whom sinus node disease is suspected but ECG has been inconclusive; (2) in patients with unexplained dizziness or syncope in whom electrocardiographic studies are nondiagnostic; and (3) in patients in whom more information is required about sinus node function and AV conduction before a pacemaker mode is selected (Table 18–3).

The results of electrophysiologic studies for sinus node disease *must always be correlated* with the clinical and ECG findings and are seldom considered finally diagnostic. The available electrophysiologic approaches are listed in Table 18–4.

SINUS NODE RECOVERY TIME

An approach based on overdrive suppression of the sinus node was pioneered by Mandel and colleagues[61] and Narula and associates.[62] The right atrium is paced beginning just above the sinus rate for a period that suppresses the sinus node in all patients. In patients with sinus node disease the recovery time is often delayed beyond that expected in normals. A typical protocol involves pacing at 80, 100, 120,

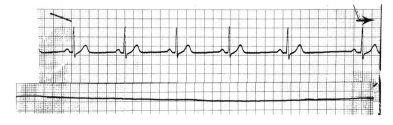

FIGURE 18–2. Electrocardiographic rhythm strip showing sinus bradycardia at 53 bpm, slowing to 43 bpm, which is then followed by sinoatrial arrest. The electrocardiographic strip is in two lines, which are continuous. There is asystole without any escape rhythm for 8 seconds.

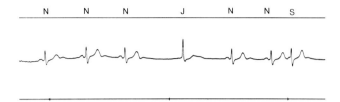

FIGURE 18–3. Rhythm strip taken from an ambulatory Holter monitor recording. This shows three complexes of sinus bradycardia followed by second-degree sinoatrial block and a junctional escape beat. Sinus bradycardia resumes with complex 5. An atrial premature beat is seen in complex 7.

TABLE 18–3. CLINICAL INDICATIONS FOR ELECTROPHYSIOLOGIC STUDIES IN PATIENTS WITH SINUS NODE DISEASE

1. Suspected sinus node disease when electrocardiography has been inconclusive
2. Unexplained syncope when sinus node disease may be the cause
3. When more information about sinus node dysfunction, its severity, extrinsic or intrinsic nature, and atrioventricular conduction prior to pacemaker mode selection or initiation of drug therapy (e.g., beta-blockers, calcium channel blockers, amiodarone) is required

140, and 160 bpm for 30 to 60 seconds at each rate, during which atrial capture must be ensured. It is important to record a multilead scalar ECG simultaneously with at least one right atrial intracavitary lead for at least 10 beats after cessation of pacing (Fig. 18–5). The initial escape rhythm may not be of sinus node origin, and there may be secondary pauses after the sinus node has reestablished itself. The time from the last stimulated atrial complex to the first sinus escape is termed the sinus node recovery time (SNRT).

The pacing period of 60 seconds is chosen to achieve stable conduction from the atria into the sinus node.[63, 64] Several pacing rates including one just above the sinus rate are chosen to attempt to overcome the possibility of sinoatrial entrance block,[65] which, if present, would prevent overdrive suppression. SNRT is prolonged with increasing pacing rates and reaches a plateau at 120 to 140 bpm in normals; the plateau usually occurs at lower rates in patients with sinus node disease.[61, 64, 66] Thus, use of very high rates, such as 180 bpm or higher, may be expected to yield little of value because of increasing sinoatrial entrance block.

SNRT requires correction for the control sinus cycle length. Corrected SNRT (CSNRT) is the SNRT minus the sinus cycle length.[61, 62, 67] The normal range for this measurement is considered to be up to 533 msec (many clinicians use a limit of <550 msec). Alternative methods consist of dividing the sinus cycle length into the SNRT and giving a percentage (normal, <150%) or to using a regression equation,[61, 68] but these methods have not reached the same level of clinical acceptance as CSNRT. Secondary pauses were analyzed by Benditt and coworkers[69] using a protocol similar to that described earlier. They found that 16 of their 39 patients sustained secondary pauses and noted a close correlation between this finding and ECG evidence of sinoatrial block or sinus pauses. The postpacing secondary pauses may be of more than one type, and the authors' explanation of this phenomenon is unclear. The total recovery time from the last paced beat to the resumption of continuous normal sinus activity should be less than 5 seconds.[70]

Peak paced cycle length (PCL_p) has been suggested as a possible means of increasing the sensitivity of SNRT.[71] This is the cycle length from which the longest SNRT is recorded. Patients without sinus node disease tend to show a PCL_p at 120 to 140 bpm. At rates above 140 bpm, the SNRT tends to decrease, probably due to the development of entrance block into the node at more rapid pacing rates and the hemodynamic consequences of the more rapid atrial pacing rate. In patients with sinus node disease peak paced cycle length tends to occur at rates less than 100 bpm.

Unfortunately, the sensitivity of SNRT is poor. Benditt and colleagues,[72] in their review in 1987, gave a range of 18% to 69%. However, the specificity of SNRT is good, ranging from 88% to 100%. The lack of sensitivity limits the role of SNRT in diagnostic confirmation of sinus node disease. This problem is most pertinent in patients who are being investigated for unexplained syncope; Benditt and colleagues found that 4% to 27% of these patients showed abnormalities of sinus node function.

SINOATRIAL CONDUCTION TIME

Sinoatrial conduction time (SACT) is the interval between the firing of the P cells and activation of the atrial muscle. Two indirect methods of determining this interval have been proposed; both are ingenious, but both can be frustrated by aspects of the disease itself. The first of these methods involves premature atrial stimulation and is known as the Strauss method.[73] The principle depends on the premature beat (inserted by the electrophysiologist) depolarizing the sinoatrial node but not altering its automaticity or conduction of the next beat of sinus origin outward from the node. From a series of increasingly premature inserted stimuli, which illustrate the resetting of the sinus node, a calculation can be made by taking the difference between the return atrial cycle length and the spontaneous cycle length. This is often given as the sum of the antegrade and retrograde conduction times. Occasionally it is divided by two, and this process makes a

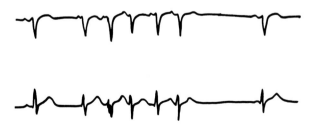

FIGURE 18–4. Rhythm strip showing sinus bradycardia on a two-channel recording. There is an escape atrial tachycardia beginning in complex 2 and terminating spontaneously with complex 6. Then there is a pause, followed by resumption of the baseline sinus bradycardia.

TABLE 18–4. ELECTROPHYSIOLOGIC ASSESSMENT OF SINUS NODE DISEASE

1. Sinus node recovery time (SNRT)
2. Sinoatrial conduction time (SACT)
3. Direct recording of the sinoatrial electrogram
4. Sinoatrial refractoriness
5. Repetition of Nos. 1 to 4 after autonomic blockade
6. Repetition of Nos. 1 to 4 after drug challenge

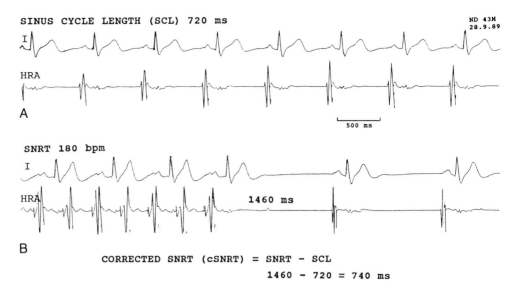

FIGURE 18–5. Surface electrocardiographic limb lead I and intracardiac recordings from the high right atrium (HRA). *A,* The patient's spontaneous sinus cycle length is 720 msec. *B,* A sinus node recovery time (SNRT) is calculated. Atrial pacing is performed at 180 bpm, and pacing is abruptly terminated. There is a 1460-msec pause before resumption of atrial activity. The corrected SNRT (cSNRT) is equal to 1460 minus 720 (the baseline sinus cycle measures 720 msec [shown in *A*]) or 740 msec. This is moderately prolonged.

further assumption that the antegrade and retrograde values are equal (Figs. 18–6 and 18–7). The range of considered normality is wide, 198 to 304 msec[74] (without dividing by two). Once again, the sensitivity of this test for sinus node dysfunction is poor. In Benditt and colleagues' review, the range of its sensitivity was 29% to 63%.[72] Even the specificity was less than that of the SNRT, ranging from 57% to 100%. Thus, this time-consuming technique has to an extent fallen out of favor in the assessment of sinus node disease.

The alternative approach to measurement of SACT is that proposed by Narula and colleagues[75] (Fig. 18–8). This is the constant atrial pacing approach in which the right atrium is paced for 8 beats less than 10 bpm above the sinus rate. SACT is calculated as the difference between the first return cycle and the mean spontaneous cycle length. Four or five determinations are made, and a mean is taken. This method has been criticized[76] because of differences in atriosinus conduction and the effect on sinus node automaticity and because of differences in the results obtained (vs. the Strauss method).

SINOATRIAL ELECTROGRAM

Direct recording of the sinoatrial electrogram promises much better results than indirect techniques. An invasive method of recording is required for precision. The difficulty of recording sinoatrial activity on the surface ECG is explained partly by the slow conduction within the sinoatrial node and partly by the presence of only approximately 5000 P cells.

The first reports of recording of the sinoatrial electrogram emanated from Cramer and colleagues.[77, 78] Investigators from the same institution later recorded the sinoatrial electrogram in humans during cardiac surgery[79] at first and then during cardiac catheterization.[80] Initial success was not great (50%[80]), but with careful positioning of the catheter and electrode very close to the sinus node and with adequate filtering success rates of more than 80% have been claimed.[81, 82] This technique has allowed comparison of direct methods with indirect methods. However, electrode position still plays an important part in the direct measurement,[83] and

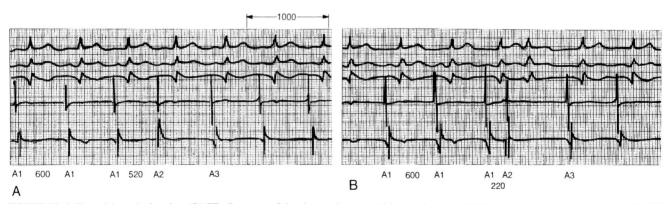

FIGURE 18–6. Sinoatrial conduction time (SACT). Response of the sinus node to an atrial extrastimulus. A1A1 is the spontaneous sinus cycle length (600 msec). *A,* The effect of an atrial extrastimulus (A2) delivered late in the cardiac cycle at a coupling interval (A1A2) of 520 msec. The sinus node is not affected by the extrastimulus as manifested by the full compensatory pause of the return cycle (A3), resulting in A1A2 + A2A3 = 2 × A1A1. *B,* An earlier extrastimulus (A1A2 = 220 msec) resets the sinus node so that the return cycle (A3) occurs earlier. The resulting A2A3 (780 msec) is longer than the sinus cycle length (A1A1 = 600 msec). The difference between the two (A2A3 − A1A1 = 180 msec) is the sum of the time taken by the extrastimulus to enter the sinus node and the time taken by the sinus impulse to propagate to the atrial tissue. This sum, divided by two, is the SACT (90 msec). (From Sutton R, Bourgeois I: The Foundations of Cardiac Pacing. Mt Kisco, NY, Futura Publishing Co., 1991.)

Strauss' Method for Sinoatrial Conduction Time

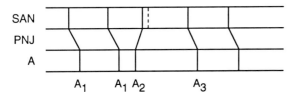

FIGURE 18–7. Strauss' method for determining sinoatrial conduction time. Ladder diagram representing conduction from the sinoatrial node (SAN) through the perinodal junction (PNJ) to the atrial muscle (A). The first two beats are spontaneous (A1, A1) and illustrate the sinus cycle length (SCL). The third beat is a premature stimulus (A2), which is conducted retrogradely into the sinus and resets it ahead of the next expected sinus beat *(dotted line)*. The next spontaneous cycle is A3. A2A3 is termed the return cycle, which represents the SCL plus the SACT (sinoatrial conduction). A2A3 minus A1A1 equals SACT. SACT is divided by 2 because the time measured here is for conduction into and out of the SAN.

the method appears to lack sensitivity.[81, 82] It has not been adopted as a routine measurement of sinus node function in electrophysiology laboratories. In general, direct recordings of sinoatrial conduction time tend to be longer than indirect methods; however, both direct and indirect methods of recording sinoatrial conduction show similar results. Based on direct recordings of the sinoatrial electrograms, it appears that sinoatrial block is an important component of the asystolic pause that occurs in patients with hypersensitive carotid sinus syndrome, and of the pauses that occur following atrial pacing. These measurements also suggest that patients with sinus node disorders who have an abnormal SNRT have marked abnormalities of sinoatrial conduction rather than depression of automaticity alone.

SINOATRIAL REFRACTORINESS

If the sinus node itself or the tissue surrounding it has prolonged refractoriness, this will influence both indirect and

Narula's Method for Sinoatrial Conduction Time

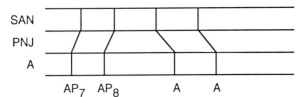

FIGURE 18–8. Narula's method for determining sinoatrial conduction time. The first two beats in this ladder diagram illustrate atrial pacing at a cycle length that is slightly shorter than the spontaneous sinus cycle length (SCL). These beats are the seventh and eighth of a series (AP7, AP8); they are conducted retrogradely into the sinus node and reset it. Pacing ceases after the eighth beat, when the spontaneous sinus rhythm resumes with two beats marked A. The postpacing sinus cycle length is used as the control cycle length to calculate the SACT with this method. The interval following termination of the atrially paced drive train and the next spontaneous atrial activation (AP8 − A) represents the sum of the basic sinus cycle length (SCL) and the SACT. The difference between the postdrive return cycle length (A-A) and the paced cycle length (AP7 − AP8) represents the SACT. Because this measurement of SACT represents conduction into and out of the sinoatrial node, SACT is divided by 2 to give half the time measured.

direct measurements of SNRT and SACT. Measurement of sinoatrial refractoriness[84] has been achieved by inserting premature atrial stimuli after a series of regular paced stimuli. As the inserted stimulus becomes increasingly premature, interpolation occurs that represents the refractory period of the sinus node. Early results suggested that this method was more reliable than SNRT and SACT,[85, 86] but it has not yet been widely applied, and it may be measurable in only 75% of patients.

AUTONOMIC BLOCKADE

In view of the possibility that measured abnormalities of sinus node function may be imposed by the autonomic nervous system rather than being representative of local pathology, it is necessary to repeat some or all of the assessments described previously after instituting autonomic blockade. This blockade can be achieved by giving a combination of atropine at a dose of 0.04 mg/kg (maximum, 3 mg) and propranolol at a dose of 0.15 mg/kg (maximum, 10 mg), administered intravenously during the electrophysiology study. The use of this drug combination was first reported by Jose in 1966[87] before the era of invasive electrophysiology, and it was later adopted by electrophysiologists.[88] This appears to be an attractive technique that permits better insight into sinus node function. Unfortunately, it is limited by the variable direct effect of atropine and propranolol on sinoatrial conduction and possibly also on the automaticity of the sinus node. Atropine should result in an increase in heart rate of about 15%, or to above 85 to 90 bpm. Propranolol should result in a 12% or more decrease in heart rate. Both of these drug effects show limited sensitivity for the diagnosis of sick sinus syndrome. The available data[67, 88–90] from application of this technique suggest that an appreciable number of patients with sinus node disease have the extrinsic form of the disease; Yee and Strauss[74] in their review suggest perhaps 25%. Autonomic blockade can be used without electrophysiology studies to define the intrinsic heart rate, as shown by Jose.[87, 91] This procedure has some diagnostic value in the identification of intrinsic sinus node abnormalities, but it is seldom used without invasive electrophysiology studies today.

DRUG CHALLENGE

Drug challenge to the integrity of AV conduction is an established although not widely used technique.[92–94] A similar approach to sinus node function can only be considered experimental because validation of its effects has not yet been published. Flecainide given intravenously during electrophysiology studies has been reported to produce significant negative effects on both AV conduction and sinus node function. It may therefore be a drug with the capability of unmasking abnormalities at both sites in patients who present with unexplained dizziness and syncope.[95] Many antiarrhythmic agents have been shown to have depressive effects on sinus node function at electrophysiology study.[96, 97]

OTHER INVESTIGATIONS

Other tests for sinus node dysfunction consist of the use of intravenous atropine, isoproterenol, and exercise to gauge their effect on the node as well as tests used for diagnosis of carotid sinus syndrome and vasovagal syndromes, which are undoubtedly related to extrinsic sinus node disease.

ISOPROTERENOL

Ferrer[11] suggested the use of isoproterenol to assess its positive chronotropic effect on the sinus node. A dose of 0.1 μg/min was given by intravenous infusion. The dose was increased progressively to achieve an effect before ventricular premature beats supervened. This test also lacks sensitivity and has fallen out of favor. The increase in heart rate that results depends on the specific dose used.

HOLTER (AMBULATORY) MONITORING

The most specific diagnostic observation is the ECG recording of the cardiac arrhythmia during the patient's symptomatic episode. Establishing a diagnosis by means of ambulatory Holter monitoring can be both expensive and frustrating. Holter monitoring is typically performed for 48 to 72 hours in either an inpatient or outpatient setting. Monitoring performed on an ambulatory basis exposes the patient to a recurrent and potentially serious symptomatic arrhythmia. On the other hand, repeated outpatient evaluation over a long period of time may be necessary because of the infrequent occurrence of the patient's symptoms.

Another diagnostic technique used in this patient population is transtelephonic recorders that are carried or worn by the patient. These recorders are typically dispensed for 1 to 2 months. The recorder is manually activated by the patient and can record from 30 seconds to 2 minutes from two ECG leads. Some models of transtelephonic recorders, continuous loop monitors, are worn continuously and have a memory that can store 30 seconds to 2 minutes of an ECG before activation of the event marker. These monitors are most useful in patients with intermittent symptoms, especially if the symptoms are not associated with abrupt syncope or if they occur with a brief prodrome.

EXERCISE TESTING

Relative exercise bradycardia was recognized early in the clinical appreciation of sinus node disease,[98, 99] although its occurrence as a marker of heart disease, especially myocardial ischemia, was noted at an even earlier stage.[50, 100] It was Ellestad and Wan[50] who first used the term chronotropic incompetence, which is now employed to describe the relative exercise bradycardia of sinus node disease. Abbott and colleagues[98] and Holden and associates[99] found exercise testing a useful adjunct to the diagnosis of sinus node disease. The emphasis has changed in recent years to the use of exercise testing to grade the severity of the condition and to select the pacing mode. The poor prognosis of chronotropically incompetent patients identified by Hinkle and colleagues[100] and Ellestad and Wan[50] is not now thought to apply particularly to patients with sinus node disease. The reasons for the poor heart rate seen with exercise in their heart disease patients were probably multiple and related to angina pectoris, dyspnea, and medication.

Chronotropic incompetence has no universally accepted definition. Ellestad and Wan[50] suggested a maximum heart rate of less than the 95% confidence limit taken from their

vast collection of exercise tests in normal individuals (see Chapter 26). In studies of sinus node disease patients, a simple rate criterion has been attractive. Simonsen[101] suggested less than 110 bpm, and Dreifus and colleagues[102] suggested less than 100 bpm. Further studies suggest that heart rate response to exercise may be variable, but in those with other clear evidence of sinus node disease it tends to deteriorate.[101, 103, 104] The pattern of heart rate change during exercise is also variable. Lau[105] has shown slow, delayed, and intermittent acceleration as well as a rapid fall in heart rate during the recovery period in patients with chronotropic dysfunction. These features determine that estimates of the incidence of chronotropic incompetence may vary from 20% to 60% of patients with sinus node disease.[104, 106, 107] The choice of exercise protocol is considered very important in assessing the heart rate response of sick sinus patients because of their age and the different patterns of heart rate change. Wilkoff and colleagues[108] have recommended a much more gently developing exercise test known as the Chronotropic Assessment Exercise Protocol (CAEP), which has come into widespread use.

CAROTID SINUS MASSAGE

Carotid sinus massage, performed according to standard techniques,[41, 42] should not be regarded as a test for sinus node disease, but a positive outcome may occur in patients with extrinsic sinus node disease. According to our present understanding, if carotid sinus massage is positive and if tests of sinus node function are abnormal, the patient is considered to have carotid sinus syndrome. With better understanding of the autonomic nervous system and its abnormalities of heart rate and peripheral vascular control, a different classification may be made.

TILT TESTING

Head-up tilt table testing, introduced in 1986[109] to diagnose vasovagal syncope, has been widely used by electrophysiologists.[110–112] A positive outcome may occur in patients with evidence of extrinsic sinus node disease. Again, as with carotid sinus syndrome, the present approach is to classify such patients as having vasovagal syndrome (see Chapter 21).

In conclusion, the diagnosis of sinus node disease must be made on the basis of findings that will always include ECG abnormalities. Electrophysiologic data can serve only to contribute to this diagnosis. That sinus node disease is symptomatic requires demonstration of the coincidence of an arrhythmia with symptoms. Ancillary tests such as exercise are used to characterize the patient rather than to diagnose the disease. It would be desirable to use the tests described not only to select immediate therapy but also to predict future developments in both symptomatic and asymptomatic patients. Gann and colleagues'[113] prospective study suggests that electrophysiology studies are also limited in this respect. However, the combination of symptoms and electrophysiologic abnormalities may be taken to support the decision for pacemaker therapy, and the presence of electrophysiologic abnormalities in asymptomatic patients is a fairly good predictor of a future need for pacing.[113]

Complications of Sinus Node Disease

Four major complications of this condition are recognized: AV block, atrial fibrillation and other atrial tachyarrhythmias, systemic embolism, and congestive heart failure.

ATRIOVENTRICULAR BLOCK

Sinus node disease is associated with disease of AV conduction.[51–53] However, AV conduction problems have not been considered serious contraindications to pacing the atrium only (AAI or AAIR mode) by some enthusiastic centers. In 1986 Sutton and Kenny's[54] literature review highlighted an apparent high incidence (8.4%) of development of clinically significant AV block over 34.2 months. This finding has since been vigorously criticized[114] on the basis of an alternative literature review. Even if the incidence is 4.5% in 4 years[115] or 8.5% in 10 years,[116] it is still appreciable because it is usually associated with symptoms, and if the AAI pacing mode has been chosen, surgical intervention is *necessary* to upgrade to DDD(R) pacing modes.

There is a considerable difference of opinion about which clinical and ECG variables best predict the development of AV block in patients undergoing AAI pacing. Several groups have argued that an intraoperative Wenckebach rate of more than 120 bpm is associated with a low likelihood of development of late AV block. Brandt and colleagues' recent study does not support this observation and suggests that only complete bundle branch block or bifascicular block is associated with a higher incidence of late development of AV block with AAI pacing.[116]

ATRIAL FIBRILLATION

Chronic atrial fibrillation is an end-point rhythm in sinus node disease. It is assumed that the presence of concomitant AV conduction system disease, the inadequacy of subsidiary cardiac pacemakers, or both lead to atrial fibrillation with a slow ventricular response. More frequently, atrial fibrillation with a rapid ventricular response is seen in this patient population. In the Sutton and Kenny review[54] development of atrial fibrillation occurred in 15.8% of patients with sick sinus syndrome over 38.2 months. The arrhythmia itself may be responsible for symptoms owing to low cardiac output or irregular heart rate, but its most important implications are the likelihood of systemic embolism and the need to abandon atrial pacing.

SYSTEMIC EMBOLISM

Patients with sinus node disease, especially those with the bradycardia-tachycardia syndrome, are at risk for systemic embolism. Sutton and Kenny[54] found an incidence of systemic embolism of 15.2% in unpaced patients, whereas in patients of similar age without sinus node disease it was 1.3%.[117]

CONGESTIVE HEART FAILURE

From the prospective study of Rosenqvist and colleagues[115] it is clear that congestive heart failure develops in some patients with sinus node disease even when they are physiologically paced.

Medical Treatment

Medical treatment for sinus node disease must be considered in two categories: first, medication to control the manifestations of the disease itself; second, medication to act as an adjunct to pacing.

The nature of sinus node disease offers an almost insuperable challenge to medical treatment. A drug is required that prevents both bradycardia and tachycardia. A conventional antiarrhythmic agent may control tachycardia but usually exacerbates bradycardia and is therefore untenable. Drugs that either block the parasympathetic or emphasize the sympathetic influences on the sinoatrial node cause intolerable side effects, fail to achieve the desired effect, and favor the initiation of atrial tachyarrhythmias. More radical approaches have been considered, notably the use of theophylline compounds to antagonize the effect of adenosine. This may have value in some patients with extrinsic sinus node disease, but experience with the drug is small, and failures have been reported.[118]

The second use of drugs in combination with pacing in patients with sinus node disease is as an aid in maximizing rhythm control and preventing complications. When the atria are stimulated, atrial tachyarrhythmias may still occur, and better control can be enforced by using an antiarrhythmic agent. In my experience, amiodarone is the drug of choice. It is associated with a long list of important side effects, but in low doses, perhaps as little as 100 mg per day, in this elderly group of patients with sinus node disease it is well tolerated, and side effects of all types are rare except for altered sleep patterns and ultraviolet sensitivity. Drugs such as flecainide and propafenone are moderately efficacious but are not free of side effects. Both these drugs adversely influence pacing and sensitivity thresholds. Once a permanent pacemaker has been implanted, patients need to be assessed by ambulatory monitoring, and if atrial tachyarrhythmias are found to remain, they should be vigorously treated. Only in this way can the physician expect to prevent chronic atrial fibrillation, systemic embolism, and congestive heart failure.

A second group of drugs to be considered is the group of anticoagulants. Many large studies on the prevention of systemic embolism in patients with atrial fibrillation have recently been reported.[119–122] The consensus of these studies is that warfarin, possibly in low doses, giving an International Normalized Ratio (INR) of 2.0 to 3.0, is superior to aspirin. If the patient continues to experience atrial tachyarrhythmias despite atrial pacing and antiarrhythmic agents, anticoagulation must be instituted.

Permanent Pacing in Patients with Sinus Node Disease

HISTORY

Pacing for sinus node disease was undertaken quite early in the history of pacing and in the understanding of the disease. The first report of ventricular pacing for management of sinoatrial block was made by Muller and Finkelstein in 1966.[123] Other reports of small series of ventricularly paced patients[124–131] followed during the next few years, reporting good control of dizziness and syncope. Ferrer[11] in 1974 recommended ventricular pacing in preference to atrial pacing, but already pioneers had selected atrial pacing with considerable success.[132–134] Early problems concerned the atrial lead, which was usually placed in the proximal coronary sinus. An excessive rise in stimulation threshold was experienced at this site.[135] By the mid-1970s small series were available for comparison with ventricular pacing[136, 137] and between different atrial pacing sites.[133, 136, 137] The hemodynamic and rhythm control advantages of atrial pacing were colored by the lead-related complications.[136]

IMPROVED TRANSVENOUS ATRIAL LEADS

At this time atrial leads underwent an important design change that eventually permitted their general use.[138, 139] This was the introduction of a J-shaped lead that allowed easy access to the right atrial appendage. Furthermore, the lead was equipped with tines close to the electrode that engaged the trabeculae in the appendage, vastly improving lead stability. Active fixation of atrial leads in the right atrial appendage also became feasible in the late 1970s.[140] The best design, that of Bisping,[141] has a retractable screw for safe passage through the venous system. J-shaped versions were made available. The screw electrode probably wraps the trabeculae in the appendage around it rather than being screwed into the thin atrial wall. Active fixation leads also permit the physician to place them at other atrial sites, for example, in the crista terminalis or interatrial septum. Tined leads are often not stable in the stump of the right atrial appendage, which remains after cardiopulmonary bypass. Active fixation leads have overcome this common clinical problem and allow the physician to map different sites in the right atrium to test pacing and sensing at various sites. A more recent study from Gross and his colleagues[142] reported a lower incidence of atrial lead–related complications. They followed 486 consecutive patients who had initial implants of transvenous DDD pacemakers between December 1981 and 1988; a 2% incidence of atrial lead dislodgments requiring a secondary operative procedure was reported in these patients.[142] Other groups have also reported a similarly low incidence of atrial lead dislodgment.

RECOGNITION OF THE BENEFITS OF ATRIAL PACING

By the mid-1980s atrial lead placement had become a widely available technique, but neither atrial nor dual-chamber pacing had been widely adopted. Literature reviews[54] and prospective studies[115] showed the clear advantages of atrial pacing over ventricular pacing in patients with sinus node disease (see Chapters 23 to 25 and Table 18–5). These have advanced the cause of more physiologic pacing modes, but worldwide their use remains limited.[143] Skeptics continue to express reservations about the ease of positioning and long-term results of atrial leads, remain concerned about atrial arrhythmias and AV block, are reluctant to expend the funds to pay for dual-chamber pacing when single-chamber ventricular pacing is cheaper, and are unconvinced by the quality of life benefits.

TABLE 18–5. THE ADVANTAGES OF PACING SYSTEMS THAT INCLUDE THE ATRIA IN SINUS NODE DISEASE

1. Normal atrioventricular sequence
2. Control of atrial arrhythmias (probable)
3. Improved quality of life
4. Greater functional capacity
5. Reduction of systemic embolism (probable)
6. Problems of retrograde atrioventricular conduction avoided
7. Less congestive heart failure (probable)
8. Lower mortality (probable)

Sutton and Kenny[54] showed a highly significant difference between 410 patients with AAI pacemakers of whom 3.9% developed atrial fibrillation over 32.8 months versus 651 VVI-paced patients who showed an incidence of 22.3% of atrial fibrillation over 39.0 months. Furthermore, systemic embolism occurred in 1.6% of 321 AAI-paced patients compared with 13% of 651 VVI-paced patients, who, however, had longer follow-up. This difference was also highly significant, but the authors emphasized that this was in no way a scientific comparison and should be considered only as a guide.

The work of Rosenqvist and colleagues[115] must be considered the most valuable published work to date because it is a nonrandomized prospective study. Two centers in Sweden, one with a VVI policy for pacing in patients with sick sinus syndrome and the other with an AAI policy for pacing in all suitable patients with this syndrome, were compared. After 4 years of follow-up the incidence of permanent atrial fibrillation in the VVI group was 47% compared to a 6.7% incidence of atrial fibrillation in the AAI group ($p < .0005$). The incidence of congestive heart failure was 37% in the VVI group compared to 15% in the AAI group ($p < .005$). The mortality in the patients with VVI pacemakers was 23% compared to only 8% in the patients with AAI pacemakers ($p < .005$). Strangely, there was no significant difference in the incidence of stroke between the two pacing modes. However, patients were not surveyed intensively after implant for atrial arrhythmias, and anticoagulation was not used. The authors advised the use of anticoagulation for patients with VVI pacemakers and sick sinus syndrome.

There now exist a large number of *retrospective* studies that compare atrial or dual-chamber pacing with single-chamber ventricular pacing. These results are shown in Figures 18–9 to 18–11, which summarize several selected studies. These studies have been recently reviewed by Lamas.[144] The majority of these studies included patients who were being paced for sick sinus syndrome, although several included patients who were being paced for AV block as well. The end-points of these studies include the development of atrial fibrillation, heart failure, stroke, and death.

With respect to atrial fibrillation, a past history of previous atrial arrhythmias is a major determinant of the development of atrial arrhythmias after implantation of a pacemaker. Many studies showed that atrial fibrillation develops more often in patients with sick sinus syndrome after implantation of a VVI pacemaker than after implantation of a DDDR or AAI pacemaker. This difference may or may not be present, depending on whether patients have a previous history of atrial tachyarrhythmias, but it is very striking in patients with a previous history of paroxysmal atrial tachyarrhythmias. Analysis of the data from multiple studies showed that the

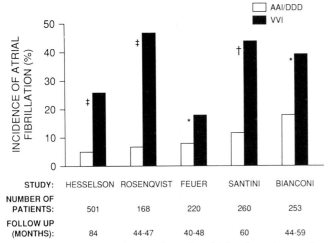

FIGURE 18–9. Comparative studies of atrial-based pacing modes (AAI/DDD) with VVI pacing mode in patients with sick sinus syndrome. The incidence of chronic atrial fibrillation developing with different pacing modes compiled from several different studies is shown. The data presented here (except for those from Feuer and colleagues) include only data from patients in whom permanent pacemakers were implanted for sinus node dysfunction. The number of patients are listed below the name of the first author of each study. The duration of follow-up is stated in months. Probabilities are as follows: *$p < .05$, †$p < .01$, and ‡$p < .005$.

average yearly rate of atrial fibrillation was 7.5% in patients with VVI pacing and 2.2% in those with DDD or AAI pacing (Fig. 18–9). There was no significant difference in the yearly incidence of atrial fibrillation in patients receiving DDD pacemakers compared to those with AAI pacemakers.

The studies examining the impact of different modes of cardiac pacing on congestive heart failure consist of two types. One group of studies compared the incidence of development of heart failure that occurred in patients with different pacing modes (Fig. 18–10). In several studies the incidence of congestive heart failure was 7.5% per year with VVI pacing versus 1.8% per year with DDD or AAI pacing. Another type of study compared the influence of preexisting congestive heart failure on mortality in patients with different pacing modes. In many studies the mortality during follow-up, which ranged from 12 to more than 84 months, in patients receiving VVI pacemakers was 7.1% compared to 3.2% in patients receiving DDD or AAI pacemakers.

Finally, the incidence of stroke and thromboembolism was measured in several studies comparing different pacing modes (Fig. 18–11). The incidence of stroke and thromboembolism was significantly higher in patients with VVI pacemakers than in those with an atrial pacing modality. The incidence of stroke was lower in patients with AAI or DDD pacing than in those with VVI pacing in two of the six studies, but there was no significant difference between the atrial and ventricular pacing modes in the other four studies in which this variable was examined.

These studies are *retrospective* analyses and fail to account for a number of shortcomings. For example, they fail to take into account the obvious selection bias favoring the less sick patients who receive the more complex DDD or AAI pacemakers, whereas sicker patients are more likely to receive VVI pacemakers. Some of these studies suffer from incomplete follow-up, inconsistent and poorly defined clinical events, failure to study quality of life, and long-term cost of care. Several studies suffer from inadequate sample size and too variable patient follow-up. Additional important concerns include the selection of older patients and those with a previous history of supraventricular tachycardia for pacing with a VVI pacemaker.

These issues are further highlighted by several recent studies. Hesselson and coworkers reviewed the experience from the Beth Israel Medical Center in Newark.[146] They found a higher incidence of chronic atrial fibrillation in patients with VVI pacemakers, whether the etiology of their conduction system disease was complete heart block or sick sinus syndrome. Their study was notable for the large number of patients studied (950), the long duration of follow-up (7 to 8 years), and the finding that survival at 7 years was lower in the VVI-paced group than in the DDD- or DVI-paced group. The differences in mortality and incidence of atrial fibrillation were most striking in patients over the age of 70 years and in those with sick sinus syndrome. The major weaknesses of this retrospective study are the obscure reasoning for selection of pacing mode and the fact that more than 40 different physicians implanted pacemakers in this series.

Sgarbossa and colleagues[147] reported findings from the Cleveland Clinic and also underscored the need for a prospective trial. They examined the total and cardiovascular mortality of 507 patients from the Cleveland Clinic who had a mean duration of follow-up of 66 months. In this study, in

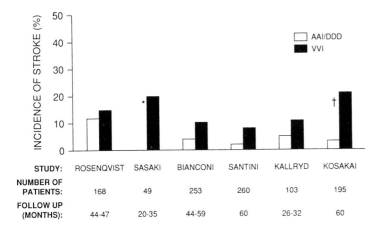

FIGURE 18–10. Comparative studies of AAI/DDD pacing modes with VVI pacing mode in patients with pacemakers implanted for sick sinus syndrome. The incidence of stroke in patients with different pacing modes from different studies is shown. The data presented here include those from patients undergoing permanent pacemaker implantation for sick sinus syndrome only. Probabilities are as follows: *$p < .05$, †$p < .01$.

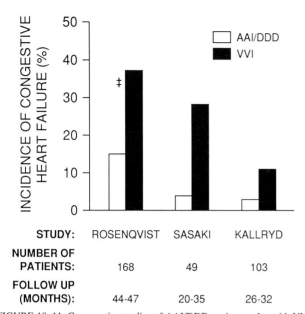

FIGURE 18–11. Comparative studies of AAI/DDD pacing modes with VVI pacing mode in patients with pacemakers implanted for sick sinus syndrome. The incidence of development of congestive heart failure from several different studies is shown. The data presented here include those from patients undergoing pacemaker implantation for sick sinus syndrome only. ‡$p < .005$.

contrast to the study from the Beth Israel hospital in Newark, the VVI pacing mode was *not* a long-term predictor of total and cardiovascular mortality using multivariate analysis. In their study (Cleveland Clinic's), the New York Heart Association (NYHA) functional class, age, peripheral vascular disease, bundle branch block, coronary artery disease, valvular heart disease, and cerebrovascular disease were the only independent predictors of mortality. Using univariate analysis, VVI pacing was associated with more than a 40% increased risk of total and cardiovascular death, but this difference was only of borderline significance ($p = .053$; confidence interval, 0.99–2.07). In another report, Sgarbossa and colleagues[148] studied the incidence of chronic atrial fibrilla-

tion and stroke in paced patients with sick sinus syndrome. In this report, the development of chronic atrial fibrillation and stroke was strongly determined, like survival in their previous reports, by clinical variables. In the case of chronic atrial fibrillation, these clinical variables were a history of paroxysmal atrial fibrillation, the use of antiarrhythmic drugs prior to implantation, age, and the presence of valvular heart disease. Clinical predictors of stroke were a history of cerebrovascular disease and a history of paroxysmal atrial fibrillation. Ventricular pacing was a significant predictor of stroke and atrial fibrillation. A tendency toward atrial fibrillation in patients who were paced by VVI devices was significant *only* in patients with a history of paroxysmal atrial fibrillation prior to implantation, especially when episodes lasted longer than 1 hour (Fig. 18–12).

NEED FOR RANDOMIZED CONTROLLED TRIALS OF ATRIAL PACING

The medical community has been calling for randomized controlled trials in this field,[144] and some of these are now underway in Canada, Europe, and the United States. The deleterious role of ventricular pacing in causing atrial fibrillation, congestive heart failure, stroke, and death is still not conclusive. The first of these trials, from Denmark, was reported at the European Congress of Cardiology in August, 1993.[145] Preliminary information obtained from this AAI versus VVI study, which meets strict scientific criteria, points to significant advantages of AAI pacing in the terms expected from the Rosenqvist work.[115] Preliminary results from this study suggest a decrease in the incidence of atrial fibrillation and cerebrovascular accidents with AAI pacing compared with VVI pacing. From these studies it is difficult to know whether AAI/DDD pacing is "antiarrhythmic" or VVI pacing is "proarrhythmic," leading to the higher incidence of atrial fibrillation seen with single-chamber ventricular pacing.

In addition to the Swedish studies,[115, 116] other valuable (although retrospective) studies supporting information about the benefits of pacing systems that include the atria have emanated from Italy,[149] Japan,[150] and the United States.[151, 152]

FIGURE 18–12. Plot of comparative incidence of chronic atrial fibrillation (CAF) according to preimplant history of paroxysmal atrial fibrillation (PAF) for each pacing modality (n = 507). (Reproduced with permission from Sgarbossa EB, Pinski SL, Maloney JD, et al: Chronic atrial fibrillation and stroke in paced patients with sick sinus syndrome. Circulation 88:1045, 1993. Copyright 1993 American Heart Association.)

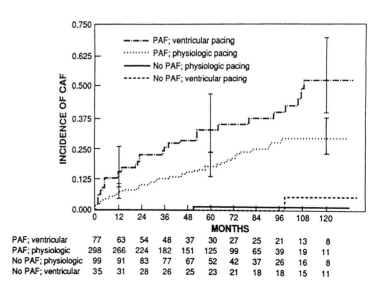

	0	12	24	36	48	60	72	84	96	108	120
PAF; ventricular	77	63	54	48	37	30	27	25	21	13	8
PAF; physiologic	298	266	224	182	151	125	99	65	39	19	11
No PAF; physiologic	99	91	83	77	67	52	42	37	26	16	8
No PAF; ventricular	35	31	28	26	25	23	21	18	18	15	11

In the presence of this evidence one is tempted to ask how much persuasion the pacing physician needs.

DUAL-CHAMBER OR ATRIAL PACING?

Controversy also continues about the need for dual-chamber pacing as opposed to simple atrial pacing. This controversy hinges on two issues. The first is the incidence of AV block, which is clearly low.[54, 115] The decision for or against the addition of a ventricular lead is founded on the psychological approach of the physician implanter and the available funds. Those who prefer to invest now to give their patients an easier time later opt for dual-chamber devices, whereas those who prefer to make a smaller investment and take a risk choose atrial pacing. The available data[48, 143] suggest that more physicians make the former choice. The second issue in this respect concerns the disadvantage of the ventricular lead. The physician has to decide how to optimally program the dual-chamber device. Ventricular stimulation will be used or not, depending on the duration of the AV delay. Selection of a long AV delay allows spontaneous conduction to the ventricle to occur with inhibition of the ventricular channel. This equates to atrial pacing and causes no problems unless ventricular stimulation actually occurs. If this happens, retrograde atrioventricular (AV) conduction and pacemaker-mediated tachycardia (PMT) may occur at some time.[153] If a shorter AV delay is selected to impose ventricular pacing, the likelihood of PMTs is less, but significant hemodynamic disadvantages are incurred[154] because ventricular pacing from the apex of the right ventricle has been shown to be negatively inotropic. Undoubtedly, this controversy will continue for some years to come and will probably be resolved only by adoption of the more sophisticated and expensive option, which allows greater programming facility.

IS ATRIAL FIBRILLATION A CURE FOR THE SYMPTOMS OF SINOATRIAL NODE DISEASE?

One additional consideration requires mention and that is whether chronic atrial fibrillation is a curative or an amelioration of sinus node disease. If it is curative, as claimed by some groups,[155, 156] with AAI pacing being irrelevant in patients with chronic atrial fibrillation, the patient would be at little or no risk. However, the relief of symptoms with the onset of chronic atrial fibrillation in sick sinus syndrome has certainly not been the impression of others,[11, 157, 158] who have observed slow ventricular rates and resumption of dizziness and syncope requiring ventricular pacing. Selection of a dual-chamber device at the outset avoids these problems.

DDD OR DDI MODE?

The next issue to be discussed is which dual-chamber mode should be selected. The possible recurrence of atrial tachyarrhythmias, which may be sensed by the atrial amplifier, resulting in high-rate ventricular stimulation, is not desirable but is likely with the DDD mode in operation. Floro and colleagues[159] in 1984 proposed the DDI mode as a means of overcoming this problem. This mode can now be programmed in nearly all dual-chamber pacemakers. It offers on-demand stimulation in the atria and the ventricles with disabling of atrial triggering of ventricular stimulation. Thus, there is no rate response of ventricular stimulation to rising atrial rates, and pacemaker-mediated tachycardia is impossible. However, problems of retrograde AV conduction[160, 161] are not avoided and in fact are probably more common because the mode can engender long AV intervals. It is certainly an attractive mode for use in sinus node disease patients with the bradycardia-tachycardia syndrome, and Bana and colleagues[162] have reported good results with its use. As Barold[160] anticipated in 1987, this mode has now been incorporated into many current dual-chamber devices to be switched on when rapid atrial rates are detected. This technique is now known as mode switching. Strictly speaking, this mode in this situation should be termed VDI because no atrial stimulation occurs except at the lower rate limit. Some manufacturers refer to it as DDI and some as VVI.

AUTOMATIC MODE SWITCHING

Mode-switching devices were introduced in the late 1980s[163] and are now widely available. They are most appropriate when a sensor is included in the dual-chamber device. This offers corroboration by another means of the physiologic or pathologic nature of the atrial tachycardia. Clinical testing of these devices is currently in an early stage, but they seem to offer symptom control of atrial tachyarrhythmias by not permitting rapid ventricular stimulation while still allowing ventricular tracking of physiologic atrial rates. Future algorithms will be fairly sophisticated, allowing the physician to program the rate and number of beats at which mode switching will occur. It is likely that these algorithms will be the ideal means for dealing with patients with paroxysmal atrial fibrillation. The function of the devices currently on the market has recently been reviewed.[164]

RATE-RESPONSIVE PACING

Nowhere is rate-responsive pacing more appropriate than in patients with sinus node disease. Pacing in patients with AV block can readily be physiologic (AV sequence plus rate response) by allowing the pacemaker to sense the normally functioning atria and pace the ventricles. In sinus node disease this normal function is frequently absent. Estimates discussed earlier of the incidence of chronotropic incompetence[50] in patients with sinus node disease range from 20% to 60%. In rate-responsive pacing a sensor is included in the pacemaker that determines the body's need for increased heart rate. Some sensors are more physiologic in their means of making this determination than others, but in theory all are suitable for this indication. A future area of research involves comparing the various sensors to the sinus node with respect to chronotropic function. Dual-sensor pacemakers are intended to mimic normal sinus node function more closely. Clearly, AAIR pacing is limited to sensors that do not require a ventricular lead (for example, stimulus-to-T or QT sensors).

Future prospective studies should be directed toward testing the hypothesis that exercise capacity is significantly improved with AAIR pacing compared with AAI pacing. A recent clinical trial surprisingly showed no significant differences in objective or subjective performance of exercise in patients with sinus node dysfunction who had pacemakers programmed to the AAI compared to the AAIR pacing mode.[165]

AAIR OR DDDR/DDIR

The capability to offer the patient a renewed ability to vary heart rate according to need fulfills the goal of emulating sinus rhythm, provided that atrial stimulation is included in the pacing mode. The availability of sensor-controlled devices reopens the argument over atrial or dual-chamber stimulation because new problems are introduced. The AAIR mode is again very attractive, but if the sensor's determination of atrial rate is not in concord with the autonomic nervous system's influence on the AV node, AV block may occur. Transient AV block, especially during sleep, has been common with AAIR pacing in my experience, but good results have been reported by Rosenqvist and colleagues,[166] with only one transient asymptomatic episode occurring in 44 patients during a mean of 12.5 months of follow-up. Aside from this problem, and without development of pathologic AV block or chronic atrial fibrillation, AAIR is the pacing mode of choice.

Carotid sinus stimulation should be performed to exclude associated carotid sinus hypersensitivity–induced AV block before AAIR pacing is implemented. Exercise evaluation should be performed to assess the need and optimal programming for sensor-driven pacing. Excessive prolongation of the PR interval (>200 to 240 msec) with exercise is a contraindication to AAIR pacing. Some investigators suggest (although significant disagreement about this issue exists) that the presence of bundle branch block or bifascicular block is a contraindication to AAIR pacing. Intraoperatively, 1:1 AV conduction should be present with atrial pacing at 120 bpm or more (also vigorously debated). Nevertheless, most practitioners would agree that these are prudent guidelines in patients in whom AAIR pacing is being considered.

Finally, another consideration also favoring the choice of AAIR pacing over dual-chamber stimulation is the likelihood that despite the best possible matching of the sensor to the patient's autonomic nervous system, some extension of the AR (e.g., paced atrial to QRS complex) interval may still occur during increased pacing rates, a phenomenon that has been well documented by Mabo and colleagues.[167] With AAIR pacing this may not have negative inotropic consequences because the ventricle is not paced, but in DDDR/DDIR pacing ventricular stimulation is likely to be brought into action as the spontaneous AR interval increases. This has important negative inotropic consequences that in some cases may be sufficient to negate the benefit of the heart rate rise. *"Reverse" hysteresis* of the AV delay is a possible means of overcoming this problem. Instead of the now widely available rate-adaptive shortening of the AV delay that is demonstrably valuable in patients with AV block,[168, 169] the AV delay is lengthened with increasing rate to preserve spontaneous AV conduction. This obviates the negative aspects of ventricular stimulation in most situations, but ventricular stimulation would still be available if complete AV block occurred. In this eventuality, ventricular pacing would take place after a long AV delay, and retrograde AV conduction could then occur and trigger a PMT. A suitable algorithm for this function would have to address this problem. Nevertheless, in many patients with sick sinus syndrome it is more advantageous to allow the AR interval to be somewhat prolonged than to let ventricular stimulation take place. The precise AR interval at which it becomes more advantageous to provide for ventricular pacing than spontaneous conduction varies depending on the patient's underlying heart disease and intra-atrial conduction time.

Despite the simplicity and attraction of AAIR pacing, physicians probably feel more comfortable with the more sophisticated and flexible dual-chamber rate-responsive devices. DDDR/DDIR devices now mostly include automatic mode switching so that ventricular stimulation can be maintained at a physiologically appropriate rate if an atrial tachyarrhythmia occurs.

INDICATIONS FOR PACING IN PATIENTS WITH SINUS NODE DISEASE

Pacing is clearly indicated for patients in whom, regardless of age, sinus node disease is found to be responsible for dizziness, syncope, or heart failure. These have been the indications for pacing for the past 25 years. Now we should think more widely than this and consider pacing for patients who have only chronotropic incompetence with or without resting sinus bradycardia that is causing minor but debilitating symptoms such as fatigue, lethargy, poor concentration, lack of memory, or dyspnea on exertion. Also, in this group we should include patients who are presenting only with palpitations but are shown to have bradycardia-tachycardia syndrome. These patients are at risk for chronic atrial fibrillation and its possible complications—stroke and heart failure. The evidence that exists now shows that atrial fibrillation can be delayed or prevented by atrial pacing (Table 18–6). We are nearer the point at which asymptomatic patients could be considered for treatment, but this must await the reports of current trials.

HEMODYNAMICS OF PACING

RETROGRADE AV CONDUCTION AND PACEMAKER SYNDROME.
The hemodynamic challenges of pacing in patients with sinus node disease were grasped in the 1970s when it was revealed that ventricular pacing was very likely to be associated with retrograde AV conduction.[170–173] This phenomenon can be regarded as a facet of normality and therefore is very common in patients with sinus node disease in whom there may be no abnormality of AV conduction. Wirtzfeld's group[171, 172] clearly showed that atrial pacing in patients with sinus bradycardia increased cardiac output by increasing heart rate without prejudice to stroke volume. In contrast, ventricular pacing at the same rate depressed stroke volume dramatically, resulting in a slightly lower cardiac output than occurred in spontaneous sinus bradycardia (Fig. 18–13). Two aspects of ventricular pacing may combine to create this effect (Table 18–7). These are the negative inotropic influence of ventric-

TABLE 18–6. INDICATIONS FOR PACING IN SINUS NODE DISEASE

PRIMARY	SECONDARY
Dizziness or syncope	Fatigue, dyspnea due to chronotropic incompetence
Heart failure	Palpitations due to bradycardia-tachycardia

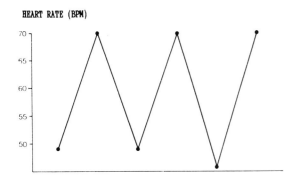

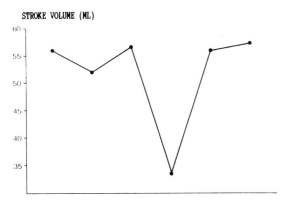

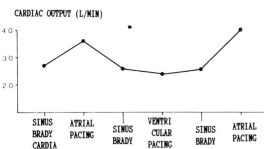

FIGURE 18–13. Heart rate (bpm), stroke volume (mL), and cardiac output (L/min) are plotted for sinus bradycardia, atrial pacing, sinus bradycardia, ventricular pacing, sinus bradycardia and atrial pacing. (After Blomer N, Wirtzfeld A, Delius W, et al: Das Sinusknotensyndrom. Erlangen, Germany, Perimed Verlag, Dr. Med. D. Straube, 1977.)

ular pacing and retrograde AV conduction. Wirtzfeld's group[172] demonstrated the striking difference that occurred in patients paced ventricularly with and without retrograde AV conduction, illustrating that this is a major factor.

Retrograde AV conduction may be intermittent and may be present only in a limited heart rate band. Thus, if VVIR pacing is employed in patients with sinus node disease, retrograde AV conduction may be absent at resting heart rates but present with exercise as catecholamines and the ventricular paced rate increase and may give rise to exercise-related symptoms.[174, 175] Ultimately, retrograde conduction may be blocked again at higher paced rates.

Atrial pacing is not completely free from the problems of pacemaker syndrome (Table 18–8). Den Dulk and colleagues[176] reported that when the AAIR mode of pacing is combined with antiarrhythmic therapy the atrial pace–spontaneous ventricular conduction interval (i.e., the AR interval) can become so prolonged that atrial contraction occurs during the ventricular systole of the previous beat.

TABLE 18–7. ADVERSE EFFECTS OF VENTRICULAR PACING IN SINUS NODE DISEASE

1. Retrograde AV conduction—pacemaker syndrome
   Reduction in cardiac output
   Atrial tachyarrhythmias
   Possible reflex vasodilation
   Atrial natriuretic peptide release
   Increased pressure in pulmonary circulation
2. Negative inotropism

Second, in patients with sinus node disease who have AAIR or DDD pacing there may be such severe abnormalities of intra-atrial conduction that left atrial activation from right atrial pacing is delayed while left ventricular activation takes place more rapidly. The result is that left atrial contraction occurs during left ventricular systole,[177] which may give rise to symptoms of pacemaker syndrome.

Indirect evidence that retrograde AV conduction favors atrial tachyarrhythmias and ultimately atrial fibrillation is provided by the literature review conducted by Sutton and Kenny.[54] More direct support of this concept comes from Curzi and associates.[178] Retrograde AV conduction, by precipitating atrial contraction during ventricular systole, causes excessive stretch of the atria. This may be a contributing factor in the incidence of atrial tachyarrhythmias. It also generates a vasodilatory reflex[179, 180] and is an important stimulus of the release of high levels of atrial natriuretic peptide,[181, 182] which is also vasodilatory at the hyperphysiologic levels recorded. Thus, hypotension occurs owing to propagation of atrial blood retrogradely into the systemic and pulmonary veins combined with peripheral vasodilation (see Chapter 25).

From this summary we must construe that ventricular pacing in patients with sinus node disease is tenable only when chronic atrial fibrillation or atrial paralysis with slow ventricular response is present because any other patient could show retrograde AV conduction with any or all of its adverse effects.

TABLE 18–8. CONTRAINDICATIONS TO AAI/AAIR PACING

Definite
1. Presence of AV block on ambulatory electrocardiogram except during sleep
2. Carotid sinus stimulation producing AV block
3. Exercise evaluation demonstrating presence of exercise-induced AV block
4. Marked PR prolongation at rest (>240 msec) or associated with low levels of exercise
5. Potential need for AV nodal blocking drugs, such as digoxin, beta-blockers, or calcium channel blockers, for management of hypertension, angina, or supraventricular tachycardias

Probable
1. Presence of bundle branch block or bifascicular block
2. Electrophysiologic study showing HV interval greater than 75–80 msec, or infra-Hisian block with atrial pacing at rates less than 120–140 bpm
3. Preoperative, intraoperative, or electrophysiologic study showing block at any site in AV conduction system at rates less than 120 bpm

Temporary Pacing

Temporary pacing is seldom required in patients with sinus node disease. Induction of general anesthesia does not seem to hold the same dangers as it does in patients with AV block, and any patient for whom it may be considered will have clear indications for permanent pacing. Temporary pacing may be employed in patients with less clear indications for permanent pacing as a clinical trial that, if successful, could be used to justify a permanent implant. Unfortunately, this type of patient will probably benefit only from DDDR/DDIR pacing, which is almost impossible to conduct accurately with an external pacing system.

Results of Pacing—Influence on Prognosis and Quality of Life

By the early 1980s survival with pacing, albeit mostly ventricular pacing, was well documented,[183, 184] and there was a generally accepted feeling that pacing did not influence prognosis.[185] Shaw's group[185] presented the most convincing evidence of this, but they used only ventricular pacemakers. During the 1980s evidence emerged continuously that atrial or dual-chamber pacing offers improved survival,[115, 151, 152] which now approaches that of the population at large of a similar age.[115] Simon and Janz[186] showed that coincident problems at initial diagnosis such as heart failure and arteriosclerotic heart disease adversely influence the prognosis. The study of Brandt and colleagues[116] of 213 consecutive patients with a mean follow-up of 60 months showed 5- and 10-year survival times that did not differ significantly from those of an age- and sex-matched general population. Other studies have also shown that atrial pacing improves survival, particularly in the elderly (>70 years).[146] In addition to improved survival, other studies have shown improvements in the neurohumoral milieu in patients with DDD/AAI pacing compared with VVI pacing, such as lower levels of atrial natriuretic peptide (ANP) and catecholamines in patients with dual-chamber pacing. Numerous studies (reviewed in Chapter 24) have shown both immediate and short-term improvements in submaximal exercise capacity following switches from the VVI to the VDD, DDD, or AAI pacing mode.

Quality of life studies have been performed relatively infrequently in patients with sinus node disease. Without using a modern questionnaire method of the type employed by Lau and coworkers[187] and Linde-Eldelstam and associates,[188] Mitsuoka and colleagues[189] found an improved quality of life in sinus node disease patients with dual-chamber pacing compared with those with ventricular pacing. Sulke and colleagues[190] compared four rate-responsive modes and found that the DDDR mode was both subjectively and objectively superior to VVIR in sinus node disease patients. This and other studies are limited by their short duration of follow-up, which ranged from several weeks to several months. Other studies are needed, particularly to test the newer modes of pacing in patients with the broader indications for pacing that are now being considered.

Programming Pacemakers for Best Results in Patients with Sinus Node Disease

Because of the large variety of pacemaker modes and devices with different sensors that are available, only generalizations are possible here. The first principle underlying management of these patients is that an individualized and active approach is needed. Telemetry information obtained from generators can provide more long-term information than Holter systems, which can provide short-term information only. Information about cardiac function during exercise or during a brief time period can be provided by telemetry from the pulse generator or from a Holter monitor placed for a short period of time. Once the full range of exercise stress testing has been explored[191] for patients with rate-responsive pacemakers, the focus is more on office-based testing,[192] and pacemaker programming can be further refined. It is now possible with many devices to clear the Holter-telemetry channel, ask the patient to undertake a standardized activity (e.g., walking down the hall or up a flight of steps), and immediately interrogate the device to assess its response to this brief exercise period. If necessary, this procedure can be repeated until the desired rate response is obtained. Newer rate-responsive algorithms include a wide variety of features that seek more closely to match normal sinus node function. One such feature in the Intermedics Relay device (Intermedics, Inc., Angleton, TX) tries to mimic the diurnal decrease in heart rate by establishing a 24-hour clock and a separate lower rate for sleep. The pacing rate is automatically and gradually decreased to the sleep rate at the programmed sleep time. The 24-hour clock is "adaptive" to take into account changes in the patient's sleep time, with a complete absence of activity being used to define sleep.

These principles apply to all rate-responsive modes, and it must be said that there is no easy way to obtain the necessary information short of investing the time needed for testing and fine-tuning the system. With careful analysis of Holter recording or telemetry, a good result can be obtained in almost all patients. Kay[193] examined the quantitation of the exercise response into quartiles and related the measured performance to the expected performance. With this approach the rate response for an individual patient can be characterized in detail and adjustments in the program made to bring it toward the ideal.

Some special considerations are necessary in some of the pacing modes used in patients with sinus node disease. For AAI and AAIR modes, far-field R-wave sensing must be avoided, and the refractory period must be set sufficiently long to allow this. For DDD and other dual-chamber modes it is advisable to program the AV delay to allow the occurrence of spontaneous AV conduction based on earlier discussion (see page 297). The question of what upper rate setting to use in these modes was vexing in the past. Some workers believed that a low upper rate should be set to avoid rapid ventricular stimulation in case of atrial tachyarrhythmias, whereas others preferred high rates and relied on drug control of the arrhythmias. This discussion is now almost invalidated by the advent of automatic mode switching and could have been avoided even with the earlier devices by using the DDI pacing mode.

Future Trends

Suggestions have already been advanced that rate-responsive atrial or dual-chamber pacing could be more effective in controlling atrial tachyarrhythmias than similar but non–rate-responsive modes.[194–197] This possibility requires thorough clinical testing and already has generated some dissenting views.[198] The trial design must take into account the fact that not all sensor-driven rate responses are the same. It may be that an aggressive rate rise such as that provided by an activity sensor[196] provides ideal overdrive of the sinus node. If rate-responsive systems that include atrial pacing are shown to be superior they will become the mode of choice for pacing and sinus node disease of all types.

Further measures to combat atrial arrhythmias may be seen. These may include antitachycardia pacing modes triggered spontaneously and even atrial cardioversion. A dual-chamber pacemaker (Medtronic 7008) was introduced in 1984 with an atrial burst pacing capability, but it was not well understood and received minimal use. Atrial burst pacing has a major limitation in that it will not convert atrial fibrillation and may precipitate atrial fibrillation in an attempt to convert other atrial tachyarrhythmias. Development of an atrial cardioverter is underway, but it will be widely adopted only when it can be shown to be effective (no ventricular tachyarrhythmias or systemic embolism) and almost painless.

Sinus node disease is associated with atrial disease, and therefore intra-atrial conduction defects may be more common than is presently realized. Right atrial pacing is associated with variable intra-atrial and interatrial conduction delays resulting in delayed left heart depolarization, and these may be sufficiently long to cause left atrial systole during left ventricular systole,[177] which may prove to be a significant clinical problem. As our aspirations toward physiologic pacing increase, the solution introduced by Daubert's group[200] of using a triple-chamber pacemaker will become a reality. The future may hold a quadruple-chamber pacing system for correct coordination of all four cardiac chambers.

Technologic advances in sensors will have the greatest effects on patients with sinus node disease. Already we have a choice of dual-sensor devices, which may offer improvement over those with only one sensor.[201] Further developments are expected in this field, including sensor adjustments that are made more automatically and that require the physician to play a smaller role in the set-up.

For patients who are adversely affected by ventricular pacing but also show a longer than physiologically optimal AR interval with AAI pacing, His bundle pacing may prove to be a solution that avoids the negative inotropism of pacing from the right ventricular apex.

Overall, we can expect great technologic sophistication tempered on the one hand by the electrophysiologic and hemodynamic problems that this may cause and, on the other, by the increasing downward pressure on health care costs.

REFERENCES

1. Lown B: Electrical reversion of cardiac arrhythmias. Br Heart J 29:469, 1967.
2. Keith A, Flack M: The form and nature of the muscular connections between the primary divisions of the vertebrate heart. J Anat Physiol 41:172, 1906–1907.
3. Flack M: An investigation of the sinoatrial node of the mammalian heart. J Physiol 41:64, 1910–1911.
4. Hoffman BF: Electrophysiology of single cardiac cells. Bull NY Acad Med 35:689, 1959.
5. West TC: Ultramicroelectrode recording from the cardiac pacemaker. J Pharmacol Exp Ther 115:283, 1955.
6. Laslett EE: Syncopal attacks associated with prolonged arrest of the whole heart. Q J Med 2:347, 1909.
7. Schott E: Ueber Vorhofsystolenausfau. Münchener Med Woch 59:292, 1912.
8. Levine SA: Observations on sino-atrial heart block. Arch Intern Med 17:153, 1916.
9. Ferrer MI: The sick sinus syndrome in atrial disease. JAMA 206:645, 1968.
10. Ferrer MI: The sick sinus syndrome. Circulation 47:635, 1973.
11. Ferrer MI: The Sick Sinus Syndrome. Mt Kisco, NY, Futura Publishing Co., 1974.
12. James TN: Cardiac conduction system, fetal and postnatal development. Am J Cardiol 25:213, 1970.
13. Hoffman BF, Cranefield PF. Electrophysiology of the Heart. New York, McGraw-Hill, 1960.
14. Davies MJ, Pomerance A: Quantitative studies of ageing changes in the human sinoatrial node and internodal tracts. Br Heart J 34:150, 1972.
15. Thery C, Gosselin B, Lekieffre J, Warembourg H: Pathology of the sinoatrial node: Correlation with electrocardiographic findings in 111 patients. Am Heart J 93:735, 1977.
16. Brooks CMcC, Lu HH: The Sinoatrial Pacemaker of the Heart. Springfield, IL, Charles C Thomas, 1972.
17. James TN: The sinus node as a servomechanism. Circ Res 32:307, 1973.
18. Bouman LN, Gerlings ED, Bierstekerpa PA, et al: Pacemaker shift in the sinoatrial node during vagal stimulation. Pfleuger Arch 302:255, 1968.
19. Goldberg JM: Intra-SA-nodal pacemaker shifts induced by autonomic nerve stimulation in the dog. Am J Physiol 229:1116, 1975.
20. Boineau JP, Miller CB, Scheussler RB, et al: Activation sequence and potential distribution maps demonstrating multicentric atrial impulse origin in dogs. Circ Res 54:322, 1984.
21. Shaw DB, Kekwick CA: Potential candidates for pacemakers. Br Heart J 40:99, 1978.
22. Bergfeldt L: HLA-B27–associated rheumatic diseases with severe cardiac bradyarrhythmias: Clinical features in 223 men with permanent pacemakers. Am J Med 75:210, 1983.
23. Maisch B, Lotze U, Schneider J, et al: Antibodies to human sinus node in sick sinus syndrome. PACE 9:1101, 1986.
24. Levander-Lindgren M, Lantz BO: Bradyarrhythmia profile and associated disease in 1,265 patients with cardiac pacing. PACE 11:2207, 1988.
25. James TN: Order and disorder in the rhythm of the heart. Circulation 47:362, 1973.
26. Bharati S, Nordenberg A, Bauerfiend R, et al: The anatomic substrate for the sick sinus syndrome in the adolescent. Am J Cardiol 46:163, 1980.
27. Lorber A, Maisuls E, Palant A: Autosomal dominant inheritance of sinus node disease. Int J Cardiol 15:252, 1987.
28. Engel TR, Meister SG, Feitusa GS, et al: Appraisal of sinus node artery disease. Circulation 52:86, 1975.
29. Shaw DB, Linker NJ, Heaver PA, et al: Chronic sinoatrial disorder (sick sinus syndrome): a possible result of cardiac ischemia. Br Heart J 58:598, 1987.
30. Rubinstein JJ, Schulman CL, Yurchak PM, et al: Clinical spectrum of the sick sinus syndrome. Circulation 46:5, 1972.
31. Moss AJ, Davis RJ: Brady-tachy syndrome. Prog Cardiovasc Dis 16:439, 1974.
32. Gurtner AP, Lenzinger HR, Dolder M: Klinik des sinusknoten Syndroms. Herz Kreislauf 8:485, 1976.
33. Lang K, Huppenbauer B, Limbourg P, et al: Die Sinusknotenerkankung. Med Welt 27:1281, 1976.
34. Rokseth R, Hatle L: Sinus arrest in myocardial infarction. Br Heart J 33:639, 1971.
35. Fluck DC, Olsen E, Pentecost BL, et al: Natural history and clinical significance of arrhythmias after acute cardiac infarction. Br Heart J 29:170, 1967.

36. Headrick J, Willis RJ: Mediation by adenosine of bradycardia in rat heart during graded global ischaemia. Pflügers Arch 412:618, 1988.

37. Watts AH: Sick sinus syndrome: An adenosine-mediated disease. Lancet 1:786, 1985.

38. Benedini G, Cuccia C, Bolognesi R, et al: Value of purinic compounds in assessing sinus node dysfunction in man: A new diagnostic method. Eur Heart J 5:394, 1984.

39. Davies MJ, Ward DE: The pathology of arrhythmias, conduction disturbances, and sudden death. *In* Julian DG, Camm AJ, Fox KM, et al (eds): Diseases of the Heart. London, Balliere Tindall, 1989, pp 486–508.

40. Leatham A: Carotid sinus syncope. Br Heart J 47:409, 1981.

41. Brignole M, Menozzi C, Gianfranchi L, et al: Neurally mediated syncope detected by carotid sinus massage and head-up tilt test in sick sinus syndrome. Am J Cardiol 68:1032, 1991.

42. Morley CA, Sutton R: Carotid sinus syncopy. Int J Cardiol 6:287, 1984.

43. Kaseda S, Zipes DP: Vagal denervation of canine sinus and atrioventricular nodes creates hypersensitive response to acetylcholine [Abstract]. J Am Coll Cardiol 11:39A, 1988.

44. Alboni P, Menozzi C, Brignole M, et al: An abnormal neural reflex plays a role in causing syncope in sinus bradycardia. J Am Coll Cardiol 22:1130, 1993.

45. Harris CL, Baldwin BJ: Permanent atrial paralysis. J Electrocardiol 9:81, 1976.

46. Williams DO, Jones EL, Nagle RE, et al: Familiar atrial cardiomyopathy with heart block. Q J Med 61:491, 1972.

47. Abdon NJ: Frequency and distribution of long-term ECG recorded cardiac arrhythmias in an elderly population. Acta Med Scand 209:175, 1981.

48. Parsonnet V, Bernstein AD: The 1989 World survey of cardiac pacing. PACE 14:2073, 1991.

49. Gillette P, Wampler DC, Shannon C, et al: Use of atrial pacing in a young population. PACE 8:94, 1985.

50. Ellestad MH, Wan MKC: Predictive implications of stress testing: Follow-up of 2700 subjects after maximum treadmill stress testing. Circulation 51:363, 1975.

51. Rosen KM, Loeb HS, Sinno MZ, et al: Cardiac conduction in patients with symptomatic sinus node disease. Circulation 43:836, 1971.

52. Narula OS: Atrioventricular conduction defects in patients with sinus bradycardia. Circulation 44:1096, 1971.

53. Mandel WJ, Hayakawa H, Allen HN, et al: Assessment of sinus node function in patients with sick sinus syndrome. Circulation 46:761, 1972.

54. Sutton R, Kenny RA: The natural history of sick sinus syndrome. PACE 9:1110, 1986.

55. Engel TR, Schaal SF: Digitalis in the sick sinus syndrome: The effects of digitalis on sinoatrial automaticity and atrioventricular conduction. Circulation 48:1201, 1973.

56. Strauss HC, Scheinmann MM, Labarre A, et al: Review of the significance of drugs in the sick sinus syndrome. *In* Bonke FIM (ed): The Sinus Node: Structure, Function, and Clinical Relevance. The Hague, Netherlands, Martinus Nijhoff, 1978, pp 103–111.

57. Davies MI, Pomerance A: Pathology of atrial fibrillation in man. Br Heart J 34:520, 1972.

58. Brodsky M, Wu D, Denes P, et al: Arrhythmias documented by 24-hour continuous electrocardiographic monitoring in 50 male students without apparent heart disease. Am J Cardiol 39:390, 1977.

59. Bjerregaard P: Mean 24-hour heart rate, minimal heart rate, and pauses in healthy subjects 40–79 years of age. Eur Heart J 4:44, 1983.

60. Talan DA, Bauernfiend RA, Ashley WW, et al: Twenty-four–hour continuous ECG recordings in long-distance runners. Chest 32:622, 1982.

61. Mandel W, Hayakawa H, Danzig R, et al: Evaluation of sinoatrial node function in man by overdrive suppression. Circulation 44:59, 1971.

62. Narula OS, Samet P, Javier RP: Significance of the sinus-node recovery time. Circulation 45:140, 1972.

63. Kerr CR, Grant AO, Wenger TL, et al: Sinus node dysfunction. Cardiol Clin 1:181, 1983.

64. Kerr CR, Strauss HC: The nature of atriosinus conduction during rapid atrial pacing in the rabbit heart. Circulation 63:1149, 1981.

65. Goldreyer BN, Damato AN: Sinoatrial node entrance block. Circulation 44:789, 1971.

66. Pop T, Fleischmann D: Measurement of sinus node recovery time after

atrial pacing. *In* Bonke FIM (ed): The Sinus Node: Structure, Function, and Clinical Relevance. The Hague, Netherlands, Martinus Nijhoff, 1978, pp 23–25.

67. Jordan J, Yamaguchi I, Mandel W: Studies on the mechanism of sinus node dysfunction in the sick sinus syndrome. Circulation 57:217, 1978.

68. Strauss HC, Bigger JT Jr, Saroff AL, et al: Electrophysiologic evaluation of sinus node funcion in patients with sinus node dysfunction. Circulation 53:763, 1976.

69. Benditt DG, Strauss HC, Scheinmann MM, et al: Analysis of secondary pauses following termination of rapid atrial pacing in man. Circulation 54:436, 1976.

70. Josephson ME, Seides SF (eds): Clinical Cardiac Electrophysiology: Techniques and Interpretations. Philadelphia, Lea & Febiger, 1979.

71. Reiffel JA, Gang E, Bigger JT Jr, et al: Sinus node recovery time related to paced cycle length in normal and in patients with sinoatrial dysfunction. Am Heart J 104:746, 1982.

72. Benditt DG, Gurnick CC, Dunbar D, et al: Indications for electrophysiological testing in the diagnosis and assessment of sinus node dysfunction. Circulation 75 (Suppl III):93, 1987.

73. Strauss HC, Saroff AJ, Bigger JT Jr, et al: Premature atrial stimulation as a key to the understanding of sinoatrial conduction in man: Presentation of data and critical review of the literature. Circulation 47:86, 1973.

74. Yee R, Strauss HC: Electrophysiologic mechanisms: Sinus node dysfunction. Circulation 75 (Suppl III):12, 1987.

75. Narula OS, Shantha N, Vasquez M, et al: A new method for measurement of sinoatrial conduction time. Circulation 58:706, 1978.

76. Breithardt G, Seipel L: Comparative study of two methods of estimating sinoatrial conduction time in man. Am J Cardiol 42:965, 1978.

77. Cramer M, Siegal M, Bigger JT Jr, et al: Characteristics of extracellular potentials recorded from the sinoatrial pacemaker of the rabbit. Circ Res 41:292, 1977.

78. Cramer M, Hariman RJ, Boxer R, et al: Electrocardiograms from the sinoatrial pacemaker recorded in vitro and in situ. Am J Cardiol 42:939, 1978.

79. Hariman RJ, Krongrad E, Boxer RA, et al: Methods for recording electrocardiograms of the sinus atrial node during cardiac surgery in man. Circulation 61:1024, 1980.

80. Hariman RJ, Krongrad E, Boxer RA, et al: Method for recording electrical activity of the sinoatrial node and automatic atrial foci during cardiac catheterization in human subjects. Am J Cardiol 45:775, 1980.

81. Reiffel JA, Gang E, Gliklich J, et al: The human sinus node electrogram: A transvenous catheter technique and a comparison of directly measured and indirectly estimated sinoatrial conduction time in adults. Circulation 62:1324, 1980.

82. Gomes JA, Kang PS, El-Sherif N: The sinus node electrogram in patients with and without sick sinus syndrome: Technique and correlation between directly measured and indirectly estimated sinoatrial conduction time. Circulation 66:864, 1982.

83. Haberl R, Steinbeck G, Luderitz B, et al: Comparison between intracellular and extracellular direct current recordings of sinus node activity for evaluation of sinoatrial conduction time. Circulation 70:760, 1984.

84. Kerr CR, Prystowsky EN, Browning DJ, et al: Characterization of refractoriness in the sinus node of the rabbit. Circ Res 47:742, 1980.

85. Kerr CR, Strauss HC: The measurement of sinus node refractoriness in man. Circulation 68:1231, 1984.

86. Kerr CR, Chung DC, Mason MA: Effect of pacing cycle length on sinus node refractoriness in man [Abstract]. Circulation 72 (Suppl III):33, 1985.

87. Jose AD: Effect of combined sympathetic and parasympathetic blockade on heart rate and cardiac function in man. Am J Cardiol 18:476, 1966.

88. Desai J, Scheinmann MM, Strauss HC, et al: Electrophysiological effects of combined autonomic blockade in patients with sinus node disease. Circulation 63:953, 1981.

89. Kang PS, Gomes JAC, El Sheriff N: Differential effects of functional autonomic blockade on the variables of sinus node automaticity in sick sinus syndrome. Am J Cardiol 49:273, 1982.

90. Sethi KK, Jaishanker S, Balachander J, et al: Sinus node function after autonomic blockade in normals and in sick sinus syndrome. Int J Cardiol 5:707, 1984.

91. Jose AD, Collison D: The normal range and determinants of the intrinsic heart rate in man. Cardiovasc Res 4:160, 1970.

92. Tonkin AM, Heddle WF, Tornos P: Intermittent atrioventricular block:

Procaineamide administration as a provocative test. Aust NZ J Med 8:594, 1978.

93. Puglisi A, Rica R, Angrisani G: The Ajmaline test in identifying patients at high risk for developing paroxysmal AV block. Ital Cardiol 12:866, 1982.

94. Bergfeldt L, Rosenqvist M, Vallin H, et al: Disopyramide-induced atrioventricular block in patients with bifascicular block: An acute stress test to predict atrioventricular block progression. Br Heart J 53:328, 1985.

95. Chamberlain-Webber R, Petersen MEV, Ahmed R, et al: Diagnosis of sick sinus syndrome with flecainide in patients with normal sinus node recovery times investigated for unexplained syncope. Eur J Cardiac Pacing Electrophysiol 2:106, 1992.

96. Vardas P, Ingram A, Theodorakis G, et al: Long-term results of diso-pyramide provocative test in syncopal patients with latent sinus node and atrioventricular conduction defects [Abstract]. PACE 16:1130, 1993.

97. Vardas PE, Kalogeropoulos CK, Kenny-Creedon RA, et al: Verapamil as a challenge to the conduction system in syncopal patients [Abstract]. PACE 10:A512, 1987.

98. Abbott JA, Hirschfield DS, Kunkel FW, et al: Graded exercise testing in patients with sinus node dysfunction. Am J Med 62:330, 1977.

99. Holden W, McAnulty JH, Rahimtoola SH: Characterization of heart rate response to exercise in the sick sinus syndrome. Br Heart J 20:923, 1978.

100. Hinkle LE, Carver ST, Plakum A: Slow heart rates and increased risk of cardiac death in middle-aged men. Arch Intern Med 129:5, 1972.

101. Simonsen E: Assessment of the need for rate-responsive pacing in patients with sinus node dysfunction: A prospective study of heart rate response during daily activities and exercise testing [Abstract]. PACE 10:1229, 1987.

102. Dreifus LS, Fisch C, Griffin J, et al: Guidelines for implantation of cardiac pacemakers and antiarrhythmic devices. J Am Coll Cardiol 18:1, 1991.

103. Vardas P, Fitzpatrick A, Ingram A, et al: Natural history of sinus node chronotropy in paced patients. PACE 14:155, 1991.

104. Gwinn N, Lemen R, Kratz J, et al: Chronotropic incompetence: A common and progressive finding in pacemaker patients. Am Heart J 123:1216, 1992.

105. Lau CP: Rate-Adaptive Cardiac Pacing: Single and Dual Chamber. Mt. Kisco, NY, Futura Publishing Co., 1993.

106. Sutton R, Citron P: Electrophysiological and haemodynamic basis for application of new pacemaker technology in sick sinus syndrome and atrioventricular block. Br Heart J 41:600, 1979.

107. Rosenqvist M: Atrial pacing for sick sinus syndrome. Clin Cardiol 13:43, 1990.

108. Wilkoff BL, Covey J, Blackburn G: A mathematical model of the cardiac chronotropic response to exercise. J Electrophysiol 3:176, 1989.

109. Kenny RA, Ingram A, Bayliss J, et al: Head-up tilt: A useful test for investigating unexplained syncope. Lancet 2:1323, 1986.

110. Fitzpatrick A, Sutton R: Tilting towards a diagnosis in unexplained recurrent syncope. Lancet 1:658, 1989.

111. Abi-Samra F, Maloney JD, Fouad-Tarazi FM, et al: The usefulness of head-up tilt testing and haemodynamic investigations in the work-up of syncope of unknown origin. PACE 11:1202, 1988.

112. Almqvist A, Goldenberg JF, Milstein S, et al: Provocation of brady-cardia and hypotension by isoproterenol and upright posture in patients with unexplained syncope. N Engl J Med 329:346, 1989.

113. Gann D, Tolentino A, Samet P: Electrophysiologic evaluation of el-derly patients with sinus bradycardia: A long-term follow-up study. Ann Intern Med 90:24, 1979.

114. Rosenqvist M, Obel IWP: Atrial pacing and the risk of AV block: Is there a time for change in attitude? PACE 12:97, 1989.

115. Rosenqvist M, Brandt J, Schüller H: Long-term pacing in sinus node disease: Effects of stimulation mode on cardiovascular morbidity and mortality. Am Heart J 117:16, 1988.

116. Brandt J, Anderson H, Fåhraeus T, et al: Natural history of sinus node disease treated with atrial pacing in 213 patients: Implications for stimulation mode selection. J Am Coll Cardiol 20:633, 1992.

117. Fairfax AJ, Lambert CD, Leatham A: Systemic embolism in chronic sinoatrial disorder. N Engl J Med 295:190, 1976.

118. Benditt DG, Benson DW Jr, Dunnigan A, et al: Drug therapy in sinus node dysfunction. In Rappaport E (ed): Cardiology Update. New York, Elsevier, 1984, pp 79–102.

119. Petersen P, Boysen G, Godtfredsen J, et al: Placebo-controlled ran-domised trial of warfarin and aspirin prevention of thrombo-

120. embolic complications in chronic atrial fibrillation. The Copenhagen Afasak Study. Lancet 1:175, 1989.

121. Connolly SJ, Laupacis A, Gent M, et al: Canadian Atrial Fibrillation Anticoagulation Study (CAFA). Circulation 82 (Suppl IV): 1990.

122. Stroke Prevention in Atrial Fibrillation Investigators: Stroke preven-tion in atrial fibrillation (SPAF). Circulation 84:527, 1991.

123. Boston Area Anticoagulation Trial for Atrial Fibrillation Investigators: The effect of low-dose warfarin on the risk of stroke in non-rheumatic atrial fibrillation. N Engl J Med 323:1505, 1990.

124. Muller OF, Finkelstein D: Adams-Stokes syndrome due to sinoatrial block. Am J Cardiol 17:433, 1966.

125. Cohen HE, Kahn M, Donoso E: Treatment of supraventricular tachy-cardias with catheter and permanent pacemakers. Am J Cardiol 20:735, 1967.

126. Cheng TO: Transvenous ventricular pacing in the treatment of parox-ysmal atrial tachyarrhythmias alternating with sinus bradycardia and standstill. Am J Cardiol 22:814, 1968.

127. Chokshi DS, Mascarenhas E, Samet P, et al: Treatment of sinoatrial rhythm disturbances with permanent cardiac pacing. Am J Cardiol 32:215, 1973.

128. Conde CA, Leppo J, Lipski J, et al: Effectiveness of pacemaker treat-ment in the bradycardia-tachycardia syndrome. Am J Cardiol 32:209, 1973.

129. Obel IWP, Cohen E, Miller RNS: Chronic symptomatic sinoatrial block: A review of 34 patients and their treatment. Chest 65:397, 1974.

130. Rokseth R, Hatle L, Gedde-Dahl D, et al: Pacemaker therapy in sino-atrial block complicated by paroxysmal tachycardia. Br Heart J 32:93, 1970.

131. Rasmussen K: Chronic sinoatrial block. Am Heart J 81:38, 1971.

132. Sigurd B, Jensen G, Meibom J, et al: Adams-Stokes syndrome caused by sino-atrial block. Br Heart J 35:1002, 1973.

133. Moss AJ, Rivers RJ, Cooper M: Long-term pervenous atrial pacing from the proximal portion of the coronary vein. JAMA 209:543, 1969.

134. Kastor JA, De Sanctis RW, Leinbach RC, et al: Long-term pervenous atrial pacing. Circulation 40:535, 1969.

135. Clarke M, Evans DW, Milstein BB: Sinus bradycardia treated by long-term atrial pacing. Br Heart J 32:458, 1970.

136. Davies JG, Sowton GE: Electrical threshold of the human heart. Br Heart J 28:231, 1966.

137. Moss AJ, Rivers RJ Jr: Atrial pacing from the coronary vein: Ten-year experience in 50 patients with implanted pervenous pacemakers. Cir-culation 57:103, 1978.

138. Ellestad MH, Messenger J, Greenberg P, et al: The use of coronary sinus pacing. In Thalen HJ, Harthorne JW (eds): To Pace or Not to Pace. The Hague, Netherlands, Martinus Nijhoff, 1978, pp 156–161.

139. Smyth NPD, Citron P, Keshishian JM, et al: Permanent pervenous atrial sensing and pacing with a new J-shaped lead. J Thorac Cardio-vasc Surg 72:565, 1976.

140. Kleinert M, Bock M, Wilhelmi F: Clinical use of a new transvenous atrial lead. Am J Cardiol 40:237, 1977.

141. Perrins EJ, Sutton R, Kalebic B, et al: Modern atrial and ventricular leads for permanent cardiac pacing. Br Heart J 46:196, 1981.

142. Bisping HJ, Kreuzer J, Birkenheier H, et al: Three-year clinical expe-rience with a new endocardial screw-in lead with introduction protec-tion for use in atrium and ventricle. PACE 3:424, 1980.

143. Gross JN, Moser S, Benedek ZM, et al: DDD pacing mode survival in patients with a dual-chamber pacemaker. J Am Coll Cardiol 19:1536, 1992.

144. Rydén L: Atrial inhibited pacing—an underused mode of cardiac stim-ulation. PACE 11:1375, 1988.

145. Lammas GA, Estes NM, III, Schneller S, et al: Does dual-chamber or atrial pacing prevent atrial fibrillation? The need for a randomized controlled trial. PACE 15:1109, 1992.

146. Andersen HR, Thuesen L, Bagger JP, et al: Atrial versus ventricular pacing in sick sinus syndrome: A prospective randomized trial in 225 consecutive patients. Eur Heart J 14(Abstract Suppl 1):252, 1993.

147. Hesselson AB, Parsonnet V, Bernstein AD, et al: Deleterious effects of long-term single-chamber ventricular pacing in patients with sick sinus syndrome: The hidden benefits of dual-chamber pacing. J Am Coll Cardiol 19:1542, 1992.

148. Sgarbossa EB, Pinski SL, Maloney JD: The role of pacing modality in determining long-term survival in the sick sinus syndrome. Ann Intern Med 119:359, 1993.

149. Sgarbossa EB, Pinski SL, Maloney JD, et al: Chronic atrial fibrillation and stroke in paced patients with sick sinus syndrome: Relevance of clinical characteristics and pacing modalities. Circulation 88:1045, 1993.

149. Santini M, Alexidou G, Ansalone G, et al: Relation of prognosis in sick sinus syndrome to age, conduction defects, and modes of permanent cardiac pacing. Am J Cardiol 65:729, 1990.

150. Sasaki Y, Shimotori M, Akahane K, et al: Long-term follow-up of patients with sick sinus syndrome: A comparison of clinical aspects among unpaced, ventricular inhibited paced, and physiologically paced groups. PACE 11:1575, 1988.

151. Stone JM, Bhakta RD, Lutgen J: Dual-chamber sequential pacing management of sinus node dysfunction: Advantages over single-chamber pacing. Am Heart J 104:1319, 1982.

152. Alpert MA, Curtiss JJ, Sanfelippo JF, et al: Comparative survival following permanent ventricular and dual-chamber pacing for patients with chronic symptomatic sinus node dysfunction with and without congestive heart failure. Am Heart J 113:958, 1987.

153. Den Dulk K, Lindemans F, Bär F, et al: Pacemaker-related tachycardias. PACE 5:476, 1982.

154. Rosenqvist M, Isaaz K, Botvinick EH, et al: The importance of a normal pattern of ventricular depolarization: A comparison between atrial AV-sequential and ventricular pacing. Am J Cardiol 67:148, 1991.

155. Cohen HE, Meltzer LE, Lattimer G: Treatment of refractory supraventricular arrhythmias with induced permanent atrial fibrillation. Am J Cardiol 28:472, 1971.

156. Vera Z, Mason DT, Awam NA, et al: Improvement of symptoms in patients with sick sinus syndrome by spontaneous development of stable atrial fibrillation. Br Heart J 39:160, 1977.

157. Perrins EJ, Sutton R, Morley C, et al: Is atrial pacing outmoded? In Feruglio G (ed): Cardiac Pacing: Electrophysiology and Pacemaker Technology. Padova, Italy, Piccin Medical Books, 1982, pp 625–626.

158. Walsh KP, Ingram A, Kenny R-A, et al: Long-term results of atrial pacing [Abstract]. PACE 8:789, 1985.

159. Floro J, Castellanet M, Florio J, et al: DDI: A new mode for cardiac pacing. Clin Prog Pacing Electrophysiol 2:255, 1984.

160. Barold SS: The DDI mode of cardiac pacing. PACE 10:480, 1987.

161. Cunningham TM: Pacemaker syndrome due to retrograde conduction in a DDI pacemaker. Am Heart J 115:478, 1988.

162. Bana G, Locatelli V, Piatti L, et al: DDI pacing in the bradycardia-tachycardia syndrome. PACE 13:264, 1990.

163. Kappenberger L, Herpers L: Rate-responsive dual-chamber pacing. PACE 9:987, 1986.

164. Sutton R: Mode-switching in DDDR pacing. In Aubert AE, Ector H, Stroobandt R (eds): Cardiac Pacing and Electrophysiology: A Bridge to the 21st Century. Dordrecht, Netherlands, Kluwer Academic Publishers, 1994, pp 363–370.

165. Haywood GA, Katritsis D, Ward J, et al: Atrial adaptive rate pacing in sick sinus syndrome: Effects on exercise capacity and arrhythmias. Br Heart J 69:174, 1993.

166. Rosenqvist M, Aren C, Kristensson BE, et al: Atrial rate-responsive pacing in sinus node disease. Eur Heart J 11:537, 1990.

167. Mabo P, Pouillot C, Kermarrec A, et al: Lack of physiological adaption of the atrioventricular interval to heart rate in patients chronically paced in the AAIR mode. PACE 14:2133, 1991.

168. Ritter P, Vai F, Bonnet JL, et al: Rate-adaptive atrioventricular delay improves cardiopulmonary performance in patients implanted with a dual-chamber pacemaker for complete heart block. Eur J Cardiac Pacing Electrophysiol 1:31, 1991.

169. Travill CM, Guneri S, Hills W, et al: The neurohumoral response to submaximal exercise in four pacing modes [Abstract]. PACE 14:621, 1991.

170. Furman S: Therapeutic uses of atrial pacing. Am Heart J 86:835, 1973.

171. Blomer H, Wirtzfeld A, Delius W, et al: Das Sinusknotensyndrom. Erlangen, Germany, Perimed Verlag Dr. Med. D. Straube, 1977.

172. Wirtzfeld A, Himmler FC, Prauer HW, et al: Atrial and ventricular pacing in patients with sick sinus syndrome. In Meere C (ed): Proceedings of the Sixth World Congress on Cardiac Pacing. Montreal, La Plante and Langevin, 1979, Chp 15-5.

173. Sutton R, Perrins J, Citron P: Physiological cardiac pacing. PACE 3:207, 1980.

174. Leibert HP, O'Donoghue S, Tullner WF, et al: Pacemaker syndrome in activity-responsive VVI pacing. Am J Cardiol 64:124, 1989.

175. Wish M, Cohen A, Swartz J: Pacemaker syndrome due to a rate-responsive ventricular pacemaker. J Electrophysiol 2:504, 1988.

176. Den Dulk K, Lindemans F, Brugada P, et al: Pacemaker syndrome with AAI rate-variable pacing: Importance of atrioventricular conduction properties, medication, and pacemaker programmability. PACE 11:1226, 1988.

177. Wish M, Fletcher RD, Gottdiener JS, et al: Importance of left atrial timing in the programming of dual-chamber pacemakers. Am J Cardiol 60:566, 1987.

178. Curzi G, Purcaro A, Molini E, et al. Deleterious clinical and haemodynamic effects of V-A retroconduction in symptomatic sinus bradyarrhythmias treated with VVI pacing: Their regression with AAI pacing. In Steinbach K, Glogar D, Laskovics A, et al (eds): Cardiac Pacing: Proceedings of the Seventh World Symposium of Cardiac Pacing. Darmstadt, Germany, Steinkopff Verlag, 1983, pp 127–134.

179. Alicandri C, Fouad FM, Tarazi RC, et al: Three cases of hypotension and syncope with ventricular pacing: Possible role of atrial reflexes. Am J Cardiol 42:137, 1978.

180. Erlebacher JA, Danner EL, Stelzer PE: Hypotension with ventricular pacing: An atrial vasodepressor reflex in human beings. J Am Coll Cardiol 4:550, 1984.

181. Ellenbogen KA, Thames MD, Mohanty PK, et al: New insights gained from hemodynamic, humoral, and vascular responses during ventriculoatrial pacing. Am J Cardiol 65:53, 1990.

182. Travill CM, Williams TDM, Vardas P, et al: Hypotension in pacemaker syndrome is associated with marked atrial natriuretic peptide (ANP) release [Abstract]. PACE 12:93, 1989.

183. Fisher JD, Furman S, Escher DJW: Pacing in the sick sinus syndrome: Profile and prognosis. In Feruglio G (ed): Cardiac Pacing: Electrophysiology and Pacemaker Technology. Padova, Italy, Piccin Medical Books, 1982, pp 519–520.

184. Hauser RG, Jones J, Edwards LM, et al: Prognosis of patients paced for AV block or sinoatrial disease in the absence of ventricular tachycardia [Abstract]. PACE 6:A123, 1983.

185. Shaw DB, Holman RR, Gowers JI: Survival in sinoatrial disorder (sick sinus syndrome). Br Med J 280:139, 1980.

186. Simon AB, Janz N: Symptomatic bradyarrhythmias in the adult: Natural history following ventricular pacemaker implantation. PACE 5:372, 1982.

187. Lau CP, Rushby J, Leigh-Jones M, et al: Symptomatology and quality of life in patients with rate-responsive pacemakers: A double-blind randomized cross-over study. Clin Cardiol 12:505, 1989.

188. Linde-Eldelstam C, Nordlander R, Undén A-L, et al: Quality of life in patients treated with atrio-ventricular synchronous pacing compared to rate-modulated ventricular pacing: A long-term double-blind crossover study. PACE 15:1467, 1992.

189. Mitsuoka T, Kenny R-A, Au Yeung T, et al: Benefits of dual-chamber pacing in sick sinus syndrome. Br Heart J 60:338, 1988.

190. Sulke N, Chambers J, Dritsas A, et al: A randomized double-blind crossover comparison of four rate-responsive pacing modes. J Am Coll Cardiol 17:696, 1991.

191. Benditt DG, Mianulli M, Fetter J, et al: Single-chamber cardiac pacing with activity-initiated chronotropic response: Evaluation by cardiopulmonary exercise testing. Circulation 75:184, 1987.

192. Benditt DG, Mianulli M, Fetter J, et al: An office-based exercise protocol for predicting chronotropic response of activity-triggered, rate-variable pacemakers. Am J Cardiol 64:27, 1989.

193. Kay GN: Quantitation of chronotropic response: Comparison of methods for rate-modulating permanent pacemakers. J Am Coll Cardiol 20:1533, 1992.

194. Kato R, Terasawa T, Gotoh T, et al: Antiarrhythmic efficacy of atrial demand (AAI) and rate-responsive atrial pacing. In Santini M, Pistolese M, Alliegro A (eds): Proceedings of the International Symposium on Progress in Clinical Pacing. Amsterdam, Excerpta Medica, 1988, pp 15–24.

195. Sutton R: DDDR pacing. PACE 13:385, 1990.

196. Bellocci F, Nobile A, Spampinato A, et al: Antiarrhythmic effects of DDD rate-responsive pacing [Abstract]. PACE 14:622, 1991.

197. Spencer III WH, Markowitz T, Alagona P: Rate augmentation and atrial arrhythmias in DDDR pacing. PACE 13:1847, 1990.

198. Feuer JM, Shandling AH, Ellestad MH: Sensor-modulated dual-chamber cardiac pacing: Too much of a good thing too fast? PACE 13:816, 1990.

199. Moura PJ, Gessman LJ, Lai T, et al: Chronotropic response of an activity-detecting pacemaker compared with the normal sinus node. PACE 10:78, 1987.

200. Daubert C, Mabo PN, Berder V, et al: Atrial tachyarrhythmias associated with high degree interatrial conduction block: Prevention by permanent atrial resynchronisation. Eur J Cardiac Pacing Electrophysiol 4(Suppl 3):35, 1994.

201. Cowell R, Morris-Thurgood J, Paul V, et al: Are we being driven to two sensors? Clinical benefits of sensor cross checking. PACE 16:1441, 1993.

CHAPTER 19

ATRIOVENTRICULAR CONDUCTION SYSTEM DISEASE

J. Marcus Wharton
Kenneth A. Ellenbogen

Historically, atrioventricular (AV) block with syncope was the first indication for cardiac pacing. Intermittent or chronic high-grade AV block still accounts for a large but variable number of permanent pacemaker implantations (e.g., between 30% and 70%), depending on the series. The site of AV block is important in that it determines to a great extent the rate and reliability of the underlying escape rhythm. Nevertheless, it is worth emphasizing that symptomatic AV block requires pacing regardless of the site, morphology, or rate of the escape rhythm.

Anatomy

It is useful to review the anatomy of the conduction system to provide insight into the structure and function of this specialized tissue (Fig. 19–1). The AV junction is a structure encompassing the AV node with its posterior, septal, and left atrial approaches as well as the His bundle and its bifurcation. The AV node is a small subendocardial structure located within the interatrial septum at the distal convergence of the preferential internodal conduction pathways that course through the atria from the sinus node.[1] Like the sinus node, the AV node has an extensive autonomic innervation and an abundant blood supply from the large AV nodal artery, which arises from either the right coronary artery (90%) or the left circumflex coronary artery (10%–15%).[2] Three regions, the transitional cell zone, the compact node, and the penetrating bundle, compose the AV node and are distinguished by functional and histologic differences. The transitional cell zone consists of cells composing the atrial approaches to the compact AV node and has the highest rate of

spontaneous diastolic depolarization. The compact node is composed of groups of cells that have extensions into the central fibrous body and the annulus of the mitral and tricuspid valves. These cells appear to be the site of most of the conduction delay through the AV node.[3] The penetrating bundle consists of cells that lead directly into the His bundle and its branching portion.

The Purkinje fibers emerging from the distal AV node converge gradually to form the His bundle, which runs beneath the membranous septum along the crest of the muscular interventricular septum until the left bundle branch and right bundle branch arise. The His bundle has relatively sparse autonomic innervation, although its blood supply, emanating from both the left and right coronary arteries, is quite ample.[4, 5] The proximal right bundle branch and the left bundle branch with its anterior fascicles receive blood from the first septal perforator branch of the left anterior descending artery and the AV nodal artery. The posterior fascicles of the left bundle receive blood from the AV nodal artery and branches of the posterior descending artery and left circumflex coronary artery. The bundle branch system is a complex network of interlacing Purkinje fibers that vary greatly among individuals.[6] These fibers generally start as one or more large fiber bands that split and fan out across the ventricles until they terminate in a vast network of strands that interface directly with the myocardium. The left bundle more commonly arises as a very broad band of interlacing fibers that spread out over the left ventricle. Although sometimes there are two or three distinct fiber tracts or fascicles branching off the left bundle branch, typically the degree of interdigitation precludes anatomic identification of either a discrete anterior or posterior fascicle.[6] The right bundle tends to

FIGURE 19–1. Diagram of the atrioventricular (AV) junction demonstrating the complexity of this region. The view is from the right side of the atrial septum along the tricuspid annulus. Three transitional cell zones connect the compact AV node cells to the atrial myocardial cells. The three zones (posterior, deep, and superficial) correspond roughly to the atrial inputs from the posterior internodal pathway, left atrium, and anterior and middle internodal pathways, respectively. The compact portion of the AV node dives into the central fibrous body as the penetrating, or His, bundle. The penetrating bundle emerges onto the crest of the interventricular septum beneath the membranous septum to form a discrete right bundle branch (RBB) and a fan-shaped left bundle branch (LBB), which are shown superimposed in this view. (From Becker AE, Anderson RH: Morphology of the human atrioventricular junctional area. *In* Wellens HJJ, Lie KI, Jause MJ, et al [eds]: The Conduction System of the Heart: Structure, Function, and Clinical Implications. Leiden, Stenfert Kroese, 1976.)

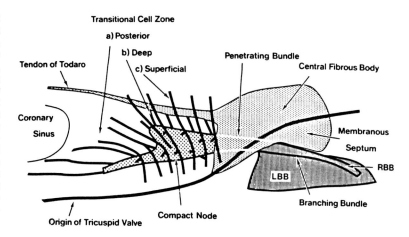

be a single distinct structure extending down the right side of the interventricular septum to the base of the anterior papillary muscle, where it divides into three or more branches. There is relatively little autonomic innervation of the bundle branch system.

Epidemiology

In complete heart block there is either a transient or a chronic absence of AV conduction, with the atrial rhythm being independent of the escape rhythm. The escape rhythm may be generated by a pacemaker in the AV junction, His bundle, bundle branches, or distal conduction system. Rarely, the underlying rhythm may arise from the ventricular myocardium or, for all practical purposes, it may be absent. The ventricular rate depends on the site of the escape pacemaker.[7] Complete AV block can be congenital or acquired. In patients with acquired complete AV block the site of block is localized distal to the His bundle in approximately 70% to 90% of patients, in the His bundle in 15% to 20%, and within the AV node in 16% to 25%.[8] In patients with congenital heart block, the escape rhythm is more often found in the proximal His bundle or AV node (see Chapter 36). Complete heart block can also be described as acute or chronic depending on its onset. Acute AV block associated with myocardial ischemia is discussed in Chapter 20. High-grade AV block is strictly defined as 3:1, 4:1, or higher AV ratios in which AV synchrony is intermittently present. As in complete AV block, block may be localized anywhere in the conduction system (Fig. 19–2). In some patients block may be present at multiple levels in the conduction system. Generically, the term high-grade AV block has been used to describe any form of AV block that suggests an increased risk of development of complete heart block or symptomatic bradycardia. This typically includes type II second-degree block, 2:1 AV block, strictly defined high-grade AV block, and complete heart block. The generic use of the term high-grade AV block should be avoided because the multiple forms of AV block included have variable pathogeneses and prognoses that blur the clinical utility of this term.

Paroxysmal AV block is defined as the sudden occurrence during a period of 1:1 AV conduction of block of the sequential atrial impulses resulting in a transient total interruption of AV conduction.[9] It is thus the onset of a paroxysm of high-grade AV block usually associated with a period of ventricular asystole before conduction returns or a subsidiary pacemaker escapes. Paroxysmal AV block may occur in a variety of clinical conditions. Patients with neurally mediated syncopal syndromes may have transient heart block, typically with associated bradycardia. It may occur in some patients with tachycardia-dependent AV block in the His-Purkinje system, during or after exertion, with the abrupt onset of bradycardia, and in type II second-degree AV block.[10]

Acquired AV block may be secondary to a number of causes of generalized myocardial scarring (Table 19–1). Causes include atherosclerosis, dilated cardiomyopathy, hypertension, infiltrative cardiomyopathies, inflammatory disorders, and infectious diseases. An entity known as idiopathic bilateral bundle branch fibrosis, *Lev's disease*, is characterized by slowly progressive replacement of specialized conduction tissue by fibrosis, resulting in progressive fascicular and bundle branch block.[11] Lev proposed that damage to the proximal left bundle branch and adjacent main bundle or main bundle alone is the result of an aging process exaggerated by hypertension and arteriosclerosis of the blood vessels supplying the conduction system.[11] Another variant of idiopathic conduction system disorder is *Lenegre's disease*, which occurs in the younger population and is characterized by loss of conduction tissue, predominantly in the peripheral parts of the bundle branch.[12]

Patients with sick sinus syndrome are known to be at risk for the development of concomitant symptomatic heart block.[13, 14] This may be due to progressive fibrodegenerative disease extending from the sinus node region to the AV

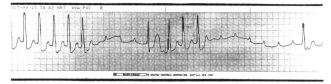

FIGURE 19–2. Rhythm strip of high-grade AV block. The baseline rhythm is sinus tachycardia in which the P wave occurs simultaneously with the T wave. After the fifth QRS complex there is an abrupt, or paroxysmal, onset of AV block with four consecutive P waves that do not conduct to the ventricles. The sixth QRS complex probably represents a junctional escape rhythm followed by three conducted complexes and then a longer episode of high-grade AV block. Prior to both episodes of high-grade AV block there is no obvious PR interval prologation nor is there slowing of the sinus rate to suggest hypervagotonia as a cause of this patient's block.

TABLE 19–1. CAUSES OF ACQUIRED COMPLETE HEART BLOCK

IDIOPATHIC FIBRODEGENERATIVE DISEASE Lev's disease Lenegre's disease	**INFECTIONS** Endocarditis Chagas' disease Lyme disease Multiple other infections: bacterial, viral, rickettsial, fungal
ISCHEMIC HEART DISEASE Myocardial infarction Ischemic cardiomyopathy	**NEUROMUSCULAR DISEASE** Myotonic dystrophy Fascioscapulohumeral dystrophy Other muscular dystrophies Kearns-Sayre syndrome Friedreich's ataxia
NONISCHEMIC CARDIOMYOPATHIES Myocarditis Idiopathic dilated cardiomyopathies Hypertensive heart disease	
CARDIAC SURGERY Coronary artery bypass Aortic, mitral, or tricuspid valve replacement Ventricular septal defect repair Septal myomectomy Ablation of septal accessory pathways	**INFILTRATIVE DISEASE** Amyloidosis Sarcoidosis Hemochromatosis Carcinoid
	NEOPLASTIC DISEASE Postradiation therapy Primary and metastatic tumors
MISCELLANEOUS Following radiofrequency and direct current His bundle ablation Exercise-induced AV block	**CONNECTIVE TISSUE DISEASE** Rheumatoid arthritis Systemic lupus erythematosus Systemic scleroderma Ankylosing spondylitis Other connective tissue diseases

conduction system. The relative frequency of this association varies between studies. Rosenqvist and Obel recently pooled the data from 28 published studies and reported a mean incidence of development of second- or third-degree AV block to be 0.6% per year (range, 0–4.5% per year) in patients in whom permanent atrial pacemakers have been implanted for symptomatic sinus node dysfunction.[15] The total prevalence of second- or third-degree AV block was 2.1% (range, 0–11%). In a retrospective review of 1395 patients with sick sinus syndrome who were followed for a mean of 34 months, Sutton and Kenny estimated that the development of conduction system disease had an annual incidence of 3%; such disease included significant first-degree AV block, bundle branch block, HV prolongation, and a low Wenckebach heart rate.[16] Thus, AV conduction system disease occurs relatively frequently in patients with sinus node dysfunction. Similarly, sinus node dysfunction, particularly chronotropic incompetence, may occur commonly in patients with acquired complete heart block.

Complete AV block may occur in a variety of clinical situations. It may occur as a consequence of coronary artery bypass surgery with an incidence of less than 1% to 2%.[17] Complete heart block occurs more commonly after aortic, mitral, or tricuspid valve replacement, given the proximity of their annuli to the AV junction.[18] Complete heart block is more common after surgical procedures to repair ventricular septal defects, tetralogy of Fallot, AV canal defects, or subvalvular aortic stenosis.[19, 20] Heart block may also occur in patients undergoing septal myomectomy for hypertrophic cardiomyopathy.[21] Finally, heart block occurs in 1% to 10% of patients undergoing surgical ablation for the Wolff-Parkinson-White syndrome when the accessory pathway is located in the anteroseptal, intermediate septal, or posteroseptal location or following surgical modification of the AV node for treatment of AV nodal reentrant tachycardia.[22]

Following discontinuation of cardiopulmonary bypass, a variety of cardiac rhythm disturbances may be seen, including sinus arrest, junctional rhythms, bundle branch block, AV block, and sinus bradycardia. Many of these rhythm disturbances are transient, resolving within 5 to 7 days. Transient bundle branch block is quite common, occurring in 4% to 35% of patients and generally resolving within 12 to 24 hours.[23] Surgery for correction of valvular heart disease may also lead to conduction defects. Conduction disturbances are particularly common in patients with aortic valve replacement, with 5% to 30% of patients experiencing some conduction abnormality following valve replacement. Most of these abnormalities are transient; however, chronic complete heart block may occur. Intraoperative heart block does not predict the need for permanent pacing.

The time course of conduction defects following bypass surgery was investigated in one study.[24] Operative technique consisted of cold, hyperkalemic cardioplegia, and conduction defects resolved partially or completely in 50% of patients. Patients with conduction defects generally had longer cardiopulmonary bypass times, longer aortic cross-clamp times, and more vessels requiring bypass. In three of the four patients with complete heart block, the heart block eventually resolved after discharge and implantation of a permanent pacemaker. Reasons for conduction abnormalities include ischemic injury to the conduction system, direct surgical manipulation or trauma to conduction tissue, traumatic disruption of the distal conduction system, or alterations in conduction caused by cardioplegia.

Complete heart block has been described in a large variety of infectious diseases. These include bacterial, viral, fungal, protozoan, and rickettsial infections. Heart block may occur with endocarditis and may be either transient or permanent. In most infectious diseases, heart block is transient and resolves with treatment of the underlying infection. In some cases, transient heart block may recur, and permanent pacing is required. This is particularly true in patients with entities such as endocarditis, in which a valve ring abscess may erode into the conduction system, and in infections such as Chagas' disease.[25, 26]

Recently, much attention has been focused on Lyme disease. This systemic illness was first described in 1975 and was characterized later as an infection caused by a spirochete, *Borrelia burgdorferi*, transmitted to humans by a tick bite. This illness is often characterized by a skin rash, erythema chronicum migrans, followed by cardiac and neurologic abnormalities and then in some cases by an arthritis.[27] Cardiac involvement may occur in 8% to 10% of patients, is generally transient, and may consist of a myocarditis or a myopericarditis.[28] Varying degrees of AV block are a common manifestation of carditis and occur in about 75% of patients. More than 50% of patients with AV block develop symptomatic high-grade or complete AV block that requires temporary pacing. Most often the site of block is localized to the AV node, although occasional cases have been reported in which the site of block is intra-Hisian or infra-Hisian.[29, 30] Continuous cardiac monitoring is recommended in all patients with second-degree AV block and a prolonged PR interval of more than 0.30 second because of the risk of developing complete AV block. Complete AV block generally resolves within 1 to 2 weeks. Recurrent AV block has not been reported. Rarely, some patients may develop symptomatic AV block as the sole manifestation of Lyme disease.[31] Permanent pacing is rarely required except when complete heart block persists, which occurs uncommonly. Two important axioms worth repeating are: (1) heart block associated with infectious disease usually resolves with appropriate and prompt antibiotic treatment, and (2) rarely is conduction disease the only presenting feature of an infectious illness.

Heart block may occur following radiation therapy or chemotherapy. Heart block may occur after radiation therapy when radiation is directed at the mediastinum, as may be the case with Hodgkin's and some non-Hodgkin's lymphomas.[32] Rarely, tumors including mesothelioma of the AV node and metastatic disease to the heart from breast, lung, or skin cancer may involve the conduction system.[33] It is unusual for toxicity to antineoplastic drugs, such as adriamycin, to result in damage to the conduction system.

Certain neuromuscular diseases also may give rise to progressive and insidiously developing conduction system disease, including Duchenne's muscular dystrophy, fascioscapulohumeral muscular dystrophy, X-linked muscular dystrophy, myasthenia gravis, myotonic dystrophy, and Friedreich's ataxia.[34] Abnormalities of conduction manifest as infranodal conduction disturbances resulting in fascicular block or complete heart block. This has been noted particularly in Kearns-Sayre syndrome (progressive external ophthalmoplegia with pigmentary retinopathy), Guillain-Barré syndrome, myotonic muscular dystrophy, slowly progressive X-linked Becker's muscular dystrophy, and fascioscapulohumeral muscular dystrophy. It is worth noting that myotonic muscular dystrophy and Kearns-Sayre syndrome are both associated with a high incidence of conduction system disease that is frequently rapidly progressive and cannot be predicted by the electrocardiogram or isolated His bundle recordings. His-Purkinje disease can culminate in fatal

Stokes-Adams attacks unless anticipated by pacemaker insertion.

Heart block may occur with amyloid and other infiltrative diseases, including hemochromatosis, porphyria, oxalosis, Refsum's disease, carcinoid, Hand-Schüller-Christian disease, and sarcoidosis.[35]

Connective tissue disorders giving rise to conduction system disease include periarteritis nodosa, rheumatoid arthritis, polymyositis, mixed connective tissue disorders, Reiter's syndrome, ulcerative colitis, scleroderma, Takayasu's aortitis, systemic lupus erythematosus, and ankylosing spondylitis.[36, 37] For example, in one study of 50 consecutive patients with scleroderma, invasive electrophysiologic studies revealed conduction abnormalities in up to 50% of patients, suggesting that a much higher degree of cardiac involvement may be present in patients than is readily apparent clinically. However, complete heart block is uncommon.[38] Most patients with AV conduction disorders have other clinical manifestations of their connective tissue disease.

Exercise-induced AV block is relatively rare, and recent studies have shown that the site of block is often in the His-Purkinje system (Fig. 19–3).[39] Donzeau and colleagues reported 14 symptomatic patients with exercise-induced AV block, of which nine patients had block localized to an infranodal site.[40] Other studies have also shown that exercise-induced AV block is primarily infra-Hisian.[41, 42] In these studies approximately 25% to 75% of patients had underlying bundle branch block. Permanent pacing is recommended in patients with exercise-induced AV block, even in the asymptomatic state, because of the high incidence of development of symptomatic AV block. Finally, several reports of patients with cardiac asystole following exertion have demonstrated postexercise sinus arrest with ventricular asystole.[43]

Vagally mediated AV block infrequently requires a permanent pacemaker. This form of AV block must be differentiated from type II second-degree AV block because these patients almost always require the implantation of a permanent pacemaker.[44] In most cases vagally induced AV block occurs at the level of the AV node and is associated with a narrow QRS complex.[45] Rarely, vagal stimulation may precipitate phase IV or bradycardia-mediated block in the His-Purkinje system.[10] AV block may occur in the setting of

Lead II at Rest

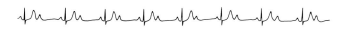

Lead II After 2 min. of Exercise

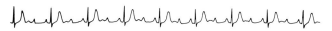

FIGURE 19–3. *Upper Panel,* Lead II rhythm strip from a patient with syncope and frequent 2:1 AV block with an incomplete right bundle branch block and a sinus rate of 97 bpm. Periods of 3:2 AV conduction were not available to determine whether the patient's 2:1 AV conduction was due to type I or type II AV block. *Lower Panel,* Rhythm strip obtained 2 minutes into treadmill testing reveals 3:1 AV conduction with an increase in heart rate to 142 bpm. The development of high-grade AV block despite exercise-induced increases in sympathetic tone and decrease in parasympathetic tone suggests infra- or intra-Hisian block and the need for permanent pacing.

increased vagal tone in response to various stimuli such as carotid sinus hypersensitivity, coughing, swallowing, or visceral distention.[46–48] As a general rule, vagally mediated AV nodal block shows obvious heart rate slowing, even if only slight, prior to the onset of block due to the concomitant effect of increased vagal tone on the sinus node.

The prognosis and natural history of individuals with primary first-degree AV block and moderate PR prolongation has been shown to be benign.[49] Progression to complete heart block over time occurred in about 4% of patients in this study. Most of the patients (66%) had only mild to moderate PR prolongation, to about 0.22 to 0.23 second. In the great majority of subjects the PR interval remained within a narrow range, changing less than 0.04 second. The natural history of 56 patients with second-degree AV block was described by Strasberg and colleagues.[50] They concluded that progression to complete heart block is also relatively uncommon. Their study is limited by the small number of subjects with structural heart disease studied. Many of their patients were under 35 years of age or were trained athletes. A more recent study by Shaw suggests that patients with type I second-degree AV block had a worse prognosis than age- and sex-matched individuals unless they had permanent pacemakers implanted.[51] In patients with type I second-degree AV block and permanent pacemakers, survival was similar to that in the age- and sex-matched normal population (see later discussion under Commentary).

Patients with bundle branch block or bifascicular block are an important clinical problem. Not infrequently, a clinician is asked to evaluate a patient with bundle branch block or bifascicular block and syncope. Most patients with chronic bifascicular block have underlying structural heart disease, the prevalence of which ranges from 50% to 80%.[52–54] Many studies have shown that chronic bifascicular block in this clinical situation is associated with substantial mortality.

Historically, it was thought that progression from chronic bifascicular block to trifascicular block was common. Retrospective studies in patients with chronic bifascicular block had suggested that the risk of progression to complete AV block was 5% to 10% per year. In the early 1980s the results of several prospective studies questioned assumptions about the incidence and clinical implications of progression of conduction system disease in this patient population. Prospective studies of groups of *asymptomatic* patients with bifascicular block and prolonged HV intervals at the time of electrophysiologic study revealed that these patients are at increased risk of developing complete heart block but that the absolute risk remains very low, about 2% per year.[52, 54] A prolonged HV interval was associated with higher total cardiovascular mortality and mortality due to sudden death. It is likely that a prolonged HV interval is associated with more extensive structural heart disease. Furthermore, these studies demonstrated that routine His bundle recordings are of *limited* usefulness in patients with bifascicular block in the *absence* of symptoms.

On the other hand, patients with *syncope* and *bifascicular block* represent a *different* clinical problem. If a thorough clinical evaluation, including a history, physical examination, and electrocardiogram (ECG) do not uncover a cause of syncope, an electrophysiologic study may be useful[55, 56] (see later discussion under Commentary). Linzer and associates[57] found that the presence of first-degree AV block or bundle

branch block increased the odds ratio of finding abnormalities suggesting risk of bradyarrhythmia (predominantly heart block) by three- to eightfold during electrophysiologic studies in patients with unexplained syncope (Table 19–2). Electrophysiologic studies may uncover other causes of syncope such as sinus node dysfunction, rapid supraventricular tachycardias, or inducible monomorphic ventricular tachycardia. In some studies, a monomorphic ventricular tachycardia was discovered in 20% to 30% of patients with bundle branch block and syncope.[55, 56] A minority of patients are found to have a markedly prolonged HV interval, abnormal or fragmented His bundle electrogram, or block distal to the His bundle with atrial pacing, suggesting the need for permanent pacemaker implantation.

Radiofrequency energy is being increasingly used to create complete AV block in patients with paroxysmal and chronic atrial fibrillation in whom the resting heart rate cannot be controlled by AV nodal blocking drugs or who are intolerant, unwilling, or unable to take drugs to maintain sinus rhythm or control the ventricular response. In these patients, an ablation catheter is placed across the tricuspid valve or, less frequently, into the left ventricle on the septum underneath the noncoronary cusp of the aortic valve to record a His bundle potential.[58] Radiofrequency current is delivered to create permanent complete AV block. Radiofrequency current ablation of the AV junction usually results in a junctional escape rhythm that has a rate generally ranging from 40 to 50 bpm. In most cases, based on limited follow-up, this escape rhythm appears to be stable. On the other hand, a direct current shock delivered through a catheter to ablate the AV junction results in a fascicular or ventricular escape

TABLE 19–2. ODDS RATIO FOR ABNORMALITY ON ELECTROPHYSIOLOGIC TESTING IN PATIENTS WITH SYNCOPE

CLINICAL VARIABLES	MULTIVARIABLE	95% CONFIDENCE INTERVAL FOR MULTIVARIABLE
Age	1.01	0.99–1.03
Duration (months)	1.00	0.98–1.02
Sex (male)	1.76	0.79–3.93
Organic heart disease	1.53	0.71–3.33
Sudden loss of consciousness	1.93	0.89–4.16
Left ventricular ejection fraction	0.99	0.93–1.06
ECG variables		
Bundle branch block	2.97†	1.23– 7.21
Sinus bradycardia	3.47†	1.12–10.71
First-degree heart block	7.89*	2.12–29.31
Premature ventricular contractions (PVCs)	1.47	0.37– 5.82
Holter variables		
Sinus bradycardia	0.68	0.21–2.23
Sinus pause	1.04	0.26–4.23
Mobitz I	0.63	0.06–6.33
PVCs	0.87	0.35–2.13

*p < .001
†p < .05

Adapted from Linzer M, Prystowsky EN, Devine GW, et al: Predicting the outcomes of electrophysiologic studies of patients with unexplained syncope: Preliminary validation of a derived model. J Gen Intern Med 6:113, 1991.

rhythm that has a rate of about 45 bpm or less, which may be unreliable.[59, 60] Overdrive pacing of the ventricle has led to prolonged ventricular asystole in these patients, and questions have been raised about the long-term stability of this escape rhythm. Until more information is available, *all patients* undergoing both radiofrequency and direct current His bundle ablation *should undergo* permanent pacemaker implantation.

Diagnosis

ELECTROCARDIOGRAPHY

First-degree AV block is usually due to conduction delay within the AV node. Much less commonly, first-degree AV block is due to intra-atrial or infra-Hisian conduction delay.[8] Localization of the site of second-degree AV block to the AV node or His-Purkinje system can be obtained by His bundle recording during invasive electrophysiologic testing, but in most cases careful analysis of the ECG and the effect of various pharmacologic agents on block may suffice.[61] Diagnosis of the site of block is particularly problematic with 2:1 AV block. As a general rule, type I second-degree AV block with a narrow QRS almost always occurs within the AV node (Fig. 19–4). However, type I second-degree AV block with concomitant bundle branch block may be associated with infra-Hisian block in up to 30% of cases.[8, 61] Wenckebach periodicity prior to the development of high-grade AV block is suggestive of an AV nodal site of block. Administration of digoxin, beta-blockers, and calcium channel blockers is also suggestive of block located in the AV node. Type II AV block is most commonly encountered when the QRS is prolonged and is generally localized within the His-Purkinje system (Fig. 19–5). Occasionally type II AV block with a narrow QRS can be localized to the His bundle (i.e., intra-Hisian), but it may also be due to type I block with relatively long Wenckebach sequences and small increases in AV nodal conduction time.

In general, the response of block, particularly 2:1 AV block, to pharmacologic agents may help to determine the site of block. Atropine generally improves AV conduction in patients with AV nodal block. However, atropine is generally expected to worsen conduction in patients with block localized to the His-Purkinje system owing to its effect on increas-

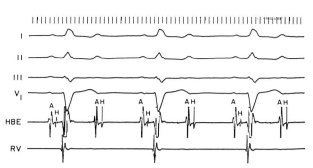

FIGURE 19–5. Intracardiac tracing of 2:1 second-degree AV block located in the His-Purkinje system. Sinus rhythm with left bundle branch block is present. The AH intervals are constant, but every other atrial complex fails to activate the ventricule even though each atrial depolarization is followed by a His bundle deflection. This shows that the site of AV block is within the His-Purkinje system. (From Josephson ME: Clinical Cardiac Electrophysiology: Techniques and Interpretations. Philadelphia, Lea & Febiger, 1979, pp 79–101.)

ing sinus rates without improving His-Purkinje conduction (Fig. 19–6). Carotid sinus stimulation is expected to worsen block localized to the AV node, whereas it has no effect or improves conduction in patients with His-Purkinje system disease by causing sinus node slowing. However, the effect of any given drug may be difficult to predict because its effect on the sinus node may be greater than its effect on the AV node. For example, atropine may improve AV node conduction, but if atropine causes excessive sinus node acceleration, AV conduction may improve marginally or not at all. The response to infusion of isoproterenol is less clear. Isoproterenol may improve conduction disorders localized in the AV node as well as occasionally in the His-Purkinje system.

Classic type I (Wenckebach) second-degree AV block has three characteristics: (1) progressive PR interval prolongation prior to the nonconducted beat, (2) progressive decrease in the increment of PR interval prolongation, and (3) progressive decrease in the RR interval, parallel to the progressive decrease in the increment of change in the PR interval.[62] All patterns of type I second-degree AV block not having this pattern are called atypical patterns, although in actuality they may occur more commonly than the classic variety.[63, 64] Lange and colleagues[65] reported on their experience with a large number of patients with transient second-degree AV block and narrow QRS complexes detected on ambulatory Holter monitoring. The authors emphasized the many ways in which second-degree AV block can be manifested. Classic type I AV block with progressive PR prolongation to more than 40 msec during at least three beats before the blocked P waves was seen in only 50% of patients. Other patterns observed included a more subtle Wenckebach periodicity with minor PR prolongation of 20 to 40 msec before a blocked P wave in 29% of patients. Another pattern, seen in 8% of patients and termed "pseudo-Mobitz" type II AV block, demonstrated nearly constant PR intervals before the blocked P wave, followed by PR shortening on the subsequent conducted beat (Fig. 19–7). Classic Mobitz type II second-degree AV block with constant PR intervals for at least three beats before the blocked P wave followed by the same PR interval after the blocked P wave was seen in 4% of patients (Fig. 19–8). A mixed type I Wenckebach and

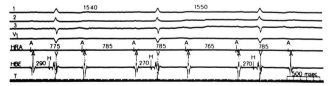

FIGURE 19–4. Spontaneous 2:1 (high-grade) AV block localized to the AV node. In this and subsequent figures, surface leads I, II, III, and V_1 are displayed with intracardiac electrograms recorded from the high right atrium (HRA), His bundle (HBE), and right ventricular apex (RV). Alternate atrial depolarizations (A) are not followed by either a His bundle or a ventricular depolarization. On the basis of a surface electrocardiogram (ECG), the finding of 2:1 AV block with a narrow QRS is compatible with a block at either the AV node or an infra-His site. The intracardiac recordings localize the site of block to the AV node. (From Josephson ME, Clinical Cardiac Electrophysiology: Techniques and Interpretations. Philadelphia, Lea & Febiger, 1979, pp 79–101.)

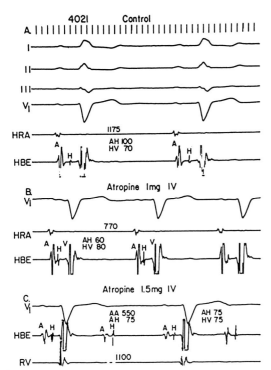

FIGURE 19–6. His-Purkinje AV block after an atropine-induced increase in sinus rate. *A,* Sinus rhythm at a cycle length of 1175 msec with 1:1 AV conduction. Left bundle branch block is present, and the HV interval is slightly prolonged to 70 msec. *B,* After injection of 1 mg of atropine, the sinus rate speeds up to 770 msec and the HV interval increases to 80 msec, but 1:1 AV conduction is still present. The AH interval shortens despite the faster sinus rate because of the direct effect of atropine on AV nodal conduction. *C,* After injection of 1.5 mg of atropine the sinus cycle length decreases further to 550 msec, and 2:1 AV block occurs below the His bundle. Atropine worsens AV conduction in this patient, not through a direct drug effect but because the improvement in AV nodal conduction caused by atropine stresses the already abnormal His-Pukinje system. (From Miles WM, Klein LS: Sinus nodal dysfunction and atrioventricular conduction distrubances. *In* Naccarelli GV [ed]: Cardiac Arrhythmias: A Practical Approach. Mt Kisco, NY, Futura Publishing Co., 1991, pp 243–282.)

pseudo-type II AV block were seen in 6% of all patients. Of all patients showing periods of pseudo-Mobitz type II block, 44% also demonstrated classic Wenckebach conduction patterns at some time as well.[65] Slowing of the sinus cycle length often preceded the blocked P wave in both classic and pseudo-Mobitz type II AV block (Fig. 19–9).

The diagnosis of complete heart block rests on demonstra-

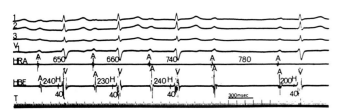

FIGURE 19–7. Example of atypical or uncommon type I second-degree AV block in the AV node. There is little alteration in the AH interval prior to the fourth atrial complex not conducting to the ventricle. The true nature of this arrhythmia is revealed by the first conducted P wave (A, atrial electrogram) after the pause, which is associated with substantial shortening of the AH interval from 230–240 msec to 200 msec. (From Josephson ME: Clinical Cardiac Electrophysiology: Techniques and Interpretations. Philadelphia, Lea & Febiger, 1979, pp 79–101.)

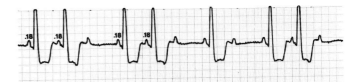

FIGURE 19–8. Example of type II second-degree AV block showing repeating episodes of block. Note that the PR interval is constant both before and after the nonconducted P wave and that there is associated bundle branch block.

tion of complete dissociation between atrial and ventricular activation. Care must be taken to distinguish transient AV dissociation due to competing atrial and junctional or ventricular rhythms with similar rates (so-called isorhythmic AV dissociation). If sufficiently long monitoring strips are available, intermittent conduction of appropriately timed atrial events will be seen. Temporary atrial pacing can be performed to accelerate the atrial rate to overdrive the competing junctional or ventricular arrhythmia, demonstrating intact AV conduction. In the presence of atrial fibrillation, complete heart block can be inferred when the ventricular rate becomes regular rather than the typical irregular ventricular response (Fig. 19–10). Digoxin toxicity may be the cause of heart block with atrial fibrillation, and this or other drug toxicity should be ruled out before one assumes that structural AV conduction disease is present.

ELECTROPHYSIOLOGIC STUDY

Invasive electrophysiologic study (e.g., His bundle recording) can be a very useful means of evaluating AV conduction in symptomatic patients in whom the need for permanent

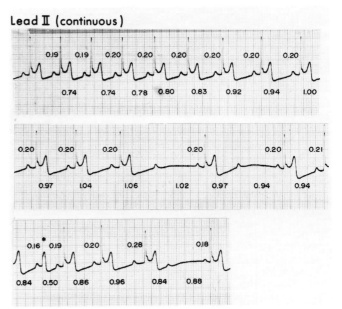

FIGURE 19–9. Rhythm strip demonstrating vagally mediated second-degree AV block. Note the progressive slowing of the heart rate prior to the first episode of block, although no change in PR interval can be discerned. During the second episode of block, there are both sinus slowing and PR interval prolongation, confirming the presence of type I second-degree AV block.

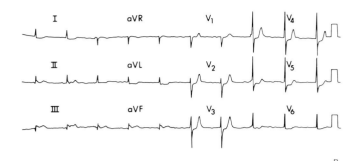

FIGURE 19–10. Twelve-lead electrocardiogram from a patient with recent aortic valve surgery and atrial fibrillation treated with digoxin. The QRS complexes are narrow and occur at a regular rate of 56 bpm, illustrating complete heart block with a junctional escape rhythm in the setting of atrial fibrillation. Despite discontinuation of digoxin, complete heart block persisted in this patient.

pacing is not obvious (Fig. 19–11). It is *not indicated* in patients with symptomatic high-grade or complete AV block recorded on surface ECG tracings, ambulatory Holter monitoring, or transtelephonic recordings because the need for permanent pacing has already been established. In addition, asymptomatic patients who have intermittent AV block associated with sinus slowing, gradual PR prolongation before a nonconducted P wave, and a narrow QRS complex also should not undergo electrophysiologic study given the benign prognosis of these findings.

As stated earlier, the incidence of progression of bifascicular block to complete heart block is variable, ranging from 2% to 6% per year. The method of patient selection will affect this incidence, with asymptomatic patients who have bifascicular block progressing to complete heart block at a rate of 2% per year, and symptomatic patients (e.g., those with syncope or presyncope) progressing at a rate closer to 6% per year.[52–54, 66] Many of these studies emphasize the high mortality associated with bundle branch block and bifascicular block. It is worth emphasizing that the mortality associated with the presence of structural heart disease predominantly reflects death due to ventricular tachyarrhythmias rather than bradyarrhythmias.

Three large studies of patients with bundle branch block have been performed to assess the role of His bundle conduction (e.g., HV interval) measurements in predicting progression to complete heart block. The measurement of the HV interval represents the conduction time through the His bundle and bundle branches until ventricular activation begins. Dhingra and colleagues[52] prospectively followed 517 patients with bundle branch block and measured the time required for progression to second- and third-degree block. In their study only 13% of patients presented with syncope; the remainder were asymptomatic. The cumulative 7-year incidence of progression to AV block was 10% in the group with a normal HV interval and 20% in the group with HV interval prolongation. The cumulative mortality at 7 years was 48% in patients with a normal HV interval and 66% in patients with a prolonged HV interval.[52] This study emphasized that despite the high mortality associated with the presence of bifascicular block, there is only a low rate of progression to trifascicular block.

McAnulty and associates[53] studied 554 patients with "high-risk" bundle branch block defined as left bundle branch block (LBBB), right bundle branch block (RBBB) and left or right axis, RBBB with alternating left and right axis, or alternating RBBB and LBBB. The cumulative incidence of AV block, either type II second degree or complete heart block, was only 4.9%, or 1% per year in patients with a prolonged HV interval and 1.9% in patients with a normal HV interval (difference not significant). HV interval prolongation did not predict a higher risk of development of complete heart block. In this study, 8.5% of patients developed syncope after entry into the study. The incidence of complete AV block was 17% in patients with syncope compared to 2% in patients without a history of syncope.

Scheinman and colleagues[54] studied 401 patients with chronic bundle branch block for approximately 30 months. Patients with an HV interval of more than 70 msec had an incidence of 12% of progression to spontaneous second- or third-degree AV block. The incidence of complete AV block was 25% for those with an HV interval of 100 msec or greater. The yearly incidence of spontaneous AV block was 3% in those with a normal HV interval compared to 3.5% in those with a prolonged HV interval. Scheinman's group included the highest percentage of patients with a history of syncope, about 40%.

Resolution of the *apparent* controversy about the clinical utility of His bundle recordings involves a realization that different patient populations are being studied. There does appear to be a relationship between a prolonged HV interval and the development of complete heart block during the ensuing years. It is also likely that this risk varies directly with the degree of HV prolongation. Demonstration of these relationships requires documentation of spontaneous high-grade complete heart block in enough patients because the absolute risk is very low overall. This can be done in one of two ways: by following a large number of patients for long

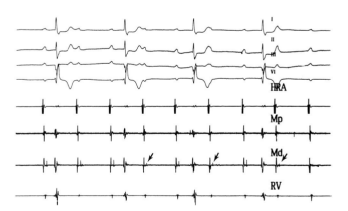

FIGURE 19–11. Surface leads I, II, III, and V₁ revealing sinus rhythm with 2:1 AV conduction, marked PR interval prolongation during conducted beats, and right bundle branch block. Intracardiac electrograms from the high right atrium (HRA), proximal and distal poles of the His bundle catheter (M_p and M_d, respectively), and the right ventricle (RV) are shown. The distal pole of the His bundle catheter registers a His bundle potential, which can be seen as a discrete sharp potential between the atrial and the ventricular electrograms on that channel. During nonconducted atrial complexes, spontaneous infra-Hisian block is apparent because the His bundle potential *(arrow)* is not followed by a ventricular electrogram.

periods of time or by including patients with symptoms of unexplained syncope. Demonstration of this relationship in an unselected, asymptomatic group of patients is difficult because the risk of complete heart block is so low. *Current recommendations are therefore not to perform electrophysiologic studies in patients with bundle branch block who are asymptomatic.*[67]

Many studies have demonstrated the clinical utility of electrophysiologic testing in patients with *bundle branch block* and *syncope.*[55, 56] In one study, 112 patients with chronic bundle branch block and syncope or near-syncope underwent electrophysiologic testing.[55] A normal electrophysiologic study result predicted a good long-term prognosis. About 25% of patients were found to have a significant conduction system disorder, underwent pacemaker implantation, and had symptoms recur at a rate of only 6%. In the study reported by Morady and associates,[56] 28% of patients (7 of 32) had sustained induced monomorphic ventricular tachycardia, whereas about 20% had conduction disturbances at electrophysiology study. Six of the seven patients who received pacemakers had no recurrent symptoms. Thus, electrophysiologic studies are useful in patients with bundle branch block or bifascicular block and syncope for several reasons. First, negative results of electrophysiologic studies identify a group of patients at low risk of cardiac events. More important, induction of sustained ventricular tachycardia during electrophysiologic testing identifies patients who are at risk of life-threatening ventricular arrhythmias and who require pharmacologic or other therapy (e.g., surgery or defibrillation). Finally, electrophysiologic testing also identifies those patients with advanced conduction system disease who require pacemaker implantation. Thus, *current recommendations are to perform electrophysiologic testing in patients with syncope or near syncope and bundle branch block.*

METHODS USED TO IDENTIFY PATIENTS AT RISK FOR AV BLOCK

In addition to measurement of HV intervals, additional electrophysiologic testing has been suggested for use in symptomatic patients with bundle branch or bifascicular block. As stated previously, a *markedly* prolonged HV interval (≥ 100 msec) is predictive of development of symptomatic heart block. HV intervals greater than 100 msec are uncommon, so although marked HV prolongation is quite specific, it is also very insensitive.

The use of atrial pacing to stress the His-Purkinje system has been suggested by some to provide additional important information. Most normal subjects will not develop second- or third-degree infra-Hisian block during atrial pacing in which the rate is gradually increased, as would occur spontaneously. However, certain pacing protocols with abrupt onset of pacing at rapid rates are more likely to induce infra-Hisian block even in normal individuals, but this rarely occurs at pacing rates below 150 bpm. Dhingra and colleagues reported a 50% rate of progression to type II or complete AV block in patients who develop block distal to the His bundle at paced rates of less than 150 bpm.[68] Because AV nodal dysfunction is frequently seen in patients with significant His-Purkinje system disease, AV nodal block may occur at lower pacing rates than those necessary to demonstrate infra-Hisian block. This "protective" effect of AV nodal dysfunc-

tion during resting states may lead to the incorrect conclusion that significant His-Purkinje disease is not present. However, repeat atrial pacing may demonstrate infra-Hisian block after administration of atropine or isoproterenol to facilitate AV nodal conduction.

Provocative drug tests have been suggested as another means of evaluating the distal conduction system (Fig. 19–12). There are only limited available data describing the experience with the intravenous type Ia antiarrhythmic drugs procainamide, ajmaline, and disopyramide and the type Ic agent flecainide.[69–72] Only intravenous procainamide is available in the United States. Administration of these agents may result in a doubling of the HV interval, a resultant HV interval greater than 100 msec, or precipitation of spontaneous type II second- or third-degree AV block, all of which indicate a higher risk of developing complete heart block. Tonkin and associates[72] administered procainamide at a dose of 10 mg/kg and produced intermittent second- or third-degree AV block in 5 of 12 patients. Progression to complete AV block over a period of 1 year was high in this group of symptomatic patients. Intravenous disopyramide has the potential benefit of facilitating AV nodal conduction by its anticholinergic properties while accentuating underlying infra-Hisian disease by its membrane-stabilizing effects.[71]

In patients with alternating bundle branch block, electrophysiologic testing almost invariably demonstrates a high degree of His-Purkinje system disease. These patients typically have very long HV intervals and are at very high risk of progression to complete heart block in a short time span. Pacing in these patients is indicated on clinical grounds, and electrophysiologic testing is unnecessary.[70]

Although electrophysiologic testing has been considered the "gold standard" for identifying significant AV nodal or His-Purkinje dysfunction, it may have its limitations.[73] In a small study conducted by Fujimura and associates,[73] 13 patients with documented symptomatic transient second- or third-degree AV block referred for implantation of a permanent pacemaker underwent AV conduction testing at the time of pacemaker insertion. These tests included facilitation of AV nodal conduction with atropine and depression of His-Purkinje conduction with low doses of procainamide. Surprisingly, only 2 of the 13 patients showed significant abnormalities in the AV conduction system (inducible infra-Hisian block in both cases) during electrophysiologic testing, yielding a sensitivity of 15.4%. Two additional patients had moderately prolonged HV intervals, although much less than 100 msec. If these two patients are included as diagnostic, then the sensitivity of electrophysiology testing is increased to 46%. Although the patient population was small, this study raises serious questions about the sensitivity of electrophysiologic testing for identifying patients at risk of developing symptomatic AV block. Further data are clearly needed in this regard. Whether other pharmacologic stressors as mentioned previously would have improved the overall sensitivity awaits further investigation.

Indications

In 1984 a committee of the American College of Cardiology (ACC) and the American Heart Association (AHA) put together a set of guidelines concerning the indications for

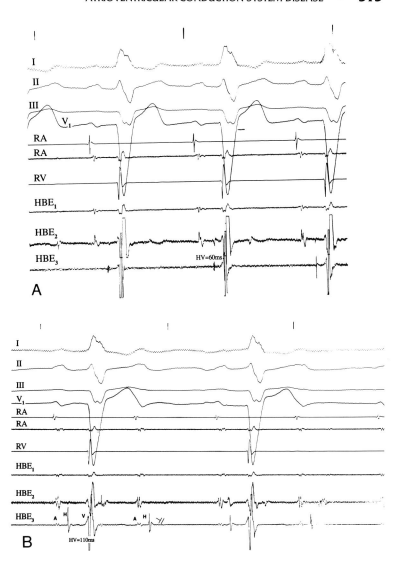

FIGURE 19–12. *A*, Electrophysiologic testing in the baseline state in a patient with syncope reveals a left bundle branch block pattern during sinus rhythm. There is 1:1 AV conduction with an HV interval of 60 msec. *B*, After a loading dose of procainamide, 2:1 AV conduction develops. The first and third atrial activations are conducted to the ventricles with an HV interval of 110 msec. The third and fourth atrial activations conduct through the AV node to generate a His bundle potential without subsequent ventricular activation. Thus, this illustrates spontaneous infra-Hisian block induced by procainamide. RA, right atrial recordings; RV, right ventricular recording; HBE$_1$, HBE$_2$, HBE$_3$, proximal, middle, and distal His bundle catheter recordings, respectively.

permanent pacing.[74] These guidelines were revised in 1991.[75] Guidelines are categorized into three classes:

CLASS I. Conditions under which implantation of a permanent pacemaker is considered necessary and acceptable. There is general agreement among physicians that a permanent pacemaker should be implanted. This implies that the condition is chronic or recurrent but not due to drug toxicity, acute myocardial ischemia or infarction, or electrolyte imbalance.

CLASS II. Conditions for which cardiac pacemakers are generally found acceptable or necessary, but there is some divergence of opinion.

CLASS III. Conditions considered unsupportable by present evidence to benefit adequately from permanent pacemakers, and there is general agreement that a pacemaker is *not* indicated.

Indications that are generally agreed on and included in the recent AHA/ACC guidelines are as follows:

PACING FOR ACQUIRED AV BLOCK IN ADULTS

CLASS I

- Permanent or intermittent third-degree AV block (at any anatomic level) with symptoms. Symptoms include (1) Syncope or presyncope, (2) congestive heart failure, (3) mental confusion improving with temporary pacing, (4) symptomatic ventricular ectopy, nonsustained or sustained ventricular tachycardia, or ventricular fibrillation related to an inadequate or slow escape rhythm, (5) asymptomatic, but with a ventricular escape rate less than 40 bpm, (6) asymptomatic, with documented asystole greater than 3 seconds, (7) chronotropic incompetence of the escape pacemaker accompanied by symptoms due to the inability to increase heart rate with exercise or stress, (8) moderate to marked exercise intolerance, (9) myotonic dystrophy

- Second-degree AV block with symptoms of syncope or presyncope: (1) type I (Mobitz I, Wenckebach), (2) type II (Mobitz II)

- Atrial flutter, atrial fibrillation, or atrial tachycardia with advanced symptomatic high-grade AV block

- Asymptomatic complete AV block with a ventricular rate greater than 40 bpm following DC (direct current) or radiofrequency ablation

- Symptomatic first-degree AV block with symptoms suggestive of pacemaker syndrome

CLASS II

- Asymptomatic complete AV block with a ventricular rate greater than 40 bpm

- Asymptomatic type II second-degree AV block
- Asymptomatic type I second-degree AV block within the His-Purkinje system (rare, requires invasive electrophysiologic study for diagnosis)

CLASS III

- First-degree AV block
- Asymptomatic type I second-degree AV block

PACING IN BIFASCICULAR AND TRIFASCICULAR BLOCK (CHRONIC)

CLASS I

- Bifascicular block with intermittent complete heart block associated with symptomatic bradycardia
- Bifascicular or trifascicular block with intermittent type II second-degree AV block without symptoms attributable to the heart block

CLASS II

- Bifascicular or trifascicular block with syncope that is not proved to be due to complete heart block, but other possible causes for syncope are not identifiable
- Markedly prolonged HV (>100 msec) interval
- Atrial pacing–induced infra-Hisian block at rates less than 150 bpm

CLASS III

- Fascicular block without AV block or symptoms
- Fascicular block with first-degree AV block without symptoms

PACING IN INTRAVENTRICULAR CONDUCTION DEFECTS

CLASS I

- Bundle branch or bifascicular block with intermittent complete heart block associated with symptomatic bradycardia
- Bundle branch block or bifascicular block with intermittent type II second-degree AV block without symptoms attributed to heart block
- Trifascicular block during 1:1 AV conduction such as alternating LBBB and RBBB, fixed RBBB with alternating left anterior hemiblock (LAH) and left posterior hemiblock (LPH) with symptoms

CLASS II

- Bundle branch block or bifascicular block with syncope that is not proved to be due to complete heart block, but other possible causes of syncope are not identifiable
- Markedly prolonged HV interval (>100 msec)
- Pacing-induced infra-Hisian block
- Trifascicular block during 1:1 AV conduction, such as alternating left and right bundle branch block and fixed RBBB with alternating left anterior and posterior hemiblock without symptoms*

---

*Represents a class I indication by some individuals.

CLASS III

- Fascicular, bundle branch or bifascicular block without AV block or symptoms
- Fascicular, bundle branch, or bifascicular block with first-degree AV block without symptoms

COMMENTARY

Barold has commented on these guidelines in a recent editorial.[76] He emphasizes that more precise definition of second-degree AV block is necessary, particularly with 2:1 AV block. He notes that second-degree AV block classified as type I should be associated with progressive prolongation of PR intervals before a blocked beat and type II with constant PR intervals before and after a single blocked beat, usually in association with a wide QRS complex. Trifascicular block is a term that is also loosely applied. Barold argues that the use of the term trifascicular block to describe the combination of bifascicular block (RBBB plus LAH, RBBB plus LPH, or LBBB) and first-degree AV block is misleading because the site of block may be located in the AV node or His-Purkinje system. Trifascicular block should only be used to refer to alternating RBBB and LBBB, RBBB with a prolonged HV interval (regardless of the presence or absence of left anterior or posterior fascicular block), and LBBB with a prolonged HV interval. In addition, trifascicular block can refer to a patient with second- or third-degree AV block in the His-Purkinje system with permanent block in all three fascicles, permanent block in two fascicles and intermittent conduction in the third, permanent block in one fascicle with intermittent block in the other two fascicles, and intermittent block in all three fascicles.[76]

Patients who present with symptomatic first-, second-, or third-degree AV block usually have symptoms of syncope, dizziness, decreased energy, palpitations, or recurrent presyncope or dizziness. Other symptoms primarily reflect inadequate cardiac output or tissue perfusion and include fatigue, angina, or congestive heart failure. The most severe symptom is recurrent Stokes-Adams attacks with documented episodes of polymorphic ventricular tachycardia. Patients with long PR intervals may have symptoms suggestive of pacemaker syndrome and may demonstrate resolution of symptoms with institution of dual-chamber pacing. It is important to emphasize that symptoms can be subtle in some patients or may be of sufficiently long duration that temporary pacing may be indicated to document improvement or reversal of long-standing problems.

The *natural history* of patients with spontaneously developing asymptomatic complete heart block in adult life dates back to the days before pacemaker therapy was available.[77, 78] Today, almost all patients with complete heart block probably eventually develop symptoms and undergo pacemaker placement. Several studies published in the 1960s emphasized the poor prognosis of patients with complete heart block. The 1-year survival of patients who developed Stokes-Adams attacks due to complete heart block and were not paced was 50% to 75%, which is significantly less than that of a sex- and age-matched control population.[77, 78] The "best" prognosis was in patients with an idiopathic or unknown cause. At least 33% of deaths were definitely related to complete heart block and Stokes-Adams attacks. These differences in survival persist even after 15 years of follow-

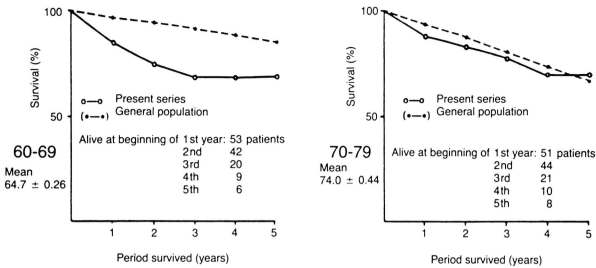

FIGURE 19–13. Survival after fixed-rate pacing in two different age groups in relation to the matched general Swedish population. (From Edhag O: Long-term cardiac pacing: Experience of fixed-rate pacing with an endocardial electrode in 260 patients. Acta Med Scand 502S:64, 1969.)

up and appear to be related to the considerably higher incidence of sudden death.[78] There is some debate about whether the presence of syncope is associated with a worse prognosis. In contrast, the prognosis for transient complete heart block is better, with a 36% 1-year mortality.[77] Edhag reported on a mean 6.5-year follow-up of 248 patients, the majority of whom had high-grade AV block.[79] The mean age at pacemaker implantation was 66, and the 1-year survival of paced patients was 86%, slightly lower than the 95% 1-year survival of an age- and sex-matched group of Swedish patients. After the first year, survival in the paced patients was similar to that in the general population. Edhag also compared survival among different age groups and found no difference in survival in elderly patients with heart block who underwent permanent pacing and the age- and sex-matched general population. In contrast, younger patients with heart block had an increased mortality even after pacing than sex- and age-matched individuals from the general population (Fig. 19–13).[79] It is likely that this higher mortality is a reflection of the underlying structural heart disease that is responsible for high-grade AV block.

Alpert and colleagues[80] compared the prognosis of 132 patients with high-grade AV block and VVI pacemakers with that of 48 patients with DDD pacemakers for high-grade AV block during a 1- to 5-year follow-up period. They showed that permanent dual-chamber pacing enhanced survival to a greater extent than permanent VVI pacing in a subgroup of patients with preexisting congestive heart failure.[80] The causes of congestive heart failure were variable; about 50% of patients had underlying ischemic heart disease, and the rest had hypertension, valvular heart disease, or idiopathic dilated cardiomyopathy. The majority of deaths in the patient group with VVI pacemakers were due to acute myocardial infarction or congestive heart failure. Linde-Edelstam and associates[81] performed a case-controlled study comparing consecutive patients who received VDD pacemakers with the first available VVI patients who fulfilled certain "predetermined characteristics." The two groups were similar with respect to other concomitant diseases and severity of congestive heart failure. They compared survival in 74 patients treated with VVI pacemakers with that in 74 patients with

VDD pacemakers over a mean follow-up period of 5.4 years. The overall survival was different between the two pacing modes and was similar to that of the age- and sex-matched general Swedish population. In a subgroup of patients with high-grade AV block and congestive heart failure, the survival rate was *lower* with VVI pacing compared to patients paced in the VDD mode (Fig. 19–14).[81] Survival was no different between patients paced in the VVI and VDD modes if congestive heart failure was absent. There are several potential explanations for the negative effects on survival of VVI pacing in this population. These include progression of heart failure due to elevated catecholamines with ventricular pacing, absence of chronotropic competence, and increased myocardial oxygen demand from ventricular pacing.

The natural history of asymptomatic patients with type II

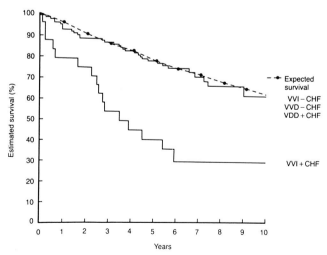

FIGURE 19–14. Expected survival rate for the general Swedish population and observed survival rates for patients with high-grade AV block and congestive heart failure (CHF) paced in fixed-rate ventricular (VVI) mode compared with (1) patients with high-grade AV block paced in atrial synchronous mode (VVD) with and without CHF and (2) patients without CHF paced in VVI mode. (From Linde-Edelstam C, Gullberg B, Nordlander R, et al: Longevity in patients with high-degree atrioventricular block paced in the atrial synchronous or fixed-rate ventricular inhibited mode. PACE 15:304, 1992.)

second-degree AV block has been addressed in only one study. In this study, from the University of Illinois, most patients were found to eventually develop symptoms within a relatively short period of time.[82] These observations form the basis for the current recommendations to institute permanent pacing in all patients with type II second-degree AV block. A more recent study showed that patients with type I second-degree AV block also did poorly if left unpaced. Shaw and colleagues[51] reported 214 patients with a mean age of 72 years who were followed over a 14-year time period. Their patient population consisted of patients with permanent AV block, who were divided into three groups: type I block (77 patients), type II block (86 patients), and 2:1 or 3:1 block (51 patients). The 3- and 5-year survival times were similarly poor regardless of the type of block. Patients who received permanent pacemakers had a survival similar to that for a control population.[51] Based on this study, elderly patients with type I AV block or 2:1 or 3:1 AV block with narrow QRS complexes should be followed closely because these electrocardiographic abnormalities may be a marker for progressive conduction system disease.

Pacing Mode Selection

The relative frequency with which single- and dual-chamber pacemakers are implanted in patients with complete or high-degree AV block varies within the United States as well as from country to country. In addition, the incidence of implantation of a dual-chamber pacemaker in patients with complete heart block varies with the age of the patient.

The rationale for implanting a dual-chamber pacemaker in patients with heart block has been heavily influenced by acute studies that show a hemodynamic benefit with AV synchrony in terms of higher cardiac output with lower right- and left-sided filling pressures (reviewed in detail in Chapters 23 and 25). Other factors include lower pulmonary pressures during dual-chamber pacing as well as lower levels of circulating catecholamines and atrial natriuretic factor (ANF). Several small randomized trials have compared DDD pacing to VVI pacing by programming different pacing modes in a single- or double-blind fashion in patients with implanted DDD pacemakers for a variable period of time. Some of these patients are reprogrammed for several days and some for as long as several months. These studies are reviewed in Chapter 24 and have consistently shown an improvement in cardiac and general symptoms during DDD pacing.

Several prospective long-term randomized studies are currently underway to determine whether pacemaker recipients achieve a better quality of life with dual-chamber pacemakers (DDDR pacing) than with single-chamber pacemakers (VVIR pacing). Studies are ongoing in Canada, Europe, and the United States. Other end-points being assessed include the incidence and severity of congestive heart failure, incidence of atrial fibrillation, incidence of stroke, cost effectiveness, and survival. Optimal pacemaker selection for the patient aged 65 years or older is being specifically studied in the PASE trial.[83] This is a prospective trial assessing a broad array of outcomes such as physical function, social function, and health perception in addition to standard clinical outcomes through measurement of quality of life with a rigorously tested questionnaire. This study differs from other blinded cross-over studies in that it will involve a large number of patients (400), who are studied prospectively over a 2-year time period. Clinical events will be measured and considered secondary end-points. These events include the incidence of atrial fibrillation, heart failure, stroke, death, and permanent reprogramming of the pacemaker to the DDDR mode due to pacemaker syndrome. A clinical event score and heart failure score also constitute additional secondary end-points.

Recently, the results of a prospective blinded trial comparing single- and dual-chamber pacing were reported in preliminary form. The Danish trial demonstrated that dual-chamber pacing was superior to single-chamber pacing for complete heart block and sick sinus syndrome. Patients with dual-chamber pacing had a lower incidence of atrial fibrillation than patients with single-chamber pacemakers. Data about mortality and incidence of cerebrovascular accidents are forthcoming.

VDDR Pacing

The development of a single lead with a series of electrodes for atrial sensing and ventricular pacing and sensing occurred over a decade ago to avoid the need for implanting two separate pacing leads. VDD or VAT pacing is an ideal mode of pacing for patients with complete heart block and normal sinus node function because it allows preservation of normal AV synchrony and rate responsiveness.[84, 85]

In the early 1970s, several groups studying different electrode configurations demonstrated clearly that a floating unipolar electrogram in the mid to high right atrium showed favorable characteristics for atrial sensing. In the 1980s, a bipolar configuration of atrial electrodes was developed to avoid sensing of myopotentials and electromagnetic interference as well as ventricular far-field signals. Various electrode configurations were studied including bipolar leads with narrow and wide spacing and orthogonal and diagonal atrial electrodes. The optimal spacing of two poles of the floating bipolar lead was found to range between 0.5 and 1 cm. In addition, atrial amplifiers capable of reliably detecting the atrial signal were developed. Factors influencing atrial electrogram detection include electrode spacing, distance from the atrial wall, orientation of electrodes relative to atrial tissue, and electrode size.

Patient selection and programming are *critical*. The ideal candidate for a single-lead VDD pacemaker is a patient with high-grade or complete AV block and normal sinus node function.[86, 87] Patients with retrograde VA conduction and sinus bradycardia may become symptomatic if their sinus rate frequently slows below the lower programmed rate leading to VVI pacing at the lower rate. This problem is avoided by obtaining a 24-hour Holter monitor recording and programming the lower rate to a rate below the slowest sinus rate. Single-lead AV pacing is also best avoided if the atrial chamber diameter of the right atrium is greater than 3 by 3 cm and if the left atrium is larger than 4 by 3 cm in the apical four-chamber view. Patients with paroxysmal supraventricular tachycardia should also probably not receive VDD pacemakers.

The implant procedure for a VDD system consists of fixing the ventricular tip to allow the atrial electrodes to lie as close as possible to the high-mid location of the midlateral atrial wall. An atrial signal should be measured at rest, during deep breathing, and during coughing as well as during arm and shoulder movements. The lowest acceptable atrial electrogram signal during any maneuver should be more than 0.5 mV during deep inspiration.[84, 85] In general, there is considerable variability between patients and within individuals from moment to moment with respect to atrial electrogram amplitude (Fig. 19–15).

Pacemaker programming should take into account atrial sensitivity as well as programming of the postventricular atrial refractory period (PVARP), AV delay, and lower rate. Some generators allow programming of the bandwidth of the atrial amplifier. This may be very helpful and allows one to attenuate interfering myopotentials as well as retrograde P waves in patients with ventricular ectopy.[88] VDDR generators with programmable atrial amplifier bandwidths allow the implanter to minimize the sensing of myopotentials and retrograde P waves, thus avoiding the need for programming long PVARPs. The PVARP should be programmed to contain retrograde P waves. The AV delay must take into account the delay in detecting atrial depolarization. The lower rate should be programmed to a value below the minimum sinus rate noted during the 24-hour Holter recording.

Clinical trials of different VDD pacing systems have shown overall good clinical performance. In one study, the mean maximum and minimum values of atrial electrogram characteristics within a whole respiratory cycle were 2.64 ± 1.05 mV and 1.65 ± 0.38 mV amplitude (maximum) and 0.31 ± 0.12 mV and 0.18 ± 0.09 mV (minimum).[85–88] Atrial oversensing during upper body isometric exercises involving the pectoral muscles was not a clinical problem. Adequate P-wave amplitude was ''easily'' obtained at the time of implantation and remained stable during follow-up. P-wave amplitude was unaffected by maneuvers that simulated daily activities such as coughing, hyperventilation, arm swinging, isometric exercises, and respiration. During a mean follow-up period of 36 months, 5 of 72 patients required conversion to the VVI mode owing to complete loss of sensing (2 patients) and to chronic atrial fibrillation (3 patients). Ninety-three percent of patients remain paced in the VDD mode. Holter monitoring confirmed AV synchrony in the majority of patients, with occasional patients showing intermittent loss of atrial sensing lasting from 4 to 5 beats to up to 3% of the monitored period. Similar results have been achieved with other systems. Ramsdale and Charles,[89] however, reported difficulty in obtaining an adequate P-wave amplitude at implantation, resulting in prolonged implantation times. In their series, almost 60% of patients showed failure of P-wave sensing. Marked fluctuations in the paced ventricular rate were noted especially during exercise, when intermittent failure to sense P waves occurred. Finally, in patients in whom sinus node dysfunction develops and a need for atrial pacing arises, upgrading to a DDDR pacing mode can be easily performed, as recently described.[90]

One of the major advantages of the VDDR pacing mode is the use of the sensor to differentiate sinus tachycardia from the tracking of myopotentials. The implanted sensor can be used to judge the appropriateness of the atrial rate. In addition, the rate-adaptive sensor allows for rate smoothing of upper rate behavior.

Enthusiasm for the VDD pacing mode has diminished as the size and experience in manipulating the new atrial leads have increased. The additional risk and work of positioning an atrial lead outweigh the disadvantage of not having atrial pacing. Studies with earlier models of atrial leads reported a high incidence of atrial lead dislodgment as well as deterioration of atrial pacing and sensing characteristics over time. With the newer designs of atrial lead, including steroid-eluting atrial leads, as well as the redesign of bandpass filters for sensing atrial activity, technical stability of the atrial lead has improved. In some series, atrial pacing and sensing are maintained in almost 90% of patients for 5 years.[91] The unpredictability in some patients of atrial chronotropic function over the long term has led some workers to favor implanting atrial leads in most individuals with complete heart block who are undergoing pacemaker implantation. Ventricular pacing can arise when the atrial rate is slower than the programmed lower rate or during exercise in a patient with chronotropic incompetence if the patient has a VDDR pacemaker and the sensor rate exceeds the P-wave rate.

Programming of the appropriate AV interval is discussed in Chapters 23 and 25. In brief, the optimal AV interval is one that provides the best timing of *left atrial* filling. There are many important factors to be considered, such as site of pacing, atrial size, ventricular function, intra-atrial and interatrial conduction times, and whether the atrial event is paced or sensed. The interatrial conduction time determines when the left atrial depolarization begins, and therefore directly determines the important left atrial–left ventricular timing interval. It is important to note that about 25% of patients undergoing DDD pacemaker implantation have high-degree intra-atrial and interatrial conduction delays.[92] Many authors have suggested that the programming of differential AV intervals for sensing and pacing may give rise to small but significant increases in cardiac output in patients with left ventricular dysfunction.[93, 94] Not only will optimal AV syn-

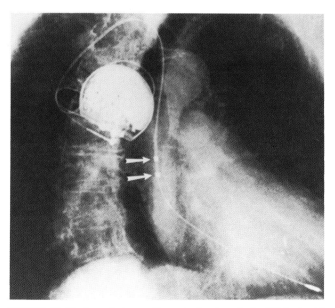

FIGURE 19–15. Lateral chest radiograph showing single AV lead with narrow-spaced AV ring electrodes connected to a LEM Biomedica/Cardiac Control Systems VDD pacemaker. The arrows denote atrial electrodes. (From Antonioli EG, Ansani L, Barbieri D, et al: Single-lead VDD pacing. *In* Barold SS, Mugica J [eds]: New Perspectives in Cardiac Pacing 3. Mt Kisco, NY, Futura Publishing Co., 1993, pp 359–381.)

chrony optimize cardiac output by increasing ventricular preload, thus lowering mean atrial pressure, it will also minimize AV valvular regurgitation. Optimal AV coupling intervals also depend on body position, catecholamine levels, interatrial conduction time, and left atrial electric-mechanical coupling times. Practically speaking, these facts lead to programming the paced AV interval and allowing the sensed AV interval to be of shorter duration.[95] The optimal AV interval varies from patient to patient, with shorter AV intervals possibly being more beneficial in patients with heart failure and valvular regurgitation and in those with hypertrophic cardiomyopathy.[96, 97] The optimal AV interval can vary considerably from patient to patient depending on many different factors and is difficult to predict a priori. The optimal AV interval can be determined by comparing the measured stroke volume at different AV intervals as measured by continuous wave cardiac Doppler, right heart catheterization, or, more recently, impedance cardiography.

Many pacemakers incorporate algorithms to mimic the effect of catecholamines to shorten the AV or PV interval during exercise. These issues become even more complex in patients with sinus node dysfunction who have intact or only mildly impaired AV conduction. In patients with sinus node dysfunction and only mild or no AV node conduction disease, the effect of the loss of ventricular synchrony during right ventricular apical pacing must also be considered. In patients with sick sinus syndrome, then, the optimal AV delay is not one that will guarantee maximal left atrial filling of the left ventricle but rather one that provides the best hemodynamic compromise between AV conduction time and a normal ventricular activation sequence. This is not an issue in patients with complete or intermittent AV block, in whom the ventricular activation sequence is not a factor and the only concern is optimizing the AV delay during rest and exercise. In a recent study using impedance cardiography to measure cardiac output at rest in patients with primarily AV block, the optimal AV delay at pacing rates of between 70 and 110 bpm was an average of less than 120 msec from the atrial stimulus to the ventricular stimulus. In this study, the cardiac output in the DDD pacing mode was similar to that in the VVI pacing mode when the AV delay was more than 200 msec. The mean difference in cardiac index comparing the best with the worst AV interval setting was $34 \pm 8\%$.

AV intervals may be shortened further during atrial tracking; when patients exercise and their heart rates increase, the sensed P wave to ventricular pacing stimulus can be shortened. This is termed rate-adaptive AV interval shortening or automatic rate-adaptive AV delay and is a programmable feature on several DDD pacemaker generators. This can be accomplished as one-step shortening or multistep shortening in discrete, nonprogrammable, or linear steps as the atrial rate increases. For example, in the Biotronik system, the sensed AV delay may be programmed to different values within a specified range of heart rates. In the Intermedics Cosmos II, the pacemaker adapts the AV delay after each sensed P wave to changes in the preceding sinus cycle length. For example, for a 20-msec shortening of the sinus cycle, the subsequent AV delay after a sensed P wave would be 2.5 msec. The minimum value below which the AV delay will not be shortened is calculated based on the programmed pacing rate, the upper ventricular rate limit, and is set to a minimum of 75 msec. The Siemens-Pacesetter models

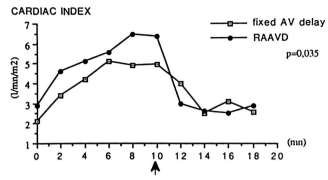

FIGURE 19–16. Comparison of an automatic rate-responsive AV delay (RAAVD) and a fixed but individually optimized (by Doppler echocardiography) AV delay in a patient with a chronically implanted DDD pacemaker for complete AV block. At each exercise level, and especially at peak exercise *(arrow)*, rate-responsive AV delay produced a significantly higher cardiac index (CI) compared with the fixed value. (From Daubert C, Ritter P, Mabo P, et al: AV delay optimization in DDD and DDDR pacing. *In* Barold SS, Mugica J [eds]: New Perspectives in Cardiac Pacing 3. Mt Kisco, NY, Futura Publishing Co., 1993, pp 259–287.)

shorten the PV interval by 25-msec steps within the limit of 75 msec less than the programmed AV delay. In the DDDR mode, the paced AV delay shortens as the pacing rate increases in response to the sensor. The Vitatron algorithm produces an exponential adaptation curve, whereas the ELA Chorus algorithm mimics physiology by adapting the sensed AV delay to the atrial rate on a beat-by-beat basis with linear shortening occurring between a maximal and a minimal value. The net result is a shortening of the total atrial refractory period, thereby allowing higher 1:1 tracking rates. The assumption behind the shortening of the PV or AV interval is that it maintains the proper timing of the atrial contraction and thereby optimizes stroke volume (Fig. 19–16). The shortened PV (or AV) intervals may result in a greater degree of ventricular pacing in patients with intermittent or catecholamine-sensitive AV conduction. If this results in fewer intrinsic beats and more ventricular pacing, there may be no improvement in hemodynamics, and potentially even a worsening of hemodynamics in certain patients.

In rare patients with high-grade interatrial conduction slowing in the presence of atrial disease and either sick sinus syndrome or heart block, optimal AV synchrony may not occur with typical AV delays of 125 to 175 msec. AV intervals of 250 to 350 msec may be required to provide effective atrial systole. This has the disadvantage of necessitating long total atrial refractory periods and limiting the upper rate possible for exercise. Second, interatrial synchrony remains widely separated, and atrial arrhythmias may be triggered by atrial pacing during the vulnerable period. Daubert and his colleagues solved this problem by using two atrial leads, one placed in the right atrium and one placed in the coronary sinus to pace and sense the left atrium.[85] This ''triple chamber'' pacemaker provides simultaneous contraction of both the right and left atria and optimizes cardiac performance with traditional values for the AV interval and PVARP. This concept has been referred to as ''permanent atrial resynchronization.''

In summary, it is likely that complete AV block will remain one of the major indications for cardiac pacing through the next decade. Most diagnoses can be made by careful analysis of the surface electrocardiogram, although electrophysiologic testing is a useful provocative tool, particularly in patients with unexplained syncope and bundle branch block. Ultimately, in the majority of cases the decision to pace a patient is based on a correlation of symptoms with an abnormal ECG (rhythm). The causes of complete heart block may change, with radiofrequency ablation of the AV junction–His bundle accounting for a larger fraction of patients with complete AV block. It is likely that DDD pacing with two separate leads will remain the major pacing modality for the majority of patients with heart block if ongoing studies demonstrate its superiority over single-chamber ventricular pacing. Mode switching will be incorporated increasingly into DDD pacemakers, and separate programming of AV intervals based on P-wave sensing or atrial pacing as well as the use of rate-adaptive AV delays will become routine.

REFERENCES

1. Becker AE, Anderson RH: Morphology of the human atrioventricular junctional area. *In* Wellens HJJ, Lie KI, Janse MJ (eds): The Conduction System of the Heart: Structure, Function, and Clinical Implications. Leiden, H.E. Stenfert Kroese BV, 1976, pp 263–286.
2. James TN: Anatomy of the Coronary Arteries. New York, Hoeber Medical Division, Harper & Row, 1961.
3. Meijler FL, Janse MJ: Morphology and electrophysiology of the mammalian atrioventricular node. Physiol Rev 68:608, 1988.
4. James TN: Cardiac innervation: Anatomic and pharmacologic relations. Bull NY Acad Sci 43:1041, 1967.
5. Frink JR, James TN: Normal blood supply to the human His bundle and proximal bundle branches. Circulation 47:8, 1973.
6. Massing GK, James TN: Anatomical configuration of the His bundle and bundle branches of the human heart. Circulation 53:609, 1976.
7. Josephson ME, Seides SF: Clinical Cardiac Electrophysiology. Philadelphia, Lea & Febiger, 1979, pp 79–101.
8. Puech P, Grolleau R, Guimond C: Incidence of different types of A-V block and their localization by His bundle recordings. *In* Wellens HJJ, Lie KI, Janse MJ (eds): The Conduction System of the Heart: Structure, Function, and Clinical Implications. Leiden, H.E. Stenfert Kroese BV, 1976, pp 467–484.
9. El-Sherif N, Scherlag BJ, Lazzara R, et al: The pathophysiology of tachycardia-dependent paroxysmal atrioventricular block after myocardial ischemia: Experimental and clinical observations. Circulation 50:515, 1974.
10. Rosenbaum MB, Elizari MV, Levi RJ, et al: Paroxysmal atrioventricular block related to hyperpolarization and spontaneous diastolic depolarization. Chest 63:678, 1973.
11. Lev M: The pathology of complete AV block. Prog Cardiovasc Dis 6:317, 1964.
12. Lenegre J: Etiology and pathology of bilateral bundle branch fibrosis in relation to complete heart block. Prog Cardiovasc Dis 6:409, 1964.
13. Narula OS: Atrioventricular conduction defects in patients with sinus bradycardia. Circulation 44:1096, 1971.
14. Evans R, Shaw DB: Pathological studies in sino-atrial disorder (sick sinus syndrome). Br Heart J 39:778, 1977.
15. Rosenqvist M, Obel IWP: Atrial pacing and the risk for AV block: Is there a time for change in attitude? PACE 12:97, 1989.
16. Sutton R, Kenny RA: The natural history of sick sinus syndrome. PACE 9:1110, 1986.
17. Caspi J, Amar R, Elami A, et al: Frequency and significance of complete atrioventricular block after coronary artery bypass grafting. Am J Cardiol 63:526, 1989.
18. Keefe DL, Griffin JC, Harrison DC, et al: Atrioventricular conduction abnormalities in patients undergoing isolated aortic or mitral valve replacement. PACE 8:393, 1985.
19. Rosenbaum MB, Corrado G, Oliveri R, et al: Right bundle branch block with left anterior hemiblock surgically induced tetralogy of Fallot. Am J Cardiol 26:12, 1970.
20. Van Lier TA, Harinck E, Hitchcock JF: Complete right bundle branch block after surgical closure of perimembranous ventricular septal defect. Eur Heart J 6:959, 1985.
21. Maron BJ, Merrill WH, Freier PA, et al: Long-term clinical course and symptomatic status of patients after operation for hypertrophic subaortic stenosis. Circulation 57:1205, 1978.
22. Ferguson TB Jr, Cox JL: Surgical treatment for the Wolff-Parkinson-White syndrome: The endocardial approach. *In* Zipes DP, Jaliffe J (eds): Cardiac Electrophysiology: From Cell to Bedside. Philadelphia, WB Saunders, 1990, pp 897–906.
23. Chu A, Califf RM, Pryor DB, et al: Prognostic effect of bundle branch block related to coronary artery bypass grafting. Am J Cardiol 59:798, 1987.
24. Baerman JM, Kirsh MM, de Buitleir M, et al: Natural history and determinants of conduction defects following coronary artery bypass surgery. Ann Thorac Surg 44:150, 1987.
25. Anderson DJ, Bulkley BH, Hutchins GM: A clinicopathologic study of prospective valve endocarditis in 22 patients: Morphologic basis for diagnosis and therapy. Am Heart J 94:325, 1977.
26. Maguire JH, Hoff R, Sherlock I, et al: Cardiac morbidity and mortality due to Chagas' disease: Prospective electrocardiographic study of a Brazilian community. Circulation 75:1140, 1987.
27. Steere AC: Lyme disease. N Engl J Med 321:586, 1989.
28. Steere AC, Batsford WP, Weinberg M, et al: Lyme carditis: Cardiac abnormalities of Lyme disease. Ann Intern Med 93(pt 1):8, 1980.
29. VanderLinde MR, Crijns HJGM, DeKoning J, et al: Range of atrioventricular conduction disturbances in Lyme borreliosis: A report of four cases and review of other published reports. Br Heart J 131:162, 1990.
30. McAlister HF, Klementowicz PT, Andrews C, et al: Lyme carditis: An important cause of reversible heart block. Ann Intern Med 110:339, 1989.
31. Kimball SA, Janson PA, LaRaia PJ: Complete heart block as the sole presentation of Lyme disease. Arch Intern Med 149:1897, 1989.
32. Cohen IS, Bharati S, Glass J, et al: Radiotherapy as a cause of complete atrioventricular block in Hodgkin's disease. Arch Intern Med 141:676, 1981.
33. Almange C, Lebrestec T, Louvet M, et al: Bloc auriculo-ventriculaire complet par métastase cardiaque: A propos d'une observation. Sem Hôp Paris 54:1419, 1978.
34. Perloff JK: The heart in neuromuscular disease. *In* O'Rourke RA (ed): Current Problems in Cardiology. Chicago, Yearbook, 1986, pp 513–557.
35. Wynne J, Braunwald E: The cardiomyopathies and myocarditides. *In* Braunwald E (ed): Heart Disease: A Textbook of Cardiovascular Medicine, 4th ed. Philadelphia, WB Saunders, 1992, pp 1349–1450.
36. Hurd ER: Extraarticular manifestations of rheumatoid arthritis. Semin Arthritis Rheum 8:151, 1979.
37. Owen DS: Connective tissue diseases and the cardiovascular system: A review. Virginia Med 110:426, 1983.
38. Janosik DL, Osborn TG, Moore TL, et al: Heart disease in systemic sclerosis. Semin Arthritis Rheum 19:191, 1989.
39. Rozanski JJ, Castellanos A, Sheps D, et al: Paroxysmal second-degree AV block induced by exercise. Heart Lung 9:887, 1980.
40. Donzeau JP, Dechandol AM, Bergeal A, et al: Blocs auriculo-ventriculaires survenant à l'effort: Considérations générales à propos de 14 cas. Coeur 15:513, 1985.
41. Woelfel AK, Simpson RJ, Gettes LS, et al: Exercise-induced distal atrioventricular block. J Am Coll Cardiol 2:578, 1983.
42. Petrac J, Gjuroić J, Vukosqvić D, et al: Clinical significance and natural history of exercise-induced atrioventricular block. *In* Belhassen B, Feldman S, Copperman Y (eds): Cardiac Pacing and Electrophysiology, Proceedings of the VIIIth World Symposium on Cardiac Pacing and Electrophysiology. Jerusalem, R & L Creative Communications, 1987, p 265.
43. Huycke EC, Card HG, Sobol SM, et al: Postexertional cardiac systole in a young man without organic heart disease. Ann Intern Med 106:844, 1987.
44. Strasberg B, Lam W, Swiryn S, et al: Symptomatic spontaneous paroxysmal AV nodal block due to localized hyperresponsiveness of the AV node to vagotonic reflexes. Am Heart J 103:795, 1982.
45. Zaman L, Moleiro F, Rozanski JJ, et al: Multiple electrophysiologic manifestations and clinical implications of vagally mediated AV block. Am Heart J 106:92, 1983.
46. Jonas EA, Kosowsky BD, Ramaswamy K: Complete His-Purkinje block produced by carotid massage. Circulation 50:192, 1974.
47. Hart G, Oldershaw PJ, Cull RE, et al: Syncope caused by cough-induced complete atrioventricular block. PACE 5:564, 1982.
48. Wik B, Hillestad L: Deglutition syncope. Br Med J 3:747, 1975.

49. Mymin D, Mathewson FAL, Tate RB, et al: The natural history of first-degree atrioventricular heart block. N Engl J Med 315:1183, 1986.
50. Strasberg B, Amat-Y-Leon F, Dhingra RC, et al: Natural history of second-degree atrioventricular nodal block. Circulation 63:1043, 1981.
51. Shaw DB, Kerwick CA, Veale D, et al: Survival in second-degree atrioventricular block. Br Heart J 53:587, 1985.
52. Dhingra RC, Palileo E, Strasberg B, et al: Significance of the HV interval in 517 patients with chronic bifascicular block. Circulation 64:1265, 1981.
53. McAnulty JH, Rahimtoola SH, Murphy E, et al: Natural history of "high risk" bundle branch block: Final report of a prospective study. N Engl J Med 307:137, 1982.
54. Scheinman MM, Peters RW, Morady F, et al: Electrophysiologic studies in patients with bundle branch block. PACE 6:1157, 1983.
55. Click RL, Gersh BJ, Sugrue DD, et al: Role of invasive electrophysiologic testing in patients with symptomatic bundle branch block. Am J Cardiol 59:817, 1987.
56. Morady F, Higgins J, Peters RW, et al: Electrophysiologic testing in bundle branch block and unexplained syncope. Am J Cardiol 54:587, 1984.
57. Linzer M, Prystowsky EN, Devine GW, et al: Predicting the outcomes of electrophysiologic studies of patients with unexplained syncope: Preliminary validation of a derived model. J Gen Intern Med 6:113, 1991.
58. Jackman WM, Wang X, Friday KJ, et al: Catheter ablation of atrioventricular junction with radiofrequency current in 17 patients: Comparison of standard and large-tip catheter electrodes. Circulation 83:1562, 1991.
59. Olgin JE, Scheinman MM: Comparison of high-energy direct current and radiofrequency catheter ablation of the atrioventricular junction. J Am Coll Cardiol 21:557, 1993.
60. Morady F, Calkins H, Langberg J, et al: A prospective randomized comparison of direct current and radiofrequency ablation of the atrioventricular junction. J Am Coll Cardiol 21:102, 1993.
61. Zipes DP: Second-degree atrioventricular block. Circulation 60:465, 1979.
62. Cabeen WR, Roberts NK, Child JS: Recognition of the Wenckebach phenomenon. West J Med 129:521, 1978.
63. Denes P, Levy L, Pick A, Rosen KM: The incidence of typical and atypical A-V Wenckebach periodicity. Am Heart J 89:26, 1975.
64. Ursell S, Habbab MA, El-Sherif N: Atrioventricular and intraventricular conduction disorders: Clinical aspects. In El-Sherif N, Samet P (eds): Cardiac Pacing and Electrophysiology, 3rd ed. Philadelphia, WB Saunders, 1991, pp 140–169.
65. Lange HW, Ameisen O, Mack R, et al: Prevalence and clinical correlates on non-Wenckebach narrow complete second-degree atrioventricular block detected by ambulatory ECG. Am Heart J 115:114, 1988.
66. Bauernfeind RA, Welch WJ, Brownstein SL: Distal atrioventricular conduction system function. Cardiol Clin 4:417, 1986.
67. Zipes DP, Gettes LS, Akhtar M, et al: Guidelines for clinical intracardiac electrophysiologic studies: A report of the American College of Cardiology/American Heart Association Task Force on Assessment of Diagnostic and Therapeutic Cardiovascular Procedures. J Am Coll Cardiol 14:1827, 1989.
68. Dhingra RC, Wyndham C, Bauernfeind R, et al: Significance of block distal to the His bundle induced by atrial pacing in patients with chronic bifascicular block. Circulation 60:1455, 1979.
69. Scheinman MM, Weiss AN, Shaffar A, et al: Electrophysiologic effects of procainamide in patients with interventricular conduction delay. Circulation 49:522, 1974.
70. Josephson ME: Clinical Cardiac Electrophysiology: Techniques and Interpretations, 2nd ed. Philadelphia, Lea & Febiger, 1992, pp 117–149.
71. Bergfeldt L, Rosenqvist M, Vallin H, et al: Disopyramide-induced second- and third-degree atrioventricular block in patients with bifascicular block: An acute stress test to predict atrioventricular block progression. Br Heart J 53:328, 1985.
72. Tonkin AM, Heddle WF, Tornos P: Intermittent atrioventricular block: Procainamide administration as a provocative test. Aust NZ J Med 8:594, 1978.
73. Fujimura O, Yee R, Klein GJ, et al: The diagnostic sensitivity of electrophysiologic testing in patients with syncope caused by transient bradycardia. N Engl J Med 321:1703, 1989.
74. Frye RL, Collins JJ, DeSanctis RW, et al: Guidelines for permanent cardiac pacemaker implantation, May 1984. A report of the Joint American College of Cardiology/American Heart Association Task Force on Assessment of Cardiovascular Procedures (Subcommittee on Pacemaker Implantation). Circulation 70:331A, 1984.
75. Dreifus LS, Fisch C, Griffin JC, et al: Guidelines for implantation of cardiac pacemakers and antiarrhythmia devices: A Report of the American College of Cardiology/American Heart Association Task Force on Assessment of Diagnostic and Therapeutic Cardiovascular Procedures (Subcommittee on Pacemaker Implantation). J Am Coll Cardiol 18:1, 1991.
76. Barold SS: ACC/AHA Guidelines for implantation of cardiac pacemakers: How accurate are the definitions of atrioventricular and intraventricular conduction blocks? PACE 16:1221, 1993.
77. Johansson BW: Complete heart block: A clinical hemodynamic and pharmacological study in patients with and without an artificial pacemaker. Acta Med Scand 180(Suppl 451):1, 1966.
78. Edhag O, Swahn A: Prognosis of patients with complete heart block or arrhythmic syncope who were not treated with artificial pacemakers. Acta Med Scand 200:457, 1976.
79. Edhag O: Long-term cardiac pacing: Experience of fixed-rate pacing with an endocardial electrode in 260 patients. Acta Med Scand 502(Suppl):64, 1969.
80. Alpert MA, Curtiss JJ, Sanfelippo JF, et al: Comparative survival after permanent ventricular and dual-chamber pacing for patients with chronic high-degree atrioventricular block with and without preexistent congestive heart failure. J Am Coll Cardiol 7:925, 1986.
81. Linde-Edelstam C, Gulberg B, Norlander R, et al: Longevity in patients with high-degree atrioventricular block paced in the atrial synchronous mode or the fixed-rate ventricular inhibited mode. PACE 15:304, 1992.
82. Dhingra RC, Denes P, Wu D, et al: The significance of second-degree atrioventricular block and bundle branch block: Observations regarding site and type of block. Circulation 49:638, 1974.
83. Lamas GA, Estes NM III, Schneller S, et al: Does dual-chamber or atrial pacing present atrial fibrillation? The need for a randomized controlled trial. PACE 15:1109, 1992.
84. Lau CP: Rate-Adaptive Cardiac Pacing: Simple and Dual Chamber. Mt Kisco, NY, Futura Publishing Co., 1993, pp 249–264.
85. Antonioli GE, Anscani L, Barbieri D, et al: Single-lead VDD pacing. In Barold SS, Mugica J (eds): New Perspectives in Cardiac Pacing 3. Mt Kisco, NY, Futura Publishing Co., 1993, pp 359–381.
86. Lau CP, Tai YT, Li JPS, et al: Initial clinical experience with a single pass VDDR pacing system. PACE 15(pt II):1894, 1992.
87. Antonioli GE, Ansani L, Barbieri D, et al: Italian multicenter study on a single-lead VDD pacing system using a narrow atrial dipole spacing. PACE 15(pt II):1890, 1992.
88. Sermasi S, Marconi M: VDD simple pass lead pacing: Sustained pacemaker-mediated tachycardias unrelated to retrograde atrial activation. PACE 15(pt II):1902, 1992.
89. Ramsdale DR, Charles RG: Rate-responsive ventricular pacing: Clinical experience with the RS4-SRT pacing system. PACE 8:378, 1985.
90. Nakata Y, Ogura S, Tokano T, et al: VDD pacing with a previously implanted single-lead system. PACE 15(pt I):1425, 1992.
91. Gross JN, Moser S, Benedek ZM, et al: DDD pacing mode survival in patients with a dual-chamber pacemaker. J Am Coll Cardiol 19:1536, 1992.
92. Wish M, Fletcher RD, Gottdiener JS, et al: Importance of left atrial timing in the programming of dual-chamber pacemakers. Am J Cardiol 60:566, 1987.
93. Daubert C, Ritter P, Mabo P, et al: AV delay optimization in DDD and DDDR pacing. In Barold SS, Mugica J (eds): New Perspectives in Cardiac Pacing 3. Mt Kisco, NY, Futura Publishing Co., 1993, pp 259–287.
94. Haskell RJ, French WJ: Physiological importance of different atrioventricular intervals to improved exercise performance in patients with dual-chamber pacemakers. B Heart J 61:46, 1989.
95. Ovsycher I, Zimlicheman R, Katz A, et al: Measurement of cardiac output by impedance cardiography in pacemaker patients at rest: Effects of various atrioventricular delays. J Am Coll Cardiol 21:761, 1993.
96. Hochleitner M, Hortnagl H, Choi-Keung N, et al: Usefulness of physiologic dual-chamber pacing in drug-resistant idiopathic dilated cardiomyopathy. Am J Cardiol 66:198, 1990.
97. Fananapazir L, Cannon RO III, Tripodi D, et al: Impact of dual-chamber permanent pacing in patients with obstructive hypertrophic cardiomyopathy with symptoms refractory to verapamil and β-adrenergic blocker therapy. Circulation 85:2149, 1992.

CHAPTER 20

Av NODE–HIS-PURKINJE SYSTEM DISEASE: AV BLOCK (ACUTE)

Maria de Guzman
David T. Kawanishi
Shahbudin H. Rahimtoola

Anatomy and Pathophysiology

The sinus node lies near the junction of the superior vena cava and the right atrium. It is supplied by the sinus nodal artery, which originates from the proximal few centimeters of the right coronary artery (RCA) in about 55% of patients and from the proximal few centimeters of the left circumflex artery (LCX) in the remainder (Fig. 20–1).[1–4]

The atrioventricular (AV) node lies directly above the insertion of the septal leaflet of the tricuspid valve just beneath the right atrial endocardium.[2–4] Van der Hauwaert and associates[5] showed that only the proximal two-thirds of the AV node is supplied by the AV nodal artery; the distal segment of the AV node has a dual blood supply in 80% of human hearts from the same AV nodal artery and the left anterior descending (LAD) artery. In 90% of patients the AV nodal artery originates from the RCA. During acute myocardial infarction (AMI), conduction disturbances in the AV node are usually the consequence of an occlusion proximal to the origin of the AV nodal artery. This arrhythmia is, therefore, usually associated with inferior myocardial infarction. The AV nodal tissue merges with the His bundle, which runs through the inferior portion of the membranous interventricular septum and then, in most instances, continues along the left side of the crest of the muscular interventricular septum. The His bundle usually receives a dual blood supply from both the AV nodal artery and branches of the LAD.[6]

The right bundle branch originates from the His bundle. It is a narrow structure that crosses to the right side of the interventricular septum and extends along the right ventricular endocardial surface to the region of the anterolateral papillary muscle of the right ventricle, where it divides to supply the papillary muscle, the parietal surface of the right ventricle, and the lower part of the right ventricular surface.[7] The proximal portion of the right bundle branch is supplied by branches from the AV nodal artery or the LAD artery, whereas the more distal portion is supplied mainly by branches of the LAD artery.

The left bundle branch is anatomically much less discrete than the right bundle branch. It may divide immediately as it originates from the bundle of His or continue for 1 to 2 cm before doing so.[4, 7] It is clinically useful to consider the left bundle as dividing into an anterior branch or fascicle and a larger and broader posterior branch or fascicle, both of which radiate toward the anterior and posterior papillary muscles of the left ventricle, respectively, even though there are many subendocardial interconnections that resemble a syncytium rather than two discrete fascicles.[8] The left bundle branch and its anterior fascicle have a blood supply similar to that of the proximal portion of the right bundle branch; the left posterior fascicle is supplied by branches of the AV nodal artery, the posterior descending artery, and the circumflex coronary artery.

Clinicopathologic studies indicate that there is a relationship between the location of the infarct and the involvement of the conduction system.[9] In most patients who develop atrioventricular (AV) block in AMI there is usually no major structural damage of the conduction system; pathologic studies have shown that significant histologic degenerative changes in the conduction system are absent in the majority of cases.[10, 11] Several mechanisms have been proposed for AV block in the presence of inferior AMI. These include

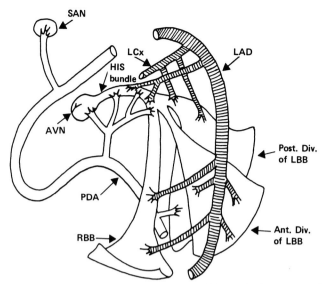

FIGURE 20–1. A diagrammatic representation of the conduction system and its blood supply. SAN, sinoatrial node; AVN, atrioventricular node, LAD, left anterior descending artery; LCX, left circumflex artery; PDA, posterior descending artery; RBB, right bundle branch; LBB, left bundle branch. (From de Guzman M, Rahimtoola SH: What is the role of pacemakers in patients with coronary artery disease and conduction abnormalities? *In* Rahimtoola SH [ed]: Controversies in Coronary Artery Disease. Philadelphia, FA Davis, 1983.)

Bezold-Jarisch reflex, reversible ischemia or injury of the conduction system, and local AV nodal hyperkalemia.

BEZOLD-JARISCH REFLEX. Stimulation of this reflex causes an abnormally increased output of vagal nerve traffic; it is initiated by ischemia of the afferent nerves in the area of the inferoposterior left ventricle. Some studies, however, show that reperfusion of the RCA with thrombolytic agents is a strong stimulus for the Bezold-Jarisch reflex.[12, 13] Despite this, the TIMI II study[14] did not show an increase in AV block in patients with inferior AMI who received thrombolytic therapy and had a patent infarct-related artery.

REVERSIBLE ISCHEMIA OR INJURY OF THE CONDUCTION SYSTEM. In inferior or posterior AMI, obstruction of the RCA produces reversible ischemia of the AV node. In patients who develop AV block, pathologic studies have demonstrated little or no necrosis in the conduction system.[10] Bilbao and colleagues,[15] however, identified a subgroup of patients with fatal inferior or posterior AMI and AV block who had necrosis of the prenodal atrial myocardial fibers. These necrotic fibers were absent in those without AV block. Clinically, the transient nature of the AV block supports the concept that the injury to the AV node is reversible.[16] The anatomic data of Bassan and associates[17] support the concept that the blood supply of the AV node is dual. In their prospective study, 11 of 51 patients who survived an inferior AMI developed some degree of transient AV block, and approximately 90% of the patients with AV block had simultaneous obstruction of the RCA (or LCA when it was dominant) and the proximal segment of the LAD artery. Moreover, patients with inferior AMI and LAD obstruction had a sixfold higher risk of developing AV block compared to those without LAD obstruction. The TIMI II data do *not* support this finding; in these patients with inferior AMI and AV block the incidence of disease of the LAD was low and was similar to that in patients with inferior AMI without AV block.[14] The TAMI study group also showed no increased incidence of LAD disease in patients with inferior AMI and complete AV block.[18]

LOCAL AV NODAL HYPERKALEMIA. An increased level of potassium was found experimentally in the lymph draining from the infarcted inferior and posterior cardiac wall of dogs after RCA occlusion.[19] Sugiura and colleagues[20] found that serum potassium was an independent predictor of the occurrence of fascicular blocks in anteroseptal AMI.

Anterior or anteroseptal AMI results from obstruction of the LAD artery. Occurrence of AV block and bundle branch block (BBB) is usually the result of necrosis of the septum and the conduction system below the AV node.[10, 21, 22] However, Wilber and colleagues[23] reported on two patients with anterior AMI and complete AV block in whom 1:1 conduction returned within minutes following late reperfusion (over 40 hours) with angioplasty. His experience suggests that reversible ischemia rather than necrosis of the conduction system occurs in some patients. Some experimental studies in dogs[24–26] with anterior AMI suggest that extensive but reversible ischemia of the infranodal conduction tissue occurs, as evidenced by recovery from complete AV block. Several clinical observations[24–28] also show that the majority of patients with anterior AMI and high-grade AV block who are discharged from the hospital return to 1:1 conduction.

Acute Myocardial Infarction

ATRIOVENTRICULAR BLOCK WITHOUT BUNDLE BRANCH BLOCK

INCIDENCE

Atrioventricular block occurs in 12% to 25% of all patients with AMI; first-degree AV block occurs in 2% to 12%, second-degree block in 3% to 10%, and third-degree block in 3% to 7%.[16, 29, 30] The onset of AV block usually occurs 2 to 3 days after the infarction but has a range of a few hours to 10 days. Its mean duration is usually 2 to 3 days and ranges from ½ hour to 16 days. In our series of 684 consecutive patients with AMI admitted to the Los Angeles County–University of Southern California Medical Center (LAC–USCMC) Coronary Care Unit (CCU) from October 1966 to July 1970, 110 developed AV block (16%);[31] 79 of 110 patients (72%) with AV block did not have BBB. The total number of patients who had first-, second-, or third-degree AV block at some time was 6%, 7%, and 4%, respectively (Table 20–1).

SITE OF INFARCTION

Of our 79 patients, 60 (76%) had an inferior infarction, 14 (18%) an anterior infarction, and 5 (6%) a combined infarction. AV block is frequently associated with inferior infarction, and in those who develop second- and third-degree block, inferior AMI is present two to four times as often as anterior AMI. The site of block in inferior infarction is above the His bundle in about 90% of patients, whereas in anterior infarction the conduction abnormality is usually localized below the His bundle in the distal conducting system[32] (Table 20–2).

TABLE 20–1. ATRIOVENTRICULAR BLOCK IN ACUTE MYOCARDIAL INFARCTION WITHOUT BUNDLE BRANCH BLOCK[a]

Incidence	(79/684 patients)	12%
First-degree AV block	(44/684 patients)	6%
Second-degree AV block	(50/684 patients)	7%
Third-degree AV block	(29/684 patients)	4%
Site of infarction		
Inferior		79%
Anterior		18%
Combined		6%
Progression		
First-degree AV block to second- or third-degree AV block		59%
Second-degree AV block to third-degree AV block		36%
Outcome		
Hospital mortality		29%
Return to 1:1 conduction in survivors		95%

[a]Data from 684 consecutive AMI patients at LAC–USCMC, Los Angeles, CA.

Adapted from de Guzman M, Rahimtoola SH: What is the role of pacemakers in patients with coronary artery disease and conduction abnormalities? *In* Rahimtoola SH (ed): Controversies in Coronary Artery Disease. Philadelphia, FA Davis, 1983, pp 191–207.

PROGRESSION OF ATRIOVENTRICULAR BLOCK

In patients with inferior AMI, progression of AV block commonly occurs in stages, whereas in those with anterior AMI it may occur in stages or third-degree AV block or ventricular asystole may develop suddenly[16] (Fig. 20–2).

Progression of AV block in the LAC–USCMC study was as follows:

INITIAL NORMAL PR INTERVAL. Of the 42 patients with AV block and no BBB who initially had a normal PR interval, 20 (48%) developed first-degree AV block. Five of the 20 (25%) stayed in first-degree AV block, eight (40%) progressed to second-degree block only, six (30%) developed second-degree block that progressed to third-degree block, and one (5%) developed third-degree block without second-degree block. Nineteen patients developed second-degree AV block without initially having first-degree block; 6 of the 19 (32%) developed third-degree AV block. Three developed sudden third-degree AV block without preceding first- or second-degree block; all three had anterior AMI.

FIRST-DEGREE AV BLOCK. Of the total 44 patients who had first-degree AV block and no BBB, 26 (59%) progressed to a higher grade of block. Twenty-four were admitted in first-degree AV block; 13 (54%) stayed in first-degree block,

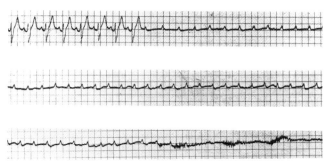

FIGURE 20–2. Lead II. Sudden ventricular asystole in a patient with AMI complicated by right bundle branch block and LAD. (From de Guzman M, Rahimtoola SH: What is the role of pacemakers in patients with coronary artery disease and conduction abnormalities? *In* Rahimtoola SH [ed]: Controversies in Coronary Artery Disease. Philadelphia, FA Davis, 1983.)

eight (33%) progressed to second-degree block, and three (13%) progressed to second-degree and then to third-degree AV block.

SECOND-DEGREE AV BLOCK. Of the total 50 patients who had second-degree AV block and no BBB, 18 (36%) progressed to third-degree AV block. Six had second-degree AV block without BBB on admission, and three went on to third-degree AV block.

THIRD-DEGREE AV BLOCK. Of the total 29 patients with third-degree AV block and no BBB, seven (24%) were admitted in third-degree block. Of the 22 who progressed to third-degree block, 18 (82%) had demonstrated second-degree AV block.

OUTCOME

Atrioventricular block complicating AMI is associated with a high mortality (24–48%), 2 to 3 times that of patients without AV block (9–16%). The major cause of death is pump failure.[30, 33] However, Tans and coworkers[30] reported that in their patients with inferior AMI, even those with high-degree AV block and no severe pump failure had a higher mortality (17%) than those without high-degree AV block (9%). In our series, the hospital mortality was 29% (32 of 110 patients); 29 of the 32 deaths (91%) were due to pump failure. Survival, therefore, is greatly influenced by the severity of the hemodynamic disturbance and is partly independent of the degree of heart block. Currently, use of AV sequential pacing may be expected to have some beneficial effect on the hemodynamic disturbance and therefore on the short-term mortality. Although death is primarily related to extensive myocardial damage, in an important minority of

TABLE 20–2. ATRIOVENTRICULAR BLOCK IN INFERIOR-POSTERIOR AND ANTERIOR ACUTE MYOCARDIAL INFARCTION

	ANTERIOR	INFERIOR-POSTERIOR
Pathophysiology	Extensive necrosis of septum	Reversible ischemia, injury of conduction system
Site of block	Infranodal	Intranodal
Frequency	Less frequent	Two to four times more frequent
Progression to complete AV block	Sudden	Gradual
Intraventricular conduction defect	Common	Rare
Escape focus	Ventricular	Junctional
Escape rate	20–40 per minute	40–60 per minute
Prognosis	High mortality	Lower mortality

patients it can be attributed to sudden ventricular asystole or severe bradycardia. In these cases, control of the cardiac rhythm by drugs or pacing may be life saving.

ATRIOVENTRICULAR BLOCK WITH BUNDLE BRANCH BLOCK

INCIDENCE

Bundle branch block is present during hospitalization in 8% to 15% of patients with AMI.[34–39] Of 2779 patients with AMI admitted to our CCU from October 1966 to March 1977, 257 (9%) had BBB. Of the 257 patients, 83 (32%) had left bundle branch block (LBBB), 80 (31%) had right bundle branch block (RBBB), 72 (28%) had RBBB plus left axis deviation, 21 (9%) had RBBB plus right axis deviation, and one had alternating (alt) BBB. The conduction abnormality was "new" in 60%—that is, the BBB developed during the infarction and was documented by serial electrocardiograms (ECGs) (definitely new) or was present on admission and was not seen on previous ECGs or reverted to normal conduction later as documented by serial ECGs (probably new). Of the 257 BBB patients, 75 (29%) had AV block (Table 20–3).

SITE OF INFARCTION

When the site of infarction was not obscured by the BBB, the block was associated with anterior AMI about 3 times as often as it was with inferior AMI. In the presence of persistent LBBB, the diagnosis of myocardial infarction is difficult and was usually made by the history and serial changes in the cardiac enzymes.

PROGRESSION OF ATRIOVENTRICULAR BLOCK

Progression of AV block occurred in 75 of our 257 patients (29%) with AMI and BBB.

INITIALLY NORMAL PR INTERVAL. Of the 28 patients with AV block and BBB who initially had a normal PR interval, 13 (46%) developed first-degree AV block. Nine of the 13 (69%) stayed in first-degree block, 2 (15%) progressed to second-degree block type II only, 1 (8%) had type II second-degree block that progressed to third-degree AV block, and 1 developed third-degree block without having second-degree block. Six patients had type II second-degree block without initially having first-degree AV block; four of the six (67%) developed third-degree AV block. One patient had type I second-degree block that progressed to third-degree block. Eight had sudden third-degree block without preceding first- or second-degree AV block; in six the infarction was anterior, and in two the site of infarction could not be determined.

FIRST-DEGREE AV BLOCK. Of the total 41 patients who had first-degree AV block and BBB, 13 (32%) progressed to high-grade block. Twenty-eight (68%) were admitted in first-degree AV block. Sixteen of the 28 (57%) stayed in first-degree block; three (11%) progressed to type II second-degree AV block, one of whom went on to third-degree block; five (18%) progressed to type I second-degree block, two of whom went on to third-degree block; and four (14%) patients developed third-degree block without preceding second-degree AV block.

TABLE 20–3. BUNDLE BRANCH BLOCK IN ACUTE MYOCARDIAL INFARCTION

Incidence	(257/2779 patients[a])	9%
LBBB	(83/257 patients)	32%
RBBB	(80/257 patients)	31%
RBBB + LAD	(72/257 patients)	28%
RBBB + RAD	(21/257 patients)	9%
Onset of BBB		
New		60%
Old		40%
Site of infarction		
Inferior		21%
Anterior		52%
Combined		4%
Indeterminate		18%
Nontransmural		5%
Incidence of AV block	(75/257 patients)	29%
First-degree	(25/257 patients)	10%
Second-degree	(13/257 patients)	5%
Third-degree	(37/257 patients)	14%
Progression of AV block		
First-degree AV block to second- or third-degree AV block		32%
Second-degree AV block to third-degree AV block		46%
Progression of high-grade AV block	(46/257 patients)	18%
Bilateral BBB + first-degree AV block		50%
New *bilateral* BBB + first-degree AV block		43%
First-degree AV block		30%
New BBB + first-degree AV block		29%
Bilateral BBB		18%
New BBB		16%
New bilateral BBB		15%
Outcome		
Hospital mortality		20%
Return to 1:1 conduction in survivors		89%

[a]Data from 2779 AMI patients seen from October 1966 to March 1977 at LAC–USCMC, Los Angeles, CA.
Adapted from de Guzman M, Rahimtoola SH: What is the role of pacemakers in patients with coronary artery disease and conduction abnormalities? *In* Rahimtoola SH (ed): Controversies in Coronary Artery Disease. Philadelphia, FA Davis, 1983, pp 191–207.

SECOND-DEGREE AV BLOCK. Of the total 24 patients who had second-degree AV block and BBB, 11 (46%) progressed to third-degree block. Six had second-degree AV block on admission; of these, type II block occurred in four, one of whom progressed to third-degree block, and type I occurred in two, one of whom progressed to third-degree block.

THIRD-DEGREE AV BLOCK. There were 37 patients with third-degree AV block and BBB, 13 (35%) of whom were admitted in third-degree block. Of the 24 who progressed to third-degree block, 11 (46%) had demonstrated second-degree block; 7 of the 11 had type II second-degree block.

PROGRESSION TO HIGH-GRADE AV BLOCK. Atrioventricular block occurs in about one third of patients with AMI and BBB.[40–43] Two large studies have developed a data bank on patients with BBB in association with myocardial infarction. One is a large collaborative multicenter study involving five centers,[28] and the other is a study conducted by our own medical center.[44] Both studies have limitations because the data were obtained retrospectively, and no protocols existed to guide decisions pertaining to pacemaker insertion, which was performed at the physician's discretion in all cases. Furthermore, the number of patients admitted to the hospital but not included in the study was not evaluated. Thus, the studies are unable to answer conclusively and definitively questions about the natural history of BBB in association with AMI. Nevertheless, very valuable clinical information is available from both.

In the *multicenter study*, reported by Hindman and co-workers,[28] high-grade AV block (second- or third-degree block with a type II pattern) occurred in 55 of 432 patients (22%). To determine which patients were at considerable risk of developing high-degree AV block while hospitalized with AMI, several variables were analyzed. Combinations of three ECG findings of first-degree AV block, bilateral BBB (if both bundle branches were involved, e.g., RBBB plus left or right axis deviation, or alternating RBBB and LBBB), and "new" BBB identified high-risk patients. The absence of all variables or the presence of only one of the three defined variables was associated with a relatively low risk (10–13%) of developing high-grade AV block during hospitalization. The risk was moderate for patients with first-degree AV block with either new BBB or bilateral BBB (19–20%), and highest (31–38%) for new bilateral BBB regardless of the PR interval (Fig. 20–3).

In the *LAC–USCMC study*,[44] high-grade AV block occurred in 46 of 257 patients (18%). The absence of the three variables or the presence of either bilateral BBB or new BBB or new bilateral BBB was associated with a relatively low risk (10–18%) of developing high-grade AV block during hospitalization with AMI. The risk was moderate for first-degree AV block with or without new BBB (29–30%) and highest (50%) for bilateral BBB plus first-degree AV block regardless of whether the BBB was old or new (Fig. 20–4).

Despite some differences in the findings between the two studies, *both studies* found that the following subgroups of patients were at high risk for high-grade AV block: (1) new

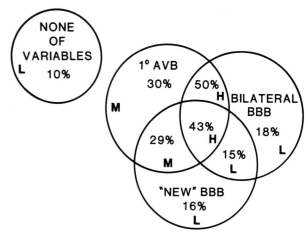

FIGURE 20–4. Venn diagram of 257 patients in the LAC-USCMC study depicting the risk of developing high-grade atrioventricular block (AVB) in patients with AMI and bundle branch block (BBB). (Reproduced with permission from de Guzman M, Rahimtoola SH: What is the role of pacemakers in patients with coronary artery disease and conduction abnormalities? *In* Rahimtoola SH [ed]: Controversies in Coronary Artery Disease. Philadelphia, FA Davis, 1983.)

bilateral BBB plus first-degree AV block (*risks*, 38% and 43% in the multicenter and LAC–USCMC studies, respectively); (2) bilateral BBB plus first-degree AV block (*risks*, 20% and 50%); and (3) new BBB plus first-degree AV block (*risks*, 19% and 29%). Thus, these subgroups of patients should be considered mandatory recipients of temporary prophylactic pacemakers during AMI. Subgroups in whom the findings of the two studies show different risks can be considered to be at moderate risk for high-grade AV block. These subgroups include patients with: (1) new bilateral BBB (*risks*, 31% and 15%) (Fig. 20–5); (2) first-degree AV block (*risks*, 13% and 30%); and (3) bilateral BBB (*risks*, 10% and 18%). Thus, these subgroups of patients can be considered as probable or possible recipients of temporary prophylactic pacemakers during AMI. The rest of the patients can be considered to have a relatively low risk (about 10%) of high-grade AV block and therefore should probably not require prophylactic temporary pacemakers during AMI. The actual clinical decision about whether to institute temporary pacing should be individualized depending on the patient-related risk factors and on the available personnel and equipment at each institution.

The data base assembled by the Multicenter Investigation of the Limitation of Infarct Size (MILIS) was used to develop a simplified method of predicting the occurrence of complete heart block. Data from 698 patients with a proven myocardial infarction were analyzed, and the presence or absence of ECG abnormalities of AV or intraventricular conduction was determined for each patient. The risk factors for the development of complete heart block were: first-degree AV block, Mobitz type I AV block, Mobitz type II AV block, left anterior hemiblock, left posterior hemiblock, RBBB, and LBBB. A risk score for the development of complete heart block was devised that consisted of the sum of each patient's individual risk factors. An incidence of complete heart block of 1.2%, 7.8%, 25%, and 36% was associated with a risk score of 0, 1, 2, or 3 or more, respectively (Fig. 20–6). The risk score was subsequently tested on the published results

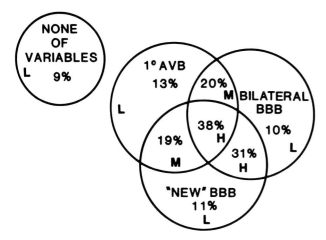

FIGURE 20–3. Venn diagram of 432 patients in the multicenter study depicting the risk of developing high-grade atrioventricular block (AVB) in patients with acute myocardial infarction (AMI) and bundle branch block (BBB). (Reproduced with permission from Hindman MC, Wagner GS, JaRo M, et al: The clinical significance of bundle branch block complicating acute myocardial infarction: 2. Indications for temporary and permanent pacemakers. Circulation 58:689, 1978. Copyright 1978, American Heart Association.)

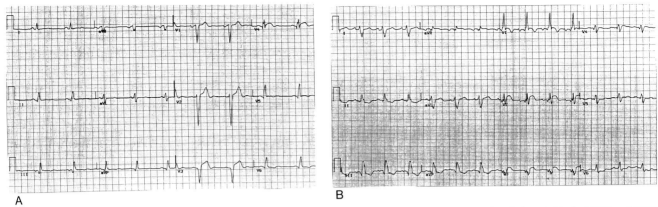

FIGURE 20–5. *A* and *B*, Electrocardiograms of a patient with anterior AMI and development of ''new'' bilateral bundle branch block (LBBB and RBBB with right axis deviation). This patient had sudden ventricular asystole.

of six studies for a combined total of 2151 patients.[45] The limitations of this scoring system include the lack of differentiation between newly appearing or old bundle branch block, a factor that has been shown to be of predictive value. It is likely that consideration of such factors would further improve the accuracy of the scoring system, but it would also add to its complexity. Another criticism of the scoring system is that it would assign a risk score of only 1 to a patient with isolated Mobitz type II AV block, a disorder usually believed to be highly predictive of progression to complete heart block. Isolated Mobitz type II AV block is however, relatively rare.

OUTCOME

Mortality in patients with AMI and BBB is higher (25–50%) than in those without BBB (15%).[30, 34–37, 41–43, 46] When the infarction is extensive and produces diffuse conduction system abnormalities progressing to high-grade AV block, it is also extensive enough to damage a large amount of myocardial muscle. Therefore, these patients often die from pump failure and from ventricular tachyarrhythmias. Nevertheless,

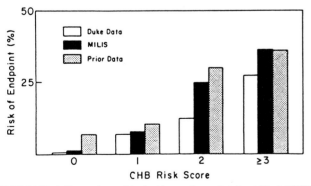

FIGURE 20–6. Comparison of the incidence of complete heart block (CHB) predicted by the CHB risk score method *(solid bars)*, the observed incidence of CHB in the Duke University myocardial infarction data base *(open bars)*, and the observed incidence of CHB or CHB and Mobitz II in six reported studies *(screened bars)*. MILIS, Multicenter Investigation of the Limitation of Infarct Size. (From Lamas GA, Muller JE, Turi AG, et al: A simplified method to predict occurrence of complete heart block during acute myocardial infarction. Am J Cardiol 57:1213, 1986.)

the conduction abnormality can be contributory and can be the major cause of death. For example, sudden third-degree AV block or asystole may be abrupt and fatal (see Fig. 20–2). It is interesting that in our study, 75% of patients with BBB and AMI had either no heart failure or, at worst, mild heart failure. Our results as well as those of the multicenter study showed that high-degree AV block influenced hospital mortality independently of pump failure.

Intracardiac electrophysiologic studies have also been evaluated as a means of predicting which patients with myocardial infarction and BBB are likely to die. Harper and associates[47] reported on 72 patients with AMI complicated by AV block or BBB, or both, who underwent His bundle recording or electrophysiologic (HBE) studies during their CCU stay. Thirty of 32 patients (94%) with AV block and narrow QRS complexes had a proximal block. Hospital mortality was low (13%), and HBE studies provided no additional information that was not obtained from the surface ECG. Of 18 patients with BBB and a normal PR interval, nine had distal block, but there were no hospital deaths in this group of patients. Of 22 patients with BBB and AV block, 5 had proximal block, 14 distal, and 3 proximal and distal blocks. Hospital mortality in these patients, who progressed to second- or third-degree AV block, was higher (9 of 12 patients, 75%) than in those who remained in first-degree AV block (2 of 10 patients, 20%). Lichstein and colleagues[48] and Lie and associates[27] also concluded that patients with BBB and AMI who had a distal block by HBE had increased hospital mortality (73% and 81%, respectively) compared with those with normal HV (or HQ) intervals (25% and 47%, respectively). Gould and coworkers,[49] on the other hand, showed that the presence or absence of a prolonged HV interval did not affect mortality.

BUNDLE BRANCH BLOCK AFTER RECOVERY FROM ACUTE MYOCARDIAL INFARCTION

It is now recognized that one major problem of patients who survive an AMI and are discharged from the hospital is late sudden death. It is also recognized that the majority of sudden deaths are likely to result from ventricular tachyarrhythmias. An important question is whether patients with coronary artery disease and persistent BBB plus transient AV block during the acute infarction have a higher risk of dying suddenly as a result of complete heart block. If so, to maximize the therapeutic benefit of permanently implanting a pacemaker in this subset of patients, those at highest risk of late sudden death resulting from AV block should be identified.

The multicenter study[28] supports the previous reports of Atkins and Ritter and their colleagues,[50, 51] who found that the subset of patients with chronic BBB and transient high-degree AV block during AMI are at increased risk of late sudden death, presumably from a bradyarrhythmia. Their data were included in the data compiled by the multicenter study. These data showed that patients who were not paced continuously had a higher incidence of sudden death or recurrent high-degree AV block during follow-up (65%) compared with those who were paced continuously (10%). These investigators suggested that implantation of a permanent pacemaker protected against sudden death in these patients. Waugh and coworkers[52] also recommended the possible role of permanent pacemaker therapy in preventing syncope or sudden death in another group of high-risk patients, those with bilateral BBB plus transient high-grade AV block (type II progression).

Other studies suggest that these patients are not at high risk of sudden death from a bradyarrhythmia.[26, 43, 47, 53, 54] In the study by Nimetz and associates[43] of 13 survivors with BBB and second- or third-degree AV block, 4 (31%) had late sudden death; 14 of 41 survivors without AV block (34%) had late sudden death. In a study by Ginks and coworkers[26] of patients with anterior myocardial infarction complicated by complete heart block with return to normal sinus rhythm but with persistent BBB, 4 of 14 hospital survivors (29%) with anterior myocardial infarction, persistent BBB, and transient AV block died, and two of four (50%) with permanent pacemakers died during a follow-up period averaging 49 months. They concluded that long-term pacing was not justified in these patients. In a study by Murphy and associates[53] of patients surviving AMI complicated by BBB, none of the deaths resulted from heart block, even in those with transient AV block during the AMI. Lie and coworkers[54] reported on a group of 47 patients who had survived an anterior infarction complicated by BBB and who were kept for 6 weeks in the monitoring area; 17 of the 47 patients (36%) sustained late hospital ventricular fibrillation. The Birmingham Trial[55] of permanent pacing in patients with persistent intraventricular defects after AMI also showed no significant difference in survival during follow-up of up to 5 years. In a prospective long-term study by Talwar and colleagues,[56] of 18 patients with anterior AMI, intraventricular defects, and transient complete AV block who were followed for a mean of 2 years, 8 had permanent pacemakers implanted and 10 did not. There was one death in the unpaced group due to a cerebrovascular accident. Therefore, at the present time, one can conclude that it has not yet been proved that in these patients sudden death is caused by heart block.

ROLE OF ELECTROPHYSIOLOGIC STUDIES IN ATRIOVENTRICULAR BLOCK IN ACUTE MYOCARDIAL INFARCTION

His bundle electrocardiography has been used to study the site of block, which has been shown to be either in the AV node (proximal block) or in the distal conduction system (distal block). The presence of a distal block may identify patients who may be at high risk for development of high-grade AV block.

It is generally accepted that in patients with inferior AMI the block is usually proximal. Harper and colleagues[57] showed that 30 of 32 patients (94%) with inferior AMI and third-degree AV block had AV nodal block during HBE; the remaining two patients were in normal sinus rhythm during the study and had a normal PR interval and normal AH and HV intervals. Thus, in this group of patients, HBE offers no additional advantage over conventional ECG criteria in localizing the site of block.

In anterior AMI the block is frequently in the distal conduction system. In Harper and colleagues' study, 50% of patients (9 of 18) with BBB and a normal PR interval on ECG had a prolonged HV interval.[57] Of their 22 patients who developed AV block and BBB, 5 had proximal block, 14 had distal block, and 3 had both proximal and distal blocks. Thus, in both groups of patients HBE was the only means of localizing the block in the proximal or distal portion of the conduction system. Distal block indicates disease in either the His bundle or the remaining bundle branches, and clinically this is a common antecedent to sudden asystole and a poorer prognosis. Despite the fact that a prolonged HV interval could identify a group of patients who may be at high risk of developing high-grade AV block, several studies have shown that this does not help in assessing the short- or long-term prognosis of patients.[57, 58] Thus, the routine use of His bundle studies is probably not helpful; however, in individual cases it may be useful.

Indications for Pacing

TEMPORARY PACING IN ACUTE MYOCARDIAL INFARCTION

Situations in which temporary pacing is recommended are listed in Table 20–4.

TABLE 20–4. TEMPORARY PACING RECOMMENDATIONS IN PATIENTS WITH ACUTE MYOCARDIAL INFARCTION

I. Atrioventricular block without bundle branch block
   A. Third-degree AV block
   B. Second-degree AV block, type II
      1. Patients with anterior AMI or with inferior AMI and wide QRS complex
      2. Patients with inferior AMI and narrow QRS complex if block recurs despite atropine administration
   C. Second-degree AV block, type I, and marked bradycardia
   D. AV block associated with marked bradycardia, hypotension, reduced cardiac output, heart failure, shock, or ventricular irritability
II. Atrioventricular block with bundle branch block
   A. Third-degree AV block
   B. Second-degree AV block
   C. Prophylactic pacing for those at high risk for high-grade AV block

ATRIOVENTRICULAR BLOCK WITHOUT BUNDLE BRANCH BLOCK

In patients with second-degree AV block, type I, those with inferior AMI and block above the His bundle (i.e., normal QRS width) normally do not require pacemaker insertion initially. These patients are not at risk for sudden asystole. However, it must be appreciated that a small number of patients with narrow QRS complexes have block in the His bundle and not in the AV node. Insertion of a pacemaker is recommended in patients with an anterior AMI or an inferior AMI with a wide QRS complex complicated by type I second-degree AV block in whom the block is presumed to be below the His bundle. This group of patients may be at risk for sudden asystole.

Regardless of the site of infarction, a temporary pacemaker should be placed whenever the AV block is associated with marked bradycardia (45 to 50 bpm), hypotension, reduced cardiac output, heart failure, shock, and ventricular irritability.

ATRIOVENTRICULAR BLOCK WITH BUNDLE BRANCH BLOCK

Prophylactic pacing is indicated for those who are considered to have a *"high risk"* of developing high-grade AV block. In both the multicenter study and our study such patients were recognized by (1) "new" bilateral BBB plus first-degree AV block; (2) bilateral BBB plus first-degree AV block; and (3) new BBB plus first-degree AV block. Those at *"moderate to high risk"* were identified by (1) new bilateral BBB; (2) first-degree AV block; and (3) bilateral BBB. These three subgroups of patients should probably receive a temporary pacemaker.

PERMANENT PACING IN PATIENTS RECOVERING FROM THE ACUTE PHASE OF MYOCARDIAL INFARCTION

Patients with persistent third-degree AV block or type II second-degree AV block, with or without BBB, should receive a permanent pacemaker. However, this situation does not occur commonly. In patients who develop second- or third-degree block in the hospital, regardless of infarct or block location, our data show a return to 1:1 conduction in 95% of patients without BBB and in 89% of patients with BBB who survive the infarction and are discharged eventually from the hospital.

A more difficult area of management pertains to patients who are survivors of an AMI complicated by persistent BBB and transient complete AV block during their hospitalization and may be at risk for serious bradyarrhythmias in the posthospitalization period. Should they be protected with a permanent pacemaker? Although some studies show that these patients have a higher incidence of late sudden death presumably caused by a bradycardia, such results must be viewed in the context of many other studies that show otherwise.

There are at least three possible ways of managing these patients: (1) all should receive permanent pacemakers; (2) only those with documented bradyarrhythmias should receive permanent pacemakers; or (3) patients should undergo left ventricular ejection fraction studies (by radionuclide study, two-dimensional echocardiography, or angiography), ambulatory 24-hour ECG monitoring, and possibly His bundle studies. Those with an ejection fraction equal to or less than 0.40, complex ventricular arrhythmias, and a greatly prolonged HV interval (65 msec or more) are at increased risk of death (including sudden death) from tachyarrhythmias, heart failure, and recurrent infarction. They should be closely followed, with performance of appropriate investigations, and therapy should be instituted accordingly. Other patients are at much lower risk for death and thus can be closely followed; insertion of permanent pacemakers may be considered in some patients.

Clearly, all patients with documented (symptomatic) bradyarrhythmias should receive a permanent pacemaker.

Selection of Pacing Mode

The selection of pacing mode for patients with acute AV block usually takes into account many of the same considerations used for mode selection for chronic AV block (see Chapter 19). However, special clinical features of acute AV block include the following: (1) if the patient was in sinus rhythm, loss of chronotropic competence will have been recent and abrupt; and (2) the loss of AV synchrony usually is associated with varying degrees of ventricular dysfunction, which may be severe. Restoration of chronotropic adaptation to activity may be achieved through VVIR and DDDR pacing in which sensor detection of changes in various physiologic stimuli are used to adjust the pacing rate. Dual-chamber pacing with sensing of the native atrial complex and synchronous pacing of the ventricle will also restore both chronotropic response to activity (providing sinus node activity is normal) and AV synchrony. Multiple factors must be considered in choosing the appropriate pacing mode, including the status and activity level of the patient, the importance of AV synchrony, the presence of chronotropic incompetence, the underlying cardiac substrate, and the estimated likelihood of the frequency and duration of pacing. The importance of each of these factors varies from patient to patient.

For *temporary* pacing of patients with acute AV block, single-chamber right ventricular VVI pacing usually provides adequate rate correction of the bradyarrhythmia. If there is no or minimal hemodynamic compromise of cardiac function, this mode of pacing may be sufficient to tide the patient over what is usually a transient period of high-grade or complete AV block. If the underlying rhythm prior to acute AV block was atrial fibrillation, single-chamber ventricular pacing should provide a satisfactory rate with no compromise of hemodynamic status because there was no preexisting AV synchrony.

In the presence of sinus rhythm, or sinus bradycardia with or without chronotropic competence, restoration of AV synchrony even in the acute situation of temporary pacing may be a desirable therapeutic goal in patients with acute AV block. Restoration of AV synchrony may result in substantial hemodynamic improvement when correction of bradyarrhythmia by ventricular pacing alone fails to increase cardiac output in the presence of acute right ventricular infarction.[59] Similar benefit has been shown for AV sequential pacing in the presence of acute anterior infarction.[60] However, it is apparent that optimization of the AV delay also is critical because an excessively long AV interval may result in deterioration with complete loss of the advantages of AV sequential pacing compared with ventricular pacing alone.[60]

In patients with acute AV block who have indications for *permanent* pacing the selection of pacing mode must take into account both the immediate condition of the patient and the possibility of future deterioration due to progression of the underlying disorder. Electrophysiologic and hemodynamic factors should be evaluated both in assessment of immediate needs and in anticipation of future problems.

The electrophysiologic factors that should be considered include: (1) the presence or absence of sinus rhythm, (2) the presence or absence of chronotropic competence, and (3) the presence of paroxysmal supraventricular arrhythmias. These may be recognized as the same general considerations used for selecting pacing mode for chronic AV block as discussed in Chapters 19 and 23. There is no clear documentary proof that the occurrence of acute AV block as described earlier predisposes the patient to any different prognosis in regard to loss of sinus rhythm, loss of chronotropic competence, or development of paroxysmal supraventricular tachycardia. The selection of pacing mode in patients with acute AV block may also be strongly influenced by the nature and severity of the hemodynamic abnormalities due to the underlying cardiac pathology. Because most of these patients have had an acute myocardial ischemic event with varying extent of infarction, the impact of the pacemaker system on acute and long-term hemodynamic factors may be a relevant concern.

For permanent pacing, the benefit of restoring the patient's ability to increase heart rate with activity (chronotropic competence) must be considered. This may be accomplished through using the VVIR, DDD (with normal sinus node function), or DDDR modes. It is clear that in the absence of an ability to increase the heart rate with activity, the only remaining mechanism for increasing cardiac output is to increase stroke volume. The magnitude of increase achieved by this mechanism is small compared to that achieved by an increase in heart rate (see Chapters 23 and 25). Furthermore, the underlying myocardial dysfunction that is present in most patients with acute AV block limits even more the contribution of change in stroke volume to the adaptive response to activity. Therefore, at the least, a VVIR system seems to be advantageous for improving cardiac output and work capacity during activity in patients with acute AV block.[61] If the indication for permanent pacing is transient advanced AV block and the patient is expected to usually be in sinus rhythm with normal AV conduction, then a simple single-chamber VVI system may be adequate as a backup to provide a reasonable minimum heart rate. The selection of a VVIR unit in preference to a VVI unit may be appropriate for patients with more frequent dependence on the pacemaker and a higher projected activity level in the anticipation that increased cardiac output with activity is a desirable and reasonable therapeutic goal. If, for example, the patient has had an associated stroke and has minimal chance of regaining even modest levels of activity, there would be little to be gained by using the more expensive rate-adaptive VVIR mode. On the other hand, although rate-adaptive VVIR pacing can achieve increases in work performance and cardiac output, the maintenance of AV synchrony is desirable, particularly at slower heart rates and in patients with impaired

ventricular function. Therefore, it has become accepted that in such patients dual-chamber pacing is advantageous[62] and the VVIR mode would seem to be appropriate only for patients with no preexisting AV synchrony, such as those with permanent atrial fibrillation on those in whom the rate and hemodynamic demands on the pacemaker system are minimal even at rest. In patients with acute complete persistent AV block and underlying intact sinus node function, dual-chamber pacing would maintain or restore AV synchrony at rest and would also allow the rate to increase with activity. If the sinus node is also diseased and chronotropically incompetent, the DDDR mode would restore both AV synchrony and rate response to activity, albeit with substitution of a physiologic parameter other than the P wave. Another consideration that might moderate the choice of pacing mode is the presence of concomitant paroxysmal supraventricular tachyarrhythmias. In such patients, an added benefit of the DDDR mode of pacing is the feature contained in several types of these units in which algorithms are used to detect and automatically change the pacing mode during such episodes. These units can automatically switch from the DDDR to VVI or VVIR mode and then, in some units, can automatically monitor the tachyarrhythmia and switch back to DDDR pacing when the supraventricular tachycardia terminates. Furthermore, the ability of many of the DDD and DDDR units to shorten the AV delay as pacing rate increases may increase the chances of providing maximum hemodynamic benefit during activity-induced rate increases.[63]

The long-term outcome of the minority of patients with acute AV block who require permanent pacing is usually most strongly affected by the extent of myocardial dysfunction or the severity of the underlying coronary disease and ischemia. In a 2-year follow-up study of 2021 permanently paced patients, the leading causes of the 249 recorded deaths were stroke (30%) and sudden cardiac death (22%).[64] The presence of BBB, which was seen predominantly in patients with AV block and myocardial infarction, was a predictor of sudden cardiac death because 28% of all patients with BBB and 35% of patients with bifascicular or trifascicular block died suddenly. In comparison, the prevalence of sudden death in the remaining 138 patients without such block was 18%. Undersensing of ectopic ventricular beats was reportedly more common in patients with, and uncommon in patients without, BBB. In 21 of 220 (10%) of the undersensed ventricular ectopic beats, the subsequent pacing impulse was "effective" or was followed by spontaneous single or repetitive ventricular arrhythmias. The authors of this study postulated that atrial sensing of dual-chamber pacing might lessen the frequency of undersensing of ventricular ectopic beats or potentially life-threatening fusion beats. However, critical analysis of the available data suggests only that intercurrent ventricular tachycardia or ventricular fibrillation remains an important cause of mortality in permanently paced patients. Whether pacemaker malfunction or the mode of pacing contributes significantly to mortality higher than that due to the coexisting cardiac disease remains an unresolved issue.[65]

A final important consideration in selection of the mode of pacing is the recognition that the extent of myocardial dysfunction in patients with ischemic heart disease may not be a permanent condition. Stunning and hibernation of the myocardium, leading to apparent dysfunction, may resolve as the ischemia resolves and after adequate time has passed for recovery.[66, 67]

Therefore, the hemodynamic benefits achieved by various modes of permanent pacing should not be employed as a substitute for reperfusion therapy of myocardial ischemia but rather as an adjunct to maximize the performance of any residual permanently injured myocardium after recovery from ischemia has been allowed to take place.

SUMMARY

The general considerations for selection of pacing mode discussed previously are summarized in Table 20–5. In general, if sinus rhythm is absent, myocardial dysfunction is minimal or clinically unimportant, the duration of pacing is expected to be brief or rare, and adaptive response of rate to activity is not needed, VVI or single-chamber ventricular pacing is adequate. If chronotropic competence is lost, due either to sinoatrial nodal disease or supraventricular arrhythmias such as atrial fibrillation, but restoration of chronotropic response is desirable, then VVIR pacing is indicated. When sinus activity is present or when AV synchrony is needed, the DDD or DDDR mode is, in general, desirable because of the high incidence of significant myocardial dysfunction in these patients.

Impact of Thrombolytic Therapy

There have been two prospective trials involving thrombolytic therapy of AMI that provide data pertaining to the impact of such therapy on the development of high-grade second- and third-degree AV block.[14, 18] Both examined the impact of thrombolytic therapy for acute inferior myocardial infarction. In one, the study was designed to examine the effect of thrombolytic therapy and adjunctive angioplasty as a treatment strategy for AMI (TAMI trial).[18] All patients had treatment initiated with thrombolytic agents within 6 hours of symptom onset. There were 373 patients with an inferior AMI, of whom 50 (13%) had complete AV block; 54% of

these patients had complete AV block on admission. In all but two patients the block was manifest within 72 hours of onset of symptoms. The duration of block was less than 1 hour in 25% and less than 12 hours in 15%; the median duration of block was 2.5 hours. There was no difference in the rate of infarct vessel patency between those with and those without AV block (90% and 91%, respectively). A precipitating clinical event—vessel reperfusion, performance of percutaneous transluminal coronary angioplasty (PTCA), or vessel reocclusion—was identifiable in 38% of instances of complete AV block. At the predischarge angiogram, the vessel patency rate was 11% lower in the AV block group than in the group without block (71% vs. 82%, respectively). Those who developed AV block showed a decrease in ejection fraction between the early post-thrombolytic angiogram and the predischarge angiogram. Also, those who developed AV block had a higher in-hospital mortality, 10 of 50 (20%) versus 12 of 323 (4%, $p < .001$). When age, left ventricular ejection fraction in the acute phase, number of diseased vessels, and grade of blood flow through the culprit lesion were entered into a multivariate model, the development of complete AV block still contributed significantly to the risk of in-hospital mortality. After a median follow-up period of 22 months, hospital survivors had equivalent mortality rates (2%) in the groups with and without AV block. These data suggest that compared with the prethrombolytic era, use of thrombolytics and angioplasty has not altered either the incidence of complete AV block or the associated greater ventricular dysfunction or in-hospital mortality.

In another study of 1786 patients with inferior AMI who received recombinant tissue-type plasminogen activator (rt-PA) within 4 hours of symptom onset, high-grade (second-or third-degree) AV block developed in 214 (12%) (TIMI II trial).[14] Of the group who had AV block, 113 (6.3% of the total or 52% of those who ever had AV block) had this finding on admission. The remaining 101 patients (5.7%) developed heart block during the 24 hours after treatment with thrombolytics. Patients who already had high-grade AV block prior to receiving thrombolytic therapy tended to be older and had a higher prevalence of cardiogenic shock than

TABLE 20–5. SELECTION OF PACING MODE FOR ACUTE ATRIOVENTRICULAR BLOCK

RHYTHM	LV FUNCTION	MODE	COMMENTS
TEMPORARY PACING			
Sinus	Normal or mild dysfunction	AV sequential, VVI	VVI if AV block is intermittent or if pacing is necessary for a short period of time only
Sinus	Depressed	AV sequential	
Atrial fibrillation, paroxysmal supraventricular tachycardia	Normal or depressed	VVI	Cardioversion or pharmacologic control of supraventricular arrhythmia may be needed if DDD pacing is desired
PERMANENT PACING			
Sinus	Normal or mild dysfunction	DDD or DDDR, VVI or VVIR[a]	If patient is chronotropically competent or need for rate-adaptivity is minimal, DDD is adequate; DDDR is needed if chronotropic incompetence is suspected
Sinus	Depressed	DDD	If chronotropically competent
		DDDR	If chronotropically incompetent (some units have added advantage of rate-adaptive AV delay and automatic mode switching for paroxysmal supraventricular tachycardia or paroxysmal atrial fibrillation)
Atrial fibrillation	Normal or abnormal	VVI or VVIR	VVIR if there is need to restore chronotropic competence (e.g., active patient with complete AV block)

[a]VVI or VVIR pacing is appropriate if pacing is expected to be infrequent and of short duration or if patient is inactive or terminally (chronically) ill; otherwise dual-chamber pacing is preferred.

those without heart block. Nevertheless, the presence of heart block did not carry an increased 21-day mortality independent of other variables such as shock, and the 1-year mortality was similar to that in the group without heart block. In this study, patients were randomly assigned to coronary arteriography 18 to 48 hours following admission. Among those who developed heart block after their admission, the infarct-related artery was less frequently patent than in those without heart block, 28 of 39 (72%) versus 611 of 723 (84.5%, $p = .04$). The RCA was the infarct-related artery more often in patients who developed heart block than in those who did not, 36 of 69 (92.3%) versus 542 of 723 (75.1%), respectively ($p = .04$). Among patients without heart block at the time of hospital admission, mortality within 48 hours was 4 of 9 (44%) in patients with and 8 of 68 (12%) in those without new heart block at 24 hours. The 21-day mortality was higher in the group with AV block than the group without block, 10 of 101 (9.9%) versus 35 of 1572 (2.2%), respectively ($p < .001$), as was 1-year mortality, 15 of 101 (14.9%) versus 65 of 1572 (4.2%), respectively ($p = .001$). A temporary pacemaker was inserted in approximately one third of patients with heart block on admission and in almost 30% of patients who developed heart block after institution of thrombolytic therapy, whereas only 6.5% of patients without heart block received temporary pacemakers. None of the patients who had heart block on admission or who developed heart block received a permanent pacemaker, but four patients without heart block at 24 hours went on to receive a permanent pacemaker. Heart block was not listed as a primary or contributing cause of death in any patient.

These data suggest that aggressive treatment with thrombolytic agents or thrombolytic therapy plus angioplasty is not associated with a lesser incidence of high-grade or complete AV block in patients with inferior AMI compared to the prethrombolytic era; the incidence remains around 12% to 13% with about half of cases appearing as new block during hospitalization. The infarct-related vessel is more often the RCA, and there is a lower vessel patency rate after thrombolysis among those who have AV block complicating their inferior AMI. In-hospital and early posthospitalization mortality is higher in patients with than in those without AV block among patients treated with thrombolytics, with or without angioplasty. It is not clear, however, that patients with acute AV block continue to be at greater risk of mortality if they survive the initial hospitalization. No causal relationship has been established between the presence of AV block and increased mortality. The presumption remains, as before the era of thrombolytic therapy, that the presence or development of AV block is associated with a higher mortality because it tends to indicate the presence of extensive infarction or injury. The impact of permanent pacing on longevity in these patients remains unknown.

REFERENCES

1. DeGuzman M, Rahimtoola SH: What is the role of pacemakers in patients with coronary artery disease and conduction abnormalities? *In* Rahimtoola SH (ed): Controversies in Coronary Artery Disease. Philadelphia, FA Davis, 1983, pp 191–207.
2. James TN: Anatomy of the coronary arteries and veins. Anatomy of the conduction system of the heart. *In* Hurst JW (ed): The Heart. New York, McGraw-Hill, 1978, pp 33–56.
3. James TN: Anatomy of the coronary arteries in health and disease. Circulation 32:1020, 1965.
4. Lev M, Bharati S: Anatomic basis for impulse generation and atrioventricular transmission. *In* Narula OS (ed): His Bundle Electrocardiography and Clinical Electrophysiology. Philadelphia, FA Davis, 1975, p 1.
5. Van der Hauwaert LG, Stroobandt R, Verhaeghe L: Arterial blood supply of the atrioventricular node and main bundle. Br Heart J 34:1045, 1972.
6. Frink RJ, James TN: Normal blood supply to the human His bundle and proximal bundle branches. Circulation 47:8, 1973.
7. Massing GK, James TN: Anatomical configuration of the His bundle and bundle branches in the human heart. Circulation 53:609, 1976.
8. Pruitt RD, Essex HE, Burchell BH: Studies on the spread of excitation through the ventricular myocardium. Circulation 3:418, 1951.
9. Hunt D, Lie JT, Vihru J, et al: Histopathology of heart block complicating acute myocardial infarction: Correlation with the His bundle electrogram. Circulation 48:1252, 1973.
10. Sutton R, Davies M: The conduction system in acute myocardial infarction complicated by heart block. Circulation 38:987, 1968.
11. Blondeau M, Maurice P, Reverdy, et al: Troubles du rythme et de la conduction auriculo-ventriculaire dans l'infarctus du myocarde récent: Considérations anatomiques. Arch Mal Coeur 60:1733, 1967.
12. Wei JY, Markis JE, Malagold M, et al: Cardiovascular reflexes stimulated by reperfusion of ischemic myocardium in acute myocardial infarction. Circulation 67:796, 1983.
13. Koren G, Weiss AT, Ben-David Y, et al: Bradycardia and hypotension following reperfusion with streptokinase (Bezold-Jarisch reflex): A sign of coronary thrombolysis and myocardial salvage. Am Heart J 112:468, 1986.
14. Berger PB, Ruocco NA, Ryan TJ, et al, and the TIMI II Investigators: Incidence and prognostic implications of heart block complicating inferior myocardial infarction treated with thrombolytic therapy: Results from TIMI II. J Am Coll Cardiol 20:533, 1992.
15. Bilbao FJ, Zabalza IE, Vilanova JR, et al: Atrioventricular block in posterior acute myocardial infarction: A clinicopathologic correlation. Circulation 75:733, 1987.
16. Rosen KM, Ehrsani A, Rahimtoola SH: Myocardial infarction complicated by conduction defect. Med Clin North Am 57:155, 1973.
17. Bassan R, Maia IG, Bozza A, et al: Atrioventricular block in acute inferior wall myocardial infarction: Harbinger of associated obstruction of the left anterior descending coronary artery. J Am Coll Cardiol 8:773, 1986.
18. Clemmensen P, Bates ER, Califf RM, et al, and the TAMI Study Group: Complete atrioventricular block complicating inferior wall acute myocardial infarction treated with reperfusion therapy. Am J Cardiol 67:225, 1991.
19. Cohen HC, Gozo EG Jr, Pick A: The nature and type of arrhythmias in acute experimental hyperkalemia in the intact dog. Am Heart J 82:777, 1971.
20. Sugiura T, Iwasaka T, Takayama Y, et al: The factors associated with fascicular block in acute anteroseptal infarction. Arch Intern Med 148:529, 1988.
21. Rotman M, Wagner GS, Wallace AG: Bradyarrhythmias in acute myocardial infarction. Circulation 45:703, 1972.
22. Hunt D, Lie JY, Vohra J, et al: Histopathology of heart block complicating acute myocardial infarction. Circulation 48:1252, 1973.
23. Wilber D, Walton J, O'Neill W, et al: Effects of reperfusion on complete heart block complicating anterior myocardial infarction. J Am Coll Cardiol 4:1315, 1984.
24. Norris RM: Heart block in posterior and anterior myocardial infarction. Br Heart J 31:352, 1969.
25. Brown RW, Hunt D, Sloman JG: The natural history of atrioventricular conduction defects in acute myocardial infarction. Am Heart J 78:460, 1969.
26. Ginks WR, Sutton R, Winston DH, et al: Long-term prognosis after acute myocardial infarction with atrioventricular block. Br Heart J 39:186, 1977.
27. Lie KI, Wellens HJ, Schuilenburg RM, et al: Factors influencing prognosis of bundle branch block complicating acute antero-septal infarction. Circulation 50:935, 1974.
28. Hindman MC, Wagner GS, JaRo M, et al: The clinical significance of bundle branch block complicating acute myocardial infarction: 2. Indications for temporary and permanent pacemakers. Circulation 58:689, 1978.
29. Forsberg SA, Juul-Moller S: Myocardial infarction complicated by heart block: Treatment and long-term prognosis. Acta Med Scand 206:483, 1979.
30. Tans AC, Lie KI, Durrer D: Clinical setting and prognostic significance

of high degree atrioventricular block in acute inferior myocardial infarction: A study of 144 patients. Am Heart J 99:4, 1980.

31. Greenfield L, DeGuzman M, Haywood LJ: Atrioventricular block and acute myocardial infarction: Factors influencing morbidity and mortality. Unpublished data, 1994.

32. Rosen KM, Loeb HS, Chiquimia R, et al: Site of heart block in acute inferior myocardial infarction. Circulation 42:925, 1970.

33. Kostuk WJ, Beanlands DS: Complete heart block with acute myocardial infarction. Am J Cardiol 26:380, 1970.

34. Bigger JT, Dresdale RJ, Heissenbuttal RH, et al: Ventricular arrhythmias in ischemic heart disease: Mechanism, prevalence, significance, and management. Prog Cardiovasc Dis 19:255, 1977.

35. Mullins CB, Atkins JM: Prognoses and management of ventricular conduction blocks in acute myocardial infarction. Mod Concepts Cardiovasc Dis 45:129, 1976.

36. Hindman MC, Wagner GS, JaRo H, et al: The clinical significance of bundle branch block complicating acute myocardial infarction. 1. Clinical characteristics, hospital mortality, and one-year follow-up. Circulation 58:679, 1978.

37. Norris RM, Croxson MS: Bundle branch block in acute myocardial infarction. Am Heart J 79:728, 1970.

38. Scheinman M, Brenman B: Clinical and anatomic implication of intraventricular conduction blocks in acute myocardial infarction. Circulation 46:753, 1972.

39. Lie KI, Wellens HJ, Schuilenburg RM: Bundle branch block and acute myocardial infarction. *In* Wellens HJ, Lie KI, Janse MI (eds): The Conduction System of the Heart: Structure, Function, and Clinical Implications. Philadelphia, Lea & Febiger, 1976, pp 662–672.

40. Godman MJ, Lassers BW, Julian DG: Complete bundle branch block complicating acute myocardial infarction. N Engl J Med 282:237, 1970.

41. Scanlon PJ, Pryor R, Blount G: Right bundle branch block associated with left superior or inferior intraventricular block. Circulation 42:1135, 1970.

42. Godman MJ, Alpert BA, Julian DG: Bilateral bundle branch block complicating acute myocardial infarction. Lancet 2:345, 1971.

43. Nimetz AA, Shubrooks SJ, Hutter AM, et al: The significance of bundle branch block during acute myocardial infarction. Am Heart J 90:439, 1975.

44. DeGuzman M, Ahmadpour H, Haywood LJ: Incidence, development, progression, and outcome of atrioventricular block in acute myocardial infarction with bundle branch block: A ten-year analysis. Circulation 64(Suppl IV):743, 1981.

45. Lamas GA, Muller JE, Turi AG, et al: A simplified method to predict occurrence of complete heart block during acute myocardial infarction. Am J Cardiol 57:1213, 1986.

46. Roos C, Dunning AJ: Right bundle branch block and left axis deviation in acute myocardial infarction. Br Heart J 32:847, 1970.

47. Harper R, Hunt D, Vohra J, et al: His bundle electrogram in patients with acute myocardial infarction complicated by atrioventricular or intraventricular conduction disturbances. Br Heart J 37:705, 1975.

48. Lichstein E, Gupta P, Liu MM, et al: Findings of prognostic value in patients with incomplete bilateral bundle branch block complicating acute myocardial infarction. Am J Cardiol 32:913, 1973.

49. Gould L, Reddy CV, Kim SG, et al: His bundle electrogram in patients with acute myocardial infarction. PACE 2:428, 1979.

50. Atkins J, Leshin S, Blomqvist CG, et al: Ventricular conduction blocks and sudden death in acute myocardial infarction. N Engl J Med 288:281, 1973.

51. Ritter WS, Atkins J, Blomqvist G, et al: Permanent pacing in patients with transient trifascicular block during acute myocardial infarction. Am J Cardiol 38:205, 1976.

52. Waugh RA, Wagner GS, Haney TL, et al: Immediate and remote prognostic significance of fascicular block during acute myocardial infarction. Circulation 47:765, 1973.

53. Murphy E, DeMots H, McAnulty J, et al: Prophylactic permanent pacemakers for transient heart block during myocardial infarction? Results of a prospective study. Am J Cardiol 49:952, 1982.

54. Lie K, Liem KL, Schuilenberg RM, et al: Early identification of patients developing late in-hospital ventricular fibrillation after discharge from the coronary care unit: A 5½-year retrospective and prospective study of 1,897 patients. Am J Cardiol 41:674, 1978.

55. Watson RDS, Glover DR, Page AJF, et al: The Birmingham Trial of permanent pacing in patients with intraventricular conduction disorders after acute myocardial infarction. Am Heart J 108:496, 1984.

56. Talwar KK, Kalra GS, Dogra B, et al: Prophylactic permanent pacemaker implantation in patients with anterior wall myocardial infarction complicated by bundle branch block and transient complete atrioventricular block: A prospective long-term study. Indian Heart J 39:22, 1987.

57. Harper R, Hunt D, Vohra J, et al: His bundle electrogram in patients with acute myocardial infarction complicated by atrioventricular or intraventricular conduction disturbances. Br Heart J 37:705, 1975.

58. Gould L, Reddy CVR, Kim SG, et al: His bundle electrogram in patients with acute myocardial infarction. PACE 2:428, 1979.

59. Topol EJ, Goldschlager N, Ports TA, et al: Hemodynamic benefit of atrial pacing in right ventricular myocardial infarction. Ann Intern Med 96:594, 1982.

60. Chamberlain DA, Leinbach RC, Vassaux CE, et al: Sequential atrioventricular pacing in heart block complicating acute myocardial infarction. N Engl J Med 282:577, 1970.

61. Nordlander R, Hedman A, Pehrsson SK: Rate-responsive pacing and exercise capacity—a comment. PACE 12:749, 1989.

62. Dreifus LS, Fisch C, Griffin JC, et al: Guidelines for implantation of cardiac pacemaker and antiarrhythmia devices: A report of the American College of Cardiology/American Heart Association Task Force on Assessment of Diagnostic and Therapeutic Cardiovascular Procedures (Committee on Pacemaker Implantation). Circulation 84:455, 1991.

63. Luceri RM, Brownstein SL, Vardeman L, et al: PR interval behavior during exercise: Implications for physiological pacemakers. PACE 13:1719, 1990.

64. Zehender M, Buchner C, Meinertz T, et al: Prevalence, circumstances, mechanisms, and risk stratification of sudden cardiac death in unipolar single-chamber ventricular pacing. Circulation 85:596, 1992.

65. Furman S: Prevalence, circumstances, mechanisms, and risk stratification of sudden cardiac death in artificial ventricular pacing. Circulation 85:843, 1992.

66. Rahimtoola SH: The hibernating myocardium. Am Heart J 117:211, 1989.

67. Braunwald E, Rutherford JD: Reversible ischemic left ventricular dysfunction: Evidence for the "hibernating myocardium." J Am Coll Cardiol 8:1467, 1986.

CHAPTER 21

CAROTID SINUS HYPERSENSITIVITY AND NEURALLY MEDIATED SYNCOPE

Fredrick J. Jaeger
Fetnat M. Fouad-Tarazi
Lon W. Castle

Carotid sinus syncope and vasovagal syncope are both examples of episodic loss of consciousness resulting from an overactive autonomic nervous system reflex with transient depression of blood pressure, heart rate, respiration, or any combination thereof. Collectively, these syndromes of adverse cardiovascular and pulmonary regulation have been categorized as neurally mediated syncope. Clinical examples of the myriad forms of neurally mediated syncope are shown in Table 21–1.

The list in Table 21–1 covers a wide spectrum of disorders of heart rate and blood pressure regulation. All can cause syncope by a final common mechanism. This mechanism is inherent in the definition of syncope itself and merits clarification. Syncope is defined as transient loss of consciousness with subsequent complete resolution without focal neurologic deficits. This loss of consciousness is a consequence of critical hypoperfusion of the brain, which deprives the brain of sufficient oxygen to maintain function. The causes of inadequate oxygen delivery to the brain are legion and are beyond the scope of this chapter.[1] Often, the causes of syncope are multifactorial. This can be especially true in the elderly patient. For example, elderly patients with a predisposition to carotid sinus syndrome may be given diuretics that cause hypovolemia, which can exacerbate the vasodepressor component.

This chapter focuses primarily on the neurocardiogenic causes of syncope and not the principal cardiac causes of syncope. The reader is referred to several comprehensive monographs addressing other forms of syncope.[1–4]

For the purpose of this chapter we limit our discussion to the most common of these neurally mediated syncope syndromes, vasovagal syncope (VVS) and to the less common carotid sinus syncope (CSS). Both of these disorders may be ameliorated by permanent pacing. Several authors have utilized the term neurally mediated syncope interchangeably with vasovagal syncope.[5, 6] However, we prefer the term VVS, partly in homage to Sir Thomas Lewis and also to be consistent with its traditional usage.[7]

TABLE 21–1. **NEURALLY MEDIATED SYNCOPE**[a]

Vasovagal syncope
Carotid sinus syncope
Tussive syncope
Glossopharyngeal neuralgia/deglutition syncope
Pallid breath-holding spells
Aortic stenosis
Hypertrophic obstructive cardiomyopathy
Pacemaker syncope
Syncope secondary to pulmonary hypertension
Micturition syncope
Mess trick
Diving reflex

[a]Syncope with atrial fibrillation, supraventricular tachycardia, and ventricular tachycardia may have a neurally mediated component.

TABLE 21–2. **VASOVAGAL SYNCOPE VERSUS CAROTID SINUS SYNCOPE**

CHARACTERISTIC	VASOVAGAL SYNCOPE	CAROTID SINUS SYNCOPE
Incidence	Common	Rare
Age of onset	Younger	Older
Prodrome	Yes	No
Associated underlying heart disease	No	Yes
Diagnosis	Head-up tilt	CSM
Predominant hemodynamic response	Vasodepressor ± cardioinhibitory	Cardioinhibitory ± vasodespressor
Untreated natural history	Spontaneous resolution	Recurrences
Treatment	None or medications ± pacemaker (see text)	Pacemaker

As can be seen from Table 21–1, there are many other forms of neurally mediated syncope, some of which can be improved with pacing. Cough syncope may be secondary to vagal reflex–induced sinus node or atrioventricular (AV) node abnormalities such as Mobitz's type I and sinus arrest, which can be improved with permanent pacing.[8, 9] However, the etiology of cough syncope may be multifactorial and involve mechanical decreases in cerebral blood flow resulting from elevated intrathoracic pressures (up to 300 mm Hg) or elevated spinal fluid pressures.

Although VVS and CSS reflect a relative hypersensitivity of a specific autonomic nervous system reflex, these disorders are quite distinct with unique clinical characteristics, demographics of patients, and pathophysiologic mechanisms (Table 21–2). Both disorders can be diagnosed by relatively noninvasive and simple tests that can be applied and interpreted with a fair amount of certainty. These tests, carotid sinus massage for carotid sinus hypersensitivity (CSH) and head-up tilt test (also called upright tilt) for VVS, are re-viewed in detail. These maneuvers are extremely valuable in the diagnosis of syncope of undetermined origin (SUO) and should be incorporated fairly early in the diagnostic algorithm for patients with low probability of an arrhythmic etiology of syncope (i.e., lack of structural heart disease) (Fig. 21–1).

That two such divergent clinical entities as CSS and VVS had common pathophysiologic etiologies was first suggested by Sir Thomas Lewis in 1932, in his intriguingly entitled paper "Vasovagal Syncope and Carotid Sinus Mechanism" in which he first proposed the term vasovagal syncope.[7] The pathophysiology of the two distinct disorders, VVS and CSS, are discussed here separately in detail. In general, several statements can be made regarding the neurally mediated syncopes. All forms involve an abnormality in the reflex arc consisting of neural afferents, the central nervous system (especially the vasomotor regions of the medulla), and the neural efferents. The specific routes of these connections vary and are shown in Figure 21–2.[10]

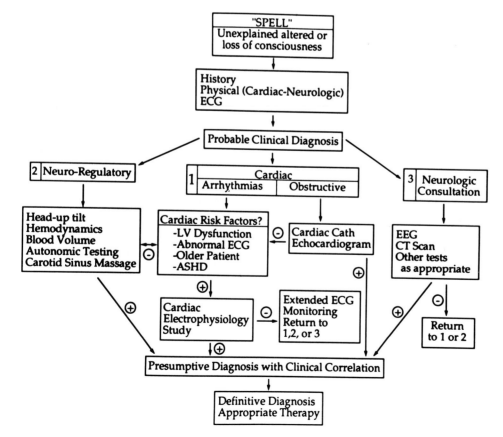

FIGURE 21–1. Algorithmic approach to syncope of unknown origin. Note incorporation of head-up tilt and carotid sinus massage when history suggests neurally mediated syncope. ECG, electrocardiogram; LV, left ventricular; ASHD, arteriosclerotic heart disease; EEG, electroencephalogram; CT, computed tomography. (From Jaeger FJ, Maloney JD, Fouad-Tarazi FM: Newer aspects in the diagnosis and management of syncope. *In* Rappaport E [ed]: Cardiology Update 1990. New York, Elsevier, 1990, pp 141–173.)

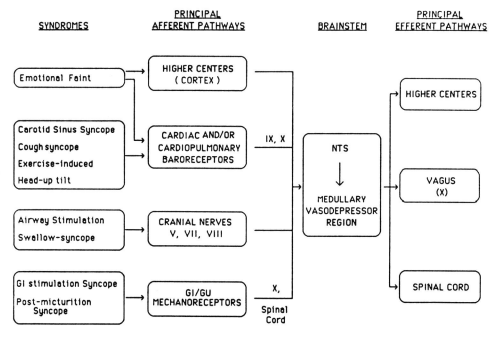

FIGURE 21–2. Schematic illustration of proposed anatomic reflex neural connections in various neurally mediated syncopes. GI, gastrointestinal; GU, genitourinary; NTS, nucleus tractus solitarius. (Adapted from Benditt DG, Remole S, Bailin S, et al: Tilt table testing for evaluation of neurally-mediated [cardioneurogenic] syncope: Rationale and proposed protocols. PACE 14:1528, 1991.)

Carotid Sinus Syndrome or Carotid Sinus Syncope

DEFINITIONS

In this chapter we use the term carotid sinus hypersensitivity to denote the abnormal responses, either cardioinhibitory, vasodepressor, or both, to carotid sinus massage (CSM). Pure cardioinhibitory response is the most common response in CSH, occurring in approximately 60% to 80%.[11] Pure vasodepressor response, on the other hand, is relatively rare, occurring in 5% to 10%.[12] The remainder of the CSM responses are of the mixed variety. The term carotid sinus syndrome or carotid sinus syncope, although used quite liberally by others, is reserved for patients with documented CSH and a consistent clinical history after elimination of all other potential causes of syncope. Historical features that strongly suggest CSS are syncope or near syncope occurring during carotid sinus stimulation, typical clinical spells reproduced during CSM, or fortuitous Holter or other documentation of asystole during syncope after maneuvers that could presumably stimulate the carotid sinus.[13–17] As discussed later, CSH is relatively common in normal individuals and patients without syncope, but true CSS is quite rare.

PATHOPHYSIOLOGY OF CAROTID SINUS HYPERSENSITIVITY

The carotid sinus reflex has been recognized for many years as an integral component of the homeostatic mechanisms of blood pressure regulation.[18] Increases in intrasinusal pressure stimulate mechanoreceptors that exit the carotid sinus via the nerve of Hering to join the glossopharyngeal (cranial nerve IX) and possibly vagus (cranial nerve X) nerves and terminate in the brain stem. These, in turn, travel to peripheral end organs both through vagal efferents that reflexly augment cardiac vagal input, slowing heart rate, and

through the spinal cord to inhibit peripheral sympathetic activity in skeletal vasculature resulting in peripheral vasodilatation. The end result, in concert with other baroreceptors, is maintenance of blood pressure within a narrow range. The carotid sinus reflex may also suppress or decrease rate and depth of respiration, although the clinical impact of this function is not known.

In certain individuals, the carotid sinus reflex may be abnormally heightened, causing exaggerated responses of heart rate and blood pressure. The exact site of the abnormality in the reflex loop is not fully understood. However, based on several studies, it appears that the major defect may reside in the central nervous system (CNS) component of the reflex arc. Evidence that the abnormality of the reflex arc does not reside in the carotid sinus or in its neural efferents is the following:

1. Histology of intima and neural terminals of the carotid sinus is essentially normal in CSH.[19]
2. Patients with CSH or CSS may have the reflex activated by other independent vagal mechanisms (e.g., micturition, defecation).[11]
3. Effects of CSM on blood pressure are prolonged and do not terminate abruptly with discontinuation of carotid pressure, although carotid sinus neural output does.[11]

It is possible that the defect may reside in the afferent limb, although patients with CSS do not demonstrate increased sensitivity to cholinesterase inhibitors.[20] However, that is not to say that cardiac abnormalities are irrelevant. Certainly, superimposed abnormalities or disease of the sinoatrial (SA) or AV node may act synergistically with abnormal neural output to create the syndrome. However, it is currently believed that the bulk of the abnormalities in CSS are present in the CNS, especially the brain stem and cardiovascular regulation centers. It has been suggested that central neuropeptides may be involved in the genesis of CSS.[19]

CLINICAL CHARACTERISTICS OF CAROTID SINUS SYNDROME

Carotid sinus syndrome, in contrast to vasovagal syncope, tends to occur in older patients and have a male predominance, as does coronary artery disease. The incidence of CSS, although difficult to state with certainty, was calculated by one center to be 35 per million population per year.[20] However, asymptomatic CSH is quite common in adult populations. Brown and colleagues[21] found a positive cardioinhibitory response to CSM in 32% of patients undergoing coronary angiography. In addition, they found that the magnitude of the exaggerated response to CSM was proportional to the severity of the underlying coronary disease. The association of CSS and CSH with coronary artery disease has been long recognized. The demonstration of CSH in an otherwise asymptomatic patient may therefore suggest the diagnosis of concomitant coronary artery disease.

In contrast to CSH, which is quite common, CSS is probably relatively rare, present in only 11% to 19% of patients with syncope of undetermined etiology.[22] The syncope in CSS tends to occur abruptly with little or no prodrome and only 50% of patients may recognize a precipitating event. Often no specific maneuver or action can be recalled to have preceded syncope. Historically, tight collars, shaving, head turning (as in looking to back up a car), coughing, heavy lifting, Valsalva maneuver, trumpet playing, or looking up (as when sitting in the front row of a theater) have been reported to initiate events. Other physiologic activities that affect the autonomic, especially vagal, milieu, can also precipitate a syncopal episode. These include swallowing, defecation, micturition, and eating.

Intrinsic anatomic distortion of the carotid sinus area, with internal carotid aneurysm, head and neck tumors, or lymphadenopathy, can predispose to CSS.[23, 24] Extrinsic deformation of the carotid sinus with episodic loss of consciousness has also been described with an orthodontic apparatus.[25] A rare cause of CSS was reported by Romano and colleagues[26] in a young patient with multiple symmetric lipomatosis, in whom lipomatous involvement of the carotid sinus region resulted in CSS. The coexistence of carotid artery stenosis and CSS has been reported. In these patients, transient ischemic attacks (TIAs) may be precipitated during episodes of CSH.[27] It should be emphasized that these structural abnormalities are unusual causes of CSS. In most cases, patients with CSS have essentially normal neck anatomy. Although rare, syncope associated with head flexion or extension can also occur with mechanical obstruction of the vertebral arteries.

Symptoms of CCS range from dizziness to profound loss of consciousness, occasionally with significant injuries. Episodes of syncope tend to occur abruptly with CSS; therefore, patients may experience injuries that can be quite severe (e.g., fractures, lacerations). Some patients may not recall losing consciousness and may present solely with unexplained falls. Kenney and Traynor[23] reported patients with CSH who did not recall episodes of loss of consciousness during CSM, presumably because of retrograde amnesia. Of seven elderly patients who had previously suffered from falls and developed loss of consciousness during CSM while undergoing upright tilt, five denied their loss of consciousness on awakening. Therefore, frequent unexplained falls in the elderly should prompt evaluation of the CSM response.

TECHNIQUE OF CAROTID SINUS MASSAGE

CSM can be performed safely and easily at the bedside, ideally with continuous electrocardiographic (ECG) monitoring. Obviously the presence of bruits or a history of cerebrovascular disease, TIAs, or endarterectomies contradicts application of pressure to the carotid area. The carotid sinus is located high in the neck below the angle of the mandible. Sequential application of carotid massage to the left and right carotid arteries should be performed with at least 10 to 20 seconds in between. Duration of carotid massage should be 5 to 10 seconds and terminated with onset of characteristic asystole. Pressure to the sinus should be nonocclusive, which can be ensured by simultaneous palpation of the ipsilateral temporal artery. In most series the predominant responses to CSM are obtained on the right.[13]

In patients undergoing CSM for syncope of undetermined etiology, comprehensive evaluation for CSH includes CSM while the patient is both supine and upright. This can be accomplished by having the patient standing erect or elevating the patient on a tilt table during CSM. This postural evaluation during CSM is critically important in unmasking an otherwise covert vasodepressor component of CSH. Occasionally the response to CSM can be augmented or accentuated by a simultaneous Valsalva maneuver. This has been particularly helpful in the termination of supraventricular tachycardia with CSM.

Responses to CSM that define CSH include cardioinhibitory and vasodepressor responses. A previously described primary cerebral type of CSH has now been disproved. The cause of syncope during CSM with this type was probably overly aggressive occlusion of the carotid artery, probably with contralateral vascular disease. This resulted in critically decreased cerebral circulation with loss of consciousness not due to a reflex mechanism.

Cardioinhibitory CSH is defined as 3 seconds or more of ventricular standstill or asystole during CSM. Ventricular asystole is usually a consequence of sinus pause but can be secondary to AV block. Utilizing continuous sinus node electrogram recordings, it has been demonstrated that CSM produces sinus pauses by initiating sinus node exit block.[28] Although the most obvious effect of CSH during asystole is on the sinus node, the profound influence of the autonomic nervous system, particularly the vagal influence, can be pancardiac and can prevent other lower escape pacemaker foci from discharging.

Typically, in patients with true CSH the onset of asystole is rapid and may produce prolonged asystolic responses with dramatic loss of consciousness. Invariably, complete recovery is also rapid after cessation of CSM.

A vasodepressor response to CSM is defined as a drop in systolic blood pressure of 50 mm Hg or more or a decrease of 30 mm Hg or more in the presence of neurologic symptoms (Fig. 21–3). In patients who have a significant concomitant cardioinhibitory component of carotid sinus massage, it may be more difficult to demonstrate the vasodepressor response. Various techniques for preventing asystole have been described and include pretreatment with intravenous atropine or temporary ventricular or AV sequential pacing during CSM.[12] Obviously, these techniques are best reserved for the electrophysiology laboratory. If temporary pacing is to be tested, it is necessary first to determine whether ventricular pacing results in hypotension because of VA conduction and

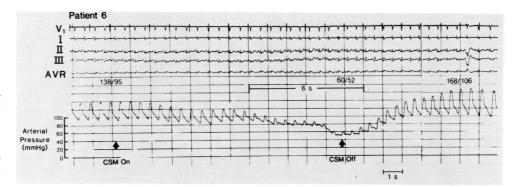

FIGURE 21–3. Pure vasodepressor response during carotid sinus massage. (From Almquist A, Gornick C, Benson W, et al: Carotid sinus hypersensitivity: Evaluation of the vasodepressor component. Circulation 71:927, 1985. Copyright 1985 American Heart Association.)

the pacemaker syndrome. In contrast to the induced cardioinhibitory component of CSH, which starts abruptly and resolves quickly with discontinuation of CSM, the vasodepressor response may have a more insidious, slower onset and a prolonged resolution (Fig. 21–4). It may be difficult to demonstrate the drop in blood pressure with standard sphygmomanometer methods and an arterial line can be placed if necessary. Others have utilized continuous digital plethysmography or the more sophisticated Finipress. Occasionally, simple palpation of the radial or brachial arteries may be sufficient to confirm suspected hypotension.

The mixed type of CSH consists of varying proportions of vasodepressor and cardioinhibitory components. The mixed type of CSS can be subdivided based on the magnitude of the vasodepressor component.[29] Type I appears to be a predominantly cardioinhibitory response, but symptoms persist after atropine administration. In type II, symptoms are late in

onset and continue after abolition of asystole with atropine, indicating a predominant vasodepressor component. We found this subclassification useful in deciding between DVI/DDD and VVI pacemaker modes. Patients with type I CSS and with no evidence of orthostatic hypotension, pacemaker syndrome, or ventriculoatrial (VA) conduction could receive VVI pacing. Patients with mixed type II CSS should always receive DVI/DDD.

ROLE OF THE ELECTROPHYSIOLOGIC STUDY

Although the demonstration of a hypersensitive carotid sinus with or without symptoms can be quite suggestive in a patient with SUO, it cannot be relied on to be wholly diagnostic. As previously mentioned, CSH is quite common, particularly in persons with coronary disease and hypertension. This is exactly the population of patients who may have

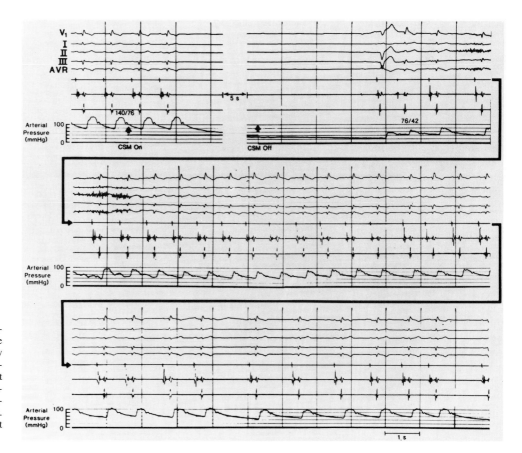

FIGURE 21–4. Combined cardioinhibitory and vasodepressor response to carotid sinus massage. Note slow return of blood pressure despite resolution of asystole. (From Almquist A, Gornick C, Benson W, et al: Carotid sinus hypersensitivity: Evaluation of the vasodepressor component. Circulation 71:927, 1985. Copyright 1985 American Heart Association.)

ventricular tachycardia as a cause of syncope. In 28 patients with SUO who were found to have CSH, 5 of 15 with coronary artery disease were found to have sustained monomorphic ventricular tachycardia provoked at comprehensive electrophysiology study.[30] Therefore, the demonstration of CSH in patients afflicted with syncope should not preclude the performance of electrophysiologic study, particularly in patients with risk factors for ventricular tachycardia: previous myocardial infarction, cardiomyopathy (dilated or hypertrophic), positive signal-averaged ECG, or left ventricular dysfunction.

In addition to excluding more potentially lethal causes such as ventricular tachycardia in patients with CSH, the electrophysiologic study can provide information on sinus node and AV node function. It is presumed that intrinsic abnormalities of these structures can be synergistic with the tendency toward increased parasympathetic activity and promote bradycardia and pauses. Also, the electrophysiologic study can be used to assess the vasodepressor component of CSH during temporary pacing of the atrium, ventricle, or both sequentially during CSM. Finally, for patients for whom a permanent pacemaker is appropriate therapy, the electrophysiologic study can be utilized to determine the optimal pacing mode. Ideally, as previously mentioned, VVI pacing should be reserved for those patients in whom no potential for pacemaker syndrome can be demonstrated.

COMPLICATIONS OF CAROTID SINUS MASSAGE

In general, CSM is safe when applied in appropriate circumstances. Rare complications include cerebrovascular accidents, and TIAs. CSM is obviously contraindicated in patients with a history of these or carotid bruits and carotid endarterectomy. Arrhythmic complications have been reported and include asystole and ventricular fibrillation.[31]

TREATMENT FOR CAROTID SINUS SYNCOPE

With determination of CSS as the likely diagnosis for syncopal spells, initial recommendations should be simple elimination of any recognized maneuvers that may precipitate an event. Discontinuation of tight collars and ties or more careful shaving may be beneficial. If possible, medications (calcium channel blockers, digoxin, and beta-blockers) that may predispose to CSH should be discontinued. Hypovolemia, resulting from diuretics or other causes, may exacerbate the vasodepressor component of CSH and should be corrected. Elimination of diuretics, addition of volume expanders such as fludrocortisone (Florinef), or high salt intake may be helpful.

In the prepacemaker era, recalcitrant cases of CSS were treated with carotid sinus denervation by a surgical technique.[32] This practice has been largely abandoned because of the development of hypertensive crisis after carotid sinus denervation. Surgery is now reserved for CSS associated with head or neck tumors or lymphadenopathy or is performed in conjunction with carotid endarterectomy or in patients with severe refractory CSS of the pure vasodepressor variety. An additional antiquated treatment for CSS was localized radiation therapy to both carotid sinus regions.

PACING FOR CAROTID SINUS SYNCOPE

For cases of recurrent, frequent, or severe CSS, permanent pacemaker implantation is the current conventional therapy, particularly for CSS of the predominantly cardioinhibitory type.[33, 34] Although permanent pacing for such cases is almost universally accepted, some controversy exists regarding the pacing mode and the role of pacing for mixed forms of CSS. Whereas CSS may have a substantial impact on the quality of life, it has not been shown to affect mortality significantly and patients with CSS who receive therapy do not appear to have a worse prognosis than the general population. In a long-term (mean, 44 months) follow-up study by Brignole and colleagues,[35] survival of patients with CSS was not significantly different from that of control patients with other causes of syncope. As expected, mortality was dependent on age, sex, and associated underlying cardiac disease (congestive heart failure, abnormal ECG). Factors related to CSS, such as the hemodynamic type, severity, and abnormalities of the SA or AV node, were not predictive of prognosis. The overall predicted 5-year survival was 73%. Treatment of these patients with CSS was nonrandomized and heterogeneous, so the results of therapy could not be interpreted to determine the best treatment modality or the impact on mortality.

A comprehensive summary of studies of pacing for CSS is shown in Table 21–3.[36–41] It is clear from these and many other studies that pacemaker implantation should be reserved for patients with recurrent symptoms and predominantly cardioinhibitory responses. Several additional points need to be emphasized. Earlier studies tended to be retrospective reports on pacing practices for CSS and therefore were inherently biased toward patients with a clear diagnosis of CSS who would truly benefit from pacing. More recently, prospective and randomized trials have been performed that examine outcome based on the presence of pacing and the mode. It is clear that in all cases of CSS, AAI pacing is contraindicated, as many patients may eventually demonstrate associated reflex AV block.[42] In general, patients benefit most from AV sequential pacing, even when a significant component of vasodepressor CSS is present. When VVI pacing is to be employed, it is critically important to ascertain susceptibility to pacemaker syndrome. Pacemaker syndrome, a form of neurally mediated vasodepression secondary to an atrial reflex, requires intact VA conduction.[43] Lack of VA conduction may, therefore, suggest that patients with CSS could receive VVI pacemakers. However, lack of VA conduction at a particular time does not ensure against its future development. Therefore, again we strongly advise DDD pacemakers for patients with CSS and normal sinus rhythm. No study has yet examined the role of rate-responsive (DDDR) pacing in CSS. As previously mentioned, many patients with CSS demonstrate evidence of sick sinus syndrome or chronotropic incompetence, either intrinsic or associated with medications. Therefore, rate-responsive pacing could be beneficial.

Ultimately, the sine qua non for the diagnosis of CSS is elimination of symptoms after pacemaker implantation. Predictors of success with permanent pacing include (1) multiple episodes before implantation, (2) episodes that occur while the person is upright or sitting, and (3) episodes that are preceded by a recognized stimulus.[44] In cases of mixed CSH,

TABLE 21–3. **PACEMAKER THERAPY FOR CAROTID SINUS SYNDROME**

AUTHORS	NUMBER OF PATIENTS	PATIENTS ASYMPTOMATIC IN FOLLOW-UP, NO. (%)	PATIENTS WITH NO SYNCOPE, NO. (%)	MEAN FOLLOW-UP (MO)	COMMENT
Sugrue et al.[38]					
No treatment	11	7 (64)	3 (73)	39	Approximately 77% of patients cardiac inhibition only
Pacing	23	16 (69)	21 (91)	23	Approximately 83% cardiac inhibition only
VVI pacing	11	8 (73)			A total of 26 patients required pacing
DVI pacing	15	13 (87)			All recurrent syncope in those with mixed CSS
Anticholinergic drugs	19	15 (79)	15 (79)	41	Approximately 90% cardiac inhibition only
Huang et al.[37]					
VVI pacing	9		9 (100)	42	All but one cardiac inhibition only
DDD pacing	4		4 (100)	42	
No treatment	8		7 (88)	42	
Morley et al.[39]					
VVI pacing	54	48 (89)		18	Five AAI converted to DDD/DVI and VVI
DVI pacing	13	12 (92)		18	Four VVI converted to DVI
DDD pacing	3	2 (66)		18	
Brignole et al.[41]					
No treatment	19	6 (32)	10 (53)	8.4	63% cardiac inhibition
Pacing	16	13 (81)	16 (100)	7.2	69% cardiac inhibition only
VVI pacing	11		11 (100)	7.2	
DDD pacing	5		5 (100)	7.2	
Randomized study: Differences between pacing and no treatment statistically significant					
Brignole et al.[40]					
VVI pacing	26	7 (27)	24 (92)	2	73% mixed CSS
DDD pacing	26	18 (69)	26 (100)	2	
Crossover study: Differences VVI/DDD statistically significant for general symptoms but not for syncope					

Adapted from Katritsis D, Ward DE, Camm AJ: Can we treat carotid sinus syndrome? PACE 14:1367, 1991.

pacing is frequently utilized for the bradycardia component and medications for the vasodepressor component. Proposed combinations include sympathomimetics, such as ephedrine, and beta-blockers,[45] although results of these medications remain generally very disappointing.

NATURAL HISTORY OF CAROTID SINUS SYNDROME

Previous reports on the natural history of medically treated patients with CSS indicated a low incidence of syncope recurrence (up to 25%).[37, 46] However, these studies were primarily retrospective analyses, involving nonpaced patients with less severe symptoms of CSS or those in whom the diagnosis was in doubt. A prospective randomized trial from a group at the hospital of Reggio, Italy, reaffirmed the important role of permanent pacing for CSS.[46] In this study, 60 patients with CSS were randomized to pacing (32 patients) and nonpacing (28 patients) therapy. During a follow-up of approximately 3 years, syncope recurred in 16 patients of the nonpaced group (51%) and in 3 (9%) of the paced group ($p = .002$). This observation confirms the efficacy of pacing for prevention of syncope in CSS.

Vasovagal Syncope

VVS is by far the most common form of all the reflex syncopes and most patients probably do not seek medical attention for rare, isolated events. Prolonged standing, sight of blood, pain, and fear have been the traditional precipitating stimuli for the "common faint" (Table 21–4). Patients develop nausea and diaphoresis with subsequent loss of consciousness resulting from hypotension with or without significant bradycardia or asystole. Recovery after several seconds is the norm, and patients recover fully. In contrast to these benign forms of VVS, we and others have used the term malignant VVS to denote the condition in patients with either little or no prodrome, no recognized precipitating stimulus, or marked bradycardia and asystole accompanying the VVS.[47–51] It is this group that has generated extensive interest in the field of electrophysiology. Again, we prefer the term

TABLE 21–4. **SITUATIONS THAT PROVOKE VASOVAGAL SYNCOPE**

Fear, anxiety, fight or flight
Pain, venipuncture
Pregnancy, standing at attention
Hypovolemia
Anemia
Hemorrhage
Prolonged bed rest, prolonged head-down tilt, microgravity
Head-up tilt, lower body negative pressure
First-dose phenomena, nitrates
Beta-blocker withdrawal

VVS to signify fainting associated with bradycardia and hypotension. Vasodepressor reactions, much less common, involve only hypotension. Other synonyms for VVS include emotional faint, reflex syncope, empty heart syndrome, neurally mediated syncope, situational syncope, vasomotor syncope, ventricular syncope, neurocardiogenic syncope, hypotension-bradycardia syndrome, and autonomic syncope. In addition, the terms convulsive syncope and venipuncture fits have been used to describe patients with VVS who develop generalized muscle movements that may mistakenly resemble epilepsy.[52, 53] The tilt table has been particularly useful in differentiating the diagnosis in these disorders.

The clinical scenario of syncope with demonstrated intermittent sinus pauses or AV block with subsequent electrophysiologic demonstration of normal AV node function may have several etiologies, such as medication effects, ischemia, and early intrinsic disease of the conduction system, but may also be due to abnormal autonomic input to the cardiac conduction system, again the so-called extrinsic sick sinus syndrome. In a study by Fujimura and associates,[54] 21 patients with syncope and the foregoing Holter findings (e.g., sinus pauses or intermittent AV block) underwent comprehensive electrophysiologic testing. Abnormalities that could explain the syncope and Holter findings were demonstrated in only 24% of patients. Head-up tilt testing was not performed in this population of patients and might have identified VVS as the cause for syncope.

PATHOPHYSIOLOGY OF VASOVAGAL SYNCOPE

Although the pathophysiology of VVS has been extensively studied for many years, multiple questions still abound.[55–57] It has been proposed that VVS that results from pain, fear, or emotion (flight or fight) originates from corticohypothalamic centers, and this has been termed the "central type,"[58] presumably independent of cardiac receptors. The potential to develop this reflex is present in all humans and also in many other mammals. The conservation-withdrawal or "playing dead" reactions may be analogous processes. A second type of vasovagal response called the peripheral type results from stimulation of cardiac receptors. The classic explanation for this type is based on animal studies demonstrating left ventricular mechanoreceptors and chemoreceptors that responded to intravenous nicotine or deformation from excessive contractions.[59] These receptors, called the C fibers, are located primarily in the inferior and posterior portions of the left ventricle and carry impulses from the heart via vagal afferents terminating in the medulla. Once stimulated, these connections reflexly decrease sympathetic output to the peripheral arteriolar vasculature, resulting in vasodilatation and hypotension. In addition, withdrawal of sympathetic innervation to the heart leaves parasympathetic, vagal, input unopposed, causing bradycardia. This reflex, called the Bezold-Jarisch reflex, would thus serve as a brake on an excessively active myocardium.[60] Stated another way, a relatively hypovolemic, vigorously contracting ventricle is the presumed trigger of the reflex. This reflex may also be important in hypotension associated with aortic stenosis, obstructive hypertrophic cardiomyopathy,[61] and hypotension-bradycardia observed in inferior myocardial infarction and during right coronary artery angiography.[60]

The end result of the reflex, once activated, is profound hypotension, bradycardia, and loss of muscle tone with subsequent collapse. It was reported that during VVS episodes, marked paradoxical vasoconstriction of the CNS vasculature occurs, which, when combined with other adverse hemodynamic effects, may act synergistically to promote syncope.[62] It has been suggested that presyncope hyperventilation may cause significant arterial hypocapnia that may produce cerebral vasoconstriction. However, we found no evidence of this.

Astronauts exposed to microgravity or patients undergoing prolonged head-down tilt (-5 degrees) may be susceptible to a vasovagal-like reaction during upright posture.[63] Attenuation of cardiopulmonary baroreceptors because of the transient central hypervolemia, as seen in space or head-down position with subsequent decrease in blood volume, may be responsible.

Evidence supporting these physiologic and autonomic changes during VVS can be obtained from a variety of studies. Wallin and Sundlöf[64] demonstrated withdrawal of sympathetic stimulation of the peripheral muscular vasculature (recorded using microneurographic techniques of the peroneal nerve) associated with the onset of VVS, consistent with the hypothesis that neurally mediated vasodilatation in the musculature occurs secondarily to sympathetic inhibition. Shalev and colleagues[65] demonstrated that left ventricular echocardiographic dimensions decrease significantly before onset of VVS during head-up tilt (HUT) and inferred that a hypovolemic ventricle may induce the reaction. Similar findings were reported by Fitzpatrick and associates,[66] who demonstrated decreased left ventricular dimensions and an increase in fractional shortening during echocardiography in patients who develop VVS during HUT. Neuroendocrine and neurohormonal aspects of VVS have also been extensively investigated. Serum epinephrine has been observed to increase significantly at the time of VVS induced by HUT,[67] the so-called epinephrine surge. This increase may be secondary to ensuing hypotension or may be a primary event that precipitates the reflex. This observation tends to support the beneficial effects of beta-blockade in preventing syncope. Evidence that elevated epinephrine was not a primary effect was reported by Calkins and colleagues.[68] Administration of intravenous epinephrine was found not to be as effective as intravenous isoproterenol in initiating vasodepressor responses in susceptible patients. Patients who develop VVS during HUT were also shown to have lower resting norepinephrine levels, which may reflect a relative heightened vagal state or simply their young age.[69] Various other neuropeptide and neurohumoral agents such as vasopressin and endorphins have also been implicated in the genesis and expression of VVS.[58, 70–72] It is an interesting historical observation that urine output after a VVS episode is minimal for several hours. This is due to the release (surge) of vasopressin during the spell.[58, 72] Vasopressin may also be responsible for the prolonged pallor after a VVS episode.[72]

That absence of appropriate vasoconstriction of the peripheral skeletal vasculature is an important component of the vasovagal response has been well established. However, whether failure of the vasoconstriction mechanism is a primary event or is secondary to the Bezold-Jarisch reflex was examined by Sneddon and coworkers.[73] Patients who eventually developed a positive tilt test (i.e., vasovagal response) were found to have significantly reduced forearm vascular resistance almost immediately after assuming the upright position on the tilt table, compared with those who had a normal tilt response. This suggests that a heretofore unobserved abnormality in primary vasoconstrictor responses may be involved in the pathophysiology of VVS. In contrast, forearm vascular resistance was similar in patients with VVS and control subjects, utilizing the postischemic reactive hyperemia technique. However, patients with VVS had paradoxical decreases of brachial artery diameter despite elevated blood pressure, suggesting an accentuated adrenergic nervous system response.[74]

The vasovagal reflex may have an important role in the genesis of hypotension and syncope in some supraventricular and ventricular tachycardias. Leitch and coworkers[75] subjected patients with supraventricular tachycardia to HUT and found no significant differences in tachycardia cycle length between those who developed syncope with tachycardia and those who did not. This suggested that syncope caused by decreased blood pressure was not related to tachycardia rate and may have been related to vasomotor factors. Huikuri and associates[76] demonstrated that some patients developed significant slowing of sinus rate during unstable ventricular tachycardia. Although there were several possible explanations for this observation, one is that the slowing was due to heightened vagal activity, suggesting that the hemodynamic instability of the ventricular tachycardia may be mediated by a reflex mechanism. It is also interesting to note that atrial fibrillation can occur as a consequence of VVS. Leitch and associates[77] reported on three patients in whom VVS, clinical syncope, and atrial fibrillation all were intimately related. During HUT-induced VVS, atrial fibrillation occurred spontaneously in two patients. The third patient had clinical atrial fibrillation after syncope and had a positive HUT test without atrial fibrillation. It is speculated that atrial fibrillation develops during VVS from marked vagal-induced alternation and nonuniformity of atrial refractoriness.

Despite these and many other studies, the ventricular mechanism proposed for provocation of the VVS reflex was significantly challenged by the report of Scherrer and colleagues[78]. These investigators reported a cardiac transplant patient who had an apparent VVS reaction while being infused intravenously with nitroprusside (Fig. 21–5). Theoretically, cardiac denervation after cardiac transplantation should have prevented the induction of VVS by eliminating left ventricular mechanoreceptors from the reflex arc. Higher CNS centers could have precipitated VVS through pain or fear, but this patient had neither. Similar results were reported by Fitzpatrick and coworkers[79] in which 7 of 10 patients with cardiac transplantation developed vasovagal reactions while undergoing HUT with saddle support. Three of these seven patients had donor heart bradycardia during VVS, suggesting cardiac vagal efferent reinnervation. These observations have yet to be explained and suggest alternative activation mechanisms for VVS.

CLINICAL CHARACTERISTICS OF VASOVAGAL SYNCOPE

Persons experiencing a typical episode of VVS can almost always identify a precipitating stimulus (e.g., venipuncture, hot room, prolonged standing) and a prodrome (nausea, anx-

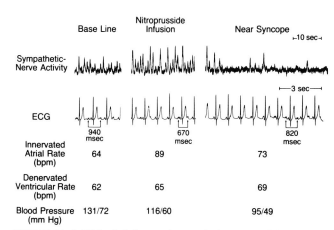

FIGURE 21–5. ECG, vital signs, and sympathetic nerve activity recording of 41-year-old heart transplant recipient who demonstrated a vasovagal response during infusion of vasodilator. Note significant attenuation of sympathetic nerve activity during near syncope and hypotension, challenging the concept that VVS induction requires intact neural connections to left ventricular mechanoreceptors. (Reprinted by permission of Scherrer V, Vissing S, Morgan BJ, et al: Vasovagal syncope after infusion of a vasodilator in a heart transplant recipient. The New England Journal of Medicine 322:602, 1990.)

iety, diaphoresis) before the faint. Common settings that may encourage the development of VVS include churches, restaurants, and dental offices. It is interesting to note that patients with a propensity for VVS frequently are susceptible to motion sickness, a phenomenon that may be related. Also, patients with VVS occasionally report that family members are similarly affected. It is not uncommon after the first episode of VVS for subsequent episodes to cluster and occur frequently. We have observed that emotional stress in patients' lives (e.g., business or marital stress) may greatly contribute to the initiation of syncopal recurrences. Female patients frequently report an association between episodes of syncope and the menstrual cycle, suggesting a relation to blood volume or endocrine influences.[66] In general, most episodes of VVS have a slow onset, with a recognized prodrome that allows the patient to remove himself or herself from harm's way. It has been said that patients with VVS "crumple" or slump to the ground instead of falling. Therefore, fractures related to VVS are uncommon. However, fractures and other severe injuries can occur, especially with the malignant form of VVS. Head injury can be particularly ominous and can result in concussions, lacerations, and postconcussion syndromes.

Spontaneous episodes of VVS and those provoked by HUT share many similar characteristics. While unconscious, which may last for up to 30 to 45 seconds, individuals may be observed to have arm or leg twitching.[80] Because of these tonic movements, it is common for bystanders to report that the victim had a "seizure" with the episode. The tilt test can be useful in differentiating loss of consciousness due to epilepsy from that due to vasovagal syncope.[52, 53] This can be especially true in the pediatric population, in whom episodes of syncope with myoclonic jerking strongly resemble seizures. This myoclonic response is a consequence of cerebral anoxia and is not epileptic in nature. We frequently evaluate children with recurrent loss of consciousness who have been given anticonvulsant medication only to demonstrate a positive HUT. Patients may then have their anticonvulsants discontinued. Electroencephalograms (EEGs) obtained during vasovagal reactions have been well documented and show generalized slowing progressing to electrocerebral silence.[47, 81] These findings are similar to those in syncope resulting from ventricular fibrillation.[82]

A subject awakening from a vasovagal episode is usually pale, drenched in sweat, and may occasionally vomit. It is not uncommon for an individual to have another episode on attempting to stand too rapidly. After awakening from a vasovagal episode, a patient may report fatigue or remain in a "twilight" state for several minutes. This period of transition from loss of consciousness to full consciousness can masquerade as a postictal state and the patient may again be mistakenly diagnosed with seizures.

It has been observed that patients with congestive heart failure demonstrate increased resistance to the provocation of VVS, presumably because of central hypervolemia, decreased cardiac inotropy, elevation of central venous pressures, and attenuation of cardiopulmonary baroreflexes.[58, 83–85]

EVOLUTION OF HEAD-UP TILT IN SYNCOPE OF UNKNOWN ORIGIN

As the modern principles of electrophysiologic testing were disseminated and applied to patients with syncope of undetermined etiology, it became apparent in the early 1980s that a significant percentage of patients remained undiagnosed despite invasive and aggressive diagnostic testing.[86] It was assumed that many of these patients were experiencing reflex forms of syncope for which no good test was available. It was at this time that the HUT test was introduced into electrophysiologic testing. The HUT test, and the equivalent lower body negative pressure, had long been a research tool for the investigation of postural influences on heart rate and blood pressure regulation, particularly in hypertension and orthostatic hypotension induced by medications or autonomic dysfunction.[87] Similarly, the tilt test was instrumental in the evaluation of patients with hypovolemia and patients with the pacemaker syndrome.[43] HUT testing had been used in the late 1970s to assess the hemodynamic impact of upright posture during ventricular tachycardia and supraventricular tachycardia.[88] Despite this long history, use of the tilt test did not mushroom until in the early 1980s, when HUT testing was incorporated in the sphere of electrophysiology and became an integral component in the evaluation of syncope, with a significant literature devoted to subtleties and applications.

METHODOLOGY OF HEAD-UP TILT TESTING

Since our initial description of HUT testing for confirmation of suspected vasovagal syncope in 1985, multiple centers evolved their own tilt protocols.[6, 89–97] Although all are similar in concept, subtle nuances in technique, related to angle and duration of tilt, abound and there is currently no uniform standard. Table 21–5 summarizes some of the reported tilt protocols. It can be seen that marked differences in methodology exist, and a letter and editorial have addressed this lack of uniformity and called for standardization of the HUT test.[98, 99] Our current technique is to perform the tilt after a 6- to 8-hour fast, usually in the morning. The HUT test exploits the potential for VVS reflex by maximizing venous pooling through elimination of the venous return contribution from active leg movement. Therefore, it is imperative to instruct the patient to remain still and especially not to move the legs. Use of the tilt table with a footboard is currently universal, as the tilt table with saddle supports has resulted in an unacceptably high incidence (60%) of positive tests in asymptomatic, normal controls.[100] Many patients may be taking medications that promote VVS reactions, such as nitrates, diuretics, and antihypertensives, and we routinely do not discontinue these medications for extended periods before their initial tilt because these drugs may be culpable for their vasovagal reactions. If the HUT test is positive, we repeat the upright tilt after discontinuation of the medication. We perform noninvasive blood pressure monitoring every minute throughout the test or more frequently, as indicated by surface ECG heart rate monitoring. Photoplethysmography with the Finipress device (Ohmeda, Englewood, CO) can be used to monitor blood pressure continuously and noninvasively.[73] During the tilt test, the light in the room is dimmed and extraneous talking and movement are minimized. Talking by the patient is discouraged except to report symptoms. The tilt test consists of a baseline supine period of approximately 30 minutes, during which baseline vital signs are obtained and intravenous access is established. This interval is followed by upright tilt to 15, 30, and 45 degrees for 2 minutes at each level and then to 60 degrees for 20 minutes. These intermediate degree steps were incorporated during early days of tilt testing to avoid profound orthostatic hypotension in patients undergoing HUT for autonomic insufficiency and were also used to grade the severity of orthostatic cardiovascular dysfunction and monitor the response to therapy.[87] Many centers do not utilize these steps, and their role for patients with SUO is probably of limited value, although we occasionally observe patients with VVS at only 15 to 30 degrees of tilt.

TABLE 21–5. HEAD-UP TILT PROTOCOLS

INSTITUTION	INITIAL TILT DURATION (MIN)	TILT ANGLE (DEG)	ISOPROTERENOL	YIELD POSITIVE IN SUO
Cleveland Clinic Foundation	20	60	Use not reported	42
Toronto	15	60	Bolus	50
Minnesota	10–15	80	1, 3, 5 μg/min for 10 min	87
Westminster	30	80	Use not reported	67
Toledo	30	80	1, 2, 3 μg/min for 30 min	60
Calgary	10	80	2 μg/min for 5 min, then 5 μg/min for 5 min	78

We use the following definitions for interpretation of tilt responses. Vasovagal response is defined by abrupt loss of consciousness accompanied by precipitous drops in heart rate and blood pressure. Vasodepressor syncope is defined by abrupt loss of consciousness with isolated drop in blood pressure but essentially preserved normal sinus rhythm. Orthostatic hypotension, although not part of the vasovagal process, is defined by a gradual drop in systolic blood pressure of 30 mm Hg or more or a diastolic drop of 10 mm Hg or more. The normal response to the HUT test is a mild decrease in systolic pressure from 10 to 20 mm Hg, a mild increase in diastolic blood pressure of approximately 10 mm Hg, and a modest increase in the heart rate of 10 beats per minute (bpm).

These additional definitions of abnormal blood pressure response are germane in that a significant number of HUTs performed in our institution are for patients with orthostatic hypotension with a variety of causes. The HUT test can be helpful in following the patient and gauging the beneficial therapeutic effects of medications and other interventions (e.g., support stockings).[101, 102]

Heart rate response during HUT can also be classified as normal, exaggerated, or blunted. Normal chronotropic responses are roughly defined as an increase of heart rate by approximately 10% above resting or by at least 10 bpm. Blunted chronotropic responses, caused by either sick sinus syndrome or negative chronotropic medications (beta-blockers), are defined by an increase of less than that. An exaggerated chronotropic response during HUT is one in which the heart rate response is 20 bpm or greater or 30% above the resting heart rate.[90] Patients who ultimately develop VVS during HUT usually have initially normal vital signs but may show a slow augmented decrease in systolic blood pressure and a heart rate that increases beyond the normal range. This heart rate increase, termed the presyncopal chronotropic response, can be quite exaggerated in some individuals.[103] Sheldon and colleagues[104, 105] described a tool that can be used to quantify nadir heart rate and blood pressure response during the tilt and define a positive test. This is the trough rate-pressure product. In their study, an abnormal tilt response was defined by a symptomatic trough rate-pressure less than or equal to 9000 mm Hg/min. Several centers in collaboration have suggested a classification schema for HUT-induced VVS.[106] In their nomenclature, HUT-induced vasovagal responses were separated into three types based on proportions of the cardioinhibitory and vasodepressor components, as recorded with digital plethysmography. This taxonomy may have practical utility in designing and reporting treatment or research protocols.

Vasovagal responses constitute the majority of positive reactions with the HUT test, while pure vasodepressor responses are probably observed in less than 10% of cases. In general, hypotension, which is universally present during a positive response, is usually observed to precede the bradycardia. ECG recording during spontaneous or HUT-induced episodes of VVS usually demonstrates some degree of bradycardia. Bradycardia may be due to atrial standstill or arrest, sinus bradycardia, AV block, or a junctional escape rhythm. We have seen many patients referred for pacemaker implantation on the basis of Holter recordings of high-degree AV block that were ultimately found to be secondary to vasovagal syncope, or VVS.

In addition to these common definitions, an additional tilt response, called the psychosomatic response, has been proposed by Linzer and coworkers.[107] These patients experience an apparent loss of consciousness during the tilt test but have adequate blood pressure and a normal heart rate.[107] In addition, during tilt-induced psychosomatic syncope, the EEG and cerebral blood flow (determined by transcranial Doppler study) were also normal. This response, although relatively rare, is due to an underlying psychiatric or neurotic disorder. Even more rare is the patient who develops a true seizure while undergoing HUT, and we have occasionally performed simultaneous EEG recording with the tilt to confirm the diagnosis.

Patients frequently report mild nausea, a hot sensation, and hyperventilation as premonitory symptoms before vasovagal reactions. It is not uncommon for patients to begin to yawn as the earliest sign. Occasionally, quizzing the patient with directed questioning about symptoms may elicit an episode and expedite the test; however, the impact on sensitivity and specificity of this action is unknown. We usually allow full expression of the vasovagal process (i.e., hypotension with or without bradycardia with syncope) before returning the patient to the supine position. Once the response is initiated it may not always be necessary to have the patient attain complete loss of consciousness in order to diagnose the response with certainty. However, the provocation of syncope may be enlightening and at times reassuring to the patient, providing finality and certainty to the diagnosis.

Much has been made in the past of questioning patients about the similarity between the HUT-induced vasovagal episode and their clinical episodes. Affirmative answers were often felt to lend support to the diagnosis. Although helpful, this practice probably lacks specificity, as provoked episodes of VVS are frequently perceived as being much slower and dissimilar in onset compared with naturally occurring ones. Ultimately, as all forms of syncope originate from decreased cerebral perfusion, any mechanism that produces syncope may feel the same to the patient.

We tend to employ screening tilts early in the diagnostic algorithm for SUO. However, other centers perform the tilts only after a negative electrophysiologic study with venous catheters and arterial line still in place.[91] Although this approach may provide important physiologic information, intravascular instrumentation has been shown to predispose and accelerate the precipitation of VVS.[108] Presumed mechanisms include fear and pain associated with invasive procedures, blood loss or sight of blood, and the length of the procedures required for insertion of venous and arterial lines.

When evaluating patients with SUO, a positive HUT result should rarely be a surprise. Predictors of positive results include normal ECG, absence of structural heart disease, young age, and a large number of spells.[105] Several studies have suggested that positive responses to CSM and ocular compression testing may also be associated with positive HUT results,[52, 109] further evidence for the overlap of neurally mediated syncopes.

ISOPROTERENOL CONTROVERSY

HUT testing may be modified by the simultaneous administration of intravenous isoproterenol, first described by Yao and coworkers.[110, 111] Administration of this beta-agonist can expedite tilt testing and provoke VVS in individuals who have a negative response during standard HUT, thereby increasing tilt testing sensitivity. It is presumed that isoproterenol augments positive tilt responses by enhancing the hemodynamic effects that initiate the Bezold-Jarisch reflex. Isoproterenol produces β_2-mediated peripheral arteriolar vasodilatation, which may act synergistically with HUT-induced sequestration of blood volume in the lower extremities. These effects result in significantly decreased venous return. Isoproterenol β_1-induced increases in myocardial inotropy and chronotropy, together with central hypovolemia, enhance the distortion and stimulate left ventricular mechanoreceptors that are thought to initiate VVS. Multiple HUT protocols have been described for isoproterenol administration, including both bolus and continuous intravenous administration.[51, 91, 104, 105, 112]

HUT testing with isoproterenol is currently a widely utilized diagnostic modality for the evaluation of syncope and many centers have adopted the protocol of the Minnesota group.[91] The Minnesota protocol consists of initiation of serial graded isoproterenol infusions of 1, 3, and 5 µg/min for 10 minutes each at 60 degrees of upright tilt with 5 minutes supine in between. Upward titration of isoproterenol is stopped if the patient develops limiting, nonsyncopal symptoms (angina, nausea, anxiety) or the heart rate reaches 140 to 150 bpm. Other centers have continued to perform their tilt testing without isoproterenol, usually with more prolonged tilts up to 45 minutes.[92] The concern about isoproterenol is that it may provoke vasovagal reactions in anyone, and this could produce a false-positive result. This hypothesis was tested in a study by Kapoor and Brant.[113] In their study, 40 control subjects and 20 patients with SUO underwent HUT protocols similar to those previously described. A positive response to HUT with isoproterenol occurred in 65% of syncope patients, which is consistent with widely reported results. However, identical HUT testing with isoproterenol resulted in positive responses in 50% of normal, control subjects. The tilt protocol used by Kapoor and Brant with the two groups was probably somewhat aggressive; isoproterenol was titrated rapidly upward in dose from 1 to 5 µg/min while the subject was upright on the tilt table after a negative 15-minute tilt. Thus, the return to the supine position after the regular tilt or between isoproterenol dose increments was eliminated and might have been more effective in precipitating a vasovagal reaction. The investigators, recognizing this possibility, performed a tilt test with an isoproterenol protocol similar to the Minnesota protocol in an additional group of control subjects and observed a 25% false-positive rate. Because of these observations, Kapoor and Brant labeled the head-up tilt with isoproterenol a nonspecific test.

In addition to the foregoing concerns regarding isoproterenol use, there is legitimate concern that the introduction of isoproterenol may increase complications with the otherwise benign HUT test. It is theoretically possible that use of isoproterenol in patients with unrecognized critical coronary artery disease may precipitate myocardial infarction or provoke malignant ventricular arrhythmias.

Despite these limitations, multiple studies have shown that isoproterenol has a role in the evaluation of patients with undiagnosed syncope. Further refinements in testing may verify its utility. Isoproterenol can greatly expedite the provocation of positive responses in susceptible patients. This pragmatic consideration can be important in busy electro-physiology laboratories where tilts are performed. Intravenous nitroglycerin has been proposed as an additional pharmacologic agent for provocation of VVS during HUT testing. Raviele and associates[114] reported 53% positive HUT responses in patients with undiagnosed syncope and a previous negative tilt and 5% positive responses in control subjects during graded, successive infusions of nitroglycerin. This approach may avoid some of the pitfalls of intravenous isoproterenol but may have other limitations, because nitroglycerin is a strong venodilator.

ASYSTOLE AND MALIGNANT VASOVAGAL SYNCOPE

One of the most dramatic aspects of vasovagal syncope is the occasional patient who develops prolonged asystole during vasovagal syncope either spontaneously or while undergoing the tilt test.[115] Several authors have commented on the incidence and implications of these unusual responses. Maloney and colleagues[47] reported a young patient who developed 73 seconds of ventricular asystole provoked by the tilt, from which he fully recovered (Fig. 21–6). Subsequent therapy with a DDD pacemaker prevented asystole but failed to prevent HUT-induced vasodepressor response with syncope. Such dramatic asystolic responses suggest an extreme form of VVS. It has been suggested that such extreme asystolic reactions to VVS, when superimposed on coexisting critical coronary or cerebral vascular disease, could result in death in susceptible individuals.[116] Sudden cardiac death in the past has been called irreversible syncope.[116] Milstein and colleagues[5] examined this relationship by performing the HUT test in six survivors of suspected asystolic sudden cardiac arrest. All six demonstrated vasovagal reactions during upright tilt, suggesting that some survivors of sudden cardiac death may succumb to this extreme form of VVS.

To investigate whether tilt-induced asystolic responses were associated with a poor prognosis, Brignole and coworkers[117] followed 28 patients with HUT-induced asystole (mean, 7.5 ± 5.9 seconds; range, 3 to 21 seconds). Compared with a control group of patients with positive tilt without asystole, patients with asystole had a higher incidence of ECG abnormalities, sinus node dysfunction, and CSH. In contrast, both groups had similar rates of syncope recurrence. These results suggested that asystole during HUT was not associated with a poorer prognosis and that the presence of associated underlying cardiac abnormalities may be responsible for the precipitation of asystolic responses.

Although asystolic responses of short duration are frequent (8 to 10 seconds), especially in pediatric or young adolescents, we have also observed some remarkably long asystolic pauses of 20 to 73 seconds in our tilt patients (Fig. 21–7). All patients had 100% recovery, rarely requiring temporary cardiopulmonary resuscitation or intravenous atropine.

It is for the patients with prolonged asystole during VVS that pacemaker therapy may be most tempting. However, patients may still experience recurrent vasodepressor episodes despite AV sequential pacing. At least, before proceeding with pacemaker implantation, the amenability to aborting VVS with pacing should be established with temporary pacing in the electrophysiology laboratory. This is discussed in further detail in the treatment section.

Prolonged episodes of asystole provoked by HUT have

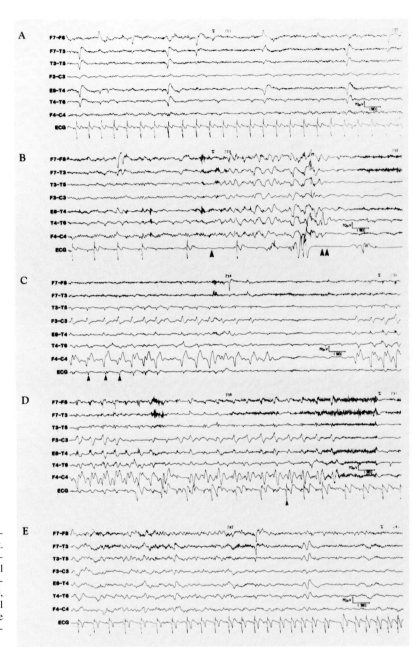

FIGURE 21–6. EEG and ECG (bottom trace) of 39-year-old patient with unexplained syncope during head-up tilt. *A*, Normal EEG and ECG. *B*, Heart block, ventricular asystole, EEG slowing. *C*, Continued asystole, electrocerebral silence during cardiopulmonary resuscitation. *D* and *E*, Recovery. Total asystole was 73 seconds. (From Maloney JD, Jaeger FJ, Fouad-Tarazi FM, et al: Malignant vasovagal syncope: Prolonged asystole provoked by head-up tilt: Case report and review of diagnosis, pathophysiology and therapy. Cleve Clin J Med 55:543, 1988.)

not been universally reported among the centers performing HUT. The origin of these episodes may be related more to the HUT protocol method than to the population of patients. The rate of descent of the tilt table may be important in normalization of blood pressure and heart rate once the VVS spell is initiated. Failure to lower the table quickly (as with motorized tables) may prevent termination of the massive vagal discharge. In our laboratories, the tilt table descent time from 60 degrees to a supine position ranges from 9 to 40 seconds. Others[50] report approximately 15 seconds descent time and still others report that HUT can be terminated immediately with manual descent. In addition, intravenous isoproterenol is widely used during HUT and may prevent some patients from developing extreme bradycardia or asystole during VVS episodes.

SENSITIVITY AND SPECIFICITY OF HEAD-UP TILT TESTING

Despite the many variations of the tilt protocol (tilt duration, angle, and type and dose of isoproterenol) the HUT appears to be moderately sensitive and reasonably specific, especially when compared with other tests performed for syncope. Reported values for sensitivity are approximately 57% to 80% and specificity has been reported to be 80% to 90%.[91, 118] Excluding the article by Kapoor and Brant,[113] the false-positive rate for the HUT is in the range of 10% to 20%. The tendency toward a positive tilt may be age related. Fouad and colleagues[118] reported that normal children and teenagers (mean age, 16 ± 2 years, n = 18) had a 17% positive response during HUT without isoproterenol. Sug-

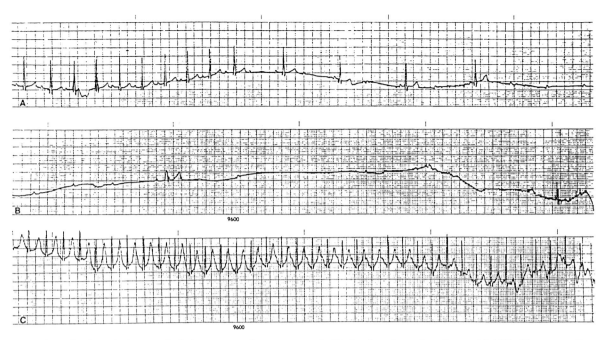

FIGURE 21–7. Example of ventricular asystole during a vasovagal response provoked by head-up tilt test in an 8-year-old child with syncope of unexplained etiology. *A*, Onset of VVS with AV block at 11 minutes of head-up tilt. *B*, Ventricular asystole during VVS. *C*, Resumption of sinus rhythm after return to supine position and administration of IV atropine with complete recovery. (From Jaeger FJ, Schneider L, Maloney JD, et al: Vasovagal syncope: Diagnostic role of head-up tilt test in patients with positive ocular compression test. PACE 13:1416, 1990.)

gested reasons include a possible immature autonomic nervous system or a heightened vagal state.

LIMITATIONS OF HEAD-UP TILT TESTING

HEAD-UP TILT REPRODUCIBILITY

As the clinical utility of HUT has been verified for patients with unexplained syncope, other ancillary issues of tilt methodology and interpretation have come under greater scrutiny. One of these issues is the concept of HUT reproducibility. Reproducibility is generally defined by the ability to demonstrate the same qualitative response, VVS, in subsequent HUT tests. The vast majority of vasovagal episodes that are observed appear to be of the mixed type, vasodepression with a component of cardiac deceleration, and it appears that the type of positive response in HUT is reasonably reproducible. That is, patients usually consistently demonstrate the same type of response to repeated tilts, such as always pure vasodepression or always mixed type. Quantitative differences, such as time of onset of VVS, heart rate, and blood pressure changes, have not been well standardized. The ability to reliably reproduce a positive response to repeated HUT tests is paramount in assessing the therapeutic efficacy of pharmacologic and pacing interventions. We have anecdotally observed over the years that a positive tilt can usually be reproduced on the same day of testing. It was assumed that after a positive vasovagal response, augmented vagal tone might predispose a patient to subsequent positive reactions. However, only recently has the reproducibility of both positive and negative HUT responses been examined in a prospective manner. Chen and associates[119] reported 80% concordance for positive tilt responses and 100% concordance

for negative tilt responses in patients undergoing two tilt tests in the same day separated by approximately 30 minutes. Similarly, Fish and colleagues[120] observed that a positive tilt response was reproducible in 67% of patients undergoing repeated tilt after previous initially positive tilt. Others have examined the reproducibility of HUT at longer intertilt time intervals. Sheldon and colleagues[104] examined the reproducibility of HUT utilizing a modified isoproterenol protocol with 46 patients. Repeated tilt tests were performed from 1 to 6 weeks on 26 patients experiencing syncope or presyncope on their initial tilt. Similar responses were provoked by repeated tilt in 23 patients (88%). Of the 20 patients with initial negative tilts, 85% remained asymptomatic when retested. Sheldon concluded that symptom outcomes and HUT variables (time to syncope, hemodynamic profile) are reproducible within 1 to 6 weeks. In contrast, some studies have failed to demonstrate adequate reproducibility. De Buitleir and coworkers[121] examined the immediate reproducibility of the HUT test in 19 patients with SUO. These investigators reported in general 77% immediate reproducibility of tilt results (5 minutes between tests). It was worrisome that an initially positive HUT result had only a 57% chance of being positive on immediate retest. This has important implications about potential limitations of assessing therapeutic efficacy both immediately and during follow-up.

No study has yet examined the reproducibility of HUT testing over much longer time periods, months or years. However, the observation that HUT testing is at least as reproducible as programmed ventricular simulation for ventricular tachycardia has many important clinical implications. First, acceptable reproducibility of positive tests is necessary to adequately assess the impact or efficacy of any therapeutic intervention. If the level of nonreproducibility was extraordinarily high, the therapeutic efficacy of any intervention (pacing, medications, or placebo) would be seriously overestimated. Second, ensuring a fair degree of reproducibility of HUT results would allow selection of patients for clinical investigation of hemodynamic, autonomic, and pathophysiologic determinants of VVS.

It is interesting to speculate about the mechanism by which 10% to 20% of previously HUT-positive patients become nonprovokable. The answer may lie in the HUT itself. It has been observed that subjects who succumb to hypotension and bradycardia during lower body negative pressure can be made more resistant to these responses by serial applications of presyncopal lower body negative pressure.[122] In this way, the stimulus becomes the treatment and allows adaptation, either physiologic or psychologic, to the repeated stimulus. HUT testing and lower body negative pressure are physiologically similar and induce vasovagal reactions by similar mechanisms, that is, sequestration of blood volume in noncardiac structures with resultant central hypovolemia and triggering of the Bezold-Jarisch reflex.[123, 124] Therefore, it is conceivable that repeated HUT testing may cause adaptation and prevention of VVS. This hypothesis has yet to be confirmed.

COMPLICATIONS AND CONTRAINDICATIONS OF HEAD-UP TILT

The HUT test is exceedingly safe, although we have observed rare complications such as prolonged asystole. We have initiated transient cardiopulmonary resuscitation in several patients with prolonged asystole and have used intravenous atropine on many occasions. Despite this, all patients invariably recovered fairly rapidly without any permanent untoward sequelae. Other complications include transient angina pectoris, particularly with isoproterenol. Therefore, as previously mentioned, patients with angina pectoris should probably not receive isoproterenol. We and others[77, 121] have also observed atrial fibrillation provoked with HUT and isoproterenol. In several thousand tilts performed over approximately 10 years at our institution, no patient has developed a permanent cardiovascular complication after HUT, although one patient may have developed a temporary focal neurologic deficit, consistent with a TIA, after demonstration of severe orthostatic hypotension on the HUT.

HEMODYNAMIC CONSIDERATIONS

The HUT test may be used to demonstrate and confirm VVS as the cause of SUO, but it provides little insight into the predisposing pathophysiologic mechanisms. In conjunction with the HUT test, we routinely investigate hemodynamic reflexes in patients with abnormal tilt responses. We have found that many patients with abnormal vasovagal responses have low intravascular blood volume or abnormalities in blood volume distribution during an upright or tilted posture.[90] These findings have also been confirmed by other centers.[125] To determine blood volume we use the radionuclide-labeled iodinated albumin technique. Excessive venous pooling is assessed by the radionuclide hemodynamic tilt test, in which serial injections of technetium 99m are administered with the patient in supine and sitting positions while undergoing radionuclide ventriculography.[90] We can then calculate the cardiac output, stroke volume, peripheral resistance, and degree of venous pooling. These "snapshots" of the patient's response to postural stress can provide useful clues on which to base therapy.

TREATMENT FOR VASOVAGAL SYNCOPE

GENERAL APPROACH

In general, most cases of VVS do not require therapy. The diagnosis can be suggested by the history and confirmed by HUT test. Patients can then be reassured about the benign nature of their illness and instructed to avoid situations that precipitate the event. The patient can be taught how to recognize a impending VVS event and can learn maneuvers to abort it. Assuming a supine position with the legs elevated and moving and rigorous repetitive coughing can be effective in stopping syncope.

For recurrent cases of VVS other treatment options may be necessary. Approaches such as use of support stockings (Jobst, Toledo, OH) or increased salt intake have historically been helpful, particularly if excessive venous pooling or hypovolemia has been demonstrated.

PACING FOR VASOVAGAL SYNCOPE

In contrast to cardioinhibitory CSS, in which permanent pacing is well established for preventing syncopal recurrences, no specific guidelines exist for the role of permanent pacing in preventing or reducing the frequency or ameliorating the effects of VVS. In the most recent American College of Cardiology and American Heart Association permanent pacemaker implantation guidelines, pacemakers for vasovagal syncope were given a class II indication and required preimplantation confirmation of benefit during a repeated tilt test with temporary pacing.[126] Few studies have examined the role of permanent pacing, and no study has examined permanent pacing in a prospective, randomized fashion. Despite this, permanent pacing could theoretically play an important role in preventing VVS, particularly if episodes are accompanied by marked bradycardia or prolonged asystole. Episodes of syncope that are partially or wholly due to a significant vasodepressor component would be expected to show little or no benefit with permanent pacing.

Sapire and coworkers[127] reported on several children who required permanent pacing for episodes of recurrent VVS. Kenny and colleagues,[92] in the initial report of pacing efficiency in adults, found that seven patients with SUO and a positive HUT test remained asymptomatic after dual-chamber pacing during a mean follow-up of 10 months.

In a further study from the same center, seven patients with syncope and tilt-provokable malignant VVS underwent detailed hemodynamic assessment to determine the effect of temporary pacing.[128] Measurements of cardiac index and mean arterial pressure were obtained during two different episodes of tilt-induced VVS, one with temporary DVI pacing and one without. Rate hysteresis of the temporary pacing system was simulated by initiating DVI pacing at 20 bpm above the resting sinus rate at the onset of VVS. All seven patients demonstrated VVS on both HUT tests. Six developed syncope during HUT and one patient developed VVS without syncope during both tests. Complete loss of consciousness during a vasovagal response was aborted by pacing in five of the remaining six, allowing the return to a supine position. In all patients, blood pressure and cardiac index were significantly improved, although only transiently, during vasovagal reactions with temporary AV sequential pacing (Fig. 21–8). However, all patients eventually required return to a supine position because of hypotension, albeit much slower in onset. Nonetheless, it is apparent from this superb study that improvement in some patients can be attained with pacing. The authors recommended DDI as an alternative to prevent atrial competition with DVI and to eliminate the possibility of pacemaker-mediated tachycardia with DDD.

In patients with VVS for whom pacemaker therapy is contemplated, the ideal approach involves characterization of the HUT response and amenability to pacer termination with temporary AV pacing.[129, 130] This is the approach reported by McGuinn and coworkers,[129] in which five patients with clinical VVS underwent HUT with temporary atrial and ventricular pacing leads in place. At the onset of VVS, pacing commenced at a rate chosen to maximize hemodynamics. Temporary pacing suppressed VVS induction in three patients. Two of these three subsequently underwent permanent pacemaker implantation with normalization to tilt on retesting.

Most trials of temporary or permanent pacemakers for VVS have used higher pacing rates, which begin before or during the episode. Interestingly, high cardiac pacing rates may marginally compensate for VVS hypotension by providing enough minimal cardiac output to the brain to prevent loss of consciousness. This approach is analogous to the proposed use of rapid atrial pacing for orthostatic hypotension.[131]

In contrast, Sra and coworkers[132] were unable to demonstrate efficacy of temporary pacing in 20 of 22 patients with VVS in whom tilt provoked bradycardia, AV block, or asystole. Twenty patients with normal sinus rhythm were temporarily AV sequentially paced and two in atrial fibrillation were ventricularly paced at 20% higher than resting supine heart rate while undergoing a repeated HUT. Although there was modest improvement in mean arterial pressure (37 ± 14 vs. 57 ± 19 mm Hg) during pacing, 20 of 22 patients still developed symptoms of syncope or presyncope.[132]

Multiple case reports have described the failure of pacing as a sole therapeutic intervention in aborting VVS on subsequent tilts.[47, 133] Although maintenance of AV synchrony may not prevent VVS episodes, some patients, particularly those with malignant VVS and prolonged asystole, may experience milder episodes. The prodrome may be lengthened or lessened and allow time for the patient to assume a supine position or self-administer a medication.

Therefore, although permanent pacing may have an as yet poorly defined role for patients with recurrent VVS attacks, it may be indicated for some patients with marked or dramatic asystole or bradycardia accompanying their episodes, optimally if confirmed by testing with temporary pacing. Patients with occupations in which VVS may be particularly hazardous, such as steelworkers, truck drivers, and pilots, may also be appropriate candidates for aggressive therapy including pacing. Initial descriptions of pacemakers with novel features such as positive rate hysteresis and search hysteresis show promise, but further work is required. Higher pacing rates can be achieved by utilization of the search options in the hysteresis mode. These options allow initiation of higher pacing rates when needed but with periodic checking for return of intrinsic rhythm at much lower rates. Previously, hysteresis modes always paced at the pacing rate and stopped pacing when the patient's intrinsic rate exceeded the pacing rate. Perhaps these features, together with new sensors that could detect an impending episode of VVS, would characterize the ultimate device. Sensors, such as for O_2 saturation, dP/dt, QT interval,[134] temperature,[135] or spectral analysis of heart rate,[136] could allow pacing to begin earlier in the VVS prodrome, preventing full-blown symptoms. Oxygen saturation sensors could monitor saturation of venous blood during VVS and could be indicators of impending syncope. Many of these approaches are being explored.

PHARMACOLOGIC THERAPY FOR VASOVAGAL SYNCOPE

In more severe cases of recurrent VVS, a variety of vasoactive pharmacologic agents have been proposed. Traditionally, anticholinergics such as hyoscyamine (Levsin), methscopolamine (Pamine), propantheline bromide (Pro-Banthine), glycopyrrolate, atropine (oral or sublingual [no longer available]), and others have been used, although most with limited success. Transdermal scopolamine has had beneficial effects; however, chronic use appears to be limited because of side effects such as skin rash and visual disturbances.[137] In the past, oral theophylline demonstrated efficacy in suppression of syncope resulting from recurrent pediatric bradycardia, presumed to be vagally mediated.[138] Theophylline has been reassessed in adults with vasodepressor (vasovagal) syncope.[139] Of 17 patients with clinical syncope and a previous positive HUT test, 82% treated with oral theophylline were tilt negative in a subsequent rechallenge. Although many patients taking oral theophylline remained syncope free during follow-up, a significant proportion discontinued the medication because of side effects or intolerances. Therefore, theophylline is another agent that has reasonable efficacy.

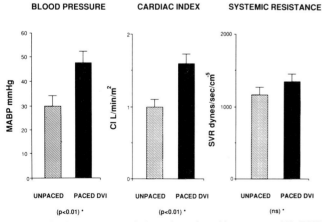

BLOOD PRESSURE   **CARDIAC INDEX**   **SYSTEMIC RESISTANCE**

FIGURE 21–8. Improvement in hemodynamics with temporary AV (DVI) pacing during vasovagal syncope. DVI pacing with stimulated rate hysteresis significantly increased blood pressure and cardiac index compared with unpaced patients, aborting syncope in five of six patients. MABP, mean arterial blood pressure. (From Fitzpatrick A, Theodorakis G, Ahmed R, et al: Dual-chamber pacing aborts vasovagal syncope induced by head-up 60 degree tilt. PACE 14:13, 1991.)

The proposed mechanism by which theophylline may exert its effects is by adenosine receptor blockade. An important role of adenosine in the genesis of VVS was suggested by the demonstration that pharmacologic doses of adenosine (20 mg) could induce a vasovagal-like reaction in susceptible individuals.[140] The Minnesota group described the use of disopyramide and beta-blockers for suppression of VVS. Disopyramide may work because of its unique anticholinergic and negative inotropic activity.[141] However, use of disopyramide can be limited because of anticholingeric side effects, as well as legitimate concerns over proarrhythmia. Negative chronotropic and inotropic effects may be the mechanism by which beta-blockers can prevent VVS.[91, 142] In addition, beta-blockade may leave the peripheral alpha receptors relatively unopposed, facilitating vasoconstriction and preventing vasodilatation. Beta-blocker efficacy can be tested at the time of the initial tilt by using intravenous esmolol. Sra and associates[143] reported that success with oral metoprolol was predicted in patients with initial positive tilt tests who were then subsequently negative on tilt retest during IV esmolol. An important caveat concerning the use of beta-blockade for the prevention of VVS was proposed by Dangovian and coworkers.[144] They reported a patient with VVS who developed prolonged asystole with HUT only when treated with oral metoprolol. Their assumption was that although beta-blockade may be effective in prophylaxis against VVS, breakthrough recurrences may be accompanied by de novo asystolic responses. Essentially, mild VVS may then be converted to the malignant variety. However, this observation requires further study and has not been reported from other centers.

Finally, antidepressant medications such as sertraline hydrochloride (Zoloft) and fluoxetine HCl (Prozac) have had some empirical success in preventing vasovagal episodes (Grubb BP, personal communication, April 1994). Presumably their prophylactic action is in the CNS, possibly involving serotonin antagonism.

Carotid Sinus Syndrome and Vasovagal Syncope: Relationship to Sick Sinus Syndrome

A CLINICAL SPECTRUM

Although sick sinus syndrome, CSS, and VVS are distinct clinical entities, it has been suspected that these disorders may have considerable overlap and common etiologies related to underlying dysfunction of the autonomic nervous system. Brignole and colleagues[145] performed CSM and HUT for 35 patients with syncope attributed to sick sinus syndrome. The syndrome was defined by persistent bradycardia, abnormal intrinsic heart rate after pharmacologic autonomic blockade, or prolonged corrected sinus node recovery time. A remarkably high percentage (80%) of these patients had abnormal responses to CSM or HUT.[145] This finding strongly suggests that abnormal cardiac neural regulation may contribute in many cases to sick sinus syndrome. These observations may also explain the failure of lower ancillary intrinsic cardiac pacemakers to discharge during periods of asystole in the tachycardia-bradycardia syndrome, possibly because of inappropriately enhanced vagal cardiac inhibition. These authors observed predominant vasodepressor re-

sponses to HUT or CSM in only 11% of patients with SSS.[145] This is consistent with the observation that the majority of patients with syncope and SSS have no recurrences after implantation of permanent pacemakers.

When syncope does recur in paced patients with SSS, it is frequently related to blood pressure dysregulation. Sgarbossa and colleagues[146] evaluated etiologies of syncope in 507 patients with sick sinus syndrome who received permanent pacemakers. Of these, 44 (9%) experienced syncopal spells during follow-up of 62 ± 38 months. Syncope was ascribed to orthostatic hypotension in 26% and VVS in 18%. Janosik and colleagues[147] also found tilt-induced vasodepressor syncope to be the most common etiology of syncope after permanent pacemaker implantation.

In contrast, Morley and associates[148] found few positive responses to CSM in patients with sick sinus syndrome.[149] Also, follow-up of a group of paced patients with CSS did not disclose emergence of sick sinus syndrome, supporting the concept that CSS is a separate entity and does not evolve or progress to manifest sick sinus syndrome.

Certainly, the presence of extrinsic neural dysregulation can affect intrinsic dysfunction of the sinus node. In dogs, supersensitivity to acetylcholine can be demonstrated in denervated SA node and AV node receptors, supporting the synergism.[149] In the extreme, VVS can be viewed as a form of extrinsic sick sinus syndrome, in contrast to the usual intrinsic variety. These syndromes overlap significantly with the electrophysiologic entity of hypervagotonia in which early AV node Wenckebach period, prolonged AV node effective refractory period, and sinus bradycardia can be corrected with intravenous atropine or other anticholinergics.[150] This tendency toward vagally induced heart block, ventricular asystole, and sinus arrest can also be evaluated using HUT, CSM, and ocular compression. Oddone and colleagues[151] evaluated 10 patients with syncope and these abnormalities on Holter monitoring. Patients had normal electrophysiologic studies and a high prevalence of positive responses to the vagal tests. Treatment with permanent pacing generally resulted in resolution of syncope. The possible relationship between this form of VVS and malignant VVS previously discussed is still uncertain.

Conclusion

In patients with well-documented symptomatic CSH and recurrent syncope (hence CSS), permanent pacemaker implantation is warranted and is associated with resolution of episodes. In contrast, permanent pacing for VVS has not been shown to be universally efficacious. Other interventions, particularly beta-blockers, should be first-line therapies. Permanent pacing should be resorted to only in recalcitrant cases with a demonstrated pronounced cardioinhibitory component. Amenability of permanent pacing to lessen the severity or frequency of VSS episodes should ideally be tested during temporary AV sequential pacing.

REFERENCES

1. Jaeger FJ, Maloney JD, Fouad-Tarazi FM: Newer aspects in the diagnosis and management of syncope. *In* Rappaport E (ed): Cardiology Update 1990. New York, Elsevier 1990, pp 141–173.

2. Benditt DG, Remole S, Milstein S, et al: Syncope: Causes, clinical evaluation and current therapy. Annu Rev Med 43:283, 1992.

3. Schaal SF, Nelson SD, Boudoulas H, et al: Syncope. Curr Probl Cardiol 17:205, 1992.

4. Kapoor WN: Diagnostic evaluation of syncope. Am J Med 90:91, 1991.

5. Milstein S, Buetikofer J, Lesser J, et al: Cardiac asystole: A manifestation of neurally mediated hypotension bradycardia. J Am Coll Cardiol 14:1626, 1989.

6. Chen MY, Goldenberg IF, Milstein S, et al: Cardiac electrophysiologic and hemodynamic correlates of neurally mediated syncope. Am J Cardiol 63:66, 1989.

7. Lewis T: A lecture on vasovagal syncope and the carotid sinus mechanism. Br Med J 1:873, 1932.

8. Baron SB, Huang SK: Cough syncope presenting as Mobitz type II atrioventricular block—An electrophysiologic correlation. PACE 10:65, 1987.

9. Choi YS, Kim JJ, Oh BH: Cough syncope caused by sinus arrest in a patient with sick sinus syndrome. PACE 12:883, 1989.

10. Benditt DG, Remole S, Bailin S, et al: Tilt table testing for evaluation of neurally-mediated (cardioneurogenic) syncope: Rationale and proposed protocols. PACE 14:1528, 1991.

11. Strasburg B, Sagie A, Erdman S, et al: Carotid sinus hypersensitivity and the carotid sinus syndrome. Prog Cardiovasc Dis 31:379, 1989.

12. Almquist A, Gornick C, Benson W, et al: Carotid sinus hypersensitivity: Evaluation of the vasodepressor component. Circulation 71:927, 1985.

13. Thomas JE: Hyperactive carotid sinus reflex and carotid sinus syncope. Mayo Clin Proc 44:127, 1969.

14. Volkmann H, Schnerch B, Kühnert H: Diagnostic value of carotid sinus hypersensitivity. PACE 13:2065, 1990.

15. Hartzler GO, Maloney JD: Cardioinhibitory carotid sinus hypersensitivity. Arch Intern Med 137:727, 1977.

16. Weiss S, Baker JP: The carotid sinus reflex in health and disease. Its role in the causation of fainting and convulsions. Medicine (Baltimore) 12:297, 1933.

17. Zee-Cheng CS, Gibbs HR: Pure vasodepressor carotid sinus hypersensitivity. Am J Med 81:1095, 1986.

18. Lown B, Levine SA: The carotid sinus. Clinical value of its stimulation. Circulation 23:766, 1961.

19. Baig MW, Kaye GC, Perrins EJ, et al: Can central neuropeptides be implicated in carotid sinus reflex hypersensitivity? Med Hypotheses 28:255, 1989.

20. Morley CA, Sutton R: Carotid sinus syncope. Int J Cardiol 6:287, 1984.

21. Brown KA, Maloney JD, Smith HC, et al: Carotid sinus reflex in patients undergoing coronary angiography: Relationship of degree and location of coronary artery disease to response to carotid sinus massage. Circulation 62:697, 1980.

22. Teichman SL, Felder SD, Matos JA, et al: The value of electrophysiologic studies in syncope of undetermined origin: Report of 150 cases. Am Heart J 110:469, 1985.

23. Kenny RA, Traynor G: Carotid sinus syndrome—Clinical characteristics in elderly patients. Age Ageing 20:449, 1991.

24. Tulchinsky M, Krasnow SH: Carotid sinus syndrome associated with an occult primary nasopharyngeal carcinoma. Arch Intern Med 148:1217, 1988.

25. Achiron A, Reger A: Carotid sinus syncope induced by an orthodontic appliance. Lancet 2:1339, 1989.

26. Romano M, Spinelli A, Feller S, et al: An unusual cause of carotid sinus syndrome: Multiple symmetric lipomatosis. PACE 15:128, 1992.

27. Solti F, Mogan ST, Renyi-Vamos F, et al: The association of carotid artery stenosis with carotid sinus hypersensitivity. J Cardiovasc Surg 31:693, 1990.

28. Gang ES, Oseran DS, Mandel WJ, et al: Sinus node electrogram in patients with the hypersensitive carotid syndrome. J Am Coll Cardiol 5:1484, 1985.

29. Brignole M, Sartore B, Barra M, et al: Ventricular and dual chamber pacing for treatment of carotid sinus syndrome. PACE 12:582, 1989.

30. Nelson SD, Kou WH, DeBuitleir M, et al: Value of programmed ventricular stimulation in presumed carotid sinus syndrome. Am J Cardiol 60:1073, 1987.

31. Alexander S, Ding WC: Fatal ventricular fibrillation during carotid sinus stimulation. Am J Cardiol 18:289, 1966.

32. Trout HH, Brown LL, Thompson JE: Carotid sinus syndrome: Treatment by carotid sinus denervation. Ann Surg 189:575, 1979.

33. Madigan NP, Flaker GC, Curtis JJ, et al: Carotid sinus hypersensitivity: Beneficial effects of dual-chamber pacing. Am J Cardiol 53:1034, 1984.

34. Stryjer D, Friedensohn A, Schlesinger Z: Ventricular pacing as the preferable mode for long-term pacing in patients with carotid sinus syncope of the cardioinhibitory type. PACE 9:705, 1986.

35. Brignole M, Oddone D, Cogorno S, et al: Long-term outcome in symptomatic carotid sinus hypersensitivity. Am Heart J 123:687, 1992.

36. Katritsis D, Ward DE, Camm AJ: Can we treat carotid sinus syndrome? PACE 14:1367, 1991.

37. Huang SKS, Ezri MD, Hauser RG, et al: Carotid sinus hypersensitivity in patients with unexplained syncope: Clinical, electrophysiologic, and long term follow-up observations. Am Heart J 116:989, 1988.

38. Sugrue DD, Gersh BJ, Holmes DR, et al: Symptomatic ''isolated'' carotid sinus hypersensitivity: Natural history and results of treatment with anticholinergic drugs or pacemaker. J Am Coll Cardiol 7:158, 1986.

39. Morley CA, Perrins EJ, Grant P, et al: Carotid sinus syncope treated by pacing. Br Heart J 47:411, 1982.

40. Brignole M, Menozzi C, Lolli G, et al: Validation of a method for choice of pacing mode in carotid sinus syndrome with or without sinus bradycardia. PACE 14:196, 1991.

41. Brignole M, Menozzi C, Loll G, et al: Natural and unnatural history of patients with severe carotid sinus hypersensitivity: A preliminary study. PACE 11:1678, 1988.

42. Probst P, Muhlberger V, Lederbauer M, et al: Electrophysiologic findings in carotid sinus massage. PACE 6:689, 1983.

43. Alicandri C, Fouad FM, Tarazi RC, et al: Three cases of hypotension and syncope with ventricular pacing: Possible role of atrial reflexes. Am J Cardiol 42:137, 1978.

44. Walter PF, Crawley IS, Dorney ER: Carotid sinus hypersensitivity and syncope. Am J Cardiol 42:396, 1978.

45. Keating EC, Burks JM, Calder JR: Mixed carotid sinus hypersensitivity: Successful therapy with pacing, ephedrine, and propranolol. PACE 8:356, 1985.

46. Brignole M, Menozzi C, Lolli G, et al: Long-term outcome of paced and nonpaced patients with severe carotid sinus syndrome. Am J Cardiol 69:1039, 1992.

47. Maloney JD, Jaeger FJ, Fouad-Tarazi FM, et al: Malignant vasovagal syncope: Prolonged asystole provoked by head-up tilt. Case report and review of diagnosis, pathophysiology and therapy. Cleve Clin J Med 55:543, 1988.

48. Sutton R: Vasovagal syncope—Could it be malignant? Eur JCPE 2:89, 1992.

49. Fitzpatrick AP, Ahmed R, Williams S, et al: A randomized trial of medical therapy in ''malignant vasovagal syndrome'' or ''neurally-mediated bradycardia/hypotension syndrome.'' Eur JCPE 2:99, 1991.

50. Fitzpatrick A, Sutton R: Tilting toward a diagnosis in recurrent unexplained syncope. Lancet 1:658, 1989.

51. Grubb BP, Temesy-Armos P, Moore J, et al: Head-upright tilt-table testing in the evaluation and management of the malignant vasovagal syndrome. Am J Cardiol 69:904, 1992.

52. Jaeger FJ, Schneider L, Maloney JD, et al: Vasovagal syncope: Diagnostic role of head-up tilt test in patients with positive ocular compression test. PACE 13:1416, 1990.

53. Grubb BP, Gerard JG, Roush K, et al: Differentiation of convulsive syncope and epilepsy with head-up tilt testing. Ann Intern Med 115:871, 1991.

54. Fujimura O, Yee R, Klein GJ, et al: The diagnostic sensitivity of electrophysiologic testing in patients with syncope caused by transient bradycardia. N Engl J Med 321:1703, 1989.

55. Weissler AM, Warren JV, Estes EH, et al: Vasodepressor syncope. Factors influencing cardiac output. Circulation 15:875, 1957.

56. Goldstein DS, Spanarkel M, Pitterman A, et al: Circulatory control mechanisms in vasodepressor syncope. Am Heart J 104:1071, 1982.

57. Glick G, Yu PN: Hemodynamic changes during spontaneous vasovagal reactions. Am J Med 34:42, 1963.

58. Van Lieshout JJ, Wieling W, Karemakar JM, et al: The vasovagal response. Clin Sci 81:575, 1991.

59. Oberg B, Thoren P: Increased activity in left A ventricular receptors during hemorrhage or occlusion of caval veins in the cat: A possible cause of the vasovagal reaction. Acta Physiol Scand 85:164, 1972.

60. Mark AL: The Bezold-Jarisch reflex revisited: Clinical implications of inhibitory reflexes originating in the heart. J Am Coll Cardiol 1:90, 1983.

61. Gilligan DM, Nihoyannopoulos P, Chan WL, et al: Investigation of a

hemodynamic basis for syncope in hypertrophic cardiomyopathy. Use of a head-up tilt test. Circulation 85:2140, 1992.

62. Grubb BP, Gerard G, Roush K, et al: Cerebral vasoconstriction during head-upright tilt induced vasovagal syncope. Circulation 84:1157, 1991.

63. Gaffney FA, Nixon JU, Karlsson ES, et al: Cardiovascular deconditioning produced by 20 hours of bedrest with head-down tilt ($-5°$) in middle-aged healthy men. Am J Cardiol 56:634, 1985.

64. Wallin BG, Sundlöf G: Sympathetic outflow to muscles during vasovagal syncope. J Auton Nerv Syst 6:287, 1982.

65. Shalev Y, Gal R, Tchou PJ, et al: Echocardiographic demonstration of decreased left ventricular dimensions and vigorous myocardial contraction during syncope induced by head-up tilt. J Am Coll Cardiol 18:746, 1991.

66. Fitzpatrick A, Williams T, Ahmed R, et al: Echocardiographic and endocrine changes during vasovagal syncope induced by prolonged head-up tilt. Eur JCPE 2:121, 1992.

67. Benditt DG, Betloff B, Bailin S, et al: Exaggerated circulating epinephrine levels during neurally mediated hypotension-bradycardia syndrome: A causal factor or secondary event. PACE 14:661, 1991.

68. Calkins H, Kadish A, Sousa J, et al: Comparison of responses to isoproterenol and epinephrine during head-up tilt in suspected vasodepressor syncope. Am J Cardiol 67:207, 1991.

69. Jaeger FJ, Fouad-Tarazi FM, Bravo EL, et al: Supine norepinephrine levels and vasovagal response during head-up tilt. Circulation 80:II-90, 1989.

70. Waxman MB, Cameron DA, Wald RW: Role of ventricular vagal afferents in the vasovagal reaction. J Am Coll Cardiol 21:1138, 1993.

71. Abboud FM: Neurocardiogenic syncope. N Engl J Med 328:1117, 1993.

72. Semple PF, Thoren P, Lever AF: Vasovagal reactions to cardiovascular drugs: The first dose effect. J Hypertens 6:601, 1988.

73. Sneddon JF, Counihan PJ, Bashir Y, et al: Impaired immediate vasoconstrictor responses in patients with recurrent neurally mediated syncope. Am J Cardiol 71:72, 1993.

74. Okabe M, Gross-Sawicka EM, Fouad FM: Vascular reactivity in patients with vasovagal syncope. Circulation 86:I-460, 1992.

75. Leitch JW, Klein GJ, Yee R, et al: Syncope associated with supraventricular tachycardia. An expression of tachycardia rate or vasomotor response? Circulation 85:1064, 1992.

76. Huikuri HV, Zaman L, Castellanos A, et al: Changes in spontaneous sinus node rate as an estimate of cardiac autonomic tone during stable and unstable ventricular tachycardia. J Am Coll Cardiol 13:646, 1989.

77. Leitch J, Klein G, Tee R, et al: Neurally mediated syncope and atrial fibrillation. N Engl J Med 324:495, 1991.

78. Scherrer V, Vissing S, Morgan BJ, et al: Vasovagal syncope after infusion of a vasodilator in a heart transplant recipient. N Engl J Med 322:602, 1990.

79. Fitzpatrick AP, Banner N, Cheng A, et al: Vasovagal reactions may occur after orthotopic heart transplantation. J Am Coll Cardiol 21:1132, 1993.

80. Schraeder PL, Pontzer R, Engel TR: A case of being scared to death. Arch Intern Med 143:1793, 1983.

81. Grossi D, Buonomo C, Mirizzi F, et al: Electroencephalographic and electrocardiographic features of vasovagal syncope induced by head-up tilt. Funct Neurol 5:257, 1990.

82. Aminoff MJ, Scheinman MM, Griffin JC, et al: Electrocerebral accompaniments of syncope associated with malignant ventricular arrhythmias. Ann Intern Med 108:791, 1988.

83. Sleight P: Cardiac vomiting. Br Heart J 46:5, 1981.

84. Sharpey-Schafer EP: Emergencies in general practice. Syncope. Br Med J 1:506, 1956.

85. Sharpey-Schafer EP, Hayter CJ, Barlow ED: Mechanism of acute hypotension from fear or nausea. Br Med J 2:878, 1958.

86. Kapoor WN, Karpf M, Wicand S, et al: A prospective evaluation and follow-up of patients with syncope. N Engl J Med 309:197, 1983.

87. Tarazi RC, Melsher HJ, Dustan HD, et al: Plasma volume changes with upright tilt: Studies in hypotension and syncope. J Appl Physiol 28:121, 1970.

88. Hammill SC, Holmes DR, Wood DL, et al: Electrophysiologic testing in the upright position: Improved evaluation of patients with rhythm disturbances using a tilt table. J Am Coll Cardiol 4:65, 1984.

89. Abi Samra FM, Maloney JD, Fouad FM, et al: Vasovagal and vasodepressor syncope—Abnormalities in blood-volume and its distribution. Circulation 72:251, 1985.

90. Abi-Samra F, Maloney JD, Fouad-Tarazi FM, et al: The usefulness of head-up tilt testing and hemodynamic investigations in the workup of syncope of unknown origin. PACE 11:1202, 1988.

91. Almquist A, Goldenberg IF, Milstein S, et al: Provocation of bradycardia and hypotension by isoproterenol and upright posture in patients with unexplained syncope. N Engl J Med 320:346, 1989.

92. Kenny RA, Ingram A, Bayliss J, et al: Head-up tilt: A useful test for investigating unexplained syncope. Lancet 1:1352, 1986.

93. Pongiglione G, Fish FA, Strasburger JF: Heart rate and blood pressure response to upright tilt in young patients with unexplained syncope. J Am Coll Cardiol 16:165, 1990.

94. Thilenius OG, Quinones JA, Husayni TS, et al: Tilt test for diagnosis of unexplained syncope in pediatric patients. Pediatrics 87:334, 1991.

95. Raviele A, Gasparini G, DiPede F, et al: Usefulness of head-up tilt test in evaluating patients with syncope of unknown origin and negative electrophysiology study. Am J Cardiol 65:1322, 1990.

96. Sra JS, Anderson AJ, Sheikh SH, et al: Unexplained syncope evaluated by electrophysiology studies and head-up tilt table testing. Ann Intern Med 114:1013, 1991.

97. Strasberg B, Rechavia E, Sagic A, et al: The head up tilt table test in patients with syncope of unknown origin. Am Heart J 118:923, 1989.

98. Cheng TO: Need for standardization of tilt-table test in evaluation of syncope. Am J Cardiol 70:1639, 1992.

99. Kligfield P: Tilt table for the investigation of syncope: There is nothing simple about fainting. J Am Coll Cardiol 17:131, 1991.

100. Fitzpatrick AP, Theodorakis G, Vardas P, et al: Methodology of head-up tilt testing in patients with unexplained syncope. J Am Coll Cardiol 17:125, 1991.

101. Jaeger FJ, Maloney JD, Castle LW, Fouad-Tarazi FM: Is absolute hypovolemia a risk factor for vasovagal response to head-up tilt? PACE 16:743, 1993.

102. Schutzman J, Jaeger F, Maloney JD, et al: Head-up tilt and hemodynamic changes during orthostatic hypotension in patients with supine systolic hypertension. PACE 15:592, 1992.

103. Jaeger FJ, Fouad-Tarazi FM, Maloney JD: Vasovagal syncope: Lack of relationship between baseline blood volume and presyncopal chronotropic orthostatic response. Clin Res 37:880A, 1989.

104. Sheldon R, Splawinski J, Killam S: Reproducibility of isoproterenol tilt-table tests in patients with syncope. Am J Cardiol 69:1300, 1992.

105. Sheldon R, Killam S: Methodology of isoproterenol–tilt table testing in patients with syncope. J Am Coll Cardiol 19:773, 1992.

106. Sutton R, Peterson M, Brignole M, et al: Proposed classification for tilt induced vasovagal syncope. Eur JCPE 3:180, 1992.

107. Linzer M, Varia I, Pontinen M, et al: Medically unexplained syncope: relationship to psychiatric illness. Am J Med 92(1A):18(S), 1992.

108. Stevens PM: Cardiovascular dynamics during orthostasis and the influence of intravascular instrumentation. Am J Cardiol 17:211, 1966.

109. Brignole M, Menozzi C, Gianfranchi L, et al: Carotid sinus massage, eyeball compression, and head-up tilt tests in patients with syncope of uncertain origin and in healthy control subjects. Am Heart J 122:1644, 1991.

110. Yao L, Cameron D, Roseman J, et al: Isoproterenol-induced vasodepressor reaction in men. Clin Invest Med 7:40, 1984.

111. Waxman MB, Yao L, Cameron DA, et al: Isoproterenol induction of vasodepressor-type reaction in vasodepressor-prone persons. Am J Cardiol 63:58, 1989.

112. Grubb BP, Temesy-Armos P, Hahn H, et al: Utility of upright tilt-table testing in the evaluation and management of syncope of unknown origin. Am J Med 90:6, 1991.

113. Kapoor WN, Brant N: Evaluation of syncope by upright tilt testing with isoproterenol. A nonspecific test. Ann Intern Med 116:358, 1992.

114. Raviele A, Gasparini G, DiPede F, et al: Usefulness of nitroglycerin infusion during head-up tilt for the diagnosis of vasovagal syncope. J Am Coll Cardiol 21:111A, 1993.

115. Fleg JL, Asante AUK: Asystole following treadmill exercise in a man without organic heart disease. Arch Intern Med 143:1821, 1983.

116. Engel GL: Psychologic stress, vasodepressor (vasovagal) syncope, and sudden death. Ann Intern Med 89:403, 1978.

117. Brignole M, Menozzi C, Gianfranchi L, et al: The clinical and prognostic significance of the asystolic response during the head-up tilt test. Eur JCPE 2:109, 1992.

118. Fouad FM, Sitthisook S, Vanerio G, et al: Sensitivity and specificity of the tilt table test in young patients with unexplained syncope. PACE 16:394, 1993.

119. Chen XC, Chen MY, Remole S, et al: Reproducibility of head-up tilt table testing for eliciting susceptibility to neurally medicated syncope in patients without structural heart disease. Am J Cardiol 69:755, 1992.

120. Fish FA, Strasburger JF, Benson DW: Reproducibility of a symptomatic response to upright tilt in young patients with unexplained syncope. Am J Cardiol 70:605, 1992.

121. De Buitleir M, Grogan W, Picone MF, et al: Immediate reproducibility of the tilt table test in adults with unexplained syncope. Am J Cardiol 71:304, 1993.

122. Lightfoot JT, Febles JS, Fortney SM: Adaptation to repeated presyncope lower body negative pressure exposures. Aviat Space Environ Med 60:17, 1989.

123. Murray RH, Thompson LJ, Bowers JA, et al: Hemodynamic effects of graded hypovolemia and vasodepressor syncope induced by lower body negative pressure. Am Heart J 76:799, 1968.

124. Epstein SE, Stampfer M, Beiser GD: Role of capacitance and resistance vessels in vasovagal syncope. Circulation 37:524, 1968.

125. Streeten DHP, Anderson GH, Richardson R, et al: Abnormal orthostatic changes in blood pressure and heart rate in subjects with intact sympathetic nervous function: Evidence for excessive venous pooling. J Lab Clin Med 111:326, 1988.

126. Dreifus LS, Fisch C, Griffin JC, et al: Guidelines for implantation of cardiac pacemakers and anti-arrhythmic devices. J Am Coll Cardiol 18:1, 1991.

127. Sapire DW, Casta A, Safley W, et al: Vasovagal syncope in children requiring pacemaker implantation. Am Heart J 106:1406, 1983.

128. Fitzpatrick A, Theodorakis G, Ahmed R, et al: Dual chamber pacing aborts vasovagal syncope induced by head-up 60° tilt. PACE 13:13, 1991.

129. McGuinn WP, Wilkoff BL, Maloney JD, et al: Treatment of autonomically mediated syncope with rapid AV sequential pacing on demand. J Am Coll Cardiol 17:271A, 1991.

130. McGuinn P, Moore S, Edel T, et al: Temporary dual-chamber pacing during tilt table testing for vasovagal syncope: A predictor of therapeutic success. PACE 14:734, 1991.

131. Moss AJ, Glanser W, Topol E: Atrial tachypacing in the treatment of a patient with primary orthostatic hypotension. N Engl J Med 302:1456, 1980.

132. Sra JS, Jazayeri MR, Avitall B, et al: Comparison of cardiac pacing with drug therapy in the treatment of neurocardiogenic (vasovagal) syncope with bradycardia or asystole. N Engl J Med 328:1085, 1993.

133. Kus T, Lalonde G, Champlain JD, et al: Vasovagal syncope: Management with atrioventricular sequential pacing and beta-blockade. Can J Cardiol 5:375, 1989.

134. Benditt DG, Yi Z, Hensen R, et al: Seemingly inappropriate QT interval changes during head-up tilt testing: A marker of imminent neurally-mediated syncope. PACE 16:861, 1993.

135. Singer I, Peavler P, Johnson B, et al: Temperature may be an ideal sensor for rate modulation in patients with posture related syncope and chronotropic incompetence. J Am Coll Cardiol 21:426A, 1993.

136. Brum J, Ribeiro M, Ferrario C, et al: Autonomic alterations preceding syncope during head-up tilt. J Am Coll Cardiol 19:75A, 1992.

137. Jaeger FJ, Fouad-Tarazi FM, Abi-Samra F, et al: Transdermal scopolamine for the treatment of vasovagal syncope. Clin Res 35:832A, 1987.

138. Benditt DG, Benson W, Kreitt J, et al: Electrophysiologic effects of theophylline in young patients with recurrent symptomatic bradyarrhythmias. Am J Cardiol 52:1223, 1983.

139. Nelson SD, Stanley M, Love CJ, et al: The autonomic and hemodynamic effects of oral theophylline in patients with vasodepressor syncope. Arch Intern Med 151:2425, 1991.

140. Flammang D, Luisy J, Waynberger M: Re-initiation and quantification of the vaso-vagal syndrome by the adenosine 5′ triphosphate (ATP) test: Assessment of the best therapy. PACE 13:539, 1990.

141. Milstein S, Buetikofer J, Dunnigan A, et al: Usefulness of disopyramide for prevention of upright tilt–induced hypotension-bradycardia. Am J Cardiol 65:1339, 1990.

142. Müller G, Deal BJ, Strasburger JF, et al: Usefulness of metroprolol for unexplained syncope and positive response to tilt testing in young persons. Am J Cardiol 71:592, 1993.

143. Sra JS, Murthy US, Jazayeri MR, et al: Use of intravenous esmolol to predict efficacy of oral beta-adrenergic blocker therapy in patients with neurocardiogenic syncope. J Am Coll Cardiol 19:402, 1992.

144. Dangovian MI, Jarandilla R, Frumin H: Prolonged asystole during head-up tilt table testing after beta blockade. PACE 15:14, 1992.

145. Brignole M, Menozzi C, Gianfranchi L, et al: Neurally mediated syncope detected by carotid sinus massage and head-up tilt test in sick sinus syndrome. Am J Cardiol 68:1032, 1991.

146. Sgarbossa EB, Pinski SL, Jaeger FJ, et al: Incidence and predictors of syncope in paced patients with sick sinus syndrome. PACE 15:2055, 1992.

147. Janosik D, Bjerregaard P, Fredman C, et al: High diagnostic yield of head-up tilt testing in patients with syncope following permanent pacemaker implantation. PACE 14:634, 1991.

148. Morley CA, Perrins EJ, Sutton R: Is there a difference between carotid sinus syndrome and sick sinus syndrome? Eur JCPE 2:62, 1991.

149. Kaseda S, Zipes DP: Vagal denervation of canine sinus and atrioventricular nodes creates supersensitive response to acetylcholine. J Am Coll Cardiol 11:39A, 1988.

150. Rubin DA, Nieminski KE, Woolf P, et al: Selective hypervagotonia isolated to the AV node. PACE 11:1529, 1988.

151. Oddone D, Brignole M, Menozzi C, et al: Spontaneous occurrence of the induced cardio-inhibitory vasovagal reflex. PACE 14:415, 1991.

CHAPTER 22

SPECIAL CLINICAL APPLICATIONS AND NEWER INDICATIONS FOR CARDIAC PACING

Kenneth A. Ellenbogen

In this chapter we review the indications for and role of various pacing modalities in selected groups of patients in whom the indications and role of cardiac pacing are currently evolving. We discuss the role of cardiac pacing in patients with orthotopic heart transplantation, hypertrophic cardiomyopathy, dilated cardiomyopathy, orthostatic hypotension, and the long-QT syndrome. These conditions have in common that cardiac pacing is generally instituted for indications other than treatment of a symptomatic bradyarrhythmia.

Cardiac Transplantation

The Registry of the International Society of Heart Transplantation reported more than 21,000 cardiac transplantation procedures performed in 230 transplantation centers by 1992.[1] The role of cardiac transplantation as treatment for patients with refractory congestive heart failure has rapidly expanded.[2] Currently, the major limitation to more widespread use of transplantation for treatment of heart failure has been the limited availability of donor organs. With the introduction of cyclosporine for the treatment of rejection, survival rates of patients after cardiac transplantation have improved to greater than 65% at 5 years and to 50% at 10 years.

The surgical procedure of orthotopic cardiac transplantation that is widely practiced today consists of retaining a large portion of the posterior wall of the right and left atria of the recipient heart.[3] The donor heart is implanted via a median sternotomy with direct end-to-end anastamoses of the aorta and pulmonary artery. The recipient heart (or remnant

atria) retains its neural innervation. Cardiopulmonary bypass is performed with moderate hypothermia, and the implantation procedure generally takes about 1 hour. Heterotopic transplantation is rarely performed today (<2% of transplants) but involves implanting the donor heart in parallel with the entire recipient heart, with left atrium to left atrium, aorta to aorta, superior vena cava to right atrium, and pulmonary artery to pulmonary artery anastomoses. This results in the donor heart functioning in conjunction with the recipient's heart.

The incidence and type of arrhythmias following cardiac transplantation vary among different studies (Table 22–1). Several large studies deserve comment. The Stanford group reported a 20-year retrospective review of their experience with 556 patients.[4] There were 41 patients (7.4%) who received permanent pacemakers. The predominant indication for pacing was a slow junctional rhythm in 46%, sinus arrest in 27%, and sinus bradycardia in 17% (Fig. 22–1). About 10% of patients had pacemakers implanted because of abnormal atrioventricular (AV) conduction, primarily heart block of various degrees. Sixty-one percent of patients with bradyarrhythmias were asymptomatic and 17% had only mild symptoms such as fatigue. The remaining 22% of patients had severe symptoms, such as syncope or near-syncope. In most patients (73%), the bradycardia was seen in the first 3 to 6 weeks after transplantation. Griffith and colleagues reported on their experience at the University of Pittsburgh with 401 patients who underwent orthotopic heart transplantation.[5] They reported a 17% (72 patients) incidence of bradyarrhythmias—heart rates less than 60 beats per minute (bpm)—by 5 days after transplantation. Only 17 of these

TABLE 22–1. CLINICAL FEATURES OF PATIENTS WITH BRADYARRHYTHMIAS FOLLOWING ORTHOTOPIC TRANSPLANTATION

STUDY	NUMBER OF PATIENTS	MEAN FOLLOW-UP (MO)	INCIDENCE OF BRADYCARDIA (%)	PACEMAKER IMPLANTATION (%)	PREDICTIVE FACTORS
Romhilt et al.[7]	13	30	46	23	
Jacquet et al.[8]	25	24	36	8	Graft ischemic time
Heinz et al.[12]	90	3	44	21	—
Miyamoto et al.[5]	401	18	18	6	Graft ischemic time
DiBiase et al.[4]	556	—	—	7.4	—
Blanche et al.[11]	41	—	—	12.2	Presence of rejection
Montero et al.[9]	52	—	27	11.5	Cardioplegia and organ storage temperature
Scott et al.[6]	154	—	—	11	—
Payne et al.[10]	46	36	—	15	Aortic cross-clamp time
Buja et al.[13]	146	25	14	7	—

patients (4.2% of the total population) had bradycardia lasting for more than 20 days. About one half of these patients were asymptomatic, but all went on to receive permanent pacemakers before hospital discharge. Scott and colleagues[6] from Newcastle upon Tyne reported on their experience with 154 patients, of which 17 (11%) went on to receive permanent pacemakers. Ten patients had sinus node dysfunction and seven experienced AV block. The pacemakers were implanted between 7 and 21 days after transplantation. In several smaller series the incidence of bradyarrhythmias leading to implantation of permanent pacemakers ranges from 8 to 23% (see Table 22–1).[7–12] In the study of Heinz and colleagues,[12] a postoperative heart rate consistently less than 70 bpm was related to a final outcome of permanent pacemaker implantation before initial hospital discharge, but was associated with an unacceptably low sensitivity (61%) and specificity (81%).

Some centers have reported a higher incidence of AV block after orthotopic transplantation. In one series, complete AV block occurred in 21 of 146 patients (14%) within 6 days of surgery.[13] Electrophysiologic studies were performed to determine the site of block. In three patients, AV block was infrahisian and permanent, and in 18 patients block was transient and suprahisian. The mean duration of AV block was 8 days. They implanted permanent pacemakers in 10

patients with persistent AV block or an infranodal site of block (8%).[13] There was no relationship between graft ischemic time, number of patients with rejection, or any other clinical variable and the presence of AV block. Dodinot and colleagues[14] also reported an incidence of heart block of 7%. This experience differs significantly from that of most other centers, where sinus node dysfunction is the major etiology for bradyarrhythmias resulting in pacemaker implantation.

The majority of patients receiving permanent pacemakers after heart transplantation have them placed for sinus node dysfunction. Electrophysiologic abnormalities of the transplanted sinus node have been demonstrated in up to 60% of various subgroups of patients after transplantation. Bexton and colleagues[15] have examined sinus node conduction and sinus node automaticity after transplantation and found the presence of relative bradycardia to be predictive of abnormal invasive electrophysiologic tests of sinus node function. They were able to separate patients into two groups, those with and without abnormal sinus node function. In their patients, abnormalities of sinus node automaticity detected by prolonged sinus node recovery times and/or secondary pauses correlated with abnormalities of sinoatrial conduction as detected by continuous pacing techniques or introduction of extrastimuli during pacing. Jacquet and coworkers[8] reported similar results. They performed serial electrophysiologic studies in a subgroup of 7 of 16 patients with sinus node dysfunction. There was a trend toward improvement in sinus node recovery times over a 3-week period. Heinz and colleagues[16] performed electrophysiologic testing in 42 patients after transplantation and showed that sinus node dysfunction is common but may improve with time. Using the technique of programmed atrial stimulation they demonstrated that sinus node refractoriness in transplant patients is similar to or shorter than that measured in control patients. This implies that most sinus node dysfunction observed in the period following orthotopic transplantation is due to impaired automaticity.

Many groups have tried to determine causes of the sinus node dysfunction seen after transplantation and its frequent improvement (Table 22–2). Two groups have shown a correlation between the presence of persistently abnormal sinus node function and prolonged donor heart ischemic times, and one group has been able to show only a correlation between donor heart ischemic time and early sinus node dysfunction.[5, 8, 16] Others, however, have not been able to correlate sinus node dysfunction with the ischemic time of the donor heart.[4, 6, 9–12, 17]

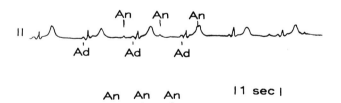

FIGURE 22–1. Limb lead rhythm strips showing rhythm commonly encountered after orthotopic heart transplantation. An is the P wave recorded from recipient (remnant, innervated) atrium and Ad is the P wave recorded from the donor (denervated) atrium. The rate of the donor atrium is about 98 bpm and the rate of the recipient is almost 60 bpm. The bottom tracing is recorded from the patient at a time of sinus node dysfunction. The atrial rate in the recipient atrium is 90 bpm, but the atrial rate of the donor heart is controlled by a junctional rhythm at 23 bpm. Permanent pacing was recommended because of the persistence of marked atrial dysfunction of the donor atrium and a slow junctional rhythm. (From Kacet S, Molin F, Lacroix D, et al: Bipolar atrial-triggered pacing to restore normal chronotropic responsiveness in an orthotopic cardiac transplant patient. PACE 14:1444, 1991.)

TABLE 22–2. PACEMAKER INDICATIONS AND LONG-TERM FOLLOW-UP

STUDY	NUMBER OF PATIENTS	PACEMAKERS IMPLANTED	INDICATIONS	PACEMAKER IMPLANTED PRIOR TO INITIAL DISCHARGE[a] (%)	BRADYCARDIA AT 1 YEAR[b] (%)
DiBiase et al.[4]	556	41 (7%)	SND, 90% AV block, 10%	73	50[c]
Miyamoto et al.[5]	401	23 (6%)	SND, 95% AV block, 5%	74	4
Scott et al.[6]	154	17 (4%)	SND, 59% AV block, 41%	100	21[d]
Payne et al.[10]	46	7 (15%)	SND, 100%	100	86
Heinz et al.[12]	90	19 (21%)	SND, 100%	89	41
Buja et al.[13]	146	12 (8%)	AV block, 100%	83	30

Abbreviation: SND, sinus node dysfunction.

[a]Refers to percent of patients in study population who had early (predischarge) pacemaker implantation compared with patients who had late pacemaker placement.

[b]<60 bpm.

[c]60–90 bpm.

[d]No patient with AV block paced.

Other explanations for the high incidence of bradycardia include surgical technique.[4, 6] Surgical trauma or distortion resulting from the atrial incision may be more likely to result in damage to the donor heart. The technique described by Lower and Shumway[3] includes ligation of the donor superior vena cava 2 cm above the junction of its entry into the atria. This was thought to protect the donor sinus node because it would be above the suture line. Another potential etiology for sinus node dysfunction is related to rejection.[11] Several case reports show a correlation of bradyarrhythmias with the onset of acute, severe rejection early after transplantation.[11, 18] It is hypothesized that acute rejection is associated with the release of adenosine, a potent negative chronotropic and dromotropic agent that may lead to sinus node slowing and AV block. The clinical response, as well as the reversal of electrophysiologic abnormalities in small numbers of patients, to low-dose theophylline (an adenosine antagonist) suggests that this agent may play a role in selected patients.[18] Use of medications that may alter sinus node function (e.g., beta-blockers or calcium channel blockers for post-transplantation hypertension) is another potential cause of sinus node dysfunction, but this is not supported by existing data. Finally, the possibility of damage to the sinus node blood supply by the surgical technique has been suggested. A comparison of coronary angiograms of unselected patients without pacemakers and patients with pacemakers has not confirmed this as a cause of sinus node dysfunction.[4] In contrast, the surgical harvesting of the heart in patients undergoing heart-lung transplantation using the domino operation may lead to a higher incidence of sinoatrial dysfunction and permanent pacemaker implantation. In this technique, the heart is harvested with preservation of only a small part of the right atrium for a single atrial anastomosis, often leading to chronotropic dysfunction of the donor heart. These investigators instead recommend harvesting the donor heart with a standard bicaval division technique to avoid sinus node damage.[19]

Multiple other factors, such as donor age, donor sex, recipient's underlying heart disease, number of rejection episodes prior to pacemaker implantation, total ischemic time, bypass time, and preoperative use of amiodarone, have not been shown conclusively by any study to be predictive of the development of sinus node dysfunction or the need for permanent pacing.[4–12] In one study, the temperature of cardioplegia or organ storage was suggested to be related to the need for pacing, with lower temperatures making it more likely for a patient to require permanent pacing.[9] Another study suggested that aortic cross-clamp time may be predictive of increased risk of sinus node dysfunction.[10] Two studies have also suggested that prolonged ischemic times of the donor heart are predictive of the need for permanent pacing, but multiple other large studies have not confirmed this finding. Interestingly, Heinz and associates[17] showed that donor ischemic time was related to early sinus node dysfunction but did not predict late or persistent sinus node dysfunction.

An important feature of sinus node dysfunction in transplant patients is that a large majority of these patients eventually appear to regain normal sinus node function (or improvement in AV conduction) (see Table 22–2). For example, in the Stanford series, pacemaker follow-up at 6 and 12 months showed persistent bradycardia in only 75% and 50% of patients, respectively.[4] In this large series, like most others, more than 70% of patients undergoing pacemaker implantation did so before discharge after transplantation. In the Pittsburgh series, 55 of 72 patients with slow heart rates after transplantation had bradycardia for less than 20 days. In fact, 50 of these 55 patients had bradycardia for a duration of less than 7 days.[5] The remaining 17 patients underwent pacemaker implantation, and 12 of 17 patients with sinus node dysfunction had sinus rhythm with a rate greater than 60 bpm between 1 and 12 months of follow-up. An additional 6 of 401 patients required pacemakers during 5 and 31 months of follow-up. In the series from Newcastle upon Tyne, only 3 of 14 patients had a rate below 50 bpm during follow-up testing at 3 to 6 months.[10] Likewise, in a series of 52 patients from Spain there were 14 patients (27%) with bradyarrhythmia at 24 hours, 11 with bradyarrhythmias at 1 week, and only 4 patients with a rate below 60 bpm by 3 weeks.[9] Two additional patients required pacemakers at late follow-up. Heinz and associates[12] found 39 of 90 transplant patients with impaired sinus node function, and only 17 still showed sinus node impairment at 3 months. In the series of patients with AV block reported by Buja and colleagues,[13] a progressive improvement in heart rate and AV conduction was observed in all the paced patients except for three with persistent complete AV block.

The clinical implications of sinus bradycardia have been a source of controversy. Several groups have suggested that sinus node dysfunction may lead to sudden unexplained death. For example, the group from Stanford reported two unexplained sudden deaths that they felt may have been related to bradycardia, especially as transplant patients often have a less reliable escape rhythm because of their loss of autonomic influence on the AV node and subsidiary pacemakers (e.g., the transplanted heart is a denervated structure).[4] Mackintosh and coworkers[20] also reported a patient with sudden death who had Holter evidence of a fatal bradyarrhythmia. Buja and colleagues[13] reported a patient who developed cardiac arrest with seizures secondary to complete infrahisian block. Grinstead and colleagues[21] reported progressive bradycardia terminating in asystole and sudden death in a transplant patient wearing a Holter monitor. The patient did not have evidence of new conduction abnormalities before death, and only minimal allograft rejection and significant coronary arteriopathy were seen at autopsy. Electrophysiologic data suggest that post-transplantation sinus node dysfunction is characterized by impaired automaticity and not abnormal refractoriness.[16] This is consistent with results of previous studies implying that abnormal automaticity of subsidiary pacemakers, as well, may lead to absence of an adequate escape rhythm in many transplant recipients with sinus node dysfunction. A major problem is the lack of data about the long-term reliability of escape rhythms (e.g., junctional rhythms) in the denervated transplanted heart because the majority of these patients receive permanent pacemakers before discharge.

Another important clinical implication of sinus node dysfunction is related to exercise ability post transplant. The peak heart rate response to exercise remains attenuated after cardiac transplantation.[22, 23] This attenuation of maximal heart rate response is seen up to several years after transplantation. In patients without frank clinical sinus bradycardia or sinus pauses, the ability to exercise may also be diminished because of chronotropic insufficiency of the denervated sinus node. Impaired sinus node chronotropic response may be a significant factor limiting rehabilitation post transplantation

(Fig. 22–2). A final reason often used to justify pacemaker implantation before discharge is related to cost. The high incidence of gradual improvement in sinus node function and AV conduction occurs over a *long* period of time. It is difficult to justify continued hospitalization of a patient for several months based on the possibility that sinus node function may eventually return, and instead most patients receive permanent pacemakers before initial hospital discharge.

In summary, the requirement for permanent pacing after heart transplantation varies from 6% to 23%. Pacemakers are generally implanted after an average of 3 weeks following the date of transplantation in the majority of cases. The primary indication for implantation is a heart rate below 60 bpm, and about 70% to 90% of patients have sinus node abnormalities. In at least 50% of patients, sinus node dysfunction resolves by 12 months as judged by routine electrocardiographic recordings or Holter monitoring. The clinical significance of asymptomatic bradycardia despite the frequent implantation of pacemakers in these patients is unknown.

The optimal mode for cardiac pacing in transplant recipients is also a source of controversy. There are some unique aspects of cardiac function in postoperative transplant recipients. The incidence of hypertension is high, approaching 70% in the first year, leading to diastolic abnormalities of the left ventricle. In addition, rejection may lead to diastolic dysfunction.

The importance of the atrial contribution to ventricular filling post transplantation was studied by Midei and associates in nine patients several weeks after transplantation.[24] They found a mean decrease in cardiac output from 5.5 ± 1.4 to 4.6 ± 1.5 L per minute ($p < .005$) for atrial compared with ventricular pacing. They measured decreases in systolic, diastolic, and mean systemic arterial pressure of 12.5%, 9.5%, and 11%, respectively, during a shift from atrial to ventricular pacing.

The importance of the atrial contribution to ventricular filling has been confirmed by Parry and colleagues.[25] They measured Doppler-derived cardiac output at rates of 90, 110, and 130 bpm in five pacing modes: right ventricular pacing, donor atrial pacing, recipient and donor atrial synchronous pacing, donor AV sequential pacing, and synchronous recipient and donor AV sequential pacing. They found that donor atrial or donor atrial-ventricular sequential pacing was asso-

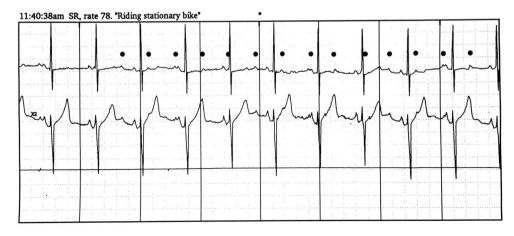

11:40:38am SR, rate 78. "Riding stationary bike"

FIGURE 22–2. Tracings from a Holter recording of a patient who underwent orthotopic heart transplantation and complained of effort intolerance and dyspnea with moderate exertion. The patient was a 42-year-old man who rode a stationary bike for 6 minutes before having to stop because of dyspnea. He was in sinus rhythm with a ventricular rate of only 78 bpm. His recipient (remnant) P wave may be seen (P waves below filled circles) at a rate of 140 bpm while his donor atrial rate is only 78 bpm. This patient had severe chronotropic insufficiency of the donor atrium. A DDDR pacemaker was implanted and his exercise tolerance improved greatly.

ciated with the highest cardiac output, 8% to 11% higher than with ventricular pacing alone. Synchronization of the recipient and donor atria did not provide additional improvement in cardiac output. This study was performed with patients at rest and these results cannot be extrapolated to exercising transplant recipients. In addition, the value of the recipient atrium as a biologic sensor to determine pacing rate was not evaluated.

Chronotropic dysfunction of the transplanted heart is the rule, rather than the exception.[23, 26] Multiple explanations for this observation include a decrease in the rise of circulating catecholamines in response to exercise, an abnormality of beta-adrenergic receptor function in the sinus node, a lack of direct sympathetic innervation of the transplanted heart or subclinical sinus node dysfunction because of graft ischemic time, blood supply, medications, rejection, or some combination of these and other factors. Implantation of rate-responsive or rate-adaptive systems has been proposed for these patients. A rate-modulated pacemaker allows patients to increase their heart rate with exercise and achieve benefits of physical conditioning.

Multiple special considerations exist when contemplating pacing in transplant patients (Table 22–3). No studies specifically compare different sensors in this population of patients. With intact AV conduction, the simplest pacing sys-

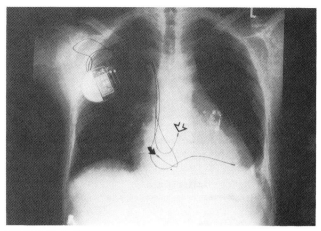

FIGURE 22–3. Chest roentgenogram showing position of two atrial leads, one in the donor atrium *(open arrow)* and one recording the recipient atrial electrogram *(filled arrow)*. The two atrial leads were connected to a DDD pacemaker and programmed to the VDD mode with an AV delay of 65 msec. A ventricular lead was inserted for safety reasons. (From Markewitz A, Osterholzer G, Weinhold C, et al: Recipient P wave synchronized pacing of the donor atrium in a heart transplanted patient: A case study. PACE 11:1402, 1988.)

TABLE 22–3. COMPARISON OF PACING MODALITIES IN ORTHOTOPIC HEART TRANSPLANT PATIENTS

VVI (R)
  Pro:
    Adequate in many patients because sinus node dysfunction or AV block disappears in majority by 3 to 6 months
    Single-lead system, simple
  Con:
    Loss of AV synchrony
    Loss of use of recipient atrium as biosensor
AAI (R)
  Atrial lead in donor atrium
  Pro:
    AV synchrony in absence of AV block
    Single-lead system, simple
  Con:
    AV block may develop later
DDD/SSI
  Two atrial leads and DDD generator (VDD mode, short AV interval) or one unipolar atrial lead connected to donor atrium and the other to recipient atrium and both leads connected together with Y connector (pacemaker programmed to triggered mode)
  Pro:
    One atrial lead senses recipient (remnant) atrial activity and other atrial lead is in donor atrium
    Remnant (recipient) atrium serves as sensor
  Con:
    Long-term stability of recipient remnant sinus node is unknown
    Atrial arrhythmias in remnant lead to upper rate pacing
    AV block may develop later
DDDR
  One atrial and one ventricular lead in donor heart
  Pro:
    Greater programming flexibility
    Chronotropic incompetence of donor heart is common
    AV block can occur later
    Does not rely on recipient atrium as sensor, concerns about reliability and development of atrial arrhythmia
  Con:
    Two leads, higher chance of dislodgement with biopsy

tem that may be implanted is an AAIR system. Loria and colleagues[26] described two patients with symptomatic sinus bradycardia during the postoperative period who had a single transvenous bipolar lead placed in the donor right atrium and connected to an activity-driven pacemaker programmed to the AAIR mode. Each patient was demonstrated to have sensor-driven increases in heart rate during exercise, but both patients eventually had enough improvement in sinus node dysfunction at late follow-up testing to obviate the need for pacing.[26] The advantages of this system are the avoidance of multiple permanent pacing leads and particularly the absence of a ventricular lead, which may be a hindrance during endomyocardial biopsy. Alternatively, with intact AV conduction, another approach involves utilizing the innervated recipient (remnant) atrium as an atrial sensor for pacing. This may be accomplished in two ways (Fig. 22–3). First, a dual-chamber device may be used with the atrial lead positioned near the recipient or remnant atrium and the lead placed in the ventricular channel positioned in the donor or denervated atrium.[27, 28] The recipient atrium serves as the sensor, and the dual-chamber pacemaker is programmed to the VDD mode with the shortest possible AV delay. A second option is to utilize a bipolar single-chamber device programmed to the triggered mode with one unipolar lead implanted near the recipient atrium and the other unipolar lead in the donor atrium and connected to the device using a Y adapter.[29] Several criteria determine the feasibility of these approaches. First, the implanter must be able to map or relatively selectively localize the electrical activity of the recipient atrium. In general, the recipient atrium abuts the posterolateral, posteromedial, and posterior aspect of the donor atrium, and the donor atrium forms the medial, anterior, and anterolateral portion of the composite atrium. Second, the recipient atrial rate must be shown to increase with exercise or isoproterenol. The implanter can record an atrial electrogram and, if it is arising from the donor (e.g., denervated) heart, there will be a one-to-one relationship with the patient's QRS unless AV block is present. If the atrial electrogram bears no relationship to the surface QRS, it most likely represents the remnant or remaining recipient atrial tissue. Bexton and colleagues[15] reported the ability to record recipient atrial activity in 87% of their patients. Three of 21 recipient atria showed no spontaneous atrial activity and two patients had persistent atrial fibrillation in the remnant, and in the remainder of patients recipient atrial activity was recorded from some region of the transplanted heart. If the donor heart exhibits complete or high-grade AV block, simultaneous recording of donor endocardial atrial electrogram from a pacing lead and another catheter is helpful in documenting capture of the donor atrium. If AV block is present in the donor heart or if atrial arrhythmias develop in the atrial remnant, this pacing approach will not be successful (e.g., leads in atrium only).

An idealized algorithm for pacing transplant patients has been suggested by Markowitz and Routh (personal communication, April 1994). This scheme covers all patients and provides for coordinated contraction of the recipient and donor atria. The functional status of the recipient sinus node, the donor sinus node, and the donor AV node must be considered. The functional status of these structures is included in the algorithm in Table 22–4, where adequate function is referred to as OK and abnormal function as X. A universal pacing mode consists of implanting a dual-chamber rate-responsive pacemaker and splitting the atrial bipolar lead into two unipolar leads. One unipolar atrial lead is placed in the donor atrium, and the other in the recipient atrium. The two atrial leads are connected together with a Y connector and placed in the generator's atrial port. If the recipient or donor atrium cycle length is shorter than the lower rate limit and faster (e.g., shorter) than the sensor-predicted rate, the faster of the two atria determines the ventricular rate. Whichever atrium is stimulated first causes the other atrium to be stimulated via the triggered mode. This is an extension of the single-chamber pacing idea of Kacet and colleagues[29] (see Table 22–4). If both atria demonstrate a cycle length below (e.g., longer than) the lower rate limit, both atria are stimulated.

There are several technical considerations. Active fixation leads are to be preferred to passive fixation leads because of the lower likelihood of displacement soon after implantation with frequent endomyocardial biopsies. The active fixation lead also allows better mapping of the atrium to find the best implantation site. The size of atrial and ventricular electrograms, as well as pacing thresholds, may change during episodes of acute rejection, as described in one patient, and unipolar pacing may lead to myopotential inhibition, described in one patient with tremors from cyclosporine.[30] In addition, unipolar atrial sensing may be problematic if there is intermittent sensing of far-field ventricular electrograms. Another potential problem with unipolar sensing is double sensing, with donor and recipient atrial activities intermittently sensed, resulting in pacing at higher rates and erratic intervals. Optimal atrial electrograms are critical, and this variability in electrogram amplitude leads many investigators to choose bipolar leads. Finally, it is recommended that pulse generators with high output be used because of the potential for changing pacing thresholds during episodes of acute rejection.[30]

It is worth noting that in several centers the trend toward use of atrial pacing (AAIR) or DDDR pacing has not become widespread. Ventricular leads are implanted in all patients at Stanford, and they reported an incidence of pacemaker-related complications of about 15%, related primarily to lead dislodgement or lead fracture related to repeated biopsy.[4] The University of Pittsburgh group implanted predominantly single-chamber ventricular pacemakers.[5] Their rationale for this practice is that bradycardia frequently resolves over time, ventricular leads are less likely to be displaced than atrial leads by repeated biopsy, it is not necessary to check for intact AV nodal conduction, and the concern about AV block in the future is avoided. The group from Loyola has also reported in a preliminary communication that the rate of pacemaker-related complications may be high, once again related to biopsy with dislodgement of leads and risk of pacemaker infection. Heinz and associates[12] reported implanting rate-responsive pacing systems in 17 of 19 patients—AAIR in 12 and VVIR in 5 patients. Indications for ventricular pacing were a history of atrial fibrillation or inability to obtain adequate atrial fixation. Payne and coworkers[10] implanted AAI pacemakers in all seven of their patients (before the advent of rate-responsive pacing). Scott and colleagues[6] implanted seven VVI pacemakers, eight VVIR pacemakers, one DDD, and one DDDR pacemaker. They report support for the concept of rate-responsive pacing but note that significant benefit from pacing may be needed for only a relatively short period of time.

Heterotopic transplantation may be useful in patients as a bridge to later orthotopic transplantation when there is a mismatch between the size of donor and recipient organs or pulmonary hypertension. In one report, a dual-chamber pacing system was used to coordinate the contraction of the recipient and donor hearts.[31] This is done by implanting a pacing lead in the right ventricle of the donor heart and connecting it to the atrial port, while the ventricular lead is placed in the atrium of the recipient heart. The AV interval

TABLE 22–4. IDEALIZED TRANSPLANT PATIENT PACING ALGORITHM

RSA	DSA	DAV	HRC AT REST	COMMENT	HRC EXERCISE	COMMENT
OK	OK	OK	DSA→APR	DSA drives both atria	RSA→APD	RSA drives both atria
X	OK	OK	DSA→APR	DSA drives both atria	APR + APD	Activity drives both atria
OK	X	OK	RSA→APD	RSA drives both atria	RSA→APD	RSA drives both atria
X	X	OK	APR + APD	Activity drives both atria	APR + APD	Activity drives both atria
OK	OK	X	DSA→APR, VP	DSA drives both atria, V	RSA→APD, VP	RSA drives both V
X	OK	X	DSA→APR, VP	DSA drives both atria, V	APR + APD, VP	Activity drives both atria, V
OK	X	X	RSA→APD, VP	RSA drives both atria, V	RSA→APD, VP	RSA drives both atria, V
X	X	X	APR + APD, VP	Activity drives both atria, V	APR + APD, VP	Activity drives both atria, V

Abbreviations: RSA, recipient SA node; DSA, donor SA node; DAV, donor AV node; APR, atrial pace recipient; APD, atrial pace donor; VP, ventricular pace; HRC, heart rate control; X, abnormal; V, ventricles; OK, normal function.

is adjusted to result in contraction of the recipient heart preceding that of the donor heart.

Future Indications

One of the major complications of cardiac transplantation remains detection of rejection. Currently, the diagnosis of rejection is based on endomyocardial biopsy. Reliable noninvasive tests for the diagnosis of rejection do not yet exist. Data on the utility of signal-averaged electrocardiography have been contradictory. One preliminary report failed to show clinical utility of time domain processing of signal-averaged electrocardiograms (ECGs).[32] Some data suggest that frequency analysis of the signal averaged ECG may be useful.[33] Another study suggests that the amplitude spectrum is changed with rejection but does not provide an increase in sensitivity or specificity above that of time domain analysis of the signal-averaged ECG.[34] These investigators detected a mean 11% decrease in the root-mean-square voltage of the high-pass filtered QRS complex with rejection and reported 87% sensitivity with 78% specificity for this criterion.

Warnecke and colleagues[35] reported on the use of intramyocardial electrogram (IMEG) recordings from a myocardial screw-in electrode connected to a pulse generator capable of transmitting IMEG amplitude. They reported that the onset of rejection could be predicted correctly with 87% sensitivity and 96% specificity based on a 10% to 20% drop in voltage. Pirolo and colleagues[36] developed this technique further in a canine model of intrathoracic heterotopic cardiac transplantation. They found a significant correlation between the severity of rejection and the unipolar peak-to-peak IMEG amplitude. They found no correlation between other electrophysiologic parameters, atrial and ventricular pacing thresholds and ventricular refractory periods, and the severity or presence of rejection. Another electrophysiologic parameter, the QT interval measured with an externalized QT-driven rate-responsive pacemaker (Rhythmyx, Vitatron Medical B.V., Dieren, The Netherlands), has been suggested to be of potential utility in diagnosing rejection.[37] The epicardial evoked T-wave amplitude during ventricular pacing was compared with the results of endomyocardial biopsy. The evoked T-wave amplitude fell significantly during rejection (at least 0.5 mV) but was unchanged in the absence of rejection. The sensitivity was 92% and the specificity 100% for the first rejection episode. The reason for the fall in the evoked T-wave amplitude is unknown, but it is presumed to be due to inflammation and edema occurring with rejection. All measurements were made less than 1 month after operation, so it is uncertain how reliable these measurements are on a longer-term basis. These preliminary results must be confirmed by larger prospective studies but may open up a new application of pacing technology. Other potential variables that may have a role in noninvasively detecting transplant rejection include monitoring of the paced evoked response, heart rate variability, and myocardial impedance.

In summary, the majority of patients who are paced after transplantation are paced for sinus node dysfunction. These patients should receive dual-chamber rate-adaptive pacemakers. I recommend the use of active fixation leads for atrial pacing, with the active fixation lead used to map the atrium to locate regions where maximal donor and recipient atrial electrograms can be recorded. It is likely that the recipient or remnant atrium is the ideal sensor when atrial activity is present and recordable, as it is in the majority of patients. Other potential pacemaker modes can be considered for individual patients. Careful attention to optimizing pacing parameters and programming is necessary in these patients. Many patients demonstrate decreased usage of their pacemakers with time; however, appropriate programming will ensure adequate early rehabilitation of the transplant recipient by providing AV synchrony and chronotropic responsiveness.

Pacing For Hypertrophic Cardiomyopathy

In 1975, there were two reports of improved hemodynamics in patients with hypertrophic cardiomyopathy who underwent dual-chamber pacing for treatment of AV block.[38, 39] The principle of P-wave–triggered ventricular pacing (VAT mode) with a shorter conduction time than the patient's intrinsic AV conduction time was that it leads to excitation of the right and left ventricles before development of obstruction at the outflow tract. Two small series were described in the German literature, but it was not until 1988 that the first prospective study of this potential mode of therapy was described. McDonald and colleagues[40] from St. Vincent's Hospital in Belfast studied 11 patients treated with DDD pacing for severe, medically refractory heart failure symptoms. Ten of the 11 patients had received beta- and/or calcium channel–blocking drugs, and 8 of the 11 patients had resting left ventricular outflow gradients ranging from 7 to 80 mm Hg. The mean duration of exercise was 7.69 minutes in sinus rhythm and 10.05 minutes in paced rhythm. Seven of the 11 patients who underwent paired exercise tests showed an improved exercise capacity with pacing. The improved exercise capacity noted at a stress test 1 week later was maintained when the patients were studied 2 years later. Finally, all patients had subjective improvement of congestive heart failure symptoms and improvement of functional status by one or two classes. Richter and coworkers[41] reported on four patients with hypertrophic cardiomyopathy and were able to show reduction in left ventricular outflow tract (LVOT) gradients by continuous-wave Doppler recordings and cardiac catheterization that was stable and reproducible 3 to 6 months after pacemaker implantation. McDonald and Maurer,[42] in reviewing these results, point out that no significant adverse effects of this intervention have been reported. These results of dual-chamber pacing are comparable both subjectively and objectively (e.g., hemodynamics) to those achieved with myectomy.

The most definitive studies in this area were published by Fananapazir and his colleagues at the National Institutes of Health.[43, 44] They studied 44 consecutive patients with obstructive hypertrophic cardiomyopathy (left ventricular outflow tract gradient >30 mm Hg at rest or >50 mm Hg after amyl nitrate inhalation) who failed to benefit from verapamil (240 to 480 mg/day) and beta-adrenergic blocking agents (propranolol at 240 to 360 mg/day or atenolol at 100 mg/day). Each patient underwent a detailed evaluation consisting of treadmill exercise tests with measurement of oxygen consumption by analysis of expired gas, echocardiographic measurement of outflow tract gradient, cardiac catheterization, and symptom questionnaire. Patients were reevaluated after 1.5 to 3 months of chronic pacing in sinus rhythm and during DDD pacing.

The impact of DDD pacing was striking, with none of the patients experiencing worsening of symptoms (Fig. 22–4). During a follow-up period of 9 months, only 1 of the 15 patients with a history of effort or postural syncope had a further episode of syncope. The New York Heart Association functional status improved by one class in 12 patients and by two or more classes in 30 patients. Treadmill exercise duration achieved during DDD pacing improved by a mean of 2.5 minutes (6.3 ± 2.3 minutes in sinus rhythm to 8.8 ± 3.3 minutes in paced rhythm). Echocardiographic evaluation of LVOT gradient showed a significant decrease in systolic anterior mitral valve leaflet motion and a decrease in peak outflow tract Doppler velocity and gradient. For example, the mean LVOT gradient was 64 ± 7 mm Hg during sinus rhythm at baseline and was 43 ± 7 during sinus rhythm at the time of the predischarge study, decreasing further to 27 ± 5 with DDD pacing at late follow-up.

The hemodynamic changes caused by AV sequential pacing were a decrease in pulmonary arterial and pulmonary capillary wedge pressures during AV sequential pacing, as well as increased cardiac output compared with atrial pacing (Fig. 22–5). Higher heart rates were associated with significant increases in systemic arterial pressure and reduction in left ventricular systolic pressure and LVOT gradients. Surprisingly, the hemodynamic measurements recorded during

sinus rhythm at the follow-up evaluation had improved significantly compared with the hemodynamic findings at baseline.

In another study, McAreavey and Fananapazir[44] demonstrated that the hemodynamic changes that occur during DDD pacing are accompanied by significant changes in R-wave and T-wave amplitude recorded by surface 12-lead electrocardiography and in duration of the total QRS and root-mean-square voltage of the QRS (of the filtered Y axis) on the signal-averaged ECG. There was no simple relationship between the changes in the LVOT gradient and changes in the ECG.

A preliminary report described DDD pacing instituted in a group of 13 patients with nonobstructive hypertrophic cardiomyopathy. The design of this study was similar to that of previous studies performed at the National Institutes of Health with dual-chamber pacing in patients with obstructive hypertrophic cardiomyopathy.[45] The authors found slightly reduced filling pressures, while filling volumes and indices of left ventricular systolic performance were unchanged with DDD pacing. The hemodynamic changes they observed were less marked than those observed in hypertrophic cardiomyopathy patients with obstructive hemodynamics. A recent report extends these findings, suggesting that there is no consistent clinical benefit to DDD pacing in patients with nonobstructive hypertrophic cardiomyopathy.

Many investigators have shown that right ventricular pacing may reduce LVOT gradients in patients with hypertrophic cardiomyopathy. This is thought to be caused by an

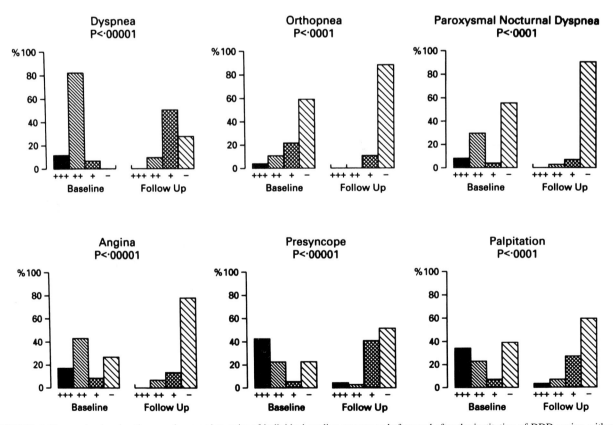

FIGURE 22–4. Bar graphs showing the prevalence and severity of individual cardiac symptoms before and after the institution of DDD pacing with a short AV interval in patients with obstructive hypertrophic cardiomyopathy. The severity of symptoms is shown as: −, symptoms absent; +, mild symptoms; + +, moderate symptoms; + + +, severe symptoms. (From Fananapazir L, Cannon RO III, Tripodi D, et al: Impact of dual-chamber permanent pacings in patients with obstructive hypertrophic cardiomyopathy with symptoms refractory to verapamil and β-adrenergic blocker therapy. Circulation 85:2149, 1992. Copyright 1992 American Heart Association.)

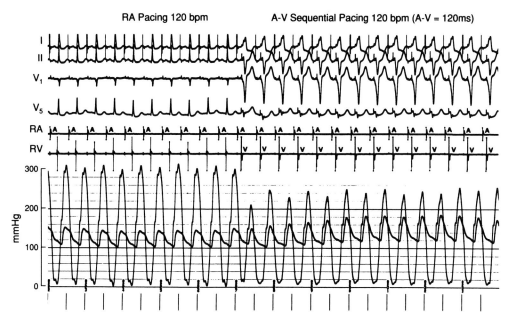

RA Pacing 120 bpm   A-V Sequential Pacing 120 bpm (A-V = 120ms)

FIGURE 22–5. Tracing showing the impact of AV sequential pacing on left ventricular and femoral arterial pressure in an individual patient. On the left, during right atrial (RA) pacing at 120 bpm, the maximum left ventricular systolic pressure is 330 mm Hg and the left ventricular outflow tract gradient is 170 mm Hg. On the right, an acute change in AV sequential pacing at the same rate is made with an AV interval of 120 msec to preexcite the ventricular septum. The left ventricular systolic pressure is reduced to 250 mm Hg, and a left ventricular outflow tract gradient to 70 mm Hg is shown. These changes were accompanied by an improvement of the femoral arterial systolic and pulse pressure. Shown from top to bottom are surface ECG leads I, II, III, V_1, and V_5; RA, right atrial intracardiac recording; RV, right ventricular intracardiac recording; A and V, atrial and ventricular intracardiac electrograms.

(From Fananapazir L, Cannon RO III, Tripodi D, et al: Impact of dual-chamber permanent pacings in patients with obstructive hypertrophic cardiomyopathy with symptoms refractory to verapamil and β-adrenergic blocker therapy. Circulation 85:2149, 1992. Copyright 1992 American Heart Association.)

altered ventricular activation sequence resulting in paradoxical septal motion or a septal activation sequence similar to that seen in patients with left bundle branch block. The altered sequence of ventricular contraction leads to an enlarged LVOT during early to midsystole and thereby reduces forces causing systolic anterior motion of the mitral valve and its apparatus. A variety of important questions still remain about the use of pacing in this population of patients (Table 22–5). A number of ongoing studies should answer these questions over the next decade.

In summary, in patients with hypertrophic cardiomyopathy and symptoms of congestive heart failure refractory to beta- and calcium channel blockers, dual-chamber pacing may be an alternative to septal myectomy (Fig. 22–6). Patients

TABLE 22–5. PACING ISSUES IN HYPERTROPHIC CARDIOMYOPATHY PATIENTS

1. Is there an optimal AV delay for these patients?
2. Do patients with left bundle branch block benefit from AV pacing?
3. Do patients need an invasive hemodynamic-pacing study before permanent pacemaker implantation to document benefit? If benefit cannot be documented by a hemodynamic study, should pacing be offered?
4. What is the mechanism for improvement after pacing is discontinued? How long does improvement continue after pacing is discontinued?
5. Does pacing lead to permanent structural or biochemical changes in the septum?
6. What roles does DDD pacing have in patients with nonobstructive hypertrophic cardiomyopathy? What testing is necessary before pacemaker implantation?
7. Comparison of medication (beta-blockers, calcium channel blockers) with pacing in patients with hypertrophic cardiomyopathy?
8. What role does pacing have in patients with mild symptoms of hypertrophic cardiomyopathy?
9. Can pacing prolong survival in patients with hypertrophic cardiomyopathy and moderate to severe symptoms?

should be selected on the basis of the presence of an LVOT gradient and in most cases the demonstration of a decrease in the LVOT gradient with AV pacing at a short AV interval resulting in ventricular septal excitation via the pacemaker rather than through the AV node. Fananapazir and colleagues have begun to utilize DDD pacing for most symptomatic patients with hypertrophic cardiomyopathy and LVOT gradients without prior hemodynamic pacing studies because of the striking and uniform success of pacemaker therapy (Fananapazir L, personal communication, April 1994). The clinician must be sure to program the AV interval to a short enough value (generally 50 to 150 msec) to maintain excitation of the septum via the pacemaker. It may be desirable to use a pacemaker that has AV delay shortening. Rate-responsive pacing is generally not needed, although it may be of use in patients with atrial arrhythmias to program separate upper rate limits for atrial tracking and the sensor.

Pacing For Dilated Cardiomyopathy

Iskandrian and Mintz[46] proposed that atrial pacing at higher rates could help decrease the end-diastolic volume of the left ventricle, which would help allow the myofibrils and sarcomeres that are distorted by the dilated left ventricle to become realigned. This would help left ventricular function in areas of decreased contractility because of dilatation rather than ischemia or fibrosis. Second, a decrease in end-diastolic volume would probably result in little decrease in stroke volume, because the patient with a dilated, failing left ventricle is functioning on the flat portion of the Starling curve. The slight decrease in stroke volume would be more than compensated for by the increased heart rate and increased cardiac output. In addition, the decrease in right ventricular end-diastolic volume by pacing might result in a lower filling pressure and further decrease left ventricular filling pressure via the common septum and pericardium. Finally, there

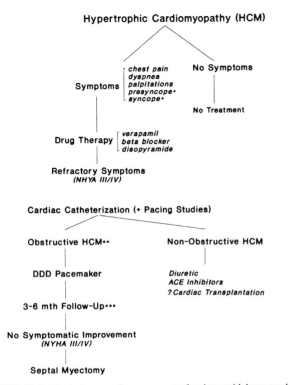

FIGURE 22–6. Chart of proposed management of patients with hypertrophic cardiomyopathy. * refers to exertional or postural symptoms; ** refers to left ventricular outflow tract gradient in the absence of all drugs greater than 30 mm Hg at rest or greater than 50 mm Hg after provocative maneuvers; *** refers to repeated treadmill exercise tests to assess symptomatic improvement and to ensure that pacemaker programming allows preexcitation of the right ventricle throughout exercise. The echocardiogram is obtained to establish a reduction in severity of anterior systolic motion of the mitral valve leaflet and left ventricular outflow tract velocities and cardiac catheterization to demonstrate hemodynamic improvement. NYHA, New York Heart Association functional class; DDD, dual chamber pacing; mth, month; ACE, angiotensin converting enzyme inhibitors. (From Fananapazir L, Cannon RO III, Tripodi D, et al: Impact of dual-chamber permanent pacings in patients with obstructive hypertrophic cardiomyopathy with symptoms refractory to verapamil and β-adrenergic blocker therapy. Circulation 85:2149, 1992. Copyright 1992 American Heart Association.)

might also be a decrease in secondary mitral and tricuspid regurgitation resulting from a decrease in end-diastolic volume and thereby an increase in cardiac output.

Hochleitner and colleagues[47] reported on 17 critically ill patients with chronic heart failure caused by dilated cardiomyopathy in whom DDD pacemakers were used to shorten the PV interval. After institution of DDD pacing (with an AV delay of 100 msec), these patients experienced improvements in functional class. All eight patients receiving continuous dopamine or dobutamine had their infusions discontinued after pacemaker implantation. A decrease in right ventricular and left atrial dimensions was shown by echocardiography, consistent with a decrease in preload. Systolic blood pressure increased by a mean of 18 mm Hg and diastolic blood pressure by a mean of 13 mm Hg. Left ventricular ejection fraction increased from $16.0 \pm 8.4\%$ to $25.6 \pm 8.6\%$. Three patients who were awaiting heart transplantation improved sufficiently to not require heart transplantation. Hochleitner and colleagues[48] reported the long-term efficacy of DDD pacing in this group of patients with follow-up to 5 years. The clinical improvement achieved

after pacemaker implantation was maintained throughout the study period or until death. No patient required rehospitalization because of worsening of heart failure, echocardiographic dimensions progressively decreased, and arterial blood pressure increased during the study. Nine patients died suddenly while at home, four patients underwent orthotopic heart transplantation, and one died of adenocarcinoma. An interruption of DDD pacing for 2 to 4 hours was followed by a decrease in left ventricular ejection fraction and an increase in left atrial and left ventricular size. This response was seen at 2 weeks after pacemaker implantation and to a smaller extent at 6 and 12 months. Hochleitner concluded that DDD pacing had long-term benefit in patients with severe congestive heart failure. The etiology of improvement was multifactorial, including preservation of atrial outflow for ventricular ejection, improvement in forward cardiac output, decrease in mitral regurgitation, enhanced myocardial contractility, better coordination of ventricular contraction with subsequent reduction in wall stress, and increased blood pressure allowing administration of higher doses of angiotensin-converting enzyme inhibitors. Katoaka[49] reported a patient who appeared to benefit from DDD pacemaker therapy in the setting of end-stage dilated cardiomyopathy. This patient had a PR interval of 240 msec or greater. A pacemaker was implanted, and the AV interval was programmed to 100 msec, resulting in an improved clinical course for 4 months. Invasive hemodynamic measurements and Doppler study were performed at a rate of 92 bpm, with AV intervals of 50, 100, 150, and 200 msec. At an AV delay of 100 msec, the cardiac output and aortic flow velocity integral were maximized. Further improvements in systemic blood pressure and cardiac output were observed 10 days after pacemaker implantation.

The rationale for the improvement of heart failure with DDD pacing has been studied by Brecker and colleagues in London.[50] They performed Doppler echocardiography on 12 patients with idiopathic dilated cardiomyopathy who underwent DDD pacing for treatment of severe heart failure. They measured cardiac output, ventricular filling time, and exercise capacity on treadmill at multiple AV delays during pacing. They reported that the duration of both mitral and tricuspid regurgitation was significantly shorter and both left and right ventricular filling times were increased with short AV intervals. An improved exercise duration correlated with an improved cardiac output, increased maximum oxygen consumption, and lessened symptoms of breathlessness at the shorter AV interval. The investigators hypothesized that the short filling time of the right or left ventricle is caused by extended functional mitral or tricuspid regurgitation caused by ventricular dysfunction, and correction of this abnormality results in the improved exercise tolerance observed. Other factors contributing to valvular regurgitation include prolonged PR intervals and intraventricular conduction defects. By changing from the longest to the shortest AV interval the degree of mitral regurgitation was reduced by a mean of 85%, and the left ventricular filling time was increased by 65 msec. In all their patients, the presystolic component of regurgitation, as well as shortening of the duration of regurgitation, was accomplished with a short AV delay. The authors concluded that a short AV delay probably improves stroke volume and exercise capacity acutely by increasing ventricular filling time and shortening the duration and degree of valvular regurgitation. These clinical studies are preliminary, and until prospective trials are performed pacing for treatment of heart failure should be considered investigational.

In summary, the use of DDD pacing for patients with idiopathic dilated cardiomyopathy refractory to medications should be considered investigational and unproven based on data from the available clinical studies. Potential candidates are patients refractory to intravenous inotropes and vasodilators awaiting heart transplantation or without other therapeutic alternatives. Significant benefit with invasive hemodynamic monitoring during temporary pacing should be demonstrated before permanent pacing is considered.

Pacing For Severe Refractory Idiopathic Orthostatic Hypotension

In 1980, Moss and colleagues[51] reported on the use of atrial pacing in a patient with severe, refractory orthostatic hypotension. Subsequently, Moss and coworkers[52] reported on five patients seen over an 11-year period with refractory idiopathic hypotension who have subsequently been treated with pacemakers. Four of the 5 patients demonstrated hemodynamic or symptomatic improvement. All patients were also being treated with fludrocortisone therapy that was continued after pacemaker implantation. An additional three patients were reported in the medical literature, two with sustained improvement resulting from atrial pacing.[53, 54]

Significant improvement in six of eight patients probably results from the absent or markedly attenuated tachycardia these patients show in response to positional hypotension. The absent or impaired chronotropic response may contribute to the orthostatic hypotension by allowing a longer time for blood to be distributed to the periphery with the low heart rate (e.g., long diastole). Increasing the heart rate with pacing (in this series, the programmed lower heart rate varied from 90 to 100 bpm) reduces the duration of diastole and allows patients with some ability to vasoconstrict to further increase their vascular tone by an increased cardiac output. Six of the eight patients had AAI pacemakers; one had a DDD and another a DDDR unit. The small size of this population does not allow any conclusions regarding pacing modality. Our own experience with three patients with this syndrome who received AAI or DDD pacemakers is that each patient experienced a moderate to significant improvement in symptoms and arterial blood pressure, in two cases allowing patients to avoid admission to nursing homes. The use of dual-chamber adaptive-rate pacing with the preejection interval sensor in a patient with refractory orthostatic hypotension has been reported. In this patient, temporary fixed-rate pacing was only minimally effective in preventing syncope during upright tilt table testing. However, during upright tilt table testing and pacing at rates of 85 bpm and then 120 bpm, he was able to remain upright for 15 minutes. A DDDR pacemaker, Precept DR (CPI, St. Paul, MN), was implanted and the patient was able to return home and carry on a normal existence. The patient's symptoms could be reproduced during DDD but not DDDR pacing. It is hypothesized that the sudden drop in venous return and right ventricular filling leads to shortening of the preejection interval and an increased pacing rate when needed during standing and that a lower rate is adequate during lying.[55]

In summary, atrial or AV pacing may be employed for patients with idiopathic orthostatic hypotension refractory to salt and steroid therapy. This therapy usually results in some clinical improvement, which varies considerably from patient to patient. Efficacy can be demonstrated by measurement of blood pressure before and after standing with and without pacing. Dual chamber and dual chamber rate-responsive pacemakers are recommended for these patients.

Long-QT-Interval Syndrome

Pacing for treatment of the long-QT interval syndrome differs from pacing for patients with either dilated or hypertrophic cardiomyopathy because pacing is instituted to prevent the development of symptomatic polymorphic ventricular tachycardia. The role of pacing in these patients has been described.[56, 57] The long-QT-interval syndrome is an uncommon disorder in which affected individuals demonstrate an abnormality of repolarization manifested as a prolonged QT or QT-U interval and have an increased risk of syncope caused by fatal or nonfatal ventricular polymorphic tachycardia. The genetics of this syndrome indicate that it may be inherited as an autosomal dominant (e.g., Romano-Ward syndrome with normal hearing) or an autosomal recessive pattern (e.g., Jervell and Lange-Nielsen syndrome and includes congenital neural deafness). Sporadic new cases without familial inheritance have also been reported. A prospective longitudinal study of 328 families demonstrated that the risk of syncope or death before age 50 (presumably due to ventricular fibrillation) can be predicted by a history of syncope, QT_c greater than 0.50 seconds, and a resting heart rate below 60 bpm.[58] As expected, arrhythmogenic syncope often occurred in the setting of physical, emotional, or auditory arousal. Therapy for these patients consists of treatment with beta-adrenergic blockers and left cardiac sympathetic denervation. Schwartz and colleagues[59] reported a large series of 85 patients with this syndrome and a history of syncope. After left stellectomy (cardiac sympathetic denervation), there was a significant decrease in the number of cardiac events (e.g., syncope, sudden death, seizure) per patient from 22 ± 32 to 1 ± 3 events and a decrease in the number of patients with five or more events from 71% to 10% over a mean follow-up period of about 6 years.[59] The incidence of sudden death was 8% over the study period. In contrast, Scheinman and colleagues at San Francisco and Stanford reported on a group of 10 patients with long QT syndrome who underwent cardiac sympathetic denervation.[60] Cardiac symptoms persisted in eight of these patients. Three patients required more extensive sympathectomy, one required an implantable cardioverter defibrillator, and three required chronic atrial pacing. Only one patient remained asymptomatic without drug or pacemaker therapy.

The role of permanent cardiac pacing in patients with the long-QT syndrome was described by Eldar and associates.[55, 60, 61] They reported on eight patients with the long-QT syndrome who underwent pacemaker implantation for recurrent syncope or seizures. Three patients were treated unsuccessfully with both a beta-blocker and cardiac sympathectomy, two were refractory or intolerant to beta-blockers, and three had pacemakers implanted because of AV block in one, aborted sudden death in one, and one patient's preference.

Pacing was instituted at a rate of 70 to 85 bpm with AAI pacing in four, VVI pacing in two, and DDD pacing in two. Only one patient had recurrent cardiac events and syncope under emotional stress, which was felt to be due to hyperventilation.

Moss and colleagues[59] reviewed the efficacy of permanent pacing in 30 patients from the international prospective study of the long-QT syndrome. The average age at pacemaker implantation was 19 ± 13 years, the mean QT_c was 0.55 ± 0.08 second, and 87% were female. The median cardiac event rate was significantly reduced by pacing. Twenty-one of 30 patients experienced no cardiac events during an average pacemaker follow-up of 49 months. Four of the other nine patients had a decrease in the yearly cardiac event rate. In this study, 43% of patients received AAI pacemakers, 37% received VVI pacemakers, 13% received DDD pacemakers, and the mode of pacing was unknown in 7%. It is emphasized that 57% of patients were receiving beta-adrenergic blockade and 10% had already undergone a left cervicothoracic sympathetic ganglionectomy.

Locati and Schwartz[61] emphasize that no evidence supports the use of pacemakers alone as therapy for the long-QT syndrome. There are insufficient data on the effect of pacing to reduce mortality, so pacemakers should be considered as adjunctive therapy only. Pacing should be considered for patients in whom beta-blockers and cervical sympathectomy have failed, beta-blockers induce bradycardia, or bradycardia-dependent polymorphic ventricular tachycardia has been demonstrated. Eldar and colleagues[62] reported on the efficacy of combination therapy with beta-blockers and cardiac pacing in 21 patients. Before combination therapy, 20 of 21 patients had experienced either cardiac arrest (n = 8) or syncope (n = 18); 9 had not responded to beta-blocker alone and 5 had not responded to left cervicothoracic sympathectomy (Fig. 22–7). All patients were treated with combined beta-blockers and long-term pacing at rates of 70 to 125 bpm, resulting in shortening of the QT_c from 541 ± 62

to 479 ± 41 msec. After a mean follow-up of 55 ± 62 months the only episode of sudden death occurred in a patient who discontinued beta-blocker therapy. Syncope occurred in four patients, caused by a lead fracture in two. In general, DDD pacing was preferred, as spontaneous or induced AV block developed in five patients. Block was infrahisian in four, occasionally functional in nature such as after a PVC resulting in a compensatory pause and increased His-Purkinje refractoriness. When functional block occurred, it tended to be self-perpetuating. Other pacing problems included prolonging long ventricular refractory periods to avoid T-wave sensing. The authors concluded that combination therapy (e.g., beta-blockers and pacing) may be highly effective for symptomatic patients with the long-QT syndrome and should be considered adjunctive therapy for patients who require insertion of an implantable defibrillator.

In summary, the author recommends consideration of permanent cardiac pacing combined with beta-blocker therapy for patients who do not respond to beta-blocker therapy alone and/or cardiac sympathectomy. I believe that permanent pacing may be reasonable alternative therapy to left cardiac sympathectomy in patients with prominent bradycardia or in patients presenting with aborted sudden death while taking beta-blockers, who refuse implantation of the implantable cardioverter defibrillator or cardiac sympathectomy. The role of cardiac pacing as sole therapy for patients with the long-QT syndrome remains unexplored, and no prospective trials exist comparing beta-blockers plus pacing to cardiac sympathectomy or implantation of a cardioverter defibrillator.

Conclusion

The principal current indication for pacemaker therapy is the presence of a symptomatic bradyarrhythmia. Potential future indications include hypertrophic cardiomyopathy, dilated cardiomyopathy, long-QT syndrome, idiopathic asymptomatic hypotension, and asymptomatic patients with sinus node dysfunction after orthotopic heart transplantation. Pacing patients with these disorders presents new challenges in pacing mode selection and lead placement. Pacing is also providing new insights into the hemodynamic and electrical pathophysiology of these conditions and is suggesting new therapeutic options that may improve future management and clinical outcomes.

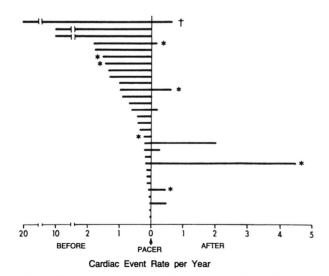

FIGURE 22–7. Graph showing cardiac event rates before (syncope or aborted cardiac arrest) and after (syncope, aborted cardiac arrest, or death) permanent pacemaker. +, cardiac death; *, left cervicothoracic sympathetic ganglionectomy. (From Moss AJ, Liu JE, Gottlieb S, et al: Efficacy of permanent pacing in the management of high risk patients with long QT syndrome. Circulation 84:1530, 1991. Copyright 1991 American Heart Association.)

REFERENCES

1. Kaye MP: The Registry of the International Society for Heart and Lung Transplantation: Ninth official report—1991. J Heart Lung Transplant 11:592, 1992.
2. Reitz BA: Heart and heart-lung transplantation. *In* Braunwald E (ed): Heart Disease: A Textbook of Cardiovascular Medicine, 4th ed. Philadelphia, W. B. Saunders, 1992, pp 520–534.
3. Lower RR, Shumway NE: Studies on the orthotopic homotransplantation of the canine heart. Surg Forum 11:18, 1960.
4. DiBiase A, Tse T-M, Schnittger I, et al: Frequency and mechanism of bradycardia in cardiac transplant recipients and need for pacemakers. Am J Cardiol 67:1385, 1991.
5. Miyamoto Y, Curtiss EI, Kormos RL, et al: Bradyarrhythmia after heart transplantation: Incidence, time course, and outcome. Circulation 82(suppl IV):IV-313, 1990.
6. Scott CD, Omar I, McComb JM, et al: Long-term pacing in heart transplant recipients is usually unnecessary. PACE 14:1792, 1991.
7. Romhilt DW, Doyle M, Sagar KB, et al: Prevalence and significance of

arrhythmias in long-term survivors of cardiac transplantation. Circulation 66(suppl I):I-219, 1982.

8. Jacquet L, Ziady G, Stein K, et al: Cardiac rhythm disturbances early after orthotopic heart transplantation: Prevalence and clinical importance of the observed abnormalities. J Am Coll Cardiol 16:832, 1990.

9. Montero JA, Anguita M, Concha M, et al: Pacing requirements after orthotopic heart transplantation: Incidence and related factors. J Heart Lung Transplant 11:799, 1992.

10. Payne ME, Murray KD, Watson KM, et al: Permanent pacing in heart transplant recipients: Underlying causes and long-term results. J Heart Lung Transplant 10:738, 1991.

11. Blanche C, Czer LSC, Trent OA, et al: Bradyarrhythmias requiring pacemaker implantation after orthotopic heart transplantation: Association with rejection. J Heart Lung Transplant 11:446, 1992.

12. Heinz G, Hirschl M, Buxbaum P, et al: Sinus node dysfunction after orthotopic cardiac transplantation: Postoperative incidence and long-term implications. PACE 15:731, 1992.

13. Buja G, Miorelli M, Livi U, et al: Complete atrioventricular block after orthotopic heart transplantation: Incidence, electrocardiographic-electrophysiological evolution and clinical importance. Eur JCPE 3:173, 1992.

14. Dodinot B, Costa AB, Godenir JP, et al: AV block after cardiac transplantation—pacing mode selection. PACE 14:692, 1991. Abstract.

15. Bexton RS, Nathan AW, Hellestrand KJ, et al: Sinoatrial function after cardiac transplantation. J Am Coll Cardiol 3:712, 1984.

16. Heinz G, Ohner T, Laufer G, et al: Clinical and electrophysiologic correlates of sinus node dysfunction after orthotopic heart transplantation. Chest 97:890, 1990.

17. Heinz G, Ohner T, Laufer G, et al: Demographic and perioperative factors associated with initial and prolonged sinus node dysfunction after orthotopic heart transplantation: The impact of ischemic time. Transplantation 51:1217, 1991.

18. Ellenbogen KA, Szentpetery S, Katz MR: Reversibility of prolonged chronotropic dysfunction with theophylline following orthotopic cardiac transplantation. Am Heart J 116:202, 1988.

19. Rosado LJ, Huston CL, Sethi GK, et al: Sinoatrial node dysfunction in recipients of domino heart transplants: Complication of a surgical harvesting technique. J Heart Lung Transplant 11:1078, 1992.

20. Mackintosh AF, Carmichael DJ, Wren C, et al: Sinus node function in first three weeks after cardiac transplantation. Br Heart J 48:584, 1982.

21. Grinstead WC, Smart FW, Pratt CM, et al: Sudden death caused by bradycardia and asystole in a heart transplant patient with coronary arteriopathy. J Heart Lung Transplant 10:931, 1991.

22. Pope SE, Stinson EB, Daughters GT, et al: Exercise response of the denervated heart in long-term cardiac transplant recipients. Am J Cardiol 46:231, 1980.

23. Quigg RJ, Rocco MB, Gauthier DF, et al: Mechanism of the attenuated peak heart rate response to exercise after orthotopic cardiac transplantation. J Am Coll Cardiol 14:338, 1989.

24. Midei MG, Baughman KL, Achuff SC, et al: Is atrial activation beneficial in heart transplant recipients? J Am Coll Cardiol 16:1201, 1990.

25. Parry G, Malbut K, Dark JH: Optimal pacing modes after cardiac transplantation: Is synchronisation of recipient and donor atria beneficial? Br Heart J 68:195, 1992.

26. Loria K, Salinger M, McDonough T, et al: AAIR pacing for sinus node dysfunction after orthotopic heart transplantation: An initial report. J Heart Transplant 7:380, 1988.

27. Markewitz A, Osterholzer G, Weinhold C, et al: Recipient P wave synchronized pacing of the donor atrium in a heart transplanted patient: A case study. PACE 11:1402, 1988.

28. Osterholzer G, Markewitz A, Authuber M, Keinkes BM: An example of how to pace a patient with a heart transplantation. J Heart Transplant 7:23, 1988.

29. Kacet S, Molin F, Lacroix D, et al: Bipolar atrial-triggered pacing to restore normal chronotropic responsiveness in an orthotopic cardiac transplant patient. PACE 14:1444, 1991.

30. Markewitz A, Kemkes BM, Reble B, et al: Particularities of dual chamber pacemaker therapy in patients after orthotopic heart transplantation. PACE 10:326, 1987.

31. Breedveld RW, van Gelder LM, Mitchell AG, et al: Optimized hemodynamics by implantation of a dual chamber pacemaker after heterotopic cardiac transplantation. PACE 15:274, 1992.

32. Keren A, Gillis AN, Freedman RA, et al: Heart transplant rejection monitored by signal averaged electrocardiography in patients receiving cyclosporine. Circulation 70(suppl I):124, 1984.

33. Haberl R, Weber M, Reichenspurner H, et al: Frequency analysis of the surface electrocardiogram for recognition of acute rejection after orthotopic cardiac transplantation in man. Circulation 76:101, 1987.

34. Lacroix D, Kacet S, Savard P, et al: Signal-averaged electrocardiography and detection of heart transplant rejection: Comparison of time and frequency domain analyses. J Am Coll Cardiol 19:553, 1992.

35. Warnecke H, Schüler S, Goetze H-J, et al: Noninvasive monitoring of cardiac allograft rejection by intramyocardial electrogram recordings. Circulation 74(suppl III):72, 1986.

36. Pirolo JS, Tweddell JS, Brunt EM, et al: Influence of activation origin, lead number, and lead configuration on the noninvasive electrophysiologic detection of cardiac allograft rejection. Circulation 84:344, 1991.

37. Grace AA, Newell SA, Cary NRB, et al: Diagnosis of early cardiac transplant rejection by fall in evoked T wave amplitude measured using an externalized QT driven rate responsive pacemaker. PACE 14:1024, 1991.

38. Johnson AD, Daily PO: Hypertrophic subaortic stenosis complicated by high degree heart block: Successful treatment with an atrial synchronous ventricular pacemaker. Chest 67:491, 1975.

39. Hassenstein P, Walther H, Dittrich J: Haemodynamische Veranderungen durch Einfach-oder Gekoppelte Stimulation bei patienten mit obstruktiver Kardiomyopathie. Verh Dtsch Ges Inn Med 81:17, 1975.

40. McDonald K, McWilliams E, O'Keeffe B, et al: Functional assessment of patients treated with permanent dual chamber pacing as a primary treatment for hypertrophic cardiomyopathy. Eur Heart J 9:893, 1988.

41. Richter T, Cserhalmi M, Lengyel M, et al: Changes in left ventricular hemodynamics of hypertrophic obstructive cardiomyopathy (HOCM) patients treated with VAT sequential pacing. In Baroldi G, Camerini F, Goodwin JF (eds): Advances in Cardiomyopathies. New York, Springer-Verlag, 1990, pp 168–174.

42. McDonald KM, Maurer B: Permanent pacing as treatment for hypertrophic cardiomyopathy. Am J Cardiol 68:108, 1991.

43. Fananapazir L, Cannon RO III, Tripodi D, et al: Impact of dual-chamber permanent pacings in patients with obstructive hypertrophic cardiomyopathy with symptoms refractory to verapamil and β-adrenergic blocker therapy. Circulation 85:2149, 1992.

44. McAreavey D, Fananapazir L: Altered cardiac hemodynamic and electrical state in normal sinus rhythm after chronic dual chamber pacing for relief of left ventricular outflow obstruction in hypertrophic cardiomyopathy. Am J Cardiol 70:651, 1992.

45. Cannon RO II, Dilsizian V, Bonow RO, et al: Symptom, hemodynamic and myocardial benefit of atrial-synchronized ventricular pacing in nonobstructive hypertrophic cardiomyopathy. J Am Coll Cardiol 19(suppl): 120A, 1992. Abstract.

46. Iskandrian AS, Mintz GS: Pacemaker therapy in congestive heart failure: A new concept based on excessive utilization of the Frank-Starling mechanism. Am Heart J 112:867, 1986.

47. Hochleitner M, Hortnagl H, Ng C-K, et al: Usefulness of physiologic dual-chamber pacings in drug resistant idiopathic dilated cardiomyopathy. Am J Cardiol 66:198, 1990.

48. Hochleitner M, Hortnagl H, Hortnagl H, et al: Long-term efficacy of physiologic dual-chamber pacing in the treatment of end-stage idiopathic dilated cardiomyopathy. Am J Cardiol 70:1320, 1992.

49. Kataoka H: Hemodynamic effect of physiological dual chamber pacing in a patient with end-stage dilated cardiomyopathy: A case report. PACE 14:1330, 1991.

50. Brecker SJD, Xiao HB, Sparrow J, et al: Effects of dual-chamber pacing with short atrioventricular delay in dilated cardiomyopathy. Lancet 340:1308, 1992.

51. Moss AJ, Glaser W, Topol E: Atrial tachypacing in the treatment of a patient with primary orthostatic hypotension. N Engl J Med 303:885, 1980.

52. Weissmann P, Chin MT, Moss AJ: Cardiac tachypacing for severe refractory idiopathic orthostatic hypotension. Ann Intern Med 116:650, 1992.

53. Goldberg MR, Robertson RM, Robertson D: Atrial tachypacing for primary orthostatic hypotension. N Engl J Med 303:885, 1980.

54. Kristinsson A: Programmed atrial pacing for orthostatic hypotension. Acta Med Scand 214:79, 1983.

55. Grubb BP, Wolfe DA, Samoil D, et al: Adaptive rate pacing controlled by right ventricular preejection interval for severe refractory hypotension. PACE 16:801, 1993.

56. Eldar M, Griffin JC, Abbott JA, et al: Permanent cardiac pacing in patients with the long QT syndrome. J Am Coll Cardiol 10:600, 1987.

57. Moss AJ, Liu JE, Gottlieb S, et al: Efficacy of permanent pacing in the

management of high risk patients with long QT syndrome. Circulation 84:1530, 1991.

58. Moss AJ, Schwartz PJ, Crampton RS, et al: The long QT syndrome: Prospective longitudinal study of 328 families. Circulation 84:1136, 1991.

59. Schwartz PJ, Locati EH, Moss AJ, et al: Left cardiac sympathetic denervation in the therapy of congenital long QT syndrome: A worldwide report. Circulation 84:503, 1991.

60. Bhandari AK, Scheinman MM, Morady F, et al: Efficacy of left cardiac sympathectomy in the treatment of patients with the long QT syndrome. Circulation 70:1018, 1984.

61. Locati EM, Schwartz PJ: The idiopathic long QT syndrome: Therapeutic management. PACE 15:1374, 1992.

62. Eldar M, Griffin JC, VanHare GF, et al: Combined use of beta-adrenergic blocking agents and long-term cardiac pacing for patients with the long QT syndrome. J Am Coll Cardiol 20:830, 1992.

CHAPTER 23

Basic Physiology of Cardiac Pacing

Denise L. Janosik
Arthur J. Labovitz

When permanent cardiac pacing was introduced in the late 1950s, the principal goal was to prevent death or syncope caused by ventricular asystole. Parallel advances in pacemaker technology and in our understanding of cardiac hemodynamics have expanded the indications for pacing and increased the expectations of patients and physicians[1-3] (Fig. 23–1). Today, in addition to relieving symptoms related to bradycardia, a major goal of pacing is to provide the most hemodynamically optimal pacing system for the individual patient.

The appreciation of the hemodynamic significance of atrial systole, along with improved pacemaker implantation techniques, resulted in the development of atrial synchronous ventricular pacemakers. Advances in atrial lead technology and programmability of pulse generators increased the utilization of dual-chamber pacemakers in the late 1970s. However, the ability of dual-chamber pacing systems to adapt to an individual's metabolic needs is dependent largely on normal sinus node function. In the early 1980s it was demonstrated that heart rate was the primary means of augmenting cardiac output during exercise in paced subjects. This observation, along with the high prevalence of sinus node dysfunction in paced patients, encouraged the development of rate-adaptive pacemakers that increase the pacing rate in response to a metabolic sensor other than the sinus node. Evidence that ventricular rate-adaptive pacing yields exercise hemodynamics equivalent to that seen with dual-chamber pacing and involves the insertion of a single pacing lead contributed to the great popularity of VVIR pacemakers in the mid-1980s. A variety of metabolic sensors were introduced and clinically validated to acutely improve exercise hemodynamics. Before the availability of dual-chamber rate-responsive pacemakers in the late 1980s, there were heated debates regarding the relative importance of rate responsiveness and atrioventricular synchrony in the hemodynamics of cardiac pacing. With the current availability of dual-chamber rate-responsive pacemakers, rate responsiveness and atrioventricular synchrony are no longer mutually exclusive features. It is now appreciated that a truly physiologic pacemaker will maintain the normal sequence and timing of atrial and ventricular activation over a wide range of heart rates, vary the heart rate in response to metabolic demands, and preserve the normal rapid synchronous sequence of ventricular activation when possible.

Hemodynamic Importance of Atrioventricular Synchrony

Although the relative contribution of atrial systole to cardiac performance may vary between individuals, it has been demonstrated to be hemodynamically beneficial in those with normal hearts as well as those with diseased ones, at rest and during exercise, and in both acute and chronic interventions. An appropriately timed atrial systole maintains a low mean atrial pressure, thus facilitating venous return; maximizes preload and cardiac performance by means of the Starling mechanism; and closes the atrioventricular valves before ventricular systole, thereby minimizing atrioventricular valvular regurgitation (Fig. 23–2). In addition, it has been appreciated that important circulatory and neurohumoral reflexes originate in the atria and are regulated, in part, by atrial volume and filling pressure.

ANIMAL STUDIES

Much of the early understanding of atrial function and its importance during cardiac pacing was derived from animal models. Sir William Harvey[4] first observed the booster pump function of the atria in the 1600s in the excised frog heart: "when the auricles alone are beating, if you cut off the tip of the heart with a scissors, you will see blood gush out at

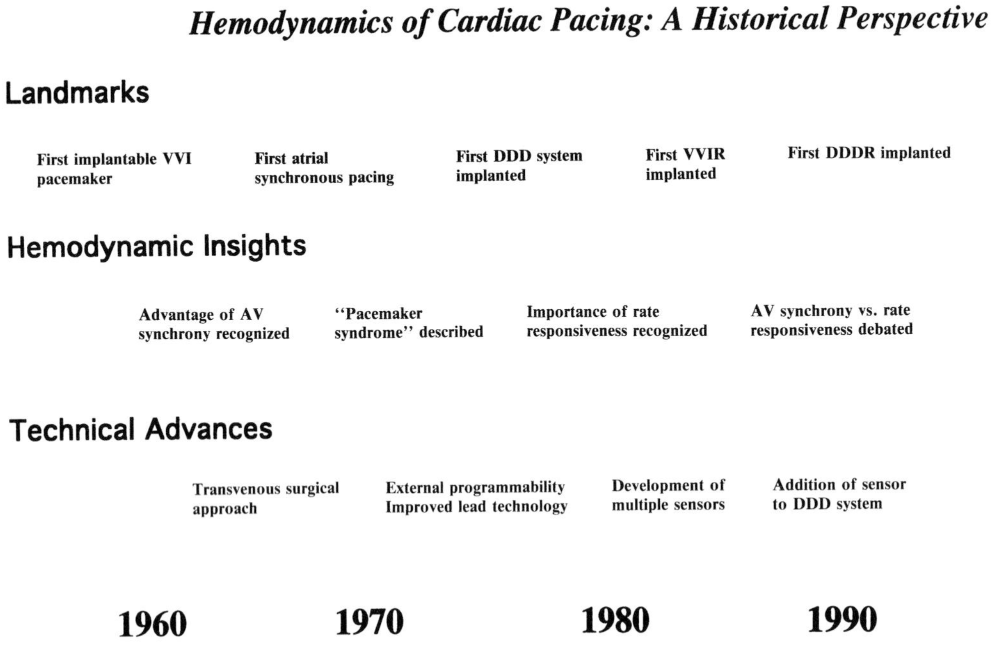

Hemodynamics of Cardiac Pacing: A Historical Perspective

Landmarks

| First implantable VVI pacemaker | First atrial synchronous pacing | First DDD system implanted | First VVIR implanted | First DDDR implanted |

Hemodynamic Insights

| Advantage of AV synchrony recognized | "Pacemaker syndrome" described | Importance of rate responsiveness recognized | AV synchrony vs. rate responsiveness debated |

Technical Advances

| Transvenous surgical approach | External programmability Improved lead technology | Development of multiple sensors | Addition of sensor to DDD system |

1960   **1970**   **1980**   **1990**

FIGURE 23–1. Historical perspective illustrating major landmarks in cardiac pacing and the parallel advances in hemodynamic insights and pacemaker technology.

each beat of the auricles." In 1910 Straub[5] described an early rapid phase of ventricular filling followed by a sudden increase in filling coincident in filling with atrial systole. Wiggers and Katz[6] further delineated and quantitated the phases of normal ventricular filling. They observed that early rapid inflow accounted for 30% to 50% of total filling and was followed by a phase of retarded filling (diastasis). The volume contributed by atrial systole was noted to vary under different conditions and accounted for 18% to 60% of total filling. In a series of experiments on dog preparations with heart block performed in the early 1900s, Gesell[7] demonstrated a 10% to 15% decrease in arterial blood pressure and an increase in venous pressure with loss of atrial systole and noted that the function of the atrium included "adequate

filling of the ventricles with a comparatively low venous pressure, thus preventing continued strain upon the venous system." He also observed that the effectiveness of atrial systole varied, depending on its temporal relationship to ventricular systole, with auricular systoles completed 0.008 to 0.02 second before the initiation of ventricular systole being most advantageous. He later demonstrated that an appropriately timed atrial systole increased ventricular fiber length and intraventricular tension and optimized the surface-volume relation, thereby increasing ventricular efficiency and output by approximately 50% over that maintained by venous pressure alone.[8]

Subsequent investigations in animals confirmed that appropriately timed atrial contraction augments ventricular fill-

Hemodynamic Effects of an Effective and Appropriately Timed Atrial Systole Concentration

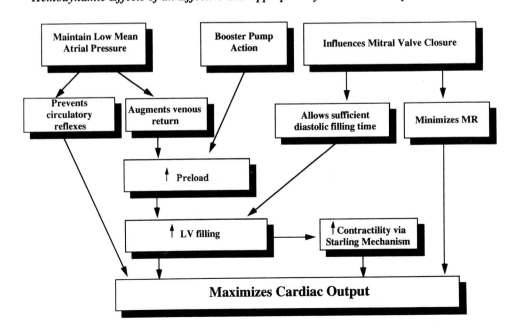

FIGURE 23–2. The hemodynamic importance of an effective and appropriately timed atrial contraction. LV, left ventricular; MR, mitral regurgitation.

TABLE 23–1. **FACTORS INFLUENCING EFFECTIVENESS OF ATRIAL CONTRACTION IN ANIMAL MODELS**

Timing relative to ventricular contraction
Vigor of atrial contraction
Autonomic nervous system
Heart rate
Left atrial volume
Left atrial pressure
Presence of pericardium
Sequence of ventricular activation
Left ventricular end-diastolic pressure
Atrial compliance

ing and cardiac output by 18% to 60%.[9–24] In addition, other factors altering the effectiveness of atrial systole were described, including the vigor of atrial contraction,[12, 14] heart rate,[12, 13] influence of the autonomic nervous system,[12, 14, 22, 23] left atrial volume[12, 17] and pressure,[12] left ventricular end-diastolic pressure-volume relationship,[9, 12, 18] and site of ventricular activation[11, 16, 19, 25–29] (Table 23–1). Using a canine heart block model, Mitchell and colleagues[12] demonstrated that cardiac output and left ventricular end diastolic pressure were higher and mean left atrial pressure lower with atrial pacing compared to ventricular pacing at the same rate (Fig. 23–3). For any given left ventricular end-diastolic pressure, the mean left atrial pressure was lower during atrial pacing than during ventricular pacing. They also demonstrated that heart rate and the vigor of atrial contraction exerted independent influences on the contribution of atrial function to cardiac performance and both were affected by the autonomic

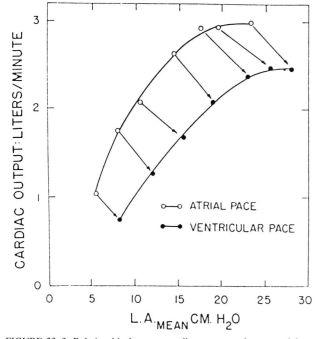

FIGURE 23–3. Relationship between cardiac output and mean atrial pressure (LA mean) during atrial pacing *(open circles)* compared with ventricular pacing *(solid circles)* in an intact dog model. For any given mean left atrial pressure, the cardiac output is higher with atrial pacing than with ventricular pacing. (From Mitchell JH, Gilmore JP, Sarnoff SJ: The transport function of the atrium. Factors influencing the relation between mean left atrial pressure and left ventricular end diastolic pressure. Am J Cardiol 9:237, 1962.)

nervous system.[12] Mean left atrial pressure was higher for any left ventricular end-diastolic pressure as heart rate increased and the relative period during which atrial emptying occurs decreased.[12] At a constant heart rate, left atrial pressure was higher at any given left ventricular end-diastolic pressure during efferent vagal stimulation because of a negative inotropic atrial effect and lower during sympathetic stimulation because of a positive inotropic effect on the atrium. In a subsequent study, Mitchell and associates[13] demonstrated that the atrial contribution to cardiac output remained significant over a wide range of heart rates, 60 to 210 beats per minute (bpm), and the percentage augmentation by atrial systole over ventricular pacing alone increased with increased rates of pacing at rest (Fig. 23–4A and B). Investigations by Gilmore[11] and Kosowsky[16] and their colleagues suggested that the temporal relationship between atrial and ventricular contraction and the sequence of ventricular depolarization were independent and additive determinants of ventricular performance during pacing. Several subsequent investigators have demonstrated that the asynchronous ventricular contraction produced by right ventricular apical pacing is deleterious to systolic and diastolic ventricular function compared with more normal sequences of ventricular activation.[19, 25–29]

Normally, the atria function as a conduit that transfers blood to the ventricle when the atrioventricular (AV) valves are open, a reservoir to accept venous inflow during ventricular ejection, and a booster pump during atrial systole. Payne and coworkers[17] investigated the effects of volume loading on left atrial contractile function in the intact dog model. They demonstrated that as left atrial diameter increased with volume loading, left atrial systolic shortening initially increased. However, the ascending limb of the function curve was short, and as volume further increased, the amplitude of atrial shortening decreased. Thus, at a critical level of distention the optimal atrial end-diastolic diameter is exceeded; the booster pump function of the atrium is diminished and conduit function dominates. Studies of a circulatory analog model indicate that cardiac output is enhanced with increased atrial compliance in the presence of constant ventricular contractility.[30]

Linderer and associates[18] examined the influence of atrial systole on the left ventricular function curve in open-chest dogs with both intact and opened pericardia. When the pericardium was closed, withdrawal of atrial systole consistently shifted the relationship between left ventricular stroke volume and end-diastolic pressure downward. When the pericardium was opened, the entire curve shifted upward and stroke volume was relatively independent of atrial contribution. Consistent with the Frank-Starling mechanism, the stroke volume increased with increased end-diastolic diameter regardless of the presence of atrial systole or an intact pericardium.

Animal studies have also defined the role of atrial systole in the initiation of mitral valve closure.[14, 15] The mitral valve closes as a result of the reversal of the atrioventricular pressure gradient before ventricular ejection. Sarnoff and colleagues[14] demonstrated in a heart block canine preparation that the timing and vigor of atrial contraction and relaxation contribute to the rate of rise of left ventricular end-diastolic pressure and the rate of decline of atrial pressure. By altering the timing of atrial contraction relative to ventricular contrac-

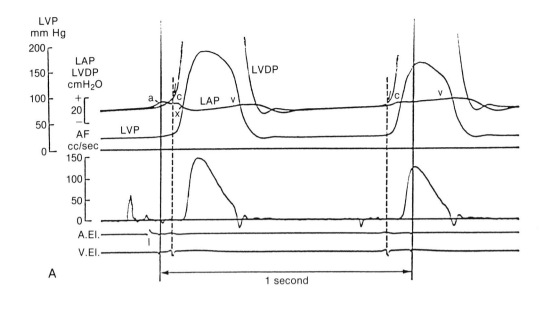

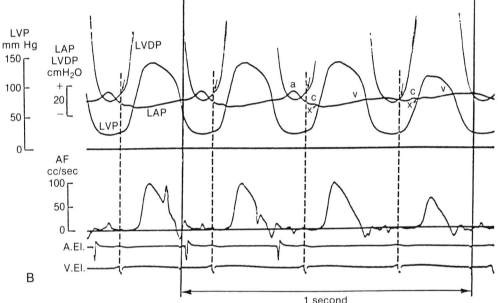

FIGURE 23–4. Hemodynamic effects of atrial systole at a low heart rate (A) and at a higher heart rate (B). The a, v, and c waves and x descent are present in ejections in which ventricular systole is preceded by atrial systole. The a wave is absent, and there is no x descent when atrial systole is absent (last beat of each panel). The loss of atrial systole diminished effective left ventricular stroke volume by 25% at the low heart rate and by almost 50% at the higher heart rate. LVP, left ventricular pressure; LAP, left atrial pressure; LVDP, left ventricular diastolic pressure; AF, aortic flow; A.EL, left atrial bipolar electrogram; V.EL, left ventricular bipolar electrogram. Time lines are at 1-second intervals. (From Mitchell JH, Gupta DN, Payne RM: Influence of atrial systole on effective ventricular stroke volume. Circ Res 17:11, 1965.)

tion, they demonstrated that closure of the mitral valve could be induced solely as a result of atrial activity.[14] They further demonstrated that when atrial contraction and relaxation were able to promote mitral valve closure, this could be abolished by diminishing the contractility of the atrium through vagal stimulation and, conversely, enhanced by augmenting contractility by sympathetic stimulation. Using a similar animal model, Skinner and associates[15] demonstrated that with a very short atrial ventricular contraction sequence or in the absence of atrial activity, the mitral valve was closed by the ventriculoatrial (VA) pressure gradient generated solely by ventricular systole and mitral regurgitation was noted to occur. If the AV interval was excessively long, they demonstrated that the pressure generated by atrial systole occurred against a closed AV valve and, if too short, occurred simultaneously with ventricular contraction.[15] In more recent animal studies, Doppler echocardiography has demonstrated that diastolic filling is interrupted and cardiac out-

put reduced by short (50 msec) AV delay intervals during AV sequential pacing.[24]

Observations in animal models have contributed to our understanding of the deleterious hemodynamic effects of ventricular pacing. In open-chest heart block dog models, ventricular pacing resulting in one-to-one retrograde VA conduction has been shown to cause significant decreases in cardiac output, left ventricular pressure, and systolic blood pressure and increases in right atrial and pulmonary venous pressures and left atrial size compared with ventricular pacing with complete retrograde VA block or random VA conduction.[19–21] An increase in left atrial size and elevation of atrial pressure during one-to-one VA conduction may be a stimulus for the abnormal atrial reflexes observed in the pacemaker syndrome in humans. Naito and associates[20, 21] evaluated the hemodynamic effects of abnormal AV sequencing in dog models of heart block by angiography and M-mode echocardiography. As the AV interval decreased

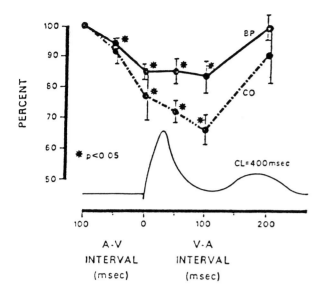

FIGURE 23–5. Relationship between atrioventricular (AV) and ventriculo-atrial (VA) intervals and cardiac output (CO) and blood pressure (BP) in intact dogs. Cardiac output and blood pressure fall at AV intervals of less than 50 msec and are lowest at VA intervals of 100 msec. (From Ogawa S, Dreifus LS, Shenoy PN, et al: Hemodynamic consequences of atrioventricular and ventriculoatrial pacing. PACE 1:8, 1978.)

from +100 to −100 msec there was a progressive decrease in cardiac output, left ventricular and aortic pressure, and left ventricular dimension and an increase in left atrial pressure. At negative AV intervals, not only was there a loss of atrial contribution to ventricular filling but also pulmonary venous regurgitation or a "negative atrial kick" occurred, resulting in further hemodynamic deterioration. Varying the AV interval from +100 to −200 msec, Ogawa and coworkers[19] found the least favorable hemodynamics to occur at a VA interval of 100 msec (Fig. 23–5).

HEMODYNAMIC EFFECTS OF VENTRICULAR PACING IN COMPLETE HEART BLOCK

Initially, permanent ventricular pacemakers were implanted in the early 1960s to prevent death or syncope caused by ventricular asystole. Appreciation of both the beneficial and the deleterious hemodynamic effects of ventricular pacing soon followed. In both animal and humans with acquired complete heart block and a slow ventricular escape, cardiac output is reduced compared with normal resting heart rates

TABLE 23–2. **HEMODYNAMIC EFFECTS OF VENTRICULAR PACING IN COMPLETE HEART BLOCK**

HEMODYNAMIC PARAMETER	CHB WITH SLOW VENTRICULAR RESPONSE	VENTRICULAR PACING IN CHB
Ventricular rate	↓	↑
Cardiac index	↓	↑
Stroke volume	↑	↓
Sympathetic tone	↑	↓
Ventricular contractility	↑	↓
Systemic vascular resistance	↑	↓
Atrial rate	↑	↓

Abbreviation: CHB, complete heart block.

despite compensatory increases in sympathetic tone and end-diastolic ventricular volume that are manifested by increased atrial rates, enhanced ventricular contractility, and augmented stroke volume (Table 23–2). In patients with acquired complete heart block, ventricular pacing produces a more physiologically appropriate resting heart rate and increased cardiac output associated with decreased sympathetic tone and a reduction in end-diastolic ventricular volume that are reflected by decreased atrial rates, diminished stroke volume, and reduced ventricular contractility.[31–36] Brockman[31] described an immediate decrease in cardiac output and increase in left ventricular stroke volume after surgically induced heart block in dogs. The canine heart adapted to the increased diastolic volume produced by bradycardia acutely by dilatation and chronically by hypertrophy. Despite compensatory mechanisms, animals remaining in heart block for over 4 months tended to manifest signs of congestive heart failure. The frequency of congestive heart failure symptoms in patients with complete heart block correlates with the duration of heart block, suggesting that the ability of ventricular dilatation and hypertrophy to compensate for chronic bradycardia in humans is also limited.[32] Congestive heart failure has been described during chronic complete heart block even in individuals with normal ventricular function. Brockman and Stoney[32] reported that in two thirds of patients with complete heart block and congestive heart failure, symptoms were relieved by ventricular pacing alone and no additional medical therapy was required.

Early studies suggested that the maximal increase in cardiac output during ventricular pacing at rest occurred at rates between 70 and 90 bpm[33–36] (Fig. 23–6). Further increases in rates resulted in either no additional increase or a decrease in cardiac output accompanied by increased peripheral vascular resistance. Sowton[34] described two patterns of hemodynamic response to increased rates of ventricular pacing. In the flat response, after an initial increase, cardiac output remained relatively constant as stroke volume decreased with increasing heart rate (Fig. 23–7A). This response occurred most often in individuals with normal cardiac function and indicates that cardiac output is relatively independent of heart rate. In the peaked response, cardiac output increased progressively until the optimal pacing rate was achieved and any

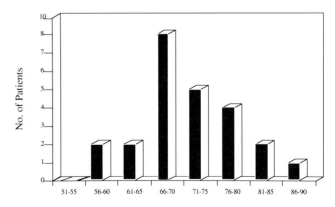

FIGURE 23–6. Histogram of optimal ventricular pacing rates at rest as defined by cardiac outputs determined by dye dilution in patients with complete heart block. (From Sowton E: Hemodynamic studies in patients with artificial pacemakers. Br Heart J 26:737, 1964.)

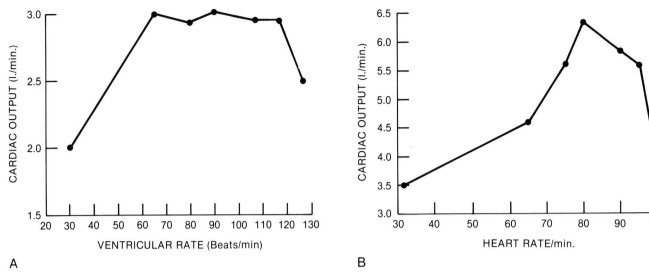

FIGURE 23–7. *A*, Example of flat response indicating a relatively constant cardiac output over a wide range of ventricular pacing rates. *B*, Example of a peaked response curve demonstrating progressive increase in cardiac output with heart rate until an optimal heart rate is achieved. After this optimal heart rate, a further increase in heart rate results in a decrease in cardiac output. (From Sowton E. Hemodynamic studies in patients with artificial pacemakers. Br Heart J 26:737, 1964.)

further increase in rate resulted in a diminution in cardiac output (see Fig. 23–7*B*). The peaked response was more commonly observed in individuals with myocardial disease, in which cardiac output is more sensitive to changes in preload, afterload, myocardial contractility, and distensibility. The major factors limiting the increase in resting cardiac output that can be achieved by pacing rate alone are shortened diastolic filling time, reduced left ventricular compliance at higher rates of ventricular pacing, and increased systemic vascular resistance.[33–36]

Rowe and colleagues[37] examined cardiac output and coronary blood flow at low (47 bpm), intermediate (77 bpm), and high (117 bpm) ventricular pacing rates in subjects with complete heart block. Cardiac output increased from the low to the intermediate rate but decreased at the higher rate. Coronary blood flow and cardiac oxygen consumption increased progressively with increasing rates. They concluded that low and intermediate heart rates yield the most efficient systemic and coronary dynamics.

Fixed-rate ventricular pacing maintains a resting cardiac output adequate for the prevention of syncope in the majority of individuals. However, VVI pacing is not physiologic in the sense of preserving an appropriate atrial-to-ventricular relationship or in terms of the ability to increase heart rate in response to metabolic demands. The importance of the atrial contribution to cardiac output has long been appreciated. Loss of an effective atrial systole because of atrial fibrillation is recognized to cause symptoms of congestive heart failure even in individuals with normal hearts and adequate control of the ventricular response of the atrial fibrillation.[38–41] During ventricular pacing for complete heart block it was noted that QRS complexes preceded by P waves resulted in higher stroke volumes and systemic pressures than QRS complexes occurring in the absence of P waves.[42–46] Observations of the hemodynamic effects of randomly distributed AV coupling intervals during ventricular pacing suggested the importance of timing between atrial and ventricular contraction.[44–46] It

was noted that very short or very long AV coupling intervals resulted in minimal hemodynamic improvement compared with ventricular pacing alone. An inverse relationship between the optimal PR interval and ventricular pacing rate was also described.[44] The relative contribution of a fortuitously timed P wave to cardiac output during ventricular pacing for complete heart block has been reported to be greater at higher ventricular pacing rates.

ADVERSE HEMODYNAMIC EFFECTS OF VENTRICULAR PACING

Samet and associates[47, 48] demonstrated increased thermodilution cardiac output during temporary AV sequential pacing and atrial demand pacing compared with ventricular demand pacing at the same heart rate. Numerous subsequent studies have demonstrated 10% to 53% increments in resting cardiac output[49–85] with AV synchronous or sequential pacing compared with VVI pacing (Table 23–3). These studies have been performed utilizing both invasive[47–59, 76, 77] and noninvasive[60–75, 78–85] (Fig. 23–8) assessment of cardiac output, during temporary pacing[47–58] as well as with acute reprogramming of permanent pacemakers,[59–84] and in individuals with diseased hearts[50, 51, 53–58] and those with normal cardiac function.[48, 49, 70, 74] Higher left ventricular end-diastolic pressures[47, 57] and volumes,[57, 63, 64, 70, 71] higher systolic and mean blood pressures,[54, 59, 60] lower venous pressures, and lower pulmonary capillary wedge pressures[52, 56, 58] have been reported with modes of pacing that maintain AV synchrony compared to ventricular pacing. The significance of the atrial contribution to resting cardiac output persists over a wide range of paced heart rates in the upright position as well as in the supine position and in the presence of inotropic stimulation. At rest, the atrial contribution to cardiac output and percentage augmentation in cardiac output with AV sequential pacing compared with ventricular pacing increases with increasing heart rate. Most

TABLE 23–3. **RESTING CARDIAC OUTPUT DURING PHYSIOLOGIC PACING MODES COMPARED TO VVI PACING**

REFERENCE	METHOD OF CARDIAC OUTPUT MEASUREMENT	PERCENTAGE INCREMENT, DDD vs. VVI
Invasive studies		
Samet[47]	Dye dilution	19
Karlof[52]	Thermodilution	10
Leinbach[53]	Dye dilution	24
Chamberlain[54]	Dye dilution	24
Hartlzer[55]	Dye dilution	34
Greenberg[56]	Thermodilution	25
Reiter[58]	Thermodilution	17
Noninvasive studies		
Nanda[61]	Doppler	18
Zugibe[62]	Doppler	19.5
Boucher[64]	Radionuclide angiography	16
Nitsch[66]	Radionuclide angiography	10
Stewart[67]	Doppler	19
Labovitz[68]	Doppler	21
Faerestrand[69]	Doppler	21
Rediker[78]	Doppler	43
Janosik[80]	Doppler	33
Lascault[81]	Doppler	27
Masuyama[85]	Doppler	26

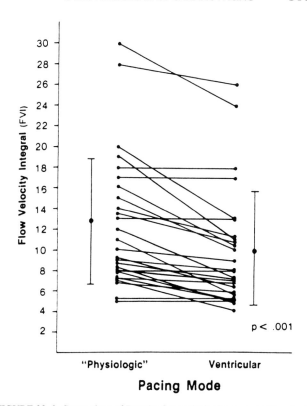

FIGURE 23–8. Comparison of Doppler flow velocity integrals in 26 patients during AV sequential physiologic pacing versus ventricular pacing at identical heart rates. A mean reduction in flow velocity integral of 21% occurred when programming from physiologic pacing mode to ventricular pacing. (From Labovitz AJ, Williams GA, Redd RM, Kennedy HL: Noninvasive assessment of pacemaker hemodynamics by Doppler echocardiography: Importance of left atrial size. J Am Coll Cardiol 6:196, 1985. Reprinted with permission from the American College of Cardiology.)

radionuclide studies indicate higher cardiac outputs but no significant change in left ventricular ejection with a dual-chamber pacing mode compared with VVI pacing at similar heart rates.[63–65, 70, 71] In fact, lower left ventricular ejection fractions have been reported with DDD pacing than with VVI pacing. This may be explained by the fact that cardiac output is increased by augmenting ventricular filling with dual-chamber pacing and that relatively higher catecholamine levels and enhanced contractility are compensatory mechanisms for the lower volume with VVI pacing. In addition to the loss of the atrial contribution to cardiac output, ventricular pacing can result in significant tricuspid or mitral regurgitation in some individuals because of asynchrony of atrial and ventricular contraction and poorly timed AV valve closure.[86, 87]

Most individuals can compensate for a reduction in cardiac output related to loss of atrial systole by baroreceptor reflexes that increase peripheral resistance and maintain systemic blood pressure. In addition, during ventricular pacing in individuals without retrograde VA conduction there is intermittent hemodynamic benefit from fortuitously timed P waves (Figs. 23–9 and 23–10). However, in some individuals the asynchrony between atrial and ventricular contraction may be poorly tolerated and induce unfavorable autonomic reflexes that further compromise cardiac output. The atrial reflexes are thought to be initiated by sudden distention of the atrium with increased volume and pressure because of contraction of the atrium against a closed AV valve or retrograde VA conduction. When activated, atrial reflexes override compensatory baroreceptor reflexes and result in an inappropriate decrease in peripheral vascular resistance despite a fall in cardiac output.[88–92] The constellation of neurologic and cardiovascular symptoms resulting from these deleterious hemodynamics has been termed the pacemaker syndrome.[91] This syndrome is discussed in detail in Chapter 25.

DIFFERENTIAL HEMODYNAMIC BENEFIT OF ATRIOVENTRICULAR SYNCHRONY

Although the hemodynamic superiority of dual-chamber pacing modes over VVI pacing has been demonstrated in a wide variety of clinical situations, it is clear that not all individuals benefit equally from the maintenance of AV synchrony during cardiac pacing. Both invasive and noninvasive

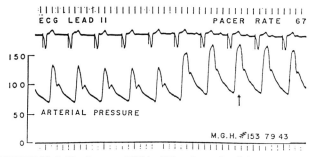

FIGURE 23–9. Simultaneous ECG lead II tracing and radial artery pressure from a patient with complete AV block during fixed-rate ventricular pacing. Arterial pressure is higher in beats preceded by dissociated P waves. The peak systolic pressure is observed when the PR interval is 270 msec. (From Leinbach RC, Chamberlain DA, Kastor JA, et al: A comparison of the hemodynamic effects of ventricular and sequential A-V pacing in patients with heart block. Am Heart J 78:502, 1969.)

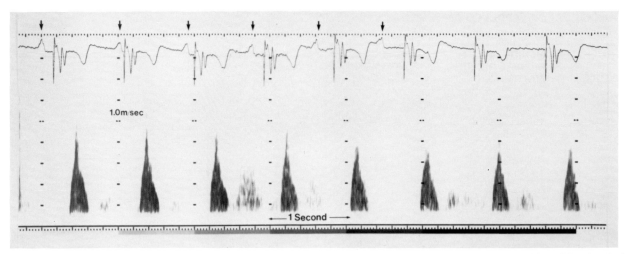

FIGURE 23–10. Doppler aortic flow velocity integrals during ventricular pacing in a patient with complete heart block. The effect of fortuitously timed P waves *(arrows)* on aortic flow is demonstrated.

studies have attempted to identify factors predictive of the greatest relative benefit of AV synchrony during pacing (Table 23–4). Discrepancies in the results may be attributed partly to the small number of subjects in each study, heterogeneous populations of patients, and variable attempts to optimize the AV delay interval during pacing.

Benchimol and colleagues[51] compared invasive hemodynamic measurements during atrial and ventricular pacing in normal control subjects, patients with compensated nonvalvular heart disease, and patients with decompensated heart failure. In normal subjects, both atrial and ventricular pacing at increasing rates resulted in progressive and comparable increases in cardiac output and decreases in stroke volume. Thus, the contribution of atrial systole to cardiac output in normal subjects did not appear to be significant. However, in subjects with heart disease, incremental atrial pacing rates resulted in a progressive increase in cardiac output, whereas with ventricular pacing at increasing rates there was a decrease in cardiac output and stroke volume. In patients with diseased hearts, the cardiac output and stroke volume were

TABLE 23–4. FACTORS ASSOCIATED WITH INCREASED HEMODYNAMIC BENEFIT OF ATRIAL SYSTOLE DURING CARDIAC PACING

Presence of clinical congestive heart failure[51]
Absence of clinical congestive heart failure[56, a]
Low baseline cardiac output and stroke volume[51, 93–95]
Pulmonary capillary wedge pressure <20 mm Hg[56]
Cardiac index <2 L/m and normal LV volume[57]
Normal LV end-diastolic and systolic dimensions[75, 81]
Retrograde VA conduction[67, 79]
Normal LA size[68, 81]
History of pacemaker syndrome[67]
Low stroke volume during VVI pacing[79]
Large increase in arterial pulse pressure from atrial systole[58]
Increased left ventricular wall thickness[81]
Presence of aortic valve disease[72]
High peak atrial to early rapid filling velocity[85]

Abbreviations: LA, left ventricular; VA, ventriculoatrial.
[a]In independent investigations, both the presence and absence of clinical congestive heart failure have been reported to result in a relatively greater benefit of AV synchrony than of ventricular pacing alone.

higher with atrial pacing than with ventricular pacing at the same heart rate. Invasive studies directly measuring the atrial contribution to left ventricular filling and stroke volume support the concept that individuals with the lowest baseline cardiac output and stroke volume derive the greatest benefit from maintenance of AV synchrony.[93–95] Braunwald and Frahm[93] studied a group of patients by means of trans-septal left heart catheterization and demonstrated that the duration of left atrial contraction is longer and the magnitude of atrial kick is greater in patients with left ventricular hypertrophy than in normal subjects. Matsuda and colleagues[94] evaluated left atrial function in normal subjects and those with remote myocardial infarction and found that the ratio of active atrial emptying to left ventricular stroke volume and the amount of left atrial work were higher in patients with previous myocardial infarction than in control subjects. Utilizing simultaneous hemodynamic and angiographic volume studies, Hamby and coworkers[95] demonstrated a higher atrial contribution to stroke volume in patients with coronary artery disease than in control subjects (33% vs. 20%, $p < .05$). They demonstrated significant negative correlations between the atrial contribution to stroke volume and baseline stroke volume and left ventricular ejection fraction, and positive correlations with left ventricular end-diastolic pressure and left ventricular end-systolic volume (Fig. 23–11). The combination of congestive heart failure and cardiomegaly was the only clinical feature associated with a significantly higher atrial contribution to stroke volume in the subgroup of patients with coronary artery disease.

Greenberg and colleagues[56] performed ventricular and AV sequential pacing in a group of patients with diverse types of heart disease and demonstrated an inverse relationship between left ventricular filling pressure and the atrial contribution to cardiac output. In this study, the atrial contribution was less effective in augmenting cardiac output when the pulmonary capillary wedge pressure exceeded 20 mm Hg or the patient clinically manifested heart failure. The apparent conflict between the results of Greenberg and associates and the data indicating that the greatest relative benefit of atrial systole occurs in patients with diseased hearts may be partially explained by examining the left ventricular pressure-

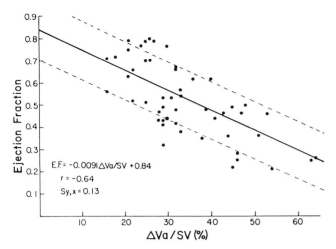

FIGURE 23–11. Relationship between left ventricular ejection fraction and atrial contribution to stroke volume (ΔVa/SV%). Shown are the regression equation *(solid line),* correlation coefficient *(r),* and one standard error of estimate (Sy,x, *dashed lines).* The percentage atrial contribution to stroke volume and resting left ventricular ejection fraction are inversely correlated. (From Hamby RI, Noble WJ, Murphy DH, Hoffman I: Atrial transport function in coronary artery disease: Relation to left ventricular function. J Am Coll Cardiol 1:1011, 1983. Reprinted with permission from the American College of Cardiology.)

volume relationship (Fig. 23–12). Regardless of left ventricular function, individuals functioning on the ascending limb of the Frank-Starling curve benefit from atrial contribution to left ventricular volume and pressure, whereas those with high filling pressure derive little benefit, as they already function on the plateau phase of the curve. Patients with systolic ventricular dysfunction may operate on a flatter curve, so the absolute increase in stroke volume when filling pressures are optimized may be quantitatively less than in patients with normal hearts. *However, this increase may represent a greater percentage increment and, therefore, result in a greater hemodynamic and clinical benefit than in individuals with normal ventricular function.* Patients with diastolic dysfunction operate on a steeper function curve and may be especially dependent on volume to optimize cardiac performance. Patients with normal left ventricular function may be able to compensate for loss of atrial systole through increased ventricular contractility and stroke volume, whereas compensatory mechanisms are less effective in patients with impaired left ventricular function. The validity of this postulation is supported by the finding of Rahimtoola's and colleagues[57] that in post–myocardial infarction patients the atrial contribution to stroke volume was significantly greater in patients with cardiac indexes less than 2 L/m compared with those with cardiac indexes greater than 2 L/m (56% vs. 31%) and in those with normal left ventricular volumes compared with those with elevated left ventricular volumes (19% vs. 10%). In other words, those deriving the greatest relative benefit were functioning on the ascending limb of a left ventricular function curve for a diseased heart. Using Doppler and M-mode echocardiographic assessment of hemodynamic responses to temporary pacing, Faerestrand and colleagues[75] demonstrated that the relative hemodynamic benefit of dual-chamber pacing over ventricular pacing diminishes as left ventricular end-diastolic and end-systolic dimension increases, placing function on the plateau phase of the left

ventricular function curve. In patients with New York Heart Association functional class III–IV failure, the increase in cardiac output with AV sequential temporary pacing compared with ventricular pacing correlated strongly with the increase in arterial pulse pressure observed when a dissociated atrial contraction preceded a ventricular paced beat by a physiologic AV interval during ventricular pacing.[58]

Noninvasive Doppler echocardiographic techniques have also been useful in identifying subgroups who derive a relatively greater hemodynamic benefit from maintenance of AV synchrony during cardiac pacing. In patients with permanent dual-chamber pacemakers, Stewart and colleagues[67] reported a 19% increase in Doppler-derived cardiac output with reprogramming from VVI to DVI pacing mode for the overall group. Patients with retrograde VA conduction or a history of the pacemaker syndrome derived the greatest increment in cardiac output (30.4% vs. 14.4%, $p < .01$). This is consistent with the fact that patients without intact VA conduction receive intermittent benefit from fortuitously timed atrial contractions, whereas those with one-to-one VA conduction are in a constant state of AV dyssynchrony and have the highest susceptibility to adverse circulatory reflexes initiated by atrial receptors. Our laboratory reported a significantly greater decrement in Doppler cardiac output when AV sequential pacing was switched to ventricular pacing alone in patients with normal-size left atria compared with those with enlarged left atria (32% vs. 11%, $p < .01$).[68] We reported a negative correlation between left atrial dimension determined from M-mode echocardiograms and the percentage decrement in stroke volume with ventricular pacing. We suggested that

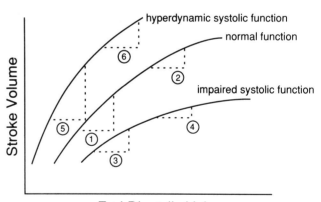

FIGURE 23–12. Left ventricular function curve indicating the relationship between left ventricular end-diastolic volume and stroke volume. In subjects with normal left ventricular systolic function on the ascending limb of the curve, increases in volume result in a substantial increase in stroke volume (1). If left ventricular filling pressures are higher (2), further increases in volume result in smaller increments in stroke volume. In individuals with impaired left ventricular systolic function on the ascending limb of the function curve (3), increases in end-diastolic volume result in an increase in stroke volume. Although the absolute increase in stroke volume may be less than that in the individual with normal systolic function (1), the relative increase in stroke volume may be greater in the individual with impaired systolic function. As left ventricular filling pressures increase in individuals with impaired left ventricular systolic function, further increases in volume result in little further augmentation of the stroke volume. Cardiac output in patients with hyperdynamic systolic function is often critically dependent on preload. Similar increases (5 and 6) result in larger increments in stroke volume than in individuals with normal function (1 and 2). (Adapted from Greenberg B, Chatterjee K, Parmley WW, et al: The influence of left ventricular filling pressure on atrial constriction to cardiac output. Am Heart J 98:742, 1979.)

enlarged and abnormally compliant atria may be less capable of generating vigorous contraction and, therefore, less effective booster pumps than normal atria.[68] Other investigators have confirmed that individuals with VA conduction and those with normal-size left atria derive greater relative hemodynamic benefits from AV synchrony than individuals lacking these factors.[79, 81] Additional factors that have been demonstrated by Doppler echocardiography to predict a relatively greater hemodynamic benefit of AV synchrony over VVI pacing include stroke volume less than 50 mL during VVI pacing independent of the presence of VA conduction,[79] normal end-systolic dimension,[81] increased left ventricular wall thickness and the presence of aortic valve disease,[72] and high peak atrial to rapid early filling velocity ratio on transmitral flow.[85] In noninvasive studies, there has been little correlation between measures of left ventricular systolic function and degree of benefit from AV synchrony. However, as is apparent from invasive studies, filling pressure plays an extremely important role in determining the relative benefit of atrial systole and cannot be measured reliably by noninvasive techniques.

In summary, it appears that the patients deriving the greatest benefit from maintenance of AV synchrony during cardiac pacing are those with poor hemodynamics with or without VA conduction during ventricular pacing alone, normal left atrial size, thick or noncompliant left ventricles that may be more dependent on atrial systole, and normal volume and filling pressure, thus placing their function on the ascending limb of the Frank-Starling left ventricular function curve. The relative importance of maintaining AV synchrony may be greatest in those with poor left ventricular function in whom compensatory hemodynamic mechanisms are impaired and in whom even a small increase in cardiac output may result in significant clinical improvement.

Timing of Atrial and Ventricular Contraction During Cardiac Pacing

The mere presence of atrial systole is not sufficient to optimize cardiac performance. It is well established that the relative timing of atrial and ventricular contraction is critical in maximizing hemodynamics during-dual chamber pacing. The appropriate timing of atrial contraction is necessary to optimize left ventricular filling, minimize atrioventricular valvular regurgitation, maintain low mean atrial pressure, and prevent unfavorable circulatory and neurohumoral reflexes. An improperly timed atrial contraction may result in no hemodynamic benefit compared with ventricular pacing alone. In fact, a poorly timed atrial contraction may activate atrial reflexes producing deleterious hemodynamic effects accompanied by symptoms of the pacemaker syndrome. Studies have demonstrated about a 25% increment in resting stroke volume, comparing the most advantageous to least advantageous AV delay interval during dual-chamber pacing.[79, 81]

INFLUENCE OF AV DELAY INTERVAL ON MITRAL VALVE CLOSURE AND LEFT VENTRICULAR FILLING

Electric and mechanical atrial activity plays an important role in the events of a normal cardiac cycle (Fig. 23–13). Atrial contraction followed by relaxation produces a negative

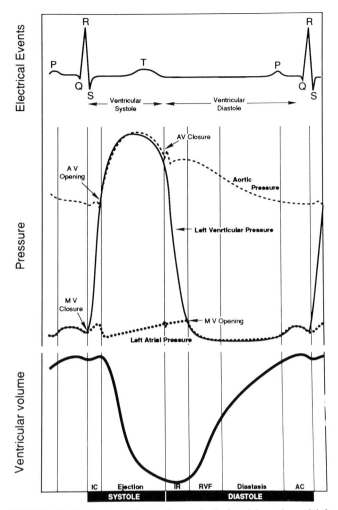

FIGURE 23–13. Events of the cardiac cycle. Left atrial, aortic, and left ventricular pressures are correlated with electric events and left ventricular volume. AC, atrial contraction; AV, aortic valve; MV, mitral valve; IC, isovolumetric contraction; IR, isovolumetric relaxation; RVF, rapid ventricular filling from 80 to 250 msec (bottom to top). (See text for description.)

pressure gradient causing a surge of blood into the ventricle at the end of diastole. Reversal of the AV pressure gradient initiates mitral valve closure because of a rapid decrease in pressure between the AV valve cusps pulling them into apposition. A brief period of isovolumetric contraction exists after mitral valve closure and before aortic valve opening during which the maximum rate of pressure change (peak dP/dt) occurs. Rapid ejection occurs during ventricular systole and is terminated when ventricular pressure falls below aortic pressure, thus closing the aortic valve. A brief period of isovolumic relaxation follows, during which the maximum rate of pressure decline (peak negative dP/dt) occurs. As left ventricular pressure continues to decline and fall below left atrial pressure, the mitral valve opens and diastolic ventricular filling begins. Normally, diastolic filling is characterized by an initial rapid increase in ventricular filling during early diastole followed by a slow phase of filling during mid-diastole. A second rapid increase in ventricular filling occurs in late diastole as a result of atrial contraction.

The presence of atrial systole and its timing relative to ventricular systole can influence mitral valve closure and dramatically influence diastolic ventricular filling pattern and

TABLE 23–5. INFLUENCE OF ATRIOVENTRICULAR DELAY ON LEFT VENTRICULAR FILLING

Appropriately timed atrial systole (optimal AV delay)
  Closure of AV valve before ventricular systole
  Minimizes AV valvular regurgitation
  Optimizes diastolic filling
Atrial systole inappropriately early (AV delay too long)
  Incomplete venous return prior to atrial contraction
  Early mitral valve closure
  AV valvular regurgitation caused by reopening of cusps
Atrial systole inappropriately late (AV delay too short)
  Atrial ejection limited
  AV valvular regurgitation

total diastolic filling time (Table 23–5). An atrial contraction, which occurs before the preejection period of the ventricle, maximizes left ventricular filling and thus cardiac output via the Starling mechanism. An optimally timed atrial contraction occurs during late ventricular diastole and initiates AV valve closure before the onset of ventricular contraction. If the AV delay interval is too long, atrial contraction and relaxation occur too early in relationship to ventricular contraction. This may result in atrial contraction before venous return is completed and thus diminish ventricular volume and contractile force. Importantly, it may also initiate early mitral valve closure, thereby limiting ventricular diastolic filling time. AV valvular regurgitation may also occur with long AV delay intervals because once closed, valve cusps may separate again before ventricular contraction. If the AV delay interval is too short, there may be insufficient time for atrial ejection to occur, thus decreasing left ventricular filling and elevating left atrial pressure. With short AV delay intervals, preclosure of the mitral valve does not occur and ventricular systole begins with the AV valves wide open, which may result in mitral or tricuspid regurgitation.

Several studies utilizing M-mode echocardiography and Doppler echocardiography have clearly demonstrated the effects of varying AV delay intervals on left ventricular filling and mitral valve closure during dual-chamber pacing. Freedman and colleagues,[96] utilizing M-mode and Doppler echocardiography, demonstrated that mitral valve closure was closely related to the P wave, indicating an atriogenic mechanism of mitral valve closure at AV delay intervals of 100 msec or greater. At AV delays shorter than 100 msec, completion of mitral valve closure occurred earlier in relationship to the P wave, suggesting a ventriculogenic mechanism of mitral valve closure. He suggested that both atrial and ventricular contraction may influence mitral valve closure and that the relative contribution of atrial and ventricular contraction to valve closure is dependent on the programmed AV delay interval. VonBibra and associates[97] reached similar conclusions utilizing M-mode echocardiograms of the mitral valve and simultaneous apexcardiograms to define ventricular systole.

With long AV delay intervals, late diastolic mitral regurgitation can result because of reopening of the mitral valve before ventricular contraction. Ishikawa and associates[98] recorded mitral valve flow at varying AV delay intervals and found that diastolic mitral regurgitation could be induced in the majority of patients with DDD pacemakers. The mean AV delay interval at which diastolic mitral regurgitation occurred was 230 msec, and the range was 140 to 260 msec. In patients with no clinical congestive heart failure, diastolic

mitral regurgitation was observed only at PR intervals exceeding 200 msec but was observed even at physiologic AV intervals in patients with congestive heart failure. There was a significant negative correlation between the pulmonary capillary wedge pressure and the critical AV delay interval for inducing diastolic mitral regurgitation. Although the clinical significance of mitral regurgitation during dual-chamber pacing has not been defined, its presence at physiologic AV delay intervals may indicate elevated left ventricular end-diastolic pressure and thus be of prognostic significance.

Because of its influence on mitral valve closure, the timing of atrial contraction can markedly alter diastolic filling time. A strong negative correlation has been demonstrated between the AV delay interval during AV sequential (DVI) and atrial synchronous (VDD) pacing and the time to mitral valve closure and total diastolic filling time.[97–99] To understand the effects of AV delay on diastolic filling, the total diastolic filling time can be divided into the time period from mitral valve opening to the ventricular pacing spike and the period from the ventricular pacing spike to the time of mitral valve closure (Fig. 23–14). VonBibra[97] and Pearson[99] and their coworkers, in independent investigations, demonstrated that as the AV delay interval is increased during dual-chamber

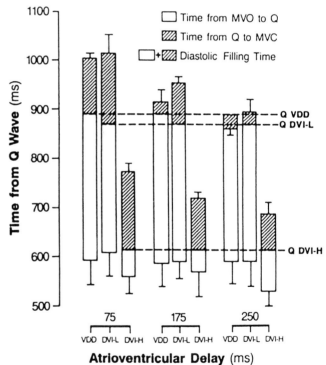

FIGURE 23–14. Effect of programmable AV delay interval on diastolic filling time. Time from the mitral valve opening (MVO) to the onset of the Q wave (Q) is represented by the white portion of the bars. The time from the Q wave to mitral valve closure (MVC) is represented by the hatched portion of the bar. The combined white and hatched segments represent the total diastolic filling time. These intervals are displayed at programmable AV delays of 75, 175, and 250 msec in the VDD, DVI low heart rate (DVI-L), and DVI high heart rate (DVI-H) modes. Time on the ordinate represents time from the previous Q wave. Horizontal dashed lines indicate the time from the Q wave in the various modes. It is apparent that increasing AV delay intervals results in abbreviated diastolic filling time regardless of mode and rate, primarily because of earlier mitral valve closure. (From Pearson AC, Janosik DL, Redd RM, et al: Doppler echocardiographic assessment of the effect of varying atrioventricular delay and pacemaker mode on left ventricular filling. Am Heart J 115:611, 1988.)

pacing, mitral valve closure occurs progressively earlier in relationship to the ventricular pacing spike. However, the time for mitral valve opening to the ventricular pacing spike is not significantly influenced by changes in AV delay interval. Thus, the total diastolic filling time progressively shortens with increasing AV delay. This was noted during AV sequential pacing as well as during atrial synchronous pacing and at physiologic (mean 69 bpm) heart rates as well as high rates (97 bpm).[99]

In addition to its effects on mitral valve closure and left ventricular filling time, variance in AV delay has been demonstrated to markedly change left ventricular diastolic filling pattern. The pattern of diastolic filling is a complex interaction between a multitude of passive and active properties of both the atria and the ventricles.[100–108] It is known to be influenced by heart rate, age, left ventricular relaxation and compliance, left ventricular and left atrial compliance and pressure, left ventricular radius to wall thickness, and, importantly, the temporal relationship between atrial and ventricular contraction. Pulsed Doppler echocardiography is a well-validated noninvasive method of recording beat-to-beat mitral valve inflow from which quantitative relationships between early and late atrial filling and indices of left ventricular diastolic compliance can be assessed.[103] The phases of diastolic filling include an initial rapid early filling phase, a slow filling phase during mid-diastole, and a second rapid filling phase in late diastole coincident with atrial contraction. Various measurements can be made from Doppler mitral valve inflow recordings to quantitate the contribution of early diastolic filling and that of atrial systole, including peak early and atrial velocities, the ratio of early to atrial velocity, the early and atrial flow velocity integral (area under the flow velocity curve), the ratio of early to atrial flow velocity integrals, and the amount of diastolic filling occurring in the first third of diastole (Fig. 23–15).

During ventricular pacing in the absence of atrial activity, mitral valve inflow recordings demonstrate only an early filling wave similar to that seen in patients with atrial fibrillation. During ventricular pacing in the presence of AV dis-

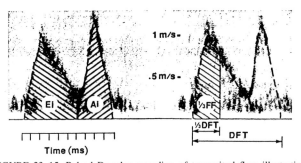

FIGURE 23–15. Pulsed Doppler recording of transmitral flow illustrating the technique utilized to measure various segments of the timed velocity integral and diastolic filling period. The relationship between early diastolic filling and that associated with atrial systole can be quantitated. Possible measurements include early and atrial velocities, the ratio of early to atrial velocity, the early (Ei) and atrial (Ai) flow velocity integral (area under the flow velocity curve), the ratio of early to atrial flow velocity integral and the amount of diastolic filling occurring in the first one third of diastole (1/3 DFT). DFT, diastolic filling time. (From Pearson AC, Janosik DL, Redd RM, et al: Doppler echocardiographic assessment of the effect of varying atrioventricular delay and pacemaker mode on left ventricular filling. Am Heart J 115:611, 1988.)

sociation, the mitral valve inflow pattern varies from beat to beat, depending on the random timing of the dissociated P waves relative to paced ventricular contraction (Fig. 23–16). During AV sequential pacing, mitral valve inflow recordings demonstrate early and atrial filling waves that vary in their relationship, depending on the rate of pacing and the AV delay interval (see Fig. 23–16B). If the AV delay interval increases, the atrial filling wave occurs progressively earlier and eventually becomes superimposed on the early rapid filling wave. Because the atrial filling wave receives a contribution from the early filling wave with long AV delay intervals, the peak atrial velocity and area under the A wave increase with increasing AV delay intervals. We have demonstrated progressive decreases in early peak velocity integral and ratio of early to atrial flow velocity integrals with increasing AV delay intervals.[99] Rokey and colleagues[102] demonstrated an inverse relationship between the atrial filling wave and early diastolic filling wave with variance of AV delay interval. As the effectiveness of atrial contraction is increased by optimization of the AV delay interval, there was a significant decrease in early mitral valve inflow velocity and peak filling rate. The authors postulated that the changes in filling pattern were a reflection of changes in left atrial volume and pressure. At shorter AV delay intervals, there may be aborted emptying of the atria resulting in larger residual volumes and higher pressure. During diastole, the left atrial volume and pressure continue to increase, resulting in a higher AV gradient at the time of mitral valve opening and increased peak early inflow. At longer AV delay intervals, atrial emptying is completed, resulting in low left atrial pressure and, therefore, decreased peak early filling rate and increased atrial filling ratio. This theory is supported by observations that early diastolic filling is increased in dilated cardiomyopathy, in which left atrial pressures are high and there is a relatively ineffective atrial contraction, whereas early diastolic filling is diminished in relation to atrial filling in conditions associated with reduced left ventricular compliance.

In summary, the timing of atrial contraction relative to ventricular contraction influences mitral valve closure and has marked effects of total diastolic filling time and the pattern of diastolic filling. Excessively long AV delay intervals may cause early mitral valve closure, thus limiting diastolic filling time primarily through reduction in early diastolic filling. Excessively short AV delay intervals fail to close the mitral valve before left ventricular systole and may result in a diminished atrial contribution to left ventricular filling because of inadequate emptying. The pattern of left ventricular filling is influenced by the AV delay interval with the relative contribution of the early filling compared with atrial filling phase decreasing with increasing AV delay interval. The clinical relevance of the AV delay interval to left ventricular filling would be expected to be most important in patients with baseline abnormalities in diastolic function and those with increased dependence on atrial contribution to cardiac output.

DETERMINATION OF OPTIMAL AV DELAY INTERVAL

Numerous investigations utilizing invasive and noninvasive measurements of cardiac output have demonstrated that an optimal AV delay interval can be determined in the ma-

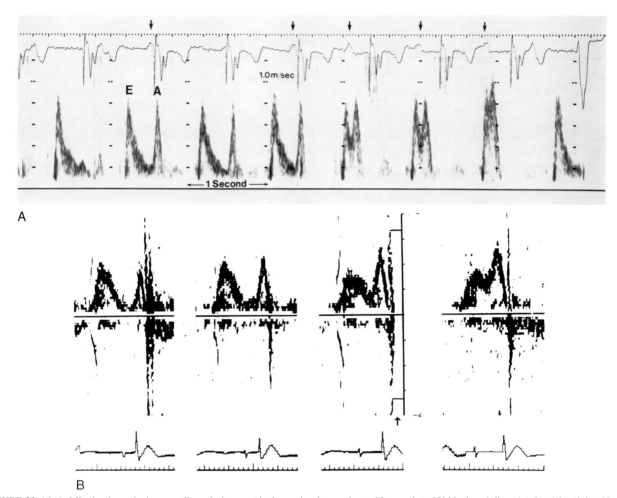

FIGURE 23–16. *A,* Mitral valve velocity recordings during ventricular pacing in a patient with complete AV block and dissociated atrial activity. Variation in the mitral flow pattern and duration of diastolic filling are evident, depending on the random occurrence of P waves. *B,* Mitral valve flow velocity pattern in a normal heart during AV sequential pacing. There is a marked variation in the temporal relationship between the A and the V waves and the magnitude of the A wave when the AV delay is modified. Note the abbreviation in total diastolic filling time and the increase in the magnitude of the A wave at longer AV delays (right side of panel) compared with the shortest AV delay (left side of panel). (*B,* From Lascault G, Bigonzi F, Frank R, et al: Noninvasive study of dual-chamber pacing by pulsed Doppler prediction of the haemodynamic response by echocardiographic measurements. Eur Heart J 10:525, 1989.)

jority of patients during dual-chamber pacing[62, 63, 66, 68–74, 76, 77, 79–84] (Fig. 23–17). Direct comparison of individual studies is difficult because most of the studies contain a relatively small number of patients with variable degrees of cardiac dysfunction and vary in the techniques utilized to measure cardiac output. In addition, most of the studies were conducted with patients at rest and in the supine position, thus limiting extrapolation of results to the clinical situation. Despite these limitations, the significance of AV delay intervals in optimizing cardiac output is apparent. The AV delay interval that maximizes resting cardiac output during dual-chamber pacing varies widely between individual patients and in most studies is reported to be between 125 and 200 msec. The AV delay interval producing optimal hemodynamics at higher pacing rates is shorter than that which is optimal at lower rates.[110] Factors that may influence the optimal AV delay interval between patients include atrial capture and sensing latencies, interatrial conduction delay, ventricular capture latency, interventricular conduction delay, the presence or absence of myocardial disease, heart rate, and catecholamine levels[111–115] (Table 23–6). In addition to interpatient variability, important factors that may influence the

optimal AV delay interval in the same individual include heart rate, paced versus sensed atrial event, catecholamine levels, drugs, and posture.[76, 80, 109, 112, 114]

It is extremely difficult to predict the optimal AV delay interval for a given patient. In some situations, AV delay intervals that are shorter than what is conventionally considered physiologic may be advantageous. AV sequential pacing for complete heart block complicating an acute myocardial infarction[54] or following cardiac surgery[55] yields optimal hemodynamics at AV delay intervals of 100 msec or less. This may be secondary to elevated catecholamine levels and reduced left ventricular compliance in these acutely stressful situations. In individuals with hypertrophic obstructive cardiomyopathy, shortening the AV delay interval so that a paced right ventricular contraction occurs has been demonstrated to decrease the intraventricular pressure gradient both acutely and chronically.[116, 117] It is believed that the altered sequence of ventricular contraction produced by right ventricular atrial pacing alters septal motion, thus increasing left ventricular outflow tract diameter and reducing the obstruction and the subaortic pressure gradient.

Most studies have demonstrated no relationship between

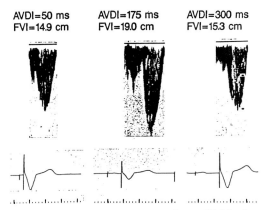

AVDI=50 ms   AVDI=175 ms   AVDI=300 ms
FVI=14.9 cm   FVI=19.0 cm   FVI=15.3 cm

FIGURE 23–17. Left ventricular outflow recording at AV delay intervals of 50, 175, and 300 msec during AV sequential pacing at identical heart rates in the same individual. The largest flow velocity integral (FVI) reflecting ventricular stroke volume occurs at an AV delay interval of 175 msec. Significant decreases are noted in stroke volume at AV delay intervals of 50 and 300 msec. (From Janosik DL, Pearson AC, Buckingham TA, et al: The hemodynamic benefit of differential atrioventricular delay intervals for sensed and paced atrial events during physiologic pacing. J Am Coll Cardiol 14:499, 1989. Reprinted with permission of the American College of Cardiology.)

left ventricular function and optimal AV delay intervals. The few that have reported a relationship between left ventricular function and optimal AV delay interval have yielded conflicting results. One small study utilizing radionuclide assessment of acute changes in left ventricular ejection fraction reported longer AV delay intervals to be more advantageous for patients with low left ventricular ejection fractions and suggested that these patients may require a longer atrial transport time.[71] In contrast, two clinical studies demonstrated significant acute and chronic hemodynamic improvement in patients with severe dilated cardiomyopathy who were physiologically paced with short AV delay intervals.[118, 119] The discrepancy between studies may be explained by differences in interatrial and/or interventricular conduction times and the presence or absence of atrioventricular valvular regurgitation between the populations of patients studied.

Although the programmable AV delay settings regulate the timing of right atrial and ventricular contraction, left atrial and ventricular contraction is most important hemodynamically.[76, 77, 115] The physiologic left-sided AV delay interval is dependent on the programmed right-sided AV delay

TABLE 23–6. POSSIBLE FACTORS INFLUENCING OPTIMAL ATRIOVENTRICULAR DELAY INTERVALS

INTERPATIENT VARIABLES
Atrial capture latency
Atrial sensing latency
Intra-atrial conduction delay
Ventricular capture latency
Intraventricular conduction delay
Underlying myocardial disease
Heart rate
Catecholamine levels
INTRAPATIENT VARIABLES
Heart rate
Paced or sensed atrial event
Catecholamine levels
Drugs

interval, latency in atrial capture and sensing, interatrial conduction time, latency in ventricular capture, and interventricular conduction time.[115] The relationship between right- and left-sided AV delay intervals during AV sequential, atrial synchronous, and atrial inhibited pacing is illustrated in Figure 23–18. It is apparent that with the same programmed right-sided AV delay interval, the left atrioventricular interval can vary by up to 200 msec, depending on whether atrial and ventricular events are paced or sensed. Wish and associates[76, 77] have demonstrated the effect of right-sided AV delay interval on the left atrial and left ventricular contraction sequence. They found a significant relationship between the optimal right-sided AV delay interval and the interatrial conduction time as measured by the time from the atrial pacing spike to the atrial depolarization on the esophageal electrogram or to the a wave on an M-mode echocardiogram. Patients with short interatrial conduction times ($\leq$ 90 msec) derived the greatest hemodynamic benefit from programmable AV delay intervals of 150 msec, and those with longer interatrial delay ($\geq$120 msec) benefited most from programmed AV delays of 200 msec or more. Wish and colleagues[76] reported some patients with interatrial conduction delays that exceeded the programmed AV delay interval, resulting in left atrial depolarization following left ventricular activation. This negative left-atrial-to-ventricular pacing sequence may produce hemodynamics equivalent to or less hemodynamically advantageous than those with VVI pacing alone.

Because of latency in atrial capture and sensing, the optimal programmable AV delay interval for sensed P waves and paced P waves may differ in an individual patient (Fig. 23–19). With a paced P wave, the programmed AV delay interval begins with the atrial pacing spike, and the physiologic PQ interval begins with atrial capture at the beginning of atrial depolarization. The physiologic PQ interval is therefore shorter than the programmed AV delay interval. The mean latency between atrial output and capture is reported to be 43 ± 10 msec; however, it may exceed 300 msec in some individuals.[111–113] With a sensed P wave, the programmed AV

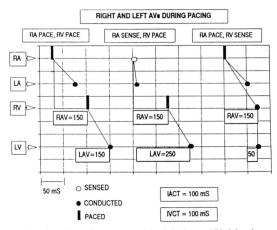

FIGURE 23–18. Effect of programmable right heart AV delay intervals on left heart AV delays during DDD pacing. RA, right atrium; LA, left atrium; RV, right ventricle; LV, left ventricle; IACT, intra-atrial conduction time; IVCT, intraventricular conduction time; RAV, right heart AV delay intervals; LAV, left heart delay intervals. (From Chirife R, Ortega DF, Salazar AI: Nonphysiological left heart AV intervals as a result of DDD and AAI "physiological" pacing. PACE 14:1752, 1991.)

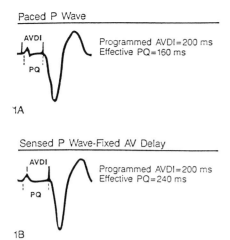

Paced P Wave

Programmed AVDI=200 ms
Effective PQ=160 ms

1A

Sensed P Wave-Fixed AV Delay

Programmed AVDI=200 ms
Effective PQ=240 ms

1B

FIGURE 23–19. Programmed AV delay interval (AVDI) and effect of PQ intervals. When a paced P wave occurs *(top)*, the effective PQ interval is shorter than the programmed AV delay because of latency in atrial capture. When a sensed P wave occurs *(bottom)*, the effective PQ interval is longer than the programmed AV interval because of latency in atrial sensing. (From Janosik DL, Pearson AC, Buckingham TA, et al: The hemodynamic benefit of differential atrioventricular delay intervals for sensed and paced atrial events during physiologic pacing. J Am Coll Cardiol 14:499, 1989. Reprinted with permission of the American College of Cardiology.)

delay interval begins when the native P wave is sensed in contrast to the physiologic PQ interval, which begins with the onset of the P wave. Thus, the physiologic PQ interval is longer than the programmed AV delay interval. In most studies, the latency from the beginning of the P wave to the time of atrial sensing is reported to be 30 to 50 msec.[112] The magnitude of atrial capture and sensing latencies varies between individuals and may be affected by the lead and pacemaker circuitry characteristics, electrode position, tissue interface, amplitude and rate of stimulation, P-wave morphology, myocardial disease, electrolytes and other metabolic factors, and drugs. It is important to recognize that the physiologic AV delay interval is never equivalent to the programmed AV delay interval for either a paced or a sensed atrial event.

Doppler echocardiography may be used to determine the difference in the timing of mechanical atrial systole when a paced compared with a sensed P wave occurs. We have found that in an individual patient, the peak A wave on the mitral valve inflow tracing occurs 40 ± 20 msec later with a paced than with a sensed P wave at similar heart rates.[84] Similarly, Alt and associates[109] have demonstrated that the peak A wave on the mitral valve M-mode recording occurs 46 ± 24 msec later with a paced P wave compared with a sensed P wave and suggested that an automatic adjustment in AV delay interval may be hemodynamically beneficial. The same investigators reported that in patients with complete heart block, short AV delay intervals of 50 to 100 msec were most hemodynamically advantageous. This was attributed to the combination of atrial sensing latency and ventricular capture latency when a paced ventricular event follows a sensed P wave, thereby yielding a physiologic AV delay interval.

Wish and colleagues[76] demonstrated that when changing from atrial pacing (DVI mode) to atrial sensing (VDD mode), a change in the timing of the left-atrial-to-ventricular sequence occurred and resulted a significant decrease in stroke

volume (Fig. 23–20). Using Doppler-derived resting cardiac output in a group of patients with DDD pacemakers, we have demonstrated that the optimal AV delay for a sensed P wave was shorter than that for a sensed P wave at similar heart rates in the same patient.[80] The mean difference between optimal AV delay intervals for a paced and a sensed P wave was 32 msec but was as great as 100 msec in some patients. At the respective optimal AV delay intervals for sensed and paced atrial events, there was no significant difference in the percentage increment over VVI pacing during AV sequential (DVI) or atrial synchronous (VDD) pacing. However, the cardiac output decreased significantly during VDD pacing at the optimal AV delay interval for a paced atrial event and during DVI pacing at the AV delay interval determined to be optimal for a sensed P wave. An additional 8% increment in cardiac output could be achieved by optimizing the AV delay interval for a sensed P wave rather than utilizing that determined to be optimal for a paced P wave. This small increment may be clinically important in individuals for whom it is critical to maximize resting cardiac output and supports the hemodynamic advantage of an automatic decrement in AV delay interval when a sensed rather than a paced P wave occurs (AV delay hysteresis) or the availability of separately programmable AV delay intervals for paced and sensed atrial events (differential AV delay intervals).

In summary, the programmed right-sided AV delay interval differs significantly from the physiologic left-sided AV delay interval. The discrepancies between right-sided and left-sided delay intervals are dependent primarily on latencies in atrial capture and sensing, interatrial conduction delay, ventricular capture latency, and interventricular conduction delay. In an individual patient, the physiologic AV delay

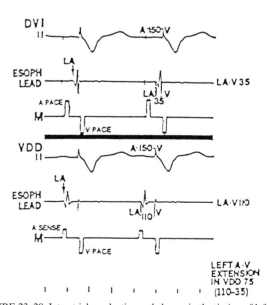

FIGURE 23–20. Interatrial conduction and change in the timing of left atrial (LA) depolarization with pacing mode change from DDD to VDD. The time delay between right atrial pacing artifact and left atrial depolarization is 115 msec, resulting in an LA-to-ventricular sequence of only 35 msec. With mode change to VDD *(bottom)* the left LA-to-ventricular sequence extends by 75 msec, resulting in an LA-to-ventricular sequence of 110 msec. (From Wish M, Fletcher RD, Gottdiener JS, Cohen AI: Importance of left atrial timing in the programming of dual-chamber pacemakers. Am J Cardiol 60:566, 1987.)

interval may vary, depending on whether a paced or a sensed atrial event and on whether a paced ventricular depolarization or intrinsic ventricular depolarization follows atrial contraction. The optimal AV delay interval for a sensed P wave is approximately 30 to 40 msec shorter than the optimal AV delay interval for a paced P wave followed by a paced QRS at a similar heart rate. Although not practical or cost-effective for every patient, fine-tuning of the AV delay interval can be performed utilizing Doppler-derived cardiac outputs at varying AV delay intervals. Alternatively, the interatrial conduction delay can be estimated noninvasively by measuring the time from the atrial pacing spike to the A wave on the M-mode echocardiogram or Doppler recording of the mitral valve and may be helpful in selecting hemodynamically advantageous AV delay intervals. These techniques may be beneficial in cases in which optimization of AV delay interval is critical to the individual's hemodynamics. Some newer dual-chamber pacemakers incorporate programmable features designed to automatically adjust the AV delay interval in response to paced versus sensed P waves and in response to the atrial rate.

RELATIVE SENSITIVITY TO AV DELAY INTERVAL

Sensitivity to changes in AV delay interval varies greatly between individuals. Whereas changes in AV delay interval of as little as 25 msec may result in significant changes in cardiac output in some patients, others are relatively insensitive to large alterations in AV delay.[55, 79, 81] We have investigated the relationship to Doppler and echocardiographic variables of systolic and diastolic ventricular function and sensitivity to variance in AV delay interval.[79] The augmentation of Doppler-derived cardiac output at the optimal AV delay interval compared with the least optimal AV delay interval was 25% during atrial synchronous pacing (VDD) and 26% during AV sequential pacing (DVI mode) (Fig. 23–21). The cardiac output at the least optimal AV delay interval was not significantly different from the cardiac output during VVI pacing. Patients with larger atrial contributions to left ventricular filling as measured from Doppler mitral valve inflow recordings derived the greatest benefit from the optimization of AV delay interval during VDD pacing. Iwase and colleagues[100] demonstrated a mean increase of 46% in mitral valve inflow from the least to the most optimal AV delay interval setting. The relative augmentation in left ventricular filling achieved by adjusting AV delay interval correlated positively with the left atrial contribution to left ventricular filling as determined by Doppler mitral valve recordings. Thus, individuals with significant atrial contributions to cardiac output, such as elderly patients and those with hypertrophied ventricles, may be particularly sensitive to changes in AV delay interval.

The data regarding the effect of left ventricular systolic function on sensitivity to AV delay interval are conflicting. Lascault and colleagues[81] reported a 25% increment in Doppler-derived stroke volume in comparing the most hemodynamically advantageous AV delay interval to the least advantageous during DDD pacing at rest. In a linear discriminate analysis of multiple factors, only the left ventricular diastolic diameter on M-mode echocardiogram predicted sensitivity to AV delay interval. Patients with normal left ventricular diastolic dimension benefited more from optimization of AV

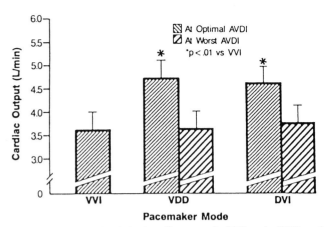

FIGURE 23–21. Doppler-derived cardiac output in VVI mode, VDD, and VDD mode at the optimal and worst AV delay intervals (AVDI). There was a 26% improvement in cardiac output from the least favorable to most favorable AV delay interval in both pacing modes. The cardiac output at the worst AV delay interval was not significantly different from that during VVI pacing in either pacing mode. (From Pearson AC, Janosik DL, Redd RM, et al: Hemodynamic benefit of atrioventricular synchrony: Prediction from baseline Doppler echocardiographic variables. J Am Coll Cardiol 13:1613, 1989. Reprinted with permission from the American College of Cardiology.)

delay interval than those with enlarged left ventricular end-diastolic dimensions. In contrast, Eugene and associates[83] used modified impedance plethysmography to assess changes in stroke volume at different AV delay intervals and suggested that patients with diseased left ventricles were more sensitive to changes in AV delay interval than those with normal left ventricular function. Individuals temporarily paced during acute myocardial infarction or a postcardiac surgery have been reported to demonstrate marked sensitivity to changes in AV delay interval.[54, 55] The apparent discrepancy in these data may be related to the diverse populations of patients and their position on the Starling function curve. Regardless of baseline left ventricular function, individuals functioning on the ascending limb of the curve would be expected to benefit most from optimizing the timing of atrial systole and those on the plateau portion of the curve would derive little additional benefit.

Effect of Exercise on Pacing Hemodynamics

EFFECT OF POSTURE ON PACING HEMODYNAMICS

The majority of studies examining the hemodynamic importance of atrial contribution to cardiac output were performed with patients at rest in the supine position. It has been demonstrated by noninvasive and invasive hemodynamic techniques that assumption of an upright posture diminishes cardiac output by up to 30% because of venous pooling and a reduction in preload.[76, 82, 120] However, the relative hemodynamic benefit of dual-chamber pacing over ventricular pacing is similar in both the upright and the supine positions.[120] Wish and associates[76] found that more patients were sensitive to changes in AV delay interval in the upright position than in the supine position and suggested that timing of contraction relative to ventricular systole may be even more significant when preload and filling pressures are low.

It appears that the same AV delay interval that maximizes cardiac output in the supine position is also usually optimal in the upright position in most individuals.

FIXED RATE VENTRICULAR COMPARED WITH ATRIAL SYNCHRONOUS PACING

Normal individuals are capable of increasing their resting cardiac output three- to fivefold during maximal exercise, depending on the level of physical fitness. In subjects with normal sinus node function, heart rate is the predominant means by which cardiac output increases during exercise, incrementing by as much as 200% to 300%. Stroke volume increases to a lesser degree with maximal increments of approximately 60% occurring in normal individuals at peak exercise[121] (Fig. 23–22). When comparing exercise hemodynamics during pacing modes capable of tracking atrial activity (VAT, VDD, or DDD) with fixed-rate ventricular pacing, physiologic pacing prolongs exercise duration, increases exercise cardiac output, reduces exercise-induced arrhythmias and hypotension, and decreases subjective complaints during exercise compared to ventricular pacing.[52, 59, 122–129] The improvement in exercise capacity with acute changes from fixed-rate ventricular pacing to physiologic pacing has been reported to be 20% to 45%. The relative improvement persists and is even more marked after more prolonged periods in the two pacing modes.[59, 123] Baseline left ventricular function, patient age, and exercise capacity during VVI pacing do not predict the relative benefit of atrial synchronous pacing compared with fixed-rate ventricular pacing during exercise.[122]

The augmentation in exercise cardiac output with physiologic pacing is due primarily to the ability to increase heart rate in response to metabolic demands without significant increases in filling pressure or stroke volume. In contrast, fixed-rate VVI pacing results in higher end-diastolic volumes and stroke volumes and left ventricular ejection fraction during exercise compared with physiologic pacing. Although partially compensatory, the augmentations in end-diastolic volume and contractility fail to achieve the degree of hemodynamic benefit derived from rate responsiveness during exercise[52] (Fig. 23–23). At steady-state submaximal workloads, physiologic pacing results in a higher exercise cardiac output and increased exercise duration with similar expenditure of myocardial oxygen consumption and coronary artery blood

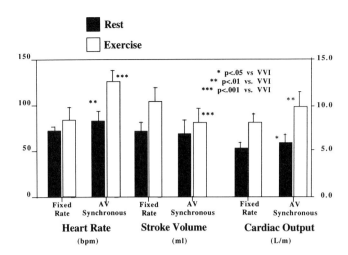

FIGURE 23–23. Comparison of exercise hemodynamics during fixed-rate ventricular pacing and atrial synchronous pacing. The exercise heart rate and cardiac output are significantly higher with atrial synchronous pacing than with fixed-rate ventricular pacing. The exercise heart rate is significantly higher with atrial synchronous pacing than with fixed-rate ventricular pacing, and the exercise stroke volume is significantly higher with fixed-rate ventricular pacing than with atrial synchronous pacing. The compensatory increase in exercise stroke volume, however, does not equal the benefit derived by the ability to increase heart rate; thus the exercise cardiac output during atrial synchronous pacing is significantly higher than during fixed-rate ventricular pacing. (From Karlöf I: Haemodynamic effect of atrial triggered versus fixed rate pacing at rest and during exercise in complete heart block. Acta Med Scand 197:195, 1975.)

flow compared with VVI pacing.[127] The increase in stroke volume during exercise that occurs with VVI pacing is due to enhanced preload from enhanced venous return during muscular contraction and, importantly, to heightened sympathetic nervous system activity resulting in greater ventricular contractility and ejection fraction.[126] Coronary sinus norepinephrine levels and arterial catecholamine levels are elevated at rest and during exercise during VVI pacing compared with physiologic pacing.[129] The heightened sympathetic activity and diminished cardiovascular reserve during fixed-rate pacing are evidenced by higher atrial rates and enhanced myocardial contractility compared with physiologic pacing at comparable workloads.

RELATIVE IMPORTANCE OF AV SYNCHRONY COMPARED WITH RATE RESPONSIVENESS

The significance of the atrial contribution to cardiac output has been demonstrated over a wide range of resting heart rates. Reiter and Hindman[58] reported that the atrial contribution to cardiac output and percentage augmentation in resting cardiac output with AV sequential compared with ventricular demand pacing increases with increasing pacing rate. However, it is now apparent that conclusions regarding the relative importance of atrial systole during pacing-induced tachycardia in the resting supine position cannot necessarily be extrapolated to tachycardia produced by upright exercise. Using Doppler assessment of left ventricular filling, Linde-Edelstam and associates[130] demonstrated that there is a significant difference in the kinetic energy of blood flow and left ventricular filling pattern with exercise-induced compared with pacing-induced increases in heart rate. Blood flow velocity and the ratio of early diastolic filling to late diastolic

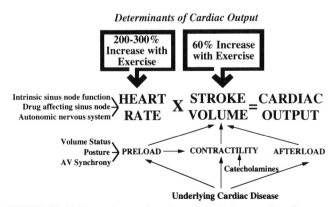

FIGURE 23–22. Determinants of cardiac output during exercise. (See text for discussion.)

filling are increased during exercise-induced tachycardia compared with atrial pacing at equivalent heart rates. This suggests that an increase in the kinetic energy of blood flow is produced by sympathetic stimulation and enhanced contractility. This increase is accompanied by a decrease in atrial contribution to left ventricular filling making the early rapid filling phase proportionally more important in exercise induced tachycardia.[130]

Several studies have compared exercise capacity and hemodynamics during atrial tracking modes (VDD or VAT pacing) with those achieved during ventricular pacing matched to the tracked atrial rate so that the peak heart rate in the two modes was equivalent.[52, 125, 131–134] These studies are reviewed in detail in Chapter 24. The authors demonstrated similar exercise capacity and cardiac output with the two pacing modes and concluded that the major determinant of exercise cardiac output in paced patients is their ability to augment heart rate. In addition, it has been demonstrated that there are no significant differences in right atrial pressure, pulmonary capillary wedge pressure, coronary sinus AV oxygen difference, or myocardial oxygen consumption between rate-matched ventricular pacing and atrial synchronous pacing during exercise.[134]

Ausubel and colleagues[133] demonstrated that atrial synchronous and ventricular rate-adaptive pacing augment cardiac output during exercise by different mechanisms. In a single-blind randomized crossover study utilizing radionuclide ventriculography during exercise, the percentage changes in stroke volume and cardiac output at peak exercise were found to be similar in the two pacing modes (Fig. 23–24). The end-diastolic and end-systolic volumes were significantly higher during atrial synchronous pacing than rate-matched ventricular pacing. Therefore, stroke volume increased mainly via the Frank-Starling mechanism, sparing myocardial contractile reserve. Conversely, rate-matched ventricular pacing was associated with lower end-diastolic volumes and end-systolic volumes but higher levels of myocardial contractility and ejection fraction, thereby yielding stroke volumes similar to those achieved during atrial synchronous pacing.

Evidence that ventricular rate-adaptive pacing yields exercise hemodynamics equivalent to that with DDD pacing and involves the insertion of only one pacing lead contributed to the enthusiasm for VVIR pacemakers in the early and mid-1980s. Various sensors that regulate heart rate were introduced and found to acutely improve exercise duration compared with ventricular pacing. Sensors utilized have included activity, right ventricular blood temperature, respiratory rate and minute ventilation, stroke volume and preejection period, and QT interval.[135–144] Buckingham and associates[141] demonstrated improved exercise duration and cardiac index with activity sensor rate-adaptive pacing compared with fixed-rate ventricular pacing utilizing Doppler echocardiography during paired-symptom limited exercise tests (Fig. 23–25). The improvement in heart rate, cardiac index, and exercise duration with VVIR pacing did not correlate with resting baseline ejection fraction. In a similarly designed study, Lau and Camm[142] found a weak negative correlation between resting left ventricular fractional shortening on M-mode echocardiograms and the percentage increase in exercise duration with VVIR compared with fixed-rate VVI pacing. Both studies demonstrated that elderly individuals and younger patients

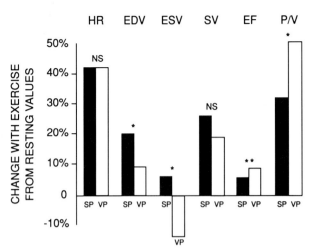

FIGURE 23–24. Percentage change in heart rate, left ventricular volume, and contractility with exercise during rate-adaptive ventricular pacing (VP) compared with atrial synchronous ventricular pacing (SP). The end-diastolic and end-systolic volumes were higher during atrial synchronous pacing, and the left ventricular ejection fraction was higher during ventricular pacing. HR, heart rate; EDV, end-diastolic volume; ESV, end-systolic volume; SV, stroke volume; EF, ejection fraction; P/V, peak systolic pressure/end-systolic volume ratio. $*p < .001$; $**p = .002$; NS, not significant. (From Linde-Edelstam CM, Juhlin-Dannfelt A, Nordlander R, Pehrsson SK: The hemodynamic importance of atrial systole: A function of the kinetic energy of blood flow? PACE 15:1740, 1992.)

derived similar benefits from rate-adaptive pacing. Thus, it appears that poor left ventricular function and advanced age do not prevent rate-adaptive pacing from improving exercise capacity and cardiac output over fixed-rate ventricular pacing.

Before the availability of dual-chamber rate-response pacemakers in the late 1980s, the relative importance of rate responsiveness and AV synchrony during cardiac pacing was disputed.[145, 146] The majority of data indicates that AV syn-

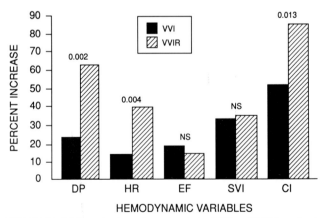

FIGURE 23–25. Exercise hemodynamics during VVI and VVIR pacing in 16 patients with activity-sensing rate-adaptive pacemakers. Percentage change in double product (DP), heart rate (HR), ejection fraction (EF), stroke volume index (SVI), and cardiac index (CI) during exercise in each pacing mode are displayed. HR, CI, and DP are significantly higher during exercise in the VVIR mode than with fixed-rate ventricular pacing. (From Buckingham TA, Woodruff RC, Pennington DG, et al: Effect of ventricular function on the exercise hemodynamics of variable rate pacing. J Am Coll Cardiol 11:1269, 1988. Reprinted with permission from the American College of Cardiology.)

chrony is most important at rest and during lower levels of exercise, whereas rate responsiveness assumes the more important role at moderate and high levels of exertion.[135, 144] It is important to realize that the effectiveness of ventricular rate-responsive pacing has been demonstrated primarily by acute exercise studies. Obvious concerns exist regarding the long-term effects of asynchronous atrial ventricular contraction on left ventricular function, atrioventricular valvular regurgitation, and even the patients' survival.[147–158] The abnormal atrial reflexes that result in pacemaker syndrome during fixed-rate ventricular pacing may also occur during ventricular rate-adaptive pacing, especially in patients with intact VA conduction. The increased incidence of atrial fibrillation and associated thromboembolic phenomena[151, 152, 154, 156–158] demonstrated with fixed-rate ventricular pacing compared with AAI or DDD pacing is also a potential problem with VVIR pacing. In addition, data suggest that there is improved survival with AV synchronous pacing compared with fixed-rate ventricular pacing, whereas no such survival benefit has been demonstrated with rate-adaptive ventricular pacing.[150, 153, 154–159]

Now that DDDR pacemakers are available, rate responsiveness and AV synchrony are no longer mutually exclusive features. Recently, Proctor and colleagues[160] demonstrated that DDDR pacing results in superior exercise hemodynamics compared with DDD or VVIR pacing in a group of patients with chronotropic incompetence. Importantly, only the DDDR pacing mode significantly increased exercise cardiac output compared with resting values, suggesting that a combination of AV synchrony and rate responsiveness is superior to either feature alone during exercise in patients with chronotropic incompetence. Other studies comparing DDDR and VVIR pacing indicate increased exercise capacity and cardiac output with DDDR pacing compared with VVIR pacing, as well as superior metabolic parameters indicating improved left ventricular efficiency during dual-chamber rate-responsive pacing.[161, 162] In patients with normal sinus node function and the ability to increase atrial rate with exercise, DDD pacing represents a physiologic pacing mode that preserves both AV synchrony and rate responsiveness. However, in patients with chronotropic incompetence DDDR pacing has been shown to yield superior exercise hemodynamics compared with DDD pacing because of the ability to achieve higher rates.[163] These data, in combination with the well-accepted hemodynamic benefits of atrial systole at rest, strongly support preservation of AV synchrony during pacing whenever possible.

AV DELAY INTERVAL DURING EXERCISE

The importance of variation in AV delay during exercise in physiologically paced patients is controversial. There are two theoretical reasons why a rate-adaptive AV delay interval would be hemodynamically beneficial. First, shortening of the AV delay interval with increasing atrial rates simulates normal physiologic PR shortening with exercise.[164–166] With an increasing heart rate, there is disproportionate shortening of diastole, and therefore the timing of atrial and ventricular contraction may become even more critical. Theoretically, shortening of the AV delay interval with increased rate of atrial sensed events would facilitate left ventricular filling and cardiac output during exercise. Second, shortening of the AV delay interval during exercise allows higher atrial track-

ing rates. Because the PR interval is part of the total atrial refractory period, shortening of the AV delay interval with exercise allows higher atrial tracking rates before two-to-one block upper rate limit behavior occurs and therefore potentially increases exercise capacity.

The physiologic relationship between PR interval and heart rate in normal, healthy individuals has been well characterized. Daubert and associates[164] demonstrated an inverse linear relationship between heart rate and PR interval that was independent of age and baseline PR interval. There is a mean decrease of 4 ± 2.1 msec in PR interval for a 10 bpm increase in heart rate. The normal PR shortening with exercise is caused by facilitation of AV nodal conduction because of increased sympathetic stimulation and diminished vagal tone. If the AV delay interval remained constant, atrial systole would occur early in diastole and result in a situation similar to that seen with unphysiologically long AV delay intervals at rest.

Initial data supporting the importance of rate-adaptive delay were obtained by examining the effects of various rates of AV sequential pacing at rest.[110] These data indicated that the most hemodynamically advantageous AV delay interval at higher rates was shorter than that which was optimal at lower rates. Ritter and associates[110] demonstrated superior cardiac hemodynamics, including increased cardiac index and left ventricular stroke work index and decreased pulmonary capillary wedge pressure and systemic vascular resistance, with rate-adaptive AV delay compared with fixed AV delay intervals during AV sequential pacing at increasing rates. They further demonstrated that when comparing two fixed rates the AV delay interval of 200 msec was more advantageous at lower pacing rates, whereas 150 msec was superior at higher heart rates. However, the hemodynamic situation during pacing-induced tachycardia and exercise varies greatly.

Because the major determinant of augmentation of cardiac output during exercise is heart rate, the contribution of atrial systole and the relative timing of atrial and ventricular contraction may diminish in significance. Studies analyzing the effects of variation in AV delay interval during exercise have yielded conflicting results.[167–173] During upright submaximal treadmill exercise in patients with complete heart block and normal left ventricular function, Mehta and colleagues[82] demonstrated that a fixed AV delay interval of 75 to 80 msec was optimal during exercise and significantly increased the Doppler-derived cardiac output compared with AV delay intervals of 150 and 200 msec. Comparing a physiologic AV delay interval (155 ± 10 msec) with a nonphysiologic AV delay interval (30 ± 29 msec) during exercise with DDD pacing, Landzberg and coworkers[169] reported a 16% increase in exercise duration, a 23% increase in time to anaerobic threshold, and a decreased level of perceived exertion with the physiologic AV delay. Lower atrial natriuretic factor levels after maximal exercise with DDD pacing at shorter AV delay intervals suggest more physiologic hemodynamics than with longer AV delay intervals during exercise.[172] Using bicycle exercise and radionuclide ejection fractions, Leman and Kratz[70] found shorter AV delay intervals to result in larger stroke volumes. Haskell and French[73] reported that both short (66 msec) and long (160 msec) AV delay intervals during AV sequential pacing during maximum bicycle exercise were superior to VVI pacing; however, no hemodynamic advantage of short over long AV delay intervals was found. Ryden and colleagues[168] found that varying the fixed AV delay interval from 50 to 200 msec on serial exercise efforts had no effect on the maximum ventricular rate, maximum oxygen uptake, minute ventilation, or perceived level of exertion during upright exercise in patients with dual-chamber pacers and normal left ventricular function.

The above studies, although varying the AV delay between exercise efforts, utilized a fixed AV delay interval during each exercise test. There is evidence that a rate-adaptive AV delay interval, which is automatically decremented in response to an increased atrial rate, is beneficial to cardiopulmonary performance during exercise. Ritter and associates[170] performed paired exercise tests, one with a fixed AV delay interval of 156 msec and one with an automatic AV delay interval ranging from 156 to 63 msec, in 23 patients with dual-chamber pacemakers implanted for high-degree AV block. Exercise duration to anaerobic threshold was significantly longer and Vo_2 and Vco_2 at anaerobic threshold and peak exercise were significantly higher with an automatic AV delay interval. The mean automatic AV delay interval was 104 ± 24 msec at anaerobic threshold and 82 ± 28 msec at peak exercise. Lower plasma norepinephrine levels during exercise with autoadaptive AV delay than with fixed AV delay intervals have been reported and suggest more efficient cardiac hemodynamics.[172] In patients with chronotropic incompetence and high-degree AV block, Sulke and colleagues[171] performed randomized double-blind crossover assessment of rate-adaptive and different fixed AV delay settings during 2 weeks of normal activity and an exercise treadmill in DDDR mode. There was subjective improvement in the sense of general well-being and patients' preference for rate-adaptive AV delay interval or fixed AV delay interval of 125 msec (Fig. 23–26). The longest AV delay interval (250 msec) was least preferred by patients and was associated with the highest symptom prevalence. Exercise

duration was not significantly different in any setting in DDDR mode but was significantly reduced in DDD mode.[171]

Although the significance of an adaptive AV delay interval during DDD and DDDR exercise is controversial, it has been demonstrated that improper and deleterious sequencing of atrial and ventricular contraction can result during AAIR pacing for chronotropic incompetence. In some individuals the AV delay interval does not adapt normally with exercise and the stimulus-to-R interval and stimulus-to-R/RR ratio may actually increase. This may result in P waves occurring immediately after or even within the R wave of the preceding cycle. The paradoxical increase in stimulus-to-R interval and stimulus-to-R/RR ratio may be related to factors intrinsic to the patient such as conduction disease, lead position, or drugs, or may represent overstimulation by the sensor-driven atrial pacemaker.[199–201] The overstimulation phenomenon occurs when the atrial sensor increases the atrial rate out of proportion to the sympathetic drive so that no corresponding decrement in PR interval occurs. This is most frequently observed in early stages of exercise and in some patients is corrected as the patient continues to exercise. In other cases, implantation of a DDDR system with more physiologic AV sequencing alleviates symptoms.

Importance of Ventricular Activation Sequence

A normal cardiac contraction depends not only on the appropriate temporal sequence of atrial and ventricular events but also on the rapid synchronous depolarization of the ventricles through the intrinsic specialized conduction system. Aberrant electric depolarization and mechanical contraction of the ventricle are produced by right ventricular pacing (VVI pacing) alone or in the presence of atrial systole as in AV sequential (DVI) or atrial synchronous (VDD) pacing.[174] In patients capable of intrinsic AV conduction, a normal or paced ventricular depolarization may occur after a P wave, depending on the programmed AV delay interval and the effects of drugs, disease, and the autonomic nervous system on intrinsic AV conduction. Atrial inhibited (AAI) pacing in individuals with intact AV conduction preserves both AV synchrony and the normal sequence of ventricular depolarization. With DDD and DDDR pacemakers representing the majority of implants in the United States, defining the relative hemodynamic significance of ventricular activation sequence is clinically important.

As early as 1925, Wiggers[25] reported that in intact dog models, artificial stimulation of the right ventricle produced a less effective ventricular contraction than activation through the normal conduction system. The greater the amount of muscle activated before activation of the His-Purkinje system, the greater the degree of dyssynchrony and the weaker the contraction. Subsequent animal studies suggested that the loss of AV synchrony and asynchrony of ventricular contraction were independent and additive factors contributing to the hemodynamic deterioration observed with ventricular pacing compared to atrial or His bundle pacing.[11, 16, 26–29] Comparing different endocardial pacing sites in the anesthetized dog, Grover and Glantz[27] demonstrated lower end-diastolic and stroke volumes with right ventricular apical

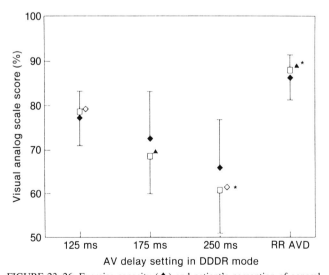

FIGURE 23–26. Exercise capacity (◆) and patient's perception of general well-being during (□) everyday activity at fixed AV delay settings of 125, 175, and 250 msec and rate-responsive AV delay (RR AVD) settings in DDDR mode. ◇, $p < .05$; ▲, $p < .03$; *$p < .01$. (Adapted from Sulke AN, Chambers JB, Sowton E: The effect of atrio-ventricular delay programming in patients with DDDR pacemakers. Eur Heart J 13:464, 1992.)

pacing compared with right atrial pacing or left ventricular pacing. In isolated canine hearts, right ventricular epicardial pacing resulted in lower left ventricular end-diastolic pressure and a compensatory decrease in oxygen consumption compared with atrial pacing at the same heart rate. In addition to diminished systolic function, the inhomogeneity of ventricular contraction during right ventricular pacing may impair diastolic relaxation and, thus, filling of the ventricle. In open-chest dogs, Zile and colleagues[29] demonstrated a decrease in regional and global indices of relaxation (isovolumetric pressure decline and relaxation time constant) with right ventricular and AV sequential pacing compared with AAI pacing that was independent of loading conditions.

Despite convincing evidence in animal models that the normal ventricular activation sequence is hemodynamically superior to asynchronous contraction, the clinical importance in humans is less clear. Comparing acute hemodynamic changes in humans during VVI, AV sequential, and AAI pacing, Samet and coworkers[50] concluded in the 1960s that asynchronicity of ventricular contraction was of minor importance compared with AV synchrony because AAI and AV sequential pacing yielded equivalent hemodynamic improvements compared with ventricular pacing. Greenberg and colleagues[56] reached similar conclusions, demonstrating that AAI and AV sequential pacings were equally beneficial and both were superior to ventricular pacing alone. However, these acute studies were performed with selected groups of patients with significant cardiovascular and pulmonary disease at rest in an intensive care unit or postoperative setting and utilized temporary pacing modalities and invasive hemodynamic measurements. Advances in noninvasive imaging techniques allow more sophisticated assessment of regional and global left ventricular systolic and diastolic function and suggest that the asynchronicity of ventricular contraction observed with a naturally occurring or pacing-induced left bundle branch block electrocardiographic pattern may produce deleterious hemodynamic effects.[174–180] Grines and colleagues[177] utilized a variety of noninvasive imaging techniques to compare left ventricular function at rest and during exercise in a group of patients with isolated left bundle branch block and a group of patients with a normal ventricular activation sequence. Patients with left bundle branch block demonstrated a reduction in global left ventricular ejection fraction both at rest and during exercise because of a regional decrease in interventricular septal ejection fraction. There was also a reduction in left ventricular diastolic filling time and an increase in the ratio of right to left ventricular filling time. Bramlet and colleagues[176] demonstrated an abrupt decrease in regional and global left ventricular ejection fraction with the development of rate-dependent left bundle branch block and no overall increase in exercise ejection fraction in a group of patients with no structural heart disease and no evidence of ischemia.

Using invasive hemodynamic measurements, Askenazi and colleagues[175] assessed the effects of AV sequential pacing and atrial inhibited pacing at constant heart rates and preload conditions on left ventricular performance. There was no significant difference in end-diastolic volume between the two modes of pacing. However, there were a significant increase in end-systolic volume and a decrease in stroke volume and ejection fraction with AV sequential pacing compared with AAI pacing. Santomauro and cowork-

ers[180] utilized radionuclide phase analysis during different pacing modes to quantitate the effects of the ventricular activation sequence on left ventricular performance. In modes resulting in a paced ventricular complex, temporal inhomogeneity of ventricular contraction and diminished global left ventricular ejection fraction occurred, whereas with atrial pacing ventricular contraction occurred through the intrinsic conduction system. There was an inverse correlation between the degree of temporal inhomogeneity and left ventricular ejection fraction. Utilizing resting radionuclide studies and rest and submaximal exercise Doppler studies during VVI, AAI, and AV sequential pacing, Rosenqvist and colleagues[174] investigated the relative hemodynamic importance of left ventricular activation sequence and AV synchrony. Ventricular pacing with or without atrial systole was associated with paradoxical septal motion, a 25% reduction in regional septal ejection fraction, and a significant reduction in global ejection fraction at rest (Fig. 23–27). In addition, peak diastolic early filling rate was decreased with AV sequential pacing compared with AAI pacing. The observed changes persisted during submaximal exercise and Doppler-derived exercise cardiac output was higher during AAI pacing than during DDD or VVI pacing. In another study comparing metabolic parameters during paired symptom-limited exercise stress tests, peak oxygen uptake and oxygen pulse were lower when a P wave was followed by a paced ventricular contraction than when it was followed by an intrinsic ventricular contraction, indicating a decrease in myocardial reserve.[179]

In addition to changes in left ventricular systolic function, there is evidence that the inhomogeneity of ventricular contraction induced by right ventricular pacing affects ventricular relaxation and diastolic function in humans. Askenazi and colleagues[175] demonstrated significant decreases in both peak dP/dt and peak negative dP/dt with a paced compared with an intrinsic ventricular contraction. They suggested that less effective contraction and relaxation occurred with asynchronously paced ventricular contractions and accounted for the diminished ejection fraction observed with AV sequential

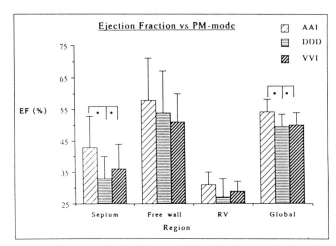

FIGURE 23–27. Regional and global ejection fractions (EF) during atrial demand pacing (AAI), synchronous atrioventricular pacing (DDD), and fixed-rate ventricular demand pacing (VVI). Septal and global ejection fractions are significantly reduced with both VVI and DDD pacing modes compared with AAI mode. (From Rosenqvist M, Isaaz K, Botvinick EH, et al: Relative importance of activation sequence compared to atrioventricular synchrony in left ventricular function. Am J Cardiol 67:148, 1991.)

pacing compared with AAI pacing. Bedotto and associates[178] presented evidence that baseline ventricular function may influence the effects of asynchronous left ventricular contraction on left ventricular relaxation. The rate of positive dP/dt and negative dP/dt and the time constant of left ventricular relaxation were measured during atrial and AV sequential pacing in a group of normal individuals and in a group of individuals with impaired left ventricular systolic function. Whereas both groups of patients demonstrated a decrease in positive dP/dt with AV sequential compared with AAI pacing, the relaxation time increased and peak negative dP/dt decreased only in patients with low baseline ejection fraction (Fig. 23–28). Impairment of left ventricular relaxation occurred independently of changes in systolic function and correlated with left ventricular wall thickness.[178]

The potential adverse hemodynamic consequences of a ventricular contraction induced by right ventricular apical pacing are summarized in Figure 23–29. Although an intrinsic ventricular contraction appears to be necessary for optimal cardiac performance, the clinical significance as it applies to cardiac pacing remains controversial. Reports of individuals experiencing symptoms related to the inhomogeneity of ventricular contraction during AV sequential pacing are rare. Some advocate programming a long AV delay interval to allow intrinsic conduction, but this must be weighed against the deleterious hemodynamic effects of a nonphysiologically long AV delay interval should intrinsic atrioventricular conduction fail. The relative importance of AV timing and synchronicity of ventricular contraction may vary between individual patients. The ability of either factor to affect pacemaker hemodynamics in the individual patient should be recognized. Although in many paced patients these factors may be of minor clinical importance, one or the other factors may significantly influence hemodynamics and produce clinical symptoms in a given individual.

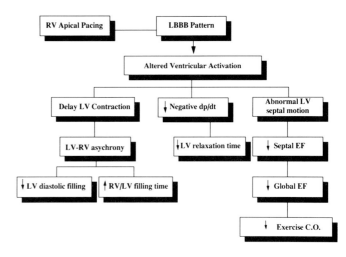

FIGURE 23–29. Potential deleterious hemodynamic consequences of a ventricular contraction induced by right ventricular apical pacing. (Adapted from Grines CL, Bashore TM, Boudoulas H, et al: Functional abnormalities in isolated left bundle branch block. The effect of interventricular asynchrony. Circulation 79:845, 1989.)

Influence of Underlying Heart Disease on Pacing Hemodynamics

Underlying cardiac disease affects the hemodynamics of pacing and influences the relative benefit of pacing mode. In certain acute conditions such as myocardial infarction or aortic insufficiency and after cardiac surgery, temporary pacing may be critical in stabilizing hemodynamics. In addition, attention to special parameters such as AV delay interval, rate, and the sequence of ventricular depolarization during temporary or permanent pacing may be extremely important in optimizing hemodynamics in specific cardiac conditions.[54, 55, 116–119, 181–192]

ISCHEMIC HEART DISEASE

Patients with ischemic heart disease who require pacing, especially those with previous myocardial infarction, benefit significantly from modes of pacing that maintain AV synchrony compared with VVI pacing alone.[54, 57, 74, 181, 186] In angiographic volume studies, Hamby and colleagues[95] demonstrated that most patients with coronary artery disease have a higher atrial contribution to resting stroke volume than normal individuals (33% vs. 20%, $p < .05$). The highest atrial contribution to ventricular filling was noted in patients with the lowest stroke volume and ejection fraction. The presence of cardiomegaly on chest x-ray study and congestive heart failure were clinical factors predictive of a relatively greater atrial contribution to stroke volume. Using a catheter tip micromanometer, Matsuda and colleagues[94] evaluated left atrial function in patients with and without remote myocardial infarction and determined that the ratio of active atrial emptying to left ventricular stroke volume and left atrial work was greater in patients with previous myocardial infarction.

Valero[181] reported clinical observations in acute myocardial infarction and noted that damaged hearts depend on atrial contribution to optimize end-diastolic volume and cardiac output. Unlike patients with normal left ventricular sys-

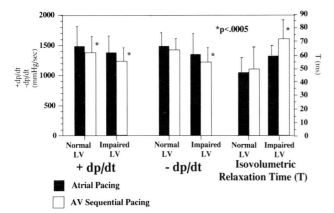

FIGURE 23–28. Hemodynamic effects of atrial and AV sequential pacing in patients with normal and impaired left ventricular (LV) systolic function. The positive dP/dt is significantly diminished in both groups of patients with AV sequential pacing compared with atrial pacing. However, the negative dP/dt is significantly lowered and the isovolumetric relaxation time significantly higher during AV sequential pacing compared with atrial pacing only in patients with impaired left ventricular systolic function. + dP/dt, maximal rate of rise in left ventricular pressure; − dP/dt, maximum rate of decline in left ventricular pressure; T, isovolumetric relaxation time. *$p < .0005$. (From Bedotto JB, Grayburn PA, Black WH, et al: Alterations in left ventricular relaxation during atrioventricular pacing in humans. J Am Coll Cardiol 15:658, 1990. Reprinted with permission from the American College of Cardiology.)

tolic function, who can compensate for effects of bradycardia and loss of AV synchrony by augmenting stroke volume and contractility, the loss of AV synchrony in acute myocardial infarction patients can result in severe hemodynamic impairment and systemic hypotension. This is particularly true in individuals suffering from a myocardial infarction with right ventricular involvement. The clinical syndrome of right ventricular infarction consists of electrocardiographic and echocardiographic evidence of right ventricular dysfunction associated with low cardiac output, hypotension, or shock.[182] The pathogenesis of the diminished cardiac output is attributed to diminished left ventricular filling resulting from right ventricular systolic dysfunction and the constraining effects of the pericardium. Maintenance of adequate cardiac output is critically dependent on maintaining adequate preload, and therapy includes aggressive administration of volume. Bradycardia and complete AV block caused by ischemia in the distribution of the right coronary artery are relatively frequent; temporary pacing is required in 45% to 75% of reported cases of right ventricular infarction.[183–185] Bradycardia, as well as the loss of atrial contribution to preload, further diminishes cardiac hemodynamics, and ventricular pacing alone is often insufficient in restoring systemic blood pressure. Temporary AV sequential pacing has been shown to reverse hypotension and shock in right ventricular infarction complicated by AV dissociation[184] (Fig. 23–30). The increases in systolic blood pressure, cardiac output, and stroke volume achieved with AV sequential pacing were significantly greater than with ventricular pacing. The relative timing of atrial and ventricular contraction is critical in influencing left ventricular filling in right ventricular infarction. With AV sequential pacing, atrial contraction during ventricular diastole increases the space in the pericardial cavity and enhances diastolic filling.[183] With AV dyssynchrony during ventricular pacing, left ventricular volume is impaired be-

cause of asynchronous atrial and ventricular contraction within a limited pericardial space.

Several studies have compared physiologic pacing modes to VVI pacing in patients requiring temporary pacing during acute left ventricular myocardial infarction and found AV sequential pacing to augment cardiac output by approximately 25% over that produced by VVI pacing alone.[54, 74, 186] In addition, Chamberlain and colleagues[54] demonstrated that a relatively short AV delay of 50 to 100 msec appears to be optimal during temporary pacing in acute myocardial infarction. This is possibly due to the relatively higher catecholamine levels and increased atrial rates during the acute infarction period. Murphy and colleagues[186] compared temporary dual-chamber pacing with fixed-rate ventricular pacing and ventricular pacing matched to the atrial rate that was tracked during DDD pacing in patients with acute myocardial infarction and high-degree AV block. Dual-chamber pacing resulted in enhanced cardiac output, increased systolic blood pressure, and reduced right atrial pressure compared with the patient's spontaneous escape rhythm, fixed-rate ventricular pacing, or ventricular pacing matched to the atrial tracked rate.

There is evidence that the hemodynamic superiority of AV sequential pacing to VVI pacing persists beyond the acute myocardial infarction period in patients with ischemic heart disease. Rahmitoola and coworkers[57] demonstrated that atrial systole made a larger contribution to left ventricular end-diastolic volume and pressure and left ventricular stroke volume in patients 3 to 6 weeks after myocardial infarction compared with normal control subjects. Although the benefit of preserving AV synchrony was noted regardless of the degree of impairment in left ventricular function, the greatest relative benefit occurred in patients with low cardiac output and normal left ventricular end-diastolic volume. In comparing AOO, DVI, and VVI pacing modes in patients with

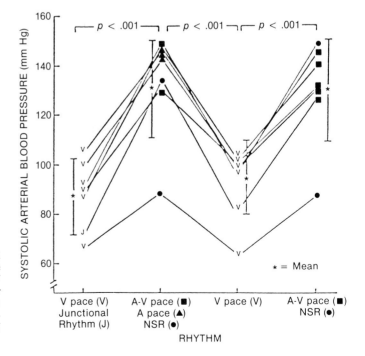

FIGURE 23–30. Effect of restoration of AV synchrony on systolic arterial blood pressure in patients with right ventricular infarction and complete heart block. The systolic blood pressure is significantly higher with AV sequential pacing compared with the underlying junctional rhythm or ventricular pacing. (From Love JC, Haffajee CI, Gore JM, Alpert JS: Reversibility of hypotension and shock by atrial or atrioventricular sequential pacing in patients with right ventricular infarction. Am Heart J 108:5, 1984.)

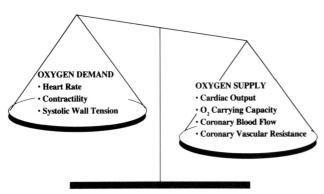

FIGURE 23–31. Factors affecting the balance of oxygen supply and demand in patients with coronary artery disease. Although physiologic pacing results in an increase in heart rate that raises oxygen demand, it is outweighed by the higher cardiac output and oxygen supply in most patients.

ischemic heart disease, Shefer and coworkers[187] showed AOO mode to be associated with the highest and VVI pacing with the lowest radionuclide indices of left ventricular function. At rates exceeding 100 bpm, left ventricular function deteriorated, probably because of pacing-induced ischemia, and the authors cautioned against higher pacing rates in patients with coronary artery disease. Although theoretically modes of pacing that allow physiologic increases in heart rate may increase myocardial oxygen consumption and exacerbate angina, most data indicate that DDD pacing is superior to fixed-rate ventricular pacing in alleviating angina.[127, 149, 188] This is probably due to the fact that the improvement in cardiac output and augmentation of coronary artery blood flow outweigh the increased oxygen demand associated with the increase in heart rate (Fig. 23–31). Also, the compensatory mechanisms of increased contractility and left ventricular dilatation associated with increasing cardiac output in VVI pacing may result in increased myocardial oxygen consumption and thus worsen angina.

TEMPORARY PACING FOLLOWING CARDIAC SURGERY

Hartzler and coworkers[55] demonstrated that temporary AAI pacing and DVI pacing were superior to ventricular pacing alone in patients with and without postoperative heart block following cardiac surgery. They further demonstrated that this subgroup was extremely sensitive to changes in AV delay interval and even small changes in AV delay interval resulted in significant changes in cardiac output. As with acute myocardial infarction patients, the optimal AV delay interval in patients after cardiac surgery was shorter than normally reported. In fact, in five of eight patients with intact AV conduction, an increase in cardiac output at AV delay intervals shorter than the patient's intrinsic AV delay interval was noted. Elevated catecholamines and changes in diastolic compliance induced by surgery may account for this observation.

ACUTE AORTIC INSUFFICIENCY

Acute severe aortic insufficiency is associated with a marked elevation in left ventricular diastolic pressure, which may exceed left atrial pressure and result in mitral valve

closure during diastole. Rapid temporary AAI and AV sequential pacings have been reported as a method of stabilizing patients with acute aortic insufficiency until definitive intervention can be performed.[189, 190] The mechanism by which rapid pacing improves hemodynamics involves shortening of diastole and therefore regurgitation, without altering forward flow. Meyer and colleagues[190] measured thermodilution cardiac output during incremental atrial pacing at rates of 72 to 140 bpm in a group of patients with severe acute aortic insufficiency. They reported that atrial pacing at a mean of 120 bpm resulted in optimal hemodynamics with a 50% reduction in left ventricular end-diastolic pressure, 43% reduction in pulmonary capillary wedge pressure, and 12% increase in cardiac index. They further demonstrated that the interval from the R wave on the electrocardiogram to the diastolic mitral valve closure point on the M-mode echocardiogram closely correlated with optimal pacing interval, allowing prediction of the optimal pacing rate in individual patients with acute aortic insufficiency.

IDIOPATHIC DILATED CARDIOMYOPATHY

Recently, the beneficial effects of DDD pacing in the treatment of end-stage idiopathic dilated cardiomyopathy were reported even in the absence of conventional indications for permanent pacemaker implantation[118, 119] (see Chapter 22). Hochleitner and associates,[118] reported dramatic hemodynamic and clinical improvement in a group of 16 patients with severe medically refractive idiopathic dilated cardiomyopathy treated with permanent DDD pacing at an AV delay interval of 100 msec. Within 3 weeks of instituting pacing, the authors observed a remarkable improvement in New York Heart Association symptomatology, diminished cardiothoracic ratio on chest x-ray study, a decreased right and left atrial size, and an increase in systolic and mean blood pressure. Normalization of heart rate occurred, with the heart rate increasing in patients with baseline bradycardia and decreasing in those with baseline tachycardia. The fractional shortening shown by M-mode echocardiography remained the same, and thus the striking improvement appeared to be related to factors influencing preload and afterload rather than changes in heart rate or contractility. It is postulated that DDD pacing with a short AV delay interval produced more hemodynamically favorable atrioventricular sequencing. In idiopathic dilated cardiomyopathy, AV diastolic valvular regurgitation commonly occurs and may be secondary to atrial relaxation before mitral valve closure. AV valvular regurgitation may result in an increase in atrial pressure and decreased forward cardiac output. The authors suggested that a prolonged delay in onset of left ventricular contraction in relation to atrial contraction may exist in dilated cardiomyopathy because of the spatial and temporal prolongation of ventricular depolarization in extreme left ventricular dilatation. Thus, a reduction in AV delay would shift ventricular contraction toward atrial systole and theoretically reduce mitral regurgitation.

HYPERTROPHIC OBSTRUCTIVE CARDIOMYOPATHY

It has long been appreciated that patients with hypertrophic obstructive cardiomyopathy who require pacing for bradycardia benefit significantly from pacing modes preserv-

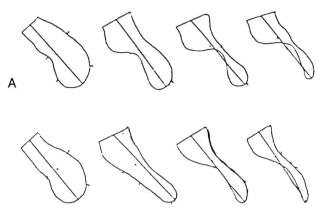

FIGURE 23–32. Schematic representation of a monoplane ventriculography in a patient with severe hypertrophic obstructive cardiomyopathy (*A*) during AAI pacing at rate of 90 bpm and (*B*) during DDD pacing at a rate of 90 bpm and AV delay interval of 50 msec. Note that the alteration in ventricular contraction pattern produced by right apical pacing results in less left ventricular outflow tract obstruction during systole. (From Jeanrenaud X, Goy JJ, Kappenberger LK: Effects of dual-chamber pacing in hypertrophic obstructive cardiomyopathy. Lancet 339:1318, 1992. © by The Lancet Ltd. 1992.)

ing AV synchrony compared with ventricular pacing.[191, 192] These patients are extremely sensitive to changes in preload, and conditions that diminish left ventricular filling result in decreased left ventricular cavity size and a subsequent increase in the intraventricular gradient. In addition, these patients have reduced left ventricular compliance and therefore derive proportionately more of their left ventricular filling from atrial systole than patients with normal hearts. Their dependence on the atrial contribution to cardiac output is manifested clinically by their poor tolerance of atrial fibrillation and ventricular pacing.

Recently it was demonstrated that individuals with hypertrophic obstructive cardiomyopathy in the absence of AV or sinus node disease may benefit acutely and chronically from the abnormal sequencing of ventricular contraction produced by right ventricular apical pacing[116, 117] (see Chapter 22). In patients with hypertrophic obstructive cardiomyopathy, systolic anterior motion of the mitral valve toward the intraventricular septum is associated with left ventricular outflow tract obstruction and often significant mitral regurgitation. Right ventricular pacing causes the septum to move away from the free wall during systole and thus increases the left ventricular outflow tract diameter and reduces the intraventricular gradient (Fig. 23–32). Fananapazir and colleagues[116] demonstrated a marked decrease in left ventricular outflow tract gradient during AV sequential pacing at short AV delay intervals compared to baseline and to AAI pacing in patients with hypertrophic obstructive cardiomyopathy refractory to medial treatment.

Chronic Hemodynamic Effects of Pacing

Although multiple studies have assessed the acute hemodynamic effects of various pacing modes and rates on left ventricular function and cardiac output, fewer data are available concerning the chronic effects of cardiac pacing. These

studies indicate, however, that the hemodynamic advantage of dual-chamber pacing over ventricular pacing persists over long-term follow-up.[69, 78, 123] In a randomized crossover study, Kruse and colleagues[123] compared resting and exercise hemodynamics acutely and after 3 months of ventricular pacing and atrial VDD synchronous pacing. At the end of the period of VDD pacing, cardiac output was significantly higher both at rest and during exercise compared with acute reprogramming to VVI mode and after 3 months of VVI pacing. There was a mean 24% increase in working capacity with chronic VDD pacing compared with chronic VVI pacing. VDD pacing produced a higher exercise cardiac output because of the capacity to increase heart rate, which outweighed the compensatory augmentation in exercise stroke volume observed during chronic VVI pacing. The AV oxygen difference and lactate production were higher during exercise with VVI pacing, indicating less myocardial efficiency and reserve. The heart size as measured by left ventricular angiography was larger after 3 months of ventricular pacing than after 3 months of VDD pacing.

In a 6-week double-blind crossover study, Rediker and associates[78] demonstrated a 43% increase in resting cardiac output, a 25% increase in left ventricular shortening fraction, and a significant increase in exercise duration with physiologic pacing compared with VVI pacing. Faerestrand and Ohm[69] measured Doppler cardiac output during VVI and AV sequential pacing in patients with DDD pacemakers before implantation and at 1, 3, 6, and 12 months after implantation. The hemodynamic superiority of DDD pacing was demonstrated acutely and persisted over 12 months of follow-up. In both modes of pacing, there was a reduction in stroke volume over the first 6 months, which was stable after that time. The authors postulated that before implantation, patients were bradycardic and therefore had compensatory increases in stroke volume that became normal after several months of pacing at higher rates. The decrease in stroke volume and cardiac output with chronic pacing compared to acute hemodynamic measurements after initiation of pacing has been noted by others.

In a similarly designed study, Faerestrand and Ohm[148] assessed Doppler cardiac output as well as M-mode measurements of left ventricular end-diastolic and end-systolic dimension and shortening fraction before and at 1, 3, and 6 months after implantation of a rate-responsive ventricular pacing system. Stroke volume and end-diastolic dimension decreased progressively over the 6-month period while end-systolic dimension remained constant. The shortening fraction decreased from 33% to 27% over the first 6 months, and the greatest reduction in end-diastolic volume and shortening fraction occurred in patients who were not previously paced. The authors suggested that these patients were now able to augment their cardiac output by increasing rate rather than by a compensatory increase in volume and shortening fraction. Thus, these observations may indicate a beneficial effect with increased contractile reserve rather than a deterioration in left ventricular function. Interestingly, the authors observed mitral regurgitation, tricuspid regurgitation, or a combination of mitral and tricuspid regurgitation to persist or develop in 9 of 13, or 69%, of the patients studied. The regurgitation was not quantitated, suggesting the need for further prospective studies assessing the effects of ventricular rate-responsive pacing on AV valvular regurgitation.

Studies assessing the symptoms and quality of life demonstrate the superiority of physiologic pacing over VVI pacing.[78, 149, 193–195] With the exception of prevention of syncope, DDD pacing was superior to fixed-rate VVI pacing in reducing symptoms of dizziness, low cardiac output, congestive heart failure, and angina and in overall sense of well-being.[149] In randomized crossover studies, patients expressing a mode preference invariably choose physiologic pacing over VVI pacing. More recently, DDD pacing has been shown to result in significant reduction in symptoms of shortness of breath, dizziness, and palpitations and improvement in cognitive function compared with VVIR pacing in randomized crossover studies assessing the two pacing modes in patients with complete heart block and preserved sinus node function.[196] In patients unable to receive dual-chamber pacing systems, VVIR pacing mode reduces symptoms and improves subjective sense of well-being compared with fixed-rate ventricular pacing.[197, 198]

An increasing amount of data suggests that physiologic pacing results in a lower incidence of permanent atrial fibrillation and thromboembolic complications, lower incidence of congestive heart failure, and lower overall mortality than with ventricular pacing alone.[149–157] In a retrospective study of patients paced for sinus node disease, there were a 1.6 times higher incidence of atrial fibrillation, 2.5 times higher incidence of congestive heart failure, and 2.9-fold increase in mortality in patients paced in the VVI mode compared with the AAI mode.[155] The differences in cardiovascular morbidity and overall mortality between the groups tended to increase with time. In another study, Hesselson and colleagues[157] studied 950 patients paced for sick sinus syndrome as well as high-degree heart block and hypersensitive carotid sinus syndrome retrospectively over 12 years. The rate of development of atrial fibrillation was more than twice as high in patients with VVI as in those with dual-chamber pacing. The incidence of atrial fibrillation was especially high in VVI-paced patients with sick sinus syndrome over the age of 70 years. The mortality rate at 7 years was higher in the VVI group than in the DDD and DVI groups. Death occurred more frequently during VVI pacing than during DDD pacing regardless of age at pacemaker implantation or the initial indication for pacing. Although these data appear to show that physiologic pacing is preferable to VVI pacing in terms of mortality and cardiovascular morbidity, it must be emphasized that these studies were retrospective nonrandomized comparisons of the pacing modes. Thus, a selective bias may have existed in terms of selecting VVI pacing mode for patients most prone to atrial fibrillation or those with a limited life expectancy.

Optimal Pacing Mode Selection

Numerous characteristics of patients must be considered in the selection of the optimal pacing system (Table 23–7). The current status of the patient's sinus node and AV node function and the possibility of future development of sinus and AV node disease are important in selection of the most appropriate pacing system. Guidelines for the selection of the optimal pacing system are outlined in Figure 23–33. Although cost effectiveness and the viability of the patient are

TABLE 23–7. PATIENT CHARACTERISTICS TO CONSIDER IN SELECTION OF PACING SYSTEM

Mechanical and electrical atrial function or arrhythmias (intermittent supraventricular tachycardia, atrial fibrillation)
Presence of retrograde VA conduction
Sinus node function
AV conduction
Medications affecting sinus/AV function
Possibility of future development of sinus and/or AV node disease
Underlying cardiac disease
  Systolic function
  Diastolic function
Age
Activity level
Concomitant illness

important factors, they are not reflected in this algorithm, which illustrates optimal pacing modes. Once the decision has been made to implant a permanent pacemaker for symptomatic bradycardia, poor resting or exercise hemodynamics, or other indications, it should be determined whether the patient has intact mechanical and electrical atrial function. If the atrium cannot be reliably paced or sensed because of chronic atrial fibrillation, mechanically silent atrium, or technical difficulty prohibiting atrial lead placement, a ventricular pacing system should be implanted. If the patient is likely to benefit from rate responsiveness, a VVIR system would be preferable to a fixed-rate ventricular pacing system. If the patient's heart rate increases adequately in response to metabolic stress or the patient has severe unstable angina making rate responsiveness undesirable, a fixed-rate ventricular pacing system may be preferable. If there is intact mechanical and electrical atrial activity and an atrial lead can be placed, implantation of a physiologic pacing system would be most desirable. If there is intact AV nodal conduction, an atrial pacing system may be placed. In chronotropically competent patients a fixed-rate AAI system may be adequate; however, in those with chronotropic incompetence an AAIR pacemaker would provide superior hemodynamics. The new development of AV nodal disease in patients paced for sick sinus syndrome is reported to be 1% to 2.8% per year over follow-up periods ranging from 2 to 5 years.[152, 153, 156] If the decision is made to implant an atrial pacing system, the potential for future development of AV nodal disease should be considered. If the patient's disease process or need for medication suggests a future possibility of impaired AV conduction, a DDD or DDDR system would be recommended. If AV nodal conduction is absent or intermittently impaired at the time of the initial implantation, a dual-chamber pacing system should be implanted. In the presence of chronotropic incompetence or a high probability that the patient will develop chronotropic incompetence in the future, a DDDR pacing system may provide optimal hemodynamics compared with DDD pacing. If the patient has adequate sinus node function, a DDD pacing system may be sufficient. In the decision to implant any physiologic pacing system, the past and future likelihood of intermittent atrial fibrillation or other supraventricular arrhythmias should be considered. If present, a DDDR or DDD system with VVIR mode, DDI mode, or automatic mode-switching capability would be preferred.

Selection of Hemodynamically Optimal Pacing System

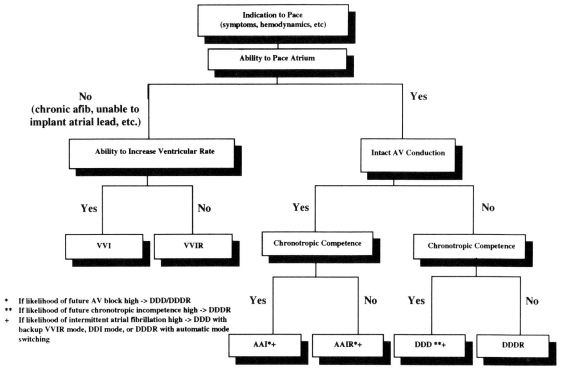

FIGURE 23–33. Algorithm demonstrating the selection of the hemodynamically optimal pacing system for an individual patient. (Adapted and reproduced with permission from Benditt DG, Milstein S, Buetikofer J, et al: Sensor-triggered, rate-variable cardiac pacing: Current technologies and clinical implications. Ann Intern Med 107:714, 1987.)

The ability of any pacing system to optimize hemodynamics is dependent on factors related to the individual patient, programmed pacemaker parameters, and the physiologic appropriateness of alternative rate sensors utilized in rate-adaptive pacing modes. The hemodynamic advantages and limitations of available pacing modes are displayed in Table 23–8. The ideal physiologic pacing system reproduces normal cardiac hemodynamics by replicating the rate responsiveness of a normal sinus node, maintaining appropriate AV sequencing over a wide spectrum of heart rates, and preserving rapid synchronous ventricular contraction when possible (Fig. 23–34). It is apparent that the ability of any pacing system to provide optimized hemodynamics is dependent on its interaction with the patient's intrinsic rhythm and conduction system. Our understanding of hemodynamics continues to evolve and lead to advances in pacemaker technology directed at providing even more sophisticated and physiologically appropriate pacing systems.

TABLE 23–8. **COMPARISON OF VARIOUS MODES IN ABILITY TO PROVIDE PHYSIOLOGIC PACING**

MODE	AV SYNCHRONY	RATE RESPONSIVENESS	SYNCHRONOUS VENTRICULAR CONTRACTION
VVI	–	–	–
VVIR	–	+ effectiveness dependent on sensor utilized	–
DDD	+ effectiveness may depend on programmed AVDI	+ if sinus node normal	± depends on programmed AVDI and intrinsic PR interval
DDI	+ effectiveness may depend on programmed AVDI	–	± depends on programmed AVDI and intrinsic PR interval
AAI	+ if AV conduction normal	–	+ assuming intact AV conduction
AAIR	+ effectiveness may depend on ability to shorten PR interval in response to atrial pacing rates	+ effectiveness dependent on sensor utilized	+ assuming intact AV conduction
DDDR	+ effectiveness may depend on programmed AVDI	+ effectiveness dependent on sensor utilized	± depends on programmed AV delay and intrinsic AV conduction

Abbreviation: AVDI, atrioventricular delay interval.

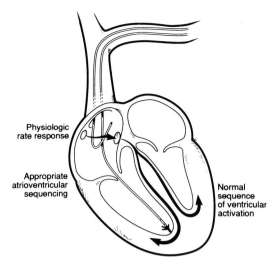

Physiologic rate response

Appropriate atrioventricular sequencing

Normal sequence of ventricular activation

FIGURE 23–34. Schematic representation of the interaction between the intrinsic conduction system and an implanted dual-chamber pacing pacemaker. The ability of the pacing system to optimize hemodynamics in an individual patient is dependent on this interaction. (See text for discussion.)

REFERENCES

1. Wirtzfeld A, Schmidt G, Himmler FC, Stangl K: Physiological pacing: Present status and future developments. PACE 10:41, 1987.
2. Baig MW, Perrins EJ: The hemodynamics of cardiac pacing: Clinical and physiological aspects. Prog Cardiovasc Dis 33:283, 1991.
3. Buckingham TA, Janosik DL, Pearson AC: Pacemaker hemodynamics: Clinical applications. Prog Cardiovasc Dis 34:347, 1992.
4. Harvey W: Movement of Heart and Blood in Animals. An Anatomical Essay (translated by D. Franklin). Oxford, England, Blackwell Scientific, 1957, p 34.
5. Straub H: The diastolic filling of the mammalian heart. J Physiol 40:387, 1910.
6. Wiggers CJ, Katz LN: The contour of the ventricular volume curves under different conditions. Am J Physiol 58:439, 1921–22.
7. Gesell RA: Auricular systole and its relation to ventricular output. Am J Physiol 29:32, 1911.
8. Gesell RA: Cardiodynamics in heart block as affected by auricular systole, auricular fibrillation, and stimulation of the vagus nerve. Am J Physiol 40:267, 1916.
9. Linden RJ, Mitchell JH: Relation between left ventricular diastolic pressure and myocardial segment length and observations on the contribution of atrial systole. Circ Res 8:1092, 1960.
10. Brockman SK: Dynamic function of atrial contraction in regulation of cardiac performance. Am J Physiol 204:597, 1963.
11. Gilmore JP, Sarnoff SJ, Mitchell JH, Linden RJ: Synchronicity of ventricular contraction: Observations comparing haemodynamic effects of atrial and ventricular pacing. Br Heart J 25:299, 1963.
12. Mitchell JH, Gilmore JP, Sarnoff SJ: The transport function of the atrium: Factors influencing the relation between mean left atrial pressure and left ventricular end diastolic pressure. Am J Cardiol 9:237, 1962.
13. Mitchell JH, Gupta DN, Payne RM: Influence of atrial systole on effective ventricular stroke volume. Circ Res 17:11, 1965.
14. Sarnoff SJ, Gilmore JP, Mitchell JH: Influence of atrial contraction and relaxation on closure of mitral valve: Observations on effects of autonomic nerve activity. Circulation 11:26, 1962.
15. Skinner NS, Mitchell JH, Wallace AG, Sarnoff SJ: Hemodynamic effects of altering the timing of atrial systole. Am J Physiol 205:499, 1963.
16. Kosowsky BD, Scherlag BJ, Damoto AN: Re-evaluation of the atrial contribution to ventricular function: Study using His bundle pacing. Am J Cardiol 21:518, 1968.
17. Payne RM, Stone HL, Engelken EJ: Atrial function during volume loading. J Appl Physiol 31:326, 1971.
18. Linderer T, Chatterjee K, Parmley WW, et al: Influence of atrial systole on the Frank-Starling relation and the end-diastolic pressure-diameter relation of the left ventricle. Circulation 67:1045, 1983.
19. Ogawa S, Dreifus LS, Shenoy PN, et al: Hemodynamic consequences of atrioventricular and ventriculoatrial pacing. PACE 1:8, 1978.
20. Naito M, Dreifus LS, Mardelli TJ, et al: Echocardiographic features of atrioventricular and ventriculoatrial conduction. Am J Cardiol 46:625, 1980.
21. Naito M, Dreifus LS, David B, et al: Reevaluation of the role of atrial systole to cardiac hemodynamics: Evidence for pulmonary venous regurgitation during abnormal atrioventricular sequencing. Am Heart J 105:295, 1983.
22. Williams JF, Sonnenblick EH, Braunwald E: Determinants of atrial contractile force in the intact heart. Am J Physiol 209:1061, 1965.
23. Wallick DW, Martin PJ, Masuda Y, Levy MN: Effects of autonomic activity and changes in heart rate on atrioventricular conduction. Am J Physiol 243:H523, 1982.
24. Ronaszeki A, Ector H, Denef B, et al: Effect of short atrioventricular delay on cardiac output. PACE 13:1728, 1990.
25. Wiggers CJ: The muscular reactions of the mammalian ventricles to artificial surface stimuli. Am J Physiol 73:346, 1925.
26. Finney JO: Hemodynamic alterations in left ventricular function consequent to ventricular pacing. Am J Physiol 208:275, 1965.
27. Grover M, Glantz SA: Endocardial pacing site affects left ventricular end diastolic volume and performance in the intact anesthetized dog. Circ Res 53:72, 1983.
28. Burkhoff D, Oikawa RY, Sagawa K: Influence of pacing site on canine left ventricular contraction. Am J Physiol 251:H428, 1986.
29. Zile MR, Blaustein AS, Shimizu G, Gaash WH: Right ventricular pacing reduces the rate of left ventricular relaxation and filling. J Am Coll Cardiol 10:702, 1987.
30. Suga H: Importance of atrial compliance in cardiac performance. Circ Res 35:39, 1974.
31. Brockman SK: Cardiodynamics of complete heart block. Am J Cardiol 16:72, 1965.
32. Brockman SK, Stoney WS: Congestive heart failure and cardiac output in heart block and during pacing. Ann NY Acad Sci 167:534, 1969.
33. Benchimol A, Li Y, Dimond EG: Cardiovascular dynamics in complete heart block at various heart rates: Effect of exercise at a fixed heart rate. Circulation 30:542, 1964.
34. Sowton E: Hemodynamic studies in patients with artificial pacemakers. Br Heart J 26:737, 1964.
35. Karlöf I, Bevegärd S, Ovenfors C: Adaption of the left ventricle to sudden changes in heart rate in patients with artificial pacemakers. Cardiovasc Res 7:322, 1973.
36. Samet P, Bernstein WH, Medow A, Nathan DA: Effect of alterations in ventricular rate on cardiac output in complete heart block. Am J Cardiol 14:477, 1964.
37. Rowe GG, Stenlund RR, Thomsen JH, et al: Coronary and systemic hemodynamic effects of cardiac pacing in man with complete heart block. Circulation 40:839, 1969.
38. Mitchell JH, Shapiro W: Atrial function and the hemodynamic consequences of atrial fibrillation in man. Am J Cardiol 23:556, 1969.
39. Philips E, Levine SA: Auricular fibrillation without other evidence of heart disease: Cause of reversible heart failure. Am J Med 7:478, 1949.
40. Kory RC, Meneely GR: Cardiac output in auricular fibrillation with observations on the effects of conversion to normal sinus rhythm. J Clin Invest 30:653, 1951.
41. Shapiro W, Klein G: Alterations in cardiac function immediately following electrical conversion of atrial fibrillation to normal sinus rhythm. Circulation 38:1074, 1968.
42. Samet P, Bernstein W, Levin S: Significance of atrial contribution to ventricular filling. Am J Cardiol 15:195, 1965.
43. Benchimol A, Duenas A, Liggett MS, Dimond EG: Contribution of atrial systole to the cardiac function at a fixed and at a variable ventricular rate. Am J Cardiol 16:11, 1965.
44. Carleton RA, Passovoy M, Graettinger JA: The importance of the contribution and timing of left atrial systole. Clin Sci 30:151, 1966.
45. Benchimol A: Significance of the contribution of atrial systole to cardiac function in man. Am J Cardiol 23:568, 1969.
46. Ruskin J, McHale PA, Harley A, Greenfield JC: Pressure-flow studies in man: Effect of atrial systole on left ventricular function. J Clin Invest 49:472, 1970.
47. Samet P, Bernstein WH, Nathan DA, López A: Atrial contribution to cardiac output in complete heart block. Am J Cardiol 16:1, 1965.
48. Samet P, Castillo C, Bernstein WH: Hemodynamic consequences of atrial and ventricular pacing in subjects with normal hearts. Am J Cardiol 18:522, 1966.
49. Samet P, Castillo C, Bernstein WH: Hemodynamic consequences of

sequential atrioventricular pacing: Subjects with normal hearts. Am J Cardiol 21:207, 1968.

50. Samet P, Castillo C, Bernstein WH: Hemodynamic sequelae of atrial, ventricular, and sequential atrioventricular pacing in cardiac patients. Am Heart J 72:725, 1966.

51. Benchimol A, Ellis JC, Dimond EG: Hemodynamic consequences of atrial and ventricular pacing in patients with normal and abnormal hearts. Am J Med 39:911, 1965.

52. Karlöf I: Haemodynamic effect of atrial triggered versus fixed rate pacing at rest and during exercise in complete heart block. Acta Med Scand 197:195, 1975.

53. Leinbach RC, Chamberlain DA, Kastor JA, et al: A comparison of the hemodynamic effects of ventricular and sequential A-V pacing in patients with heart block. Am Heart J 78:502, 1969.

54. Chamberlain DA, Leinbach RC, Vassaux CE, et al: Sequential atrioventricular pacing in heart block complicating acute myocardial infarction. N Engl J Med 282:577, 1970.

55. Hartzler GO, Maloney JD, Curtis JJ, Barnhorst DA: Hemodynamic benefits of atrioventricular sequential pacing after cardiac surgery. Am J Cardiol 40:232, 1977.

56. Greenberg B, Chatterjee K, Parmley WW, et al: The influence of left ventricular filling presure on atrial contribution to cardiac output. Am Heart J 98:742, 1979.

57. Rahimtoola SH, Ehsani A, Sinno MZ, et al: Left atrial transport function in myocardial infarction: Importance of its booster pump function. Am J Med 59:686, 1975.

58. Reiter MJ, Hindman MC: Hemodynamic effects of acute atrioventricular sequential pacing in patients with left ventricular dysfunction. Am J Cardiol 49:687, 1982.

59. Fananapazir L, Srinivas V, Bennett DH: Comparison of resting hemodynamic indices and exercise performance during atrial synchronized and asynchronous ventricular pacing. PACE 6:202, 1983.

60. Schuster AH, Nanda NC: Doppler echocardiography and cardiac pacing. PACE 5:607, 1982.

61. Nanda NC, Bhandari A, Barold SS, Falkoff M: Doppler echocardiographic studies in sequential atrioventricular pacing. PACE 6:811, 1983.

62. Zugibe FT, Nanda NC, Barold SS, Akiyama T: Usefulness of Doppler echocardiography in cardiac pacing: Assessment of mitral regurgitation, peak aortic flow velocity and atrial capture. PACE 6:1350, 1983.

63. Coskey RL, Feit TS, Plaia R, Zicari T: AV pacing and LV performance. PACE 6:631, 1983.

64. Boucher CA, Pohost GM, Okada RD, et al: Effect of ventricular pacing on left ventricular function assessed by radionuclide angiography. Am Heart J 106:1105, 1983.

65. Romero LR, Haffajee CI, Levin W, et al: Noninvasive evaluation of ventricular function and volumes during atrioventricular sequential and ventricular pacing. PACE 7:10, 1984.

66. Nitsch J, Seiderer M, Büll U, Lüderitz B: Evaluation of left ventricular performance by radionuclide ventriculography in patients with atrioventricular versus ventricular demand pacemakers. Am Heart J 107:906, 1984.

67. Stewart WJ, Dicola VC, Harthorne JW, et al: Doppler ultrasound measurement of cardiac output in patients with physiologic pacemakers: Effects of left ventricular function and retrograde ventriculoatrial conduction. Am J Cardiol 54:308, 1984.

68. Labovitz AJ, Williams GA, Redd RM, Kennedy HL: Noninvasive assessment of pacemaker hemodynamics by Doppler echocardiography: Importance of left atrial size. J Am Coll Cardiol 6:196, 1985.

69. Faerestrand S, Ohm OJ: A time-related study of the hemodynamic benefit of atrioventricular synchronous pacing evaluated by Doppler echocardiography. PACE 8:838, 1985.

70. Leman RB, Kratz JM: Radionuclide evaluation of dual-chamber pacing: Comparison between variable AV intervals and ventricular pacing. PACE 8:408, 1985.

71. Videen JS, Huang SK, Bazgan ID, et al: Hemodynamic comparison of ventricular pacing, atrioventricular sequential pacing, and atrial synchronous ventricular pacing using radionuclide ventriculography. Am J Cardiol 57:1305, 1986.

72. Forfang K, Otterstad JE, Ihlen H: Optimal atrioventricular delay in physiologic pacing determined by Doppler echocardiography. PACE 9:17, 1986.

73. Haskell RJ, French WJ: Optimum AV interval in dual-chamber pacemakers. PACE 9:670, 1986.

74. DiCarlo LA, Morady F, Krol RB, et al: The hemodynamic effects of

ventricular pacing with and without atrioventricular synchrony in patients with normal and diminished left ventricular function. Am Heart J 114:746, 1987.

75. Faerestrand S, Øie B, Ohm OJ: Noninvasive assessment by Doppler and M-mode echocardiography of hemodynamic responses to temporary pacing and ventriculoatrial conduction. PACE 10:871, 1987.

76. Wish M, Fletcher RD, Gottdiener JS, Cohen AI: Importance of left atrial timing in the programming of dual-chamber pacemakers. Am J Cardiol 60:566, 1987.

77. Wish M, Gottdiener JS, Cohen AJ, Fletcher RD: M-mode echocardiograms for determination of optimal atrial timing in patients with dual-chamber pacemakers. Am J Cardiol 61:317, 1988.

78. Rediker DE, Eagle KA, Homma S, et al: Clinical and hemodynamic comparison of VVI versus DDD pacing in patients with DDD pacemakers. Am J Cardiol 61:323, 1988.

79. Pearson AC, Janosik DL, Redd RM, et al: Hemodynamic benefit of atrioventricular synchrony: Prediction from baseline Doppler echocardiographic variables. J Am Coll Cardiol 13:1613, 1989.

80. Janosik DL, Pearson AC, Buckingham TA, et al: The hemodynamic benefit of differential atrioventricular delay intervals for sensed and paced atrial events during physiologic pacing. J Am Coll Cardiol 14:499, 1989.

81. Lascault G, Bigonzi F, Frank R, et al: Noninvasive study of dual-chamber pacing by pulsed Doppler: Prediction of the haemodynamic response by echocardiographic measurements. Eur Heart J 10:525, 1989.

82. Mehta D, Gilmour S, Ward DE, Camm AJ: Optimal atrioventricular delay at rest and during exercise in patients with dual-chamber pacemakers: A noninvasive assessment by continuous wave Doppler. Br Heart J 61:161, 1989.

83. Eugene M, Lascault G, Frank R, et al: Assessment of the optimal atrioventricular delay in DDD paced patients by impedance plethysmography. Eur Heart J 10:250, 1989.

84. Janosik DL, Pearson AC, Labovitz AJ: Applications of Doppler echocardiography in cardiac pacing. Echocardiography 8:45, 1991.

85. Masuyama T, Kodama K, Vematsu M, et al: Beneficial effects of atrioventricular sequential pacing on cardiac output and left ventricular filling assessed with pulsed Doppler echocardiography. Jpn Circ J 50:799, 1986.

86. Morgan DE, Norman R, West RO, Burggraf G: Echocardiographic assessment of tricuspid regurgitation during ventricular demand pacing. Am J Cardiol 58:1025, 1986.

87. Mark JB, Chetham PM: Ventricular pacing can induce hemodynamically significant mitral valve regurgitation. Anesthesiology 74:375, 1991.

88. Alicandri C, Fouad FM, Tarazi RC, et al: Three cases of hypotension and syncope with ventricular pacing: Possible role of atrial reflexes. Am J Cardiol 42:137, 1978.

89. Johnson AD, Laiken SL, Engler RL: Hemodynamic compromise associated with ventriculoatrial conduction following transvenous pacemaker placement. Am J Med 65:75, 1978.

90. Erlebacher JA, Danner RL, Stelzer PE: Hypotension with ventricular pacing: An atrial vasodepressor reflex in human beings. J Am Coll Cardiol 4:550, 1984.

91. Ausubel K, Furman S: The pacemaker syndrome. Ann Intern Med 103:420, 1985.

92. Ellenbogen KA, Thames MD, Mohanty PK: New insights into pacemaker syndrome gained from hemodynamic, humoral, and vascular responses during ventriculoatrial pacing. Am J Cardiol 65:53, 1990.

93. Braunwald E, Frahm CJ: Studies on Starling's law of the heart. IV. Observations on the hemodynamic functions of the left atrium in man. Circulation 24:633, 1961.

94. Matsuda Y, Toma Y, Ogawa H, et al: Importance of left atrial function in patients with myocardial infarction. Circulation 67:566, 1983.

95. Hamby RI, Noble WJ, Murphy DH, Hoffman I: Atrial transport function in coronary artery disease: Relation to left ventricular function. J Am Coll Cardiol 1:1011, 1983.

96. Freedman RA, Yock PG, Echt DS, Popp RL: Effect of variation in PQ interval on patterns of atrioventricular valve motion and flow in patients with normal ventricular function. J Am Coll Cardiol 7:595, 1986.

97. VonBibra H. Wirtzfeld A, Hall R, et al: Mitral valve closure and left ventricular filling time in patients with VDD pacemakers: Assessment of the onset of left ventricular systole and the end of diastole. Br Heart J 55:355, 1986.

98. Ishikawa T, Kimura K, Nihei T, et al: Relationship between diastolic

mitral regurgitation and PQ intervals on cardiac function in patients implanted with DDD pacemakers. PACE 14:1797, 1991.

99. Pearson AC, Janosik DL, Redd RM, et al: Doppler echocardiographic assessment of the effect of varying atrioventricular delay and pacemaker mode on left ventricular filling. Am Heart J 115:611, 1988.

100. Iwase M, Sotobata I, Yokota M, et al: Evaluation by pulsed Doppler echocardiography of the atrial contribution to left ventricular filling in patients with DDD pacemakers. Am J Cardiol 58:104, 1986.

101. Pauletti M, Raugi M, Bini G, et al: Pulsed Doppler verification of atrial contribution to ventricular filling in sequential pacing. PACE 10:333, 1987.

102. Rokey R, Quinones MA, Zoghbi WA, et al: Influence of left atrial systolic emptying on left ventricular early filling dynamics by Doppler in patients with sequential atrioventricular pacemakers. Am J Cardiol 62:968, 1988.

103. Rokey R, Kuo LC, Zoghbi WA: Determination of parameters of left ventricular filling with pulsed Doppler echocardiography: Comparison with cineangiography. Circulation 71:543, 1985.

104. Bahler RC, Vrobel TR, Martin P: The relation of heart rate and shortening fraction to echocardiographic indexes of left ventricular relaxation in normal subjects. J Am Coll Cardiol 2:926, 1983.

105. Arora RR, Machac J, Goldman ME, et al: Atrial kinetics and left ventricular diastolic filling in the healthy elderly. J Am Coll Cardiol 9:1255, 1987.

106. Pearson A, Labovitz A, Mrosek D, et al: Assessment of diastolic function in normal and hypertrophied hearts: Comparison of Doppler echocardiography and M-mode echocardiography. Am Heart J 113:1417, 1987.

107. Thomas JD, Weyman AE: Echocardiographic Doppler evaluation of left ventricular diastolic function. Circulation 84:977, 1991.

108. Ishidu Y, Meisner JS, Tsujioka K, et al: Left ventricular filling dynamics: Influence of left ventricular relaxation and left atrial pressure. Circulation 74:187, 1986.

109. Alt EU, VonBibra H, Blömer H: Different beneficial AV intervals with DDD pacing after sensed or paced atrial events. J Electrophysiol 1:250, 1987.

110. Ritter P, Daubert C, Mabo P, et al: Haemodynamic benefit of a rate-adapted AV delay in dual chamber pacing. Eur Heart J 10:637, 1989.

111. Ausubel K, Klementowicz P, Furman S: Interatrial conduction during cardiac pacing. PACE 9:1026, 1986.

112. Catania SL, Maue-Dickson W: AV delay latency compensation. J Electrophysiol 3:242, 1987.

113. Grant SCD, Bennett DH: Atrial latency in a dual chambered pacing system causing inappropriate sequence of cardiac chamber activation. PACE 15:116, 1992.

114. Sutton R: The atroventricular interval—what considerations influence its programming? Eur JCPE 3:169, 1992.

115. Chirife R, Ortega DF, Salazar AI: Nonphysiological left heart AV intervals as a result of DDD and AAI ''physiological'' pacing. PACE 14:1752, 1991.

116. Fananapazir L, Cannon RO, Tripodi D, Panza JA: Impact of dual-chamber permanent pacing in patients with obstructive hypertrophic cardiomyopathy with symptoms refractory to verapamil and β-adrenergic blocker therapy. Circulation 85:2149, 1992.

117. Jeanrenaud X, Goy JJ, Kappenberger LK: Effects of dual-chamber pacing in hypertrophic obstructive cardiomyopathy. Lancet 339:1318, 1992.

118. Hochleitner MH, Hörtnagl H, Ng CK, et al: Usefulness of physiologic dual-chamber pacing in drug-resistant idiopathic dilated cardiomyopathy. Am J Cardiol 66:198, 1990.

119. Brecker SJD, Xiao HB, Sparrow J, Gibson DG: Effects of dual-chamber pacing with short atrioventricular delay in dilated cardiomyopathy. Lancet 340:1308, 1992.

120. Hoeschen RJ, Reimold SC, Lee RT, et al: Effect of posture on response to atrioventricular synchronous pacing in patients with underlying cardiovascular disease. PACE 14:756, 1991.

121. Epstein SE, Beiser D, Stampfer M, et al: Characterization of the circulatory response to maximal upright exercise in normal subjects and patients with heart disease. Circulation 35:1049, 1967.

122. Kruse IB, Ryden L: Comparison of physical work capacity and systolic time intervals with ventricular inhibited and atrial synchronous ventricular inhibited pacing. Br Heart J 46:129, 1981.

123. Kruse I, Arnman K, Conradson TB, Ryden L: A comparison of the acute and long-term hemodynamic effects of ventricular inhibited and atrial synchronous ventricular inhibited pacing. Circulation 65:846, 1982.

124. Kappenberger L, Gloor HO, Babotai I, et al: Hemodynamic effects of atrial synchronization in acute and long-term ventricular pacing. PACE 5:639, 1982.

125. Pehrsson SK: Influence of heart rate and atrioventricular synchronization on maximal work tolerance in patients treated with artificial pacemakers. Acta Med Scand 214:311, 1983.

126. Pehrsson SK, Astrōm H, Bone D: Left ventricular volumes with ventricular inhibited and atrial triggered ventricular pacing. Acta Med Scand 214:305, 1983.

127. Nordlander R, Pehrsson SK, Astrōm H, Karlsson J: Myocardial demands of atrial-triggered versus fixed-rate ventricular pacing in patients with complete heart block. PACE 10:1154, 1987.

128. Karpawich PP, Perry BL, Farooki ZQ, et al: Pacing in children and young adults with nonsurgical atrioventricular block: Comparison of single-rate ventricular and dual-chamber modes. Am Heart J 113:316, 1987.

129. Pehrsson SK, Hjemdahl P, Nordlander R, Astrōm H: A comparison of sympathoadrenal activity and cardiac performance at rest and during exercise in patients with ventricular demand or atrial synchronous pacing. Br Heart J 60:212, 1988.

130. Linde-Edelstam CM, Juhlin-Dannfelt A, Nordlander R, Pehrsson SK: The hemodynamic importance of atrial systole: A function of the kinetic energy of blood flow? PACE 15:1740, 1992.

131. Fananapazir L, Bennett DH, Monks P: Atrial synchronized ventricular pacing: Contribution of the chronotropic response to improved exercise performance. PACE 6:601, 1983.

132. Kristensson BE, Arnman K, Ryden L: The hemodynamic importance of atrioventricular synchrony and rate increase at rest and during exercise. Eur Heart J 6:773, 1985.

133. Ausubel K, Steingart RM, Shimshi M, et al: Maintenance of exercise stroke volume during ventricular versus atrial synchronous pacing: Role of contractility. Circulation 72:1037, 1985.

134. Linde-Edelstam C, Hjemdahl P, Pehrsson SK, et al: Is DDD pacing superior to VVIR? A study on cardiac sympathetic nerve activity and myocardial oxygen consumption at rest and during exercise. PACE 15:425, 1992.

135. Benditt DG, Milstein S, Buetikofer J, et al: Sensor-triggered, rate-variable cardiac pacing: Current technologies and clinical implications. Ann Intern Med 107:714, 1987.

136. Lau CP: The range of sensors and algorithms used in rate-adaptive cardiac pacing. PACE 15:1177, 1992.

137. Donaldson RM, Rickards AF: Rate-responsive pacing using the evoked QT principle: A physiological alternative to atrial synchronous pacemakers. PACE 6:1344, 1983.

138. Alt E, Hirgstetter C, Heinz M, Blömer H: Rate control of physiologic pacemakers by central venous blood temperature. Circulation 73:1206, 1986.

139. Benditt DG, Mianulli M, Fetter J, et al: Single-chamber cardiac pacing with activity-initiated chronotropic response: Evaluation by cardiopulmonary exercise testing. Circulation 75:184, 1987.

140. Faerestrand SF, Breivik K, Ohm OJ: Assessment of the work capacity and relationship between rate response and exercise tolerance associated with activity-sensing rate-responsive ventricular pacing. PACE 10:1277, 1987.

141. Buckingham TA, Woodruff RC, Pennington DG, et al: Effect of ventricular function on the exercise hemodynamics of variable rate pacing. J Am Coll Cardiol 11:1269, 1988.

142. Lau CP, Camm J: Role of left ventricular function and Doppler-derived variables in predicting hemodynamic benefits of rate-responsive pacing. Am J Cardiol. 62:906, 1988.

143. Iwase M, Hatano K, Saito F, et al: Evaluation by exercise Doppler echocardiography of maintenance of cardiac output during ventricular pacing with or without chronotropic response. Am J Cardiol 63:934, 1989.

144. Gammage M, Schofield S, Rankin I, et al: Benefit of single-setting rate-responsive ventricular pacing compared with fixed-rate demand pacing in elderly patients. PACE 14:174, 1991.

145. Wish M, Fletcher RD, Cohen A: Hemodynamics of AV synchrony and rate. J Electrophysiol 3:170, 1989.

146. Markewitz A, Hemmer W: What's the price to be paid for rate response: AV sequential versus ventricular pacing? PACE 14:1782, 1991.

147. Hull RW, Snow F, Herre J, Ellenbogen KA: The plasma catecholamine responses to ventricular pacing: Implications for rate-responsive pacing. PACE 13:1408, 1990.

148. Faerestrand S, Ohm OJ: A time-related study by Doppler and M-mode echocardiography of hemodynamics, heart rate, and AV valvular function during activity-sensing rate-responsive ventricular pacing. PACE 10:507, 1987.

149. Stone JM, Bhakla RD, Lutgen J: Dual-chamber sequential pacing management of sinus node dysfunction: Advantages over single-chamber pacing. Am Heart J 104:1319, 1982.

150. Alpert MA, Curtis JJ, Sanfelippo JF, et al: Comparative survival after permanent ventricular and dual-chamber pacing for patients with chronic high degree atrioventricular block with and without preexistent congestive heart failure. J Am Coll Cardiol 7:925, 1986.

151. Alpert MA, Curtis JJ, Sanfelippo JF, et al: Comparative survival following permanent ventricular and dual-chamber pacing for patients with chronic symptomatic sinus node dysfunction with and without congestive heart failure. Am Heart J 113:958, 1987.

152. Sutton R, Kenny RA: The natural history of sick sinus syndrome. PACE 9:1110, 1986.

153. Rosenqvist M, Brandt J, Schüller H: Atrial versus ventricular pacing in sinus node disease: A treatment comparison study. Am Heart J 111:292, 1986.

154. Byrd CL, Schwartz SJ, Gonzales M, et al: DDD pacemakers maximize hemodynamic benefits and minimize complications for most patients. PACE 11:1911, 1988.

155. Rosenqvist M, Brandt J, Schüller H: Long-term pacing in sinus node disease: Effects of stimulation mode on cardiovascular morbidity and mortality. Am Heart J 116:16, 1988.

156. Santini M, Alexidou G, Ansalone G, et al: Relation of prognosis in sick sinus syndrome to age, conduction defects, and modes of permanent cardiac pacing. Am J Cardiol 65:729, 1990.

157. Hesselson AB, Parsonnet V, Bernstein AD, Bonavita GJ: Deleterious effects of long-term single-chamber ventricular pacing in patients with sick sinus syndrome: The hidden benefits of dual-chamber pacing. J Am Coll Cardiol 19:1542, 1992.

158. Kubica J, Stolarczyk L, Krzyminska E, et al: Left atrial size and wall motion in patients with permanent ventricular and atrial pacing. PACE 13:1737, 1990.

159. Lau CP, Wong CK, Leung WH, Liu WX: Superior cardiac hemodynamics of atrioventricular synchrony over rate-responsive pacing at submaximal exercise: Observations in activity-sensing DDDR pacemakers. PACE 13:1832, 1990.

160. Proctor EE, Leman RB, Mann DL, et al: Single-versus dual-chamber sensor-driven pacing: Comparison of cardiac outputs. Am Heart J 122:728, 1991.

161. Vogt P, Goy J, Kuhn M, et al: Single- versus double-chamber rate-responsive cardiac pacing: Comparison by cardiopulmonary noninvasive exercise testing. PACE 11:1896, 1988.

162. Jutzy RV, Florio J, Isaeff DM, et al: Limitations of testing methods for evaluation of dual-chamber versus single-chamber adaptive rate pacing. Am J Cardiol 68:1715, 1991.

163. Capucci A, Boriani G, Specchia S, et al: Evaluation by cardiopulmonary exercise test of DDDR versus DDD pacing. PACE 15:1908, 1992.

164. Daubert C, Ritter P, Mabo P, et al: Physiological relationship between AV interval and heart rate in healthy subjects: Applications to dual-chamber pacing. PACE 9:1032, 1986.

165. Luceri RM, Brownstein SL, Vardeman L, Goldstein S: PR interval behavior during exercise: Implications for physiological pacemakers. PACE 13:1719, 1990.

166. Barbieri D, Percoco GF, Toselli T, et al: AV delay and exercise stress tests: Behavior in normal subjects. PACE 13:1724, 1990.

167. Haskell RJ, French WJ: Physiological importance of different atrioventricular intervals to improve exercise performance in patients with dual-chamber pacemakers. Br Heart J 61:46, 1989.

168. Rydén L, Karlsson O, Kristensson BE: The importance of different atrioventricular intervals for exercise capacity. PACE 11:1051, 1988.

169. Landzberg JS, Franklin JO, Mahawar SK, et al: Benefits of physiologic atrioventricular synchronization for pacing with an exercise rate response. Am J Cardiol 66:193, 1990.

170. Ritter PH, Vai F, Bonnet JL, et al: Rate-adaptive atrioventricular delay improves cardiopulmonary performance in patients implanted with a dual-chamber pacemaker for complete heart block. Eur JCPE 1:31, 1991.

171. Sulke AN, Chambers JB, Sowton E: The effect of atrioventricular delay programming in patients with DDDR pacemakers. Eur Heart J 13:464, 1992.

172. Theodorakis GN, Kremastinos D, Markianos M, et al: Total sympathetic activity and atrial natriuretic factor levels in VVI and DDD pacing with different atrioventricular delays during daily activity and exercise. Eur Heart J 13:1477, 1992.

173. Igawa O, Tomokuni T, Saitoh M, et al: Sympathetic nervous system response to dynamic exercise in complete AV block patients treated with AV synchronous pacing with fixed AV delay or auto-AV delay. PACE 13:1766, 1990.

174. Rosenqvist M, Isaaz K, Botvinick EH, et al: Relative importance of activation sequence compared to atrioventricular synchrony in left ventricular function. Am J Cardiol 67:148, 1991.

175. Askenazi J, Alexander JH, Koenigsberg DI, et al: Alteration of left ventricular performance by left bundle branch block simulated with atrioventricular sequential pacing. Am J Cardiol 53:99, 1984.

176. Bramlet DA, Morris KG, Coleman RE, et al: Effects of rate-dependent left bundle branch block on global and regional left ventricular function. Circulation 67:1059, 1983.

177. Grines CL, Bashore TM, Boudoulas H, et al: Functional abnormalities in isolated left bundle branch block: The effect of interventricular asynchrony. Circulation 79:845, 1989.

178. Bedotto JB, Grayburn PA, Black WH, et al: Alterations in left ventricular relaxation during atrioventricular pacing in humans. J Am Coll Cardiol 15:658, 1990.

179. Harper GR, Pina IL, Kutalek SP: Intrinsic conduction maximizes cardiopulmonary performance in patients with dual-chamber pacemakers. PACE 14:1787, 1992.

180. Santomauro M. Fazio S, Ferraro S, et al: Fourier analysis in patients with different pacing modes. PACE 14:1351, 1991.

181. Valero A: Atrial transport dysfunction in acute myocardial infarction. Am J Cardiol 16:22, 1965.

182. Cohn JN, Guitia NJ, Broder MI, Limas CJ: Right ventricular infarction: Clinical and hemodynamic features. Am J Cardiol 33:204, 1974.

183. Topol EJ, Goldschlager N, Ports TA, et al: Hemodynamic benefit of atrial pacing in right ventricular myocardial infarction. Ann Intern Med 96:594, 1982.

184. Love JC, Haffajee CI, Gore JM, Alpert JS: Reversibility of hypotension and shock by atrial or atrioventricular sequential pacing in patients with right ventricular infarction. Am Heart J 108:5, 1984.

185. Matangi MF: Temporary physiologic pacing in inferior wall acute myocardial infarction with right ventricular damage. Am J Cardiol 59:1207, 1987.

186. Murphy P, Morton P, Murtagh JG, et al: Hemodynamic effects of different temporary pacing modes for management of bradycardias complicating acute myocardial infarction. PACE 15:391, 1992.

187. Shefer A, Rozenman Y, Ben David Y, et al: Left ventricular function during physiological cardiac pacing: Relation to rate, pacing mode, and underlying myocardial disease. PACE 10:315, 1987.

188. Kenny RA, Ingram A, Mitsuoka T, et al: Optimum pacing mode for patients with angina pectoris. Br Heart J 56:463, 1986.

189. Laniado S, Yellin EL, Yoran C, et al: Physiologic mechanisms in aortic insufficiency. I. The effect of changing heart rate on flow dynamics II. Determinants of Austin Flint murmer. Circulation 66:226, 1982.

190. Meyer TE, Sareli P, Marcus RH, et al: Beneficial effect of atrial pacing in severe acute aortic regurgitation and role of M-mode echocardiography in determining the optimal pacing interval. Am J Cardiol 67:398, 1991.

191. Shemin RJ, Scott WC, Kastl DG, Morrow AG: Hemodynamic effects of various modes of cardiac pacing after operation for idiopathic hypertrophic subaortic stenosis. Ann Thorac Surg 27:137, 1979.

192. Gross JN, Keltz TN, Cooper JA, et al: Profound "pacemaker syndrome" in hypertrophic cardiomyopathy. Am J Cardiol 70:1507, 1992.

193. Perrins EJ, Morley CA, Chan SL, Sutton D: Randomized controlled trial of physiological and ventricular pacing. Br Heart J 50:112, 1983.

194. Pehrsson SK, Aström H: Left ventricular function after long-term treatment with ventricular inhibited compared to atrial triggered ventricular pacing. Acta Med Scand 214:295, 1983.

195. Kristensson BE, Arnman K, Smedgård P, Ryden L: Physiological versus single-rate ventricular pacing: A double-blind cross-over study. PACE 8:73, 1985.

196. Linde-Edelstam C, Nordlander R, Unden AL, et al: Quality of life in patients treated with atrioventricular synchronous pacing compared to

rate modulated ventricular pacing: A long-term, double-blind, cross-over study. PACE 15:1467, 1992.

197. Lipkin DP, Buller N, Freeneaux M, et al: Randomised crossover trial of rate responsive Activitrax and conventional fixed-rate ventricular pacing. Br Heart J 58:613, 1987.

198. Candinas RA, Gloor HO, Amann FW, et al: Activity-sensing rate responsive versus conventional fixed-rate pacing: A comparison of rate behavior and patient well-being during routine daily exercise. PACE 14:204, 1991.

199. Irnich W, Conrady J: A new principle of rate-adaptive pacing in patients with sick sinus syndrome. PACE 11:1823, 1988.

200. Mabo P, Pouillot C, Kermarrec A, et al: Lack of physiological adaptation of the atrioventricular interval to heart rate in patients chronically paced in the AAIR mode. PACE 14:2133, 1991.

201. DenDulk K, Lindemans FW, Brugada P, et al: Pacemaker syndrome with AAI rate-variable pacing: Importance of atrioventricular conduction properties, medication, and pacemaker programmability. PACE 11:1226, 1988.

CHAPTER 24

CLINICAL TRIALS AND EXPERIENCE

E. J. Perrins
P. S. Astridge

Early pacing systems were designed simply to correct bradycardia and abolish Stokes-Adams attacks, but modern multiprogrammable physiologic and rate-modulating units aim to restore normal heart rate response and exercise tolerance. A large number of clinical studies have been performed to compare exercise capacity and quality of life with different pacing modes, sensors, and algorithms for rate adaptation, and this chapter reviews the results and conclusions of these clinical trials.

Clinical assessment of the benefits of pacing involves balancing the convenience and reproducibility of laboratory exercise testing protocols and simulating activities relevant to the subject's everyday life. In addition, the patient's physical condition, age, and ambition should be taken into account.

Clinical Assessment of Pacemaker Function

In assessment of exercise capacity and comparison of different pacemaker modes with normal physiology, the objectives of pacemaker therapy should be considered. Are perfect restoration of atrioventricular (AV) synchrony and simulation of normal chronotropism essential for maximum benefit to the patient? Although theoretical maximum heart rates for normal individuals at any age may be calculated from Wilkoff's mathematical model or derived from previously reported series,[1, 2] in practice most patients and indeed normal individuals may never achieve these levels during everyday life. In pacemaker patients in particular, underlying cardiac disease and intercurrent medication may mean that a theoretically maximal heart rate is irrelevant and achievement of such a rate an unrealistic test of a physiologic pacing system. It is well established that cardiac output increases when heart rates are returned from 40 to 70 beats per minute (bpm), regardless of AV synchrony. Sowton's[3] early work on hemodynamics in paced patients suggested a median optimal heart rate of 66 to 70 bpm. Whether additional rate adaptation, by either P-wave tracking or sensor-mediated rate response, increases exercise tolerance and the patient's well-being may be assessed by comparing the performance of patients with rate-adaptive units and fixed-rate units and by comparing paced patients with normal age- and sex-matched subjects.[4] The hemodynamics of AV synchrony and rate response are reviewed in Chapter 23.

Clinical Comparisons of Physiologic and Rate-Adaptive Pacing

Exercise capacity depends on the ability to increase cardiac output during exertion. This is normally achieved by a combination of increases in stroke volume and increases in heart rate (Fig. 24-1). In normal subjects, cardiac rate may increase fourfold between rest and maximum exercise and stroke volume by 50%.[5] Patients with complete heart block achieve only a fraction of the desirable increase in work capacity by increasing stroke volume,[6] although moderately high levels of exercise may be supported by two- to threefold increases in cardiac output at fixed pacing rates.[3] In patients with implanted cardiac pacemakers, an increase in heart rate during exertion may be achieved either by ventricular tracking of atrial rate in subjects with normal sinus node function or by sensor-mediated rate-adaptive pacing in those with sinus node disease or chronic atrial fibrillation. The normal sinus response remains the "gold standard" by which rate modulation may be compared.

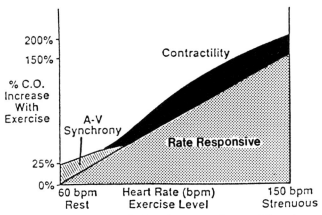

FIGURE 24–1. Relative contribution of rate responsiveness, AV synchrony, and cardiac contractility to augmentation of cardiac output with upright exercise. The ordinate shows the approximate increase in cardiac output over baseline resting values. The abscissa displays a heart rate ranging from 60 bpm at rest to 150 bpm during strenuous exercise. (Reproduced with permission from Benditt DG, Milstein S, Buetikofer J, et al: Sensor-triggered rate-variable cardiac pacing: Current technologies and clinical implications. Ann Intern Med 107:714, 1987.)

BENEFITS OF PHYSIOLOGIC (ATRIOVENTRICULAR SYNCHRONOUS) PACING

The hemodynamic advantages of AV synchrony are well proven at lower heart rates.[7, 8] Samet and colleagues[9] also showed significant benefits with AV synchrony, whether it was due to sinus rhythm or to sequential AV pacing, over ventricular pacing at matched rates up to 140 bpm in subjects with normal hearts. These findings were, however, not confirmed by Benchimol and coworkers.[10] Although at rest significantly higher stroke volumes are seen in paced patients with intact AV synchrony than in patients with fixed-rate ventricular pacing, these differences disappear during exercise, suggesting that AV synchrony may be less important than heart rate in determining exercise capacity.[8]

Many clinical studies of pacing modes have investigated the clinical advantages of physiologic pacing. Some of these studies were small, and in many the conclusions were based not only on exercise capacity but also on subjective elements such as patients' well-being and the presence of symptoms of pacemaker syndrome. The results of these trials are summarized in Table 24–1.

The exercise performance of 16 patients with an atrial synchronous ventricular inhibited unit in VDD and VVI modes during bicycle ergometry was compared by Kruse and Rydén.[11] Exercise was commenced at 30 W (women) or 50 W (men) and increased incrementally until limited by patients' symptoms. Because of continuous electrocardio-

graphic (ECG) monitoring the trial was single blind, but efforts were made to ensure that the tests were performed under strictly standardized conditions. Exercise capacity was increased by 20% when paced in the physiologic mode (i.e., VDD mode), regardless of the patient's age (Fig. 24–2). These findings were confirmed with the same group during an invasive hemodynamic study of the benefits of physiologic pacing, when a 24% improvement in exercise tolerance was observed.[12]

Fananapazir and colleagues[13] compared the treadmill performance of 14 patients with a multiprogrammable DDD pacemaker in a double-blind crossover study. An increase in work done of 44% was noted in atrial synchronous mode compared with fixed-rate ventricular pacing. Lightheadedness, postural hypotension, and dyspnea were more frequent in the latter group.

Perrins and colleagues[14] compared physiologic and asynchronous ventricular pacing in 13 patients over 1-month intervals in the first double-blind study of physiologic pacing. During each period the patients kept a symptom diary, and at the end of the trial they performed a maximal bicycle exercise test. Dizziness, breathlessness, and palpitations were significantly more frequent during the VVI stage, and exercise capacity was increased by 27% with pacing in the VDD mode. Sutton and coworkers[15] demonstrated that the improvements in exercise tolerance were sustained over an average of 33 months. Comparison of bicycle ergometry in VVI and VDD modes soon after implantation showed a 43% improvement in effort tolerance. After prolonged follow-up, exercise testing still showed a 34% advantage in VDD mode, suggesting that improvements in work capacity are maintained.

The long-term benefits of physiologic pacing were confirmed by Kristensson and coworkers,[16] who investigated 44 patients who had had AV synchronous pacemakers for more than 1 year. The subjects, randomly assigned to either VVI pacing at 70 bpm or VDD pacing mode, performed bicycle stress tests after 3 weeks. Exercise capacity was 14% greater and the incidence of palpitations, neck pulsations, and breathlessness reduced in the VDD mode. At the conclusion of the study, all but six patients either favored VDD over VVI pacing or expressed no preference. However, three of those left in the VVI pacing mode at the conclusion of the study later requested reprogramming to the VDD pacing mode. More recently, VVI pacing at 70 bpm has been compared with physiologic pacing in 19 patients with dual-chamber pacemakers.[17] The subjects spent 6 weeks in each mode before performing a modified Balke treadmill test. Exercise time was increased by 18% with AV synchrony. Eight patients insisted on early crossover from VVI pacing because

TABLE 24–1. **TRIALS OF PHYSIOLOGIC VERSUS FIXED-RATE PACING**

AUTHOR(S)	NUMBER OF PATIENTS	EXERCISE MODE	IMPROVEMENT (%)
Kruse and Rydén[11]	16	Bicycle	20
Kruse et al.[12]	16	Bicycle	24
Fananapazir et al.[13]	14	Treadmill	44
Perrins et al.[14]	13	Bicycle	27
Sutton et al.[15]	53	Bicycle	34
Kristensson et al.[16]	44	Bicycle	14
Rediker et al.[17]	19	Treadmill	18

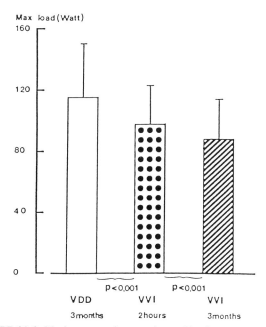

FIGURE 24–2. Maximum exercise capacity on bicycle ergometry after 3 months in DDD mode, after acutely programming to VVI mode, and after chronic pacing in VVI mode for a period of 3 months. Exercise during VVI pacing results in a further decrease in exercise capacity. (From Kruse I, Arnman K, Conradson T-B, et al: A comparison of the acute and long-term haemodynamic effects of ventricular inhibited and atrial synchronous ventricular inhibited pacing. Circulation 65:846, 1982.)

of unacceptable symptoms; this group had a high incidence of ventriculoatrial (VA) conduction and a low intrinsic heart rate and a proportionally greater gain in effort tolerance on exercise. Generally, all patients were symptomatically better with physiologic pacing.

In light of a large retrospective study showing no excess of pacemaker complications by Byrd and associates[18] in patients with dual-chamber systems, there is clear evidence that physiologic pacing increases exercise capacity and well-being compared with fixed-rate pacing, without increasing the hazards of pacemaker implantation.

CLINICAL ADVANTAGES OF SENSOR-DRIVEN RATE-MODULATED PACING

Rate modulation is now widely available, incorporated in both single- and dual-chamber units. However, until recently the choice was restricted to non–rate-responsive dual-chamber systems or sensor-driven single-chamber rate-modulated pacing. Work by Færestrand and colleagues[19] on activity-sensing rate-adaptive pacemakers showed a positive correlation between exercise duration and the increase in heart rate during exercise. If exercise capacity depends largely on increase in heart rate, patients with rate-adaptive pacemakers will outperform those with fixed-rate devices. In addition, some subgroups of patients may perform as well with P-wave asynchronous VVIR pacing as with physiologic P-wave tracking (in the absence of complications related to VA conduction). In many instances, patients are unsuitable for dual-chamber devices because of frequent, refractory, or chronic atrial arrhythmias or inexcitable atria.[20]

COMPARISON OF FIXED-RATE AND RATE-ADAPTIVE VENTRICULAR PACING

A wide variety of sensors to detect exercise and modulate heart rate are available. The most widely available is vibration-driven activity sensing, and many of the studies comparing VVI and VVIR pacing involve this sensor.[21] Twenty-one patients with Activitrax vibration-sensing pacemakers were investigated by Smedgård and coworkers.[22] Patients underwent both treadmill exercise testing and bicycle ergometry after a week in either fixed-rate or rate-responsive mode, in random order. Heart rate increase was predictably greater on the treadmill than on the bicycle, because of the greater thoracic vibrations generated during walking than cycling. Exercise capacity on the bicycle ergometer was increased by an average of 10%, and exercise duration on the treadmill increased by 18%. Similarly, Færestrand and coworkers[19] demonstrated significant prolongation of treadmill exercise time in rate-responsive mode compared with fixed-rate ventricular pacing in 15 patients with the same sensor. The improvement was particularly dramatic in the subgroup of patients who were 100% ventricularly paced, in whom exercise time was increased by 38%, compared with 17% in the intermittently paced group. Benditt and colleagues[20, 21] also showed an increase in treadmill exercise duration of 33% in activity-sensing VVIR mode over VVI mode in 12 patients. Lindemans and colleagues[23] published data from a multicenter study on 222 patients who had received Activitrax pacemakers for a variety of indications. Exercise duration on a modified Naughton protocol was prolonged by 32% overall in the VVIR pacing mode and by 52% in the subgroup of pacemaker-dependent patients. The subjects kept diaries, scoring for the presence of cardiac symptoms daily. The only significant symptomatic difference between modes was a decrease in "problems with physical effort" in the VVIR group.

Lau and colleagues[24] compared the exercise performance of 50 patients with rate-adaptive pacemakers in VVI and VVIR modes. Sensors used included two types of activity sensing, two types of respiratory sensors, QT sensor, and one pacemaker utilizing right ventricular dP/dt. The subjects underwent two treadmill exercise tests using a Bruce protocol, once in rate-adaptive mode and once with a fixed rate of 70 bpm, in random order. Highly significant and consistent improvement in duration of exercise capacity by 26% to 49% was seen, despite significant differences in rate response characteristics between the various pacemaker models.

Potential advantages of activity-sensing rate-adaptive pacing during everyday activities were investigated in 21 patients by Candinas and coworkers.[25] VVI and VVIR modes were compared in a double-blind fashion with patients performing an outdoor exercise routine involving walking on a flat surface and up a slope and climbing stairs, then repeating the circuit in reverse (i.e., downhill). In the presence of typical activity sensor limitations (e.g., prompt increase in heart rate at the start of exercise, failure to increase heart rate further with increasingly strenuous exercise followed by nonphysiologic decrease with increasing exhaustion), half of the patients with completely ventricularly paced rhythms subjectively preferred rate-adaptive pacing, but only two of nine patients with only intermittent ventricular pacing expressed a preference. Objective measurement of time to complete the exercise protocol showed no significant difference between the VVI and the VVIR pacing modes. This sort of indeterminate result for brief informal exercise with a subjective end point demonstrates the advantages to investigators and manufacturers of formal statistically supported exercise testing to demonstrate benefits of new technology.

The benefits of rate responsiveness were elegantly demonstrated noninvasively before pacemaker upgrade by McGoon and Fetter[26] by setting the currently implanted pacemaker to triggered mode, driving the ventricular rate by chest wall stimulation with an external Activitrax unit. The single patient studied improved his exercise capacity from 30% to 58% of predicted functional aerobic capacity on a Naughton treadmill protocol with rate modulation. The weight of evidence for the benefits of rate-adaptive pacing, however, probably makes individual justification of upgrading unnecessary in practical terms, unless the patient has personal objections to the increased cost of the pulse generator.

Surprisingly, a small double-blind crossover study of elderly patients with Medtronic activity-sensing pacemakers failed to show any significant difference in exercise times between rate-adaptive and fixed-rate modes.[27] However, the patients were asked to perform a gentle Naughton protocol handicapped by a face mask for oxygen consumption estimation. Overall, the study claimed a positive result because of the demonstration of raised anaerobic thresholds, but it cannot be said to be relevant to the performance of either patient or pacemaker in the real world, where most daily activities are performed at relatively low intensity. Further comparison of fixed-rate and rate-responsive pacing from comparative clinical trials is summarized in Table 24–2.

Overall, the benefits of rate-adaptive ventricular pacing over fixed-rate ventricular pacing are inescapable. The implantation procedure is neither longer nor more complicated than for a VVI system, and follow-up need not be significantly more time-consuming or arduous. If a single-chamber unit has been selected for the patient, there can be very few

situations—for example, severe immobility because of non-cardiac disease or terminal illness—when it is justifiable to implant a fixed-rate rather than a rate-responsive unit. Rate-responsive units are more expensive than VVI units, but considering the strong evidence for benefits from rate modulation in the absence of increased risk, the ethics of denying the more advanced technology are doubtful.

WHO WOULD BENEFIT FROM RATE-ADAPTIVE PACING?

Heinz and associates[28] exercised 107 pacemaker patients from a typical pacemaker population, with indications including sick sinus syndrome (47%), complete heart block (35%), and various other bradyarrhythmias (11%). With pacemakers programmed to VVI mode at 70 bpm, all patients showed a reduction in exercise capacity compared with age-matched control subjects. Excluding subjects limited by factors other than fatigue and discounting those with complete AV block more suitably treated with DDD pacing, it was estimated that 46% of all pacemaker patients might benefit from the addition of rate-adaptive pacing.

PHYSIOLOGIC COMPARED WITH VENTRICULAR RATE-ADAPTIVE PACING

Investigation of cardiac hemodynamics demonstrates superior cardiac performance with AV synchronous compared with ventricular rate-adaptive pacing, during rest, exercise, and immediately after exercise, because of enhanced stroke volume.[29] Radionuclide ventriculography suggests that left ventricular function is inferior during ventricular compared with AV sequential pacing.[30] Clinically, the patient's performance and preference during formal exercise testing or informal day-to-day activities is more relevant. A Glasgow study of 10 patients with Synergyst pacemakers (Medtronic) for third-degree AV block, and with normal sinus node func-

TABLE 24–2. TRIALS OF RATE-ADAPTIVE VERSUS FIXED-RATE VENTRICULAR PACING

AUTHOR(S)	NUMBER OF PATIENTS	SENSOR	EXERCISE MODE	IMPROVEMENT (%)
Donaldson et al.[58]	5	QT	Treadmill	57
Lindemans et al.[23]	222	Activity	Treadmill	32
Benditt et al.[21]	12	Activity	Treadmill	32
Faerestrand et al.[19]	15	Activity	Treadmill	38
McGoon and Fetter[26]	1	Activity	Treadmill	30–58
Smedgård et al.[22]	15	Activity	Treadmill	19
			Bicycle	7
Den Dulk et al.[39]	31	Activity	Treadmill	37
Lau et al.[46]	11	Activity	Treadmill	26
Lau et al.[77]	9	Minute vent.	Treadmill	33
Rossi et al.[76]	143	Resp. rate	Treadmill	30
Fearnot et al.[94]	31	Temperature	Treadmill	28
Hedman et al.[59]	18	QT	Bicycle	9
Kay et al.[83]	10	Minute vent.	Treadmill	23
Lau et al.[80]	9	Minute vent.	Treadmill	24
Lau et al.[85]	21	Resp. rate	Treadmill	29
		Minute vent.	Treadmill	32
Lau et al.[24]	46	Activity QT, dP/dt Resp. rate Minute vent.	Treadmill	24–49
Bennett et al.[100]	12	dP/dt	Treadmill	12
Santomauro et al.[73]	27	Resp. rate	Treadmill	56

TABLE 24–3. **TRIALS OF PHYSIOLOGIC VERSUS RATE-ADAPTIVE VENTRICULAR PACING**

AUTHOR(S)	NUMBER OF PATIENTS	SENSOR	EXERCISE MODE	IMPROVEMENT (%)
Menozzi et al.[35]	14	Activity	Bicycle	NS
Oldroyd et al.[31]	10	Activity	Treadmill	NS
Linde-Edelstam et al.[32]	17	Activity	Treadmill	NS

Abbreviation: NS, not significant.

tion, compared symptoms and exercise performance during maximal treadmill exercise on a fixed gradient with incrementally increasing walking speed in DDD and VVIR modes.[31] Even though patients spent a month in each pacing modality, no significant difference in the degree of breathlessness, fatigue or mood disturbance, exercise duration, and maximal oxygen consumption was found between modes. Overall the authors concluded that there was no advantage in DDD over VVIR pacing, except in one subject who developed pacemaker syndrome.

In a study from Stockholm by Linde-Edelstam and colleagues,[32] submaximal exercise capacity in VVIR and DDD modes was assessed in 17 patients with Siemens Sensolog or Synchrony pacemakers (Siemens-Elema, Solna, Sweden and Siemens Pacesetter, Sylmar, CA) implanted for high-degree AV block. All patients had a normal atrial chronotropic response to exercise demonstrated before inclusion. The slope settings in VVIR mode were set to obtain a satisfactory rate response with exertion and a reasonable decline in rate on resting for each patient, assessed during brief episodes of on-the-spot jogging and rest. The patients performed submaximal treadmill exercise tests, at their normal walking pace, with freely swinging arms until a submaximal limit was reached, subjectively estimated at Borg symptom scale 5/10 (strenuous). Heart rate increase during exercise was significantly higher in DDD than in VVIR mode, and heart rate during the first 10 minutes of recovery was higher in the DDD group. Despite this, there were no significant discrepancies in exercise time, respiratory rate, or ratings of perceived breathlessness or fatigue between DDD and VVIR modes. Of these patients, nine preferred DDD mode, three preferred VVIR, and five had no preference; there were no predictors of the patients' choices.

That benefits from rate increase outweigh benefits from maintaining AV synchrony, provided that symptoms associated with lack of AV synchrony do not arise, was confirmed by Batey and associates.[33] Eighteen patients with dual-chamber (DDD) pacemakers and chronotropic incompetence underwent Sheffield protocol treadmill tests, once in DDD mode and once in externally triggered VVIR mode using a piezoelectric crystal vibration sensor. Default settings for response slope and activity threshold were used. Fourteen patients failed to achieve intrinsic heart rates greater than 100 bpm with exercise, and all but one of these exercised significantly longer in VVIR than DDD mode. The remaining subject developed symptoms consistent with pacemaker syndrome.

Fananapazir and colleagues[13] compared atrial synchronous (VAT) pacing with chest wall–stimulated VAT pacing at rates above the intrinsic atrial rate (hence without AV synchrony) and VOO pacing. There was significant and equal improvement in exercise performance during both modes of

VAT pacing compared with asynchronous ventricular pacing, supporting the hypothesis that the superiority of physiologic pacing depends on heart rate increase rather than maintenance of AV synchrony. Ausubel and coworkers[34] showed that during upright exercise equal increases in stroke volume were seen in both the presence and the absence of AV synchrony. In P-wave asynchronous pacing, maintenance of stroke volume required an increase in myocardial contractility, regarded as a less optimal but effective route to increased cardiac output.

Exercise capacity alone, however, does not predict patients' tolerance of pacing mode. Patients with asynchronous ventricular pacing are at risk for developing pacemaker syndrome (see Chapter 25). This was demonstrated in a longer-term study of patients' tolerance of DDD and VVIR modes by Menozzi and colleagues.[35] Fourteen patients with AV block and Medtronic Synergyst pacemakers (Medtronic Inc., Minneapolis, MN) spent 6 weeks in each mode in a random-order double-blind crossover study. At the end of each period, patients performed a bicycle stress test and filled in a simple symptoms questionnaire. Although there was no significant difference in exercise capacity between pacing modes, patients were significantly more symptomatic in the VVIR mode, complaining of dyspnea, palpitations, and abnormal neck pulsations. One third of the subjects requested early switch-over to dual-chamber pacing.

Dual-chamber pacing does not appear to confer any additional gains in exercise capabilities over rate-responsive ventricular pacing, even in patients with normal atrial chronotropic function (Table 24–3). However, other factors such as the risk of pacemaker syndrome and greater risk of atrial arrhythmias with ventricular pacing make DDD pacing the better choice for patients with relatively normal sinus node function.

Desirable Properties of Sensors

In general terms, the ideal sensor would closely mimic the rate acceleration and deceleration of the normal sinus node during exercise, would respond as the sinus node to nonexercise requirements (i.e., postural changes, fever, mental stress, circadian rhythm), and would not be triggered by spurious interference. Some of these requirements are more important than others; for example, no benefit has been shown from simulating a posture sensor in a rate-adaptive ventricular pacemaker by accelerating the heart rate immediately before standing.[36]

In practice, the available sensors vary widely in their profiles during exercise and in their ability to respond to other physiologic stimuli. Each pacemaker model incorporates a range of programmable slope settings, allowing some adjustment of rate response to exercise. In addition, the threshold and sensitivity of the sensor may be variable. Many studies have been performed to assess the clinical performance of these sensor algorithms.

Clinical Studies With Individual Sensor Systems

ACTIVITY-SENSING PACEMAKERS

Pacemakers sensing body vibrations during activity are the most widely employed rate-adaptive pacemakers in clinical practice, as they do not require specialized leads, the sensor being situated inside the pacemaker can. Devices incorporating piezoelectric crystals and accelerometers are in widespread clinical use. The activity sensors are reviewed in detail in Chapter 8.

CLINICAL PERFORMANCE OF PIEZOELECTRIC CRYSTAL DEVICES

The Medtronic Activitrax/Legend (Medtronic Inc., Minneapolis, MN) is one of the most common sensors in clinical use. The crystal is fixed to the inner surface of the pacemaker casing and detects low-frequency thoracic vibrations. Sensor-mediated response appears unaffected by body constitution[37] or by site of implantation.[38]

Den Dulk and coworkers[39] investigated Activitrax pacemakers in 31 patients, most of whom had AV block and 10 of whom had evidence of sick sinus syndrome. Slopes were set to achieve a heart rate of 100 bpm during casual walking. In nine patients with complete heart block, atrial rate during treadmill exercise was compared with the paced rate by briefly inhibiting the pacemaker to allow visualization of P waves. At onset of exercise the pacemaker accelerated faster than the underlying sinus rate, and during exercise it maintained rates approximately 8% lower than the sinus node. After exercise, the pacemaker decelerated much more quickly than the sinus node, without causing symptoms.

Moura and colleagues[38] were generally more enthusiastic about the Activitrax's ability to mimic normal physiology. They compared the rate response profiles of implanted units in 12 patients and external units in 6 normal volunteers. The pacemaker responses were assessed twice, with medium activity and response settings and with high activity and maximum rate response, during Naughton exercise protocols. Although the rate response curves were different, with more rapid acceleration by the pacemaker than with the sinus node early in exercise, there were no significant differences at any point during exercise. The authors concluded that the Activitrax can achieve physiologic pacing rates during daily activities, given appropriate programming.

Lau and coworkers[40] assessed the limitations of this sensor in different forms of activity. Six normal subjects performed exercise tests with an external Activitrax strapped to the chest wall, to compare sinus and paced heart rate profiles. Fifteen patients with Activitrax pacemakers completed treadmill exercise tests according to the Bruce protocol, jogged on the spot, climbed and descended stairs, and performed the Valsalva maneuver, isometric hand grip, and changes in posture. The latter three activities were associated with only small increases in heart rate, involving little body movement. Jogging and treadmill exercise were associated with prompt heart rate increases. Paced heart rate depended on walking speed and, unlike sinus rate in normal control subjects, did not increase further with increasing gradient. Similarly, the greater stress of climbing rather than descending stairs was not reflected in greater rate acceleration. After cessation of exercise, Activitrax rate declined to baseline more quickly than the sinus rate.

The comparison between the sinus rate in normal subjects and the response of external Activitrax units was further examined.[41] The study involved exercise testing at a fixed treadmill speed but at four different step frequencies guided by a metronome, treadmill testing at different gradients at two constant speeds, and a comparison of different forms of exercise stress including walking and running on a treadmill, weight lifting, and bicycle ergometry. The rate response of the Activitrax did not correspond closely to the sinus rate. During varying stepping frequencies, the paced rate was greater with higher step rates, unlike the sinus rate, which was lowest at the maximum step rate. During graded exercise testing, at the higher speed the pacemaker overresponded compared to its reponse at lower gradients. Comparing different forms of exercise, the sensor matched the sinus rate best during walking on the level. Pacemaker rates were lower than sinus rates during bicycling and running (Fig. 24–3).

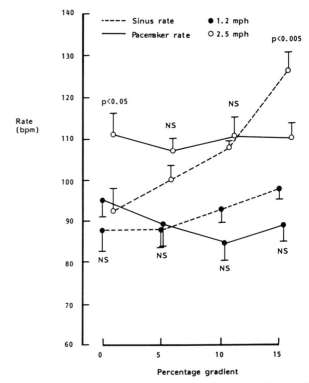

FIGURE 24–3. Pacing rate of six subjects with an externally attached Activitrax (Medtronic) pacemaker during treadmill exercises at different speeds and gradients. Each point represents 3-minute exercise on the treadmill at a combination of two speeds (1.2 and 2.5 mph) and four gradients (0% to 15%). Although there is an increase in pacing rate as the patients walked faster, there is no increase in rate as the subjects walked at higher gradients. The sinus rate, on the other hand, shows an increase in rate to walking upslope and to walking at a faster speed. (From Lau CP, Stott JRR, Toff WD, et al: Selective vibration sensing: A new concept for activity-sensing rate-responsive pacing. PACE 11:1299, 1988.)

McAlister and colleagues[42] compared the mean sinus node response of healthy volunteers with rate response profiles from external units on the same volunteers and from implanted units in four patients. All subjects underwent multiple treadmill exercise tests with a variety of rate response and activity threshold settings, in a single-blind randomized fashion. Despite repetitive exercise testing allowing fine-tuning of the programmable parameters to approximate as closely as possible sinus node function, the Activitrax rarely achieved maximum paced rate despite vigorous exercise, and the intrinsic shortcomings of the sensor with overrapid initial response and insensitivity to grade were not overcome.

The limitations of the Activitrax system are related to the detection of vibrations generated by exercise, which are only loosely related to the physical and metabolic demands of that exercise. In the third-generation models (Legend, Medtronic Pacemakers), the rate response algorithm has been altered to improve the physiologic response, with a linear response to exercise. However, a comparison of external Activitrax and Legend devices strapped to 10 control subjects did not reveal any advantages of the new algorithm's performance, with no device reaching the programmed upper rate.[43]

The rate response performance of external devices programmed to nominal values was compared with intrinsic heart rate in 10 normal subjects, who performed chronotropic assessment exercise protocol (CAEP) treadmill exercise tests, bicycle ergometry, and stair walking.[44] Despite the algorithm improvements, on treadmill testing the Legend achieved a mean maximal pulse rate of only 105 bpm, 24 bpm less than the maximal sinus rate. On stair ascent and during bicycle exercise, the Legend's heart rate was again lower than sinus rhythm. Bellamy and colleagues[45] also found limited improvement in the performance of the updated algorithm in the Legend. Although there was rapid rate modulation at the onset and offset of exercise, the response reached a plateau despite increasing workload, and unsurprisingly the device remains insensitive to gradient changes.

The Sensolog (Siemens-Elema, Solna, Sweden) pacemaker employs a similar piezoelectric crystal in the can to detect vibrations. The algorithm integrates the vibration signals rather than counting peaks above a preset threshold as in the Activitrax system.

Lau and coworkers[46] investigated the clinical performance of the new activity-based rate-adaptive pacemaker, the Sensolog 703, 1 month after implantation in 11 patients with complete heart block and atrial arrhythmias. The slope was adjusted to achieve 100 bpm by the end of Bruce protocol stage 1. Results were compared with the rate response curve of an external Activitrax strapped to the subjects during exercise. Patients underwent four brief treadmill exercise tests using different gradients and speeds, bicycle ergometry, and Valsalva maneuver, isometric arm exercise, and climbing and descending stairs. Limitations similar to those seen with the Activitrax were seen with the Sensolog; no response to Valsalva or isometric exercise was seen, heart rate increased with walking speed but not gradient, and there was no distinction by the pacemaker between the relative metabolic demands of climbing and descending stairs. There was a nonsignificant trend for the Sensolog to pace faster than the Activitrax during stair ascent and bicycle ergometry. The rate acceleration by the Sensolog at exercise onset is slower than for the Activitrax, reflecting algorithm differences including

a programmable speed of onset of rate response. Similar results were found by Kubisch and coworkers[47] in 35 patients, with satisfactory rate profiles achieved during exercise testing but algorithm insensitivity to gradient changes. Programming performed according to the treadmill results caused the pulse generator to overrespond to day-to-day activities, shown by follow-up Holter monitoring.

The responses to exercise of the Activitrax and Sensolog systems were compared by Stangl and colleagues[48] in a total of 20 patients. This clinical investigation involved constant gradient–variable speed followed by constant speed–variable gradient treadmill testing. The first stress test was used for standardization, all pacemakers being programmed to reach the same response to two walking speeds. The Activitrax was more sensitive than the Sensolog to step changes, rapidly reached maximum pacing rate at low gradient, and appeared insensitive to further gradient increases. The Sensolog, however, showed a superior ability to discriminate workload, with progressive increments in paced rate with increasing gradient, although maximum attained rate fell well short of the sinus rate. Using a Borg symptoms scoring system, there were no distinctions between the perceived levels of exertion in the two groups. Johnson and colleagues,[49] however, having programmed the units in 10 patients to achieve the same rate in response to the same stress, found that although neither system achieved sinus rhythm rates during modified Bruce treadmill testing, the Activitrax response correlated well with sinus rhythm but the Sensolog did not. Neither pacemaker responded to postural change.

The Sensolog incorporates an autoprogrammability function allowing automatic adjustment of rate modulation settings. Mahaux and coworkers[50] reviewed the clinical performance of the Sensolog after automatic programming. Eleven patients were investigated over 10 months after implantation by treadmill and bicycle exercise tests, Holter monitoring, and external telemetric recording during everyday activities. In 6 of the 11 patients the autoset functions were unacceptable, with a tendency for the system to act on-off, achieving peak heart rates soon after the onset of exercise.

The piezoelectric crystal–based rate-adaptive pacemakers respond more promptly than the normal sinus node to the onset and offset of exercise. The devices rely on sensed body vibrations that are not proportional to metabolic stresses of the exercise undertaken, and this causes some major limitations in these devices, with lack of response to isometric and mental exercise and overresponse at the beginning of exercise.

CLINICAL PERFORMANCE OF ACCELEROMETERS

The accelerometer detects movement from resistance changes within a piezoelectric crystal suspended within the pacemaker canister, rather than fixed to the inside surface. The suspended mass moves under gravity in concert with bodily movement and independent of the can. In theory, this should reflect the pacemaker recipient's physical demands better than a conventional fixed-vibration sensor. The accelerometer sensor is reviewed in detail in Chapter 16.

Bacharach and associates[44] compared the performance of an accelerometer-based device (Excel VR, CPI, St. Paul, MN) with sinus rhythm in normal volunteers during treadmill and bicycle stress testing and stair walking. Results were compared with those for Legend pacemakers, incorporating an orthodox piezoelectric vibration sensor. Both pacemakers were programmed to nominal settings for response time, threshold, and recovery period on the grounds that this provided a method of comparing the systems under identical conditions, although whether two manufacturers' nominal settings are genuinely similar appears unproven. Heart rates from the accelerometer-driven device correlated more closely with the sinus rate than those from the piezoelectric device during treadmill exercise. During bicycling, the Excel generated higher rates than the Legend but still fell well short of the sinus rate, as little upper body movement is generated by stationary cycling. The paradoxical rate increase on descending rather than on ascending stairs seen with the conventional piezoelectric device was not reflected with the accelerometer; the Excel heart rate paralleled the intrinsic heart rate.

The Excel VR was also investigated by Borst and coworkers.[51] Eight patients with sinus rhythm, chronotropically competent sinoatrial nodes, and intermittent AV block were selected to compare intrinsic and paced heart rate. Changes in posture and Naughton exercise treadmill tests in fixed-rate and rate-adaptive mode, with nominal settings, were examined. Unlike the case of the fixed crystal vibration sensors, change in posture, from supine to sitting to standing, was associated with prompt rate acceleration on each maneuver. At nominal settings, the paced rate correlated well with the sinus rate. Typical everyday activities, including posture change, corridor walking, stair ascent and descent, window cleaning, and floor mopping, have also been observed in patients with this system.[52] Posture change was associated with prompt modest rate increases, as was window cleaning with either arm, although predictably the rate increase during this activity was greater when using the arm ipsilateral to the pulse generator. Rapid ascent of stairs induced a rate increase greater than either slow ascent or descent. Overall, the response to exertion appeared roughly proportional to the physical demands of that exercise, despite a lack of correlation between paced rate and sinus rhythm in normal control exercise testing.

Lau and colleagues[53] examined the clinical performance of an alternative accelerometer-mediated system, the Relay DDDR (Intermedics Inc., Angleton, TX), in 11 patients. The algorithm incorporates a triphasic rate-acceleration curve, with steep slopes during gentle and vigorous exercise. The performance of the Relay was compared with that of an external Legend pacemaker during daily activities and treadmill testing. The Relay's rate response was "tailored" during gentle exercise according to the manufacturer's instructions. No comparison with "normal" sinus rhythm was made. With the Relay, improved rate stability and higher rate response to jogging and standing were achieved, although responses to Valsalva, corridor walking, and treadmill testing did not differ significantly from those with the Legend. As with the conventional vibration sensor, the paced rate increased with increasing treadmill speed but not gradient.

A variation on the accelerometer is the tilt-switch principle. A mercury droplet in a sealed container with an electric switch activated by movement of the mercury is incorporated in the single-chamber Sorin Swing 100 (Sorin Biomedica, Saluggia, Italy). A multicenter clinical evaluation of this system in 89 patients involved treadmill assessment of the algorithm's response to exercise and Holter monitoring during

daily activities.[54] Rise slope was normal and fall slope slow in the absence of clinical indications for other settings. During Bruce protocol treadmill testing, there was progressive heart rate increase during exercise, but no comparison was made with sinus rhythm or non–rate-adaptive pacing. The sensor was insensitive to external noise from tapping or mechanical vibrations. The rate modulation from this sensor-algorithm combination was compared with sinus rhythm in six normal volunteers by Soussou and coworkers.[55] The subjects performed three Bruce exercise tests and a discontinuous exercise protocol with an external device strapped to the chest, programmed to a different rate response curve (fast, slow, normal) each time. Paced rate rose rapidly in the first minute of the Bruce protocol, followed by a slower increase. In all three rate response settings, the paced rate correlated poorly with the sinus rate, which was more rapid than the Excel rate throughout the exercise protocol. However, the rate increase by the pacemaker appeared prompt and appropriate, and during the discontinuous activity testing the paced rate was closer to the sinus rate than in progressively graded exercise. As with all models of movement sensor, the gravitational accelerometer appears more sensitive to stepping rate than to gradient.

Overall, accelerometers appear to detect movement signals that, although still nonphysiologic, equate more closely than the vibrations assessed by fixed piezoelectric crystal devices to human activities. However, the limitation of all movement detection devices is the inability to distinguish the different neurohumoral-metabolic stresses of more and less demanding exercise tasks if the bodily acceleration and motion patterns are identical.

QT-SENSING PACEMAKERS

During exercise, a combination of heart rate increase and direct catecholamine effects causes shortening of the QT interval. In 1981 this effect was incorporated into a physiologic sensor for estimation of exercise stress.[56] The algorithm measures the interval from the pacing stimulus to the maximum negative deflection of the first derivative of the endocardial T wave. If the interval falls within the T-wave sensing window, rate modulation occurs. As the QT interval is itself affected by rate modulation, the neurohumoral effects on QT provide an influence independent of paced rate and allow sensitivity to non–exercise-related stress.[57] The QT sensor is reviewed in detail in Chapter 14.

Initial experience with an early QT-sensing rate-adaptive system showed an increase in exercise capacity of 57% over fixed-rate pacing, associated with heart rate increases from 66 to 120 bpm.[58] Hedman and Nordlander[59] also demonstrated clinical advantages of QT-sensing rate-modulated pacing. Eighteen patients with TX pacemakers (Vitatron Medical B.V., Dieren, The Netherlands) took part in a double-blind randomized crossover comparison of QT sensing versus fixed-rate ventricular pacing. The patients' performance during bicycle ergometry and mental arithmetic was observed, and a simple scaled score for assessment of symptoms was collected. In rate-adaptive mode, symptom-limited exercise tolerance was increased by 9% and an average of 6.5 minutes was taken to reach maximum pacing rates, and heart rate increased by 10% during mental arithmetic. Symptom scoring showed a small but statistically significant improvement in VVIR mode, although frequency of chest pain was increased. Eleven of the subjects preferred the rate-responsive mode. Five-year follow-up of a small number of patients showed that the physiologic advantages of rate adaptation, shown by prolongation of treadmill exercise time, are present several years after pacemaker implantation.[60]

The rate response of the TX pacemaker was compared to the sinus response in a group of patients with AV block by Fananapazir and coworkers.[61] Atrial synchronized ventricular (VAT) pacing was possible using temporary electrodes and an external pacemaker. Symptom-limited exercise duration on a Bruce protocol was comparable in VVIR and VAT modes. However, peak heart rates achieved were 148 ± 5 bpm in the VAT group compared with 124 ± 9 bpm in VVIR. Considerable intra- and interpatient variation was seen in ventricular response in rate-adaptive mode. For the patient for whom curves of atrial and ventricular rates in VVIR mode are published, it is obvious that paced rate lagged well behind the sinus rate, taking 4 to 10 minutes to catch up.

Despite the commercial success of the early models of QT-sensing pacemaker, criticisms of the rate response profile of the algorithm showed a significant delay before rate acceleration is initiated, which may result in inappropriate tachycardia after brief episodes of exercise, the peak pacing rate actually occurring during recovery.[62] The initial algorithm employed a linear relationship between stimulus to T interval and pacing rate. However, Baig and colleagues[63] demonstrated a curvilinear relationship, with a lesser degree of QT change at low heart rates, and this relationship was incorporated into subsequent models.

Several clinical studies subsequently compared the performance of the new algorithm. Baig and associates[64] simulated the new algorithm in 10 subjects with implanted or external TX pacemakers using external software. In nine of the subjects, the time taken to achieve maximum pacing rate was significantly reduced, and the maximum rate reached was significantly higher, with the new dynamic algorithm. Comparison with sinus rhythm in the seven subjects with normal chronotropic responses showed a much closer correlation to sinus rate with the newer algorithm. Further work with 11 patients showed that the major difference in function between the two algorithms was a faster initial acceleration in pacing rate with the dynamic algorithm, because of higher values of the slope setting at the lower rate limit.[65] Less rate instability and oscillation was seen with the improved algorithm, but both showed a dip in pacing rate at the onset of exercise.

A multicenter study further investigated the initial response to exercise with the dynamic algorithm.[66] This showed an increased initial response to exercise compared with the linear algorithm, with reduced gain in response time as the upper rate limit is approached, resulting in better rate smoothing at higher heart rates.

Despite the improvements with the dynamic algorithm, the response of the QT-sensing pacemaker is still too slow, probably reflecting the reliance on QT change resulting from relatively slow fluctuations in catecholamine levels with exercise.

VENTRICULAR DEPOLARIZATION GRADIENT

The ventricular depolarization gradient is derived from the integral of the QRS complex and reflects activation sequence and spatial dispersion of activation in the ventricular myocardium. The gradient increases with increasing heart rate but falls with increased catecholamine levels. An intrinsic negative feedback control mechanism maintains a constant depolarization gradient in the healthy heart.[67] The Prism-C1 pacemaker (Telectronics-Cordis, Englewood, CO) uses a closed-loop system for rate-adaptive pacing, maintaining a constant paced ventricular depolarization gradient. Because of physiologic feedback, no response curves or thresholds are necessary. The ventricular depolarization gradient is reviewed in detail in Chapter 15.

The performance of the system in five subjects was examined by Singer and coworkers.[68] Testing involved emotional stress and mental arithmetic, graded treadmill testing (modified Bruce protocol), and Holter monitoring. During treadmill testing, reasonable maximum paced heart rates were achieved (120 to 150 bpm), but rate profile was not described. Similarly, appropriate rate response appeared to be achieved during daily activities by Holter recording. During mental stress, all three patients examined exhibited a rate increase, with considerable intersubject variability. Paul and colleagues[69] reported on the clinical characteristics of the Prism in 10 patients during treadmill, burst and isometric exercise, and mental activity. The time to initial increase in rate was less than 10 seconds for both treadmill and burst maximal activity. Once the pacemaker reached maximum pacing rate, there was a tendency for the rate to decay despite increasing work load. Correlation with P-wave activity in the patients in sinus rhythm was good. Recovery time was longer after burst than treadmill testing. During isometric exercise and mental stress the heart rate response was slower and smaller, with marked variation between patients. Again, correlation between sinus and paced rates during mental activity was good. Heart rate also increased promptly on posture change.

Use of the paced ventricular depolarization gradient for control of rate response is attractive in requiring no time-consuming and potentially inaccurate individual programming of rate response curves and thresholds. Clinically, the device provides prompt rate response with exercise and appropriate reaction to emotional stress.

Techniques Dependent on Thoracic Impedance

RESPIRATORY RATE–DEPENDENT PACING

Ventilatory parameters bear a strong correlation to heart rate and oxygen consumption during exercise.[70, 71] Respiratory rate bears a linear relationship to heart rate, although baseline and slope vary considerably between individuals.[71] Minute volume also correlates very closely, in a linear fashion, with heart rate during vigorous exercise. During brief exercise, however, minute ventilation and tidal volume are closely related to heart rate increases but respiratory rate reflects low-level exercise poorly, even falling at exercise onset.[72] The respiratory sensors are reviewed in detail in Chapter 12. Two types of respiratory sensing pacemakers have been developed: respiratory rate sensing and minute ventilation sensing.

PERFORMANCE OF RESPIRATORY RATE–DEPENDENT PACEMAKERS

Three generations of Biorate pacemaker (Biotech Technologie Biomediche, Bologna, Italy) depend on respiratory rate for heart rate modulation. Respiratory rate is assessed from impedance changes with chest movement in an auxiliary pacing lead tunneled subcutaneously across the upper precordium. Santomauro and coworkers[73] followed up 27 patients with Biorate RDP-3 pacemakers. Three months after implantation, the patients underwent symptom-limited treadmill testing and Holter monitoring to assess response to everyday activities. There was significant prolongation of exercise time (from 8.2 ± 1.5 to 12.8 ± 2 minutes) in rate-adaptive mode but no heart rate response to mental stress. Swinging of the arm ipsilateral to the pacemaker caused a heart rate increase of 30 bpm. This inappropriate response was also noted by Webb and coworkers,[74] who assessed the contribution made by arm movements to the overall rate response in five patients with Biorate RDP-3 pacemakers. The study involved corridor walking at the subject's normal pace with arms swinging or free and a period of hyperventilation. In three patients, hyperventilation and walking both elicited a brisk increase in heart rate. The increase was greater with freely swinging arms (44 ± 5 vs. 26 ± 4 bpm). In the remaining two, neither hyperventilation nor walking with fixed arms caused any significant heart rate response. In these subjects, the accessory impedance sensing lead had not been inserted across the sternum, reducing sensitivity.

The performance of this system in comparison with physiologic AV synchronous pacing was assessed by Rossi and colleagues[75] in nine patients with the initial (RD) model of pulse generator. Physiologic sensitivity of the system was assessed from measurements of oxygen uptake and aerobic threshold rather than by exercise profile. During maximal exercise testing on a modified Bruce-like protocol with 6-minute stages, atrial rate was consistently higher than the paced rate in VVIR mode, although the differences were not statistically significant. Hemodynamic measures of performance were similar.

Rossi and colleagues[76] followed up a large cohort of patients with this pacemaker over 4 years. Assessment again depended on hemodynamic measurements. Ten patients from this group with sick sinus syndrome attained significantly higher peak heart rates during treadmill testing in rate-adaptive mode than in sinus rhythm (131 ± 9 vs. 106 ± 16 bpm). Holter monitoring showed rate increases that appeared appropriate to the perceived exertion, although the point was made that patients' estimation of exercise stresses may not be accurate. Patients with left ventricular dysfunction showed heart rate increases at low exercise levels, which is fitting.

MINUTE VENTILATION–SENSING PACEMAKERS

Transthoracic impedance rises and falls with inspiration and expiration, and amplitude varies with tidal volume. The Meta single- and dual-chamber rate-responsive pacemakers (Telectronics, Englewood, CO) measure minute ventilation using intrathoracic impedance changes related to a sourcing current passed regularly between the pacemaker can and the pacing electrode ring. The response can be altered by programming the respiratory response factor. The recommended

slope number is obtained by telemetry from the pulse generator during maximal exercise, following a period of rest.

Lau and coworkers[77] examined the performance of patients with this system. Optimal settings were chosen for this study according to the manufacturers' directions. During Bruce protocol exercise testing, the duration of exercise was prolonged by 33%, and patients recorded significant improvements in dyspnea and fatigue. No correlation with normal sinus node function was performed. A more thorough evaluation of the clinical rate response characteristics of this model was made by Mond and colleagues[78] in 12 patients in the VVIR pacing mode. Although no correlation with sinus rate was performed, initial heart rate response to exercise appeared brisk and the rise to peak rate depended on the length of exercise and workload. Compared with external Activitrax units, with a medium rate response setting, the minute ventilation device did not accelerate as rapidly as the overresponding Activitrax, which attained peak pacing rate in less than a minute, but reached maximum pacing rate at peak exercise. Pacing rate of the vibration-sensing device returned to baseline within 1 minute of exercise cessation. The Meta MV maintained maximum pacing rate for up to another 2 minutes before rapid return to base rate. Jordaens and associates,[79] however, showed that the heart rate response to exercise in the first minute was small with the Meta, about 6% above the basal rate. Lau and colleagues[80] also compared the Meta MV with an external Activitrax and suggested that minute ventilation sensing improved submaximal exercise capacity; during light and heavy domestic activities the implanted Meta more closely compared with the sinus rate of normal volunteers than did the Activitrax systems. However, there was a delay before initiation of rate response with the Meta systems, and in brief bursts of exercise the maximal pacing rate at times occurred during recovery.

The performance of the algorithm during informal and formal exercise testing was studied by Lau and coworkers.[81] Eleven patients with Meta MV VVIR pacemakers performed symptom-limited treadmill tests and corridor walking, climbed stairs, coughed, and hyperventilated. Exercise duration was 33% longer in VVIR than VVI mode. During brief bursts of exercise, increases in heart rate proportional to the workload were observed, and the greater stress associated with climbing rather than descending stairs was recognized, with a correspondingly higher heart rate during ascent. Pacing rate increased slightly during maneuvers interfering with respiration, such as coughing and hyperventilation, and swinging the ipsilateral arm, and the rate response was attenuated by constant talking.

The Meta MV exercise response may be adjusted to cope with the exercise demands of pediatric patients; changes in paced rate proportional to workload are seen, with rate modulation commencing within the first 30 seconds of exercise.[82] The system is unsuitable for children younger than 6 years of age, as respiratory rates above 60 bpm are not recognized.

Use of respiration sensing for rate modulation in rate-adaptive pacing allows close conformity to physiologic demands of the work performed. The linear association of minute ventilation, and respiratory rate during aerobic respiration, with heart rate is well maintained by these commercially available systems.[76, 83] Unlike activity-sensing pacemakers, the respiratory-driven pacemakers are not insensitive to gradient and physical fitness. Respiration is not the perfect sensor, however; ventilation-dependent pacemakers respond inappropriately to arm movement, and dual-chamber units may track electrocautery and myopotentials.[84] Both respiratory rate and minute ventilation sensing provide equally good correlation with aerobic ventilatory parameters, although the Biorate systems are handicapped by the requirement for an accessory lead and by sensitivity to myopotential inhibition.[85] Rate response has a medium speed, requiring up to 1 minute to commence, and is without the initial over-response and on-off profiles of activity sensors and the severe delay associated with QT sensing.

RIGHT VENTRICULAR STROKE VOLUME AND PREEJECTION INTERVAL

Right ventricular volume may be simply measured by injecting current between electrodes within the cavity. Changes in impedance are related to variation in ventricular blood volume, which carries most of the injected current.[86] A negative feedback control system for rate modulation, maintaining a constant stroke volume by increasing heart rate, has been described.[87] The ventricular impedance sensor is reviewed in detail in Chapter 13.

The Precept DR pacemaker (CPI, St. Paul, MN) utilizes either stroke volumetry or systolic preejection interval measurement for rate modulation.[88] Ten patients with single- or dual-chamber Precept pacemakers performed step tests to determine the optimal rate response slope, performed bicycle ergometry in fixed-rate and rate-adaptive modes, and underwent postural changes.[89] During exercise, the rate response curve appears relatively flat at low workloads, with more rapid rate acceleration at higher exercise workloads. Considerable intrapatient variability in preejection interval with change in posture was noted and, in two patients, resulted in palpitations. The problem could not be resolved by switching to right ventricular volume sensing, and rate response had to be discontinued in these patients. Further experience with this system and further development of the algorithm to cope with postural change are required.

Temperature Sensing

At the initiation of exercise there is an initial fall in temperature as blood is exposed by peripheral vasodilatation to the cold exterior before passing back to the right heart. Thereafter, core temperature increases with exercise because of increasing skeletal muscle heat production with work. The initial dip may be taken as a marker of exercise onset but is blunted by repeated exercise without adequate intervening rest. Following exercise, temperature slowly returns to baseline.[90] The temperature sensor is reviewed in detail in Chapter 10.

Temperature sensing is incorporated as the rate sensor in the Nova MR pacemaker (Intermedics Inc., Angleton, TX), sensing right ventricular temperature with a thermistor placed distally on the pacing electrode. The clinical performance of the rate-adaptive algorithm, including comparison with an external Activitrax, was investigated by Alt and colleagues.[91] The Activitrax was programmed to achieve a high rate increase with high sensitivity and the Nova with an average slope and sensitivity. Compared with fixed-rate pacing, exercise capacity on bicycle ergometry was improved by 36% with temperature-directed rate modulation and heart rate increase to 118 ± 20 bpm, compared with 6% increase in exercise capacity and 98 ± 19 bpm heart rate using activity sensing. This discrepancy with the usual well-documented performance of the Activitrax, with its tendency to overresponse, is due to the inappropriate use of the static bicycle as exercise mode; results may have been much more comparable with an exercise treadmill. Comparison of rate profiles showed that the majority of rate modulation occurred early in the exercise period with the Activitrax, but with the Nova MR there was a delay before heart rate rose significantly and rate increase was still occurring as the subject became exhausted. Highly inappropriate rate profiles in patients with heart failure were subsequently demonstrated by Baig and Perrins,[92] and the Nova MR was eventually abandoned.

Another model of rate-adaptive pacemaker employing temperature sensing, the Kelvin 500 (Cook Pacemakers Corporation, Leechburg, PA), was assessed by Fearnot and Evans.[93] A proportion of the patients studied had normal sinus node function, allowing comparison between the rate profiles of pacemaker and sinus node. The subjects performed symptom-limited Bruce treadmill tests, and a close correlation with the sinus response was achieved (correlation coefficient 0.92) during exercise and recovery. The mean time to onset of rate adaptation was 16 seconds. In a larger multicenter study of 45 patients receiving this system, response time compared well with previous findings at 22 ± 19 seconds.[94]

Temperature sensing acts as a medium-speed physiologic sensor with reasonable correlation to physical stress. Problems may arise in patients with congestive cardiac failure because of a prolonged temperature fall at exercise initiation,[95] and although the sensor responds to nonexercise physiologic change such as fever, it may be confounded by unexpected physical changes, such as occur in a hot bath.

Oxygen Saturation Sensing

At the onset of physical exercise, the rate of oxygen extraction from the peripheral blood rapidly increases, and the oxygen saturation of the venous blood returning to the right heart falls. This discrepancy is related to the level of activity and can be detected by an optical sensor mounted on a pacing electrode and hence utilized for the detection of physical stress for rate-adaptive pacing.[96] Variation throughout the cardiac cycle is overcome by coordinating sampling with the pacemaker spike. Such a system is at risk for erroneous sensing because of sensor drift and overgrowth.[97] The oxygen saturation sensor is reviewed in detail in Chapter 9.

Early experience with the use of a mixed venous oxygen saturation sensing system was reported by Stangl and colleagues[98] in only two patients with modified pacemakers (Siemens Pacesetter, Sylmar, CA). The system responded promptly to exercise on both bicycle and treadmill, with 10% of the total gain in heart rate achieved within 6 to 17 seconds. Heart rate increased linearly in relation to workload. The rate decay during recovery depended on the previous workload because of hemodynamic feedback. Longer-term follow-up (average, 15 months) of 14 patients showed appropriate rate adaptation during formal and informal exercise with a mean peak heart rate of 116 bpm, and no sensor dysfunction was detected.[99]

Mixed venous oxygen saturation sensing potentially offers a highly physiologic system, with potential for rapid response to physical activity and nonphysiologic stress and good correlation with workload. However, the need for a specialized sensor threatens potential chronic problems with drift and sensor overgrowth, and further study is required.

Right Ventricular dP/dt

Changes in right ventricular contractility caused by preload and afterload and the inotropic state of the heart are reflected in changes in right ventricular dP/dt, and significant changes occur secondary to both exercise and emotional stress. Hence, dP/dt max has been evaluated as a sensor for rate-adaptive pacing. The right ventricular dP/dt sensor is reviewed in detail in Chapter 11.

Twelve patients with an implanted investigational pacemaker (model 2503, Medtronic, Inc., Minneapolis, MN) and pressure-sensing right ventricular electrode (Medtronic model 6220), and five with an external rate adaptive device, were investigated by Bennett and associates.[100] A linear relationship between heart rate and dP/dt max was programmed, with a basal rate of 70 bpm, to achieve 130 bpm at submaximal exercise. Mean heart rate for all patients undergoing incremental treadmill exercise testing in VVIR mode rose from 71 ± 11 to 115 ± 24 bpm. There was no significant rate change during Valsalva or tilt-table studies, and Holter monitoring showed appropriate rate fluctuation throughout the day. In the patients with the external devices, peak atrial rate was higher than the peak pacing rate at peak exercise (140 ± 35 vs. 119 ± 13 bpm). Ovsyshcher and colleagues[101] examined the same unit, with the slope adjusted to give a heart rate increase of 20 to 30 bpm after a short walk, implanted in 10 patients. Subjective evaluation by the patients showed symptomatic improvement in VVIR mode, improving New York Heart Association (NYHA) class from 2.7 ± 0.78 to 1.3 ± 0.45. Holter recording detected rate increases during periods of emotional upset. "Adequate" heart rate response to exercise was noted, with a decay time in recovery of 5 to 6 minutes.

At this early stage of development and with the available published data, it is impossible to say more than that the dP/dt sensor probably provides an adequate and physiologic response to exercise. Because of the need for a specialized lead, the system runs the risk of chronic sensor malfunction.

Sensors: Limitations and the Future in Combination

The ideal sensor has not yet been developed; all currently have limitations in optimizing exercise performance, and none comes close to simulating normal sinus node function. For patients with normal chronotropic function, the best rate modulation is achieved by tracking the P wave. Activity sensors cause overresponse to stair descent, external vibrations, and at the initiation of exercise and are insensitive to gradient changes and non–motion-related stresses. QT and minute ventilation physiologic systems respond too slowly to rapid bursts of exertion or emotion, and the lag produces paradoxical maximal pacing during recovery. The paced ventricular depolarization gradient responds rapidly to exertion, but suffers rate decay later in exercise, and is beset by technical charge balancing, threshold, and capture problems. Temperature sensing, although prompt, can be confounded by the presence of heart failure and environmental change. Other sensors have not been widely studied.

Sulke and coworkers[102] published a comparison of the normal sinus node with seven types of rate-responsive pacemaker during day-to-day activities. Thirty-three patients had received rate-adaptive pacemakers, including the Sensolog, Meta, Activitrax, and TX II. Twenty-six patients had dual-chamber systems, including the Medico Phymos VDD, and DDD and activity-sensing DDDR units. Patients were compared with 20 normal control subjects 23 to 76 years of age. Optimal rate programming was attained in all rate-adaptive units according to the manufacturers' instructions. Assessment included CAEP treadmill tests, posture change, mental arithmetic, suitcase lifting, corridor walking, and stair ascent and descent (Figs. 24–4 and 24–5). During treadmill testing, the activity-sensing systems and Meta overresponded early

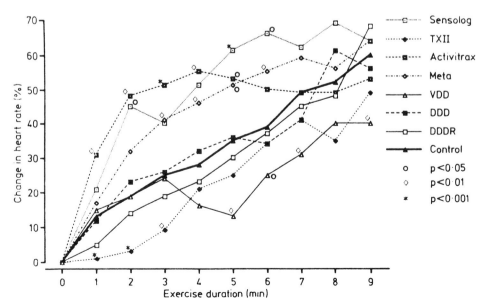

FIGURE 24–4. Comparison by the graded exercise treadmill test of seven different types of rate-responsive pacemakers. (From Sulke AN, Pipilis A, Henderson RA, et al: Comparison of the normal sinus node with seven types of rate-responsive pacemaker during everyday activity. Br Heart J 64:25, 1990.)

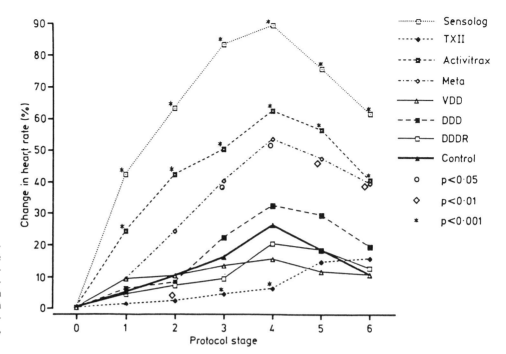

FIGURE 24–5. Effects of walking acceleration and deceleration on heart rate with seven different types of rate-responsive pacemakers. (From Sulke AN, Pipilis A, Henderson RA, et al: Comparison of the normal sinus node with seven types of rate-responsive pacemaker during everyday activity. Br Heart J 64:25, 1990.)

in exercise, but all systems simulated sinus function well at the later stages. In recovery, all systems imitated the sinus node well except the TX, in which rate decay was delayed. The Activitrax, Meta, and TX responded poorly to posture changes. DDD pacemakers responded normally to mental stress; DDDR, VDD, and TX pacemakers responded slowly; and the rest showed no change. During corridor walking, only the P-wave tracking systems responded appropriately to changes in walking speed. On staircase ascent, Meta and TX pacemakers responded with a significant lag in response, and the activity-sensing systems overresponded during descent. This extensive and thorough study concluded that all rate-adaptive systems respond appropriately to exercise but that simulation of the normal chronotropic response curve is poor.

The physiologic failings of individual sensors and associated algorithms might be overcome in part by combining sensors to take advantage of the best features and overcome the disadvantages of each.

A system incorporating activity and QT sensing was described by Landman and coworkers.[103] Patients with an implanted QT-sensing pacemaker were exercised on a treadmill, with an external Activitrax in situ. The patients were stressed during activity sensing, QT sensing, and combination sensing modes in random order. With combination sensing, the paced rate followed a pattern similar to the sinus rate, with the main rate increase over the first 2 minutes of exercise, followed by a more limited rate response over the remainder of exercise. The Topaz model 515 pacemaker (Vitatron Medical B.V., Dieren, The Netherlands) combines QT and activity sensing in a single-chamber pacemaker. The pacemaker can be programmed to receive equal contributions from each sensor or predominantly activity or QT. The response of this model to exercise was studied in 10 patients.[104] Patients performed a CAEP treadmill test with equal activity and QT sensing, and this was repeated in 3 weeks if rate response was unsatisfactory. In seven patients this configuration was acceptable, with a 33% rise in heart rate by 1 minute and 78% gain by peak

exercise. Analysis of rate modulation early and late in exercise suggested that the activity sensor contributed most in the first 3 minutes of exercise, and the QT sensor in the later stages. Cross checking between the sensors obliterated the usual (and desirable) heart rate increase secondary to mental stress seen with the QT sensor.

Other combinations of sensors for rate-adaptive pacing have been described and tested in animals and volunteers but have not so far been utilized in commercial devices.[105, 106] A dual-sensor unit employing complementary physiologic and mechanical parameters would enhance pacing. However, the use of such systems may be complicated by size, cost, and power consumption.

DDDR PACING—THE ULTIMATE STRATEGY?

Technologic evolution has led to the introduction of dual-chamber rate-responsive pacing. In theory these devices should prove advantageous to patients with regular atrial activity but abnormal chronotropism by combining the benefits of AV synchrony with those of rate adaptation. In addition, in patients in whom full atrial tracking may not be desirable, these units permit the use of DDI or DVI pacing with rate response, maintaining AV synchrony but avoiding tracking of pathologic atrial rates.

Reviewing a population of patients with long-term DDD pacemakers, Leman and coworkers[107] exercised 20 patients, 15 of whom had been paced for AV block and 5 of whom had sick sinus syndrome. Patients performed a treadmill exercise test, wearing an activity-sensing pacemaker strapped to their chests. Heart rate achieved by the subject was compared with what would have been generated by the pacemaker. Seven of the patients had a lower triggered ventricular rate during exercise than was achieved by the rate-adaptive pacemaker. Only one of these patients had been previously identified as suffering from sinus node disease. In this study, the absence of data about sinus node function in patients in both groups before original pacemaker implantation makes prediction of potential beneficiaries from additional rate modulation difficult. However, there is evidence that a significant number of patients with implanted DDD units might achieve higher heart rates during exercise with a rate-adaptive unit.

Dual-chamber rate adaptive pacing is associated with increased cardiac efficiency.[108] Vogt and colleagues[109] compared activity-sensing VVIR and DDDR pacing in a small number of patients. Exercise capacity was assessed in each mode using bicycle ergometry. Although the general trend was in favor of DDDR mode, there were no significant differences in heart rate increase, exercise duration, respiratory rate, oxygen consumption, and rate-pressure product. Overall efficiency was slightly improved by DDDR pacing. Only three of the seven subjects found the challenge easier in DDDR than in VVIR mode, using a Borg symptoms scoring method. Unfortunately, this study is handicapped by its small number of subjects and the use of bicycle ergometry, a suboptimal exercise mode for the assessment of piezoelectric vibration-sensing pacemakers. Jutzy and coworkers[110] studied a larger number of patients (14) with DDDR pacemakers and chronotropic incompetence and showed that despite significant increases in hemodynamics in DDDR over VVIR and DDD modes, CAEP treadmill exercise duration was prolonged by only 10% and 4%, respectively. The authors claim an improvement in patients' subjective feelings of well-being in DDDR mode, but no details of the time spent in each mode or the method of symptomatic assessment are provided.

Sulke and colleagues[111] thoroughly compared four rate-responsive pacing modes (DDDR, VVIR, DDD, DDIR), both subjectively and objectively, in a randomized double-blind crossover study of 22 patients with activity sensing rate-adaptive dual-chamber pacemakers (14 Pacesetter Synchrony, 8 Siemens Multilog). All subjects had received pacemakers for AV block and chronotropic incompetence. Rate response slopes were not altered during the study. Patients spent 4 weeks in each mode and, at the completion of each stage, performed a series of tests, including treadmill exercise testing using the CAEP protocol,[112] postural changes, mental arithmetic, suitcase lifting, and staircase ascent and descent. The patients' well-being was assessed using a visual analog scale and specific symptoms scoring. During exercise testing, there was no significant difference in exercise tolerance between VVIR, DDIR, and DDD modes, but tolerance was significantly prolonged during DDDR pacing. During mental stress, heart rate increase was predictably greatest in the modes with atrial tracking preserved (i.e., DDD and DDDR). During all other tests, excluding staircase descent, no significant difference between modes was seen. High thoracic vibration during staircase descent caused initial overresponse in all rate-adaptive modes compared to DDD pacing. The DDDR mode was preferred by 59% of patients, and VVIR was least favored. Five subjects requested early termination of the VVIR limb because of pacemaker syndrome. The preference for DDDR mode was associated with greater increases in stroke volume when paced in DDD rather than VVI mode at baseline (Fig. 24–6). Overall, this study provides convincing evidence of the superiority of DDDR pacing both objectively and subjectively, during everyday life and during formal exercise testing, for patients with chronotropic incompetence requiring a pacemaker. These results are condensed in Table 24–4.

IS ACCURATE RATE PROGRAMMING NECESSARY?

The rate response slopes of pacemakers evaluated in these comparative studies of pacing modes have been appropriately programmed according to manufacturers' instructions to achieve the optimal exercise response, and heart rate decline at rest, for each system. This does not reflect everyday life in

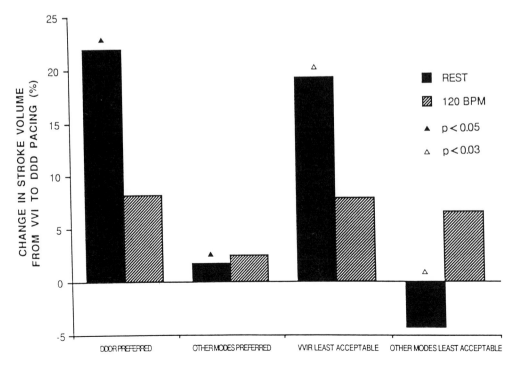

FIGURE 24–6. Changes in stroke volume as a predictor of pacing mode preference. The patients preferring the DDDR pacing mode or finding the VVIR pacing mode the least acceptable have significantly greater increases in stroke volume when paced in a dual-chamber mode than when paced in the VVI mode (at rest). (From Sulke AN, Chambers J, Dritsas A, et al: A randomised double-blind cross-over comparison of four rate-responsive pacing modes. J Am Coll Cardiol 17:696, 1991. Reprinted with permission from the American College of Cardiology.)

TABLE 24–4. **TRIALS OF DUAL-CHAMBER VERSUS VENTRICULAR RATE-ADAPTIVE PACING**

AUTHOR(S)	NUMBER OF PATIENTS	SENSOR	EXERCISE MODE	IMPROVEMENT (%)
Vogt et al.[109]	7	Activity	Bicycle	NS
Jutzy et al.[110]	14	Activity	Treadmill	NS
Sulke et al.[111]	22	Activity	Treadmill	11

Abbreviation: NS, not significant.

the pacemaker clinic, in which many of the pacemakers are found left in the manufacturer's factory settings. This may in part reflect the fact that these settings represent a reasonable average, but it also reflects lack of time and inclination to tailor the pacing response to an individual patient's need. McAlister and associates[42] showed that multiple exercise tests may be required to define the slope setting that most closely approximates sinus rhythm, although the hemodynamic advantages of such fine adjustment are not proved. Does fine-tuning make a difference?

Sulke and coworkers[113] investigated the results of under- and overprogramming activity-sensing DDDR and VVIR units. VVI pacing in pacemaker-dependent patients and DDD pacing in patients with an abnormal chronotropic response were compared to VVIR and DDDR with appropriate rate acceleration and to DDDR and VVIR programmed to overrespond with maximal slope settings. Objective treadmill exercise testing showed underachievement only in the group with fixed-rate ventricular pacing. However, overresponse was generally symptomatically least acceptable, with 33% to 50% of patients requesting early crossover from that phase of the study. All but one patient chose appropriate programming as the preferred mode of pacing. Despite improvements in exercise capacity, overresponsive programming of rate-adaptive pacemakers appears even less acceptable to patients than fixed-rate pacing, making the extra investment required for rate-adaptive pacing a waste of time and money.

A similar comparison was made using minute ventilation–sensing rate-adaptive pacemakers (Meta MV, Telectronics Cordis).[114] Subjects performed three exercise tests: one with fixed rate and one with a high and finally one with an average rate response factor. Slight changes in slope programming could change submaximal heart rate responses to normal chronotropic function, causing a significant improvement in exercise capacity, suggesting that appropriate individualized programming of slope is desirable.

RATE-ADAPTIVE ATRIOVENTRICULAR DELAY

In normal subjects, AV conduction is accelerated by exercise stress. There is a linear relationship between heart rate and AV interval,[115] and there may be a short latent phase at the beginning of exercise without alteration in the AV interval before acceleration of AV conduction occurs.[116] During cardiac pacing, a short AV interval is associated with a reduced cardiac output,[117] and maximal cardiac performance is obtained with intrinsic AV conduction in patients with dual-chamber pacemakers.[118] "Overstimulation" pacing at greater than physiologic heart rates is associated with paradoxical lengthening of the AV delay.[119] In cardiac pacing, rate modulation of the AV delay should improve cardiac function, and there is much convincing evidence of the hemodynamic ben-

efits of rate modulation.[120–122] However, there is little evidence of the clinical benefits of optimizing AV delay for heart rate.

Clinical advantages of a "normal" AV delay over a shortened interval were demonstrated by Landzberg and colleagues.[123] Twelve patients with normal sinoatrial function and dual-chamber pacemakers performed Balke exercise treadmill tests with pacemakers programmed to a normal AV delay of 150 msec or to the minimum possible (0 to 75 msec). Ten subjects exercised for longer with the physiologic AV interval and two with the short AV delay. Exercise time was increased by an average of 16%. Rydén and coworkers[124] investigated exercise capacity in patients with dual-chamber pacemakers. The subjects performed bicycle stress tests with pacemakers programmed to AV intervals of 50, 100, 150, and 200 msec. There was no significant difference in exercise duration at various AV intervals, nor were there differences between the levels of perceived exertion, using a Borg symptoms scale. Haskell and French[125] compared the effects of ventricular inhibited pacing to physiologic pacing with a short (66 msec) or a long (168 msec) AV delay. Although physiologic pacing was superior to ventricular pacing, there was no significant difference between the peak workloads achieved at bicycle ergometry at the two AV intervals.

Patients with dilated cardiomyopathies may benefit from pacing with a short AV delay, even in the absence of conventional indications for pacing, by reducing the time available for mitral regurgitation occurring before ventricular systole. Brecker and coworkers[126] demonstrated an increase in exercise duration by 33% in 12 patients with poor ventricular function physiologically paced with an AV delay of 6 to 31 msec.

Many DDDR pacemakers incorporate a rate-adaptive AV delay algorithm capable of approximating the normal physiologic response to exercise.[127, 128] The effects on exercise capacity and subjective well-being of AV delay rate modulation was assessed by Sulke and colleagues.[129] Ten patients with Pacesetter 2020T Synchrony or Siemens P51T Multilog pacemakers spent 2 weeks in each of three fixed AV delays (125, 175, and 250 msec) and in rate-responsive AV delay mode. After each study period, a symptoms questionnaire was completed and treadmill exercising performed. One patient had to be excluded because of pacemaker-mediated endless-loop tachycardia when her pacemaker was programmed to the longest fixed AV delay. Subjective well-being was significantly better with a rate-responsive AV delay or a fixed AV interval of 125 msec than at the longest AV delay. However, there was no significant variation in exercise capacity at any AV setting.

Although evidence of clinical advantages of rate modulation of the paced AV delay is sparse, the hemodynamic advantages suggest that these algorithms should prove a useful adjunct to dual-chamber rate-responsive pacing during everyday activity.

Problems With Exercise Testing and Choice of Test

For the results of investigation of clinical performance of pacemaker systems and pacing modes to be understood and validated, manufacturers and investigators employ standardized exercise testing, using protocols familiar to a wide audience. Bruce, Naughton, Balke, and CAEP protocols and bicycle ergometry are widely used, and the readership comprehend differences in exercise performance using such regimens. Furthermore, effort tolerance on treadmill and bicycle correlates well with the physician's assessment of functional class.[130, 131] The test selected to examine the properties of various systems must be chosen with care to highlight the benefits of the system under review but without causing unreasonable disadvantage to the comparator. Unfair comparison risks excessive skepticism about the study results.

For example, investigation of fixed crystal vibration-sensing rate-adaptive pacemakers may be severely affected by choice of testing. The limitations of the Activitrax system, with a tendency to on-off pacing with rapid initial overresponse, have been well documented. The sensor depends on thoracic vibrations; hence exercise in which the upper body is fixed blunts response and obscures the behavior of the system in day-to-day life. Lau and coworkers[41] compared the exercise performance of patients with this model of pacemaker on the treadmill and exercise bicycle. During treadmill exercise, pacing and sinus rates were similar, but during bicycle ergometry pacing rate lagged behind sinus rate. Matula and colleagues[132] showed that bicycling under street conditions, with body sway and road vibration, corresponded more closely to intrinsic rate than did stationary bicycle ergometry.

Small interpatient idiosyncrasies in treadmill technique may affect results. Grasping the treadmill rails, as some subjects prefer for security, tends to restrict upper body movement and may affect rate modulation. During a comparison of QT- and activity-sensing pacemakers, a greater rate response was seen in some subjects in activity-sensing mode during a brief corridor walk for slope setting than during vigorous treadmill exercise, and this was judged to be due to greater arm swinging during free walking.[45]

Clinical exercise capacity may be affected by variables other than the efficiency of the pacing system under review. Particularly in the elderly, stress testing limited by symptoms may well be affected by additional factors such as intercurrent disability, making exercise level and duration potentially unreliable end points. During Holter monitoring of daily activity, the patient's diary is an imperfect guide to the stress of the tasks undertaken. It is for these reasons that many studies perform objective hemodynamic measurements, although the relevance of these to practical application can be argued.

Clinical comparison of pacing system and mode is an imperfect art. Apart from the activity-sensing pacemakers, devices are generally unsuitable for external assessment. Many studies employ external activity devices because of

this convenience. Doubts have been expressed regarding the comparability of these with an implanted system. However, Zarling and colleagues[133] have demonstrated a high correlation between the rate responses of implanted and external accelerometer-based units. Intrapatient comparisons are widely made because of multiprogrammable units, and this allows some objectivity, although the effects of training during multiple stress tests should be remembered. The desire for comparison of rate response profiles with normal sinus node function causes study design problems. The relevance of comparing the performance of normal (often unmatched for age and usually unmatched for cardiac disease) volunteers' sinus nodes with the performance of pacemaker patients is disputable, and comparison with intrinsic atrial rates may be affected by the possibility of undetected sinus impairment in the pacemaker population.

Study of sensors is also affected by algorithm performance. This is illustrated by the history of the QT pacemaker, with significant improvement in rate response profile with the updated algorithm employing the curvilinear rather than linear relationship. A sensor is only as effective as the algorithm mediating its responses.

QUALITY-OF-LIFE ASSESSMENT

Assessment of new therapies should not be limited to biomedical measures but should include effects on the quality of life of the patients, encompassing productivity, everyday function, social and sexual factors, emotional stability, and intellectual capability. Despite the wealth of evidence of prolongation of life, hemodynamic improvement, and augmentation of exercise capacity, relatively little investigation of the subjective benefits of pacemaker implantation has been performed. Many of the studies of pacemaker mode try to assess the patients' individual benefits from improved technology, but there is little standardization of approach. Many centers employ in-house questionnaires of variable complexity, and the results of comparison are often badly reported as an overall subjective improvement. Some homogeneity is achieved in the use of NYHA and Borg symptom scores,[134, 135] which at least allow some substantiation of patients' responses. In addition, it can be difficult to separate out the effects of the intensive follow-up with frequent personalized attention that the subjects of these studies receive.

Even in the early days of cardiac pacing, before the introduction of multiprogrammable physiologic and rate-adaptive units, there was a high degree of acceptability associated with pacemakers. In a study of 60 patients, 80% showed pacemaker acceptance and had increased their activities within 6 months of implantation.[136] The authors concluded that most patients gained a "rejuvenating lease on life." Hervé and colleagues[137] showed that this contentment was, however, accompanied by a reduction in activities in 70% of 361 patients questioned.

More recently, Mickley and coworkers[138] attempted to assess the subjective consequences of permanent pacemaker therapy in 81 preretirement patients. A semistructured questionnaire was completed by 98.6% of the subjects approached. Improvement or relief from prepacing symptoms were reported by 93%; this was particularly noted in those with preceding syncope or dizziness. Only 11% expressed anxiety about being a pacemaker carrier. Most patients suffered no discomfort from the pacemaker, but 24% complained of mechanical discomfort from the pulse generator, awareness of pacing impulses, or nonspecific worries about external interference from machinery or the presence of an internal foreign body. Only 8% of patients described a deterioration in their sexual life, although 15% failed to answer the question. Eighty-five percent felt that the implantation of their pacemaker had improved or at least not harmed the quality of their life. It is interesting that only one subject was said to complain of unease related to pacemaker syndrome.

Catipovic-Veselica and coworkers[139] followed up an unselected sample of 80 patients with indwelling pacemakers over 1 to 4 years. Perceived quality of life was assessed using the Emotions Profile Index compiled by Plutchik to measure the strengths of eight basic emotions (protection, destruction, rejection, incorporation, deprivation, reproduction, exploration, orientation). This involves a 62-item forced-choice test with 12 emotional trait terms deployed in all possible combinations (e.g., ''Are you more shy or gloomy?''). The majority of subjects were in NYHA functional class II, free from health worries, leading unrestricted lives, and considered themselves as capable and clever as their peers. Most had failed to return to work after pacemaker implantation, but this was felt to reflect local conditions in Yugoslavia at the time, where income was the same for workers and nonworkers alike.

Little has been published concentrating specifically on lifestyle in various pacing modes. Most quality-of-life information is obtained as a rider to studies of objective clinical performance. Lau and coworkers[140] reported a nonsignificant improvement in quality of life with rate-adaptive pacing using the non–disease-specific Nottingham Health Profile. Oto and colleagues[141] compared fixed-rate pacing and rate modulation in only 11 patients with Meta MV pacemakers. A questionnaire derived in Turkey, the Halcettepe Quality-of-Life Questionnaire, was employed; this consists of 43 questions relating to general aspects of work, health, sleep, and sexual function. Quality-of-life scores were significantly higher in rate-adaptive mode, with improvement in general well-being, activity, and work, sleep, and sexual function.

The results of these studies show that pacemaker implantation is a well-tolerated procedure associated with positive improvements in lifestyle, with few emotional and psychosocial penalties. Comparison of studies is impossible because of the use of diverse methods of assessing quality of life. Many questionnaires are nonspecific for cardiac disease and may therefore lack sensitivity, and questionnaires of obscure local origin are unvalidated.

INFORMAL EXERCISE TESTING

Many pacemaker patients cannot manage conventional treadmill testing or bicycle ergometry because of age or intercurrent disability. In this situation, simple informal walking and stepping tests may be substituted. Treadmill and bicycle ergometry require complicated equipment in dedicated spaces and are relatively time consuming. Informal testing is convenient and less expensive than formal exercise testing and, if the subject's daily activity is more closely simulated, is more relevant.

Langenfeld and coworkers[142] assessed a simple 6-minute walk previously described in patients with pulmonary dis-

ease. Walking speed was determined by the subject, and lower performance and dyspnea scores, and exercise heart rates showed the tests to be submaximal. In elderly patients, the walk was preferred to other forms of exercise testing, results correlated well with those of both treadmill and bicycle testing, and the test probably reproduced daily activities more appropriately than formal exercise protocols. However, in younger patients, the exercise level achieved was criticized as too easy, and differences in performance appeared between the walk and conventional testing. In this subgroup, a maximal test may be preferable.

Lau and colleagues[24] compared standard Bruce exercise protocols with simple submaximal exercise testing in the comparison of fixed-rate with rate-adaptive ventricular pacing. The informal testing involved simple ascent and descent of four flights of stairs. The authors concluded that formal maximal studies are probably unnecessary in clinical practice and that the simple tests adequately assessed rate response and slope setting for everyday activities. In addition, functional algorithm and sensor problems, such as the delayed response of the QT-sensing pacemakers, and inability of activity-sensing pacemakers to distinguish the differing stresses associated with ascent and descent of stairs were appropriately highlighted.

An exercise protocol for use in the office with restricted space and no exercise machinery for the programming of activity-sensing pacemakers was investigated by Benditt and coworkers.[143] They demonstrated that walking-on-the-spot and arm exercise produced consistent results that underestimated, but bore a constant relationship to, steady-state treadmill exercise. Hence, pacing rate during simple activities predicted pacing responses during exercise and could be used for selection of pacemaker settings.

Standardization of informal exercise testing would encourage uptake in busy clinics and probably reduce the usage of manufacturers' settings in implanted rate-adaptive pacemakers. A method of standardization has been described by Hayes and associates.[144] Four age groups of volunteers between 20 and more than 70 years old without conduction system disease were tested with metronome-guided casual and brisk walks to determine the expected heart response for these levels of exercise. There were no significant differences between resting, casual, and brisk heart rates in the four groups. In the elderly, although increased exercise levels require greater metabolic reserves, this is not reflected by higher heart rates due to diminished heart rate response with increasing age. The authors suggest that rate modulation should be set in rate-adaptive units to achieve a heart rate of 85 to 100 bpm for casual exercise, and 100 to 110 bpm for brisk walking in patients with good ventricular function.

The elderly are a relatively difficult group to assess, and traditionally there has been a tendency to deprive them of rate-adaptive pacing in favor of fixed-rate units because of their relative immobility. In addition, traditional assessments of maximal exercise capacity and effects on hemodynamics are irrelevant to their requirements. This subset may be assessed using tailored exercise protocols reflecting normal activities, such as rising from a chair 30 times and walking on a flat surface and up stairs at slow and brisk rates. Gamage and colleagues[145] employed time taken to achieve these tasks with a Borg scale symptom score to compare fixed-rate with single-setting rate-responsive ventricular pacing in 12 post-retirement patients with Activitrax pulse generators. They demonstrated small but statistically significant reductions in times taken to perform all tasks except slow corridor walking. The subjects were significantly less breathless and symptomatic overall. Hence, even elderly patients appear to benefit from rate-adaptive pacing and should not be excluded on the grounds of age or complexity of follow-up. Benefits accrued may be assessed despite inability to perform standard exercise tests.

Conclusions

The results of many small studies have been reviewed in this chapter. Most studies have shown some benefits for the particular mode or sensor being evaluated, but observer bias, small numbers, and lack of randomization limit the usefulness of these studies. The clinical benefits offered by dual-chamber and rate-adaptive pacemakers compared with fixed-rate ventricular pacemakers are no longer in doubt, but the magnitude and exact clinical relevance of some of these advantages are unclear. There is an urgent need for large prospective cooperative multicenter clinical trials in pacing. Until these are done, the impact of sophisticated pacing therapies on long-term morbidity and, particularly, mortality will never be known. Without these data, unsophisticated pacing practices will continue to the ultimate detriment of the patient.

REFERENCES

1. Sheffield LT, Maloof JA, Sawyer JA, et al: Maximal heart rate and treadmill performance of healthy women in relation to age. Circulation 57:79, 1978.
2. Astrand I: Aerobic exercise capacity in men and women with special reference to age. Acta Physiol Scand [Suppl] 169:49, 1960.
3. Sowton E: Haemodynamic studies in patients with artificial pacemakers. Br Heart J 26:737, 1964.
4. Sowton E: Exercise testing in the indication and evaluation of pacemaker treatment. Eur Heart J 8(Suppl D):155, 1987.
5. Epstein SE, Beiser GD, Stampfer M, et al: Characterisation of the circulatory response to maximal upright exercise in normal subjects and patients with heart disease. Circulation 35:1049, 1967.
6. Karlöf I: Haemodynamic effect of atrial triggered versus fixed rate pacing at rest and during exercise in complete heart block. Acta Med Scand 197:195, 1975.
7. Gesell RA: Auricular systole and its relation to ventricular output. Am J Physiol 29:32, 1911.
8. Kristensson B-E, Arnman K, Rydén L: The haemodynamic importance of atrioventricular synchrony and rate increase at rest and during exercise. Eur Heart J 6:773, 1985.
9. Samet P, Castillo C, Bernstein WH: Hemodynamic consequences of sequential atrioventricular pacing: Subjects with normal hearts. Am J Cardiol 21:207, 1968.
10. Benchimol A, Ellis JG, Dimond EG: Hemodynamic consequences of atrial and ventricular pacing in patients with normal and abnormal hearts: Effects of exercise at fixed atrial and ventricular rate. Am J Med 39:911, 1965.
11. Kruse I, Rydén L: Comparison of physical work capacity and systolic time intervals with ventricular inhibited and atrial synchronous ventricular inhibited pacing. Br Heart J 46:129, 1981.
12. Kruse I, Arnman K, Conradson T-B, et al: A comparison of the acute and long-term haemodynamic effects of ventricular inhibited and atrial synchronous ventricular inhibited pacing. Circulation 65:846, 1982.
13. Fananapazir L, Bennett DH, Monks P: Atrial synchronised ventricular pacing: Contribution of the chronotropic response to improved exercise performance. PACE 6:601, 1983.
14. Perrins EJ, Morley CA, Chan SL, et al: Randomised controlled trial of physiological and ventricular pacing. Br Heart J 50:112, 1983.

15. Sutton R, Perrins EJ, Morley C, et al: Sustained improvement in exercise tolerance following physiological cardiac pacing. Eur Heart J 4:781, 1983.
16. Kristensson B-E, Arnman K, Smedgård P, et al: Physiological versus single-rate ventricular pacing: A double-blind cross-over study. PACE 8:73, 1985.
17. Rediker DE, Eagle KA, Homma S, et al: Clinical and hemodynamic comparison of VVI versus DDD pacing in patients with DDD pacemakers. Am J Cardiol 61:323, 1988.
18. Byrd CL, Schwartz SJ, Gonzales M, et al: DDD pacemakers maximize haemodynamic benefits and minimize complications for most patients. PACE 11:1911, 1988.
19. Færestrand S, Breivik K, Ohm O-J: Assessment of the work capacity and relationship between rate response and exercise tolerance associated with activity-sensing rate-responsive ventricular pacing. PACE 10:1277, 1987.
20. Benditt DG, Milstein S, Buetikofer J, et al: Sensor-triggered rate-variable cardiac pacing: Current technologies and clinical implications. Ann Intern Med 107:714, 1987.
21. Benditt DG, Mianulli M, Fetter J, et al: Single-chamber cardiac pacing with activity-initiated chronotropic response: Evaluation by cardiopulmonary testing. Circulation 75:184, 1987.
22. Smedgård P, Kristensson B-E, Kruse I, et al: Rate-responsive pacing by means of activity sensing versus single rate ventricular pacing: A double-blind cross-over study. PACE 10:902, 1987.
23. Lindemans FW, Rankin IR, Murtaugh R, et al: Clinical experience with an activity-sensing pacemaker. PACE 9:978, 1986.
24. Lau C-P, Butrous GS, Ward DE, et al: Comparison of exercise performance of six rate adaptive right ventricular cardiac pacemakers. Am J Cardiol 63:833, 1989.
25. Candinas RA, Gloor HO, Amann FW, et al: Activity-sensing rate-responsive versus conventional fixed-rate pacing: A comparison of rate behaviour and patient well-being during routine daily exercise. PACE 14:204, 1991.
26. McGoon MD, Fetter J: Non-invasive conversion of a fixed-rate demand pacemaker to activity mode: A method for assessing the clinical effect of rate-responsiveness. Mayo Clin Proc 62:882, 1987.
27. Humen DP, Kostuk WJ, Klein GJ: Activity-sensing, rate-responsive pacing: Improvement in myocardial performance with exercise. PACE 8:52, 1985.
28. Heinz M, Wörl HH, Alt E, et al: Which patient is most likely to benefit from a rate-responsive pacemaker? PACE 11:1834, 1988.
29. Lau C-P, Wong C-K, Leung W-H, et al: Superior cardiac haemodynamics of atrioventricular synchrony over rate-responsive pacing at submaximal exercise: Observations in activity-sensing DDDR pacemakers. PACE 13:1832, 1990.
30. Markewitz A, Hemmer W: What's the price to be paid for rate response: AV sequential versus ventricular pacing? PACE 14:1782, 1991.
31. Oldroyd KG, Rae AP, Carter R, et al: Double-blind cross-over comparison of dual-chamber pacing (DDD) and ventricular rate-adaptive (VVIR) pacing on neuroendocrine variables, exercise performance, and symptoms in complete heart block. Br Heart J 65:188, 1991.
32. Linde-Edelstam C, Nordlander R, Pehrsson SK, et al: A double-blind study of submaximal exercise tolerance and variation in paced rate in atrial synchronous compared to activity sensor modulated ventricular pacing. PACE 15:905, 1992.
33. Batey RL, Sweesy MW, Scala G, et al: Comparison of low rate dual-chamber pacing to activity-responsive rate-variable ventricular pacing. PACE 13:646, 1990.
34. Ausubel K, Steingart RM, Shimshi M, et al: Maintenance of exercise stroke volume during ventricular versus atrial synchronous pacing: Role of contractility. Circulation 72:1037, 1985.
35. Menozzi C, Brignole M, Moracchini PV, et al: Intrapatient comparison between chronic VVIR and DDD pacing in patients affected by high-degree AV block without heart failure. PACE 13:1816, 1990.
36. Leitch JW, Arnold JM, Klein GJ, et al: Should a VVIR pacemaker increase the heart rate with standing? PACE 15:288, 1992.
37. Schuchert A, Kuck K-H, Bleifeld W: Effects of body constitution and age on maximum pacing rate of activity-modulated rate-responsive pacemakers. PACE 14:1467, 1991.
38. Moura PJ, Gessman LJ, Lai T, et al: Chronotropic response of an activity-detecting pacemaker compared to the normal sinus node. PACE 10:78, 1987.
39. Den Dulk K, Bouwels L, Lindemans F, et al: The Activitrax rate-responsive pacemaker syndrome. Am J Cardiol 61:107, 1988.

40. Lau C-P, Mehta D, Toff WD, et al: Limitations of rate response of an activity-sensing rate-responsive pacemaker to different forms of exercise. PACE 11:141, 1988.

41. Lau C-P, Stott JRR, Toff WD, et al: Selective vibration sensing: A new concept for activity-sensing rate-responsive pacing. PACE 11:1299, 1988.

42. McAlister HF, Soberman J, Klementowicz P, et al: Treadmill assessment of an activity-modulated pacemaker: The importance of individual programming. PACE 12:486, 1989.

43. Mond H, Line P, Hunt D: A third-generation activity pacemaker: Is the rate response algorithm superior? (Abstract.) PACE 13:514, 1990.

44. Bacharach DW, Hilden TS, Millerhagen JO, et al: Activity-based pacing: Comparison of a device using an accelerometer versus a piezo-electric crystal. PACE 15:188, 1992.

45. Bellamy CM, Roberts DH, Hughes S, et al: Comparative evaluation of rate modulation in new-generation evoked QT and activity-sensing pacemakers. PACE 15:993, 1992.

46. Lau C-P, Tse W-S, Camm AJ: Clinical experience with Sensolog 703: A new activity-sensing rate-responsive pacemaker. PACE 11:1444, 1988.

47. Kubisch K, Peters W, Chiladakis I, et al: Clinical experience with the rate-responsive pacemaker Sensolog 703. PACE 11:1829, 1988.

48. Stangl K, Wirtzfeld A, Lochschmidt O, et al: Physical movement sensitive pacing: Comparison of two activity-triggered pacing systems. PACE 12:102, 1989.

49. Johnson SL, Bradding P, Watkins J: A simultaneous noninvasive comparison with sinus rhythm of two activity-sensing rate-adaptive pacemakers in an elderly population. PACE 14:20, 1991.

50. Mahaux V, Waleffe A, Kulbertus HE: Clinical experience with a new activity-sensing rate-modulated pacemaker using autoprogrammability. PACE 12:1362, 1989.

51. Borst U, Siekmeyer G, Maisch B, et al: A new motion-responsive pacemaker: First clinical experience with an acceleration sensor pacemaker. PACE 15:1809, 1992.

52. Erdelitsch-Reiser E, Langenfeld H, Millerhagen J, et al: New concept in activity-controlled pacemakers: Clinical results with an accelerometer-based rate-adaptive pacing system. PACE 15:2245, 1992.

53. Lau C-P, Tai Y-T, Fong P-C, et al: Clinical experience with an activity-sensing DDDR pacemaker using an accelerometer sensor. PACE 15:334, 1992.

54. Bongiorni MG, Soldati E, Arena G: Multicentre clinical evaluation of a new SSIR pacemaker. PACE 15:1798, 1992.

55. Soussou AI, Helmy MG, Guindy RR, et al: A new acceleration-driven pacemaker: Rate modulation versus normal sinus rhythm—comparison during treadmill exercise. PACE 15:1804, 1992.

56. Rickards AF, Norman J: Relation between QT interval and heart rate: New design of physiologically adaptive cardiac pacemaker. Br Heart J 45:56, 1981.

57. Hedman A, Nordlander R: Changes in QT and Q-aT intervals induced by mental and physical stress with fixed-rate and atrial-triggered ventricular-inhibited cardiac pacing. PACE 11:1426, 1988.

58. Donaldson RM, Fox K, Rickards AF: Initial experience with a physiological, rate-responsive pacemaker. Br Med J 286:667, 1983.

59. Hedman A, Nordlander R: QT-sensing rate-responsive pacing compared to fixed-rate ventricular-inhibited pacing: A controlled clinical study. PACE 12:374, 1989.

60. Bloomfield P, Macareavey D, Kerr F, et al: Long-term follow-up of patients with the QT rate-adaptive pacemaker. PACE 12:111, 1989.

61. Fananapazir L, Rademaker M, Bennett DH: Reliability of the evoked response in determining the paced ventricular rate and performance of the QT or rate responsive (TX) pacemaker. PACE 8:701, 1985.

62. Mehta D, Lau C-P, Ward DE, et al: Comparative evaluation of chronotropic responses of QT-sensing and activity-sensing rate-responsive pacemakers. PACE 11:1405, 1988.

63. Baig MW, Boute W, Begemann MJS, et al: Nonlinear relationship between pacing and evoked QT intervals. PACE 11:753, 1988.

64. Baig MW, Wilson J, Boute W, et al: Improved pattern of rate responsiveness with dynamic slope setting for the QT-sensing pacemaker. PACE 12:311, 1989.

65. Baig MW, Green A, Wade G, et al: A randomised double-blind cross-over study of the linear and nonlinear algorithms for the QT-sensing rate-adaptive pacemaker. PACE 13:1802, 1990.

66. Den Heijer P, Nagelkerke D, Perrins EJ, et al: Improved rate-responsive algorithm in QT-driven pacemakers—evaluation of initial response to exercise. PACE 12:805, 1989.

67. Callaghan F, Vollman W, Livingston A, et al: The ventricular depolar-

68. Singer I, Olash J, Brennan F, et al: Initial clinical experience with a rate-responsive pacemaker. PACE 12:1458, 1989.

69. Paul V, Garratt C, Ward DE, et al: Closed-loop control of rate-adaptive pacing: Clinical assessment of a system analyzing the ventricular depolarisation gradient. PACE 12:1896, 1989.

70. McElroy PA, Janicki JS, Weber KT: Physiologic correlates of the heart rate response to upright isotonic exercise: Relevance to rate-responsive pacemakers. J Am Coll Cardiol 11:94, 1988.

71. Rossi P, Plicchi G, Canducci G, et al: Respiration as a reliable sensor for controlling cardiac pacing rate. Br Heart J 51:7, 1984.

72. Vai F, Bonnet JL, Ritter PH, et al: Relationship between heart rate and minute ventilation, tidal volume and respiratory rate during brief and low-level exercise. PACE 11:1860, 1988.

73. Santomauro M, Fazio S, Ferraro S, et al: Follow-up of a respiratory rate modulated pacemaker. PACE 15:17, 1992.

74. Webb SC, Lewis LM, Morris JA, et al: Respiratory-dependent pacing: A dual response from a single sensor. PACE 11:730, 1988.

75. Rossi P, Rognoni G, Occhetta E, et al: Respiration-dependent ventricular pacing compared with fixed ventricular and atrial-ventricular synchronous pacing: Aerobic and haemodynamic variables. J Am Coll Cardiol 6:646, 1985.

76. Rossi P, Prando MD, Magnani A, et al: Physiological sensitivity of respiratory-dependent cardiac pacing: Four-year follow-up. PACE 11:1267, 1988.

77. Lau C-P, Antoniou A, Ward DE, et al: Initial clinical experience with a minute ventilation–sensing rate-modulated pacemaker: Improvements in exercise capacity and symptomatology. PACE 11:1815, 1988.

78. Mond H, Strathmore N, Kertes P, et al: Rate-responsive pacing using a minute ventilation sensor. PACE 11:1866, 1988.

79. Jordaens L, Berghmans L, van Wassenhove E, et al: Behavior of a respiratory-driven pacemaker and direct respiratory measurements. PACE 12:1600, 1989.

80. Lau C-P, Wong C-K, Leung W-H, et al: A comparative evaluation of minute-sensing and activity-sensing adaptive rate pacemakers during daily activities. PACE 12:1514, 1989.

81. Lau C-P, Antoniou A, Ward DE, et al: Reliability of minute ventilation as a parameter for rate-responsive pacing. PACE 12:321, 1989.

82. Yabek SM, Wernly J, Chick TW, et al: Rate-adaptive cardiac pacing in children using a minute ventilation biosensor. PACE 13:2108, 1990.

83. Kay GN, Bubien RS, Epstein AE, et al: Rate-modulated cardiac pacing based on transthoracic impedance measurements of minute ventilation: Correlation with exercise gas exchange. J Am Coll Cardiol 14:1283, 1989.

84. Lau C-P, Tai Y-T, Fong P-C, et al: The use of implantable sensors for the control of pacemaker-mediated tachycardias: A comparative evaluation between minute ventilation sensing and acceleration sensing dual-chamber rate-adaptive pacemakers. PACE 15:34, 1992.

85. Lau C-P, Ward DE, Camm AJ: Single-chamber cardiac pacing with two forms of respiration-controlled rate-responsive pacemaker. Chest 95:352, 1989.

86. Baan J, Jong TT, Kerkof PM, et al: Continuous stroke volume and cardiac output from intraventricular dimensions obtained with an impedance catheter. Cardiovasc Res 15:328, 1981.

87. Salo RW, Pederson BD, Olive AL: Continuous ventricular volume assessment for diagnosis and pacemaker control. PACE 7:1267, 1984.

88. McGoon MD, Shapland JE, Salo RW, et al: The feasibility of utilising the systolic pre-ejection interval as a determinant of pacing rate. J Am Coll Cardiol 14:1753, 1989.

89. Ruiter JH, Heemels JP, Kee D, et al: Adaptive rate pacing controlled by the right ventricular pre-ejection interval: Clinical experience with a physiological pacing system. PACE 15:886, 1992.

90. Sellers TD, Fearnot NE, Smith HJ, et al: Right ventricular blood temperature profiles for rate-responsive pacing. PACE 10:467, 1987.

91. Alt E, Völker R, Högl B, et al: First clinical results with a new temperature-controlled rate-responsive pacemaker: Comparison of Activitrax and Nova MR pacemakers with VVI/AAI pacing. Circulation 78 Suppl:III-116, 1988.

92. Baig MW, Perrins EJ: Anomalies of the temperature profiles and rate response in patients with heart failure and an implanted temperature-sensing pacemaker. Eur JCPE 2:87, 1991.

93. Fearnot NE, Evans ML: Heart rate correlation, response time, and effect of previous exercise using an advanced pacing rate algorithm for temperature-based rate modulation. PACE 11:1846, 1988.

94. Fearnot NE, Smith HJ, Sellers D, et al: Evaluation of the temperature response to exercise testing in patients with single-chamber rate-adaptive pacemakers: A multicentre study. PACE 12:1806, 1989.

95. Shellock FG, Rubin SA, Ellrodt AG, et al: Unusual core temperature decrease in exercising heart failure patients. J Appl Physiol 52:544, 1983.

96. Wirtzfeld A, Heinze R, Liess HD, et al: An active optical sensor for monitoring mixed venous oxygen saturation for an implantable rate-regulating pacing system. PACE 6:494, 1983.

97. Seifert GP, Moore AA, Graves KL, et al: In vivo and in vitro studies of a chronic oxygen saturation sensor. PACE 14:1514, 1991.

98. Stangl K, Wirtzfeld A, Heinze R, et al: First clinical experience with an oxygen saturation controlled pacemaker in man. PACE 11:1882, 1988.

99. Færestrand S, Ohm O-J: Long-term follow-up of a rate-variable pacemaker controlled by central venous oxygen saturation. (Abstract.) J Am Coll Cardiol 17:289A, 1991.

100. Bennett T, Sharma A, Sutton R, et al: Development of a rate-adaptive pacemaker based on the maximum rate-of-rise of right ventricular pressure (RV dP/dt max). PACE 15:219, 1992.

101. Ovsyshcher I, Guetta V, Bondy C, et al: First derivative of right ventricular pressure, dP/dt, as a sensor for a rate-adaptive VVI pacemaker: Initial experience. PACE 15:211, 1992.

102. Sulke AN, Pipilis A, Henderson RA, et al: Comparison of the normal sinus node with seven types of rate-responsive pacemaker during everyday activity. Br Heart J 64:25, 1990.

103. Landman MAJ, Senden PJ, van Rooijen H, et al: Initial clinical experience with rate-adaptive cardiac pacing using two sensors simultaneously. PACE 13:1615, 1990.

104. Provenier F, Van Acker R, Backers J, et al: Clinical observations with a dual-sensor rate-adaptive single-chamber pacemaker. PACE 15:1821, 1992.

105. Sugiura T, Kimura M, Mizushina S, et al: Cardiac pacemaker regulated by respiratory rate and blood temperature. PACE 11:1077, 1988.

106. Alt E, Theres H, Heinz M, et al: A new rate-modulated pacemaker system optimized by a combination of two sensors. PACE 11:1119, 1988.

107. Leman RB, White JK, Kratz JM, et al: The potential utility of sensor-driven pacing in DDD pacemakers. Am Heart J 118:919, 1989.

108. Proctor EE, Leman RB, Mann DL, et al: Single- versus dual-chamber sensor-driven pacing: Comparison of cardiac outputs. Am Heart J 122:728, 1991.

109. Vogt P, Goy JJ, Kuhn M, et al: Single- versus double-chamber rate-responsive pacing: Comparison by cardiopulmonary noninvasive exercise testing. PACE 11:1896, 1988.

110. Jutzy RV, Florio J, Isaeff DM, et al: Comparative evaluation of rate-modulated dual-chamber and VVIR pacing. PACE 13:1838, 1990.

111. Sulke AN, Chambers J, Dritsas A, et al: A randomised double-blind cross-over comparison of four rate-responsive pacing modes. J Am Coll Cardiol 17:696, 1991.

112. Wilkoff BL, Corey J, Blackburn G: A mathematical model of the cardiac chronotropic response to exercise. J Electrophysiol 3:176, 1989.

113. Sulke N, Dritsas A, Chambers J, et al: Is accurate rate response programming necessary? PACE 13:1031, 1990.

114. Brachmann J, MacCarter D, Frees U, et al: Is accurate programming of the rate adaptive slope necessary? (Abstract.) PACE 14:643, 1991.

115. Daubert C, Ritter P, Mabo P, et al: Physiologic relationship between AV interval and heart rate in healthy subjects: Applications to dual-chamber pacing. PACE 9:1032, 1986.

116. Barbieri D, Percoco GF, Toselli T, et al: AV delay and exercise stress tests: Behaviour in normal subjects. PACE 13:1724, 1990.

117. Ronaszeki A, Ector H, Denef B, et al: Effect of short atrioventricular delay on cardiac output. PACE 13:1728, 1990.

118. Harper GR, Pina IL, Kutalek SP: Intrinsic conduction maximizes cardiopulmonary performance in patients with dual-chamber pacemakers. PACE 14:1787, 1991.

119. Irnich W, Conrady J: A new principle of rate-adaptive pacing in patients with sick sinus syndrome. PACE 11:1823, 1988.

120. Ritter P, Daubert C, Mabo P, et al: Haemodynamic benefit of a rate-adapted AV delay in dual-chamber pacing. Eur Heart J 10:637, 1989.

121. Eugene M, Lascault G, Frank R, et al: Assessment of the optimal atrio-ventricular delay in DDD paced patients by impedance plethysmography. Eur Heart J 10:250, 1989.

122. Mehta D, Gilmour S, Ward DE, et al: Optimal atrio-ventricular delay at rest and during exercise in patients with dual-chamber pacemakers: A non-invasive assessment by continuous wave Doppler. Br Heart J 61:161, 1989.

123. Landzberg JS, Franklin JO, Mahawar SK, et al: Benefits of physiologic atrioventricular synchronization for pacing with an exercise rate response. Am J Cardiol 66:193, 1990.

124. Rydén L, Karlsson Ö, Kristensson B-E: The importance of different atrioventricular intervals for exercise capacity. PACE 11:1051, 1988.

125. Haskell RJ, French WJ: Physiological importance of different atrioventricular intervals to improved exercise performance in patients with dual-chamber pacemakers. Br Heart J 61:46, 1989.

126. Brecker SJ, Xiao HB, Sparrow J, et al: Effects of dual-chamber pacing with short atrioventricular delay in dilated cardiomyopathy. Lancet 340:1308, 1992.

127. Limousin M, Ripart A, Girodo S, et al: Automatic atrioventricular delay algorithm: A guarantee for an optimal exercise capacity. PACE 11:817, 1988.

128. Antonioli GE, Barbieri D, Percoco GF, et al: Clinical experience using a DDD-RR pacemaker with rate-adaptive AV delay. PACE 12:1572, 1989.

129. Sulke AN, Chambers JB, Sowton E: The effect of atrioventricular delay programming in patients with DDDR pacemakers. Eur Heart J 13:464, 1992.

130. Patterson JA, Naughton J, Pietras RJ, et al: Treadmill exercise in the assessment of the functional capacity of patients with cardiac disease. Am J Cardiol 30:757, 1972.

131. Franciosa JA, Ziesche S, Wilen M: Functional capacity of patients with chronic left ventricular failure. Am J Med 67:460, 1979.

132. Matula M, Alt E, Fotuhi P, et al: Influence of varied types of exercise to the rate adaptation of activity pacemakers. (Abstract.) PACE 15:578, 1992.

133. Zarling J, Belott P, Brown D, et al: A comparison of external rate-responsive pacemakers with identical implanted units. PACE 15:1886, 1992.

134. Goldman L, Hashimoto B, Cook EF, et al: Comparative reproducibility and validity of systems for assessing cardiovascular functional class: Advantages of a new specific activity scale. Circulation 64:1227, 1981.

135. Borg GA: Psychosocial bases of perceived exertion. Med Sci Sports Exerc 14:377, 1982.

136. Greene WA, Moss AJ: Psychosocial factors in the adjustment of patients with permanently implanted cardiac pacemakers. Ann Intern Med 70:897, 1969.

137. Hervé L, Farge C, Guize L, et al: Quality of life of paced patients. PACE 2:A-53, 1979.

138. Mickley H, Petersen J, Nielsen BL: Subjective consequences of permanent pacemaker therapy in patients under the age of retirement. PACE 12:401, 1989.

139. Catipovic-Veselica K, Skrinjaric S, Mrdenovic S, et al: Emotion profiles and quality-of-life of paced patients. PACE 13:399, 1990.

140. Lau C-P, Rushby J, Leigh-Jones M, et al: Symptomatology and quality-of-life in patients with rate-responsive pacemakers. Clin Cardiol 12:505, 1989.

141. Oto MA, Müderrisoglu H, Ozin MB, et al: Quality of life in patients with rate-responsive pacemakers: A randomised cross-over study. PACE 14:800, 1991.

142. Langenfeld H, Schneider B, Grimm W, et al: The six-minute walk—an adequate exercise test for pacemaker patients? PACE 13:1761, 1990.

143. Benditt DG, Mianulli M, Fetter J, et al: An office-based exercise protocol for predicting chronotropic response of activity-triggered rate-variable pacemakers. Am J Cardiol 64:27, 1989.

144. Hayes DL, Von Felt L, Higano ST: Standardized informal exercise testing for programming rate-adaptive pacemakers. PACE 14:1772, 1991.

145. Gamage M, Schofield S, Rankin I, et al: Benefit of single-setting rate-responsive ventricular pacing compared with fixed-rate demand pacing in elderly patients. PACE 14:174, 1991.

CHAPTER 25

PACEMAKER SYNDROME

Kenneth A. Ellenbogen
Bruce S. Stambler

Pacemaker syndrome is best defined as a constellation of signs and symptoms resulting from the selection of a suboptimal pacing mode or the programming of inappropriate pacing parameters. For example, pacemaker syndrome may arise as a result of choosing the VVI or VVIR pacing mode in a patient with hypertrophic cardiomyopathy and intact retrograde ventriculoatrial (VA) conduction. Pacemaker syndrome may also arise in a patient being paced in the AAI mode who develops progressive atrioventricular (AV) conduction delay resulting in AV nodal conduction times greater than 200 msec. The symptoms and signs associated with pacemaker syndrome are multiple, subtle, and often quite nonspecific. The pathophysiology of this syndrome results from a complex interplay between the cardiac conduction system, the autonomic nervous system, and humoral factors. The incidence, clinical manifestations, causes, association with various pacing modes, and treatment of pacemaker syndrome are discussed in this chapter.

Incidence and Epidemiology

In 1969, Mitsui and colleagues[1] described a patient who was intolerant of ventricular pacing as manifested by complaints of chest pain, dizziness, shortness of breath, cold sweats, and facial flushing. The authors attributed these symptoms to the pacing rate rather than to the mode of pacing. They described this phenomenon as "pacemaking syndrome" and attributed it to a suboptimal cardiac output. A number of case reports appeared in subsequent years describing patients who were unable to tolerate ventricular pacing.[2-4] These patients had a variety of types of structural heart disease and presented with a wide spectrum of clinical signs and symptoms.

Ausubel and Furman[5] reviewed the incidence and clinical manifestations of pacemaker syndrome in 1985. They reported that pacemaker syndrome occurs in 7% to 21% of patients with VVI pacemakers. They emphasized that patients presenting with severe symptoms are easily recognized, but pacemaker syndrome may be quite subtle in patients with milder symptoms.

Pacemaker syndrome occurs in both sexes and in patients of all ages. Patients undergoing pacemaker implantation for a variety of causes (e.g., sinus node dysfunction, complete heart block) and with a variety of types of structural heart disease may develop pacemaker syndrome.[5, 6] Symptoms attributable to pacemaker syndrome may occur immediately after implantation or may be delayed for months or years.

The "true" incidence of pacemaker syndrome has become clearer from recent studies that have abandoned "rigid" definitions of pacemaker syndrome. Instead, these studies have compared single- versus dual-chamber pacing modes based on subjective (e.g., quality of life, symptom questionnaires) and objective criteria (e.g., exercise duration, Doppler stroke volume measurements) and have sought to identify patients who were intolerant or symptomatic during periods of VVI pacing. The Mayo Clinic reported that 20% of a group of 50 patients were at "risk" for developing pacemaker syndrome during VVI pacing, based on a mean decrease in systolic blood pressure of 24 ± 11 mm Hg during VVI pacing compared with DVI pacing or sinus rhythm.[7] Ten patients in this study experienced dizziness in the standing position during VVI pacing, whereas no patient experienced symptoms in the supine position during pacing.

In another study, Heldman and colleagues[8] reported an incidence of pacemaker syndrome of 83% in 40 unselected patients with DDD pacemakers based on the answers to symptom questionnaires during various pacing modes. Symptoms evaluated included shortness of breath, fatigue, dizziness, apprehension, cough, pulsations in the neck or abdomen, orthopnea, palpitations, headaches, chest pain, and several other related cardiac symptoms. Symptoms in this trial were assessed by asking the patients to complete a questionnaire comparing the relative severity of each of 16 different symptoms on a severity scale ranging from 0 to 10 during 1 week each of VVI and DDD pacing. Eighteen percent of patients experienced mild symptoms, 28% reported moderate symptoms, and 37% had severe symptoms during VVI pacing. Only 17% of patients in this study experienced no new or worsened symptoms during VVI pacing. Forty-two percent of patients were unable to tolerate VVI pacing for 1 week. No readily identifiable clinical, hemodynamic, or electrophysiologic variable predicted which patients would develop pacemaker syndrome.

Sulke and colleagues[9, 10] reported on 22 patients programmed to the DDD, VVIR, and DDIR pacing modes. Comparisons based on subjective (e.g., symptomatic, functional class, health perception, and exercise tolerance) and objective (e.g., maximal exercise treadmill test time, and echocardiographic assessment) criteria found that the VVIR mode was the least acceptable pacing mode in 73% of patients (Fig. 25–1). Functional assessment of physical capability was assessed with an activity grading scale ranging from class I (unlimited physical capacity) to class IV (grossly incapacitated). Quality of life was assessed by using visual analog scales to assess patient-perceived general well-being and exercise capacity. General well-being, functional status, perceived exercise capacity, and specific symptom scores (shortness of breath) were lower with the VVIR pacing mode compared to DDD, DDDR, and DDIR pacing modes. Exercise treadmill time was longer in the DDDR mode. Five patients paced in the VVIR mode demanded early crossover to a dual-chamber pacing mode owing to symptoms of dyspnea, dizziness, tiredness, and palpitations. Among these five patients, symptoms resolved within 24 hours of being programmed to a dual-chamber pacing mode.

In another study the same investigators studied 16 patients with VVI pacemakers who had felt ''generally well'' for at least 3 years. These patients had an atrial lead inserted at the time of generator change for upgrading to a dual-chamber pacemaker. The authors used the same methodology to quantitate subjective and objective responses during the pacing mode changes. Seventy-five percent of patients preferred the DDD mode, and 68% of patients found the VVI mode the least acceptable; only 12% expressed no preference. Perceived general well-being, symptom scores, and exercise treadmill time were better with DDD pacing. The authors concluded that most patients who are asymptomatic with long-term VVI pacing will derive symptomatic benefit from upgrading to DDD pacing. This suggests that a ''subclinical'' pacemaker syndrome may be present in up to 75% of patients with VVI pacemakers who do not have overt symptoms of pacemaker syndrome. Many other investigators have also performed similar studies comparing various pacing modes immediately after reprogramming or weeks to months later. Their results are fairly consistent and suggest that a majority of patients demonstrate symptomatic and objective evidence of hemodynamic improvement with AV synchrony. The studies are reviewed in Chapter 24.

Description of the Clinical Syndrome

The most prominent symptoms arising from pacemaker syndrome are attributable to a decrease in cardiac output and

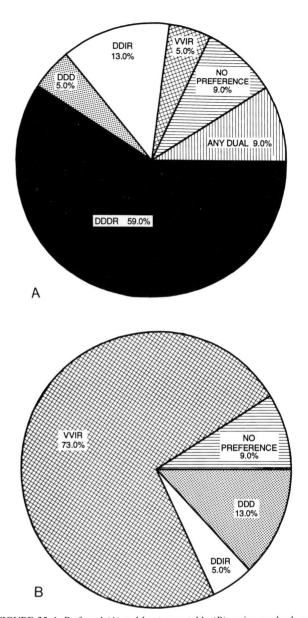

FIGURE 25–1. Preferred *(A)* and least acceptable *(B)* pacing modes based on symptom questionnaire. (From Sulke AN, Chambers J, Dritsas A, Sowton E: A randomized double-blind crossover comparison of four rate-responsive pacing modes. J Am Coll Cardiol 17:696, 1991. Reprinted with permission from the American College of Cardiology.)

arterial pressure, but some symptoms may also arise from reflexes elicited by increases in pulmonary artery and pulmonary venous pressures. In many patients, however, symptoms and signs are subtle and nonspecific (Table 25–1). Elderly patients may have symptoms that are incorrectly attributed to a variety of other constitutional or chronic medical conditions. In Heldman and colleagues' study, 65% of patients with pacemaker syndrome had moderate to severe symptoms.[8] Based on their patient questionnaires, the following symptoms were worse during VVI pacing: shortness of breath, fatigue, dizziness, apprehension, cough, pulsations in neck or abdomen, orthopnea, headache, palpitations, chest pain, choking sensation, and confusion. In Sulke and associates' study, patients with intolerance to VVI pacing complained of effort dyspnea, palpitations, dizziness, and tired-

TABLE 25–1. **SYMPTOMS OF PACEMAKER SYNDROME**

MILD
Pulsations in neck, abdomen
Palpitations
Fatigue, malaise, weakness
Cough
Apprehension
Chest fullness or pain, jaw pain
Headache
MODERATE
Shortness of breath on exertion
Dizziness, tiredness, vertigo
Orthopnea, paroxysmal nocturnal dyspnea
Choking sensation
Confusion or alteration of mental state
SEVERE
Presyncope
Syncope
Shortness of breath at rest, pulmonary edema

Diagnosis

In our clinical experience, the diagnosis of pacemaker syndrome requires a high degree of suspicion and a willingness to evaluate all patient complaints thoroughly. Diagnosis is best confirmed by correlating the patient's cardiac rhythm with his or her symptoms after excluding the possibility of intermittent pacemaker malfunction. This demonstration may require the use of Holter or transtelephonic monitoring (Fig. 25–2). These techniques may show ventricular pacing, echo beats, or the presence of retrograde VA conduction during ventricular pacing associated with patient symptoms. The demonstration of retrograde VA conduction increases the likelihood that pacemaker syndrome may be responsible for the patient's symptoms and justifies a careful search for pacemaker syndrome. The finding on Holter or transtelephonic monitoring of relief of the patient's symptoms with resumption of sinus rhythm or sinus bradycardia (e.g., restoration of AV synchrony) also suggests the diagnosis of pacemaker syndrome.

On physical examination, the findings that aid in the diagnosis of pacemaker syndrome include cannon A waves in the jugular venous pulse or palpable liver pulsations (Fig. 25–3). A frequently performed test is the measurement of arterial pressure in the supine and upright positions during ventricular and atrial or AV pacing. In some cases, arterial pressure during ventricular pacing is compared to arterial pressure in sinus rhythm. In general, a significant drop in arterial pressure (usually considered greater than 20 mm Hg) implies that pacemaker syndrome is present. However, the absence of a significant drop in arterial pressure does not eliminate the possibility that pacemaker syndrome is responsible for the patient's symptoms because symptoms may be secondary to

ness. Other symptoms identified in some clinical studies or case reports include syncope, confusion or decreased ability to concentrate, near-syncope, dizziness, headaches, vertigo, jaw pain, paroxysmal nocturnal dyspnea, and a sensation of a lump in the throat or neck. It is important to realize that in some patients symptoms may be mild or their development may be subacute. Rarely, patients may have severe symptoms if pacemaker syndrome results in syncope or pulmonary edema and requires removal of a VVI pulse generator. It has recently been suggested that patients with hypertrophic cardiomyopathy may be particularly susceptible to more severe clinical deterioration during ventricular pacing, and AV synchrony is strongly advocated in this group of patients.

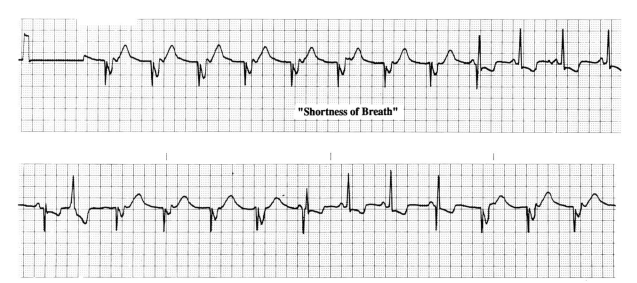

"Shortness of Breath"

FIGURE 25–2. Continuous rhythm strips recorded with a transtelephonic cardiac monitor in a 65-year-old farmer with pacemaker syndrome. This patient's underlying rhythm disorder was sick sinus syndrome with sinus bradycardia and multiple episodes of atrial fibrillation 1 year earlier. His sinus bradycardia was exacerbated by treatment with quinidine, verapamil, and digoxin. After implantation of a VVIR device he returned to his physician complaining of fatigue, weakness, dizziness, malaise, and shortness of breath 1 month later. Following documentation of this rhythm by a cardiac event monitor, he underwent further testing. During VVI pacing, ventriculoatrial (VA) dissociation occurred. During VVI pacing at 90 bpm his blood pressure dropped to 90/68 mm Hg, and during AAI pacing it was 160/90 mm Hg (at 90 bpm). During sinus rhythm at 58 to 64 bpm, the blood pressure measured 136/70 mm Hg. A DDDR pacemaker was implanted, and within 48 hours the patient's symptoms were abolished. He has returned to his active, vigorous lifestyle and has had no subsequent episodes of atrial fibrillation for 1 year. (From Ellenbogen KA, Wood MA, Stambler B: Pacemaker syndrome: Clinical, hemodynamic, and neurohumeral features. *In* Barold SS, Mujica J [eds]: New Perspectives in Cardiac Pacing 3. Mt Kisco, NY, Futura Publishing Co., 1992.)

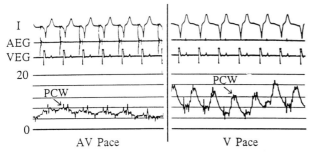

FIGURE 25–3. Surface electrocardiographic lead I, atrial electrogram (AEG), ventricular electrogram (VEG), and pulmonary capillary wedge pressure (PCW) recordings from a single patient during AV pacing (AV Pace) and ventricular pacing (V Pace) at 80 bpm with an AV interval of 150 msec. The cannon A wave is noted *(arrow)* on the PCW tracing. (From Reynolds DW: Hemodynamics of cardiac pacing. *In* Ellenbogen KA [ed]: Clinical Cardiac Pacing. Cambridge, Blackwell Scientific, 1992, pp 120–161. Reprinted by permission of Blackwell Scientific Publications, Inc.)

an elevation of pulmonary pressures. We recommend that blood pressure be checked immediately after the institution of the new pacing mode and then at 30 seconds and several minutes after the pacing mode change. In some patients, blood pressure decreases further 10 to 20 seconds after ventricular pacing is instituted.

Ocular pneumoplethysmography, Doppler echocardiography, and other noninvasive techniques may be useful for documenting the changes in stroke volume or cardiac output that occur during pacing mode changes. In some cases, documentation of significant changes in cardiac output is important for demonstrating the physiologic benefit of DDD pacing and may be required by insurers to justify pacemaker upgrade. The majority of studies consistently show that patients with the greatest decreases in stroke volume during ventricular pacing are the ones most likely to develop symptoms of pacemaker syndrome. In some cases, measurement of forearm vascular resistance with venous occlusion plethysmography may be performed to show a patient's failure to maintain forearm vascular resistance during ventricular pacing.

Table 25–2 presents a summary of some of the clinical measures that have been found to predict the development of pacemaker syndrome.

Pathophysiology of Pacemaker Syndrome

The pathophysiology of pacemaker syndrome is complex and multifactorial. This clinical syndrome arises from a complex interplay of hemodynamic, neurohumoral, and vascular factors.

At first glance, the loss of AV synchrony appears to be the major hemodynamic change that occurs with pacemaker syndrome. More accurately, not only is AV synchrony lost, but also in many cases hemodynamic compromise is produced by simultaneous atrial and and ventricular contraction. Atrial contribution to ventricular filling is discussed elsewhere in detail (see Chapter 23). To briefly summarize, the atrium functions as a booster pump to contribute 15% to 25% of cardiac output. In patients with a stiff or noncompliant left ventricle, the contribution of the atrial kick may be even greater. This occurs in disease states such as restrictive cardiomyopathies, hypertensive heart disease, and hypertrophic cardiomyopathies. In patients with dilated cardiomyopathy, some investigators have suggested that the atrial contribution to ventricular filling is negligible, primarily because these patients are on the "flat" portion of their Starling curve.[19–23] More recent investigations, however, have demonstrated that these patients do benefit significantly from the atrial contribution to ventricular filling.[24, 25] The change in cardiac index, the percentage change in cardiac index, and the change in pulmonary capillary wedge pressure during a change in pacing mode from DDD to VVI were similar in a group of patients with normal cardiac function and a group with New York Heart Association (NYHA) class III and class IV congestive heart failure. Finally, the atrial contribution to ventricular filling depends on many factors, including heart

TABLE 25–2. CLINICAL CORRELATES OF PACEMAKER SYNDROME

STUDY	NO. PATIENTS	PREDICTIVE	NOT PREDICTIVE
Nishimura[7]	50	VA conduction	CHF present or absent Cardiomegaly
Heldman[8]	40	None	LV function VA conduction SSS vs. AV block
Sulke[9, 10]	22	% increase in SV with DDD pacing	LA size EF, VA conduction FS
Pearson[15]	24	% atrial contribution to LV filling VA conduction SV during VVI pacing <50 mL	FS, LA size LV size
Stewart[16]	29	VA conduction % change in CO with DDD pacing	LV function
Rediker[17]	19	VA conduction SSS	LV size LA size FS
Erlebacher[18]	20	Cannon A waves VA conduction	Baseline SV or PCW pressure

CO, cardiac output; EF, ejection fraction; FS, fractional shortening; SV, stroke volume; CHF, congestive heart failure; VA, ventriculoatrial; LV, left ventricular; LA, left atrial; PCW, pulmonary capillary wedge pressure; SSS, sick sinus syndrome.

rate, myocardial systolic and diastolic function, the presence of valvular heart disease, and left ventricular contractility.

Several studies have shown that patients with pacemaker syndrome tend to experience greater decreases in cardiac output when changing from DDD to VVI pacing than do patients without pacemaker syndrome. In one study of 29 patients with DDD pacemakers, the mean cardiac output decreased from 5.0 ± 0.3 L/min to 4.3 ± 0.3 L/min during a mode switch from DDD to VVI pacing. In patients with pacemaker syndrome, the decrease in cardiac output during VVI pacing was 30% compared to a 14% decrease in cardiac output in patients without retrograde conduction or absent pacemaker syndrome (Fig. 25–4).[16] There was no significant correlation between left ventricular function and change in cardiac output during a shift from VVI to DDD pacing. Pearson and colleagues[15] used echocardiography to show that patients with a stroke volume of less than 50 mL had a significantly higher percentage increase in stroke volume during AV sequential pacing than during VVI pacing. Other studies have shown a correlation between the presence of retrograde conduction and greater decreases in cardiac output during VVI pacing (see Table 25–2).[5, 7, 11–18] Sulke and colleagues[9] showed that subjects who found the VVI mode least acceptable had the greatest increases in stroke volume when paced in the DDD mode compared to the VVI mode.

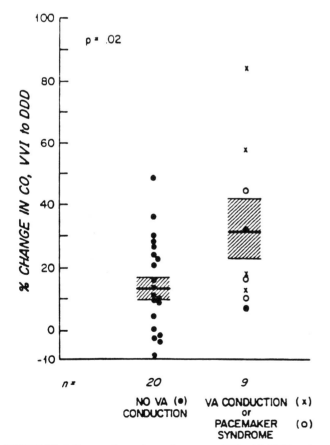

FIGURE 25–4. Percent change in cardiac output (CO) with DDD pacing according to the presence (x) or absence (●) of ventriculoatrial (VA) conduction or the presence of pacemaker syndrome (○). VA conduction is assessed at the time of pacemaker implant. (From Stewart WJ, Dicola VC, Hawthorne JW, et al: Doppler ultrasound measurement of cardiac output in patients with physiologic pacemakers. Am J Cardiol 54:308, 1984.)

Similar results have been demonstrated by several other groups of investigators.[9, 10, 15]

Although changes in cardiac output and blood pressure are often the primary focus of discussions about AV synchrony, it is likely that in many patients hemodynamic alterations in these variables are responsible for only the most severe cases of pacemaker syndrome. In most cases, increased atrial pressure during ventricular pacing is probably a more common mechanism by which symptoms are produced. During ventricular pacing, increases in mean and phasic right and left atrial pressures as well as pulmonary venous and arterial pressures are seen.[24, 26, 27] These elevations in atrial pressures, especially when manifest by cannon A waves (e.g., reflection of atrial contraction against a closed mitral or tricuspid valve), may be further transmitted to the jugular, hepatic, and pulmonary veins. Symptoms such as headaches, fullness in the head or neck, pulsations in the neck or abdomen, cough, and jaw pain may arise as a result of these pressure changes.

Another hemodynamic consequence of VA conduction is the production of VA "dyssynchrony." In patients with intact VA conduction, compared to those in whom it is absent, there is a greater decrease in cardiac output and blood pressure as well as a greater increase in right atrial, pulmonary artery, and pulmonary capillary wedge pressures during ventricular pacing. Studies by Reynolds and Ellenbogen and their colleagues[24, 26] have demonstrated that simultaneous pacing of the ventricle and the atrium (to simulate VA conduction) with a VA interval of 100 to 150 msec produces greater decreases in blood pressure and cardiac output and greater increases in right and left ventricular filling pressures than ventricular pacing when retrograde VA conduction is absent. Nishimura and associates[7] also reported that patients with intact VA conduction showed a much greater decrease in systolic blood pressure with VVI pacing (24 ± 11 mm Hg) compared to those with VA dissociation (-4 ± 15 mm Hg, $p < .005$).

The altered pattern of ventricular activation resulting from ventricular pacing leads to a variable but generally small change in ventricular performance.[28, 29] In a dog model, both atrial and AV sequential pacing led to a marked improvement in cardiac performance compared with ventricular pacing. These investigators also noted a slight but further reduction in pulmonary capillary wedge pressure, mean right atrial pressure, and systemic vascular resistance and a simultaneous increase in mean arterial pressure and stroke volume during atrial pacing compared with AV sequential pacing. The mean systolic ejection rate (milliliters per second) is an index of the rate of myocardial fiber shortening. Ventricular pacing results in a somewhat lower mean systolic ejection rate, but there is also a lower mean systolic ejection rate during AV sequential pacing compared with atrial pacing with intact AV conduction. This results directly from the less coordinated myocardial contraction that occurs with ventricular pacing because excitation is initiated at a site in the right ventricular apex where the pacing lead is implanted. In humans, the impact of the ventricular activation sequence on cardiac output is thought to be considerably less than that measured in dogs. In one study 12 patients with AV sequential pacemakers and intact AV conduction underwent radionuclide studies at rest and Doppler echocardiographic studies at rest and during submaximal exercise.[28] Cardiac output was about 10% higher during AAI pacing than during AV sequential pacing. The duration of LV contraction among patients was more homogeneous during AAI pacing, and the peak filling rate was higher. Finally, Doppler evaluation showed higher peak aortic blood velocity, mean aortic blood acceleration, and systolic time integrals during rest and submaximal exercise during AAI pacing than during DDD pacing. Similar findings have been reported by Askenazi and colleagues.[29] It is likely that the altered pattern of ventricular activation that occurs with ventricular pacing may play a small role in the development of pacemaker syndrome in some patients.

It was widely thought that pacing modes that do not restore AV synchrony are associated with an increased incidence and degree of mitral and tricuspid valve regurgitation.[30–32] This theory has been specifically studied by several investigators. Furman and Cooper reported tricuspid valve insufficiency in 9 of 13 patients with VVIR pacemakers over a 6-month period.[31] There was, however, no evidence of an increase in atrial size in patients with valvular regurgitation. The role of AV valvular regurgitation in producing the increased atrial pressures noted during ventricular pacing is unclear. Reynolds and his colleagues[24] used left ventricular cineangiography in patients during AV and VA pacing to assess mitral regurgitation. Only 30% of patients had slight or mild worsening of mitral regurgitation during ventricular pacing. Of the five patients with worsening mitral regurgitation, two developed trace mitral regurgitation and three developed mild mitral regurgitation. There are, however, several reports of patients with marked increases in mitral regurgitation. Naito and associates were able to demonstrate angiographic evidence of retrograde blood flow into the pulmonary venous system but no mitral regurgitation.[32]

In another study of patients with DDDR pacemakers, the presence and severity of mitral or tricuspid regurgitation were assessed by color flow Doppler echocardiography.[9, 10] The presence of tricuspid (TR) and mitral regurgitation (MR) was greater during VVI pacing than in any dual-chamber mode (e.g., VVI, 73% with TR and 75% with MR; DDD, 57% with TR and 34% with MR). These changes did not reach statistical significance, and the extent of mitral regurgitation assessed by color flow Doppler imaging was similar during VVI and DDD pacing. Importantly, the extent of TR was greater during VVI than DDD pacing. The presence of TR did not correlate with the development of symptoms suggestive of pacemaker syndrome. Thus, based on these studies, it appears unlikely that valvular regurgitation plays an important role in the acute production of increased atrial pressure and the development of pacemaker syndrome in most patients. Whether long-term hemodynamic effects facilitate further chamber enlargement and valvular regurgitation is still not known.

Role of Retrograde Conduction

Five studies have identified the presence of retrograde VA conduction during ventricular pacing as predictive of development of pacemaker syndrome.[7, 15–18] VA conduction occurs over the AV node and His-Purkinje system and cannot be predicted from the presence or absence of antegrade AV conduction. Several generalizations can be made.[33] In patients with normal AV conduction, VA conduction is intact in almost 70%. The incidence of retrograde block in the AV node is significantly higher in patients with evidence of AV nodal conduction system disease. The frequency of VA block increases from 62% in patients with first-degree AV block to 80% in patients with second-degree AV (nodal) block and to 100% in patients with third-degree AV block. The incidence of VA block ranges from 50% in patients with second-degree block (infranodal) to 85% in patients with third-degree infranodal block. This implies that retrograde conduction is more likely to be intact in patients undergoing pacemaker implantation for sinus node dysfunction than for AV block.

In patients with intact AV conduction, the VA intervals range from 100 to 400 msec.[34, 35] The VA conduction time is primarily dependent on the site of measurement of the atrial and ventricular electrograms and baseline autonomic tone. Retrograde conduction is dynamic, and patients may have absent VA conduction during pacemaker implantation but demonstrate VA conduction during exercise.[35, 36] Facilitation of VA conduction can occur with appropriately timed premature ventricular contractions (PVCs) following AV sequential pacing due to facilitation of conduction in the AV node or His-Purkinje system.[36] Finally, the presence of type Ia, Ic, and III antiarrhythmic drugs such as procainamide, flecainide, sotalol, and beta-blocking or calcium channel blocking drugs may affect retrograde VA conduction as well.[37]

Retrograde conduction has two important clinical corollaries. First, the hemodynamic consequences of retrograde conduction are a greater elevation of right-sided and pulmonary filling pressures. Second, retrograde conduction is associated with a higher incidence of cannon A waves and greater atrial distention, which may elicit reflex mechanisms originating from the atria.[18, 25–27, 32] Erlebacher and coworkers studied 20 patients following coronary artery bypass surgery with indwelling pulmonary artery catheters and temporary atrial and ventricular pacing wires.[18] They noted a greater decrease in stroke volume index during ventricular pacing in patients with cannon A waves (defined as new V waves >4 mm Hg on the pulmonary capillary wedge pressure tracing). There was a decrease in mean systemic blood pressure only in patients with cannon A waves. Ten of 13 patients with cannon A waves had retrograde conduction.

Atrial and Vascular Reflexes

Atrial receptors and cardiopulmonary reflexes have been the subject of several recent in-depth reviews. Briefly, the atria and the cardiopulmonary circulation are innervated by afferents from the vagus nerve. Myelinated vagal afferents are present primarily at the venoatrial junctions, and in animals their selective activation results in parasympathetic activation and diuresis. Nonmyelinated vagal afferents are also present throughout the cardiopulmonary area, posteriorly over both atria, pulmonary veins, and the venoatrial junctions. In response to cardiac or atrial distention, a vasodepressor response occurs with a decrease in mean arterial blood pressure and heart rate as well as withdrawal of sympathetic vasoconstriction.[28, 29]

The vascular response to ventricular pacing has important consequences. In Erlebacher and associates' study, patients without cannon A waves had a significant rise (22.8%) in total peripheral vascular resistance during ventricular pacing, whereas those with cannon A waves had a much smaller increase in total peripheral vascular resistance (4.9%, $p <$ .002).[18] Therefore, the response to ventricular pacing in patients with cannon A waves was less than 25% of the response in patients without cannon A waves. The authors argued that the vasoconstrictor response to ventricular pacing is modified by inhibitory atrial reflexes, which are stimulated during increases in atrial pressure or stretch.

Other data supporting the role of the atrium were compiled by Alicandri and colleagues from the Cleveland Clinic.[40] These investigators carefully studied three patients with hypotension and near-syncope during ventricular pacing. They measured arterial pressure, cardiac output, right atrial pressure, and total peripheral vascular resistance. They noted a small but variable decrease in cardiac output during shifts from ventricular pacing to sinus rhythm, which was similar to that observed in a small group of control subjects without pacemaker syndrome. The striking difference between the control subjects and the three patients studied was the approximately 20% increase in peripheral resistance in the control patients and the failure of peripheral resistance to increase in the patients with pacemaker syndrome (Fig. 25–5). Another study in a group of patients with intact VA conduction showed similar results in that peripheral resistance failed to rise in seven patients with VVI pacemakers who ultimately underwent pacemaker upgrade to the DDD pacing mode.[41]

Ellenbogen and colleagues at the Medical College of Virginia measured the changes in forearm blood flow and forearm vascular resistance during atrial, ventricular, and VA pacing with a VA interval of 100 to 150 msec.[26] Forearm blood flow was measured by venous occlusion plethysmography, which provides accurate measurement of changes in regional blood flow, reflecting changes in regional vasomotor tone. During ventricular pacing with simulated VA conduction (e.g., VA pacing) but not during ventricular pacing striking increases in forearm vascular resistance occurred within 30 seconds. These changes were blocked by intra-arterial phentolamine, an alpha-sympathetic antagonist, suggesting that vasoconstriction is mediated by the sympathetic nervous system. Further documentation of these reflex changes is provided by more recent experiments in our laboratory with peroneal microneurography. This technique allows measurement of local postganglionic muscle sympathetic nerve activity to the leg.[42] We have been able to demonstrate greater increases in local sympathetic nerve activity during ventricular pacing than during atrial pacing. These observations confirm that sympathetic nervous system activation is a normal physiologic response to ventricular pacing.

Based on this body of work, we hypothesize that during ventricular pacing, especially in the presence of retrograde VA conduction, regional vasomotor tone increases in most patients in response to the decreased cardiac output or increased filling pressures. The changes in sympathetic tone correlate well with the change in systolic pressure and are probably mediated by the arterial baroreceptors. In the upright position, blood is pooled in the extremities, and arterial baroreceptors are further activated to compensate for the decreased cardiac output and systolic pressure. In some patients pacemaker syndrome results from an inability to further compensate for the upright position by augmentation of autonomic tone. In other patients pacemaker syndrome results from the modification of these vascular responses by the effect of drugs (e.g., vasodilators, diuretics, centrally acting sympathetic antagonists), underlying organic heart disease, volume status, and autonomic defects. In still other patients, pacemaker syndrome results from activation of inhibitory atrial and cardiopulmonary reflexes that counteract the vasoconstrictor response. These responses may also be further modified by the production of catecholamines and atrial natriuretic peptide (ANP) (Fig. 25–6) (see later discussion).

Neurohumoral Factors

We and others have studied the humoral changes that take place during different modes of pacing. These studies have shown that plasma norepinephrine and epinephrine levels increase markedly in patients during shifts from sinus rhythm to ventricular pacing.[43–45] In one report, coronary sinus norepinephrine was found to be higher during VVI pacing at rest and exercise than during ventriculoatrial triggered (VAT) or AV synchronous pacing.[44] Arterial concentrations of catecholamines also increase more during exercise in the VVI mode, but the differences are less striking than those measured from the coronary sinus. The measurement of cardiac norepinephrine spillover, calculated as the difference between coronary sinus and arterial plasma concentrations multiplied by coronary sinus blood flow, is a reasonable measure of cardiac sympathetic nerve activity. This study demonstrated for the first time that VVI pacing causes a greater increase in cardiac sympathetic activity than AV synchronous pacing. In our study, the increase in plasma norepinephrine levels correlated best with the decline in systolic blood pressure observed during ventricular pacing. In other studies, plasma norepinephrine increased only slightly with VVI pacing but increased by greater amounts during ventricular pacing in the presence of retrograde VA conduction.[45]

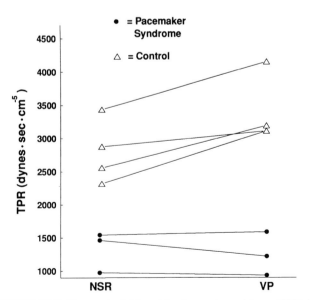

FIGURE 25–5. Changes in total peripheral vascular resistance (TPR) in dynes•sec•cm^{-5} during normal sinus rhythm (NSR) and ventricular pacing (VP) in four control patients and three patients with pacemaker syndrome. (Data from Alicandri C, Fowad FM, Tarazi RC, et al: Three cases of hypotension and syncope with ventricular pacing: Possible role of atrial reflexes. Am J Cardiol 42:137, 1978.)

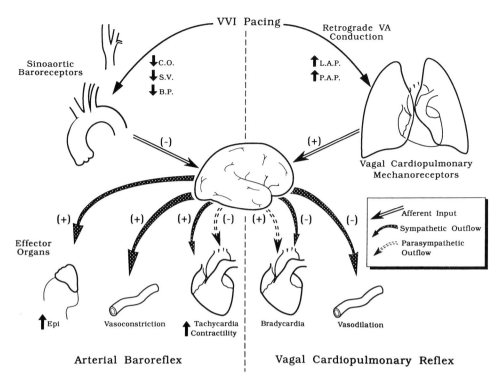

FIGURE 25–6. Diagrammatic representation of multiple reflex pathways involved in pacemaker syndrome. See text for discussion. The arterial baroreflexes detect a decrease in stroke volume when atrioventricular (AV) dyssynchrony occurs, leading to sympathetic activation and vasoconstriction. Conversely, AV dyssynchrony leads to increased atrial wall tension and activation of reflex pathways leading to vagally mediated vasodilation as well as release of humoral substances such as atrial natriuretic peptide (ANP), which further facilitate these reflexes (e.g., counteracting baroreflex-mediated vasoconstriction). LAP, left atrial pressure; PAP, pulmonary artery pressure; CO, cardiac output; SV, stroke volume; BP, blood pressure; EPI, epinephrine.)

There are several limitations of these studies, including the observation that plasma catecholamines give only a rough approximation of overall sympathetic activity because they are influenced by the rate of release and clearance from different vascular beds. Plasma catecholamine levels may poorly reflect cardiac sympathetic activity during non–steady-state conditions, such as changes in pacing modes. Overall, the general consistency of elevated plasma or coronary sinus catecholamine measurements during VVI pacing probably reflects the response of the sympathetic nervous system to the decrease in cardiac output or systolic blood pressure that occurs with AV dyssynchrony.

ANP is a 28-amino acid polypeptide produced primarily by granules located in the cardiac atria. ANP functions as an arterial and venous vasodilator and as a natriuretic hormone, and in rats it also results in a vagally mediated inhibition of regional sympathetic nervous system activation.[46] Plasma ANP levels are increased when atrial pressure or atrial volume is elevated. Lower ANP levels during rest are seen in DDD than in VVI pacing in both the acute situation and over the long term.[47] Stangl and colleagues[47] also showed that ANP levels increase during exercise in both DDD and VVI pacing modes, but the increase with VVI pacing was greater. Peak ANP levels also occur later after exercise is stopped with VVI than with DDD pacing. Ventricular pacing with retrograde VA conduction causes striking elevations of ANP levels. Other studies have also demonstrated higher ANP levels during VVI than DDD pacing.[48–51] In one study, ANP release was higher during rate-matched VVI pacing with exercise than during DDD pacing. These studies confirm that AV synchrony leads to less atrial distention and less ANP release, both during exercise and at rest. A report on five patients with pacemaker syndrome showed a higher plasma concentration of ANP during shifts from sinus rhythm to VVI pacing than during shifts from sinus rhythm to DDD pacing in this group.[52] Whether ANP plays a causative role in producing symptoms during nonatrioventricular synchronous pacing or is a secondary factor is unclear.[52b] Future experiments with ANP inhibitors should be able to answer this question more clearly.

"Newer" Forms of Pacemaker Syndrome

When pacemaker syndrome was first recognized, it was attributed to ventricular pacing and recognized primarily as a problem of single-chamber ventricular pacemakers. The development of rate-responsive pacing and newer pacing modes has led to a recognition that pacemaker syndrome is more accurately termed AV dyssynchrony syndrome[53] (Table 25–3).

Pacemaker syndrome has been described during VVIR pacing. In some patients, retrograde VA conduction is absent during baseline testing at pacemaker implantation in the resting or sedated state, but increased sympathetic tone can facilitate retrograde conduction during exercise or stress. Development of VA conduction increases the likelihood that pacemaker syndrome will become manifest. Second, VVIR pacing may occur abruptly during DDDR pacing due to "inappropriate" mode switching (see later discussion).

The development of pacemaker syndrome during AAI or AAIR pacing has also been described and underscores the importance of AV dyssynchrony. During AAI pacing at typical rates of 60 to 70 bpm, pacemaker syndrome is rarely seen because the AR interval is usually less than 200 msec. During AAIR pacing at higher rates, AV conduction may be sufficiently lengthened (>225 to 250 msec) to lead to AV dyssynchrony. AV dyssynchrony may also occur in patients with dual AV node pathway physiology during shifts in conduction from a fast pathway to the slow pathway with longer AV nodal conduction times.[54] AV nodal blocking

TABLE 25–3. PACEMAKER SYNDROME WITH OTHER PACING MODES

AAIR

Long A-R intervals due to slow AV node conduction or dual AV nodal pathways

Inappropriately "aggressive" programming of rate response slope leading to increased atrial rate before effect of catecholamines on AR interval is seen

Solution: Stop drugs with negative dromotropic effects; reprogram rate response slope; upgrade by implanting ventricular lead

VDDR

Pacemaker syndrome occurs only when atrial rate falls below lower rate

Solution: Stop drugs with negative chronotropic effects; program lower rate to a slower heart rate; begin trial of low-dose theophylline to increase atrial rate; implant ventricular lead

DDIR

Pacemaker syndrome occurs whenever spontaneous atrial rate exceeds lower rate or sensor-indicated rate

Solution: Program to DDDR and have separate upper rates for atrial tracking and sensor; begin antiarrhythmic drugs to suppress atrial arrhythmias, then reprogram to DDD or DDDR mode

FALLBACK AND RATE-SMOOTHING IN DDD OR DDDR MODE, CONDITIONAL VENTRICULAR TRACKING LIMIT (CVTL) IN DDDR MODE

Pacemaker syndrome occurs during paroxysmal tachycardias and abrupt heart rate changes, or with divergence of information between sensor and sinus node

Solution: Program parameters so that fallback and rate-smoothing occurrences are limited and short in duration; use stress testing in patients to observe sensor response during rest and exercise; avoid CVTL behavior

MODE-SWITCHING IN DDDR

Pacemaker syndrome occurs with "inappropriate" mode switching

Solution: Use newer algorithms that allow greater programmability and avoid mode-switching for single PACs, sinus tachycardia, and PVCs with retrograde conduction; shorten PVARP; give antiarrhythmic drugs to suppress PACs, PVCs, and atrial tachyarrhythmias; reprogram to DDD mode if possible

DDD

Pacemaker-mediated or endless loop tachycardia occurs

2:1 block occurs during exercise

AV interval misprogramming is present

Repetitive nonreentrant ventriculoatrial synchrony

Solution: Reprogram pacemaker; use pacemaker algorithms to avoid endless loop tachycardia (PVARP extension after PVC, etc.), rate-responsive AV delay, and PVARP that allows tracking at higher rates. Intra-atrial conduction time may need to be measured and accounted for with AV interval programming

MISCELLANEOUS

Reset from the DDD or DDDR mode to the VVI or VOO mode due to noise reversion or end-of-life generator behavior

PVARP, postventricular atrial refractory period; PVC, paroxysmal ventricular contractions; PAC, premature atrial contraction.

drugs (digoxin, beta-blockers, calcium channel blockers, amiodarone, flecainide) can also prolong AV nodal conduction. Pacemaker syndrome may also occur with AAIR pacing if the slope determining the rate of sensor response is too great, leading to an increased pacing rate prior to the expected elevation of catecholamine levels during exercise (Fig. 25–7). The paced atrial to QRS (AR) interval leading to the expression of pacemaker syndrome varies depending on the intra-atrial conduction times, autonomic tone, level of exercise, and latency between the stimulus artifact and atrial activation. Choosing an AAIR pacemaker requires individualization and assessment of the AR interval during different levels of exercise.

During dual-chamber pacing in the VDD, DDI, or DDD mode, pacemaker syndrome may also occur. The VDD pacing mode functions like the DDD mode but without atrial pacing. In the absence of sensed atrial activity, the VDD mode effectively becomes a VVI pacemaker at the lower rate. In one report, a patient with a VDD pacemaker developed pacemaker syndrome when his sinus rate dropped below the lower rate and VVI pacing ensued.[55] The VDD mode, previously out of favor, has recently been revived by the introduction of single-pass leads for VDD pacing.[56] The increased popularity of VDD pacing with these new leads should lead to increased vigilance for detection of pacemaker syndrome in these patients.

The DDI and DDIR pacing modes are useful in patients with paroxysmal supraventricular tachycardias such as paroxysmal atrial fibrillation. In the DDI pacing mode practically no tracking of P waves occurs unless the atrial rate is identical to the programmed lower rate. When the atrial rate is above the lower rate limit, there is no atrial tracking. If the ventricular rate is below the lower rate, ventricular pacing occurs at the lower rate. When the atrial rate is above the lower rate, variable sensed P wave to paced ventricular complex interval (PV) relationships occur, leading to discoordination of the atrium and paced ventricle (Fig. 25–8). In the DDIR pacing mode, the pacemaker increases its rate only in response to sensor input. Likewise, if the atrial rate exceeds the sensor-driven ventricular pacing rate, atrial dissociation from the ventricular paced rhythm occurs. In DDI or DDIR pacing, repetitive episodes of AV dyssynchrony may result from ventricular pacing with retrograde or anterograde P waves marching through the pacing cycle with variable PV relationships.[57, 58] In patients with DDI or DDIR pacemakers implanted following AV node–His bundle ablation for paroxysmal atrial arrhythmias, the DDI and DDIR pacing modes offer the advantage of avoiding tracking of the atrial arrhythmias at the programmed upper rate. However, when the patient is not in atrial fibrillation or flutter, he or she may experience relatively long and intolerable periods of AV dyssynchrony if the sinus rate exceeds the programmed lower or sensor-determined rate.

AV dyssynchrony may also occur during DDD pacing with rate-smoothing or fallback, programmable features available in some DDD and DDDR pacemakers (CPI Delta and Precept, Intermedics Relay). Rate-smoothing is designed to eliminate pronounced variations in paced rate due to paroxysmal atrial tachycardias. Rate-smoothing distinguishes between pathologic and physiologic heart rates by analyzing the absolute heart rate and the rate of change. Fallback is a feature that limits the time the ventricular rate remains at the programmed upper rate and may also be useful in patients who cannot tolerate a sustained upper rate due to paroxysmal palpitations or angina (see Chapter 31). Fallback and rate-smoothing may both give rise to AV dyssynchrony as the ventricular paced rate is being altered.[59]

The Intermedics Relay DDDR pacemaker (Intermedics, Freeport, TX) responds to "nonphysiologic" atrial rates by a sudden change in the pacing rate *without* a change in pacing mode.[60] This response is termed the conditional ven-

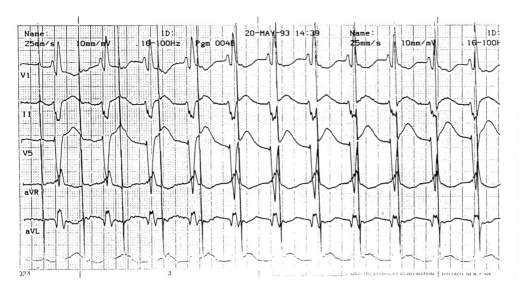

FIGURE 25–7. AAIR pacemaker recording in a patient receiving beta-blockers who developed pacemaker syndrome while walking. His heart rate increased from 70 to 90 bpm and his paced atrial to sensed QRS (AR) interval increased from 180 msec to more than 500 msec, resulting in shortness of breath. Discontinuing beta-blockers and reprogramming the pacemaker to a less "aggressive" slope resulted in a much shorter prolongation of the AR interval with exercise.

tricular tracking limit (CVTL). This algorithm thus limits the paced ventricular rate when the sensor determines that the atrial rate is nonphysiologic (see Chapter 16). The CVTL is 35 bpm above the lower rate. If the sensor determines that the sensed atrial rate is faster than the CVTL, the ventricular response is limited to the CVTL rate. This algorithm is more accurately considered an advanced fallback system, receiving input from both the atrium and the sensor. Pacemaker syndrome may arise in patients if at the end of exercise, with the abrupt loss of sensor input, a persistent increase in sinus rate results in activation of the CVTL algorithm, leading to loss of AV synchrony.

The Meta 1250 DDDR (Telectronics) utilizes an algorithm that allows mode switching from DDDR to VVIR pacing when successive atrial sensed events fall within the postventricular atrial refractory period (PVARP) but outside the 100-msec absolute atrial refractory period (Fig. 25–9).[60, 61] To avoid excessive mode switching, a number of cycles without a P wave during the PVARP are required before the pace-

maker switches back to DDDR pacing. The VVIR pacing mode is temporary and was designed to avoid dual-chamber pacing during atrial fibrillation. AV dissociation leads to AV dyssynchrony, and pacemaker syndrome may occur if mode switching occurs during sinus tachycardia, premature atrial ectopic beats, far-field sensing of the R or T wave in the atrial channel, and PVCs with long retrograde VA conduction times. Programming factors that may precipitate mode switching have been shown to be a low rate-response factor, a low upper rate setting, a long base PVARP, and a long AV delay (see Chapter 12).[61] In some patients up to 50% of the time was spent with VVIR pacing instead of with DDDR pacing. The authors recommended that until further improvements in the mode-switching algorithm become available, patients with intact sinus node function who are at risk for inappropriate mode switching should be programmed to the DDD mode.

In the DDD mode, pacemaker-mediated or endless loop tachycardia occurs whenever a retrograde P wave occurs after the PVARP is sensed. This occurs after a loss of atrial sensing, failure to capture the atrium, or a PVC with retrograde conduction when a short PVARP is programmed. Pacemaker-mediated tachycardia may then result with ventricular pacing at or below the programmed lower rate as long as retrograde conduction is maintained. Pacemaker-mediated tachycardia is relatively uncommon today, however, because of the many programmable values for the PVARP and other features such as automatic extension of the PVARP following a PVC (see Chapters 31 and 33). Pacemaker syndrome, a result of AV dyssynchrony, can also occur when long AV intervals and PVARPs are programmed. This limits the maximal tracking rate. If after exercise a patient subsequently goes into 2:1 AV block, a marked decrease in cardiac output ensues. In this case, pacemaker syndrome results from the decrease in cardiac output and is treated by shortening the AV and PVARP intervals to allow tracking at higher rates.

A DDD pacemaker senses from a site in the right atrium and paces from the right ventricle; however, the timing relationships on the left side of the heart determine the hemodynamic performance. Wish and colleagues[63] performed M mode echocardiograms to determine the optimal left atrial

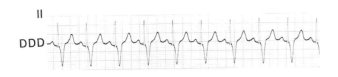

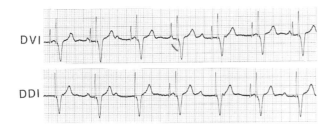

FIGURE 25–8. Demonstration of transient periods of AV dyssynchrony during DVI and DDI pacing in a patient whose atrial rate is above the programmed lower rate. AV dyssynchrony may be present for relatively long periods of time with this pacing mode. In the DVI pacing mode, there is no atrial sensing or tracking, whereas in the DDI mode sensed P waves inhibit atrial pacing, but there is no tracking of P waves.

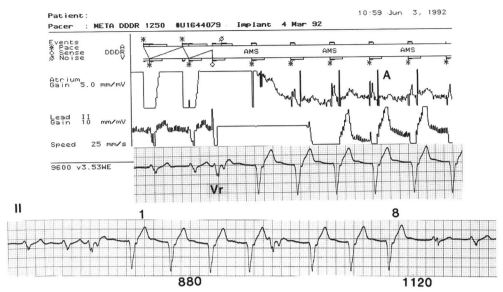

FIGURE 25–9. Automatic mode switching (AMS) and the retrograde sequence triggered by a ventricular extrasystole with the Meta DDDR device, programmed to the DDDR mode. There is bipolar atrial and ventricular sensing. The Telectronics 9600 programmer printout of the event recording demonstrates atrial pacing and the sensed ventricular extrasystole with retrograde conduction causing AMS, which continues because of retrograde atrial depolarization (A) following ventricular pacing. The symbol ø denotes the sensing of noise or atrial electric activity within the PVARP; if this is appropriately timed it will trigger AMS. There are three ECG recordings, all of lead II. The top two are simultaneous recordings, one from the programmer and the other a high-quality surface recording. They demonstrate atrial and ventricular (fusion) pacing, the ventricular extrasystole (Vr) and ventricular pacing with retrograde P waves. The bottom nonsimultaneous ECG recording demonstrates the 8-beat sequence with the terminal 240 msec extension of the atrial escape or pacemaker VA interval. Following the ventricular ectopic beat, AMS is triggered for 8 ventricular paced beats provided that retrograde conduction occurs. Note that a sensed ventricular ectopic beat is included in the count because it too has retrograde conduction. After the eighth beat, the pacemaker VA interval is extended from 880 msec to 1120 msec, allowing atrial pacing (or atrial sensing) to occur and break the retrograde sequence. (From Mond H: Mode switching. In Barold SS, Mujica J [eds]: New Perspectives in Cardiac Pacing 3. Mt Kisco, NY, Futura Publishing Co., 1992.)

timing in patients with dual-chamber pacemakers. They showed that pacemakers should automatically shorten the AV delay when the pacing mode switches from atrial pacing to atrial sensing. These investigations also demonstrated that there was considerable variation in interatrial conduction delays, and in the presence of long interatrial conduction times (e.g., >150 msec), a programmed AV delay of 150 msec could result in left atrial activity occurring after the ventricular pacing spike. Poorly timed left atrial activity leads to a lower stroke volume and no sequential atrial and ventricular activity. One may hypothesize that the presence of severe atrial disease or antiarrhythmic drugs can result in increased latency between the pacing spike and atrial activation as well as slower interatrial conduction times resulting in the development of pacemaker syndrome despite the presence of apparently normal DDD pacemaker function. A case of pacemaker syndrome was reported by Toressani and associates[58] in a patient with hypersensitive carotid sinus syndrome when the AV interval was programmed to less than 100 msec.

Prevention

Pacemaker syndrome is a preventable condition that can be avoided when the correct type of pacemaker is implanted and appropriately programmed. The British Pacing and Electrophysiology Group, in an important position paper on pacemaker choice and pacemaker mode, recommended that "the atrium be paced and sensed unless contraindicated.[64] The only indication for VVI and VVIR pacing modes is the presence of chronic atrial fibrillation or flutter and a slow

ventricular response. A VVI pacemaker programmed to a lower rate may be justifiable in the occasional patient with rare transient episodes of bradycardia. Another instance when a VVI pacemaker may be indicated is in an elderly, inactive or incapacitated, bedridden patient with a short life expectancy. Otherwise, dual-chamber or atrial pacing should be the mode of choice for permanent pacing in the majority of patients. Furthermore, the pacemaker should be programmed to avoid development of AV dyssynchrony.

Treatment

The treatment of pacemaker syndrome is straightforward. Once the diagnosis has been made, symptoms may be ameliorated by switching from single-chamber ventricular pacing to dual-chamber AV synchronous pacing (Table 25–4). In patients with AAI or AAIR pacing and long AR intervals, symptoms will resolve after a ventricular lead has been implanted and upgrade to a dual-chamber pacemaker with AV intervals shorter than 200 to 250 msec has been completed. It is important to note that many third-party payers require documentation of pacemaker syndrome, which can be done by performing Doppler measurement of cardiac output, ocular plethysmography, pulmonary artery catheterization for measurement of the right and left heart pressures, or blood pressure measurement in the supine and upright positions during ventricular pacing and sinus rhythm (e.g., for sick sinus syndrome) or dual-chamber pacing (e.g., for complete heart block). Other, less commonly used diagnostic techniques include measurement of finger pulse amplitude and

TABLE 25–4. TREATMENT OF PACEMAKER SYNDROME

Avoid problem by ensuring appropriate selection of pacemaker and optimal programming

Make diagnosis by maintaining a high level of suspicion

Document symptoms of AV dyssynchrony by recording blood pressure measurements, transtelephonic event monitoring, Holter monitoring, Doppler measurement of stroke volume, or other objective testing

Upgrade from VVIR to DDDR pacemaker by implanting atrial lead; ensure appropriate programming

Decrease lower rate or program hysteresis to decrease frequency of VVI pacing if upgrade to DDD is not possible or is not selected

Begin trial of antiarrhythmic drugs to eliminate retrograde conduction in selected cases

Begin trial of theophylline to increase sinus rate and improve AV nodal conduction to decrease frequency and duration of ventricular pacing or AV dyssynchrony

Schedule explantation if indictions are unclear of if there are minimal symptoms from bradycardia

cardiopulmonary exercise testing. Clearly, it is preferable to identify which patients are at risk for developing pacemaker syndrome by carefully evaluating candidates for VVIR pacing prior to pacemaker implantation.

In some patients with relatively mild pacemaker syndrome and sick sinus syndrome, other potential alternatives should be explored. First, the lower rate of the VVIR pacemaker can be decreased to limit the amount of time spent pacing the ventricle. This can also be accomplished by programming hysteresis on. Hysteresis allows initiation of ventricular pacing only after a pause longer than the programmed lower rate. A second strategy in these patients is to prescribe low-dose theophylline to increase sinus node automaticity, thereby indirectly leading to less ventricular pacing. Antiarrhythmic drugs may be used to block retrograde VA conduction, which may lead to better tolerance of ventricular pacing. Both of these approaches are probably most applicable in mildly symptomatic patients or elderly patients who may be unenthusiastic about undergoing another surgical procedure for pacemaker upgrade. Finally, in the rare patients who are very symptomatic with pacemaker syndrome, the original indications for pacemaker implantation may be unclear or undocumented. It is conceivable that these rare patients might best be managed by pacemaker explantation.

In summary, pacemaker syndrome is a common and often overlooked clinical problem in patients in whom pacing or programming is suboptimal. Careful attention to the patient's symptoms and programmed mode and parameters will help avoid suboptimal pacemaker therapy.

REFERENCES

1. Mitsui T, Hori M, Suma K, et al: The "pacemaking syndrome." *In* Jacobs JE (ed): Proceedings of the Eighth Annual International Conference on Medical and Biological Engineering. Chicago, Association for the Advancement of Medical Instrumentation, 1969, pp 29–33.
2. Haas JM, Strait GB: Pacemaker-induced cardiovascular failure. Am J Cardiol 33:295, 1974.
3. Patel AK, Yap VU, Thomsen JH: Adverse effects of right ventricular pacing in a patient with aortic stenosis: Hemodynamic documentation and management. Chest 72:103, 1977.
4. Edhag O, Fagrell B, Lagergren H: Deleterious effects of cardiac pacing in a patient with mitral insufficiency. Acta Med Scand 202:331, 1977.
5. Ausubel K, Furman S: The pacemaker syndrome. Ann Intern Med 103:420, 1985.
6. Travill CM, Sutton R: Pacemaker syndrome: An iatrogenic condition. Br Heart J 68:163, 1992.
7. Nishimura RA, Gersh BJ, Vliestra RE, et al: Hemodynamic and symptomatic consequences of ventricular pacing. PACE 5:903, 1982.
8. Heldman D, Mulvihill D, Nguyen H, et al: True incidence of pacemaker syndrome. PACE 13:1742, 1990.
9. Sulke N, Chambers J, Dritsas A, et al: A randomized double-blind crossover comparison of four rate-responsive pacing modes. J Am Coll Cardiol 17:696, 1991.
10. Sulke N, Dritsas A, Bostock J, et al: "Subclinical" pacemaker syndrome: A randomized study of symptom-free patients with ventricular demand (VVI) pacemakers upgraded to dual-chamber devices. Br Heart J 67:57, 1992.
11. Reynolds DW: Hemodynamics of cardiac pacing. *In* Ellenbogen KA (ed): Cardiac Pacing. Boston, Blackwell Scientific, 1992, pp 120–161.
12. Levine PA, Mace RC: Pacing Therapy: A Guide to Cardiac Pacing for Optimum Hemodynamic Benefit. Mt Kisco, NY, Futura, 1983, pp 3–18.
13. Cohen SI, Frank HA: Preservation of active atrial transport: An important clinical consideration in cardiac pacing. Chest 81:51, 1982.
14. Miller M, Fox S, Jenkins R, et al: Pacemaker syndrome: A non-invasive means to its diagnosis and treatment. PACE 4:503, 1981.
15. Pearson AC, Janosik DL, Redd RM, et al: Hemodynamic benefit of atrioventricular synchrony: Prediction from baseline Doppler echocardiographic variables. J Am Coll Cardiol 13:1613, 1989.
16. Stewart WJ, Dicola VC, Hawthorne JW, et al: Doppler ultrasound measurement of cardiac output in patients with physiologic pacemakers. Am J Cardiol 54:308, 1984.
17. Rediker DE, Eagle KA, Homma S, et al: Clinical and hemodynamic comparison of VVI versus DDD pacing in patients with DDD pacemakers. Am J Cardiol 61:323, 1988.
18. Erlebacher JA, Danner RL, Stelzer PE: Hypotension with ventricular pacing: An atrial vasodepressor reflex in human beings. J Am Coll Cardiol 4:550, 1984.
19. Baig MW, Perrins EJ: The hemodynamics of cardiac pacing: Clinical and physiological aspects. Prog Cardiovasc Dis 33:283, 1991.
20. Mitchell JH, Gilmore JP, Sarnoff SJ: The transport function of the atrium: Factors influencing the relation between mean left atrial pressures and left ventricular end-diastolic pressure. Am J Cardiol 9:237, 1962.
21. Samet P, Castillo C, Bernstein WH: Hemodynamic consequences of sequential atrioventricular pacing: Subjects with normal hearts. Am J Cardiol 21:207, 1968.
22. Greenberg B, Chatterjee K, Parmley WW, et al: The influence of left ventricular filling pressure on atrial contribution to cardiac output. Am Heart J 98:742, 1979.
23. Buckingham TA, Janosik DL, Pearson AC: Pacemaker hemodynamics: Clinical implications. Prog Cardiovasc Dis 34:347, 1992.
24. Reynolds DW, Wilson MF, Burow RD, et al: Hemodynamic evaluation of atrioventricular sequential vs. ventricular pacing in patients with normal and poor ventricular function at variable heart rates and posture. J Am Coll Cardiol 1:636, 1983.
25. Mukharji J, Rehr R, Hastillo A, et al: Comparison of atrial contribution to cardiac hemodynamics in patients with normal and severely compromised cardiac function. Clin Cardiol 13:639, 1990.
26. Ellenbogen KA, Thames MD, Mohanty PK: New insights into pacemaker syndrome gained from hemodynamic, humoral, and vascular responses during ventriculoatrial pacing. Am J Cardiol 65:53, 1990.
27. Ogawa S, Dreifus LS, Shenoy PN, et al: Hemodynamic consequences of atrioventricular and ventriculoatrial pacing. PACE 1:8, 1978.
28. Rosenqvist M, Isaaz K, Botvinick EH, et al: Relative importance of activation sequence compared to atrioventricular synchrony in left ventricular function. Am J Cardiol 67:148, 1991.
29. Askenazi J, Alexander JH, Koenigsberg DI, et al: Alteration of left ventricular performance by left bundle branch block simulated with atrioventricular sequential pacing. Am J Cardiol 53:99, 1984.
30. Morgan DE, Norman R, West RO, et al: Echocardiographic assessment of tricuspid regurgitation during ventricular demand pacing. Am J Cardiol 58:1025, 1986.
31. Furman S, Cooper JA: Atrial fibrillation during AV-sequential pacing. PACE 5:133, 1982.
32. Naito M, Dreifus LS, Mardelli TJ, et al: Echocardiographic features of atrioventricular and ventriculoatrial conduction. Am J Cardiol 46:625, 1980.
33. Akhtar M: Retrograde conduction in man. PACE 4:548, 1981.

34. Hayes DL, Furman S: Atrioventricular and ventriculoatrial conduction times in patients undergoing pacemaker implant. PACE 6:38, 1983.

35. Webb CR, Spielman SR, Greenspan AM, et al: Improved method for evaluating ventriculoatrial conduction before implantation of atrial-sensing dual-chamber pacemakers. J Am Coll Cardiol 5:1395, 1985.

36. Mahmud R, Denker S, Lehmann M, et al: Functional characteristics of retrograde conduction in a pacing model of "endless loop tachycardia." J Am Coll Cardiol 3:1488, 1984.

37. Akhtar M, Gilbert C, Mahmud R, et al: Pacemaker-mediated tachycardia: Underlying mechanisms, relationship to ventriculoatrial conduction characteristics, and management. Clin Prog 3:90, 1985.

38. Hainsworth R: Atrial receptors in reflex control of the circulation. *In* Zucker IH, Gilmore JP (eds): Reflex Control of the Circulation. Boca Raton, FL, CRC Press, 1991, pp 273–290.

39. Mary DASG: Electrophysiology of atrial receptors. *In* Hainsworth R, McGregor KH, Mary DASG (eds): Cardiogenic Reflexes. Oxford, Oxford Scientific, 1987, pp 3–11.

40. Alicandri C, Fouad F, Farazi RC, et al: Three cases of hypotension and syncope with ventricular pacing: Possible role of atrial reflexes. Am J Cardiol 42:137, 1978.

41. Witte J, Bundke H, Muller S: The pacemaker syndrome: A hemodynamic complication of ventricular pacing. Cor Vasa 30:393, 1988.

42. Ellenbogen KA, Wood MA, Stambler B: Pacemaker syndrome: Clinical, hemodynamic, and neurohumoral features. *In* Barold SS, Mugica J (eds): New Perspectives in Cardiac Pacing 3. Mt Kisco, NY, Futura, 1993, pp 85–112.

43. Hull RW, Snow F, Herre J, et al: The plasma catecholamine responses to ventricular pacing: Implications for rate-responsive pacing. PACE 13:1408, 1990.

44. Pehrrson SK, Hjemdahl P, Nordlander R, et al: A comparison of sympathoadrenal activity and cardiac performance at rest and during exercise in patients with ventricular demand or atrial synchronous pacing. Br Heart J 60:212, 1988.

45. Oldroyd RG, Rae AP, Carter R, et al: Double-blind crossover comparison of the effects of dual-chamber pacing (DDD) and ventricular rate-adaptive (VVIR) pacing on neuroendocrine variables, exercise performance, and symptoms in complete heart block. Br Heart J 65:188, 1991.

46. Bishop VS, Haywood JR: Hormonal control of cardiovascular reflexes. *In* Zucker IH, Gilmore JP (eds): Reflex Control of the Circulation. Boca Raton, FL, CRC Press, 1991, pp 253–271.

47. Stangl K, Weil J, Seitz K, et al: Influence of AV synchrony on the plasma level of atrial natriuretic peptide (ANP) in patients with total AV block. PACE 11:1176, 1988.

48. Ellenbogen, KA, Kapadia K, Walsh M, et al: Increase in plasma atrial natriuretic factor during ventriculoatrial pacing. Am J Cardiol 64:236, 1989.

49. Blanc JJ, Mansourati J, Ritter P, et al: Atrial natriuretic factor release

50. during exercise in patients successively paced in DDD and rate matched ventricular pacing. PACE 15:397, 1992.

50. Vardas PE, Travill CM, Williams TDM, et al: Effect of dual-chamber pacing on raised plasma atrial natriuretic peptide concentrations in complete atrioventricular block. Br Med J 296:94, 1988.

51. Noll B, Krappe J, Goke B, et al: Influence of pacing mode and rate on peripheral levels of atrial natriuretic peptide (ANF). PACE 12:1763, 1989.

52. Travail CM, Williams TDW, Vardas P, et al: Pacemaker syndrome is associated with very high plasma concentrations of atrial natriuretic peptide (ANF). J Am Coll Cardiol 13:111, 1989.

52b. Clemo HF, Baumgarten CM, Stambler BS, et al: Atrial natriuretic factor: Implications for cardiac pacing and electrophysiology. PACE 17:70, 1994.

53. Barold SS: Repetitive reentrant and non-reentrant ventriculoatrial synchrony in dual-chamber pacing. Clin Cardiol 14:754, 1991.

54. Den Dulk K, Lindemands FW, Brugada P, et al: Pacemaker syndrome with AAI rate variable pacing: Importance of atrioventricular conduction properties, medication, and pacemaker programmability. PACE 11:1226, 1988.

55. Levine PA, Seltzer JP, Pirzada FA: The "pacemaker syndrome": In a properly functioning physiologic pacing system. PACE 6:279, 1983.

56. Curzio G, and the Multicenter Study Group: A multicenter evaluation of single-pass lead VDD pacing system. PACE 14:434, 1991.

57. Cunningham TM: Pacemaker syndrome due to retrograde conduction in a DDI pacemaker. Am Heart J 115:478, 1988.

58. Torresani J, Ebagosti A, Allard-Latour G: Pacemaker syndrome with DDD pacing. PACE 7:1148, 1984.

59. Barold SS, Falkoff MD, Ong LS, et al: Upper rate response of DDD pacemakers. *In* Barold SS, Mugica J (eds): New Perspectives on Cardiac Pacing. Mt Kisco, NY, Futura, 1988, pp 121–172.

60. Barold SS, Mond HG: Optimal antibradycardia pacing in patients with paroxysmal supraventricular tachyarrhythmias: Role of fallback and automatic mode-switching mechanisms. *In* Barold SS, Mugica J (eds): New Perspectives in Cardiac Pacing 3. Mt Kisco, NY, Futura, 1993, pp 483–518.

61. Pitney MR, May CD, Davis MJ: Undesirable mode switching with a dual-chamber rate-responsive pacemaker. PACE 16:729, 1993.

62. Wish M, Fletcher RD, Gottdiener JS, et al: Importance of left atrial timing in the programming of dual-chamber pacemakers. Am J Cardiol 60:566, 1982.

63. Wish M, Gottdiener JS, Cohen AL, et al: Use of M mode echocardiograms for determination of optimal left atrial timing in patients with dual-chamber pacemakers. PACE 9:290, 1986.

64. Clarke M, Sutton R, Ward D, et al: Pacemaker prescription for symptomatic bradycardia: Report of a working party of the British Pacing and Electrophysiology Group. Br Heart J 66:185, 1991.

CHAPTER 26

CARDIAC CHRONOTROPIC RESPONSIVENESS

Bruce L. Wilkoff

God, as described in the biblical account of Genesis, gave humans the challenge of naming and measuring all that is on the earth. Subsequently, we have been occupied with nomenclature, descriptions, and definitions of every type. Even so, description of the normal and pathologic cardiac chronotropic responses to exertion began only in the 20th century after the development of sensor-driven rate-modulated pacemakers. This chapter provides the historical, physiologic, and practical context by which the concept of chronotropic responsiveness can be applied to patients with and under consideration for rate-modulated pacemakers.

History of Exercise Testing

Monitored exertion for the purpose of clinical or physiologic evaluation is a 20th century phenomenon. The initial descriptions of electrocardiographic (ECG) changes during exercise were made by Bousfield in 1918.[1] Ten years later, Feil and Siegel produced a pivotal observation when they documented the fact that exertion could produce pain and ST changes that resolved with rest.[2] Maximal stress testing by climbing stairs was first advocated by Missal in 1938 but was not widely accepted until 1955, when Master and his coworkers simplified the procedure.[3] The Master's step test was the first protocol specifically proposed as a means of evaluating functional capacity, including measurements of heart rate and blood pressure.[4, 5]

Further developments were necessary to overcome the limitations of low exercise intensity and the inability to observe the subject's heart rate and ECG during stress. In 1956, Robert Bruce described a treadmill stress test that categorized patients according to their New York Heart Association

(NYHA) class.[6] During the same decade, Astrand and Rhyming teamed up and established the progressive exercise test as a tool for physiologic evaluation.[7] They observed that maximal oxygen uptake, or aerobic capacity, is correlated with maximal heart rate during maximal exercise.[7] This foundational concept has become the basis for the development and evaluation of rate-modulated pacemakers. Balke and Ware added to these developments by producing a method of estimating oxygen uptake during treadmill exertion.[8] At about the same time, Hellerstein and Hornsten safely applied treadmill exercise to patients who had had a myocardial infarction. This initiated the concept of cardiac rehabilitation and sending cardiac patients back to work.[9] Since that time, coronary artery disease has clearly dominated the development of exercise testing. Exercise stress testing today continues to be used primarily in the screening and management of patients with coronary artery disease. Applications include the physiologic assessment of angiographic lesions, detection of postinterventional restenosis, response to medical therapy, postmyocardial infarction risk stratification, and guiding cardiac rehabilitation exercise prescriptions. Exercise stress testing has also become useful in the assessment of systolic and diastolic cardiac dysfunction, cardiovascular fitness, dyspnea of unclear etiology, exercise-induced arrhythmias, cardiac disability, valvular heart diseases, aortic outflow tract obstruction in hypertrophic cardiomyopathy, and evaluation of chronotropic responsiveness.

History of Chronotropic Evaluation

Originally used for descriptive purposes in the study of exercise physiology, the recording of heart rate during clinical exercise testing has become a standard procedure. As maximal exercise testing became routine, the normal maximal heart rate response during exertion was determined to be an age-related value. Although frequently calculated as 220 minus age, the origin of this accurate formula for the maximal predicted heart rate (MPHR) is obscure. This unquestionably useful calculation provides the most frequent measure of maximal exertional effort, reaching 85% of MPHR. In addition to effort, the chronotropic response has been viewed predominantly in terms of the patient's ability or inability to reach the MPHR during maximal exertion. Rate-modulated pacemaker technology has provided the impetus for the development of methods of evaluating the appropriateness of heart rate response for submaximal exertion, specifically in the range of activities of daily living. The premise has developed that if a pacemaker is to respond at a specific rate with a certain amount of sensor stimulation, a predetermined rate must be specified as being appropriate for that amount of exertion.[10] Despite the attractiveness and relative simplicity of this approach, other factors, including patient symptoms, other diseases, and impact on device longevity, also need to be calculated. Therefore, the techniques discussed in this chapter must be considered preliminary and descriptive rather than definitive.

Relation of Heart Rate to Hemodynamics

The delivery of oxygen for metabolism by the tissues in adequate quantity is the bottom-line principle in the evaluation of clinical hemodynamics. Factors affecting this process are multiple, including inspired FiO_2, alveolar gas exchange, respiratory muscle mechanics, pulmonary vascular resistance, systemic regional blood flow shifts, and oxygen-carrying capacity, which in turn is affected by hemoglobin concentration, hemoglobinopathies, and local tissue factors. Certainly the heart's ability to generate cardiac output and its appropriate rise with exercise is central to the principle of oxygen delivery and is the core of this chapter.

Cardiac output is the product of heart rate and stroke volume. Augmentation of these two factors during exertion is produced by reduced parasympathetic and increased sympathetic activity, increased circulating catecholamines, the Bainbridge reflex (increased venous return producing right atrial distention), increased myocardial contractility, and probably also a drop in left ventricular afterload. During low-intensity exercise, both a rise in stroke volume and a rise in heart rate contribute to the increase in cardiac output. Above heart rates of 110 to 120 bpm there are no further increases in stroke volume. Therefore, heart rate alone contributes to further elevations in the cardiac output. Throughout exercise, heart rate increments are linearly related to increases in maximal ventilatory oxygen uptake ($\dot{V}O_2$).[11] Near peak exercise, an increase in oxygen extraction provides the major adaptive mechanism. The heart rate increments continue but tend to level off. The anaerobic threshold is crossed when oxygen demand exceeds supply and further activity is accomplished at the expense of lactate accumulation. Sometimes, depending on the condition of the ventricles and valves, stroke volume decreases as heart rate increases. The net result can

be an undesirable reduction in cardiac output with increased heart rate and myocardial oxygen consumption.

The capacity to increase oxygen delivery is designated the oxygen delivery reserve. To achieve this increase in oxygen delivery, the changes in cardiac output and oxygen extraction are multiplied. Normally, the cardiac output reserve is 6 times the baseline value. In an athletic subject it rises from 5 to 6 L/min at baseline to about 36 L/min during maximal exercise. Arterial oxygen saturation is about 95%. Owing to oxygen consumption, this drops to a mixed venous oxygen saturation of 75% under resting conditions. During exertion, oxygen extraction triples and yields a mixed venous oxygen percentage saturation of 35%. Therefore, the total oxygen delivery reserve is the oxygen delivery reserve times the cardiac output reserve, or 3×6, which yields 18 times the baseline oxygen delivery. Because heart rate is only one factor in the equation governing exercise capacity, the role played by each factor in any given patient's symptoms can become quite confusing. Furthermore, resting cardiac output, ejection fraction, and left ventricular filling pressure do not correlate well with $\dot{V}O_2$max and therefore fail to reliably predict cardiac output reserve. Estimates of heart size by chest radiograph and echocardiography also correlate poorly with cardiac output and thus with oxygen delivery reserve.[12]

Problems and Assumptions

To assess adequately any patient's chronotropic response to the metabolic stress of exercise, the patient and testing environment must be free from confounding variables that may alter the heart rate response. The presence of fever, active infection, emotional stress, pain, metabolic derangements, severe anemia, dehydration, or a hot testing environment all may contribute to a premature and excessive rise in chronotropic response for any given level of exercise. Likewise, the pharmacologic milieu, including the presence of beta-blocking agents, blunts the intrinsic chronotropic response. Absolute contraindications to chronotropic exercise testing are the same as those used for any exercise test and include the acute stage of myocardial infarction, unstable angina, severe aortic stenosis, severe hypertension, acute systemic illness, and uncompensated congestive heart failure. Care should be taken to choose an exercise testing situation within the musculoskeletal ability of the patient. The quality of the testing environment will affect the interpretability of the response.

Clinical end-points for exercise testing usually assume a normal chronotropic response. However, achievement of a heart rate response above or below 85% of the maximally predicted heart rate for age at maximal exertion does not always indicate an inappropriate chronotropic response. On the other hand, chronotropic abnormalities disqualify heart rate as the variable used to determine the end-point of the exertional assessment. Unrealistic expectations by the observer can produce evaluations that produce misleading conclusions about the cardiopulmonary response.

The anaerobic threshold has been defined as the oxygen uptake prior to the systematic increase in the ventilatory equivalent for oxygen ($\dot{V}E/\dot{V}O_2$) without a concomitant increase in the ventilatory equivalent for carbon dioxide ($\dot{V}E/\dot{V}CO_2$).[13] However, recent publications have cast doubt on both the validity of this concept and the relationship between blood lactate levels and gas exchange indices of the anaerobic threshold.[14, 15] Because of this, it is preferable to call the oxygen uptake prior to the increase in $\dot{V}E/\dot{V}CO_2$ the ventilatory threshold.[16] Simple exercise testing, which monitors only heart rate and blood pressure, does not detect when the patient's anaerobic threshold is crossed or measure the magnitude of the subject's effort. In every subject there is a point at which oxygen delivery is outstripped. The crossing of the anaerobic threshold, also termed the lactate or ventilatory threshold, is the most reproducible indicator of this condition. Exercise testing without the collection and measurement of inspired and expired gases relies on estimated oxygen consumption, usually recorded as METs (calculated metabolic equivalents). This estimate assumes the presence of normal physiology and tends to overestimate the measured or actual METs achieved during metabolic stress testing, which is used for testing patients with left ventricular dysfunction and ischemic heart disease.

Cardiac Chronotropism

Although there is a tremendous desire on the part of physicians, pacemaker manufacturers, and the Food and Drug Administration to define chronotropic incompetence, we must first be able to recognize chronotropic competence. This is a fundamental issue that is not easily solved. Although age-related maximally predicted heart rates have been recognized since the 1950s, assessment of heart rate at submaximal exercise intensities is poorly defined. Until recently, chronotropic insufficiency has been defined mainly as an inability to achieve an age-specific maximally predicted heart rate. In 1991, the American College of Cardiology and the American Heart Association published a joint paper that indicated that rate-modulated pacemakers are used appropriately in patients who fail to achieve a heart rate of 100 bpm at maximal exertion.[17] Although this definition may be high in specificity, it is quite lacking in sensitivity, failing to account for age or other clinical characteristics. Because rate response is not the only indication for or benefit to be derived from rate-modulated pacemakers, the application of this standard would prevent the beneficial use of pacemakers in many individuals. Another reasonable method uses a statistical approach, defining age- and protocol-specific heart rate responses in terms of one and two standard deviations around a mean heart rate for each stage. Ellestad and Wan used such an approach, defining mild chronotropic incompetence as one standard deviation below the mean heart rate and more severe chronotropic incompetence as two standard deviations below the mean heart rate. In doing so, they coined the term chronotropic incompetence.[18]

Normal Chronotropic Response

Cardiac output, in a normally adaptive individual, varies directly in proportion to oxygen consumption ($\dot{V}O_2$). During exertion, this cardiac output response is produced by a cooperative rise in heart rate, sympathetic stimulation, and use of the Frank-Starling mechanism. Augmentation of cardiac output during low-intensity exercise is mediated through an increase in both stroke volume and heart rate. However, the

increase in stroke volume soon levels off, and further increases are primarily mediated by heart rate. As the maximal heart rate is approached, the rate of rise of heart rate slows and levels off, producing a linear relationship between $\dot{V}O_2$ and heart rate up to near maximum oxygen consumption.[7]

The trained athlete has a lower resting heart rate and, during progressive exercise testing, a decreased rate of change in heart rate as exercise intensity increases. This produces a lower heart rate at any given level of exercise compared with matched untrained controls. Circulating catecholamines are also lower at any given submaximal exercise load. Sinoatrial node responsiveness to catecholamine stimulation is unaffected by training.[19] The final result, despite relative bradycardia, is that the cardiac output response is preserved and augmented owing to left ventricular hypertrophy and an increase in end-diastolic ventricular volume.

In the average 20-year-old, heart rate increases from 65 bpm at rest to 200 bpm during maximal exercise. The difference between maximal age-predicted heart rate and resting heart rate can be expressed as the heart rate reserve (HRR). The maximal heart rate is age related and reproducible and decreases linearly with advancing age. The resting heart rate is quite variable depending on various factors including autonomic tone, volume status, and environmental temperature. In our laboratory, the resting heart rate in 537 normal subjects was found to be 65 ± 10 bpm.[20] Another, more reproducible measure of a baseline heart rate is the intrinsic heart rate, defined as the resting heart rate during complete pharmacologic autonomic blockade. Total blockade is usually accomplished by administration of intravenous atropine (1 mg) and propranolol (10 mg) and is not only reproducible to within a few beats per minute but also declines linearly with age, similar to the maximal exercise heart rate.[21] Despite its reproducibility, intrinsic heart rate is elevated compared with the measured resting heart rate and therefore is an unattractive index of the "normal" resting heart rate.

At the onset of exercise, heart rate increases within 0.5 second, probably secondary to an abrupt withdrawal of vagal tone. A sawtooth effect has been observed in the first few seconds of exercise. This probably reflects a flux in the autonomic nervous system tone before steady state is again achieved.[22] Bates,[23] in studying cardiac output as a limiting factor on exercise, demonstrated that heart rate, cardiac output, and oxygen consumption increased in a linear fashion up to an oxygen uptake of 1500 mL/min. Above approximately 80% of maximal capacity, both heart rate and cardiac output tended to level off. Further increase in peripheral oxygen consumption was achieved through widening of the arterial-venous oxygen gradient. The overall effect is that submaximal exercise heart rates increase in a linear fashion with $\dot{V}O_2$.

The oxygen uptake of a seated individual is approximately one MET.[24] The term metabolic equivalent (MET) was coined as the quantity of oxygen consumed by the body-inspired air under basal conditions and is equal on the average to 3.5 mL of O_2/kg per minute. Oxygen consumption ($\dot{V}O_2$) can be translated into METs by dividing by 3.5, thus providing a unit-less, convenient, and accurate reference for exercise capacity. MET levels can be used for writing exercise prescriptions and for estimating levels of disability by using tables listing the demands of most common activities[25] (Table 26–1). The maximal MET value minus the baseline or resting MET value is defined as the metabolic reserve (MR). Using

TABLE 26–1. ESTIMATED ENERGY REQUIREMENTS OF SELECTIVE ACTIVITIES[a]

MILD	METs
Baking	2.0
Billiards	2.4
Bookbinding	2.2
Canoeing (leisurely)	2.5
Conducting an orchestra	2.2
Dancing, ballroom (slow)	2.9
Golf (with cart)	2.5
Horseback riding (walking)	2.3
Playing a musical instrument:	
Accordion	1.8
Cello	2.3
Flute	2.0
Horn	1.7
Piano	2.3
Trumpet	1.8
Violin	2.6
Woodwind	1.8
Volleyball (noncompetitive)	2.9
Walking (2 mph)	2.5
Writing	1.7
MODERATE	
Calisthenics (no weights)	4.0
Croquet	3.0
Cycling (leisurely)	3.5
Gardening (no lifting)	4.4
Golf (without cart)	4.9
Mowing lawn (power mower)	3.0
Playing drums	3.8
Sailing	3.0
Swimming (slowly)	4.5
Walking (3 mph)	3.3
Walking (4 mph)	4.5
VIGOROUS	
Badminton	5.5
Chopping wood	4.9
Climbing hills	
No load	6.9
With 5-kg load	7.4
Cycling (moderately)	5.7
Dancing	
Aerobic or ballet	6.0
Ballroom (fast) or square	5.5
Field hockey	7.7
Ice skating	5.5
Jogging (10-minute mile)	10.2
Karate or judo	6.5
Roller skating	6.5
Rope skipping	12.0
Skiing (water or downhill)	6.8
Squash	12.1
Surfing	6.0
Swimming (fast)	7.0
Tennis (doubles)	6.0

[a]These activities can often be done at variable intensities, assuming that the intensity is not excessive and that the courses are flat (no hills) unless so specified. Categories are based on experience of tolerance; if an activity is perceived to be more than indicated, it should be judged accordingly. MET, metabolic equivalent (3.5 mL/kg^{-1}/min^{-1} oxygen uptake).
Reproduced with permission from Fletcher FF, Froelicher VF, Hearley LH, et al: Exercise standards: A statement for health professionals from the American Heart Association. Circulation 82:2307, 1990. Copyright 1990 American Heart Association.

an identical approach, the predicted HRR is defined as the difference between the age-predicted maximal heart rate (220 minus age) and the resting heart rate. Wilkoff and colleagues[26] first described the mathematical relationship be-

tween heart rate and oxygen consumption termed the metabolic chronotropic relation. This mathematical model has now been refined and defines the normal chronotropic response during exercise as being primarily dependent on age, resting heart rate, and peak functional capacity. Previously it had been shown that heart rate is a linear function of oxygen consumption. However, this new model demonstrates that the percentage of HRR achieved during exercise equals the percentage of metabolic reserve achieved when a normally functioning adult exercises on an exercise treadmill. Regardless of the exercise protocol, subjects exhibited a linear rise in the percentage of HRR equal to the percentage of MR. Therefore, the model suggests that when the percentage of HRR is plotted against the percentage of MR, a linear response with a slope of close to 1.0 and a y-intercept of 0.0 is to be expected (Fig. 26–1). This physiologic concept was confirmed by exercising 537 normal adults on one of two exercise protocols. One was the standard Bruce protocol (n = 234), and the other was the chronotropic assessment exercise protocol (CAEP, n = 303) (Table 26–2). Each subject demonstrated this linear relationship despite varying ages, resting heart rates, and peak functional capacities. The mean slope of this relation was 1.058 ± 0.134 with an R^2 value of 0.982 ± 0.016 for the CAEP subjects and 1.044 ± 0.112 with an R^2 value of 0.992 ± 0.012 for the Bruce protocol subjects. The mathematical expression of this metabolic chronotropic relation is expressed as follows:

Eq 1 $\quad HR_{stage} = \dfrac{(220 - age - HR_{rest}) \times (METs_{stage} - 1)}{(METs_{peak} - 1)} + HR_{rest}$

Or, when simplified:

Eq 2 $\quad HR_{stage} = (HRR \times \%MR) + HR_{rest}$

By using this formula, the heart rate achieved at any point of exercise can be classified as consistent or inconsistent with normal chronotropic function. To classify the entire metabolic chronotropic response, the slope of this relation must

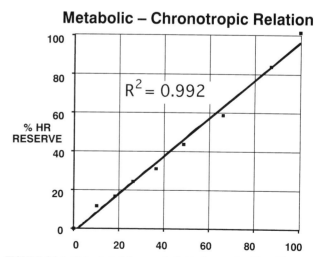

Metabolic – Chronotropic Relation

$R^2 = 0.992$

% HR RESERVE

FIGURE 26–1. Data plotted from an individual normal subject. The metabolic-chronotropic relation (MCR) plots normalized heart rate response (percentage heart rate reserve) versus normalized oxygen consumption (percentage metabolic reserve). The response is linear ($R^2 = 0.992$), with an MCR slope of 1.0 and a y-intercept of 0.0. This response is consistent regardless of age, peak functional capacity, resting heart rate, and exercise protocol for all normal subjects.

TABLE 26–2. CHRONOTROPIC ASSESSMENT EXERCISE PROTOCOL

STAGE	SPEED (MPH)	GRADE (%)	TIME (MIN)	CUMULATIVE TIME	METs
Warmup-Stage 0	1.0	0	—	—	1.5
Stage 1	1.0	2	2.0	2.0	2.0
Stage 2	1.5	3	2.0	4.0	2.8
Stage 3	2.0	4	2.0	6.0	3.6
Stage 4	2.5	5	2.0	8.0	4.6
Stage 5	3.0	6	2.0	10.0	5.8
Stage 6	3.5	8	2.0	12.0	7.5
Stage 7	4.0	10	2.0	14.0	9.6
Stage 8	5.0	10	2.0	16.0	12.1
Stage 9	6.0	10	2.0	18.0	14.3
Stage 10	7.0	10	2.0	20.0	16.5
Stage 11	7.0	15	2.0	22.0	19.0

CAEP was designed to test physiologic and chronotropic responses to exercise at submaximal and maximal exertional levels. Since the protocol incorporates gradual increases in elevation and treadmill velocity, subjects with rate-modulated pacemaker sensors that are sensitive to stepping frequency (i.e., activity sensors) can be compared with other sensor responses. This protocol is well suited for the evaluation of patients with limited functional capacity or mild orthopedic difficulties with treadmill exercise.

be measured and classified as being within the 95% confidence intervals of the normal response (Fig. 26–2).

Chronotropic Dysfunction

ABNORMAL SINUS RHYTHM

When the sinus node is the controlling natural pacemaker, the presumption is that a homeostatic negative feedback loop mechanism metabolically couples cardiac output to need. Abnormal chronotropic function results in a heart rate that is too fast or too slow for the demands of the situation. As an example, tachycardia due to reentrant or automatic focus

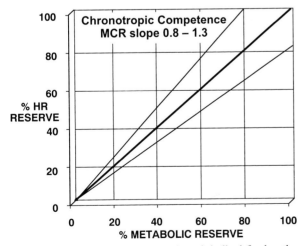

Confidence Intervals

FIGURE 26–2. Chronotropic competence is statistically defined as the response to physical exertion that provides a metabolic chronotropic relation (MCR) slope between 0.8 and 1.3. The normal essential characteristic of the MCR is a y-intercept of 0.0 and a linear MCR slope of 1.0. Instead of calculating the heart rate achieved at a particular level of exertion, the MCR slope provides the best statistical method for identification of chronotropically incompetent patients.

mechanisms is clearly abnormal and represents a situation in which there is an uncoupling between oxygen demand and supply.

Recognition of chronotropic dysfunction is difficult because it is inconsistently manifest as either intermittent or continuous bradycardia and or tachycardia. There may be a sinus pause, a conduction disturbance producing varying degrees of heart block, or a sinus mechanism that is firing too slowly because of intrinsic or extrinsic disease. In many patients bradycardia may be present only at rest, whereas during exertion the response reaches the age-predicted maximal heart rate. However, other subjects with normal resting heart rates demonstrate relative bradycardia during exercise and an inappropriately low maximal heart rate at peak exercise. Finally, some patients have symptoms of dyspnea on exertion and easy fatigability with early exercise, but as they warm up, they are able to perform prolonged exertional tasks without difficulty. This result may be due to an inappropriately slow chronotropic mechanism during early exercise that eventually "warms up." To illustrate these phenomena, 52 subjects with symptomatic sinus node dysfunction that was severe enough to require a permanent pacemaker were tested by treadmill exercise in an effort to define the exertional chronotropic manifestations of this disease.[27] The data were compared with data compiled from 100 normal subjects using the metabolic chronotropic relation analysis described earlier in equations 1 and 2. Despite the need for permanent pacemakers, only 18 of the 52 patients (33%) failed to reach the maximum age-predicted heart rate (Fig. 26–3). These patients also lost the linear response described in normals (Fig. 26–4). Thus, abnormal sinus function can be a periodically manifest problem, sometimes requiring a pacemaker to prevent syncope, sometimes providing a normal linear heart rate response to exercise, and sometimes producing a nonlinear response to exercise.

Although sinus bradycardia can be defined as a sinus rate that is less than 60 bpm, it is not always apparent when a heart rate is inappropriately slow. For example, a well-trained athlete may be asymptomatic with a resting heart rate in the 40s, due in part to an increase in stroke volume. An octogenarian may feel fatigued and washed out with a heart rate in the 50s. Clinically, a significant problem is present when the "bradycardia" produces clinical symptoms.

Sick sinus syndrome, the major cause of a clinically inappropriate chronotropic response, is a collection of various clinical heart rate patterns.[28] These include persistent sinus bradycardia, sinus arrest, sinoatrial node exit block, and the "tachycardia-bradycardia" syndrome. Carotid sinus hypersensitivity (CSH) is usually defined as ventricular asystole lasting at least 3 seconds or a decrease in systolic blood pressure of at least 50 mm Hg after a 5-second carotid sinus massage.[29–31] Carotid sinus syndrome (CSS) refers to symptoms such as bradycardia, dizziness, presyncope, or syncope resulting from hypersensitivity of the carotid sinus reflex.[32] This differentiation is of obvious clinical importance because hypersensitivity is a sign that is found in asymptomatic individuals. CSH may be found in up to 30% of patients with hypertension or ischemic heart disease.[33] The incidence of CSS among patients investigated for syncope is unknown, and the reported numbers vary considerably, from 0.5%[34] to 41%.[35] There is rarely evidence of abnormalities of the sinus node or of chronotropic responsiveness in patients with a

Percent Maximal Predicted Heart Rate
Sinus Node Dysfunction

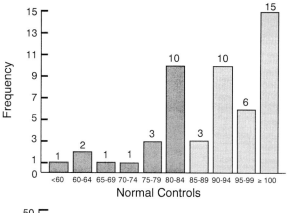

Normal Controls

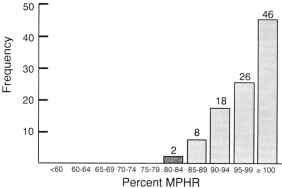

Percent MPHR

FIGURE 26–3. Histogram of the response to exercise of patients with a history of pacemaker implantation for the primary indication of sinus node dysfunction shows that only 33% failed to achieved 85% of the age-predicted maximal heart rate (MPHR). Their response is compared with that of 100 control subjects.

accurate; however, when they are normal or borderline normal, they do not rule out sick sinus syndrome. There is a large overlap between the findings in normal subjects and the findings in subjects with this diagnosis. Furthermore, there are varying degrees of severity of sick sinus syndrome; the natural course is usually progression over time. Because of the various presentations of sick sinus syndrome, the different degrees of severity, and the lack of sensitivity of electrophysiologic testing, exercise stress testing can be a valuable instrument in the evaluation of this condition.

In 1978 Holden and colleagues[40] compared the heart rate response to exercise in seven subjects with sick sinus syndrome with that in seven normal age-matched controls and seven young athletically trained subjects. They found that the subjects with sick sinus syndrome had a lower maximum heart rate and a reduced rate of change of heart rate as exercise intensity increased compared with age-matched control subjects. The sick sinus syndrome subjects did, however, reach a peak oxygen consumption ($\dot{V}O_2$max) that was equivalent to that of age-matched controls but much lower than that reached by well-trained subjects. When the velocity of HRR to exercise in sick sinus syndrome subjects was measured as the change in heart rate versus change in $\dot{V}O_2$ per kilogram, the HRR demonstrated a lower slope than that reached by age-matched controls but equivalent to that seen in the younger well-trained subjects. This suggests that patients with sick sinus syndrome may have circulatory adaptations similar to those seen in well-trained athletes, such as an exaggerated increase in stroke volume with exercise, a widening of the arterial-venous oxygen difference, and an increased efficiency of perfusion to the peripheral exercising muscles.[40] Similar responses have been seen in the dener-

hypersensitive carotid sinus.[36] The pathophysiology of CSH is not clear, and the site of hypersensitivity with the reflex arc is unknown. Denervation-like acetylcholine sensitivity of the efferent limb[37] and, especially, inappropriately high vagal response to baroreceptor stimulation have been proposed as possible explanations. Because up to 70% of patients with CSS may have reflex atrioventricular (AV) block,[31] AAI pacing is obviously contraindicated. VVI pacing should be considered only if preimplantation assessment has confirmed the absence of retrograde ventriculoatrial (VA) conduction and pacemaker syndrome symptomatology.[38] If permanent pacing is chosen, a DDD pacemaker is indicated. If the patient has retrograde conduction with a long VA time, DDI or, ideally, DDIR pacing is advocated.[39]

Very seldom are all of these characteristics present in any one patient, but one or more may be evident. Although most patients with sick sinus syndrome have resting bradycardia, this is not always the case. There are many ways of evaluating patients with suspected sick sinus syndrome, but none has perfect sensitivity and specificity. Although Holter monitoring remains a key tool in correlating symptoms with rhythm disturbances, symptoms and Holter findings are often sporadic and infrequent. Provocative means such as electrophysiologic testing and exercise stress testing are often useful. When these tests are abnormal, they are diagnostically

Sinus Node Dysfunction

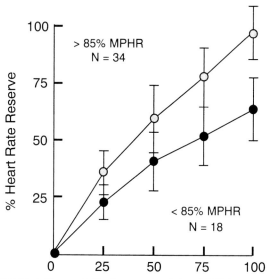

FIGURE 26–4. The metabolic chronotropic relation (MCR) in patients with sinus node dysfunction and pacemakers has been plotted for 18 patients *(dark circles)* who failed to achieve and 34 patients *(shaded circles)* who achieved 85% of the age-predicted maximal heart rate (MPHR) during exercise testing. Note the nonlinear response of both groups.

vated heart[41] as well as in subjects with AV block or during atrial pacing at a fixed rate,[42] in whom the changes in cardiac output are mediated primarily through changes in stroke volume.

Abbott and associates[43] had previously demonstrated in 1977, using 16 subjects with sick sinus syndrome, that individuals with sick sinus syndrome were unable to achieve maximum heart rates comparable to those reached by age- and sex-matched controls. However, their patients attained a lower $\dot{V}O_2$max than their controls, a finding different from the findings of Holden and colleagues.[40] This difference, according to Holden, is most likely attributable to the presence of coexisting heart disease as a confounding variable in 8 of the 16 subjects with sick sinus syndrome in the Abbott study.

Chronotropic incompetence in some individuals is related to ischemic heart disease. These individuals tend to have appropriate resting heart rates but during exercise fail to achieve an adequate heart rate response. Ellestad described a subgroup of patients who, in spite of being deconditioned, had an inadequate heart rate response to stress testing.[44] This has been associated with a poor prognosis.[18] Ellestad also described a 51-year-old man with a similar heart rate response that became normal after successful coronary artery bypass revascularization, implicating ischemia as the major cause of his chronotropic insufficiency.[44] Hinkle and colleagues confirmed this concept when they reported an increased incidence of sudden death in middle-aged men who had "sustained relative bradycardia" in response to exercise and daily activities.[45]

Chin, Ellestad, and their colleagues retrospectively evaluated 25 patients with mild chronotropic insufficiency whose peak heart rate fell 1 standard deviation below the predicted mean for age and sex, and 28 patients with more severe chronotropic incompetence whose peak heart rate fell 2 standard deviations below the predicted mean for age and sex. There were 45 controls. Coronary angiograms were performed in all 98 patients after maximum treadmill exercise testing. Of note is the finding that 72% of the patients with chronotropic incompetence alone without ST-segment depression had significant coronary disease.[46] A prospective study in which coronary angiograms are performed in all patients with chronotropic incompetence has yet to be done to demonstrate the true prevalence of significant coronary disease in this subgroup of patients.

Distinguishing primary chronotropic abnormalities from adaptive or maladaptive responses to various disease states is a significant problem. In a study similar to the one done by Ellestad and his colleagues relating chronotropic dysfunction to ischemia, we compared the chronotropic responses of 48 normal controls to those of 12 patients with severe ventricular dysfunction and no ischemia.[47] These patients had an elevated resting heart rate, a depressed maximal heart rate, and a linear percentage HRR response to exercise (Fig. 26–5). In patients with both ischemia and severe ventricular dysfunction, it can be argued teleologically that the responses that occur are protective, minimizing the opportunity for ischemia and optimizing cardiac output. If this is so, then a rate-modulated pacemaker tuned to produce the "normal" chronotropic response would produce a maladaptive balance. In contrast, it is rare to see a rate-modulated pacemaker produce angina despite the frequent coexistence of coronary artery disease in pacemaker patients over the age of 65.

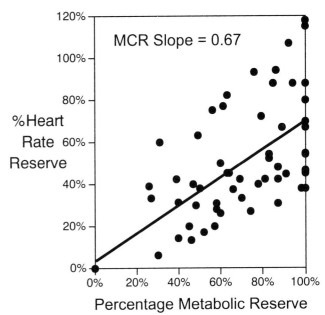

FIGURE 26–5. The metabolic chronotropic response (MCR) is plotted for 12 patients with left ventricular dysfunction who are being considered for cardiomyoplasty. The responses were linear, with a mean MCR slope of 0.67.

ATRIAL FIBRILLATION

Despite many similarities in the exertion-related response of patients with atrial fibrillation to that of subjects with a sinus node abnormality, the chronotropic response is quite different. Some of the similarities include catecholamine release, autonomic response, and an increase in venous return. Each of these factors exerts its major chronotropic influence on the AV node in subjects with atrial fibrillation, whereas the site of action is the sinus node in patients with a sinus mechanism. The sinus node usually functions as the primary natural pacemaker, generating depolarizations at its own autonomous rate and accelerating and decelerating as indicated. The AV node also is capable of functioning as a depolarization-initiating pacemaker but at a slower rate than the sinus node, resulting in a junctional escape rhythm if sinus pauses occur that are long enough. In patients with atrial fibrillation the AV node is not the primary initiator of depolarizations but rather the gatekeeper and conduit, controlling the frequency of depolarization entry into and the rate of transit through the AV node. The rate of repolarization and the effective refractory period are variables that help to determine the rate at which the AV node may conduct impulses to the His-Purkinje system. Furthermore, the pharmacologic milieu of the AV node, specifically AV nodal-depressing drugs, plays a large role in altering the chronotropic response. These drugs are usually present in patients with atrial fibrillation to prevent an inappropriately rapid ventricular response and may also occasionally influence sinoatrial node activity in subjects with normal sinus rhythm and paroxysmal atrial fibrillation.

Early work in evaluating the heart rate response to exercise in atrial fibrillation was described by Knox in 1949.[47a] Using the step test as the mode of exercise, several important ob-

TABLE 26–3. **CHRONOTROPIC ABNORMALITIES OF ATRIAL FIBRILLATION PATIENTS DURING EXERCISE**[a]

	EARLY STAGE	LATE STAGE	EITHER STAGE	BOTH STAGES	NEITHER STAGE
Slow	21	53	58	16	42
Fast	74	32	74	32	26
Normal	5	16	21	0	79
Slow or Fast	95	84	100	21	0

[a]Data expressed as percentage.

The chronotropic response of patients with pacemakers due to inadequate heart rate during atrial fibrillation is divided into quartiles. The early stage represents exercise at 25% and 50% of metabolic reserve. The late stage represents chronotropic responsiveness at 75% and 100% of metabolic reserve. All patients demonstrated inappropriate chronotropic responsiveness during exercise.

From Corbelli R, Masterson M, Wilkoff BL: Chronotropic response to exercise in patients with atrial fibrillation. PACE 13:179, 1990.

servations were made. At first, the heart rate falls in comparison with the pretest value, unlike the normal anticipatory response to heart rate acceleration. Second, a delayed acceleration occurs in very early exercise, followed by an exaggerated heart rate response. Last, prolonged tachycardia persists well into the recovery period.

Corbelli and associates[48] described some additional patterns of chronotropic response in 19 patients with chronic atrial fibrillation, VVI demand permanent pacemakers, and medication-controlled ventricular responses. Heart rate and metabolic reserve were calculated as described previously in the section on the normal cardiac chronotropic response (see equations 1 and 2). The percentage of HRR was tabulated for the end of each quartile of metabolic reserve. The metabolic chronotropic relation plot for each patient with atrial fibrillation was compared with the averaged data from 100 normal subjects. Subjects who had a percentage of HRR of more than 1 standard deviation above or below the mean of the control population were considered abnormal. The quartile heart rate response was divided into the early and late exercise response. Early exercise response data were defined as the percentage of HRR observed at 25% and 50% of metabolic reserve. Late exercise response data were calculated at 75% and 100% of metabolic reserve. No patient in chronic atrial fibrillation had a normal heart rate response during both early and late exercise (Table 26–3). Three distinct patterns were established: relative tachycardia throughout exercise, relative bradycardia throughout exercise, and relative tachycardia early with a plateauing of the heart rate response at either a normal or bradycardic rate (Fig. 26–6). During early exercise, 95% of patients had an abnormal chronotropic response (21% slow, 74% fast), and during late exercise, 84% of patients had an abnormal chronotropic response (53% slow, 32% fast). In terms of maximal heart rate achieved, 16% exceeded 115% (2 standard deviations) of their age-predicted maximal heart rate, and 42% did not reach 85% (2 standard deviations) of their age-predicted maximal heart rate. Therefore, chronotropic incompetence in patients with chronic atrial fibrillation can be categorized as tachychronotropism, bradychronotropism, and a mixed chronotropic response.[48] From these data, it appears that very few patients with chronic atrial fibrillation have appropriate chronotropic responses throughout the entire spectrum from rest to maximal exertion.

Goals of Exercise Testing for Chronotropic Assessment

Exercise testing can be used as a diagnostic and therapeutic tool in the adjustment of rate-modulated pacers. The first step is to identify who might be an appropriate candidate for chronotropic exercise testing. For patients with symptoms, such as syncope, lightheadedness, dyspnea on exertion, or easy fatigability, exercise testing can be used as a diagnostic test.

The documented correlation of symptoms with an inadequate heart rate response to exercise should lead to implantation of a sensor-driven rate-modulated pacemaker in these patients. For other patients who have already demonstrated a need for pacing, exercise stress testing can be performed before a permanent pacemaker is implanted. This test can help to determine whether the sensor-driven pacing option, with its added expense, would significantly improve the patient's quality of life.

Once a permanent pacemaker with rate-modulated pacing capacity has been implanted, exercise testing is useful for evaluating pacemaker behavior as well as for optimizing the pacemaker response. Each situation has its unique aspects, and an ability to simulate different activities is essential in

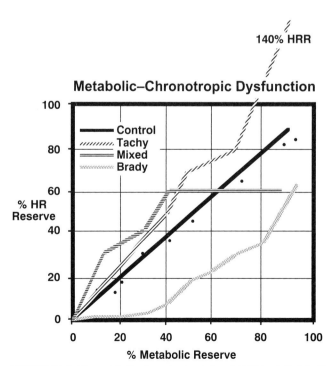

FIGURE 26–6. The metabolic chronotropic relation (MCR) is plotted for 3 of 19 patients with atrial fibrillation and compared with the response in 100 control subjects. All 19 patients demonstrated inappropriate bradycardia (brady), inappropriate tachycardia (tachy), or both tachycardia and bradycardia (mixed) responses.

comparing the responses of different sensors, pacemakers, programmed settings, and sensor algorithms. For example, because stationary bicycle exercise tends to underestimate the response of systems using piezoelectric activity sensors, the mode of exercise must be appropriate to both the patient and the pacing system. Exercise testing also helps to improve our understanding of the physiology of exercise and provides direction for future advancements in the development of rate-modulated pacing.

Last, exercise testing is essential in documenting improvements in measurable end-points with improved chronotropic responsiveness to exercise after placement of a rate-modulated pacemaker. The exercise test documents what degree of chronotropic insufficiency is present at baseline, and what magnitude of improvement is provided by the pulse generator. Even though the exercise response is an important index of rate-modulated pacemaker systems, the value of these systems is not completely described by exercise duration, oxygen uptake, anaerobic threshold, or achievement of a particular chronotropic goal. When a pacing system consistently meets all the present and future symptomatic and physiologic needs of the patient, the medical community will have succeeded. Even so, proper exercise evaluation tools are an essential component in producing the perfect pacing system.

Techniques of Exercise Testing

The major modality used for chronotropic testing in North America continues to be the treadmill exercise test. The wide range of protocols available make this a convenient test for the young and elderly, trained and untrained individuals alike. Continuous ECG monitoring is extremely valuable for identifying tachyarrhythmias or bradyarrhythmias as well as the heart rate response during each stage of exercise. To obtain near steady-state heart rate data, the stage durations should be long enough or the increments in exercise intensity small enough to collect heart rate data that are representative of the subject's physiology. Heart rate is usually recorded during the last 15 seconds of each test stage. Steady-state heart rate is reached by 2 minutes in most individuals but is completely dependent on the appropriateness of the exercise protocol to the patient's degree of fitness.

Obtaining multiple heart rate data points prior to exhaustion is advantageous in evaluating chronotropic response, especially in the range of activities of daily living. Blackburn and colleagues developed the CAEP protocol specifically with these points in mind (see Table 26–2).[49] This protocol allows formation of plots of heart rate versus exercise intensity, with multiple data points between rest and peak exertion. The resultant graph allows analysis of the heart rate response at rest, at submaximal exertion, and at maximal exertion. Selection of a protocol with smaller work increments and shorter stages is ideal for producing more data points and a more complete chronotropic assessment (Fig. 26–7).

To adequately evaluate maximal heart rate response, exhaustion should be produced by an adequately large workload rather than by generalized fatigue or boredom from an excessively prolonged test. Therefore, selection of the proto-

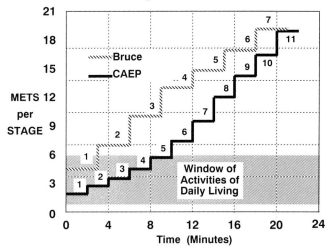

Choosing Exercise Protocols

FIGURE 26–7. The chronotropic assessment exercise protocol (CAEP) is compared to the most commonly employed Bruce protocol. The strength of the CAEP is demonstrated in this graph, which illustrates several stages at work intensities reflecting activities of daily living. Chronotropic and metabolic assessments of submaximal levels of work require this type of analysis whether or not the patient has a pacemaker.

col should be suited to the characteristics of the patient being tested.

Proper administration of the treadmill test is also very important. If a subject is allowed to hold onto the front rail, side arm rail, or the test supervisor during exercise, the estimated workload for that stage will be falsely elevated. The oxygen uptake and heart rate will also be reduced compared with a test performed without arm support. Furthermore, running rather than walking at the same speed and grade produces a higher oxygen uptake and a higher heart rate.[50]

Cycle ergometry has more frequently been used in Europe, during metabolic testing, and when an individual subject is unable to adequately ambulate on a treadmill. However, when physical impairment prevents an individual from ambulating, the use of alternative modalities such as arm or leg ergometry to test cardiac chronotropic responsiveness is probably a moot point. Heart rate response is not likely to be the most limiting factor for that individual.

For a cycle ergometer, the mechanical work rate, in oxygen consumption (in milliliters per minute), is relatively fixed, being dependent on cycle resistance and revolutions per minute. It is independent of body weight except for extremely obese or frail individuals. However, when METs are calculated (in milliliters per kilogram per minute), the larger the individual, the smaller the relative $\dot{V}O_2$ becomes. Oxygen consumption can be estimated relatively accurately for work rates between 50 and 200 W for leg ergometry and for work rates between 25 and 125 W for arm ergometry. When evaluating chronotropic response by cycle ergometry, it is important to remember that the heart rate response to arm ergometry is higher than that seen in response to leg ergometry for the same submaximal work rate; however, the peak heart rate achieved with arm ergometry is lower than that achieved with leg ergometry. Cycle stages are typically 2 to 3 minutes long, and the heart rate is measured during the last 15 seconds of each stage. The peak heart rate attained by a cycle ergometer is only 65% to 70% of the age-adjusted maximal heart rate, making the cycle stress test less optimal than the treadmill for chronotropic evaluation.[51]

In recent years, a call for "optimizing" exercise testing, including customizing the test given with respect to the specific conditions, patient, and test purpose has been made. Other forms of exercise can be attempted. Formal tests such as the Harvard step test or the Master's test are not calibrated into stages to evaluate submaximal heart rates and workloads. Furthermore, maximal stress produced with step testing tends to produce lower oxygen consumption than treadmill testing. Some physicians have used these tests to evaluate how long a person can exercise at a single workload, but this can also be done on treadmills. Although these two tests were once popular, their use has rapidly declined, and they are scarcely used today because of the advantages of other modalities.

Informal stress testing such as walking in place, hallway ambulation, or climbing up and down flights of stairs and individualized ramp treadmill tests[52] may be useful for general screening; however these approaches have many disadvantages. These include lack of calibration in terms of work expenditure, lack of continuous monitoring, lack of hard copy rhythm strips, lack of proper supervision, and lack of proper emergency equipment. However, the importance of these techniques increases in patients needing postimplantation adjustment of rate-modulated parameters in pacemakers. The advantages of these informal tests are their simplicity and their ability to reproduce the symptoms and activities that are similar to those experienced by the subject on a day-to-day basis.

Exercise Protocols

The treadmill remains the most widely used instrument for exercise evaluation of chronotropic response. There are many treadmill protocols available, each varying in factors such as incline, treadmill velocity, and duration of each stage. In choosing an exercise protocol, important factors to consider are the maximal speed that can be reasonably achieved by the individual subject and whether they can be expected to trot or run. If treadmill speed is a limitation, incline increase should be the major variable for adjusting the treadmill work intensity. Nagle and coworkers,[53] Naughton and associates,[54] and Fox and associates[55] advocate a constant speed with a gradual increase in grade (Fig. 26–8). The modified Astrand protocol also has a constant speed with progressive grade step increases. However, the speed selected is between 5 and 8½ miles per hour based on the individual subject's ability to run.[56] The Bruce[57] and Ellestad[58] protocols have stepwise increases in both grade and speed, the modified Bruce (or Sheffield) protocol adding two lower workload, 3-minute stages onto the beginning of the standard Bruce protocol.[59] The CAEP protocol also has progressive stepwise increases in both grade and speed and was developed specifically with chronotropic evaluation in mind (see Fig. 26–7). Its main advantage is the use of 2-minute stages, which produce multiple data points at low levels of exercise within the range of the activities of daily living. This protocol also has one other valuable feature. Protocols for chronotropic assessment should allow people with moderate functional aerobic im-

pairment or orthopedic limitations an opportunity to produce data at several stages of exercise before the velocity of the treadmill requires the subject to jog. Comparison of the Balke, Bruce, Ellestad, and modified Astrand protocols by Pollock demonstrated a linear rise in $\dot{V}O_2$ and heart rate over time, though at different slopes, with similar peak $\dot{V}O_2$ attainment for each of these protocols.[60] A similar result has been obtained with the CAEP protocol.[49] If the assumptions of the exercise protocol for steady-state measurements are met, any protocol that produces enough data points is acceptable for chronotropic assessment.

Cycle ergometer protocols typically increase workload in 2- to 3-minute stages, increasing workload 25 to 50 W per stage. Alt has proposed a cycle stress protocol designed for pacemaker patients that has 25-W incremental stages.[61] This protocol allows multiple low MET points of assessment, which is ideally suited for pacemaker patients. A ramp cycle protocol also exists that increases workload slowly in a continuous manner and can be used for chronotropic assessment.[62] The advantage of the ramp approach, on either a bicycle or a treadmill is a nearly continuous direct relationship between oxygen consumption, heart rate, and steady state. The assumption is that the ramp does not increase faster than the rate of the patient's adaptation to it.

Metabolic Stress Testing

There are certain situations in which a standard exercise test may be inadequate for full evaluation of a given subject. For example, an individual with mixed pulmonary and cardiac pathology may have symptoms that may be difficult to attribute to one specific disease process or another. Other individuals may have vague nonspecific symptoms such as easy fatigability or dyspnea on exertion that could be due to chronotropic incompetence, pulmonary disease, congestive heart failure, coronary artery disease, pericardial disease, pulmonary hypertension, anxiety with hyperventilation, malingering, or other processes. The metabolic cart breath-by-breath analyzer is a very useful instrument for assessing these difficult patients. It allows simultaneous measurement of exhaled oxygen and carbon dioxide, respiratory rate, and minute ventilation during exercise.

The subject with advanced pulmonary disease tends to develop oxygen desaturation during exercise, limiting peak oxygen consumption due to a premature anaerobic threshold. The respiratory quotient (RQ) is the ratio of carbon dioxide produced to oxygen consumed during metabolism. Normal subjects have RQ of approximately 0.85 at low levels of exertion. The quotient increases to above 1.0 and usually above 1.2 at the termination of exercise. This ratio rises further in the postexercise period.[63] An RQ of greater than 1.0 indicates a near maximal effort; failure to reach an RQ of 1.0 indicates a submaximal exercise test owing to inadequate effort, malingering, musculoskeletal limitation, claudication, or congestive heart failure.

Patients with heart failure do not alter their arterial blood gases during exercise. Although normal individuals reach a plateau in oxygen consumption, this plateau is rarely achieved by patients with heart failure[64] because these individuals stop exercising owing to symptoms such as malaise or generalized fatigue. Minute ventilation increases with

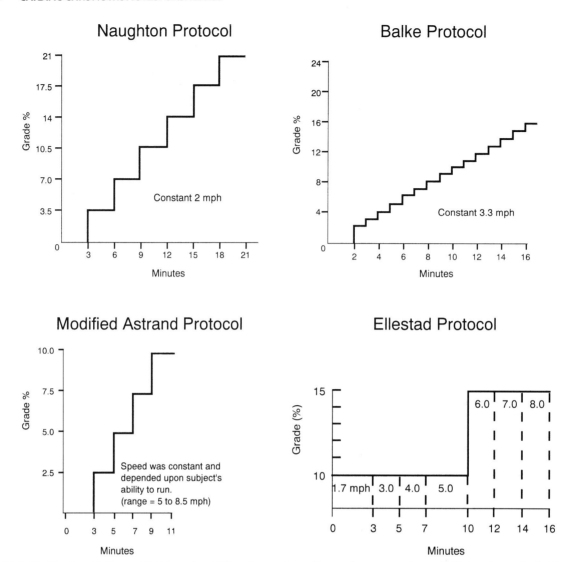

FIGURE 26–8. The Naughton, Balke, modified Astrand, and Ellestad protocols are illustrated to compare the treadmill elevations and velocities required by each. The protocols hold constant either the treadmill velocity or the treadmill elevation for large portions of the study. Sometimes large increases in elevation or velocity require significant adjustments by the patient. This presents problems in making patient-to-patient comparisons of submaximal exercise unless the patient group is homogeneous.

maintenance of a normal carbon dioxide tension, whereas anaerobic metabolism leads to a progressive metabolic acidosis due to inadequate cardiac output.[65] Higginbotham and coworkers demonstrated that heart failure patients have a heart rate response similar to that of normal subjects for a given workload; however, the heart failure patients terminated exercise before achieving the age-predicted maximal heart rate response.[66] Therefore, it appeared that these patients had a significant heart rate response to exercise. However, they terminated exercise prematurely owing to an inadequate rise in stroke volume and hence cardiac output, leading to increased metabolic acidosis. Additional insights arise from the metabolic chronotropic relation analysis described in previous paragraphs. The exercise data obtained from 12 patients with severe left ventricular dysfunction who were under consideration for cardiomyoplasty were evaluated and compared with the responses achieved by 48 normal control patients.[47] Compared with controls, the resting heart rate was elevated and the peak heart rate was reduced. As in the control patients, the responses remained linear, but the

average slope was reduced by one-third (see Fig. 26–5). The question, which is unanswered at this time, is whether this altered but apparently balanced chronotropic response is optimally adaptive or not. Perhaps the stroke volume would fall if heart rate increased to the age-predicted maximal heart rate. Certainly it is necessary to hold a different standard of chronotropic dysfunction for these patients than for people with normal ventricular function.

Practical Aspects of Cardiac Chronotropism

PROGRAMMING RATE-MODULATED PACEMAKERS

Despite the complexity of the descriptions in this chapter, once the rate-modulated pacemaker has been implanted, only three or four programming decisions need to be made to define the chronotropic responsiveness of the patient. These parameters are the lower rate, the upper rate, the sensor threshold to heart rate response, and the slope or incremental response desired for increased sensor activation. With the exception of sensor threshold, each of these parameters has a closely correlative physiologic parameter that is useful in programming the pacemaker response.

The sensor threshold should be conceived as the calibration parameter between the patient and the pacemaker. The smallest sensor response to an increase in activity or metabolic demand above the sensor threshold should initiate the chronotropic response. Ideally, the sensor threshold should be used to distinguish inactivity from minimal activity (Fig. 26–9). Another way of looking at the situation is that the sensor threshold is the parameter designed to distinguish false activity (noise) from true activity. Noise is the variation in sensor output intrinsic to the sensor and not produced by a response to patient activity. Optimally, as incorporated in some of the current pacemakers, the pacemaker should recognize the ''noise'' sensor activity and automatically set the sensor threshold at just above that level. If the pacemaker algorithm is unable to distinguish rest from activity, then the sensor threshold should be set at the level that causes some heart rate response with a minimal amount of activity but no response when the subject is at complete rest.

The other three parameters can be appropriately programmed only if the pacemaker expert understands chronotropic physiology. The lower rate of the pacemaker corresponds to the desired resting heart rate of the patient. Of 537 normal patients, the average resting heart rate was 65 ± 10 bpm. This is a good starting point, but adjustments should be made up or down to address the specific symptoms and issues facing the patient. If the patient is experiencing lightheadedness at rest or while standing still, then the lower heart rate should be increased by between 5 and 25 bpm. However, if all the patient's symptoms are related to significant exertion, reducing the lower rate to promote pacemaker longevity is advisable. Be careful to consider whether changing the lower rate will prevent or increase the incidence of atrial fibrillation.

The upper rate of the pacemaker should be programmed according to the age-predicted maximal heart rate. Subtracting the patient's age from 220 yields the expected sinus heart rate ± 2 standard deviations from the mean. Since an individual patient with a normal chronotropic response may be 2 standard deviations below the mean, calculation of 85% of predicted maximal heart rate (220 − age) and initially programming the upper rate to this value is appropriate. This relatively conservative upper rate value is significantly higher than the values in frequent use around the world. However, for every beat per minute below this value there is a reduction in cardiac output in proportion to the stroke volume. For a 67-year-old person, the upper rate should be initially programmed to 130 bpm, and for a 50-year-old patient it should be programmed to 145 bpm. If the patient has symptoms during significant exertion, the response should be increased by 15% to 20%. However, if the patient has symptoms related to angina or significant ventricular, pulmonary, or orthopedic dysfunction, the response should be reduced by about 10%.

The goal of the sensor slope, which is the parameter that determines the incremental heart rate response to a change in sensor activation, is to produce a linear heart rate increase with exercise that is directly related to the percentage of exercise capacity achieved. To simplify this description, the sensor slope should provide an appropriate change in heart rate from the lower to the upper rate over the entire range of patient activities. The more the patient can do, the smaller the desired slope. Patients with the smallest functional capacity should be given a very steep sensor slope (Fig. 26–10). Because the sensor threshold has been set to detect the smallest amount of activity, one way of setting the sensor slope is to maximally exercise the patient and set the slope at the smallest value that produces the upper rate. Usually, once the sensor threshold and the lower and upper heart rates are programmed, a moderate sensor slope can be empirically programmed, decreased if the patient is active, increased if the patient is inactive, and only finely tuned in patients that show further symptoms.

In summary, the lower rate, upper rate, and sensor slope can be appropriately programmed by empiric methods and

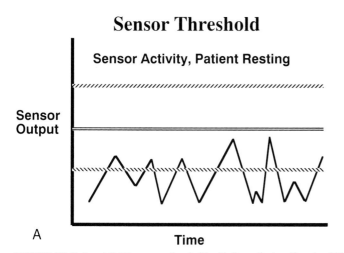

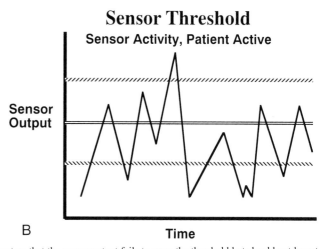

FIGURE 26–9. *A* and *B*, The sensor threshold with the patient resting should be set so that the sensor output fails to cross the threshold but should not be set so high that large increases in output are needed to cross the threshold. The middle horizontal line represents the appropriate choice for the activity shown in these figures. If the lower threshold was chosen, the patient would experience sensor-driven rate increases during inactivity. If the higher threshold was chosen, the patient might not experience a rate increase during activities of daily living.

Rate Responsiveness

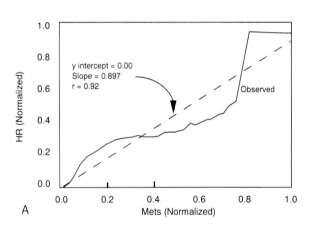

FIGURE 26–10. The sensor slope, which may be nonlinear, produces rate increases from the sensor threshold to maximum exertion when properly adjusted. The same level of exertion (sensor activation) provides different rate responses related to the sensor slope. Since resting heart rate and peak heart rate are not related to peak functional capacity, it is necessary to adjust for functional capacity by adjusting the sensor slope. The most unfit patient needs the highest (most aggressive) slope, whereas the most fit patient requires a more gentle sensor slope.

produce a physiologic response. However, the sensor threshold should either be automatically determined by the pulse generator or determined experimentally. An understanding of chronotropic physiology permits the physician to use a ra-

tional method for programming pacemaker rate responsiveness without intensive exercise testing.

EVALUATING THE CHRONOTROPIC RESPONSE

Evaluation and optimization of a sensor-driven rate-modulated pacemaker response is the ultimate clinical goal of understanding chronotropic physiology. Knowing what to expect is the first step, but evaluating the actual response is critical in evaluating the relationship between the patient, the pacemaker, and his or her activities. Kay[67] described three methods of evaluating the chronotropic response of rate-modulated pacemaker systems. Employing the concepts of heart rate and metabolic reserve, the metabolic chronotropic response was plotted, and linear regression analysis provided a line with a y-intercept and slope. It was clear from the analysis of his 10 patients that the response was not well described by linear regression (Fig. 26–11A). He then divided exercise into quartiles of exertion, calculating the difference between the expected and observed heart rate responses at the midpoint and end of each quartile (see Fig. 26–11B). This analysis allowed the possibility of variations in the slope of the curve during various stages of exercise. However, it also tended to overemphasize transient deviations of the metabolic chronotropic response curve. Finally, he integrated the area under the response curve, compared it with the area under the expected response, and reported this calculation for the entire response and for the four quartiles of response. This final method seemed to summarize the

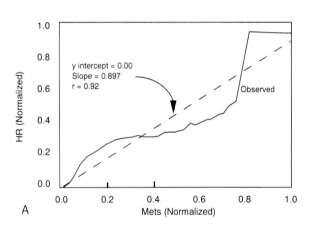

FIGURE 26–11. Kay uses normalized heart rate and normalized metabolic equivalents (METs) instead of percentage heart rate and metabolic reserve, but the process is the same. Method 1 *(A)* calculates the metabolic chronotropic relation (MCR) slope of 0.897 (r = 0.92) but clearly incompletely describes the rate response of the pacemaker. Method 2 *(B)* divides the exertion into four quartiles of response. The heart rate is measured at the midpoint and end of each quartile and is expressed as the percentage of the expected response. Method 3 *(C)*, compares the area under the expected and observed MCR curves during each quartile and for the entire exertion. The patient achieved only 89% of the expected heart rate area but, during early and late exercise, demonstrated excessive responses with a lag in response during the second and third quartiles. (From Kay GN: Quantitation of chronotropic response: Comparison of methods for rate-modulating permanent pacemakers. J Am Coll Cardiol 20:1534, 1992. Reprinted with permission from the American College of Cardiology.)

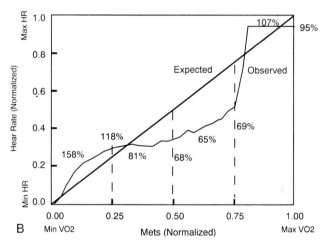

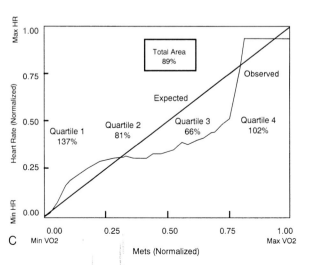

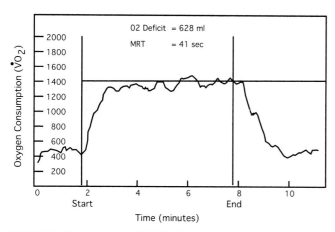

FIGURE 26–12. During low (35 W/min) but constant-intensity exercise, oxygen consumption ($\dot{V}O_2$) is measured. During the plateau phase, a horizontal line is drawn, and the area is integrated between this line and the observed $\dot{V}O_2$ from the initiation of exercise to the plateau. The mean response time (MRT) and O_2 deficit *(integrated area)* are calculated. (Unpublished data, used by permission of Thorsten Lewalter, M.D.).

differences between the observed and expected responses best (see Fig. 26–11C).

Lewalter and colleagues[68] propose another method for evaluating the chronotropic responsiveness of patients with pacemakers. During low-intensity, fixed-workload treadmill exercise, oxygen consumption is measured. When steady-state $\dot{V}O_2$ is obtained, the area between the actual and the ideal $\dot{V}O_2$ response is integrated. The goal is to program the rate response to minimize the metabolic difference (O_2 deficit) (Fig. 26–12).

It is interesting to analyze the responses of Kay's 10 VVIR patients and compare their responses to the reported responses in normal subjects, heart failure patients, and patients with atrial fibrillation. Normals provide the standard, which is a purely linear response ($R^2 = 0.95$) with a slope of 0.99. Similarly, the heart failure patients produced a linear response ($R^2 = 0.75$) with a slope of 0.67. In contrast, the atrial fibrillation patients produced responses that are extremely similar to the responses provided by rate-modulated pacemakers. Some of the responses were too slow throughout, others too fast, and some were too fast at low-intensity exertion but too slow at higher exertional intensities.

In summary, analysis of the metabolic chronotropic responsiveness of a patient and his or her pacemaker should include measurement of linearity and slope and quantification of the contribution of each quartile of response to expected behavior. Even so, heart rate reflects only one of the two components of cardiac output and fails to reflect the adequacy of the response in regard to oxygen consumption. However, expired gas analysis exercise testing as described previously validates the use of heart rate as the measure of a metabolically appropriate response.

Summary

Cardiac chronotropic analysis has just begun to develop into a clinically relevant science. In the past, formal exercise testing was usually reserved for assessment of ischemia or cardiac rehabilitation. The establishment of rate-modulated

pacemakers as a potentially effective treatment for chronotropic incompetence forced investigators to define cardiac chronotropism and assessment of the pacemaker response. Very little is known about the normal chronotropic response, and less has been established about patients with ventricular dysfunction or ischemia, but standards are being set, and modern pacemakers have produced the ideal clinical laboratory for investigation. Advanced telemetry, including sensor and actual rate trends, histograms, and sensorgrams produce previously unobtainable clinical data. Now scientific inquiry demands that chronotropic evaluations seek to match the pacemaker-augmented response of the chronotropically incompetent patient to the metabolic requirements of his or her body. Only with formal exercise testing will this goal be defined and achieved. Once the physiology has been completely defined, the lessons learned can be implemented with less formal techniques.

REFERENCES

1. Bousfield G: Angina pectoris: Changes in electrocardiogram during paroxysm. Lancet 2:457, 1918.
2. Feil H, Siegel M: Electrocardiographic changes during attacks of angina pectoris. Am J Med Sci 175:225, 1928.
3. Missal ME: Exercise tests and the electrocardiograph in the study of angina pectoris. Ann Intern Med 11:2018, 1938.
4. Master AM, Oppenheimer EJ: A simple exercise tolerance test for circulatory efficiency with standard tables for normal individuals. Am J Med Sci 177:223, 1929.
5. Master AM, Jafe HL: The electrocardiographic changes after exercise in angina pectoris. J Mt Sinai Hosp 7:629, 1941.
6. Bruce RA: Evaluation of functional capacity and exercise tolerance of cardiac patients. Mod Concepts Cardiovasc Dis 25:321, 1956.
7. Astrand PO, Rhyming I: Nomogram for calculation of aerobic capacity (physical fitness) from pulse rate during submaximal work. J Appl Physiol 7:218, 1954.
8. Balke B, Ware RW: An experimental study of physical fitness of Air Force personnel. US Armed Forces Med J 10:675, 1959.
9. Hellerstein HK, Hornsten TR: The coronary spectrum: Assessing and preparing a patient for return to a meaningful and productive life. J Rehabil 32:48, 1966.
10. Wilkoff BL: Criteria for optimal pacemaker function. J Cardiovasc Electrophysiol 2:416, 1991.
11. Astrand PO, Cuddy TE, Saltin B, et al: Cardiac output during submaximal and maximal work. J Appl Physiol 19:268, 1964.
12. Franciosa JS, Park M, Levine B: Lack of correlation between exercise capacity and indices of left ventricular performance in heart failure. Am J Cardiol 47:33, 1981.
13. Wasserman K, Whipp BJ: Exercise physiology in health and disease. Am Rev Respir Dis 112:219, 1975.
14. Green HJ, Hughson RL, Orr GW, Ranney DA: Anaerobic threshold, blood lactate, and muscle metabolites in progressive exercise. J Appl Physiol 54:1032, 1983.
15. Simon J, Young JL, Gutin B, et al: Lactate accumulation relative to the anaerobic and respiratory compensated threshold. J Appl Physiol 54:13, 1983.
16. Hughes EF, Turner SC, Brook GA: Effects of glycogen depletion and pedaling speed on anaerobic threshold. J Appl Physiol 53:58, 1982.
17. Dreifus LS, Fisch C, Griffin JC, et al (eds): Guidelines for implantation of cardiac pacemakers and antiarrhythmic devices: A report of the ACC/AHA task force on assessment of diagnostic and therapeutic cardiovascular procedures. Circulation 84:455, 1991.
18. Ellestad MH, Wan M: Predictive implications of stress testing: Follow-up of 2700 subjects after maximum treadmill stress testing. Circulation 51:363, 1975.
19. Blomqvist CG, Saltin B: Cardiovascular adaptations to physical training. Annu Rev Physiol 45:169, 1983.
20. Wilkoff BL, Beck G, Pashkow F, et al: Confidence interval calculation of chronotropic incompetence [Abstract]. PACE 13:1215, 1990.
21. Jose AD, Collison D: The normal range and determinants of the intrinsic heart rate in man. Cardiovasc Res 4:160, 1970.

22. Fagraeus L, Linnarsson D: Autonomic origin of heart rate fluctuations at the onset of muscular exercise. J Appl Physiol 40:679, 1976.
23. Bates DV: Commentary on cardiorespiratory determinants of cardiovascular fitness. Can Med Assoc J 96:704, 1967.
24. Jette M, Sidney K, Blunchen G: Metabolic equivalent (METS) in exercise testing, exercise prescription, and evaluation of functional capacity. Clin Cardiol 13:555, 1990.
25. Fletcher GF, Froelicher VF, Hartley LH, et al: Exercise standards: A statement for health professionals from the American Heart Association. Circulation 82:2286, 1990.
26. Wilkoff BL, Corey J, Blackburn G: A mathematical model of the cardiac chronotropic response to exercise. J Electrophysiol 3:176, 1989.
27. Wilkoff BL, Blackburn G, Pashkow F, et al: Exercise testing in the identification of sinus node dysfunction. Euro-pace '93: 6th European Symposium on Cardiac Pacing, 1993, pp 105–111.
28. Ferrer MI: The sick sinus syndrome in atrial disease. JAMA 206:645, 1968.
29. Sugrue DD, Gersh BJ, Holmes DR, et al: Symptomatic "isolated" carotid sinus hypersensitivity: Natural history and results of treatment with anticholinergic drugs or pacemaker. J Am Coll Cardiol 7:158, 1986.
30. Morley CA, Perrins EJ, Grant P, et al: Carotid sinus syndrome treated by pacing: Analysis of persistent symptoms and role of AV sequential pacing. Br Heart J 47:411, 1982.
31. Almquist A, Gornick C, Benson W, et al: Carotid sinus hypersensitivity: Evaluation of the vasodepressor component. Circulation 5:927, 1985.
32. Strasberg B, Sagie A, Erdman S, et al: Carotid sinus hypersensitivity and carotid sinus syndrome. Prog Cardiovasc Dis 5:379, 1989.
33. Thomas JE: Hyperactive carotid sinus reflex and carotid sinus syncope. Mayo Clin Proc 44:127, 1969.
34. Kapoor WN, Karpf M, Wieand S, et al: A prospective evaluation and follow-up of patients with syncope. N Engl J Med 309:197, 1983.
35. Volkmann H, Sehnerch B, Kuhnert H: Diagnostic value of carotid sinus hypersensitivity. PACE 13:2065, 1990.
36. Vardas PE, Fitzpatrick A, Ingram A, et al: Natural history of sinus node chronotropy in paced patients. PACE 14(2):155, 1991.
37. Gang ES, Oseran DS, Mandel WJ, et al: Sinus node electrogram in patients with the hypersensitive carotid sinus syndrome. J Am Coll Cardiol 5:1484, 1985.
38. Brignole M, Menozzi C, Lolli G, et al: Validation of a method for choice of pacing in carotid sinus syndrome with or without sinus bradycardia. PACE 14:186, 1991.
39. Ketritsis D, Ward DE, Camm AJ: Can we treat carotid sinus syndrome? PACE 14:1367, 1991.
40. Holden W, McAnulty JH, Rahimtoola SH: Characterization of heart rate response to exercise in the sick sinus syndrome. Br Heart J 40:923, 1978.
41. Donald DE, Shepherd JT: Response to exercise in dogs with cardiac denervation. Am J Physiol 205:293, 1963.
42. Ross JJ Jr, Linhart JW, Braunwald E: Effects of changing heart rate in man by electrical stimulation of the right atrium. Circulation 32:549, 1965.
43. Abbott JA, Hirshfeld DS, Kunkel FW, et al: Graded exercise testing in patients with sinus node dysfunction. Am J Med 62:330, 1977.
44. Ellestad MH: Parameters to be measured. In Stress Testing: Principles and Practice, 3rd ed. Philadelphia, FA Davis, 1986.
45. Hinkle LE, Carver ST, Plakun A: Slow heart rates and increased risk of cardiac death in middle-aged men. Arch Intern Med 129:732, 1972.
46. Chin CF, Messenger JC, Greenberg PS, et al: Chronotropic incompetence in exercise testing. Clin Cardiol 2:12, 1979.
47. Hamer DS, Wilkoff BL, Blackburn CG, et al: Chronotropic incompetence during exercise in patients with severe left ventricular dysfunction. J Am Coll Cardiol 2:329A, 1993.
47a. Knox JAC: The heart rate with exercise in patients with auricular fibrillation. Br Heart J 11:119, 1949.
48. Corbelli R, Masterson M, Wilkoff BL: Chronotropic response to exercise in patients with atrial fibrillation. PACE 13:179, 1990.
49. Blackburn G, Harvey S, Wilkoff B: A chronotropic assessment exercise protocol to assess the need and efficacy of rate-responsive pacing [Abstract]. Med Sci Sports Exerc 20:S21, 1988.
50. Astrand PO: Principles in ergometry and their implications in sports practice. Sport Med 1:1, 1984.
51. Hansen JE, Casaburi R, Cooper DM, Wasserman K: Oxygen uptake as related to work rate increment during cycle ergometer exercise. Eur J Appl Physiol 57:140, 1988.
52. Myers J, Buchman N, Smith D, et al: Individualized ramp treadmill: Observations on a new protocol. Chest 101(5):236s, 1992.
53. Nagle FJ, Balke B, Naughton JP: Graduation step tests for assessing work capacity. J Appl Physiol 20:745, 1965.
54. Naughton J, Balke B, Nagle F: Refinements in methods of evaluation and physical conditioning before and after myocardial infarction. Am J Cardiol 14:837, 1964.
55. Fox SM, Naughton JP, Haskell WL: Physical activity and the prevention of coronary artery disease. Ann Clin Res 3:404, 1971.
56. Astrand PO, Rodahl K: Textbook of Work Physiology. New York, McGraw-Hill, 1970.
57. Bruce RA, McDonough JR: Stress testing in screening for cardiovascular disease. Bull NY Acad Med 45:1288, 1969.
58. Ellestad MH, Allen W, Wan M, et al: Maximal treadmill stress testing for cardiovascular evaluation. Circulation 39:517, 1969.
59. Sheffield LT, Roitman D: Stress testing methodology. Prog Cardiovasc Dis 19:33, 1976.
60. Pollock ML: A comparative analysis of 4 protocols for maximal exercise testing. Am Heart J 93:39, 1976.
61. Alt E: A protocol for treadmill and bicycle stress testing designed for pacemaker patients. Stimucoeur 15:33, 1987.
62. Whipp BJ, Davis JA, Torres F: A test to determine parameters of aerobic function during exercise. J Appl Physiol 50:217, 1981.
63. Jones NL, Campbell EJM: Physiology of exercise. In Clinical Exercise Testing, 2nd ed. Philadelphia, WB Saunders, 1982.
64. Poole-Wilson PA: Exercise as a means of assessing heart failure and its response to treatment. Cardiology 76:347, 1989.
65. Franciosa JA, Leddy CL, Wilen M, et al: Relation between hemodynamic and ventilatory responses in determining exercise capacity in severe congestive heart failure. Am J Cardiol 53:127, 1984.
66. Higginbotham MB, Morris KG, Conn EH, et al: Determinants of variable exercise performance among patients with severe left ventricular dysfunction. Am J Cardiol 51:52, 1983.
67. Kay GN: Quantitation of chronotropic response: Comparison of methods for rate-modulating permanent pacemakers. J Am Coll Cardiol 20:1533, 1992.
68. Lewalter T, Jung W, MacCarter D, et al: Heart rate and oxygen uptake kinetics: A goal of rate-adaptive pacemakers? PACE 16(pt 2):852, 1993.

CHAPTER 27

PERMANENT PACEMAKER IMPLANTATION

Peter H. Belott
Dwight W. Reynolds

The approach to cardiac pacemaker implantation has undergone considerable evolution over the past 40 years.[1] From the initial epicardial implants of Senning[2] and transvenous implantation by Furman and Schwedel,[3] cardiac pacemaker implantation has seen radical change not only in the implanted hardware but also in the preoperative planning, anatomic approach, personnel, and implantation facilities. The early trend from the epicardial approach to the simpler transvenous cutdown has led the way to the percutaneous technique developed by Littleford and Spector.[4] Preoperative planning and in particular device selection, once simple, has become complex. The pacemaker system, both device and electrodes, must be individualized to the patient's particular clinical and anatomic situation. The implantation procedure, previously the exclusive domain of the cardiovascular surgeon, has also become the purview of the invasive cardiologist. Similarly the procedure has undergone a transition from the operating room to the cardiac catheterization laboratory or special procedures room. The luxury of an anesthesiologist has, except in special instances, disappeared, with the implanting physician assuming additional responsibilities. Finally, driven by concerns over cost containment, the usual in-hospital postoperative observation period has been dramatically reduced or replaced by an ambulatory approach to pacemaker implantation. All of these changes have not been without a price; new techniques have brought new problems and concerns. This chapter attempts to explore all aspects of modern pacemaker implantation from a practical point of view. It also addresses these new problems and concerns.

Personnel

Traditionally, pacemaker implantation procedures have been performed exclusively by a thoracic or cardiac surgeon.

The skills were acquired during a residency or fellowship. Early pacemaker implantations involved more extensive surgery and, at times, an open-chest procedure for epicardial electrode placement. The pulse generator and electrodes were large, requiring considerable dissection and surgical skill. Over the past decade, decreasing pacemaker size has limited the more extensive surgery previously required. Today the knowledge and skills required for dual-chamber pacing are well suited for the physician trained in cardiac catheterization. It has become generally well accepted that the implanting physician may be either a thoracic surgeon or an invasive cardiologist.[5] At times the two may even act as a team, with the surgeon isolating the vein and the cardiologist positioning the electrodes. With the current reimbursement structure and the changing economic environment, however, this team approach is rapidly becoming burdensome and in any event is frequently unnecessary. Today the credentialing for pacemaker implantation procedures poses a dilemma. The trainee in thoracic surgery is subject to an ever-diminishing exposure to pacemaker implantation as the procedure becomes more the responsibility of the cardiologist. At the same time, the cardiologist has little or no exposure to proper surgical technique, the use of surgical instruments, or pre- and postoperative care. There is considerable controversy about what constitutes an appropriate implantation experience and over what length of time that experience should extend. One thing that appears certain is that physicians with limited training and ongoing experience have unacceptable complication rates.[6] It has been suggested that in order to remain proficient one must perform a minimum of 12 cases per year. There is a definite need for formal training programs specifically designed to teach cardiac pacing.[7–9] Such programs should be offered to both cardiologists and surgeons interested in cardiac pacing. The ideal program should be comprehensive and integrated, involving not only all implantations but also follow-up and trouble-shooting. To be an effective implanter, one must understand the problems of follow-up and trouble-shooting. A formal didactic experience as well as "hands-on" exposure should be included. Although a formal, year-long, comprehensive, integrated training program is ideal, consideration of physicians who are out of formal training programs requires, at times, combining more intensive didactic programs with extended, supervised hands-on experience. Even this latter approach should involve a requirement for involvement in nonimplantation aspects of pacing. It has been our frequent experience that there is substantially less enthusiasm for mastering these aspects of pacing. We ardently believe such mastery to be critical to becoming an effective implanter.

Regardless of how one has become trained to implant pacemakers, careful review (by those responsible for credentialing in a given institution) of the training and experience of individuals in pacing will assist in preventing inadequately trained individuals from performing independent, unsupervised pacemaker implantation. Criteria for adequate training and experience should include a minimum number of pacemaker procedures, including single- and dual-chamber implantations, lead replacements, pulse generator replacements, and "upgrades" to dual-chamber from single-chamber systems. Also, some documentable experience in an active pacemaker service-clinic should be required.[10]

Support personnel are critical to the success and safety of any pacemaker procedure. Historically, whether in a large medical center or a small community hospital, the procedure was performed in the operating room. This had its drawbacks because each case could be a first-time experience for the operating room staff. Pacemaker procedures were frequently added at the end of a busy operating room schedule and were placed in the first available room with support personnel who changed from procedure to procedure. Personnel not familiar with the procedure can interrupt the flow of the case. Even with the transition to the cardiac catheterization laboratory for pacing procedures, the same problems can exist. Conversely, depending on the volume of procedures in the operating room and the cardiac catheterization laboratories, there may be more of an opportunity for consistent, recurrent availability of cardiovascular technicians, nurses, and x-ray personnel in the latter. These more focused staff members tend to have a certain appreciation for the procedure and are better equipped to deal with the unique problems that may be encountered in a pacemaker procedure. Whether in the operating room or catheterization laboratory, the minimal personnel required are the same and include a scrub nurse or technician familiar with each operator's surgical preferences, a circulating nurse to support the personnel who have scrubbed (with this generally involving delivering supplies and equipment to the sterile field as needed and patient monitoring and medication administration, although this is somewhat limited in the operating room when an anesthesiologist is present), and an individual responsible for the performance of electric testing. It is also useful to have access to an experienced cardiovascular radiology technician, which generally is more easily accomplished in the cardiac catheterization laboratory than in the operating room.

The presence of an anesthesiologist or nurse anesthetist is becoming something of a luxury. Initially an essential member of the implant team, an anesthesiologist in many centers is now involved only in special situations requiring airway support in an unstable or otherwise problematic patient. Anesthesiology staff should always be available for emergency situations and consulted if problems are anticipated.

The participation of the pacemaker manufacturer's representative support personnel has always been a subject of debate. His or her role varies from center to center.[11] At one extreme he or she merely delivers the pacemaker and leads to the hospital. At the other extreme, he or she is a critical member of the support team, retrieving threshold data, filling out registration forms and, at times, offering technical advice. The latter is particularly true in smaller institutions with less pacemaker activity. A well-trained, experienced pacemaker representative can be an important member of the support team. An experienced representative dedicated to cardiac pacing frequently has a broad experience and knowledge base in problems especially unique to his or her company's products. Although such a representative of industry can be helpful, such a person, no matter how experienced or knowledgeable, should not be considered an acceptable alternative to a knowledgeable, skilled, and experienced physician implanter. If an industrial representative is to be used during implantations for support, hospital approval is advisable.

When comparing the support personnel requirements of the operating room and the catheterization laboratory, there are the previously noted general advantages in the latter. There is one other important concern that relates to sterile technique. The regular operating room personnel tend to be more keenly aware of sterile technique and are scrupulous in this regard. In contrast, the cardiac catheterization laboratory personnel are not routinely trained in operating room and sterile technique, and if these procedures are not strongly reinforced, they can be disastrously neglected.

Implantation Facility and Equipment

The cardiac catheterization laboratory and special procedures room appear well suited for permanent pacemaker procedures.[12, 13] Early concerns over safety and sterility have been shown to be unfounded when these issues are appropriately addressed prospectively. The unique capabilities from a radiologic point of view are invaluable. High-resolution images, unlimited projections, and angiographic capabilities can be extremely helpful in venous access and electrode placement, not to mention variable image magnification, digital image acquisition, and image imposition techniques and storage. In addition, these facilities tend to be equipped for ready access with all of the catheters, guide wires, sheaths, and angiographic materials that might be required for special situations. It is also generally the location of the most sophisticated physiologic monitoring and recording equipment (Fig. 27–1), offering both continuous surface and endocardial electric recordings as well as extensive hemodynamic monitoring capabilities. Staffing with qualified cardiovascular nurses and technicians has already been mentioned. Concerns over the potential for infection must be addressed. These facilities are designated as intermediate sterile areas. The sterile precautions tend to be less rigid than in the operating room. The cardiac catheterization laboratory also tends to be a high-traffic area. A rigid protocol for sterile technique must be

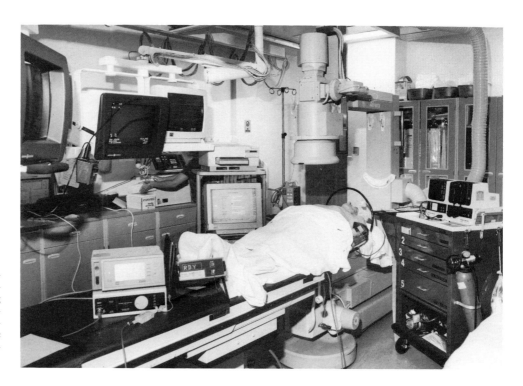

FIGURE 27–1. Cardiac catheterization laboratory. The patient is surrounded by sophisticated monitoring equipment that includes a pulse oximeter, a physiologic recorder, an external defibrillator, an automatic blood pressure cuff, and an emergency crash cart.

established and the room sealed from traffic after it has been cleaned for the surgical procedure. All personnel entering this area must wear scrub clothing, a hat, and a mask. The ventilation system should also meet the standards for an intermediate sterile area.

The cardiac catheterization laboratory and special procedures room generally have another drawback. Most do not allow the patient to be placed in the Trendelenburg position, which can be so important in the percutaneous approach to pacemaker implantation. This problem, however, can be obviated by use of a wedge under the legs early in the procedure.

Of course, the ideal is a dedicated room or suite for pacemaker procedures containing all of the capabilities previously noted as well as skilled staffing as previously described. The ability to maintain sterility as well as dedicated equipment and staff in such a room is attractive, although it is clearly the exception at present. As growth occurs in the numbers of transvenously implantable defibrillators, the establishment of rooms dedicated to pacemaker and defibrillator implantation will likely also increase.

The strongest arguments for implanting a pacemaker in the operating room are sterility and patient control. It is typically the area of best sterility and sterile technique. A pacemaker represents a foreign body and, therefore, one prime concern is infection. A procedure in the operating room generally offers the maximum in protection from infection. In addition, patient control is better because most operating rooms, as a matter of policy, require an anesthesiologist to be available. This allows for more effective airway control and ventilation in the unstable or uncooperative patient. The anesthesiologist is available to intubate and even administer general anesthesia if necessary. Another small advantage is the seemingly endless availability of surgical instruments and supplies. It can also be argued that if a catastrophe should occur requiring more extensive surgery, such as an open-chest procedure,

one is already in the operating room. Conversely, in our independent experience, this is only a theoretical advantage.

The biggest pitfall of the operating room is the fluoroscopy equipment. It is usually of lesser quality and of limited capability when compared with that available in the catheterization laboratory. In addition, it is frequently shared with other services, such as orthopedics. Frequent conflicts can occur when more than one service is trying to use it at the same time. Further, the lack of immediate access to angiographic materials and catheterization equipment is another drawback to using the operating room for pacemaker procedures. Unless pacemaker implantation is given special consideration and is performed in a specific operating room with equipment and supplies under the control of a pacemaker physician and staff, there is a tendency to be unprepared technically. This disrupts the flow of the procedure and can adversely affect the outcome. This same caveat holds, however, for a busy catheterization laboratory as well.

The monitoring equipment used for a pacemaker procedure is quite variable. A multichannel electrocardiographic recording system is frequently recommended; such systems are able to monitor and record a minimum of three surface and one intracardiac electrocardiograms (ECGs).[14] From a more practical point of view, all that is absolutely required is continuous electrocardiographic monitoring on an oscilloscope. The electrocardiographic pattern need only be clear. Electrocardiographic lead selection should demonstrate adequate atrial and ventricular morphology for defining underlying rhythm, arrhythmias, and atrial and ventricular capture. Threshold information can be obtained from the combined use of a pacing system analyzer (PSA) (see further on) and an oscilloscope. Sensing data can be obtained from a reliable PSA alone. Multichannel recorders provide more thorough evaluation and documentation and occasionally are extremely valuable in discerning arrhythmias, capture, capture morphology, timing, and so on. The multichannel recorder also allows retrieval of intracardiac signals, precise wave form analysis, and assessment of ventriculoatrial conduction. High-quality hard copy for analysis is also generally available with these more sophisticated recording devices, which tend to be ubiquitous in the catheterization laboratory but uncommon in the operating room.

Patient monitoring should also include a reliable means for blood pressure and arterial oxygen saturation determinations. This can usually be accomplished adequately by use of an automatic noninvasive blood pressure cuff and a transcutaneous oxygen saturation monitor (some institutions place indwelling arterial lines for blood pressure monitoring, although this is generally not necessary and has some associated morbidity). These devices are of particular value when an anesthesiologist is not in attendance. Continuous oxygen saturation monitoring can detect hypoventilation from sedation, pneumothorax, and air embolization. A direct current (DC) defibrillator and complete emergency cart should be in the room where the pacemaker procedure is performed. The cart must include an ambu bag and intubation equipment.

The surgical instruments for a pacemaker procedure usually call for something akin to a "minor surgical" set-up (Fig. 27–2). At times, depending on the institution, the contents of a minor surgical set-up can be rather overwhelming. This is particularly true for the nonsurgeon-implanting physician. The rows of unnamed clamps and retractors would suggest that some major body cavity might have to be entered. Actually, a pacemaker procedure can be performed efficiently with only a few, well-selected instruments,[15] and there are many acceptable variations and personal preferences. Problems can occur, however, with the nonsurgeon-implanting physician who is unfamiliar with the instruments and their appropriate uses. The contents of a basic acceptable surgical tray for pacemaker implantations are outlined in Table 27–1. There are several valuable retractors worthy of individual comment. The Gilpey or Weitlander (see Fig. 27–2) retractors, or both, can be used throughout the procedure

TABLE 27–1. PACEMAKER SURGICAL INSTRUMENT TRAY

Two Adson forceps with teeth
One mouth-tooth forceps
One smooth forceps
One medium blunt Weitlander retractor
One small Weitlander retractor
Two Senn retractors
One Army-Navy retractor
Four baby towel clips
Five curved mosquito clamps
One Peers clamp
Two curved Kelly clamps
One small Metzenbaum scissors
One curved Mayo scissors
One No. 3 knife handle
Two small needle holders
One Goulet retractor
One Bozeman uterine dressing forceps

One package of 1–0 silk 18-inch suture material
One package of 2–0 polyglactin mesh nonabsorbable suture material
One package of 4–0 polyglactin mesh nonabsorbable suture material
No. 3 or 4 F eye needle
No. 10 scalpel blade

for improved visual exposure. The Senn retractor is used for more delicate retraction (see Fig. 27–2). One end is shaped in an L and the other end has tiny claws. This instrument allows the more delicate lifting of tissue edges. Another useful retractor is the Goulet retractor (see Fig. 27–2), which can be replaced with a Richardson retractor. It is extremely helpful in retraction when creating the pacemaker pocket. Unlike other large retractors, the smooth, scalloped ends of these retractors are gentle to the tissues while affording a generous area of exposure. Army-Navy retractors can also be helpful for this purpose. Other instruments such as forceps (with or without "teeth"), hemostats, scissors (tissue and other), needle holders, and clamps are a necessity, but their uses do not require explanation here. It is important to add that proper use and care of the instruments is critical and replacement of worn-out instruments mandatory in avoiding frustration, delays, and suboptimal work.

Pacemaker procedures performed in the operating room benefit from typically excellent lighting. Multiple high-intensity lamps light the surgical field. This is not the case for pacemaker procedures performed in the catheterization laboratory or special procedures room. Frequently, lighting is marginal at best. One solution to this problem is the use of a high-intensity head lamp (Fig. 27–3). This is extremely useful when creating the pocket and inspecting for bleeders, particularly when the operator's head blocks out other light. The use of the head lamp initially can be frustrating and requires practice. Once the operator is facile with its use, it will become the major light source for creating the pocket. Even in the operating room, despite all the lighting, the head light can be very helpful.

The final piece of equipment to be discussed is the electrocautery. This device can be useful, and some experienced implanters consider it essential to any pacemaker procedure. Its use, however, has been the subject of controversy.[16–18] Historically, the use of electrocautery equipment for cutting or coagulation during a pacemaker procedure was considered taboo. Concerns have been raised with respect to its causing

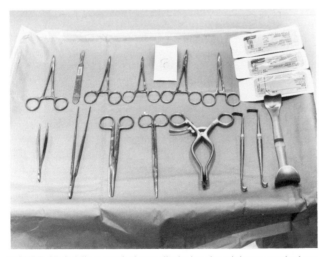

FIGURE 27–2. Minor surgical tray displaying the minimum required surgical instruments and supplies. From the top left and clockwise: needle holder, scalpel, four sizes of curved hemostats and clamps, Goulet retractor, two Senn retractors, Weitlander self-retaining retractor, Metzenbaum scissors, suture scissors, nontoothed forceps, toothed forceps. The four packages include "free needles" and three packages of resorbable and nonresorbable suture.

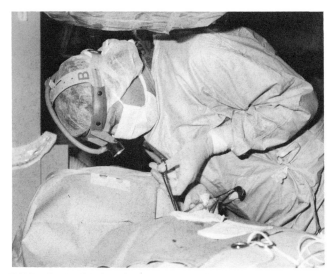

FIGURE 27–3. High-intensity head lamps optimize visualization in situations of limited lighting frequently experienced in the catheterization laboratory and sometimes in the operating room.

burns at the myocardium-electrode interface, destruction of the pulse generator, and damage to the pacemaker leads. There is a growing consensus that the use of an appropriately grounded electrocautery is safe if one takes a couple of precautions. First, active cautery should never touch the exposed proximal pin of the electrode. Second, the use of all electrocautery should cease once the pulse generator is on the surgical field.

During pulse generator changes, the use of electrocautery can be extremely useful. Cutting with electrocautery expedites the freeing up of the pulse generator and leads at the same time, avoiding the misfortune of cutting the lead. At times, even in the most experienced hands, a tedious dissection ends with the scalpel or scissors nicking or cutting the electrode insulation. Use of rapid strokes with cautery avoids the build-up of heat, avoiding injury to leads.

Experience leads us to believe that there are no important untoward effects on the myocardium if the cautery touches the pulse generator. There is, however, a risk of causing a permanent no-output situation by destroying the pulse generator. This appears to be particularly true in certain pulse generators. The risk to the patient of sudden lack of output can be completely avoided by placing a temporary pacemaker in patients who are pacemaker-dependent. This is a consideration that is fundamental to all pacemaker procedures whether electrocautery is used or not.

The PSA is extremely valuable during pacemaker procedures. Even when stimulators and recorders are available, a PSA, whose circuitry (especially sensing) mimics that of the planned pulse generator, will more accurately predict the performance of the pulse generator. In some institutions, the PSA is provided by the pacemaker manufacturer. The early PSAs were simple and designed to measure the pacing and sensing thresholds for single-chamber ventricular pacing. They were unable to perform (or were cumbersome when performing) the tasks required for atrial and dual-chamber pacing.[19] Today's PSA should be able to perform all of the measurements required for any pacemaker procedure for both the pulse generator and the pacing electrode. At the same

time, it should offer back-up pacing support during parameter measurements. The modern PSA should be able to function in any mode and measure from either chamber, offering a clear digital display as well as extensive programmability. It should have emergency capabilities of high output and high rate. The capacity to generate a hard copy for analysis and record keeping is also desirable. The first of the new generation of PSAs is the Medtronic 5311 (Medtronic, Inc., Minneapolis, MN) (Fig. 27–4). A summary of its desirable features is provided in Table 27–2. Some of the sensor-driven pacemakers—for example, temperature and oxygen sensors—require special additional sensor analysis by a specialized PSA tool. Whether supplied by the institution or the manufacturer, a good PSA is a must.

It sometimes seems that there are never enough spare parts during a pacemaker procedure. It is certainly common that just when you need it, the key spare part is unavailable. Most manufacturers offer service kits containing splice kits, stylets, lead adapters, wrenches, lubricant, lead caps, wire cutters, and so on (Table 27–3). It is advisable to set up a pacemaker cart stocked with all the supplies one is likely to need. This cart should include (1) a temporary pacemaker tray that contains the materials for venous insertion as well as the temporary pulse generator and leads; (2) an assortment of sheath sets, dilators, and guide wires; (3) the service kits of the manufacturers most commonly used; (4) the equipment for lead retrieval; and, if they are used, (5) a supply of polyester (Parsonnet) pouches (Fig. 27–5). Someone should be designated to make sure supplies are reordered and up to date.

There are other, rarely used supplies that can be obtained from the operating room or central supply facility. An example would include a Jackson-Pratt drain (Fig. 27–6) for

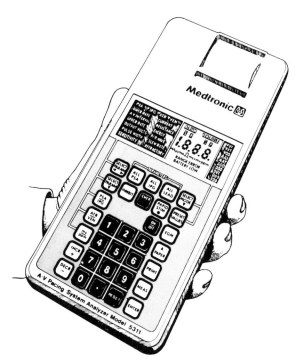

FIGURE 27–4. The multifunction hand-held Medtronic 5311 (Medtronic Inc., Minneapolis, MN) pacemaker system analyzer. This device determines the pacing and sensing functions of the electrode and the pulse generator as well as the electric integrity of the electrode. (From Barold S [ed]: Modern Cardiac Pacing. Mt Kisco, NY, Futura Publ. Co, Inc., 1985, p 444.)

TABLE 27–2. **5311 PSA OPERATING FEATURES**

PROGRAMMABLE PARAMETERS MODE	ADJUSTABLE RANGE (VVI/T/O, AAI/T/O, VDD, DDD, DVI, DOO)
Lower rate	30–180 ppm
AV interval	25–250 msec
Upper rate	100–180 ppm
Output volts	0.1–10 V
Pulse width	0.05–2 msec
Sensitivity	
Atrium	0.75–1 mv
Ventricle	1.0–10 mv
MEASURABLE PACING ELECTRODE PARAMETERS	
Output volts	0.5–10.2 V
Output current	0.1–25 ma
Resistance	100–1900 ohms
Energy	1–1000 μJ
P-wave amplitude	0.5–25.4 mv
R-wave amplitude	0.5–25.4 mv
Slew rate	0.1–7.5 V/sec
MEASURABLE PULSE GENERATOR PARAMETERS MODE	
Lower rate	20–1999 ppm
AV interval	1–500 msec
Upper rate	100–180 ppm
Output volts	1–10 V
Pulse width	0.05–19.99 msec
Sensitivity	0.5–10 mv
Current	0.2–20 ma
Energy	1–1000 μJ
Refractory period	50–1000 msec
SPECIAL FEATURES	
Rapid stimulations—AOO, BOO, DOO modes	800 ppm
Print out	
All electrode programmed and measured data	
All pulse generator measured data	
Endocardial electrogram—VA conduction system atrium, ventricular	

managing hematomas and various sizes of Penrose drains that may be used for tunneling.

Preoperative Planning

The planning that goes into a pacemaker procedure is important if the case is to proceed smoothly. It starts with the evaluation of the patient. A history elucidating patient symptoms, medications the patient is taking, and associated

TABLE 27–3. **PACEMAKER SUPPLIES AND SPARE PARTS**

Lead Stylets
Varying lengths
Variable stiffness
Straight and variable J curve
Silicone oil
Helical coil adaptor with 5-mm pin
Sterile medical adhesive
Wire crimper-cutter
Lead connector caps, 3.2, VS-1, and 5-mm sizes
Step-up and step-down adapters
Adapter sleeves
Screwdriver kit and torque wrenches
One set of connecting cable introducer sets, 11 and 12 F

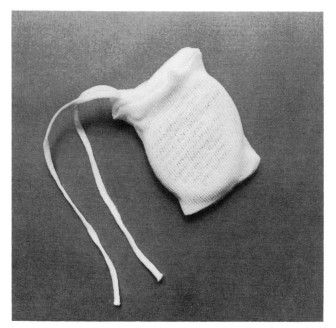

FIGURE 27–5. The polyester (Dacron) Parsonnet pouch is useful in patients with little subcutaneous tissue. The pouch is usually soaked in povidone-iodine (Betadine) before inserting the pacemaker into the pouch, and then into the pacemaker pocket.

conditions is essential. The physical examination may demonstrate the effects of bradycardia, including altered vital signs, evidence of cardiac decompensation, or neurologic deficits. Anatomic issues potentially affecting the implant can also be uncovered. One of the most important preoperative considerations is the documentation of the bradyarrhythmia. This can be accomplished with the 12-lead ECG, Holter monitor, event recordings, as well as in-hospital critical care unit and telemetry unit monitoring. Supporting laboratory data, such as digitalis levels, thyroid panels and chemistries, help document the nontransient nature of the problem. The work-up of the patient should substantiate the indications outlined by the American College of Cardiology–American

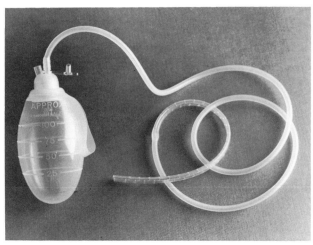

FIGURE 27–6. The Jackson-Pratt drainage system allows for sterile closed wound drainage. The negative-pressure squeeze bulb has a one-way valve that prevents drainage from returning to the wound.

TABLE 27–4. **AMBULATORY AND EARLY DISCHARGE: TEN-YEAR ANNUAL ANALYSIS**

	YEAR									
	1983	1984	1985	1986	1987	1988	1989	1990	1991	1992
Total procedures (N)	99	102	112	110	112	123	100	107	135	119
Total ambulatory (N)	34	34	56	60	78	87	70	87	124	94
Discharge same day (N)	8	16	44	56	78	86	68	83	124	90
Discharge next morning (N)	26	18	12	4	0	1	2	4	0	4
Ambulatory (%)	34	34	50	60	69	70	70	77	91	78

Heart Association joint task force.[20] The documentation should be readily available and generally affixed to the patient's chart.

With all of the documentation obtained and indications met, the next step is the scheduling of the pacemaker procedure. Today the pacemaker surgery can be performed on either an inpatient or an outpatient basis.

Traditionally, pacemaker procedures have been performed on an inpatient basis, which involves formal admission of the patient to the hospital for the procedure. The preoperative evaluation (in most cases), the pacemaker procedure, and early postoperative care are carried out in the hospital. Generally, the patient has already been admitted to the hospital because of symptoms (i.e., syncope) and the diagnosis of a bradyarrhythmia subsequently established. The pacemaker procedure is then scheduled. Alternatively, some or most of the work-up is completed prior to admission, and once the need for a pacemaker is determined the patient is admitted for the pacemaker procedure and postoperative care. In some cases, this inpatient approach is inefficient and cost-ineffective.

The early pacing systems were large, had brief longevity, and were prone to catastrophic complications, such as lead dislodgment, perforation, and wound infection. Postoperatively, patients were managed with extreme caution because of these concerns, and an abbreviated hospital stay seemed radical, whereas the concept of an ambulatory procedure was unthinkable. Today, complications are rare, the pacemakers are small, venous access is easy and quick by the introducer technique, and the surgery is relatively minor. Refinements of the electrode systems with active and passive fixation have reduced the dislodgment rate to near zero. In addition, the indications have been expanded to include more patients who are less pacemaker-dependent. Finally, and perhaps most directly, there is an increasing mandate for cost-containment. The very technology that has made cardiac pacing physiologic, reliable, and safe has resulted in higher cost. For all these reasons, it seems logical that an ambulatory approach for pacemaker procedures could at once be safe and effective as well as less expensive.

Today there is a trend toward performing pacemaker procedures on an ambulatory basis. The experiences at several centers, both in Europe and the United States, have clearly supported the safety and efficacy of this approach.[21, 22] Concerns with respect to potential complications continue to be expressed.[23–25] Questions about lead selection, the timing of discharge, and the intensity of follow-up are raised frequently. In addition, the economic impact has yet to be fully appreciated. Although we believe that more pacemaker procedures are being performed on an ambulatory basis, this has not been reflected in the pacing literature. Since the original

reports of Zegelman and colleagues[21] and Belott,[22] Haywood and associates have reported a randomized, controlled study of the feasibility and safety of ambulatory pacemaker procedures.[26] Although the study group was small (50 patients), the results were similar to the experience of one of us (PHB). There was good patient acceptance, no evidence of a higher complication rate, and cost savings of £540 (1 pound sterling = $1.50). Since the initial report of 181 new pacemaker implants in 1987, our own ambulatory experience continues to be gratifying. Over the past 10 years, that experience now includes performance of 1139 pacemaker procedures, 658 (58%) of which were performed on an ambulatory basis. This experience includes pulse generator changes, all of which have been performed on an ambulatory basis since 1987. Based on this experience, it appears that between 60% and 75% of new pacemaker implantations can be successfully performed on an ambulatory basis (Table 27–4). There have been no additional ambulatory failures and pacemaker-related emergencies or deaths. An ambulatory failure is a case that is initiated on an ambulatory basis, but the hospital stay is extended to an admission because of a complication. The complications encountered in ambulatory cases included one hemothorax detected 2 weeks after discharge. This was successfully managed by hospitalization and chest tube drainage. Three hematomas were managed on an ambulatory basis by reoperation, control of bleeding, and drain placement. Two small pneumothoraces, not requiring chest tubes, occurred fortuitously in hospitalized patients not intended for an ambulatory procedure.

These experiences underscore the safety of the ambulatory approach. At present, one of us (PHB) approaches all elective pacemaker procedures (new implants, electrode repositioning, upgrade procedures, electrode extractions, and pulse generator changes) on an ambulatory basis. A simple protocol is used, and the patients often go home 1 to 2 hours after the procedure. They are seen the following day in the pacemaker clinic. A simple outpatient protocol is outlined in Table 27–5.

It is important to note that in most places, patients can

TABLE 27–5. **OUTPATIENT PROTOCOL**

Surgery scheduled as outpatient with outpatient number assigned
Preoperative blood work, ECG, and chest x-ray study performed as an outpatient within 24 hours prior to admission
Patient instructed to fast after midnight of the evening prior to the procedure
Patient instructed to report to the outpatient department in the morning
Postoperative ECG and chest x-ray film
Discharged when fully awake and vital signs stable
Instructed to report to the pacemaker center the following morning

TABLE 27–6. DEFINITION OF AMBULATORY SURGICAL PROCEDURES

> When a patient with a known diagnosis enters a hospital for a specific minor surgical procedure or treatment that is expected to keep him in a hospital for only a few hours (less than 24) and this expectation is realized, he will be considered an outpatient regardless of the hour of admission, whether or not he occupied a bed, and whether or not he remained in the hospital past midnight.

From Health Care Financing Administration; Hospital manual, publication 10, section 210A.

remain in the hospital overnight and still be considered outpatients. This conforms to the present Health Care Financing Administration definition of ambulatory surgery for reimbursement in the United States (Table 27–6). An important caveat of ambulatory pacemaker procedures is that if there is any doubt or concern about the patient's well-being, the stay can be extended.

In order for ambulatory procedures to become more widely practiced, reasonable and equitable reimbursement schedules will have to be instituted. To date, such schedules are lacking, and this fact may be contributing to a slower than optimal transition toward more ambulatory procedures.[27]

The preoperative patient assessment relates to the synthesis of all patient information, including history, physical examination, old records, rhythm strips, and laboratory data. With this information, appropriate decisions can be made pertaining to the pacemaker mode, leads, and general approach.

The first such decision is whether the patient requires a single- or dual-chamber pacemaker. As a rule, if the patient has intact atrial function, every effort is made to preserve atrial and ventricular relationships. Single-chamber ventricular pacing is usually reserved for the patient with chronic atrial fibrillation or atrial paralysis. A device is selected with acceptable size, longevity, and programmability. If the patient is chronotropically incompetent, a device that offers some form of rate adaptation is considered. Just as important is the lead selection. The issue of lead selection is more completely addressed in another chapter (Chapter 3). One necessary decision is whether to use passive or active fixation leads. Generally, an active fixation electrode is selected when problems of dislodgment are expected, such as in the patient with a dilated right ventricle or amputated atrial appendage. Active fixation leads are one of several factors that enhance removability of the lead, if it is necessary in the future. Also important is the pacing configuration (unipolar vs. bipolar). This decision relates to both electrodes and the pulse generator. Although bipolar pacing and sensing has definite advantages, bipolar leads have historically been more complicated and prone to problems. Bipolar leads are also larger in diameter. The compatibility of electrodes and the pulse generator is extremely important, particularly when using an older existing electrode with a modern new pulse generator. If incompatibility exists, an appropriate adapter must be obtained.

If an ambulatory approach is a consideration, the patient is assessed with respect to the risk of this approach. An unstable patient should always be admitted to the hospital. If the patient is critically ill, pacemaker-dependent, or unstable, a temporary pacemaker is considered. It is frequently better to take the few extra minutes and place a temporary pacemaker. It can avoid moments of "terror" during the procedure if asystole occurs. This is particularly true in patients with complete atrioventricular (AV) block in whom an apparently stable escape rhythm can suddenly disappear, a common situation once initial pacing has been established.

The timing of the procedure usually relates to the stability of the patient. In the critically ill patient in whom there are concerns over the stability of the cardiac rhythm or temporary pacemaker, an early permanent procedure is in order. Conversely, in a patient whose survival is in doubt, one may appropriately decide to wait for stabilization. At times the procedure is delayed because of systemic infection or sepsis. A permanent pacemaker implantation performed on a septic patient may lead to the seeding of bacteria on the pacemaker or electrode. It has been our approach that if there is active infection, the procedure is deferred until the patient is afebrile and no longer septic to reduce the risk of a pacemaker system infection.

Decisions with regard to the implant site are not as important today as they were when only large pulse generators were available. The currently available devices, weighing less than 30 g, make the implant site, in most situations, moot. They tend to be tolerated well in almost any location. There are, however, special circumstances that deserve mention. These are hobbies, recreational and occupational activities, cosmetic issues, and previous medical conditions. The hunter, for instance, should have the pacemaker placed on the side opposite where the rifle butt is placed. Similar considerations are appropriate for the tennis enthusiast or golfer (although, in our experience, it is variable for the golfer as to whether the backswing or follow-through side is better). In a young person, placement of the pacemaker under the breast (women) or in the axilla may be more desirable from a cosmetic point of view. Medical conditions, such as previous surgery, radiation therapy, or skeletal or other anatomic abnormalities, should be considered. In the patient who is small with little subcutaneous tissue, a subpectoral implant may be required. This calls for the use of a bipolar system to avoid skeletal muscle stimulation.

The preoperative orders are generally quite simple. The patient fasts for at least 6 hours prior to the procedure. If the implant is being performed on an ambulatory basis, the patient is instructed to report to the hospital on the day of the procedure, allowing enough time to obtain the necessary preoperative testing. Generally 2 hours prior to the procedure is adequate. The preoperatives includes posteroanterior (PA) and lateral chest x-ray films, an ECG, a complete blood count, prothrombin time, partial thromboplastin time, and electrolytes, blood urea nitrogen, and creatinine determinations. Because the patient is fasting, adequate hydration is maintained with a stable intravenous (IV) line. Hydration is extremely important for subsequent venous access and prevention of air embolization during the procedure. It can be frustrating and dangerous to try to gain venous access in a patient who is dehydrated after prolonged fasting without IV hydration. We generally request that the IV be started on the side of the planned procedure to facilitate venography during attempts at venous access if this becomes a problem. If the patient undergoes anticoagulation with warfarin, the protime can be lowered to the 15-second range, or the International Normalized Ratio (INR) below 1.75, without an excessive risk of bleeding. Alternatively, the patient can be given heparin, which is discontinued 4 to 6 hours before the start of the procedure and reinstituted subsequent to the procedure. The patient is instructed to continue maintenance oral medications, which may be taken with small sips of water. Patients taking hypoglycemic agents are instructed to reduce the preoperative dose by 50%. The administration of prophylactic antibiotics is controversial. Both of our individual preferences call for a broad spectrum cephalosporin such as cefazolin to be given intraoperatively. Many others use vancomycin, which covers all the gram-positive potentially pathogenic organisms. We also have the patient scrub chest, neck, shoulders, and supraclavicular fossae with a povidone-iodine (betadine) sponge the evening and the morning before the procedure. In most instances, skin shaving is carried out in the procedure room. Finally, we ask the patient to void before coming to the procedure room.

Pacemaker Implantation: General Information

On arrival at the procedure room, the patient is transferred to a radiography table. In the catheterization laboratory or special procedures area, the table's radiolucent properties are expected. In the operating room, prior arrangements are made for a special radiolucent operating table. In this latter situation, it is advisable to test the fluoroscopy equipment's ability to penetrate the table. It is also helpful to establish proper x-ray tube orientation. Attention to these details can avoid considerable hassle later when it is discovered that the patient is on the wrong table, the x-ray equipment is inoperative, or the image is upside down or backwards, or both. Almost immediately, the patient is connected to physiologic monitoring (electrocardiograph, pulse oximetery, and automatic blood pressure cuff). If it has not already been accomplished, a reliable venous line is established, preferably on the side of the operative site. The circulating nurse must have easy access to the IV line for drug administration or introduction of radiographic materials, or both. Oxygen can be administered by nasal cannula or mask. If a temporary pacemaker is to be placed, the appropriate site is shaved and prepared and the temporary pacemaker is placed using the Seldinger technique. It is important to adequately secure the lead and sheath to maintain accessibility so that it can be easily removed at the end of the procedure.

Once effective patient support has been established, focus turns to the operative site. If not already accomplished, skin shaving and cleansing is carried out, which should be generous in scope and include the neck, supraventricular fossae, shoulders, and chest. The operative site, shaved and cleansed, is now formally prepared and draped. There are several ways to accomplish this. One can use a povidone-iodine scrub, followed by alcohol, followed by povidone-iodine solution, with skin drying before the final povidone-iodine solution is applied. This older, more-time consuming, although effective, scrub can be replaced by the use of povidone-iodine solution gel, which is a gelatinous preparation of povidone-iodine. It is spread liberally over the operative site. Within 30 seconds, an optimal bactericidal effect is achieved. With this approach, scrubbing the area is not required. In the case of patients who are allergic to povidone-iodine, a chlorhexidine (Hibiclens) or hexachlorophene (phisoHex) scrub can be carried out. The draping process is a matter of personal preference. One of us (DR) applies a sterile, see-through plastic adhesive drape (impregnated with an iodoform solution) over the entire operative area. The other (PB) uses one or more sterile plastic drapes with adhesive along one side (Fig. 27–7). The adhesive surface is applied from shoulder to shoulder at the level of the clavicle, which serves to create a sterile barrier from the shoulder level down. Depending on the situation, other barriers can be created. In both cases, the use of the plastic drape is to optimize sterility. After establishing some form of sterile barrier, the operative site is then draped with sterile towels, and one or more large sterile

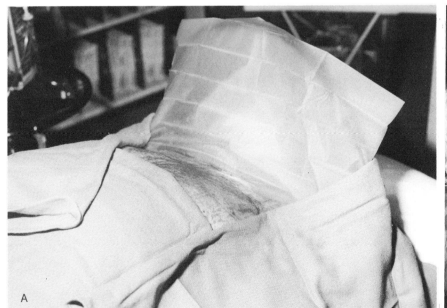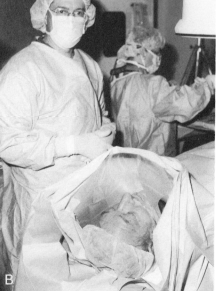

FIGURE 27–7. *A,* Application of a 3M 10/10 drape (Minneapolis, MN) to create a sterile barrier. *B,* The drape folds over the common house wire (Romex wire) support, creating an effective sterile barrier and preventing patient claustrophobia.

surgical sheets are applied. Care is taken to avoid smothering the patient or causing claustrophobia. This is best achieved by keeping the drapes off the patient's face and maintaining the cephalic aspect of the main drape perpendicular to the patient's neck. This allows unrestricted access to the patient's head and neck. The main drape is clipped to some form of support on both sides of the patient. This support can consist of IV poles placed on each side of the patient. This arrangement may not be possible in laboratories where it interferes with radiographic equipment. In this case, the drape may be fixed to the C-arm or image intensifier. This solution is less than optimal, as the drapes pull away every time the C-arm or radiographic table is repositioned. This increases the risk of contamination and breaks in sterile technique. More recently, a simple, cost-effective solution to this problem has been developed. A length of common house wire (8/3-gauge Romex) is shaped into an arc over the patient's neck. The ends of the wire are bent at right angles to the arc and tucked under the x-ray table padding at the level of the patient's shoulders (Fig. 27–8). The weight of the patient's shoulders supports the wire arc. The wire can be shaped to fit any patient. The wire positioned under the shoulder is checked under fluoroscopy to avoid interference with the radiographic field of view. The Romex wire is strong enough to maintain its shape under the weight of the surgical drape. This offers optimal patient comfort and a very reliable sterile barrier. There is no interference with the C-arm, and claustrophobia is avoided. The traditional use of a Mayo stand over the patient's face is problematic in that it can cause claustrophobia, makes access to the patient's airway difficult in an emergency, and may interfere with the x-ray equipment.

Finally, it should be pointed out that from the moment the catheterization laboratory or special studies room is cleaned, it must be treated as a surgical suite. All personnel must wear surgical clothing, hats, and masks. There should be an attempt to seal the room, limiting traffic and restricting access to those participating in the procedure.

The majority of pacemaker procedures are performed with local anesthesia and the addition of some form of sedation and pain reliever.[28] Local anesthesia alone is inadequate for optimal patient comfort. Even in the best circumstances, the effect of local anesthesia does not avoid the discomfort associated with the creation of the pacemaker pocket. For this reason, the additional combination of a narcotic and sedative is recommended. The use of sedation alone is frequently inadequate. The challenge to the physician in charge is the achievement of patient comfort without risking oversedation or respiratory depression. If an anesthesiologist or nurse anesthetist is part of the implantation team, patient comfort is usually achieved easily and safely. In this situation, if respiratory depression occurs, the patient can easily be ventilated. In the circumstance in which the implanting physician orders the sedation and narcotics, the patient must be carefully monitored by the circulating nurse. It is recommended that the medications be administered slowly.

The selection of the local anesthetic and the dose delivered are also important considerations. The use of a local agent in therapeutic concentration that provides rapid onset of action and sustained duration is desirable. Local agents can be used in combination to achieve the desired effect. An example is the use of lidocaine, for its rapid onset, and bupivacaine for its sustained action. There is also an upper limit of total local anesthetic dose that should not be exceeded. Toxic blood levels of commonly used local anesthetics can result in profound neurologic abnormalities, including obtundation and seizures. A number of local anesthetic agents are listed in Table 27–7.

The selection of sedative and narcotic is dependent on personal preference. We currently use midazolam and fentanyl. The operator should become familiar with one or more sedative agents as well as an analgesic, preferably a narcotic. There are many newer agents available. The selection of a benzodiazepine in combination with a semisynthetic narcotic can achieve ideal sedation, amnesia, and analgesia. A cooperative, relaxed, and pain-free patient is fundamental to the success of the procedure and the avoidance of complications. Pentathol and nitrous oxide have been used to effect brief periods of complete sedation at times of anticipated maxi-

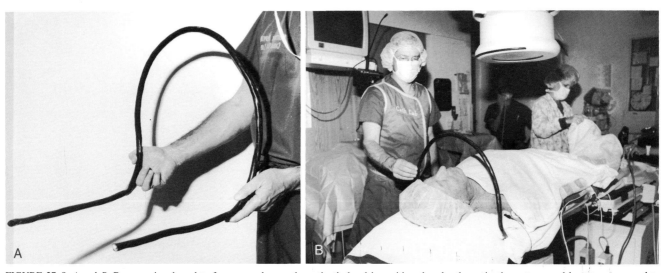

FIGURE 27–8. A and B, Romex wire shaped to form an arch over the patient's head is positioned under the patient's mattress and bent to accommodate differences in patients and circumstances.

TABLE 27–7. PHARMACOLOGIC PROPERTIES OF COMMONLY USED LOCAL ANESTHETIC AGENTS

	ONSET (MIN)	DURATION (HR)	PROTEIN BINDING	MAXIMUM ADULT DOSE
ESTERS				
Chloroprocaine (Nesacaine)	Slow (5–10)	Short (0.5–1.5)	5%	800 mg (11 µg/kg)
Procaine (Novocain)	Fast (5–15)	Short (0.5–1.5)		800 mg (11 µg/kg)
Tetracaine	Slow (20–30)	Long (3–5)	85%	200 mg
AMIDES				
Bupivacaine (Marcaine)	Moderate (10–20)	Long (3–5)	82–96%	100 mg
Lidocaine (Xylocaine)	Fast (5–15)	Moderate (1–3)	55–65%	300 mg (4 µg/kg)

mum discomfort, but the use of these drugs requires the expertise of an anesthetist, as temporary respiratory support is frequently required.

In the United States, the Joint Commission of Hospital Accreditation mandates that institutions establish a policy and protocol for patients receiving conscious sedation. Pacemaker procedures would be included in such a protocol. In essence, the protocol requires formal patient assessment prior to sedation. The sedation and recovery areas must have resuscitation equipment present at all times, and patients undergoing conscious sedation must be monitored with pulse oximetry, continuous electrocardiographic rhythm monitoring, and automatic blood pressure recordings. Monitoring of the patient should continue for at least 30 minutes after the last intravenous sedative drug administration and for at least 90 minutes after intramuscular sedative drug administration. There are also strict discharge criteria. A common conscious sedation drug protocol is shown in Table 27–8.

The use of prophylactic antibiotics to reduce the incidence of postoperative wound infection in a pacemaker procedure is controversial.[29] It is important to point out that they are not a substitute for good infection control practices, an adequate surgical environment, and good surgical technique. The use of antibiotics in a pacemaker procedure follows the principle of prophylaxis in which the risk of infection is low but the monetary penalty or morbidity is high.[30–32] The selection of antibiotics is based on site-specific flora for wound infection and the spectrum, kinetics, and toxicity of the antimicro-

bial agent. The risk factors for infection have been well defined. The National Research Council for Wound Classification places the risk of infection from an elective procedure closed primarily at less than 2%. One important factor to be considered is the increased risk of infection in operations lasting longer than 2 hours. Although not formally studied, the use of prophylactic antibiotics in the low-risk, high-morbidity group, such as patients receiving pacemakers, appears justified. It should be pointed out that there are no specific references in the literature to antibiotic prophylaxis for pacemaker procedures, only for prosthetic devices. The spectrum of the antibiotic prophylaxis need only cover the gram-positive skin flora, primarily *Staphylococcus epidermidis* and *Staphylococcus aureus*. In the case of pacemakers and cardiac procedures, the cephalosporins appear ideal (i.e., 1 to 2 g cefazolin IV, preanesthesia). If an institution has a high incidence of methicillin-resistant *S. aureus* or *S. epidermidis*, vancomycin should be considered (i.e., 1 g vancomycin IV slowly preoperatively). Postoperative doses are left to clinical judgment. Generally, 1 g of either drug may be given intravenously up to 8 hours postoperatively. Occasionally, the postoperative doses of cephalosporin are given orally for several days. These drug guidelines are also reflected in the *Medical Letter* of January 1992.[33] It is interesting to note that the *Medical Letter* specifically does not recommend antibiotic prophylaxis for pacemaker procedures.

An additional strategy in the prevention of infection is topical antibiotic prophylaxis or antibiotic wound irrigation.[34] It is important to note that controlled trials evaluating the benefit of antibiotic irrigations is lacking. The concept of irrigation is to provide a high concentration of antibiotic at the site of potential infection at the time of contamination. The technique has proved most efficient in the absence of established infection. It calls for the use of nonabsorbable antibiotics. Historically, aminoglycosides and bacitracin combinations have been used, but there are many regimens that are varied in number, type, concentration, and duration of antibiotic use. Systemic toxicity with antibiotic irrigation is a major concern. When large volumes of irrigating solutions are used in combination with systemic antibiotics, the therapeutic range can be greatly exceeded. The superiority of irrigation over systemic antibiotic administration has never been proved, and given the potential toxicity, caution is recommended. Some popular antibiotic irrigation protocols are shown in Table 27–9.

TABLE 27–8. CONSCIOUS SEDATION DRUG PROTOCOLS

DRUG NAME	ROUTE OF ADMINISTRATION	DOSAGE RANGE	MAXIMUM DOSE	COMMENTS
Meperidine	IM or IV	25–100 mg	100 mg	Long acting
Morphine	IM or IV	1.5–15 mg	20 mg	Long acting
Fentanyl	IM or IV	50–100 µcg	100 mg	Short acting, very potent
Valium	IV	2–10 mg	10 mg	
Droperidol	IV	8–17 µg/kg	17 µg/kg	
Midazolam	IV	1–2.5 mg	5 mg	
Nitrous oxide	Inhalation	30–50%	50%	
Thiopental	IV	1–4 mg/kg		Temporary loss of consciousness
Ketamine	IV	0.5 mg/kg	0.5 mg/kg	Temporary loss of consciousness

Abbreviations: IM, intramuscular; IV, intravenous.

TABLE 27–9. COMMON ANTIMICROBIAL IRRIGATION PROTOCOLS

AGENT	CONCENTRATION
Bacitracin	50,000 units in 200 mL of saline
Cephalothin	1 g/L of saline
Cefazolin	1 g/L of saline
Cefuroxime	750 mg/L of saline
Vancomycin	200–500 mg/L of saline
Povidone-iodine	Concentrated or diluted in aliquots of saline

TABLE 27–10. VENOUS ACCESS FOR SINGLE- AND DUAL-CHAMBER PACING

Venous cutdown: Isolate one or two veins
Percutaneous: Two separate sticks and sheath applications
Percutaneous: Two electrodes down one large sheath
Percutaneous: Retained guide wire (Belott technique)
Percutaneous access to the extrathoracic portion of the subclavian vein (Byrd technique)
Cutdown with cephalic vein guide wire (Ong-Barold technique)

Despite the controversial nature of prophylactic systemic antibiotics and topical irrigation, the E1 Cajon experience has been very gratifying. A protocol of intravenous antibiotics and wound irrigation has been followed since 1978. In each case, 1 g of cefazolin was given intraoperatively followed by cefadroxil monohydrate, 500 mg, twice daily for 4 days. A sponge soaked in povidone-iodine is placed in the pacemaker pocket just after pocket formation and is removed at the time of wound closure. In more than 1500 pacemaker procedures, there have been two wound infections. A similar low incidence of infection has occurred at the University of Oklahoma where, since 1980, our regimen has included a preoperative dose of cefazolin, 1 g IV, followed by 1 g IV for one to five more doses every 8 hours (depending on length of stay), as well as pocket irrigation with a solution of bacitracin, gentamycin, and polymyxin. Although the issue is admittedly controversial, all one needs is one pacemaker infection with all of its problems to become convinced that infection should be avoided at all cost.

There are two basic anatomic approaches for the implantation of a permanent pacemaker.[35, 36] From a historical perspective, the first is the epicardial and the second is the transvenous approach. The epicardial approach calls for direct application of pacemaker electrodes on the heart. This requires general anesthesia and surgical access to the epicardial surface of the heart. The transvenous approach is usually performed with local anesthesia and IV sedation. Each approach can be accomplished by several unique techniques. Today, 95% of all pacemaker implantations are performed transvenously.

The epicardial approach is generally reserved for patients who cannot undergo safe or effective pacemaker implantation via the transvenous route. The epicardial techniques (Fig. 27–9) include applying the electrode or electrodes directly to a completely exposed heart or performing a limited thoracotomy via a subxiphoid incision. A third technique places the leads by mediastinoscopy. There is even a fourth technique that is a combination of both epicardial and endocardial lead placement.

Several techniques are used for the transvenous approach. All involve a venous surgical "cutdown" or percutaneous venous access, or a combination of both (Table 27–10). The pros and cons of the various approaches and techniques are reviewed.

A thorough knowledge of the anatomic structure of the neck, upper extremities, and thorax is essential for cardiac pacing (Fig. 27–10). The precise location and orientation of the internal jugular, innominate, subclavian, and cephalic veins is important for safe venous access.[37] Their anatomic relation to other structures is crucial in avoiding complications. The location of the subclavian vein may vary from a normal lateral course to an extremely anterior or posterior orientation in elderly patients. Byrd has described the subclavian venous anatomy of two distinct deformities.[38] Both conditions make venous access more difficult and hazardous. The first deformity involves a posteriorly displaced clavicle (Fig. 27–11). This is commonly seen in patients with chronic lung disease with anteroposterior chest enlargement. These patients can be identified by a horizontal deltopectoral groove and the posteriorly displaced clavicle. The second deformity is an anteriorly displaced clavicle (Fig. 27–12), which is found occasionally, especially in elderly women. In

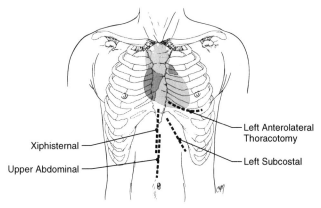

FIGURE 27–9. Location of surgical incisions for the placement of epimyocardial systems.

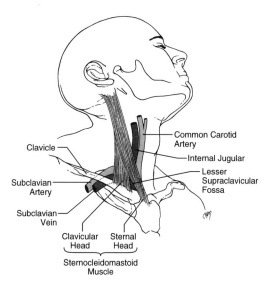

FIGURE 27–10. Anatomic relationship of the vascular structures in the neck and superior mediastinum.

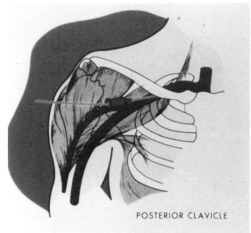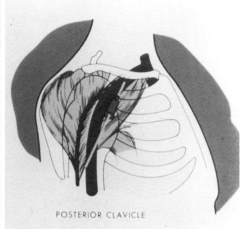

POSTERIOR CLAVICLE POSTERIOR CLAVICLE

FIGURE 27–11. Posterior displacement of the clavicle, recognized by a horizontal rather than oblique position of the deltopectoral groove. (From Byrd CL: Current clinical applications of dual-chamber pacing. *In* Zipes DP [ed]: Proceedings of a Symposium. Minneapolis: Medtronic, Inc., 1981, p 71.)

this situation, the clavicle is anteriorly bowed or actually displaced anteriorly. It is important that these variations are recognized to avoid complications of pneumothorax and hemopneumothorax when approaching the patient percutaneously.

It is assumed that the implanting physician is also completely familiar with the anatomy of the heart and great vessels.[39] However, their spatial orientation is at times confusing. This is particularly true with respect to the right atrium and ventricle. It is recalled that in the frontal plane, the border of the right side of the heart is formed by the right atrium. The border of the left side of the heart is composed of the left ventricle. Importantly, the right ventricle is located anteriorly (Fig. 27–13) and is triangular. The apex of the right ventricle is the generally accepted initial "target" for ventricular lead placement. Unfortunately, the location of the apex of the right ventricle can be variable. Its normal location, distinctly to the left of midline, depends on the rotation of the heart, which is affected by various pathologic and anatomic conditions. At times, it may be located directly anterior to or even to the right of midline. A lack of appre-

ciation of these variances can lead to considerable difficulty in electrode placement.

The choice of site for pacemaker implantation is also occasionally important anatomically. This decision is typically made most appropriately based on the patient's "handedness," occupation, recreational activities, and medical conditions. The decision should not be made based on the handedness of the implanting physician. There are, however, some fundamental differences in the anatomy of the right side compared with that of the left side. Such differences can result in frustration when one is passing a pacemaker electrode. Although for some it seems to be easier for a right-handed individual to work on the right side of the patient (and vice versa), from a surgical point of view catheter manipulation from the right can be a frustrating experience. When entering the central venous circulation from the left upper limb, the pacemaker electrode tracks along a smooth arc to the right ventricle. There are generally no sharp angles or bends (Fig. 27–14A). Conversely, when approaching from the right, the electrode is forced to negotiate a sharp angle or bend at the junction of the right subclavian and internal

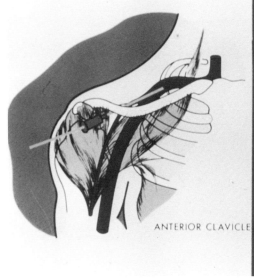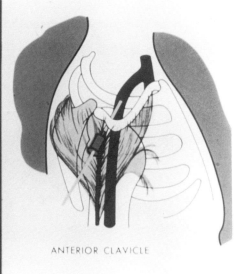

ANTERIOR CLAVICLE ANTERIOR CLAVICLE

FIGURE 27–12. Anterior displacement of the clavicle. The deltopectoral groove is nearly vertical. (From Byrd CL: Current clinical applications of dual-chamber pacing. *In* Zipes DP [ed]: Proceedings of a Symposium. Minneapolis: Medtronic, Inc., 1981, p 71.)

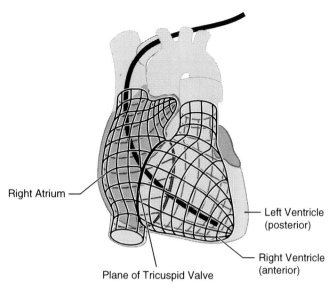

Right Atrium

Left Ventricle
(posterior)

Right Ventricle
(anterior)

Plane of Tricuspid Valve

FIGURE 27–13. The spatial orientation of the right ventricle as an anterior structure in relationship to the left or posterior ventricle or coronary sinus, which is also posterior.

jugular veins where the innominate vein is formed (see Fig. 27–14B). This acute angulation can make the manipulation of the pacemaker electrode difficult when a curved stylet is fully inserted. Another anatomic pitfall occurs when there is a persistent left superior vena cava, making passage to the heart from the left more difficult and, if there is no right superior vena cava, from the right impossible. These situations will be considered when ventricular electrode placement is discussed further on.

Transvenous Pacemaker Placement

The right or left cephalic vein is the most common vascular entry site for insertion of pacemaker electrodes by the cutdown technique.[40] The cephalic vein is located in the deltopectoral groove (Fig. 27–15). This is a groove formed by the reflections of the medial head of the deltoid and the lateral border of the greater pectoral muscles. It can be precisely located by palpating the coracoid process of the scapula. The dermis along the deltopectoral groove is infiltrated with local anesthetic, encompassing the anticipated length of the incision. A vertical incision is made adjacent to and at the level of the coracoid process. It is extended for approximately 2 to 5 cm. Care is taken to keep the scalpel blade perpendicular to the surface of the skin. Smooth skin edges are created by making an initial single stroke that carries through the dermis to each corner of the wound. The subcutaneous tissue is infiltrated with local anesthetic along the edges of the incision. The Weitlander retractor is applied to the edges of the wound, and the subcutaneous tissue is placed under tension. The tension is released by light strokes of the scalpel from corner to corner of the wound in the midline. As the subcutaneous tissue falls away, tension is restored by reapplying the Weitlander retractor. This process is continued down to the surface of the pectoral fascia. The fascia is left intact. At this level, the borders of the pectoral and deltoid muscles forming the deltopectoral groove are identified. A Metzenbaum scissors is used to dissect along the groove by separating the muscles' fibrous attachments. The Weitlander retractor is reapplied deeper to retract the muscle. Gradual release of the fascial tissue between the two muscle bodies will expose the cephalic vein. At times, the cephalic vein is diminutive or atretic and unable to accommodate a pace-

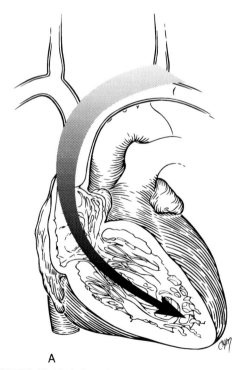

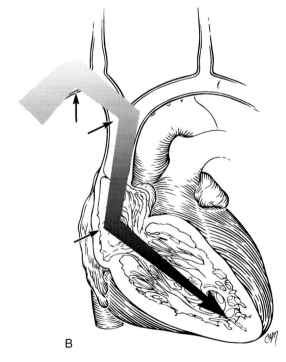

A

B

FIGURE 27–14. A, Smooth course of an electrode entering from the left side. B, Acute angulation of the catheter course when the lead enters the venous system from the right.

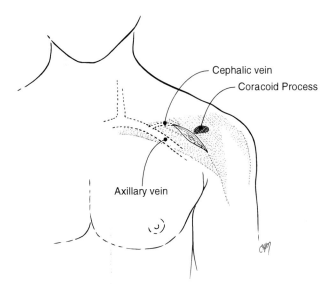

FIGURE 27–15. Anatomy of the deltopectoral groove.

maker lead. In this case, the cephalic vein can be dissected, centrally, to the axillary vein and this larger vein catheterized. Once the vein to be catheterized is localized, it is freed of all fibrous attachments. Ligatures are applied proximally and distally (Fig. 27–16A). The distal ligature is tied and held by a small clamp. The proximal ligature is not tied but is kept under tension with another clamp. An arbitrary entry site is chosen between the two ligatures. The anterior half of the vein at this site is grasped with a smooth forceps, and the vein is gently lifted. A small horizontal venotomy is made using iris scissors (see Fig. 27–16B) or a No. 11 scalpel

blade. The vein is continuously supported by the forceps. The venotomy is held open by any of several means: a mosquito clamp, forceps, or vein pick. Gentle traction is applied on the distal ligature while tension is released on the proximal ligature. With the venotomy held widely open, the electrode or electrodes are inserted and advanced into the central venous circulation (see Fig. 27–16C).

For many years, vascular access has been achieved for many purposes by use of the Seldinger technique. This simple approach calls for the percutaneous puncture of the vessel with a relatively long, large-bore needle; passage of a wire through the needle into the vessel; removal of the needle; and passage of a catheter or sheath over the wire into the vessel with removal of the wire. An 18-gauge thin-walled needle 5 cm in length is commonly used, although smaller needles are available. These needles come prepackaged with most introducer sets (Fig. 27–17), but an extra supply should be available. The historical problem limiting the use of this technique in cardiac pacing was the inability to remove the sheath from the pacemaker lead. The development of a ''peel-away'' sheath by Littleford solved this problem.[41–44]

Use of the percutaneous approach calls for a thorough knowledge of both normal and abnormal anatomy to avoid complications. The subclavian vein is generally the intended venous structure used for percutaneous venous access in cardiac pacing. Given the previously discussed anatomic variations, it is recommended that the subclavian vein puncture be made near the apex of the angle formed by the first rib and clavicle.[45] This defines the ''subclavian window'' (Fig. 27–18). At this puncture site (and following both skin infiltration with local anesthetic and a 1-cm incision at the site, which generally is 1 to 2 cm inferolateral to the point where the clavicle and first rib actually cross), the needle is aimed in a

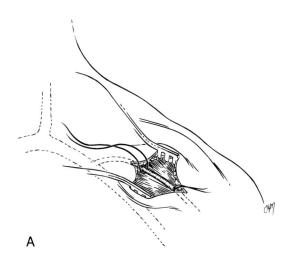

A

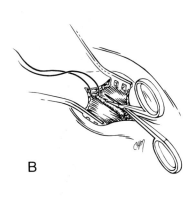

B

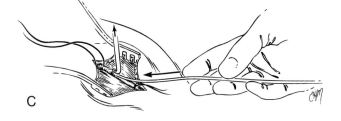

C

FIGURE 27–16. A, Introduction of a lead into the cephalic vein. The cephalic vein is isolated and tied off distally. B, Venotomy performed with iris scissors. C, Lead inserted while venotomy is held open with a vein pick.

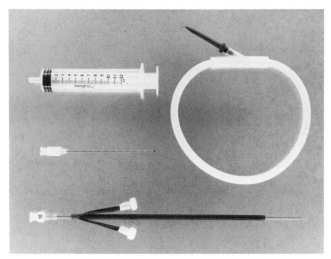

FIGURE 27–17. Prepackaged introducer set with 18-gauge needle, guide wire, and sheath with rubber dilator.

medial and cephalic direction. It is important to make the puncture with the patient in a "normal" anatomic position. The infraclavicular space or costoclavicular angle should not be artificially opened by maneuvers such as extending the arm or by placing a towel roll between the scapulae. These maneuvers can open a normally closed or tight space and result in undesirable puncture of the costoclavicular ligament or subclavius muscle, which can result in lead entrapment and crush. With the patient in the normal anatomic position, access to the "subclavian window" is medial yet usually avoids the costoclavicular ligament. The more medial puncture and needle trajectory of this approach vastly increases the success rate and dramatically reduces the risks of pneumothorax and vascular injury compared with a more lateral

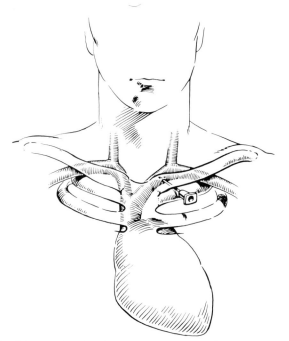

FIGURE 27–18. The subclavian window. (From Barold SS, Mugica J [eds]: New Perspectives in Cardiac Pacing 1. Mt Kisco, NY, Futura Publ. Co., Inc., 1988, p 257.)

approach. With this medial position, the vein is a much larger target and the apex of the lung is more lateral. It should be pointed out that this safer approach is a departure from the conventional subclavian venous puncture, which calls for introduction of the needle in the middle third of the clavicle.

There are legitimate concerns that this medial approach, although safer, results in a later increase in the complication rate of failure from conductor fracture and insulation damage.[46] It is postulated that the extreme medial position results in a tight fit, subjecting the lead to compressive forces, causing binding between the first rib and the clavicle. Occasionally this binding can even crush the lead and today is called "the subclavian crush phenomenon." This phenomenon is more common in larger, complex leads of the "in-line" bipolar, coaxial design. Fortunately, the incidence of this complication is low. Fyke first reported insulation failure of two leads placed side by side via the percutaneous approach through the subclavian vein where there was a tight costoclavicular space.[47, 48] More recently, this issue has been addressed thoroughly by two independent groups. Jacobs and associates analyzed a series of failed leads for the mechanism of failure.[49] They correlated the anatomic relationship of lead position to compressive forces by autopsy study (Fig. 27–19). These autopsy data demonstrated a significant increase in pressure generated when leads were inserted in the costoclavicular angle as compared with that occurring with a more lateral puncture. They concluded that the tight costoclavicular angle should be avoided. Magney and colleagues derived similar data from cadaveric studies and suggest that lead damage is caused by soft tissue entrapment by the subclavius muscle rather than bony contact.[50] This soft tissue entrapment causes a static load on the lead at that point, and repeated flexure around the point of entrapment may be responsible for the damage. Concern about this problem also has been communicated by pacemaker manufacturers in company literature.[51, 52] Reduction in lead diameter and, perhaps, modification of lead technology may be required to eliminate this problem. In the meantime, technique modification appears to be effective at reducing the occurrence of this problem. It has been our experience that if a pacemaker lead feels "tight" in the costoclavicular space, it is more susceptible to being crushed, and it has become our practice at the University of Oklahoma to remove the lead from the vein in this situation and repuncture the vein in a slightly different location with reintroduction of the lead. We believe that this has reduced the incidence of "crush," although more substantial modifications in technique, described further on, may be indicated.

Addressing this issue, along with other introducer- or percutaneous-related complications, Byrd has described a "safe introducer technique."[53] This technique consists of a "safety zone" associated with precise conditions ensuring a safe puncture. Also described is a new technique for cannulating the axillary vein if this safety zone cannot be entered. Byrd's safety zone is defined as a region of venous access between the first rib and the clavicle, extending laterally from the sternum in an arc (Fig. 27–20A). As a condition for puncture, the site of access must be adequate for ease of insertion to avoid friction and puncture of bone, cartilage, or tendon. With this technique, subclavian vein puncture should never be made outside the safety zone or in violation of the preceding conditions. If the safety zone is inaccessible, or the pre-

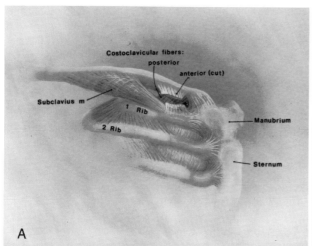

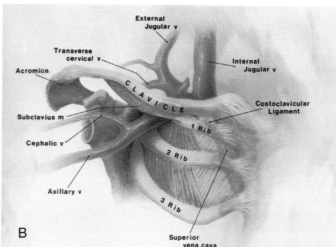

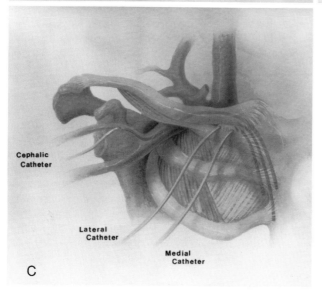

FIGURE 27–19. *A,* Musculoskeletal anatomy of the infraclavicular space. *B,* The relationship of the venous structures to clavicle, first rib, and costoclavicular ligaments. *C,* Course of leads through the venous structures demonstrating how the pacemaker electrode can become entrapped. (*A* to *C* from Jacobs DM, Fink AS, Miller RP, et al: Anatomical and morphological evaluation of pacemaker lead compression. PACE 16:434, 1993.)

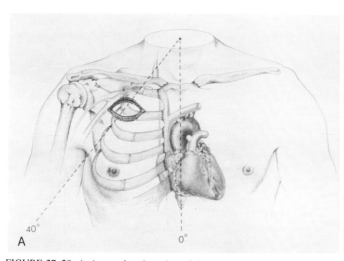

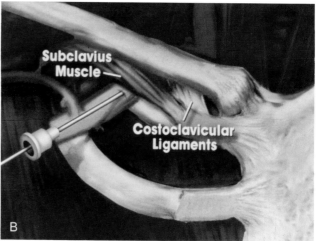

FIGURE 27–20. *A,* Anatomic orientation of the ''safety zone'' for intrathoracic subclavian vein puncture. *B,* Safe access to the extrathoracic portion of the subclavian vein as described by Byrd. (*A* from Barold SS, Mugica J [eds]: New Perspectives in Cardiac Pacing 2. Mt Kisco, NY, Futura Publ. Co., Inc., 1991, p 108. *B* from Byrd CL: Recent developments in pacemaker implantation and lead retrieval. PACE 16:1781, 1993.)

ceding conditions are not met, an axillary vein puncture is recommended. (Byrd uses the term extrathoracic portion of the subclavian vein synonymously with the continuation of the subclavian vein as the axillary vein.) The axillary vein puncture is performed as a modification of the standard subclavian vein procedure without repositioning the patient (see Fig. 27–20*B*). The introducer needle is guided by fluoroscopy directly to the medial portion of the first rib. The needle is held perpendicular to, and touches, the first rib. The needle, held perpendicular to the rib, is "walked" laterally and posteriorly, touching the rib with each change of position. Once the vein is punctured, as indicated by aspiration of venous blood into the syringe, the guide wire and the introducer are inserted using standard technique. This approach essentially guarantees a successful and safe venipuncture without compromising the leads if the conditions for entering the safety zone are adhered to and if the first rib is touched to maintain orientation. The only complication not prevented by this approach is inadvertent puncture of the axillary artery.

The axillary vein approach actually is not new. In 1987, based on cadaveric studies that established reliable surface landmarks, Nichalls[54] and Taylor and Yellowlees[55] reported this approach as an alternative safe route of venous access for large central lines. The axillary vein has a completely infraclavicular course. The needle path must always be anterior to the thoracic cavity, avoiding risks of pneumothorax and hemothorax. The suggested landmarks for this infraclavicular course of the axillary vein (Fig. 27–21) are as follows: The axillary vein starts medially at a point below the aspect of the clavicle where the space between the first rib and clavicle becomes palpable. The vein extends laterally to a point approximately three fingerbreadths below the inferior aspect of the coracoid process. The skin is punctured along the medial border of the smaller pectoralis muscle at a point above the vein as it is defined by the surface landmarks. The

axillary vein is punctured by passing the needle anterior to the first rib, maneuvering posteriorly and medially corresponding to the lateral to medial course of the axillary vein. The needle never passes between the first rib and the clavicle, staying lateral to this juncture. It is recommended that the arm be abducted 45 degrees to use this approach.

For a more conventional subclavian vein approach, Lamas and colleagues have even recommended fluoroscopic observation of the needle trajectory for achieving a successful and safe subclavian vein puncture.[56] They initially identify the clavicle on the side of puncture, noting its course and landmarks. The skin is entered approximately 2 cm inferior to the junction of the medial and lateral halves of the clavicle, aiming with fluoroscopic guidance for the caudal half of the clavicular head.

Whether using the techniques of the subclavian window, the safety zone, the axillary vein puncture, or fluoroscopic guidance, there are some common features. Needle orientation is always medial and cephalad, almost tangential to the chest wall. All needle probing should use a forward motion. Lateral needle probing should be avoided because it could cause laceration of important structures. Anatomic landmarks are defined and the puncture is made, with rare exception, with the patient in the anatomic position. The costoclavicular angle is not artificially opened by maneuvers. Although the essence of the (nonaxillary) approaches is medial to avoid the lung, the undesirable puncture of the costoclavicular ligament should be avoided. In the obese patient, the tendency is to orient the needle more perpendicular to the chest wall in an attempt to pass between the clavicle and first rib. This perpendicular angle is to be avoided, as it is associated with a higher incidence of pneumothorax. In this circumstance, a more inferior skin puncture is recommended, allowing the needle to slip between the first rib and clavicle. The needle is, therefore, maintained almost tangential to the chest wall, avoiding the lung. Some implanters will bend the needle in an attempt to slip under the clavicle. We do not recommend this because of a higher incidence of pneumothorax and vascular trauma. In the morbidly obese patient, it is recommended that the subclavian puncture be carried out after direct visualization of the pectoral muscle. This can be done only by making an initial skin incision and carrying it down to the pectoral muscle. Once the anatomic landmarks are defined, the needle is slipped between the first rib and the clavicle with a trajectory that is nearly tangential to the chest wall directed cephalad and medial.

This raises the question of whether the skin incision should routinely be made first, with percutaneous venous access carried out through the incision, or whether an initial percutaneous venous puncture should be performed, followed by the incision. It is possibly better not to commit oneself with an initial pocket-length incision and subsequent venipuncture. This avoids the embarrassment of having to explain matching incisions if venous access could not be achieved through the initial incision and one is forced to move to the other side. It is difficult enough explaining multiple unsuccessful skin punctures. As an acceptable alternative, and one that we regularly use at the University of Oklahoma, a 1 cm–long "stab wound" can be made initially, through which the venipunctures can be accomplished. This allows easy incorporation of the puncture sites (especially if two separate punctures are used for a dual-chamber pacing system) into a

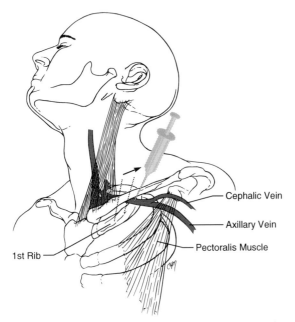

FIGURE 27–21. The anatomic landmarks for axillary vein (extrathoracic subclavian vein) puncture.

Cephalic Vein

Axillary Vein

Pectoralis Muscle

1st Rib

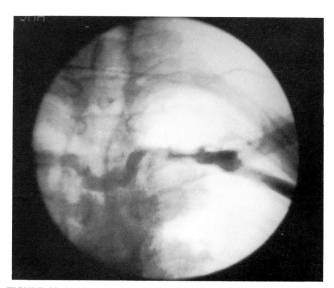

FIGURE 27–22. Contrast venography–guided venipuncture. With contrast material, the needle is guided under fluoroscopy directly to the vein.

contrast material. The contrast material injection is performed by a nonsterile assistant. Ten to 20 ml of contrast material (nonionic or ionic) is injected rapidly into the intravenous line in the forearm. This should be followed by a saline bolus flush. The contrast medium moves slowly in the peripheral venous system and can be moved along by massaging the arm through or under the sterile drapes. The venous anatomy is observed under fluoroscopy in the pectoral area and, if possible, recorded for repeated viewing (Fig. 27–22). The needle trajectory and venipuncture are guided by the contrast material in the subclavian vein. In more sophisticated radiologic laboratories, a mask or map can be made for guidance after the contrast medium has dissipated. The process can be repeated as necessary.

The actual percutaneous stick is carried out with a syringe attached to the 18-gauge needle. A common practice is to partially fill the syringe with saline. The theory behind this practice is that if a pneumothorax occurs, it will be detected by air bubbles aspirated through the saline. In addition, the saline can be used to flush out tissue plugs that may obstruct the needle and prevent aspiration. We avoid this practice. One does not need air bubbles to detect an inadvertent pneumothorax. More importantly, the syringe even partially filled with saline makes it difficult to differentiate between arterial and venous blood. This is because when blood (arterial or venous) mixes with the saline it takes on the color of oxygenated blood. If saline is not used, it is more readily apparent which vascular structure has been entered.

When proceeding with a percutaneous venipuncture, the syringe should be held in the palm of the hand with the dorsal aspect of the hand resting on the patient. This gives support and control as the needle is advanced. With the needle held this way, tactile sensation is enhanced, and one can frequently feel the needle enter the vein. Once the vessel is entered, the guide wire is inserted and the tip advanced to a position in the vicinity of the right atrium (Fig. 27–23). We

single incision that is extended after successful venipuncture. The author of the safe introducer technique and many other implanters use a full incision to the greater pectoral fascia before gaining venous access to the subclavian vein.

The subclavian puncture can also be facilitated by the use of contrast venography.[57] This is helpful in patients in whom venous access can be anticipated to be a problem. It should be considered prior to any puncture in which venous patency is in doubt or abnormal anatomy is suspected. The technique has been described by Hayes and colleagues.[57] A venous line is established in the arm on the side of planned pacemaker venous access. The line should be reliable and 20-gauge or larger. The patient should not have an allergy to radiographic

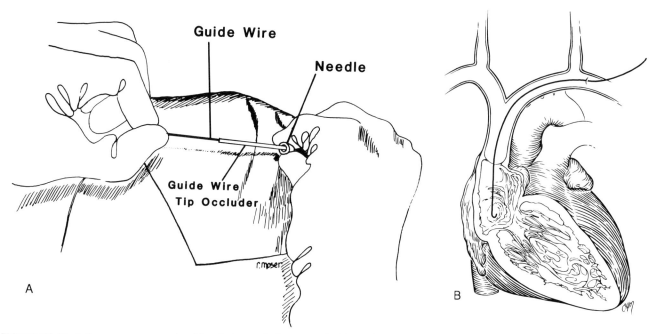

FIGURE 27–23. *A*, Once venous access is achieved, the needle is supported with one hand and the guide wire with tip occluder advanced with the other hand. *B*, Guide wire tip advanced to the middle right atrium. (*A* from Belott PH: Retained guide wire introducer technique, for unlimited access to the central circulation. Clin Prog Pacing Electrophysiol 1:59, 1983.)

prefer to use curved-tip guide wires for safety concerns. If resistance is encountered, the wire is withdrawn slightly and readvanced. If the resistance persists, the wire position is checked under fluoroscopy. If the wire just outside the tip of the needle is coiled, it is probably extravascular. In this case, the wire and needle are removed and a new venous stick carried out. Extremely rarely, one may not be able to reenter the vein. This may be due to collapse of the vein by a resultant hematoma caused by a small tear in the vein from the misdirected guide wire. In this case, one should probably proceed to an alternative approach or site of venous access, avoiding an unnecessary waste of time and increasing the risk of pneumothorax with multiple subsequent unsuccessful percutaneous punctures. Occasionally the guide wire tracks up the internal jugular vein. By changing the angle of the needle slightly to a more medial and inferior direction while the guide wire is still in the internal jugular vein, withdrawal of the guide wire back into the needle and readvancing usually results in passage of the guide wire through the innominate vein and superior vena cava into the right atrium. At times this maneuver has to be repeated several times with varying needle angulations. Care must be exercised to avoid tearing the vein. The application of a 5 or 6 F dilator can sometimes help steer the guide wire in the right direction. In rare instances, the guide wire and needle must be removed and a new puncture site selected. The key point here is that once venous access has been achieved, every effort is made to retain it.

If air is withdrawn through the needle during attempted venipunctures, suggesting lung puncture and raising the possibility of a pneumothorax, our practice has been to withdraw the needle, wait a moment or two to make certain that a rapid-onset, large, markedly symptomatic pneumothorax is not occurring, and then proceed (obviously with a different needle trajectory) with reattempts at venipuncture. In our experience, most lung punctures occurring with forward (not lateral!) needle motion do not result in a clinically apparent (by chest radiography) pneumothorax. If a pneumothorax does develop, it may do so in this setting over a matter of hours and may not even be apparent radiographically at the end of the procedure. If a lung puncture has occurred, repeating the postoperative upright chest x-ray study 6 hours after completion of the procedure is advisable. If a pneumothorax has developed, a chest tube or catheter evacuation procedure may be necessary, although frequently a small to moderate pneumothorax that is not expanding can be managed conservatively without evacuation.

Similarly, if an arterial puncture occurs inadvertently, removal of the needle, compression at the site of the puncture for 5 minutes or so, followed by repeated venipuncture attempts with a different needle path has been our approach. It is rare for such arterial punctures to result in a hemothorax provided that no tearing of the artery has occurred (avoidance of lateral needle motion is critical here also). Follow-up chest x-ray films 6 to 18 hours following the procedure are advisable, and postoperative hemoglobin-hematocrit measurements are suggested. The most important problem to avoid if the artery has been punctured is nonrecognition and placement of a sheath into the artery. If there is any doubt about whether the artery has been punctured, a blood sample withdrawn through the needle and subjected to oximetric analysis should clarify the situation.

Once the wire is successfully in the vein, some implanters place a pursestring type of suture in the tissue around the point of entry of the wire into the tissue. Alternatively, a figure-of-eight stitch can be applied (Fig. 27–24). This can be helpful later for hemostasis.[58] These sutures require that an incision be made beginning at the needle and extending inferiorly to the depth of the pectoral fascia.

Once the guide wire or wires are in the subclavian vein, it is usually a simple procedure to advance the appropriate sized dilator and peel-away sheath over the wire into the venous circulation. Occasionally, there is substantial resistance to dilator-sheath advancement, and repetitive dilatation with progressively larger dilators is necessary. Alternatively, a 15- to 20-degree bending of the tip of the full-sized introducer will frequently facilitate advancement over the wire. If difficulty with advancement occurs, we generally remove the sheath from the dilator and use only the dilator to initially dilate the track into the vein. This protects these rather "sensitive" sheaths from damage. After successfully advancing the dilator alone over the wire, the dilator can be withdrawn, the sheath added, and both then advanced over the wire. We have found that gentle back-pressure on the guide wire when advancing the dilator-sheath also facilitates advancement in difficult or tortuous vessel situations.

Once the sheath has been successfully passed over the guide wire to the vicinity of the superior vena cava, the dilator and guide wire can be removed and the lead advanced through the sheath. Problems can be encountered when passing the lead through the sheath. Occasionally, in the process of introduction the sheath will buckle at a point in the venous system where there is a bend (Fig. 27–25).[59] This usually occurs after the removal of the dilator. This can also occur if the sheath is advanced against the lateral wall of the superior vena cava. If a buckle occurs, the lead will not pass this point. Forcing the lead can result in damage to the cathode and insulation. This kink can usually be observed on fluoroscopy. There are several solutions to this problem. If the guide wire and dilator have both been removed, both can be re-

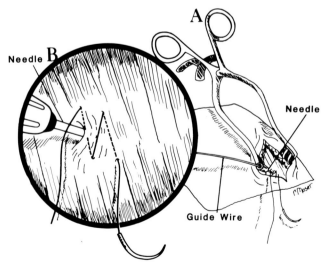

FIGURE 27–24. Placement of the "figure-of-eight" stitch to enhance hemostasis. (From Belott PH: Retained guide wire introducer technique, for unlimited access to the central circulation. Clin Prog Pacing Electrophysiol 1:59, 1983.)

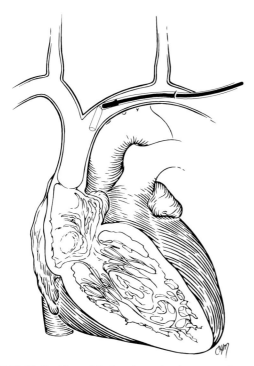

FIGURE 27–25. Buckling of the introducer sheath prevents the passage of the electrode.

placed down the sheath. The dilator with wire inside is now functioning not only to stiffen the sheath but also as a tip occluder, and both can be passed back down the sheath. The tapered tip of the dilator will straighten the buckle. The position of the buckle point can be changed by either slightly advancing or retracting the sheath. The dilator is removed but the guide wire can be retained. It is hoped that the retained guide wire will act as a stent, preventing the buckle from recurring and thus allowing the electrode to pass completely down the sheath. Another option when this buckling of sheath occurs is to advance the lead to within a couple of centimeters of the buckle and then slowly withdraw the sheath, holding the lead position stationary. The sheath, including the buckle point, may occasionally be easily withdrawn over the tip of the lead, and the lead can be cautiously advanced. In this situation, it is sometimes necessary to withdraw the stylet from the tip of the lead to allow easy advancement of the lead beyond the buckle point. Inexperienced implanters should be cautious with this technique because distal electrode damage can occur. If these maneuvers fail, the guide wire and dilator are reinserted and the sheath and dilator are removed, leaving the guide wire in the vein. Tissue compression or traction is applied to the pursestring suture for hemostasis. The sheath is inspected for buckling. At this point, one should consider advancing the next larger sized sheath over the retained guide wire. The application of the same sized sheath usually results in recurrence of the same problem. Again, the important point is that despite this frustrating experience, one must be reluctant to relinquish the vein once it has been catheterized. Generally the larger sheath is less likely to buckle, especially if the guide wire is retained to act as a stent. With successful electrode introduction, the sheath is briskly pulled back out of the circulation, and skin compression or traction is applied to the pursestring or figure-of-eight suture for hemostasis.

The risk of air embolization is substantial with the percutaneous approach. This issue has been addressed by the recommendation that the Trendelenburg position be used. With the shift of the pacemaker procedure to the cardiac catheterization laboratory or special procedures room, however, it is frequently impossible to place the patient in the Trendelenburg position. Consequently, the patient is at greater risk for air embolization if the percutaneous approach is used. It is most important that the implanting physician be aware of the danger and take steps necessary to avoid this potential catastrophe (Table 27–11). The physician must be aware that removal of the sheath dilator in a patient who is fasting and somewhat volume-depleted can rapidly cause aspiration of large quantities of air. Since the luxury of the Trendelenburg position is unlikely to be available in the catheterization laboratory, other steps must be taken. Contrary to some practices, the preoperative pacemaker patient should be maintained in a euvolemic or even a relatively volume-overloaded state if there is no contraindication. Instead of administering intravenous fluids at a restricted rate, adequate hydration should be maintained. We routinely place a large wedge sponge under the patient's legs to enhance blood return and increase central venous pressure. An assessment of the state of hydration can be carried out during the procedure. With the sheath in the central venous circulation one can "take a peek." By carefully withdrawing the dilator from the sheath, the state of hydration and venous pressure can be observed.

Once the dilator is withdrawn in the hydrated patient with adequate venous pressure, there is continuous blood flow out of the sheath despite the cycle of respiration. In the case of the dehydrated patient, withdrawal of the dilator results in little or no flow of blood. The blood meniscus is barely visible. More importantly, on inspiration the blood meniscus is observed to move substantially inward. If this is observed, the dilator can be rapidly advanced back into the sheath or, alternatively, the sheath can be pinched and additional precautions taken to avoid air embolization. If a wedge has not been placed under the patient's legs, this can be done now and is frequently quite helpful. Also, at this point it is most important to have the cooperation of the patient. If the patient is sleeping, he or she should be aroused. The patient should be coached to reduce the depth of respirations and avoid the sudden large inspiration that can result in the aspiration of a lethal volume of air. At the same time, administration of intravenous fluids is increased to enhance hydration. Having

TABLE 27–11. **PREVENTION OF AIR EMBOLISM DURING PERMANENT PACEMAKER PROCEDURES**

Awareness of the potential problem
A well-hydrated patient, avoiding long periods of nothing by mouth
Awareness of when patient is at greatest risk—open sheath in vein
Assess hydration: (Take a peek)
High-risk patient
    Increase hydration—wide open IV lines
    An awake, cooperative patient
    Elevate lower extremities, place wedge under legs
    Trendelenburg position (if available)
    Expeditious lead placement and sheath removal
    Check for introduction of air
    Continuous monitoring (vital signs, oxygen saturation, blood pressure)
In an extremely high-risk, uncooperative patient, intubation and sedation causing temporary loss of consciousness may be required

the patient hold the breath following maximal inspiration offers the greatest latitude in time, as the patient will have to exhale prior to pulling negative intrathoracic pressure and aspirating air. This gives the implanter time to insert the lead. Pinching of the sheath with the lead going through it to avoid air embolization is ineffective and gives a false sense of security. A peel-away sheath with a nonrebleed valve would be useful. In the patient who is substantially sedated or uncooperative, adequate hydration and elevation of the lower extremities are the only solutions. Careful planning of the lead insertion procedure will also help. Expeditious lead insertion is important. For example, positioning the electrodes with the sheath in situ is unwise because it may result in air embolism or unnecessary blood loss.

Once the lead has been inserted, the introducer should be rapidly withdrawn. The practice of peeling away the sheath while part of it is in an intravascular location should be avoided, as it is a waste of time and increases the risk of air embolization and blood loss. In this regard, the actual peeling away of the sheath is not even a necessity at this point as long as it is completely extravascular. It can be peeled away later at one's convenience. In fact, the tabs of the unpeeled sheath can be used to pin the lead to the drapes during threshold testing, preventing inadvertent dislodgment of the lead onto the floor. With the sheath withdrawn completely from the circulation, hemostasis is achieved by applying tension to the pursestring or figure-of-eight suture or by applying skin compression over the entry site.

A variation of the introducer technique involves retaining the guide wire. Instead of removing the guide wire together with the dilator, it is left in place so that the lead is passed through the sheath alongside the guide wire. The sheath is subsequently removed and peeled away (Fig. 27–26). Occa-sionally the size of the electrode and the sheath preclude the passage of the lead alongside the guide wire. In this case, the guide wire is removed, the lead is passed down the sheath, and the guide wire is reinserted behind the electrode. The reason this can work is that in most cases it is the electrode that will not pass alongside the guide wire, whereas the lead body is thinner and leaves enough room to accommodate both guide wire and lead body. Certain leads (especially those with bipolar electrodes) and sheath combinations are too tight to allow passage of both electrode and guide wire. In this case, a larger sized sheath can be used. When reintroducing the guide wire, the tip occluder is not used, as it can wind up in the central circulation fairly easily. It works well to reuse the dilator as a tip occluder when reinserting the guide wire. The retained guide wire may provide unlimited venous access and the ability to exchange or introduce additional electrodes by simply applying another sheath set to the guide wire. The retained guide wire should be held to the drape by a clamp to avoid inadvertent dislodgment. The retained guide wire can serve as a ground for unipolar threshold analysis instead of a grounding plate. It can also be used as an intracardiac lead for recording of the atrial electrogram (to confirm atrial capture) or as an electrode for emergency pacing. It is our routine practice to retain an intravascular guide wire in both single- and dual-chamber procedures until a satisfactory lead position is obtained.

The percutaneous approach is particularly useful in dual-chamber pacing and has eliminated the earlier dilemma of having to introduce two leads into a vein exposed by cut-down that may barely accommodate a single lead and the resultant need for a second venous access site. The options for dual-chamber venous access are shown in Table 27–10. For dual-chamber pacing, there are now at least four methods

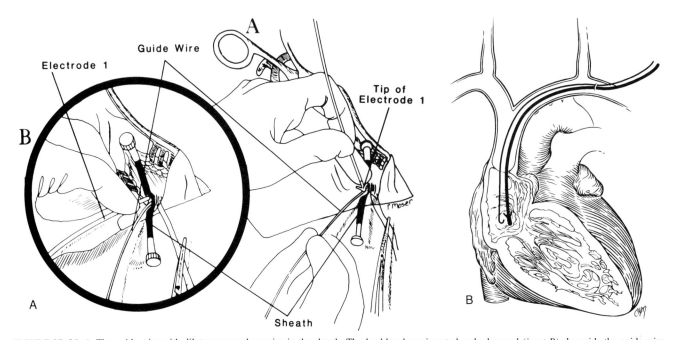

FIGURE 27–26. *A,* The guide wire with dilator removed remains in the sheath. The lead has been inserted and advanced *(inset B)* alongside the guide wire. *B,* Both the guide wire and the lead are advanced to the vicinity of the middle right atrium. Additional introducers can be advanced over this retained guide wire to place additional leads. *(A from Belott PH: Retained guide wire introducer technique, for unlimited access to the central circulation. Clin Prog Pacing Electrophysiol 1:59, 1983.)*

that involve the percutaneous approach. These techniques, except for the fourth, can be used with any of the previously described percutaneous approaches.

1. *Two separate percutaneous sticks and the use of two sheath sets.*[60] Two separate punctures increase the risk of complications related to the venipuncture process, and there is also the possibility of not finding the vessel the second time. The advantage of this method (which one of us [DWR] preferentially uses) is that even relatively large bipolar leads can be easily and independently manipulated after introduction, with little risk of unwanted and frustrating movement of the other lead.

2. *One percutaneous stick and the use of a large sheath with the passage of both electrodes.*[61, 62] The passage of two electrodes down one sheath reduces the risk of two separate punctures, but the large sheath may increase the risk of substantial air embolism and blood loss. In our experience, there is also frequent frustration from lead interaction, entanglement, and dislodgment.

3. *The retained guide wire technique.*[63, 64] This procedure can be used alone as a method for the introduction of two leads or can be incorporated into any of the other techniques for the introduction of two leads. One of us (PHB) uses this technique alone, preferentially for dual-lead introductions and the other of us (DWR) uses it as back-up in combination with the two separate puncture techniques described previously. This approach is most desirable because it provides unlimited access to the central circulation. The implanter using this technique can easily add and exchange leads. This is important in dual-chamber pacing in which the initially chosen atrial lead is occasionally unacceptable for a given anatomic situation. Less commonly, it is also helpful to be able to exchange ventricular leads. When using the retained guide wire technique for dual-chamber implantation, the ventricular electrode is usually positioned first. This is practical and safe. The ventricular electrode can be more easily stabilized and is less susceptible to dislodgment from positioning of the second electrode. The ventricular electrode can then be stabilized by leaving the stylet pulled back in the lead in the vicinity of the lower right atrium (Fig. 27–27). A stitch should be placed proximally around the lead and suture sleeve and secured approximately 1 to 2 cm from the puncture site in the subcutaneous tissue on the surface of the pectoral muscle. After ventricular electrode stabilization, a second sheath can be advanced over the retained guide wire. The atrial electrode is introduced, positioned, tested, and secured. Alternatively, the retained guide wire technique can be employed to introduce both leads into the superior vena cava, right atrium, or inferior vena cava areas before positioning either of the electrodes. This may eliminate some of the risk of dislodgment of the initially positioned electrode that is incurred by introduction of the second sheath. Regardless of variation, the guide wire is removed only after a satisfactory procedure (Fig. 27–28). A pursestring or figure-of-eight suture can be tied loosely to achieve hemostasis around the puncture site.

4. *The sheath set technique can also be used in conjunction with the cutdown approach.*[65, 66] Ong and Barold and their associates described a modified cephalic vein guide wire technique for the introduction of one or more electrodes.

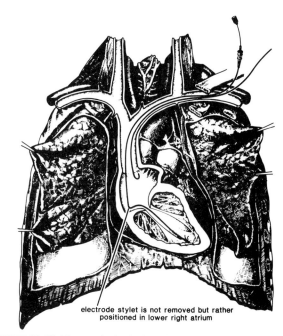

electrode stylet is not removed but rather positioned in lower right atrium

FIGURE 27–27. The ventricular lead has been placed first. The guide wire has been retained, and the lead stylet is positioned in the lower right atrium for stability.

The Ong-Barold technique appears safe and a reasonable alternative to the percutaneous subclavian vein introducer technique. It is particularly recommended for the inexperienced implanter. It is also recommended in patients at high risk of complication from the percutaneous approach and in situations in which one can anticipate the percutaneous approach to be difficult if not impossible. This requires an initial cutdown to the cephalic vein as previously described. For a single-lead introduction, the size of the vein is irrelevant. All that is necessary is the introduction of the guide wire, which is accomplished using needle puncture under direct visualization. The cephalic vein is sacrificed, as it seems to invaginate into the subclavian vein with advancement of the sheath set over the guide wire (Fig. 27–29). Hemostasis is achieved by pressure or the application of a figure-of-eight stitch. Despite sacrificing the cephalic vein, there have been no reported venous complications. When two leads are required, the retained guide wire technique and sheath set technique can be used in this approach.

Ventricular Electrode Placement

There are many techniques for placing the ventricular electrode described throughout the published pacing literature,[67] essentially reflecting the approach with which any particular author has facility. There is no one correct technique. Ventricular electrode placement is largely independent of the route of venous access. The implanting physician must draw on experience to deal with the variety of situations that will be encountered in any given patient. In time, one develops one's own technique. There are some fundamental principles and maneuvers that are common to all: (1) simultaneous

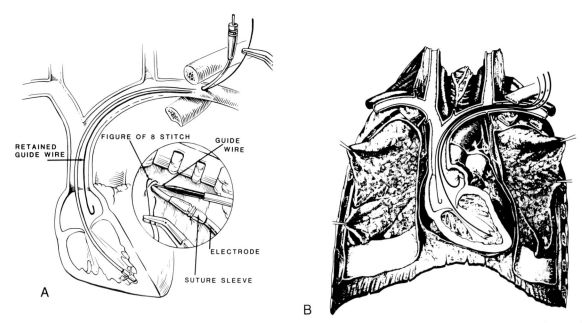

FIGURE 27–28. *A* The ventricular electrode and retained guide wire are demonstrated in the main drawing. The *inset* demonstrates the ventricular lead anchored by suture about its suture sleeve and the second sheath advancing over the retained guide wire. A hemostat on the figure-of-eight suture maintains hemostasis. *B*, The atrial and ventricular electrodes have been positioned, yet the guide wire is still retained. (*A* from Barold SS, Mugica J [eds]: New Perspectives in Cardiac Pacing 2. Mt Kisco, NY, Futura Publ. Co., Inc., 1991, p 110.)

manipulation of lead and stylet, (2) documentation of passage into the right side of the heart, and (3) manipulation of the electrode into the apex or other desired location of the right ventricle.

It is necessary to grasp the concept that pacemaker electrode placement involves a "symphony" of lead and stylet movement. Without the two working together, proper electrode positioning is impossible. The lead without stylet is somewhat like a limp piece of spaghetti. When positioning the ventricular electrode, the lead must negotiate a course through the chambers of the right side of the heart and ultimately to the apex of the right ventricle. This is typically

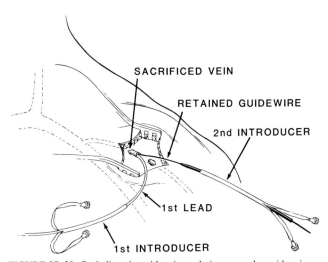

FIGURE 27–29. Cephalic vein guide wire technique uses the guide wire as access to the vein for one or more electrodes. The distal connection of the cephalic vein is sacrificed (Ong-Barold technique). (From Barold SS, Mugica J [eds]: New Perspectives in Cardiac Pacing 2. Mt Kisco, NY, Futura Publ. Co., Inc., 1991, p 112.)

accomplished by preforming the lead stylet. This enables easier manipulation of the lead and is probably the best way to effectively position a pacemaker electrode. A curve is applied to the distal aspect of the stylet. The size or tightness of the curve and how it is created are a personal preference. As a rule a curve that is too gentle will fail to negotiate the tricuspid valve, making passage into the pulmonary artery difficult. Conversely, a curve that is too tight may fail to negotiate the venous structures in the superior mediastinum, such as the innominate vein and superior vena cava. At times, however, unusual circumstances will call for extremes of wire curvature to effectively position the electrode. In every case, the ideal curve will be slightly different. There are several ways to form the curve on the stylet. Some implanters choose to use a blunt instrument, such as the tip of a clamp or scissors. The stylet is pulled between the thumb and the blunt instrument with a rotary motion of the wrist forming the curve. Another method is to form the curve by pulling the guide wire between the thumb and index finger, gently shaping the curve. Whatever method is used, the curve should be a bend that is not sharp, because a sharp bend in a stylet will generally preclude its passage through the lead. In making the curve, the aim is that the curved stylet will direct the electrode to the appropriate position.

Unlike diagnostic catheters, the pacemaker lead cannot be steered or torqued into position. Positioning of a pacemaker electrode is solely dependent, therefore, on the manipulation of lead and stylet together. The basic technique of lead positioning involves advancing the electrode, with curved stylet in place, through the chambers of the right side of the heart. A more sophisticated variation of this technique involves simultaneous advancement of the electrode while retracting and readvancing the stylet. The retraction of the stylet renders the lead tip floppy. Using a slightly retracted although curved stylet and pointing the electrode body in the proper direction, the lead, with 1 to 2 cm of its floppy tip, in some instances can make for more precise and expeditious electrode placement. An alternative, related technique, and one that can expedite ventricular lead implantation, although it is clearly more difficult to master, involves the use of a straight stylet. The stylet is retracted to allow the floppy lead tip to "catch" on a structure in the right atrium with subsequent advancement of the lead. The lead body then prolapses through the tricuspid valve into the right ventricle. The stylet can then be cautiously advanced to stiffen the lead body and, generally, free the tip from the "catch."

The fluoroscope should be used for the entire lead positioning process and can be used initially in the PA projection or in the right anterior oblique (RAO) projection. The latter helps delineate the apex of the right ventricle to the left of the spine and toward the left lateral chest wall. The RAO projection creates the illusion that our "mind's eye" expects with respect to the location of the apex of the right ventricle—specifically, that the right ventricular apex is near the apex of the cardiac silhouette. In many patients, however, the right ventricular apex tends to be more anterior than leftward. Much time can be wasted trying to position a ventricular electrode to the left of the spine toward the apex of the cardiac silhouette (in the PA projection) when in reality the right ventricular apex is directly anterior to the spine. This anterior position results in an electrode position that is over the spine or nearly so and appears in the PA projection to be erroneously placed in the right atrium or in the less desirable proximal aspect of the right ventricle. Rotating the image intensifier unit into the RAO projection in this situation superimposes the right ventricular apex over the apex of the cardiac silhouette in the left side of the chest, confirming the appropriate position (Fig. 27–30). Whether or not the initial choice of projection is the RAO, it should be used freely to facilitate ventricular lead placement.

We recommend that the electrode be passed initially across the tricuspid valve and then out into the pulmonary artery (Fig. 27–31A to C). This maneuver confirms passage into the right side of the heart and precludes erroneous placement in the coronary sinus. The RAO projection also is helpful in making certain the lead is not in the coronary sinus. If the lead is appropriately in the apex of the right ventricle, there will be no posterior component of the course of the lead in the RAO projection. If the lead is in the coronary sinus, it will have a posterior course in this projection. If it courses down the middle cardiac vein, it will have a posterior course as it traverses the coronary sinus and then an anterior course as it traverses this branch.

There are several techniques for the actual placement of the electrode into the right ventricular apex. They involve the combined manipulation of the lead stylet and electrode body. If one chooses to pass the electrode to the pulmonary artery as an indicator of being across the tricuspid valve, the next maneuver is to advance the stylet to the tip of the electrode. With the stylet advanced to the electrode tip and the electrode tip in the pulmonary artery, the electrode is slowly withdrawn from the pulmonary artery, dragging the tip down along the interventricular septum. This may result in premature ventricular contractions or runs of nonsustained ventricular tachycardia. When the electrode tip has reached the lower third of the septum, the stylet may be retracted about 2 to 3 cm, making the tip floppy. This can be done with a curved or straight stylet (Fig. 27–31D). The lead tip can be observed to move up and down with the flow of blood, the motion of the tricuspid valve, and the contractions of the right ventricle. As it does so, it will intermittently point toward the apex of the right ventricle. If one coordinates the advancing of the lead body (with or without stylet fully inserted, although generally only straight stylets should be fully inserted at this point) with the appropriate lead trajectory, the tip can be gently seated in the right ventricular apex. This maneuver can be repeated by withdrawing and readvancing the electrode until the desired fluoroscopic location is achieved for threshold testing. After satisfactory electrode tip placement, the curved stylet is withdrawn and replaced with a straight stylet if a curved stylet was initially used and if it was not already replaced (some implanters replace the curved stylet with a straight one while the lead tip is still in the pulmonary artery). The straight stylet is advanced to the electrode tip, and the electrode with stylet in place is gently advanced toward the right ventricular apex until it is fully inserted and resistance is encountered. Care should be taken not to dislodge the electrode tip with the straight stylet. This is a common occurrence, especially in patients with an enlarged right atrium. In the process of advancing the straight stylet to the electrode tip, the stylet can force the electrode body inferiorly to the lower right atrium and inferior vena cava, consequently dragging the tip of the electrode out of the right ventricular apex back into the right atrium. This phenomenon can obviously be extremely frustrating. Hints for avoiding this problem include using a more flexible stylet that will be guided more easily by the electrode coil than will the stiff stylet. Also, before advancing the stylet, the lead body is straightened as it crosses the tricuspid valve by gently pulling back on the lead. This usually avoids the looping of lead in the lower right atrium. Right ventricular lead fixation can be validated by gently pulling on the electrode until resistance, both tactile and visual, is encountered. This is a good method for assuring reliable fixation if a tined or other passive fixation lead is being used. In the case of an active fixation lead, the best method for determining that reliable fixation is accomplished is a subject of debate. Some believe that threshold measurements, and not retraction of the lead tip to the point of resistance, is a better way of validating fixation. It is argued that the strength of fixation in the tissue with a screw-in electrode is impossible to gauge by the sen-

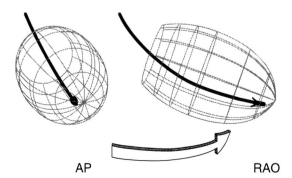

AP   RAO

FIGURE 27–30. Wire frame demonstrating the orientation of the lead in the right ventricular apex in the anteroposterior (AP) and right anterior oblique (RAO) projections. Note that in the AP projection the electrode appears to be vertical, whereas in the RAO the lead is horizontal from right to left.

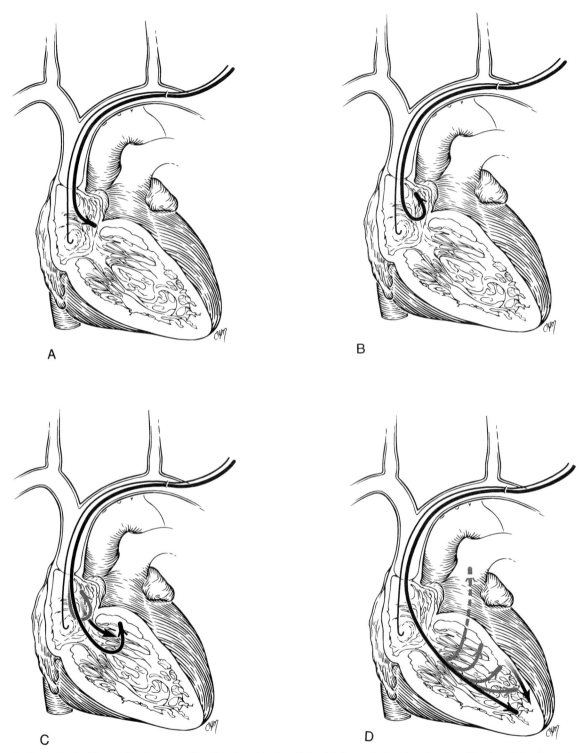

FIGURE 27–31. *A*, Lead with curved stylet approaching the tricuspid valve. *B*, Lead being pushed against the tricuspid valve. *C*, Lead snapping across the tricuspid valve into the right ventricle. *D*, Lead passed to the pulmonary artery, then withdrawn to the right ventricular apex.

sation of resistance on retraction and that all too often the bond is disrupted by pulling back on the screw-in electrode to the point of resistance. Conversely, others argue that the same gentle lead retraction, coupled with achievement of acceptable thresholds, is more appropriate validation for achievement of active fixation. The argument here is that acceptable thresholds may be achieved without adequate fixation and that adequate fixation easily prevents the disruption of an acceptable bond by gentle retraction. If the initial stylet choice was straight, or after the electrode with the curved stylet has been passed to the pulmonary artery and is replaced with a stiff, straight stylet, the tip of the straight stylet can be positioned just across the tricuspid valve. It will usually point to the right ventricular apex. Simultaneous advancement of the stylet and retraction of the electrode will drag the electrode tip down the interventricular septum to the end of the stylet, which is tracking toward the right ventricular apex. Once the electrode tip has snapped into a straight position, now in line with the trajectory of the stylet, both are advanced to the right ventricular apex. In both cases, when seating the electrode in the right ventricular apex, perforations can be more easily avoided by simultaneously advancing the electrode body while retracting the stylet. Thus, the stylet is not acting as a battering ram but is merely pointing the way. In all cases, if there is any doubt as to the location of the electrode in the right ventricular apex, the fluoroscope is merely rotated into the steep RAO or lateral projection. As previously noted, a correctly placed electrode will be observed to curve anteriorly, with the electrode tip appearing to almost touch the sternum. If the electrode curves posteriorly toward the spine, it is likely in the coronary sinus.

Although the means of venous access has little bearing on electrode placement, there is some difference when comparing left and right sides. Placement of the ventricular electrode

after venous access has been achieved from the left side generally seems to be more expeditious. The ventricular lead with a curved stylet in place will track in a gentle curve from the point of venous entry through to the superior vena cava, right atrium, right ventricle, and pulmonary outflow tract (see Fig. 27–14A). Typically, little or no difficulty is encountered. There are generally no acute bends or angles. The only occasional impediment is the tricuspid valve, which can be negotiated using one of several techniques. One may be able to simply advance the tip across the valve without hang-up. If the lead tends to hang up on the valve, retracting the stylet and using the floppy tip technique already described will frequently avoid this impasse. There is also the possibility of using a technique in which the curved tip of the electrode is pushed across the valve by building a loop. Whatever technique is used, because of the anatomic configuration, passage from the left typically presents little difficulty. One exception is the elderly patient with an extremely tortuous left subclavian–innominate venous system. In this case, the venous structure may have one or more sharp angles or bends in the superior mediastinum prior to entry into the right atrium. It would be a truly extreme case for such tortuosity to preclude passage of the electrode from the left.

Passage and placement of the ventricular electrode after right venous access may be much more challenging. Intrinsic to this approach is one acute angle or bend in the venous system (see Fig. 27–14B). This bend occurs at the junction of the right subclavian vein and internal jugular vein, where the innominate vein is formed. More important is the fact that this bend is ''clockwise.'' Because of this, when a lead with a curved stylet is placed in the vein from the right, the electrode typically is directed clockwise or to the lateral right atrial wall (Fig. 27–32A). In this situation, routing the tip across the tricuspid valve, which is in the other direction,

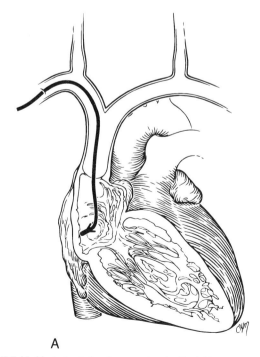
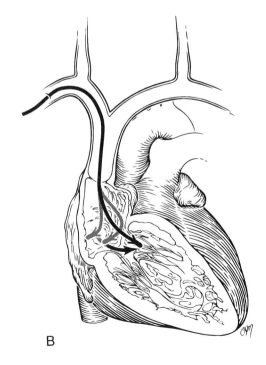

A   B

FIGURE 27–32. *A,* Acute bends encountered with right venous access orient the lead to the lateral wall of the right atrium when a stylet with a modest curve is inserted into the electrode. *B,* The lead must be backed into the right ventricle, across the tricuspid valve when approaching from the right. Rotating or partial withdrawal of the stylet is sometimes helpful in getting the electrode across the valve.

may call on all of one's skill, ingenuity, and luck. One method involves building a loop in the right atrium in an attempt to prolapse the lead and back the electrode across the valve, with the tip ultimately flipping into the right ventricle (see Fig. 27–32B). If the lead has tines, they may get caught on the tricuspid valve and prevent transit to the right ventricle. Another method of crossing the tricuspid valve that is somewhat more successful uses the floppy tip technique. If the curved stylet is withdrawn to the high right atrium, with the lead tip in the lower right atrium, the lead will no longer point to the lateral atrial wall. Its trajectory may now be medial toward the tricuspid valve. Advancing the body of the lead, even though the tip is floppy, will frequently allow the lead tip to cross the tricuspid valve into the right ventricle. With this approach, it is important to avoid extreme stylet curves, as they serve to increase the tendency for the lead tip to move toward the lateral right atrial wall. It is hoped that future lead designs will incorporate some steering mechanism in either the stylet or the lead.

One of the benefits of modern lead design is the various fixation mechanisms that have resulted in a near zero dislodgment rate. One should become familiar with the lead handling characteristics of the various active and passive fixation designs. It is important to become familiar with the passive fixation mechanism of tines. Learning to recognize when tines are stuck on an endocardial structure and not be intimidated by the resistance encountered when traction is applied is a must. There has yet to be a reported case of endocardial trauma from a tined electrode, even though one may occasionally get the impression that the tines have permanently attached themselves to an endocardial structure during attempts at lead placement. It is this same feeling of resistance that assures us that the electrode will not dislodge once an ideal location is found. When the tip of a tined lead becomes caught on a structure in an undesirable position, it is usually impossible to advance the lead. The lead must be pulled free and usually withdrawn to the right atrium, no matter what force must be applied. Sometimes it may take multiple electrode advances and withdrawals with the tines hanging up and preventing placement in the right ventricular apex. Subtle adjustments in the stylet manipulation as well as persistence will ultimately overcome this problem.

The active fixation leads offer a new set of problems. There are some unique problems in placement directly related to design. There are basically two types of active fixation leads currently in use, both involving a helix or "screw" as the fixation mechanism. First, there is the fixation tip design with an exposed or fixed screw. Since the screw is continually exposed, its tip may catch onto any endocardial structure. As one would expect, this type of helix has a high propensity for getting caught, particularly on the chordae of the tricuspid valve. Unlike tines, the screw, when caught, cannot be pulled free without some fear of damaging endocardial structures. It can usually be freed easily by counterclockwise rotation of the lead body, which results in unscrewing the tip (the available screws are made with a clockwise helix). Some manufacturers have attempted to resolve this problem by coating the exposed screw with a sugar compound that ultimately dissolves, exposing the screw. This can work well provided that one is consistently able to place the lead in an "optimal" position quickly. This requires significant skill and experience among other things, including

luck. Once the coating has dissolved, the screw can hook endocardial structures if there is a difficult positioning or a need to reposition or withdraw to the right atrium. The exposed screw does, however, offer a reliable fixation mechanism. The second type of active fixation lead employs an extendible-retractable screw that is mechanically extended from its "resting" retracted position. This lead is generally easier to work with, as the problem of helix hangup is avoided. In fact, the extendible-retractable screw-in type of leads may be the easiest of all leads to position. Placement of both types of fixation mechanisms use the stylet techniques previously described.

Once one is satisfied with electrode placement, the stylet may be withdrawn to the vicinity of the lower right atrium (Fig. 27–33)[68] or, alternatively, completely removed. Threshold testing is then carried out. If thresholds are acceptable, the ventricular electrode may be secured. Some implanters leave the stylet in the lead with the tip in the lower right atrium and secure the lead with the anchoring sleeve. This reduces the risk of ventricular lead dislodgment during placement and positioning of the atrial lead. Other implanters remove the stylet completely for testing and securing the lead but not for atrial lead placement and positioning, as there is general agreement that the stylet helps stabilize the ventricular lead during atrial lead manipulation, which can frequently dislodge the ventricular lead otherwise.

The suture sleeve is advanced down the shaft of the lead body to the vicinity of venous entry. One to three ligatures are applied around the suture sleeve and lead, incorporating a generous amount of pectoral muscle (Fig. 27–34). It has been our experience that multiple ligatures that are not excessively tight make lead slippage as well as lead damage less likely compared with one tightly applied ligature. Securing the ventricular electrode immediately after satisfactory posi-

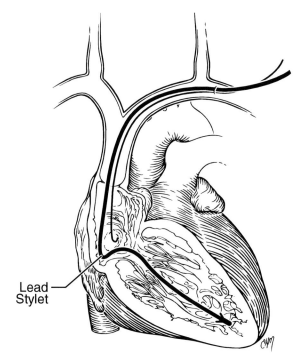

FIGURE 27–33. The stylet of the ventricular electrode is left in the lead but is withdrawn to the lower right atrium to permit threshold testing and assessment of the appropriate amount of lead redundancy.

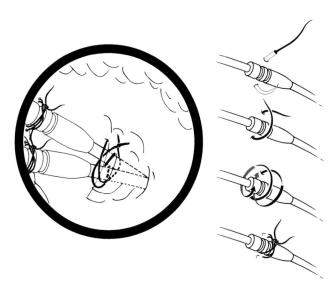

FIGURE 27–34. Securing the ventricular electrode to the pectoral muscle using the suture sleeve.

tioning is important. Early securing helps prevent inadvertent dislodgment whether or not an atrial electrode is to be placed. The ventricular electrode should be oriented somewhat horizontally in a plane roughly parallel to the clavicle. This avoids excessive bending of the lead at the point it exits the vein.

Atrial Electrode Placement

Atrial electrode placement can be extremely easy but has been the nemesis of many an implanting physician. It has even been responsible for many resisting the dual-chamber approach to cardiac pacing. This, we believe, is largely because the clinician has not been exposed to proper placement technique. Once again, it must be appreciated that the proper placement of any pacemaker electrode is a symphony of lead and stylet. The lead, by itself, cannot be steered or twisted into place. There are two fundamental techniques that directly relate to lead design. The first is placement of an electrode with a preformed curve or atrial J electrode.[69] This electrode can have either active or passive fixation mechanisms. More commonly, a lead with passive fixation tines is used. After insertion into the venous system, the lead tip is positioned with straight stylet fully inserted in the middle to lower right atrium. The preformed J has been straightened with the straight stylet. Fluoroscopy can be in either the PA or the RAO projection. Under fluoroscopic observation, the straight stylet is withdrawn several centimeters. The atrial lead tip can be observed to begin assuming its J configuration with the tip beginning to point upward. The lead body is then slowly advanced at the venous entry site (Fig. 27–35). On fluoroscopy, the lead tip will be observed to continue its upward motion, eventually seating in the atrial appendage. If the lead tip is too low in the right atrium, it may catch on or cross the tricuspid valve as the stylet is withdrawn. In this case, the lead is simply withdrawn a bit and the maneuver repeated slightly higher in the right atrium. If the lead tip is too high in the right atrium or is in the superior vena cava, the tip will not move upward adequately. In this case, the

electrode is repositioned more inferiorly. As one gains comfort with this maneuver, it can be repeated over and over. With experience, the act of retracting the stylet slightly can be performed briskly. This "snaps" the lead tip into the atrial appendage, at times resulting in better electrode-endocardial contact. Frustration and failure may occur if atrial placement is attempted by briskly removing the entire stylet and expecting the electrode to jump into the atrial appendage. This maneuver usually results in the electrode coiling on itself in the superior vena cava or right atrium. Further attempts at positioning are impossible until the stylet has been reinserted and the process begun again.

Good atrial positioning consists of a generous J loop, with the tip moving medial to lateral in a to-and-fro fashion in the PA radiographic projection (Fig. 27–36).[70, 71] In the lateral projection, the tip should be anterior and observed to "bob" up and down. With the firmly seated tip in the atrial appendage, the lead body should be twisted or torqued to the left and right to establish a position of neutral torque. Sometimes in the process of positioning, torque can build up. If it is not released, electrode dislodgment could result. This same maneuver of twisting can also result in better electrode-myocardial contact. With experience, one gets a sense of the proper J or loop size. This can be a source of frustration. Too much or too little loop can result in dislodgment. This may vary somewhat with the lead model. Another frustration can occur in relation to conformational changes in the vasculature with postural movement. With the patient supine, just the right loop appears to have been created, but as soon as the patient becomes upright, the conformational change occurs and it seems as though the mediastinal vasculature shifts inferiorly, pulling up on the lead, and obliterating the loop. Unfortunately, this situation may not be discovered until the postimplantation chest x-ray film is seen. Attempts at gauging the loop size by having the patient take deep inspirations is

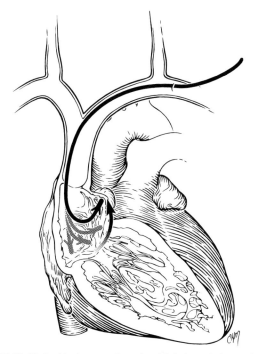

FIGURE 27–35. Positioning a preformed atrial J electrode by partial withdrawal of the lead stylet.

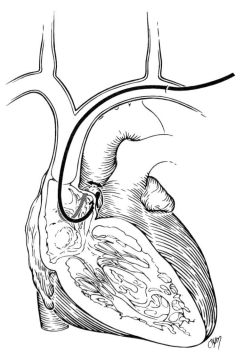

FIGURE 27–36. The to-and-fro, medial-to-lateral motion of a well-placed atrial lead in the atrial appendage when viewed in the PA projection.

frequently unrewarding. As a general rule, it is better to create a more generous loop.

Positioning the performed J atrial lead with an active fixation screw-in mechanism uses the same basic technique described earlier. After positioning in the atrial appendage, however, the active fixation mechanism must be activated. This usually involves the extension of a screw or helix. The exposed or fixed screw described previously is not available in a preformed atrial J configuration.

The second technique of placing an atrial electrode involves the use of a straight or nonpreformed lead. This lead is positioned in the atrium by use of a stylet that is preformed into a J and can be modified into other configurations. The stylets typically come with the lead already preformed into the J shape or, if desired, a straight stylet can be shaped into the J or other configurations using the same technique described for curving the ventricular lead stylet. It can then be positioned in the atrium, frequently in the atrial appendage, although it has become increasingly evident that other locations in the atrium, especially the anterior and lateral free walls, can be easily and safely targeted.[72] Manipulation of the stylet is required to gain access to the various atrial locations. Not uncommonly, modification of the preformed stylet shape is required. At the University of Oklahoma, we have found that modification of the J stylet into a shape similar to that of an Amplatz coronary artery catheter (several varieties) is most helpful in gaining access to a number of positions in the right atrium. The principal advantage of the nonpreformed leads (using various shapes of stylets) with active fixation mechanisms is that one is not restricted to the atrial appendage. This is discussed in more detail further on. With a straight or nonpreformed active fixation lead, either a fixed screw or an extendible-retractable screw can be used.

There are reports of successful placement of a straight, tined lead in the atrial appendage without dislodgment, but because of the risk of dislodgment and the high success rate of both the active fixation and preformed atrial J leads, this is not recommended, especially early in one's experience. The use of an active fixation lead in the atrium is ideal for patients who have undergone open heart surgery during which the atrial appendage was amputated. There are several other advantages to using an active fixation lead in the atrium. The first, as already noted, is the ability to choose the placement site or to map the atrium for optimal electric threshold, or both. By extending and retracting an extendible-retractable screw or attaching and detaching a fixed screw, multiple positions can be analyzed. The straight active fixation lead can be placed essentially anywhere in the atrium. On the contrary, the preformed atrial J lead can typically and easily be placed only in the atrial appendage. The second advantage of the active fixation lead is its ease of retrievability. The ability to remove a chronically implanted lead, if it becomes necessary in the future, is probably more easily accomplished with this lead.

Proper or adequate placement of active fixation leads is reflected by good electric threshold measurements. As discussed in the section on ventricular electrode placement, there are differences of opinion as to whether, in addition to achieving optimal electric parameters, a gentle tug on the lead after fixation is helpful in determining that good mechanical fixation is achieved. Although some implanters use a ''floppy tip'' technique for unusual or precise lead placement, or both, some types of active fixation leads (especially of the extendible-retractable variety) require full insertion of the stylet to activate the screw-in mechanism. The floppy tip approach obviously will not be effective in this situation. The fixed screw and some of the extendible-retractable screws do not have this problem.

Occasionally, difficulty is encountered while attempting placement of leads in the atrial appendage with the preformed atrial J stylet. In certain situations, the lead with J stylet in place will not assume an adequate J shape to enter the atrial appendage or make contact with atrial muscle. This may be because the stylet is too limp, does not have enough curve, or the atrium is large. In this situation, one may have to use a stiffer stylet and preform it with an exaggerated curve or J. Problems can be encountered trying stiffer stylets down through the electrode as well as during negotiation of the venous system in the superior mediastinum. Trial and error with multiple stylet configurations is almost always ultimately rewarded by success.

The side of venous access has little effect on atrial electrode placement. Whether placement is from the right or left, the preformed J electrode or straight electrode with preformed J stylet can generally provide easy access to the atrial appendage. Venous access may affect placement of the electrode in unusual atrial positions. Precise placement by use of stylet and electrode manipulation may be more difficult from the right side. As discussed with ventricular lead placement, the electrode, depending on the shape of the stylet curve, may seek a right lateral orientation.

Securing the atrial lead is similar to that of the ventricular lead. When securing the atrial lead after percutaneous venous access and placement, like the ventricular lead it should be oriented in a generally horizontal plane, roughly parallel to the clavicle. If the pocket has not already been made, the infraclavicular space is opened via dissection with Metzenbaum scissors. Dissection is carried to the surface of the greater pectoral muscle near its attachment point under the clavicle. The fibers of the platysma muscles are severed. A 1–0 silk suture is placed in a generous "bite" of the pectoral muscle under the anticipated site of attachment. The suture sleeve is advanced down the lead to the vicinity of the suture. Care should be taken not to dislodge or change the atrial lead position in the process. Occasionally, the suture sleeve will bind to the electrode, making it difficult to position. This is best managed by lubricating the lead with sterile saline or other fluid and using smooth forceps to then slide the sleeve into position. Once in position, the suture is secured around the suture sleeve. Many implanters first put a knot in the suture on the surface of the muscle. The two ends of the suture are then wrapped around the suture sleeve and tied. This second tie is directly around the lead and is designed to prevent lead slippage. Some implanters use multiple sutures rather than a single one, as discussed in the section on Ventricular Electrode Placement. Care must be taken to make the tie snug and yet avoid injury to the lead. It is important to orient the electrode horizontally. As with ventricular leads, this orients the lead in a plane similar to the axillary vein, reduces the bend of the lead, and may decrease the likelihood of the crush phenomenon or other stress-related lead damage.

If venous access and electrode placement have been achieved by venous cutdown, there is essentially no risk of the classic crush injury. Generally, the suture sleeve and lead are anchored to the pectoral muscle parallel to the vein. Similar precautions concerning lead injury should be observed. The securing process is the same, and one should avoid acute angulation of the lead and the creation of points of lead stress.

Upgrading Techniques

An upgrading procedure is necessary in patients with the pacemaker syndrome. With the increasing acceptance of dual-chamber pacing, all patients with initial VVI systems who have intact atrial function are now being considered for a pacemaker system upgrade with the addition of an atrial lead. Generally, this is deferred until the time of pulse generator power depletion, but increased awareness of the pacemaker syndrome has resulted in earlier pacemaker system upgrades. The upgrade procedure requires new venous access for the introduction of an atrial lead. It may also involve the introduction of a new ventricular lead because of problems with the chronic lead. Most pacemaker system upgrades require the replacement of the pulse generator, although occasionally the chronic pulse generator used in the ventricle can be used for atrial pacing. Most of the time, upgrade procedures involve a conventional approach using one of the previously described percutaneous techniques or a venous cutdown. If the patient has had an initial ventricular lead placed via the cephalic vein, the percutaneous approach is almost mandatory for the upgrade. Conversely, patients with an initial percutaneous subclavian approach can have the atrial lead introduced either by cutdown of the cephalic vein or percutaneous venous access. In the case of an initial percutaneous approach, the ventricular electrode can serve as a map. Using fluoroscopy, the trajectory of the percutaneous needle is guided by the chronic ventricular electrode. Care should be taken not to touch or damage the first lead with the needle.

The lead should be used as a reference landmark for the expected location of the subclavian vein. Bognolo and associates have described a technique to reestablish venous access using the old ventricular lead.[73, 74] The patency of the venous structures can be assessed as previously described with the injection of radiographic contrast material.[57]

If access to the subclavian vein cannot be obtained using the axioms of the "safe introducer technique" previously described by Byrd,[51] an extrathoracic puncture of the axillary vein can be carried out. The puncture of the vein can be expedited by a simple technique. A guide wire or catheter is passed to the vicinity of the subclavian vein via a vein in the arm. The guide wire or catheter can be palpated or viewed fluoroscopically, or both, thus serving as a reference for venous access. In the case of a cutdown on a previously unused cephalic vein, the Ong-Barold percutaneous sheath set technique can be used.[65]

Lead compatibility is important when considering a pacemaker system upgrade. To avoid embarrassment, one must be aware of the new pulse generator's compatibility with the chronic lead system.

Occasionally, ipsilateral venous access is impossible. Either the vessel is thrombosed or there is some form of obstruction that precludes the addition of a second (atrial) lead from the same side. In this case, contralateral venous access can be achieved and the lead tunneled back to the original pocket (Fig. 27–37). Early injection of radiographic contrast material may expedite the decision to use this approach. The use of the contralateral subclavian (rather than cephalic) vein is recommended for this approach.[75] The distance to the original pocket is less, and the new lead is not as susceptible to dislodgment. The same percutaneous techniques and precautions are used as previously described for the percutaneous approach. The only difference is the size of the skin incision, which is limited to about 1 to 1.5 cm. The incision need only be large enough to allow anchoring of the lead and securing of the suture sleeve. Similar to an initial implantation, the incision should be carried down to the pectoral fascia. Once the lead has been positioned and secured, it can be tunneled to the original pocket.

The maneuver of passing an electrode or catheter through tissue from one location to another is referred to as tunneling. It always involves the passage of a catheter from one wound through tissue to a second wound remote from the first. An example is the placement of a pacemaker lead via the internal jugular vein. The lead is passed from the jugular incision through the tissue over (or under) the clavicle to the pacemaker pocket in the pectoral area. Recently, with the development of nonthoracotomy-implantable defibrillator lead and patch systems, tunneling has become popular and necessary.

There are a number of techniques available for tunneling. They differ in the degree of trauma to the tissue and lead. As a rule, the least traumatic technique is desirable. A popular technique is to place the proximal end of the lead or leads to be tunneled in a ¼-inch Penrose drain (Fig. 27–38A). A gentle, nonconstricting tie is applied around the drain just distal to the lead connector (see Fig. 27–38B). The tract of the tunnel is infiltrated with local anesthesia using an 18-gauge spinal needle from the satellite wound to the pocket. The free end of the Penrose drain is then brought to the receiving wound from the satellite wound in the subcutaneous tissue. This can be accomplished by several tech-

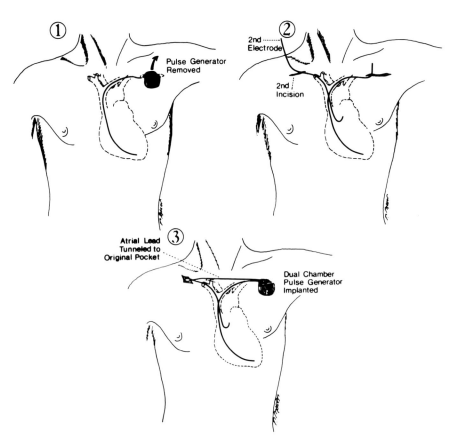

FIGURE 27–37. Pacemaker upgrade using the contralateral subclavian vein: (1) the pacemaker pocket is opened, and the old pulse generator and lead are dissected free, externalized, and disconnected; (2) the second lead is inserted via the contralateral subclavian vein; and (3) the second lead is tunneled back to the initial pocket. (From Belott PH: Use of the contralateral subclavian vein for placement of atrial electrodes in chronically VVI paced patients. PACE 6:781, 1983.)

niques. The first technique involves the use of a Kelly clamp or uterine packing forceps. The tip of the clamp is pushed bluntly in the subcutaneous tissue from the receiving wound directly to the satellite wound. Care is taken to keep the tunnel as deep as possible, usually on the surface of the muscle. The free end of the Penrose drain is grasped and pulled back from the satellite wound to the receiving wound. The remainder of the Penrose drain containing the electrode connector pin is pulled through the tract to the receiving wound. The tie is released and the Penrose drain is removed.

A second technique delivers the Penrose drain to the receiving wound by use of a "passer," usually a knitting needle or dilator. In this technique, the free end of the Penrose drain is fixed to the back end of the passer by use of a tie. The pointed tip of the passer is inserted into the satellite wound and pushed to the receiving wound. The tip of the passer is grasped and pulled into the receiving wound with the Penrose drain attached. The remainder of the Penrose drain with the lead is pulled into the receiving wound.

A variation of this technique uses the percutaneous technique to establish the tunnel. After infiltrating the tract of the tunnel with an 18-gauge spinal needle, the needle is passed from the wound of origin to the receiving wound. A guide wire is passed through the needle into the receiving wound.

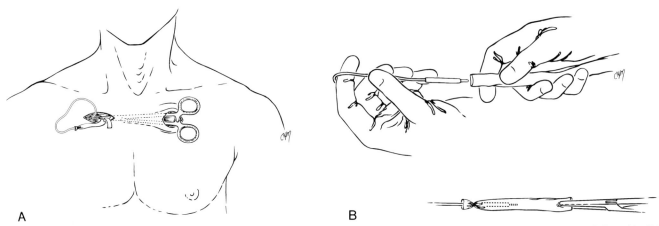

FIGURE 27–38. *A*, Penrose drain and lead grabbed by clamp that has been passed from the recipient wound to the donor site. The Penrose drain and lead(s) are pulled back to the recipient wound. *B*, Tunneling from one wound to another by placing the electrode(s) in a Penrose drain. The lead(s) are placed in a ¼-inch Penrose drain and tied. The Penrose drain is then grabbed with a long clamp.

A standard peel-away introducer is then passed over the guide wire from the satellite incision to the receiving wound, and the sheath can then be used to pass the lead, with the sheath eventually being removed and peeled.

Another variation uses the dilator of the sheath set to tunnel and the guide wire to pull the Penrose drain from wound to wound. After tunneling from one wound to the other with the dilator, the guide wire is passed through the dilator. The dilator is removed and the guide wire attached to the loose end of the Penrose drain. The Penrose drain is then brought to the receiving wound by pulling the guide wire.

A technique that is similar in principle to the use of the Penrose drain, but may be more traumatic, involves the use of a small chest tube and Pean clamp. The size of the chest tube is determined by the size and number of leads to be tunneled at one time. The length is determined by the distance from the initial wound to the receiving wound. The tube may be cut to size and the end beveled to a point. The leads at the wound of origin are placed in the back end of the chest tube. The Pean clamp is bluntly passed from the receiving wound to the wound containing the leads. The pointed end of the chest tube is grasped by the Pean clamp and is pulled into and through the receiving wound. Although more traumatic to tissue, the technique is protective of the electrodes.

Another related technique involving the use of a chest tube requires blunt passage of the chest tube, with trocar in place, through the subcutaneous tissue from the site of origin to the receiving wound with the lead or leads placed in the "back end" of the tube after removal of the trocar. The tube can be then be pulled through into the receiving wound.

Finally, new tunneling tools have been developed for use with implantable defibrillators. These tools may be used for pacemaker lead tunneling also.

The preceding techniques and principles are used whenever tunneling is required. Tunneling with a clamp and directly grasping the lead should always be avoided because of the risk of damage to the lead.

Epicardial Electrode Placement

Epicardial pacemaker implantation was the earliest, and once the most common, implantation technique, but it has limited use and utility today. This is largely due to the unparalleled success of transvenous implantation. Today, epicardial implantation is reserved mainly for patients undergoing cardiac surgery. In fact, in many centers, even patients undergoing cardiac surgery who also need permanent pacing have temporary epicardial electrodes applied with subsequent permanent transvenous pacing systems implanted. Modern transvenous leads have largely eliminated the problems of exit block and dislodgment. These leads have proved more reliable than epicardial leads. In addition, the abdominal pacemaker location of epicardial systems may cause more discomfort than a prepectoral one. Today, only unusual circumstances mitigate an epicardial implant. These circumstances include (1) patients undergoing cardiac surgery for another indication (with the preceding caveat), (2) patients with recurrent dislodgments of transvenous systems, and (3) patients with prosthetic tricuspid valves or congenital anomalies such as tricuspid atresia.

Although this chapter has dealt extensively with transvenous electrode placement, epicardial placement will be treated more superficially.

There are several epicardial surgical approaches. The most common is probably the median sternotomy performed as a secondary procedure at the time of other related cardiac surgery. In this case, both atria and ventricles are mapped for optimal pacing thresholds and other electrophysiologic parameters. The electrodes are attached directly to the epicardium. The electrode is tunneled by the chest tube technique to a subcutaneous pocket in the upper abdomen.

As a primary procedure, there are three distinct approaches: the subxiphoid, left subcostal, and left anterolateral thoracotomy. The first two avoid a "formal" thoracotomy. The pericardium is entered through an abdominal incision that is supradiaphragmatic. The subxiphoid approach exposes the diaphragmatic surface of the heart and mainly the right ventricle. The right ventricle can be thin, and care should be taken to avoid laceration that can require urgent thoracotomy and possibly cardiopulmonary bypass. The left subcostal approach exposes more of the left ventricle. The left lateral thoracotomy favors left ventricular electrode placement. With this approach, an incision is made in the fifth intercostal space. The incision extends from the left parasternal border to the left anterior axillary line. Care must be taken to avoid the phrenic nerve.

All of the epicardial pacemaker implantation techniques require general anesthesia. The median sternotomy and left lateral implantation procedures generally require chest tube placement. The epicardial procedures are performed in an operating room by a thoracic surgeon trained specifically in epicardial pacemaker implantation.

Securing Leads, Pocket Creation, and Closure

Once all electrodes are in position, it is time to establish permanent venous stasis and secure the leads. These maneuvers pertain to the transvenous approach only. In the epicardial procedures, the electrodes have already been secured directly to the heart, and no vascular structure has been entered that requires comparable attainment of venous stasis. In the case of the transvenous approach, one or more leads must be secured and the venous port of entry permanently sealed. If the cutdown approach has been used, the proximal and distal ligatures must be tied. Care should be taken not to injure or cut the lead when securing the ligature around the vein containing the lead. The venous ties are merely to effect hemostasis, not to secure the lead. These ties should be "gentle" and as nonconstricting as possible. The securing process using the anchoring sleeves has already been described. It is reiterated that the leads should be secured and oriented in a plane that is roughly parallel to the subclavian or axillary vein to reduce the risk of subclavian crush injury (Fig. 27–39). As with the ligatures around the leads, the suture sleeves should be secured snugly but not overtightened.

If the figure-of-eight or pursestring suture has been used in conjunction with the percutaneous approach, it can be tied after all leads are in position and no further venous entry is desired. Also at this time, the retained guide wire can be

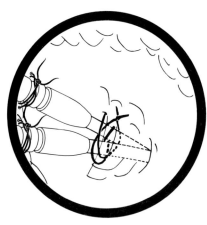

FIGURE 27–39. Secured atrial and ventricular electrodes using the suture sleeves. Hemostasis is effected at the puncture site, when necessary, with a loose nonconstricting tie.

removed, although it is not essential to do so. The retained guide wire can be removed later, just prior to wound closure. In this case, if the figure-of-eight or pursestring suture has been tied properly, there will be no back-bleeding. The guide wire should, in any case, be retained until the last moment when no further venous access is required. It should be removed only after one is completely satisfied with electrode placement and there is no need for replacement or exchange. Like the venous ligatures used in the cutdown technique, the figure-of-eight or pursestring suture requires only enough tension to collapse the vein or the tissue surrounding the leads near the point of entry of the leads into the vein. It is not intended to anchor the leads. If tied too tight, it may injure the lead or leads. It is not essential that the retained guide wire be removed prior to tying the figure-of-eight stitch. The retained guide wire can be removed much later, just prior to wound closure. In this case, if the figure-of-eight stitch has been tied properly, there will be no back-bleeding.

Once the leads have been secured, it is time to create the pacemaker pocket if this has not already been accomplished. Traditionally, this is performed at the end of the procedure. The actual timing of the pocket creation, however, is at the discretion of the implanting physician. Some implanters prefer to create the pocket early in the procedure, even as the initial step in a pacemaker implantation. In this case, a rudimentary pocket is created and packed with gauze, allowing time for natural hemostasis. Toward the end of the procedure, the packing is removed and the pocket is reinspected for hemostasis and surgically modified as necessary. The alternative approach involves creation of the pacemaker pocket after the lead or leads have been secured. There are arguments for both approaches. Proponents of the early pocket approach argue that bleeding is more easily controlled, and the risk of damage to leads is lower. Proponents of the late pocket approach will argue that to make the pocket early is "putting the cart before the horse" and that the highest priority is to establish pacing early to protect the patient. Creation of the pacemaker pocket is of lower priority. In addition, early creation of the pocket may result in embarrassment if the pocket is not used because of unsuccessful venous access.

A reasonable modification of the early pocket approach exists that avoids the risk of embarrassment should the vein on that side not be used for access. It involves percutaneous venous access with placement and maintenance of an intravenous guide wire prior to pocket creation, which, in turn, precedes placement of the leads using the guide wire. This approach assures venous access prior to formation of the pocket and achieves the advantages of early pocket formation noted previously.

Prior to creation of the pacemaker pocket, the area is generously infiltrated with a local anesthetic agent, assuming local anesthesia is used. If an earlier incision has already been made to facilitate lead placement and securing the lead, anesthesia is best achieved by infiltrating along the edge of the incision directly into the subcutaneous tissue. The incision is carried down to the anterior surface of the pectoral fascia. The pacemaker pocket is best formed predominantly inferior and medial to the incision, although many implanters also form a small portion of the pocket superior and lateral to an incision directed from the venipuncture site in an inferolateral vector. The advantage of this approach is that the pulse generator, with leads coiled deep, can then be placed directly under the incision, making subsequent pacing procedures, such as pulse generator replacement, both easy and safe with an incision at the same site. A plane of dissection is created at the junction of the subcutaneous tissue and pectoral fascia. This is best achieved by putting the subcutaneous tissue under slight tension with some form of retraction. This maneuver better defines the plane of dissection. Initially, the Senn retractor can be used and then replaced by the Goulet retractor. The plane of dissection can be started by using the Metzenbaum scissors or the cutting function of electrocautery. Once a plane of dissection has been established, the remainder of the pocket can be created by blunt dissection. Some argue that blunt dissection is less traumatic to the tissues. The problems with blunt dissection are there is no good visualization and there is a lack of control with respect to tissue depth. Optimally, the pacemaker pocket should be as deep as possible, right on top of the fascia of the pectoral muscle. This offers the optimal subcutaneous tissue thickness necessary to avoid erosion. Unfortunately, with blunt dissection, this ideal plane can be lost, creating inconsistent pocket thickness with its increased risk of erosion. Today's pacemaker is small, limiting the amount of dissection required and the pocket size needed. The pocket can easily be created by direct visualization instead of blindly. As previously noted, the subcutaneous tissue is held under gentle tension, defining the plane of dissection. Sharp dissection with Metzenbaum scissors or the cutting function of electrocautery, or both, is then used to completely form the pocket. This technique is less traumatic than blunt dissection. The pocket created by precise dissection over the pectoral muscle provides optimal tissue thickness. Thus, the pocket is created by visual inspection, and the plane of dissection is well controlled. The head lamp as a light source can be helpful here. There is less risk of hematoma, as all bleeding is directly visualized and managed with electrocautery.

Occasionally a patient will have little or no subcutaneous tissue. In this situation, a subpectoral muscle implant should be considered. Fortunately, with the dramatically reduced size of today's pacemakers and the availability of the Parsonnet pouch (see Fig. 27–5), this approach is rarely necessary.[76]

If required, the placement of the pacemaker under the pectoral muscle represents only a slight departure from the techniques already described. The one major concern using this approach is with the increased bleeding that is typically encountered, causing an increased risk of hematoma formation. In subpectoral implantation, the incision has already been carried down to the surface of the pectoral muscle and the leads secured. An incision is made through the muscle parallel to the muscle fibers. The muscle is separated and a plane of dissection is established on the chest wall. This pocket is best created by blunt dissection. As already described, considerable bleeding can be encountered with subpectoral implants. This bleeding is best controlled with electrocautery. Careful visual inspection using a Goulet retractor and good lighting is important. All bleeding sources should be identified and either sutured or coagulated. Pocket drainage is frequently required.

Use of electrocautery has been a traditional taboo in cardiac pacing.[15] It can cause fibrillation or burns at the myocardium-electrode interface and can reprogram or even irreparably damage the pulse generator. However, electrocautery can be extremely useful in a pacemaker procedure in both coagulation and cutting modes. It is the surest and most expeditious way to control bleeding and create the pacemaker pocket. It can be used safely provided that one is aware of the dangers and takes a few precautions. Today's electrocautery systems are extremely safe from an electric hazard point of view. There are built-in mechanisms protecting against improper grounding. Modern electrocautery equipment will not function if not grounded correctly. A few simple rules should be followed that are specific to the use of electrocautery systems in pacemaker implantation procedures. First, the use of electrocautery should be avoided when the pulse generator is in the surgical field. Second, the cautery must never touch the exposed pin of the pacemaker lead. Finally, the cautery must never touch the retained guide wire if it is in the heart.

Wound drainage is required in patients who manifest excessive bleeding. The term wet pocket has been used to describe this condition. This situation is encountered more frequently today with the increasing use of anticoagulants. Patients taking aspirin, warfarin, or heparin will frequently manifest a wet pocket. Not rarely, medical indications preclude cessation of such drugs. If a patient is taking warfarin, a prothrombin time 1 to 1½ times the control level is less likely to cause a problem than if it is greater than 1½ times the control level. In the latter situation, the procedure should be postponed until the prothrombin time reaches a more reasonable level. Heparin or platelet antagonists seem to cause the greatest problem. Despite diligent efforts to establish hemostasis, the pockets may continue to ooze diffusely. In this circumstance, some implanters have resorted to the topical application of thrombin.

Patients taking anticoagulants and those receiving a subpectoral implant should be considered for some form of drainage. As a general rule, if reasonable hemostasis cannot be achieved, the pacemaker pocket should be drained (although drainage should not be considered an alternative to adequate attempts at attaining hemostasis). This is accomplished by placing a Jackson-Pratt drain or Hemovac system. A trocar connected to the drainage tubing is passed from the inferior aspect of the pacemaker pocket to a satellite exit wound remote from the pacemaker pocket. The distal end of the tubing in the pacemaker pocket is specially designed of soft rubber with multiple drainage ports. This end can be cut to desired size to avoid excessive tubing in the pocket. Once the pacemaker pocket is closed, the proximal end of the drainage tubing is connected to a closed suction system. The Jackson-Pratt system is preferred, as it has a one-way valve that allows emptying yet prevents inadvertent flushing of old drained fluids back into the pocket. It is small and of little encumbrance to the patient. To avoid infection, the drainage system is removed within 24 hours. If drainage is copious, a longer period may be required. In the case of persistent bloody drainage, the wound should be reexplored and the culprit bleeder ligated or cauterized.

Wound irrigation is largely a personal preference, with no clearly established mandate by investigations to do so. There is a spectrum from simple saline lavage to concentrated solutions of multiple antibiotics. It is likely that such antibiotic solutions are unnecessary, especially if systemic antibiotics are used. This issue has been previously addressed. In addition to irrigation of the wound, some implanters place antibiotic-soaked gauze pads in the pocket early to achieve not only antibiosis but also hemostasis by compression with the pads.

Closure of the pacemaker pocket consists of initial approximation of the subcutaneous tissue and subsequent skin closure. The subcutaneous tissue can be approximated by single or multiple layers of interrupted or running sutures. The number of layers is a function of the thickness of the subcutaneous tissue. The suture material used by most implanters for subcutaneous closure is an absorbable semisynthetic that is fairly strong, usually 2–0 or 3–0. There are several techniques of skin closure. The choice of technique relates to the desired cosmetic effect and time spent. An ideal cosmetic effect can be achieved by use of the subcuticular suture. This is best accomplished using 4–0 semisynthetic absorbable suture material, which does not require removal. The use of interrupted sutures has the least cosmetic result, and the sutures require removal. The resulting scar may have visible crosshatches. Many skin closures today are performed with surgical staples or clips. This closure is cosmetically appealing and extremely fast. The only drawback to the use of staples is that they require removal in 7 to 10 days. After closure of the skin, the wound can be coated with an antiseptic ointment, and a dry sterile dressing applied. Since a pocket has been created that can fill with blood, some form of pressure dressing may be used, although maintaining the pressure is frequently not easily accomplished in an ambulatory or otherwise active patient.

Immediate Postoperative Care

There is considerable center to center variability in the intensity of monitoring following implantation. There is general agreement that intensive care monitoring postoperatively is not usually required. Patients who were in the intensive care unit before implantation may be transferred to a bed on a nursing unit for continuous cardiac rhythm monitoring postoperatively unless, of course, there is another reason for the patient to be in an intensive care setting. Other patients electively admitted to the hospital specifically for pacemaker implantation are also returned to a cardiac monitoring area. Basic rhythm monitoring would appear to be all that is necessary. The activity level of the patient in immediate postoperative period is subject to personal preference and philosophy. In the early days of pacing, the patient was kept on strict bed rest with restricted activity for many days. Today's lead systems with both active and passive fixation mechanisms offer a new dimension of security. The earlier dislodgment rates of nearly 20% have been dramatically reduced. In most centers, the current philosophy is to have the patient active immediately or shortly after arrival at the monitoring area. The intention is early detection of patients with potential pacemaker system malfunctions. The patient with a precariously placed electrode who is kept on strict bed rest may not demonstrate malfunction, giving a false sense of security at the time of discharge. The active patient will give a better indication that reliable pacemaker sensing and capture are occurring. This approach is important in the patient being managed on an ambulatory basis. If the patient is to stay in the hospital postoperatively, noninvasive pacemaker evaluation and programming may be carried out. This might include reevaluation of sensing and pacing thresholds as well as initial activation and set-up of the rate-adaptive system. If the patient is to be managed as an outpatient, these functions can be carried out at the time of the initial postoperative visit to the pacemaker clinic.

The documentation of the pacemaker procedure is crucial from both a clinical and a medicolegal point of view. An operative report that identifies indications; pacemaker and lead manufacturer, make, and model; details of the implantation procedure; and pacemaker-programmed settings is essential. A clear description of the procedure, including problems encountered as well as electric testing data, is important. Copies of the operative report should be sent to the pacemaker clinic as well as to the referring and follow-up physicians. Further documentation includes the manufacturer's registration form and, in the United States, the hospital registry or log required by the Food and Drug Administration. Copies of the manufacturer's registration form should also be forwarded to the pacemaker clinic and any physician following the patient. It is extremely important to have multiple resources for retrieving pacemaker implantation information. Many manufacturers supply convenient stickers containing pulse generator and lead data for the patient's chart.

A postoperative chest x-ray study is extremely important for documentation of the lead position immediately following surgery. It can be used for comparison if subsequent dislodgment is suspected. In the case of a percutaneous procedure, it is essential to rule out a pneumothorax. Generally, it is useful to obtain both PA and lateral films for documentation of lead position. We ask that the postoperative x-ray film be overpenetrated and that the patient's arms not be raised above shoulder level.

Similarly, a 12-lead ECG with and without magnet application is essential to document initial appropriate pacemaker sensing and capture. The chest x-ray film and electrocardiographic documentation also have medicolegal value should a question arise subsequently.

The timing of discharge is controversial, with considerable variability among institutions. Today, there is a trend toward a more abbreviated hospital stay. For example, at the University of Oklahoma patients are now discharged routinely the day after implantation unless there is a specific reason for prolonging the hospital stay. During the short hospital stay, the patient ambulates within 2 hours of completion of the procedure, a chest x-ray study and ECG are performed, and preliminary interrogation, threshold testing, and programming are accomplished. Even markedly pacemaker-dependent patients are approached this way. We have experienced no complications or morbidity following discharge that would have been averted by longer hospitalization. Some centers use the first and second postoperative days for more extensive testing of the pacemaker system and the patient-pacemaker system interface. Such testing might include Holter monitoring, extensive reprogramming with particular attention to pacing and sensing thresholds, and exercise testing to adjust rate-adaptive parameters. In some centers, the pacemaker-dependent patient may be hospitalized longer. At the other end of the spectrum is a completely ambulatory approach. Patients are discharged on the same day immediately after the pacemaker procedure regardless of whether they are pacemaker-dependent or not. This has been the approach at the El Cajon Pacemaker Center. This experience in the United States, in addition to a large series of ambulatory procedures in Europe, has been very encouraging. The El Cajon experience is now longer than 10 years and includes 658 ambulatory pacemaker procedures. There have been no postoperative pacemaker deaths or pacemaker emergencies. The El Cajon experience suggests that between 70% and 75% of pacemaker procedures can be safely conducted on an ambulatory basis. It is likely that patients referred for a pacemaker on an ambulatory basis are at no greater risk from the bradyarrhythmia than they were before they entered the hospital in the unlikely event the entire system were to fail postoperatively. If there are specific concerns about the pacemaker-dependent patient, the hospital stay can always be extended. As previously noted, it is important to have ambulatory-based patients active during the monitored postoperative period so that potential problems can be detected. This philosophy also applies to any patient who is considered to have a higher risk of a problem or complication developing.

The timing of initial follow-up varies depending on the timing of discharge and which physician is going to perform follow-up of the pacing system. If the implanting physician is to discharge the patient and perform the follow-up, there should be excellent continuity of care. Parenthetically, we have a strong bias that implanting physicians must be involved substantially in both acute and chronic follow-up of pacemaker patients in order to understand and appreciate many important aspects of the process as they relate to implantation.

Even if the discharging physician did not perform the procedure but is responsible for the follow-up, there may again be good continuity of care. Of concern is the situation in which the implanting physician discharges the patient to someone else for follow-up. In this case, there is the possibility that ideal pacemaker follow-up will not take place. This is common when a patient is discharged to a nursing home. In this case, it is imperative that the implanting or discharging physician arrange some form of reliable follow-up. It is important that patients whose procedure has been performed on an ambulatory basis be seen the following day for an initial follow-up visit. At the other extreme are patients who have been hospitalized and evaluated intensively for days postoperatively with Holter monitoring and extensive reprogramming. These patients may not need to be seen for a week or even a month.

Special Considerations and Situations

If initial venous access is unsuccessful, jugular venous access may be considered.[77] This is less desirable than subclavian, axillary, or cephalic vein placement because of the increased risk of lead fracture and the potential for erosion. An acute bend must be created in the lead after it exits the venous structure and is brought down to the pacemaker pocket under or over the clavicle. In addition, some form of tunneling is required to bring the lead to the pacemaker pocket. If one tunnels under the clavicle, there is increased risk of vascular injury. If the lead is tunneled over the clavicle, the tissue is typically thin and there is a greater chance of erosion.

Both the internal and external jugular veins have been used. Generally, the right jugular approach is preferred (Fig. 27–40). For a jugular venous approach, two separate incisions are required, above and below the clavicle. There are many published detailed descriptions of anatomic dissection including both the internal and external jugular veins. In these, there is particular attention paid to precise anatomic landmarks. An alternative percutaneous technique is proposed that is simple, requiring little attention to anatomic landmarks or dissection. Additionally, an initial supraclavicular incision is not required. This approach involves the percutaneous access of the right internal jugular vein. Once the decision is made to place the electrodes via the jugular vein, the neck must be prepared and draped in a sterile fashion accordingly. To save time, this may be performed in the initial preparation. If done in such a manner, the sterile field can be moved directly to the right supraclavicular area. If not, an effective sterile barrier can be created by use of an iodoform-impregnated see-through plastic drape. Access to the internal jugular vein is best obtained with the patient in

the normal anatomic position, with the head facing anteriorly. Turning the head to the left should be avoided, as this may distort the anatomy. The carotid artery is palpated in the lower third of the neck. The internal jugular vein is lateral to the common carotid artery. The two structures are parallel and lie side by side. Standing on the right side of the patient (for a right jugular vein approach), the implanting surgeon places the left middle finger along the course of the common carotid artery. The course of the internal jugular vein will be under the index finger. In fact, the index and middle fingers are, side by side, generally analogous in size and orientation on the surface of the skin to the internal jugular vein and common carotid artery as they run side by side underneath the skin. A puncture anywhere along this course should enter the internal jugular vein. The higher the puncture is in the neck, the less the risk of pneumothorax. Some prefer to make the needle puncture roughly perpendicular to the plane of the neck rather than angled. This also will help avoid a pneumothorax. Once the vein is entered, the needle and syringe can be gently angled inferiorly for passage of the guide wire. If the carotid artery is inadvertently punctured, the needle is removed, pressure over the puncture site is maintained briefly, and a reattempt at venipuncture is made a little lateral to the initial stick. The remainder of the lead placement technique is essentially identical to the previously described percutaneous technique. A small incision is carried laterally down the shaft of the needle to the surface of the muscle (sternocleidomastoid). If more tissue depth is required, the muscle can be split and the incision carried down to the vein. A small Weitlander retractor is used for retraction. A figure-of-eight or pursestring suture can be applied for hemostasis. Two leads for dual-chamber pacing can be placed by the retained guide wire technique. After the leads have been placed, the hemostasis suture is tied and the leads anchored to the muscle using the anchoring sleeve. A second incision for pocket formation is made infraclavicularly. A pacemaker pocket is created with conventional techniques. The leads are then tunneled to the pocket by the techniques previously described. If the electrodes are tunneled under the clavicle, care must be taken to avoid vascular trauma. Conversely, when tunneling over the clavicle, every effort should be made to ensure optimal tissue thickness.

Ellestad and French reported a 90-patient experience using the iliac vein as an alternative source of venous access for both single- and dual-chamber pacemaker implantation (Fig. 27–41).[78, 79] It can be used for transvenous lead placement when an abdominal pocket is desired, such as when patients have little pectoral tissue, in bilateral radical mastectomy patients following surgery, in patients with extensive pectoral radiation damage, and for a variety of cosmetic reasons. A small incision is made just above the inguinal ligament over the vein (just medial to the palpable artery) and carried down to the fascia above the vein. The vein is punctured by the sheath set technique with the guide wire retained for dual-chamber implants. A figure-of-eight or pursestring suture is placed for hemostasis through the fascia around the lead as it enters the vein. Long (85-cm) leads are positioned in a conventional manner and secured to the fascia by use of a tie around the suture sleeve and lead. A second horizontal incision is made lateral to the umbilicus and is carried to the surface of the rectus sheath. A pacemaker pocket is created by blunt dissection. Preparations are made to tunnel the leads

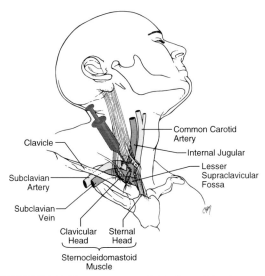

FIGURE 27–40. Venous anatomy of right internal jugular approach.

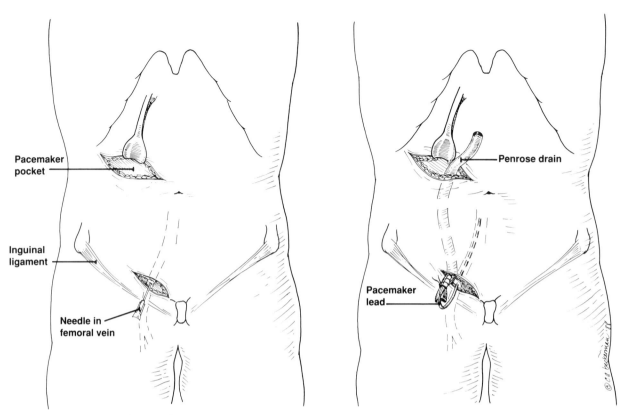

FIGURE 27–41. Use of the right iliac vein for placement of pacemaker lead(s). Percutaneous capture of the iliac vein is performed, and the lead is tunneled up to an upper-quadrant pacemaker pocket with the use of a Penrose drain. (From Ellestad MH, French J: Iliac vein approach to permanent pacemaker implantation. PACE 12:1030, 1989.)

from the initial incision to the pacemaker pocket by use of one of the previously described techniques.

Active fixation leads are recommended for both atrial and ventricular lead placement. Lead dislodgment is the major weakness of this approach, with 9 of 42 (21%) of the atrial and 5 of 67 (7%) of the ventricular leads in the Ellestad and French experience requiring repositioning. Lead fracture and venous thrombosis do not seem to be problems, although the published experience with this approach is relatively small and the latter especially could be difficult to discern. The complication of pneumothorax essentially does not exist.

If major patient concern occurs about the negative cosmetic effects of standard pacemaker pocket location, at least two alternatives exist.[80] Both can be performed with local anesthesia, but may best be performed with general or modified general anesthesia for patient comfort, as these procedures involve more extensive surgery. Both of these procedures lend themselves well to the percutaneous approach for both single- and dual-chamber pacing. In both procedures, after the subclavian vein is accessed, a limited (1.5-cm) initial skin incision is made. The incision is carried to the surface of the pectoral muscle, allowing only enough room to secure the lead or leads. A second incision is then made. For one of the alternative pocket locations, an incision is made under the breast along the breast fold or reflection. A standard pacemaker pocket is created under the breast with care taken to stay on the pectoral fascia (Fig. 27–42). The pocket is carefully inspected for hemostasis. Similarly, for another alternative pocket location, a second incision can be made in the axilla with the arm abducted 60 degrees. This incision can be carried to a depth that exposes the muscle

fascia, where a pocket can be formed with appropriate attention to hemostasis. With either of these approaches, tunneling of leads can be carried out using the previously described techniques.

The pulse generator and the lead or leads are connected and the incisions closed. A polyester (Dacron) or Parsonnet

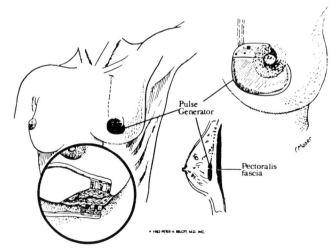

FIGURE 27–42. Inframammary placement of pulse generator after percutaneous lead placement for optimal cosmetic effect. A small incision is made near the clavicle, and the pocket incision is made in the hidden fold under the breast. The lead is tunneled deep to the breast, between the incisions. (From Belott PH, Bucko D: Inframammary pulse generator placement for maximizing optimal cosmetic effect. PACE 6:1241, 1983.)

pouch (see Fig. 27–5) (C. R. Bard, Inc., Billerica, ME) can be used to avoid rotation of the pulse generator and leads in the tissue. To avoid the problems of diaphragmatic stimulation, a bipolar system should be used, especially with the inframammary pocket.

Historically, the predominance of epicardial pacing has persisted substantially longer in pediatric patient populations than it has in adolescent and adult populations. Explanations for this are manifold. Much of the need for pacemaker implantation during infancy and childhood has occurred as a comorbidity of cardiac surgery for congenital heart disease.[81] In this context, epicardial implantation at the time of surgery has been typical. Additionally, certain forms of congenital heart disease (e.g., tricuspid atresia) make transvenous pacing difficult if not impossible. Expertise in transvenous pacing in pediatric patients has also been difficult to acquire because of the relatively smaller number of patients in this age group who require pacemaker therapy.[82] Also, there has been a perception that the relatively rapid growth in body size that occurs in childhood makes transvenous pacing problematic with respect to the intravascular length of leads. There has also been a reluctance by parents and physicians to place pacemakers in the traditional prepectoral area in children with, instead, a preference for abdominal pulse generator implantation. Finally, the lead diameters for transvenous pacemaker system implantation and pulse generator sizes have been felt to be excessive for conventional techniques of transvenous implantation. Conversely, as problems with epicardial pacemaker implantation have been more clearly elucidated, especially the problems of epicardial lead fracture and epicardial exit block, transvenous approaches have been appropriately reconsidered.[83] Encouraging in this reconsideration is the evolution of transvenous pacemaker implantation expertise by pediatric cardiologists or in concert between pacemaker implantation experts and pediatric cardiologists. More sophisticated lead placement techniques coupled with smaller diameter leads and pulse generators have also encouraged this relatively recent trend toward transvenous implantation in this age group.[84] New technologies in electrodes that help prevent the ever-concerning exit block problem have also been a motivator for the trend toward transvenous systems. Finally, the clear capacity to successfully implant transvenous pacing systems in patients in a variety of pediatric age groups with a variety of congenital cardiac problems has been a critical factor. With all of these considerations, especially with anticipated future developments in pacing technology, there is little question that transvenous pacing will become progressively dominant in the pediatric population as it has in adolescent and adult populations.

As noted previously, the relative infrequency of pediatric pacemaker implantation, compared with the frequency in the adult population, makes acquisition of expertise in implantation difficult. It is, perhaps, ideal when individuals specifically expert in pediatric implantation can be used, although the degree of regionalization necessary to accomplish this might be unrealistic. A team approach is a reasonable alternative, pairing an expert in pacemaker implantation (adult cardiologist or cardiac surgeon) with an invasive pediatric cardiologist or pediatric electrophysiologist. Although generally this type of redundancy in physician services is inefficient and not often well compensated, it may be the most attractive of a variety of options.

Pediatric pacemaker implantation can be carried out with local anesthesia and relatively substantial intravenous sedation and pain control without the services of an anesthesiologist. Conversely, although uncommon in the pediatric age group, excessive sedation must be monitored closely by someone experienced in doing so. It is appropriate to consider general anesthesia for pediatric pacemaker implantation, and in many cases general anesthesia is the safest approach to use.[84]

For transvenous pacemaker implantation, the techniques of venous access are precisely those described for adults. Smaller venipuncture needles and guide wires are available, although typically are not necessary except, perhaps, for infants. An important consideration in the pediatric population is blood loss. Generally speaking, the younger and smaller the patient, the more critical blood loss is. Special attention to this is warranted in young patients in comparison to their older counterparts.

The choice of pacemaker leads for pediatric implantation is also worthy of brief discussion. The five most important considerations in this regard involve the choice of bipolar or unipolar leads, the lead diameters, the fixation mechanisms (active versus passive), the higher incidence of exit block in the pediatric age group, and lead length. Although bipolar leads and the resulting bipolar (and optional unipolar) pacing systems have distinct advantages, in small infants or in certain situations in which maximal lead flexibility is necessary, unipolar leads and pacing systems may be appropriately chosen. Most small children beyond infancy tolerate not only the thicker bipolar systems but also dual-chamber bipolar systems. As lead (and pulse generator) technology moves toward smaller diameters, bipolar dual-chamber systems may be more comfortably used in even smaller patients. The fixation mechanism is another important consideration. The advantages of the types of fixation are not categorically different from those previously discussed. The flexibility for placement of leads in a variety of locations using active fixation leads is attractive. It is also an unproven hypothesis that active fixation leads may be less likely to become dislodged than their passive counterparts in a population of patients not able to understand the importance of temporary immobilization of the shoulder and arm following implantation. In contrast, electrode technologies such as that of steroid elution have proved useful in reducing the problem of exit block, which occurs in substantially greater frequency in the pediatric population. This steroid elution technology has been married, to date, more effectively with passive fixation leads. Finally, and possibly most importantly, lead length is a critical issue for this patient population. Excessive lead that must be coiled in the pacemaker pocket beneath the pulse generator creates formidable bulk for these small patients. Leads of variable lengths should be available and the choices for a specific patient carefully made. In this regard, it should be remembered that these patients will grow significantly and an adequate extra length of lead to accommodate this growth is desirable. In this context, one of the advantages in unipolar lead technology is that leads can be shortened or lengthened by splicing techniques, although this is certainly an imperfect solution to this vexing problem.

Once the lead or leads have been positioned, one may secure them (if such a procedure is desired) in the manner previously described using the anchoring sleeve. Alternatively, one may use an absorbable suture material for securing the leads using the anchoring sleeve. This approach has the advantage of good security of the lead during the time when the electrode-myocardium interface is unstable and dislodgment is most likely; it also provides for eventual elimination of the fixation to the pectoral fascia and muscle by dissolution of the suture material, facilitating movement of the lead through the anchoring sleeve and into the vein as growth occurs. Another alternative is to use active fixation leads and avoid the anchoring sleeve completely.

The formation of the pacemaker pocket follows the same guidelines outlined previously. There has been greater enthusiasm for the subpectoral muscle implant in pediatric patients, although as pulse generators decrease in size, this trend may wane.

There are certain unusual situations, especially those that relate to congenital anomalies and their surgical correction, that mitigate creativity. One example of this involves the need to pace the left ventricle or atrium, or both, in patients who have undergone a Mustard-type baffle procedure for transposition of the great arteries. Another example is successful transvenous pacing in patients with tricuspid atresia. This can be accomplished by passage of a transvenous lead through the right atrium into the coronary sinus and, respectively, into one of the posterior ventricular veins such as the middle cardiac vein. A caveat here relates to the higher risk of diaphragmatic pacing, especially if a unipolar system is employed. In pediatric patients with congenital heart disease, intracardiac shunting creates the need for special concern about the risks of systemic embolization related to placement of endocardial pacing systems. Normally, placement of endocardial systems should not be the procedure of choice in these patients prior to surgical correction of the shunts.

Although a question often arises as to the minimum age or size that would be considered acceptable for transvenous pacing, the answer is not easily provided. At the University of Oklahoma (and in many other medical centers) transvenous implantation is considered appropriate for infants weighing 10 pounds or more, although it is likely that as lead and pulse generator technologies are progressively downsized, this minimum size will also decrease.

The use of radiography may be problematic in certain situations such as during pregnancy. The prospect of implanting a pacemaker in such patients becomes particularly challenging. Guldal and colleagues have described an implantation technique for single-chamber (ventricular) pacemakers using two-dimensional echocardiography and intracardiac electrocardiography.[85] The technique involves subcostal visualization of the structures of the right side of the heart and the lead by two-dimensional echocardiography. The electrode position is verified by recording an intracardiac electrogram, and adequate capture is assured by intermittent pacing. More recently, Lau and Wong used ultrasound to position an electrode in severe pulmonary tuberculosis.[86] In this patient, collapse of the right side of the chest caused deviation of the heart to the right, making fluoroscopic visualization impossible. A passive fixation lead was introduced via a left cephalic cutdown and was passed with fluoroscopic visualization to an ill-defined cardiopulmonary shadow in the right side of the chest. The lead could then apparently no longer be visualized adequately by fluoroscopy. Two-dimensional echocardiography identified the lead in relation to the anat-

omy and assisted in final placement. Lead placement was verified by the intracardiac electrogram.

Repositioning of a malpositioned or dislodged permanent pacemaker electrode traditionally requires a surgical procedure. The pacemaker pocket must be surgically reopened. The pacemaker and leads are freed of adhesions and disconnected. A nonsurgical approach has been described by Morris and associates.[87] The technique uses principles similar to those of lead extraction via the femoral vein. The malpositioned lead is hooked and pulled into the inferior vena cava using a 3-mm J-shaped deflecting wire passed through a catheter placed in the femoral vein. This is accomplished by forming a closed loop in the deflecting wire and "capturing" the lead tip with the loop. The lead tip in the inferior vena cava is snared by a loop formed with a 300 cm–long 0.021 exchange wire. The loop is passed through an 8 F catheter with a 2-cm radius curve steamed at its tip. The snared lead tip is then repositioned in the apex of the right ventricle. Iatrogenic repeated dislodgment is avoided by releasing the snare, which is accomplished by advancing one end of the 0.021 guide wire, forming a large loop, while retracting the other end of the wire from the catheter.

Transvenous endocardial lead placement is occasionally contraindicated, impractical, or impossible. Westerman and Van Devanter described a transthoracic technique requiring general anesthesia and a limited thoracotomy for electrode placement.[88] The electrodes are passed and positioned transatrially through the sixth intercostal space (Fig. 27–43). The right atrium is identified and the electrode is passed transatrially through an incision or by using a sheath set. Hemostasis is effected by a pursestring suture around the entry site. Fluoroscopy can be used for the ventricular placement of a tined or screw-in electrode. All of the electrodes are secured to the endocardial surface. A tined electrode can be directly secured to the atrial endocardium. Double-needle–ended sutures are tied around the leads under the tines of the electrode. Prior to introduction of the lead, the needles are driven

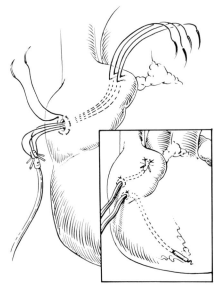

FIGURE 27–43. Transatrial endocardial lead placement during thoracotomy allows low-threshold transvenous leads to be implanted at the time of thoracic surgery. (From Barold SS, Mugica J [eds]: New Perspectives in Cardiac Pacing. Mt Kisco, NY, Futura Publ. Co., Inc., 1988, p 271.)

through the atriotomy into the atrial cavity and then out of the atrial muscle at the point of desired endocardial atrial fixation. The electrode is then pulled through the incision into the atrium and "snugged" to the endocardium by retracting and tying the double-ended suture. In many situations, this approach may have more merit than the epicardial approach, as better chronic electric thresholds are typically achieved. This technique may be useful for some pediatric implantations.

Hayes and colleagues described a similar technique of endocardial atrial electrode placement at the time of corrective cardiac surgery (Fig. 27–44),[89] avoiding atrial epicardial pacing because of poor pacing and sensing thresholds. In this description, a dual-chamber pacemaker patient with severe tricuspid regurgitation and chronic endocardial electrodes required removal of all four previously implanted endocardial leads and placement of a prosthetic tricuspid valve. New epicardial electrodes were placed on the ventricle. Stable atrial pacing and sensing were achieved by a transatrial endocardial placement in the right atrial appendage. In this case, the lead was secured by pursestring ligatures around the incision.

Byrd described another epicardial approach based on experience in five patients.[90] The technique also allows conventional transvenous leads to be implanted in patients requiring an epicardial approach, including those with superior vena cava syndrome or anomalous venous drainage and young patients with one innominate vein occluded by thrombosis. The technique uses a limited surgical approach with general anesthesia. The right atrial appendage is exposed through a 4-to 5-cm incision. The third and fourth costal cartilages are excised. A sheath set is placed inside an atrial pursestring suture and secured in a vertical position. The atrial and ventricular leads are passed down the sheath into the atrium

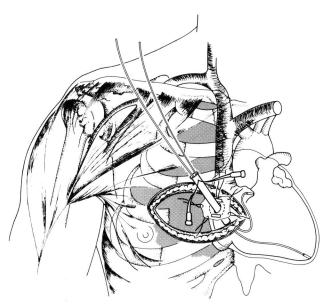

FIGURE 27–45. Endocardial lead placement via limited thoracotomy with removal of only the third and fourth costal cartilages. Standard fluoroscopy and peel-away introducer techniques are used with transatrial access. (From Byrd CL, Schwartz SJ, Siviona M, et al: Technique for the surgical extraction of permanent pacing leads and electrodes. J Thorac Cardiovasc Surg 89(1):142, 1985.)

(Fig. 27–45). Using standard techniques, including fluoroscopy, the electrodes are positioned. Once the electrodes are positioned, the sheath is removed and the pursestring suture around the atriotomy is secured. The pacemaker is placed in a pocket created at the incision on the anterior chest wall. The advantage of this technique for patients in whom conventional transvenous systems are contraindicated or impossible is that it provides for implantation of a more conventional transvenous pacing system with minimal morbidity compared with a standard epicardial implantation. The chest is not entered (except for the atrium), and the time required is similar to that required for transvenous implantation. The disadvantages (although not necessarily in relation to other nonstandard transvenous techniques) include the requirement of general anesthesia, violation of the pericardia and epicardia, and the necessity of a right-sided approach (this may not be possible because of prior infection, mastectomy, and so on).

Occasionally, one encounters a persistent left superior vena cava. Normally, the left superior vena cava becomes atretic embryologically. However, in 0.5% of the population, this structure persists and remains patent, connecting with the coronary sinus. Ten to 15% of these patients will also have no right superior vena cava. This precludes venous access to the right atrium and ventricle from the right side. Despite the fact that there are reported classic physical and radiographic signs, the diagnosis is traditionally discovered unexpectedly at the time of pacemaker implantation. Placement of electrodes via a persistent left superior vena cava can prove to be extremely challenging.[91–95] A thorough knowledge of anatomy and radiographic orientation is required. How one proceeds is determined by the initial side of approach.

If one proceeds from the left and is confronted with a persistent left superior vena cava, it must be appreciated that

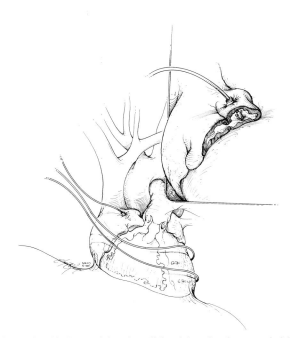

FIGURE 27–44. Transatrial endocardial atrial pacing in congenital heart disease. The ventricular leads were epicardial, since the patient required a prosthetic tricuspid valve. (From Hayes DL, Vliestra RE, Puga FJ, et al: A novel approach to atrial endocardial pacing. PACE 12:125, 1989.)

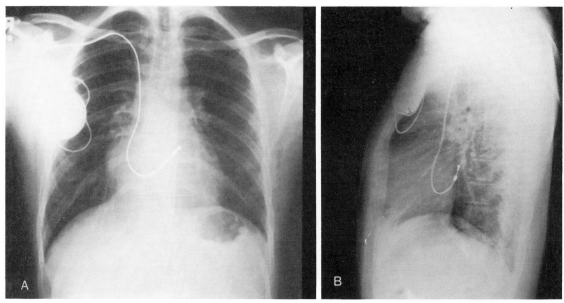

FIGURE 27–46. *A*, PA chest x-ray film of a patient with a coronary sinus permanent pacemaker electrode. The lead tip is superior and to the left side across the midline. *B*, Lateral film shows that the coronary sinus and the lead curve posteriorly and superiorly, precluding right ventricular placement. (Used by permission of Hayes.)

the lead actually advances into the coronary sinus and out its ostium into the right atrium. The lead must then negotiate an acute angle to cross the tricuspid valve and advance to the right ventricular apex. This is best accomplished by having the lead form a large loop on itself, using the lateral right atrial wall for support. Occasionally, such efforts to use a persistent left vena cava prove unsuccessful, and changing the side of venous approach is necessary. At this point, it is prudent to assess the patency of the right vena cava with radiographic contrast material. A standard end-hole catheter (on the introducer sheath) can be passed via the left superior vena cava to the vicinity of the right superior vena cava and contrast material injected. If there is no right superior vena cava, the iliac vein approach described by Ellestad or one of the epicardial approaches may be used.

With the left vena cava approach, an atrial electrode is required—a positive fixation screw-in type is recommended.[96] Passage of a preformed atrial J will prove difficult if not impossible. Dislodgment of the preformed J is also a concern. When using the positive fixation electrode, care should be taken to avoid pacing the right phrenic nerve.

When an absent right superior vena cava is discovered from a right-sided approach, the side of approach must be changed. In this case, the expected venous tortuosity of the persistent left superior vena cava should alert one to request longer leads. At times, an 85-cm lead is required. Again it is advisable to use positive fixation leads in anticipation of dislodgment problems.

The coronary sinus has been used for pacing both by design and by accident (Fig. 27–46). It is unreliable for ventricular pacing and should generally be avoided. It can be an acceptable location for atrial pacing.[97, 98] The problem with coronary sinus atrial pacing has been access and lead stability. Prior to the development of reliable atrial electrodes, the coronary sinus was a popular site of lead placement for atrial pacing. The best place for atrial pacing is the proximal coronary sinus. It is also the least stable location. Special coronary sinus leads have been developed to enhance position stability. These leads have a flexible, elongated tip that reaches deep into the coronary sinus wedging in the great cardiac vein for stability. Gaining access to the coronary sinus requires experience (unless one is trying to avoid it, in which case it seems to be routinely entered). With the growing number of implanting electrophysiologists who use the coronary sinus routinely for diagnostic studies, this experience becomes a moot point. In addition, as more implants are performed in the catheterization laboratory, which is equipped with sophisticated x-ray equipment, including biplane fluoroscopy, the required beneficial fluoroscopic projections for placement are easily achieved.[99]

Placement of a coronary sinus lead is easier from the left side. A generous curve is required on the lead stylet. Coronary sinus placement is confirmed by a posterior lead position on lateral fluoroscopy. In addition, lead placement will not be associated with ventricular ectopy.

Although it was once a popular approach to atrial pacing, the coronary sinus is used infrequently today. This is largely due to extremely reliable atrial leads equipped with fixation devices and tips that preclude dislodgment and ensure effective capture.

REFERENCES

1. Schecter DC: Modern era of artificial cardiac pacemakers. *In* Schecter DC: Electrical Cardiac Stimulation. Minneapolis, Medtronic, 1983, pp 110–134.
2. Senning A: Discussion of a paper by Stephenson SE Jr, Edwards WH, Jolly PC, Scott HW: Physiologic P-wave stimulator. J Thorac Cardiovasc Surg 38:639, 1959.
3. Furman S, Schwedel JB: An intracardiac pacemaker for Stokes-Adams seizures. N Engl J Med 261:948, 1959.
4. Littleford PO, Spector SD: Device for the rapid insertion of permanent endocardial pacing electrode through the subclavian vein: Preliminary report. Ann Thorac Surg 27:265, 1979.

5. Parsonnet V, Furman S, Smyth NP, Bilitch M: Optimal resources for implantable cardiac pacemakers. Pacemaker Study Group. Circulation 68(1):226A, 1983.
6. Parsonnet V, Bernstein AD, Lindsay B: Pacemaker implantation complication rates: An analysis of some contributing factors. J Am Coll Cardiol 13:917, 1989.
7. Harthorne JW, Parsonett V: Seventeenth Bethesda Conference: Adult cardiac training. Task Force VI: Training in cardiac pacing. J Am Coll Cardiol 7:1213, 1986.
8. Parsonnet V, Bernstein AD: Pacing in perspective: Concepts and controversies. Circulation 73:1087, 1986.
9. Parsonnet V, Bernstein AD, Galasso D: Cardiac pacing practices in the United States in 1985. Am J Cardiol 62:71, 1988.
10. Hayes DL, Naccarelli GV, Furman S, et al: Training requirements for permanent pacemaker selection, implantation, and follow-up. PACE 17:6, 1994.
11. Bernstein AD, Parsonnet V: Survey of cardiac pacing in the United States in 1989. Am J Cardiol 69:331, 1992.
12. Stamato NJ, O'Toole MF, Enger EL: Permanent pacemaker implantation in the cardiac catheterization laboratory versus the operating room: An analysis of hospital charges and complications. PACE 15:2236, 1992.
13. Hess DS, Gertz EW, Morady F, et al: Permanent pacemaker implantation in the cardiac catheterization laboratory: The subclavian approach. Cathet Cardiovasc Diagn 8:453, 1982.
14. Anderson FH, Crossland, Alexander MB: Use of a three-channel electrocardiographic recorder for limited intracardiac electrocardiography during single- and double-chamber pacemaker implantation. Ann Thorac Surg 39:485, 1985.
15. Sutton R, Bourgeois I: Techniques of implantation. *In* Sutton R, Bourgeois I (eds): The Foundations of Cardiac Pacing: An Illustrated Practical Guide to Basic Pacing, vol I, pt 1. Mt Kisco, NY, Futura Publishing, 1991.
16. Levine PA, Balady GJ, Lazar HL, et al: Electrocautery and pacemakers: Management of the paced patient subject to electrocautery. Ann Thorac Surg 41:313, 1986.
17. Belott PH, Sands S, Warren J: Resetting of DDD pacemakers due to EMI. PACE 7:169, 1984.
18. Chauvin M, Crenner F, Brechenmacher C:: Interaction between permanent cardiac pacing and electrocautery: The significance of electrode position. PACE 15:2028, 1992.
19. Hauser RG, Edwards LM, Guiffe VW: Limitation of pacemaker system analyzers for evaluation of implantable pulse generators. PACE 4:650, 1981.
20. Dreifus LS, Fisch C, Griffin JC, et al (eds): Guidelines for implantation of cardiac pacemakers and antiarrhythmic devices: A report of the ACC/AHA task force on assessment of diagnostic and therapeutic cardiovascular procedures. Circulation 84:455, 1991.
21. Zegelman M, Kreyzer J, Wagner R: Ambulatory pacemaker surgery—medical and economical advantages. PACE 9:1299, 1986.
22. Belott PH: Outpatient pacemaker procedures. Int J Cardiol 17:169, 1987.
23. Dalvi B: Insertion of permanent pacemakers as a day case procedure. Br Med J 300(6717):119, 1990.
24. Hayes DL, Vliestra RE, Trusty JM, et al: Can pacemaker implantation be done as an outpatient? J Am Coll Cardiol 7:199, 1986.
25. Hayes DL, Vliestra RE, Trusty JM, et al: A shorter hospital stay after cardiac pacemaker implantation. Mayo Clin Proc 63:236, 1988.
26. Haywood GA, Jones SM, Camm AJ, et al: Day case permanent pacing. PACE 14:773, 1991.
27. Belott PH: Ambulatory pacemaker procedures [editorial]. Mayo Clin Proc 63:301, 1988.
28. Philip BK, Corvino BG: Local and regional anesthesia. *In* Wetchler BV (ed): Anesthesia for Ambulatory Surgery, 2nd ed. Philadelphia, JB Lippincott, 1991, pp 309–334.
29. Page CP, Bohnen JMA, Fletcher R, et al: Antimicrobial prophylaxis for surgical wounds: Guidelines for clinical care. Arch Surg 128:79, 1993.
30. Muers MF, Arnold AG, Sleight P: Prophylactic antibiotics for cardiac pacemaker implantation: A prospective trial. Br Heart J 46:539, 1981.
31. Ramsdale DR, Charles RG, Rowlands DB: Antibiotic prophylaxis for pacemaker implantation: A prospective randomized trial. PACE 7:844, 1984.
32. Bluhm G, Jacobson B, Ransjo U: Antibiotic prophylaxis in pacemaker surgery: A prospective trial with local and systemic administration of antibiotics at pulse generator replacement. PACE 8:661, 1985.
33. Antimicrobial Prophylaxis in Surgery. Med Let 34(862):5–8, 1992.
34. Golightly LK, Branigan T: Surgical antibiotic irrigations. Hosp Pharm 24:116, 1989.
35. Smyth NPD: Techniques of implantation: Atrial and ventricular, thoracotomy and transvenous. Prog Cardiovasc Dis 23:435, 1981.
36. Smyth NPD: Pacemaker implantation: Surgical techniques. Cardiovasc Clin 14:31, 1983.
37. Netter FH: Atlas of Human Anatomy, fifth printing. West Caldwell, Ciba Geigy Medical Education, 1992, pp 174–176, 186, 200, and 201.
38. Byrd C: Current clinical applications of dual-chamber pacing. *In* Zipes DP (ed): Proceedings of a Symposium. Minneapolis, Medtronics, 1981, p 71.
39. Netter FH: The Ciba Collection of Medical Illustrations, vol 5. Heart. Summit, NJ, Ciba Medical Education Division 1981, pp 22–26.
40. Furman S: Venous cutdown for pacemaker implantation. Ann Thorac Surg 41:438, 1986.
41. Feiesen A, Kelin GJ, Kostuck WJ, et al: Percutaneous insertion of a permanent transvenous pacemaker electrode through the subclavian vein. Can J Surg 10:131, 1977.
42. Littleford PO, Spector SD: Device for the rapid insertion of permanent endocardial pacing electrodes through the subclavian vein: Preliminary report. Ann Thorac Surg 27:265, 1979.
43. Littleford PO, Parsonnet V, Spector SD: Method for rapid and atraumatic insertion of permanent endocardial electrodes through the subclavian vein. Am J Cardiol 43:980, 1979.
44. Miller FA Jr, Homes DR Jr, Gersh BJ, Maloney JD: Permanent transvenous pacemaker implantation via the subclavian vein. Mayo Clinic Proc 55:309, 1980.
45. Belott PH, Byrd CL: Recent developments in pacemaker implantation and lead retrieval. *In* Barold SS, Mugica J (eds): New Perspectives in Cardiac Pacing. 2. Mt Kisco, NY, Futura Publishing, 1991, pp 105–131.
46. Stokes K, Staffeson D, Lessar J, et al: A possible new complication of the subclavian stick: Conductor fracture. PACE 10:748, 1987.
47. Fyke FE III: Simultaneous insulation deterioration associated with side by side subclavian placement of two polyurethane leads. PACE 11:1571, 1988.
48. Fyke FE III: Infraclavicular lead failure: Tarnish on a golden route [editorial comment]. PACE 16:445, 1993.
49. Jacobs DM, Fink AS, Miller RP, et al: Anatomical and morphological evaluation of pacemaker lead compression. PACE 16:373, 1993.
50. Magey JE, Flynn DM, Parsons JA, et al: Anatomical mechanisms explaining damage to pacemaker leads, defibrillator leads, and failure of central venous catheters adjacent to the sternoclavicular joint. PACE 16:445, 1993.
51. Subclavian venipuncture reconsidered as a means of implanting endocardial pacing leads. Angleton, TX, Issues Intermedics, December, 1987, pp 1–2.
52. Subclavian puncture may result in lead conductor fracture. Minneapolis, MN, Medtronic News 16:27, 1986–1987.
53. Byrd CL: Safe introducer technique for pacemaker lead implantation. PACE 15:262, 1992.
54. Nichalls RWD: A new percutaneous infraclavicular approach to the axillary vein. Anesthesia 42:151, 1987.
55. Taylor BL, Yellowlees I: Central venous cannulation using the infraclavicular axillary vein. Anesthesiology 72:55, 1990.
56. Lamas GA, Fish DR, Braunwald NS: Fluoroscopic technique of subclavian venous puncture for permanent pacing: A safer and easier approach. PACE 11:1398, 1987.
57. Higano ST, Hayes DL, Spittell PC: Facilitation of the subclavian-introducer technique with contrast venography. PACE 15:731, 1992.
58. Belott PH: Implantation techniques—new developments. *In* Barold SS, Mugica J (eds): New Perspectives in Cardiac Pacing. Mt Kisco, NY, Futura Publishing, 1988, pp 258–259.
59. Bognolo DA: Recent advances in permanent pacemaker implantation techniques. *In* Barold SS (ed): Modern Cardiac Pacing. Mt Kisco, NY, Futura Publishing, 1985, pp 206–207.
60. Parsonnet V, Werres R, Atherly T, et al: Transvenous insertion of double sets of permanent electrodes. JAMA 243:62, 1980.
61. Bognolo PA, Vijayanagar RR, Eckstein PR, et al: Two leads in one introducer technique for A-V sequential implantation. PACE 5:217, 1982.
62. VanderSalm TJ, Haffajee CI, Okike ON: Transvenous insertion of double sets of permanent electrodes through a single introducer: Clinical application. Ann Thorac Surg 32:307, 1981.

63. Belott PH: A variation on the introducer technique for unlimited access to the subclavian vein. PACE 4:43, 1981.

64. Gessman LJ, Gallagher JD, MacMillan RM, et al: Emergency guide wire pacing: New methods for rapid conversion of a cardiac catheter into a pacemaker. PACE 7:917, 1984.

65. Ong LS, Barold S, Lederman M, et al: Cephalic vein guide wire technique for implantation of permanent pacemakers. Am Heart J 114:753, 1987.

66. August DA, Elefteriades JA: Technique to facilitate open placement of permanent pacing leads through the cephalic vein. Ann Thorac Surg 42:112, 1986.

67. Hayes DL, Holmes R Jr, Furman S: A Practice of Cardiac Pacing, 3rd ed. Mt Kisco, NY, Futura Publishing, 1993, pp 271–274.

68. Belott PH: Retained guide wire introducer technique, for unlimited access to the central circulation: A review. Clin Prog Electrophysiol Pacing 1:59, 1981.

69. Bognolo DA, Vijayanagar R, Ekstein PF, et al: Anatomical suitability of the right atrial appendage for atrial J lead electrodes. *In* Proceedings of the Second European Pacing Symposium, Florence, Italy. Cardiac Pacing. Padova, Italy, Piccin Medical Book, 1982 p 639.

70. Bognolo DA, Vigayanagar R, Ekstein PF, et al: Implantation of permanent atrial J lead using lateral fluoroscopy. Ann Thorac Surg 316:574, 1981.

71. Thurer RJ: Technique of insertion of transvenous atrial pacing leads— the value of lateral fluoroscopy. PACE 4:525, 1981.

72. Jamidar H, Goli V, Reynolds DW: The right atrial free wall: An alternative pacing site. PACE 16:959, 1993.

73. Bognolo DA, Vijaranagar RR, Eckstein PF, Janss B: Method for reintroduction of permanent endocardial pacing electrodes. PACE 5:546, 1982.

74. Bognolo DA, Vijay R, Eckstein P, Jeffrey D: Technical aspects of pacemaker system upgrading procedures. Clin Prog Pacing Electrophysiol 1:269, 1983.

75. Belott PH: Use of the contralateral subclavian vein for placement of atrial electrodes in chronically VVI paced patients. PACE 6:781, 1983.

76. Parsonnet V: A stretch fabric pouch for implanted pacemakers. Arch Surg 105:654, 1972.

77. Said SA, Bucx JJ, Stassen CM: Failure of subclavian venipuncture: The internal jugular vein as a useful alternative. Int J Cardiol 35:275, 1992.

78. Ellestad MH, French J: Iliac vein approach to permanent pacemaker implantation. PACE 12:1030, 1989.

79. Antonelli D, Freedberg NA, Rosenfeld T: Transiliac vein approach to a rate-responsive permanent pacemaker implantation. PACE 16:1637, 1993.

80. Belott PH, Bucko D: Inframammary pulse generator placement for maximizing optimal cosmetic effect. PACE 6:1241, 1983.

81. Young D: Permanent pacemaker implantation in children: Current status and future considerations. PACE 4:61, 1981.

82. Smith RT Jr: Pacemakers for children. *In* Gillette PC, Garson A Jr (eds): Pediatric Arrhythmias: Electrophysiology and Pacing. New York, Grune & Stratton, 1990, pp 532–558.

83. Smith RT Jr, Armstrong K, Moak JP, et al: Actuarial analysis of pacing system survival in young patients [abstract]. Circulation 74(Suppl II):120, 1986.

84. Gillette PC, Zeigler VL, Winslow AT, Kratz JM: Cardiac pacing in neonates, infants, and preschool children. PACE 15(11 pt 2):2046, 1992.

85. Guldal M, Kervancioglu C, Oral D, et al: Permanent pacemaker implantation in a pregnant woman with guidance of ECG and two-dimensional echocardiography. PACE 10:543, 1987.

86. Lau CP, Wong CK, Leung WH, et al: Ultrasonic assisted permanent pacing in a patient with severe pulmonary tuberculosis. PACE 12:1131, 1989.

87. Morris DC, Scott IR, Jamesson WR: Pacemaker electrode repositioning using the loop snare technique. PACE 12:996, 1989.

88. Westerman GR, Van Devanter SH: Transthoracic transatrial endocardial lead placement for permanent pacing. Ann Thorac Surg 43:445, 1987.

89. Hayes DL, Vliestra RE, Puga FJ, et al: A novel approach to atrial endocardial pacing. PACE 12:125, 1989.

90. Byrd CL, Schwartz SJ: Transatrial implantation of transvenous pacing leads as an alternative to implantation of epicardial leads. PACE 13:1856, 1990.

91. Dosios T, Gorgogiannis D, Sakorafas G, et al: Persistent left superior vena cava: A problem in transvenous pacing of the heart. PACE 14:389, 1991.

92. Hussaine SA, Chalcravarty S, Chaikhouni A: Congenital absence of superior vena cava: Unusual anomaly of superior systemic veins complicating pacemaker placement. PACE 4:328, 1981.

93. Ronnevik PK, Abrahamsen AM, Tollefsen J: Transvenous pacemaker implantation via a unilateral left superior vena cava. PACE 5:808, 1982.

94. Cha EM, Khoury GH: Persistent left superior vena cava. Radiology 103:375, 1972.

95. Colman AL: Diagnosis of left superior vena cava by clinical inspection: A new physical sign. Am Heart J 73:115, 1967.

96. Hellestrand KJ, Ward DE, Bexton RS, Camm AJ: The use of active fixation electrodes for permanent endocardial pacing via a persistent left superior vena cava. PACE 5:180, 1982.

97. Moss AJ, Rivers RJ Jr: Atrial pacing from the coronary vein: Ten-year experience in 50 patients with implanted pervenous pacemakers. Circulation 57:103, 1978.

98. Greenberg P, Castellanet M, Messenger J, Ellestad MH: Coronary sinus pacing. Circulation 57:98, 1978.

99. Hewitt MJ, Chen JTT, Ravin CE, Gallagher JJ: Coronary sinus atrial pacing: Radiographic considerations. Am J Radiol 136:323, 1981.

CHAPTER 28

Management of Implant Complications

Charles L. Byrd

Implantable electrophysiologic devices for controlling bradyarrhythmias, tachyarrhythmias, or a combination of both have components that are implanted in the chest and abdominal wall, transvenously in the right side of the heart, or in the pericardial tissues. Management of complications from an implanted device has become a subspecialty of cardiology and cardiovascular surgery. Special training is required to acquire the skills in cardiovascular surgery and invasive cardiology that are needed to achieve a successful result. Most complications result from tissue injury inflicted by the implanter and by the interaction of the device with the tissue. Understanding the causes of tissue injury and the associated inflammatory reaction is important in preventing and managing these complications.

Treatment includes managing both the soft tissue and intravascular portions of the device, including removal of all foreign material. In the early 1980s, prior to the development of successful low-morbidity techniques for extracting leads, every attempt was made to salvage the chronic pacemaker site. The alternative was to abandon the site, removing all foreign material including chronically implanted leads. Abandonment of the site was considered only when the risk of a recurrent complication (e.g., septicemia) exceeded the risk of lead extraction.

During the past decade, effective low-morbidity techniques for extracting leads transvenously have been developed. Consequently, the drive to salvage an implant site has dwindled, and abandonment of the site has become the procedure of choice. As successful experiences with lead extraction increase, the indications for extraction have expanded to include the prophylactic removal of some leads.

Tissue Injury and Inflammatory Reaction

TISSUE INJURY

A pacemaker or an implantable defibrillator and its leads are routinely placed in a subcutaneous or submuscular tissue pocket. Tissue injury caused by the incision and dissection of the pocket (tissue disruption) initiates an inflammatory reaction. Tissue injury caused by device-related mechanical stresses, such as pressure exacerbated by motion, continues the inflammatory reaction. Normally, the incision heals by the normal wound healing process, and tissue around the device heals by encapsulation. Ideally, this fibrous tissue sheath protects the surrounding tissue from further injury. The goal is to maintain this accord between the encapsulated device and the surrounding tissue indefinitely.

Poor tissue nutrition, tissue reaction to the implanted materials, excessive pressure, infection, and recursive reactions may cause further tissue injury and a device-related complication (Fig. 28–1). Tissue nutrition associated with device implants is directly related to the adequacy of the blood supply. Poor nutrition is caused by tissue ischemia; the resultant injury ranges from dissolution of fatty tissue to cellular necrosis (gangrene). Except for extremely rare immunologic reactions, a reaction to implanted materials is associated only with conditions such as the thrombogenic properties of lead insulation (e.g., surface texture, silicone rubber vs. polyurethane).[1] Excessive pressures are associated with implantation of large pulse generators and large stiff leads. Both the reaction to materials and excessive pressures are device perform-

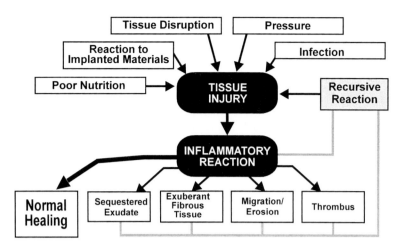

FIGURE 28–1. Tissue is injured by a variety of causes. Once tissue is injured an inflammatory reaction ensues. Depending on the magnitude of the injury and its duration, tissue heals "naturally" or "unnaturally," developing one of the recursive reactions. A recursive reaction is defined as part of the inflammatory reaction that further injures the tissue and perpetuates the inflammatory reaction.

ance issues. Infection is not related to a specific device but to tissue contamination by bacteria. However, the tissue's susceptibility to infection is probably related to the device-tissue reaction. The term recursive was originally a mathematical term referring to an equation in which the solution is part of the equation (e.g., $yn = yn - 1 + 1$). Some of the products of an inflammatory reaction may cause more tissue injury; this process may be called a recursive reaction. For example, sequestered exudate, exuberant fibrous tissue, migration or erosion, and thrombus formation, all of which are products of an inflammatory reaction, may cause further injury to the surrounding tissue and perpetuate the inflammatory reaction. These factors, acting individually or together, may alter the accord between the encapsulated device and the surrounding tissue, resulting in a complication.

PROPERTIES OF AN INFLAMMATORY REACTION

An inflammatory reaction is a localized protective response elicited by injury or destruction of tissues. It is an

integral part of the body's biologic defense system and serves to destroy (e.g., bacteria), dilute (e.g., toxins), or wall off (e.g., foreign bodies) the injurious agent. Inflammatory reactions cover a broad spectrum but are usually separated into acute and chronic reactions. In acute reactions, vascular and exudative processes predominate. Acute reactions often mature into chronic reactions, in which the formation of stable fibrous tissue predominates. Figure 28–2 summarizes the inflammatory reaction processes.

EXUDATIVE RESPONSE (NATURAL OR UNNATURAL)

The exudative process is secondary to the vascular effects of the injury and results in a collection of blood plasma, cells, and cellular debris. Depending on the magnitude of the injury and the cellular response, the exudate ranges from an inflammatory edema to pus. Based on the exudative response, I further subdivide inflammatory reactions into natural and unnatural reactions. A natural reaction matures with-

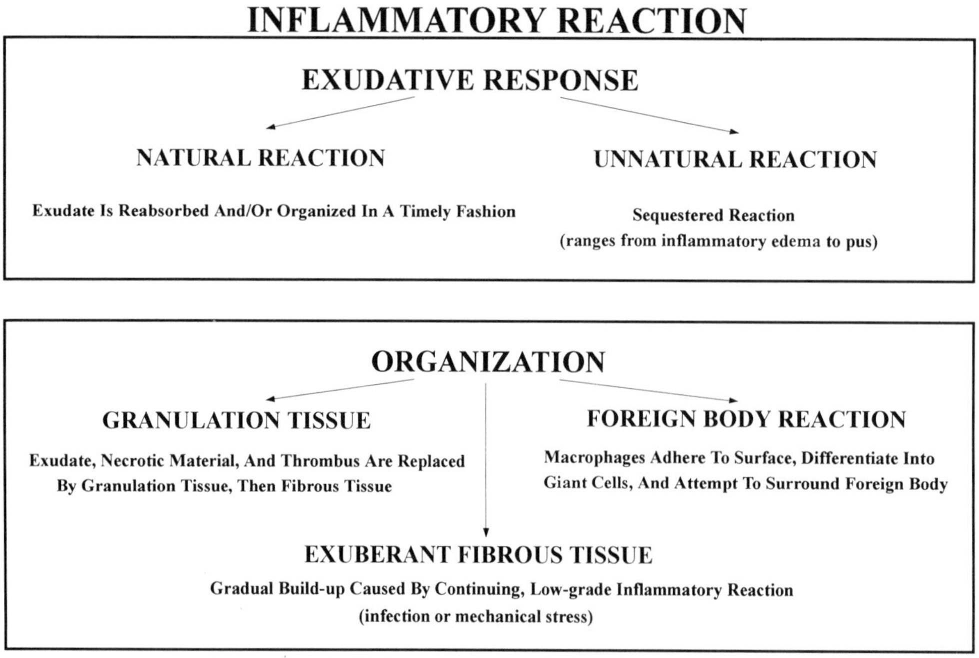

INFLAMMATORY REACTION

EXUDATIVE RESPONSE

NATURAL REACTION

Exudate Is Reabsorbed And/Or Organized In A Timely Fashion

UNNATURAL REACTION

Sequestered Reaction
(ranges from inflammatory edema to pus)

ORGANIZATION

GRANULATION TISSUE

Exudate, Necrotic Material, And Thrombus Are Replaced By Granulation Tissue, Then Fibrous Tissue

FOREIGN BODY REACTION

Macrophages Adhere To Surface, Differentiate Into Giant Cells, And Attempt To Surround Foreign Body

EXUBERANT FIBROUS TISSUE

Gradual Build-up Caused By Continuing, Low-grade Inflammatory Reaction
(infection or mechanical stress)

FIGURE 28–2. The initial response to tissue injury is the exudative response. If the exudate is absorbed or organized in a timely fashion, it is classified as natural. If the exudate is sequestered, it is classified as unnatural. All unnatural reactions represent a complication of wound healing.

Organization of the exudate and inflammatory debris begins with the formation of granulation tissue. In natural reactions the granulation tissue matures into fibrous tissue. In most unnatural reactions, some granulation tissue persists. The foreign body reaction begins in the initial stages of the inflammatory reaction with macrophages adhering to the surface of the foreign body. During maturation of the organization process, giant cells are formed that attempt to surround the foreign body. If the inflammatory reaction is chronic (with infection, mechanical injury, etc.), exuberant fibrous tissue is formed.

out the formation of a sequestered exudative effusion. The exudate is reabsorbed or organized in a timely fashion. In an unnatural reaction the exudative process predominates, causing sequestration of the exudative effusion. Unnatural reactions are caused by excessive production, poor reabsorption, or retarded organization of the exudate. For example, the exudative effusion formed by tissue injured by virulent bacteria or collections of necrotic tissue may progress to an abscess or discharge spontaneously. The accumulation of exuberant inflammatory tissues (fibrous and granulation tissue) caused by smoldering infections or mechanical stresses occurring over an extended period of time may form a sequestered exudative effusion. These chronic effusions usually contain less cellular debris. Retarded organization also includes cases in which a space large enough to prevent organization of the exudate is created by the device. For example, leads coiled in some configurations may create a space. The unnatural reaction encapsulates this space, causing a cyst usually filled with edematous fluid. For a given tissue type, the difference between a natural and an unnatural reaction is a matter of the magnitude and duration of the inflammatory reaction and the presence of ''dead space'' around the device.

ORGANIZATION

Organization refers to the replacement of the exudate, necrotic material, and thrombus first with granulation tissue and then with fibrous tissue. Granulation is the beginning of the healing phase of an inflammatory reaction. It is the reddish, granular, collagenous tissue formed by elongated fibroblasts and buds of endothelial cells forming fibrous tissue and capillaries. The amount of granulation tissue present depends on the magnitude and duration of the tissue injury. In a natural inflammatory reaction associated with an uncomplicated device implant, the granulation tissue is rapidly replaced by fibrous tissue. The incision and pacemaker pocket may appear pink for a few weeks following the implant, but exuberant granulation tissue is not present.

A foreign body reaction occurs when any durable foreign body (too large for phagocytosis) injures the tissue. A foreign body reaction is characterized by macrophages that adhere to the surface, differentiating into foreign body giant cells and attempting to surround the foreign body. For example, a foreign body reaction occurs when the pacemaker pulse generator and lead (or leads) are placed within the disrupted tissue (pacemaker pocket) and when an electrode is implanted in the heart. The chronic pacemaker pocket is the encapsulation of the pacemaker and leads by fibrous tissue and foreign body giant cells, which result from the organization process and foreign body reaction.

EXUBERANT FIBROUS TISSUE

A gradual build-up of exuberant fibrous tissue is caused by a continuing low-grade chronic inflammatory reaction. This is caused by a smoldering or occult infection or by mechanical stress. Over time, the scar tissue increases both in mass and in tensile strength; it may even calcify after 8 to 10 years in an adult or after 3 to 4 years in a child.[4, 5] Although the role of fibrous tissue is to form a protective barrier or increase the tissue's tensile strength, aging exuberant fibrous tissue may cause further injury to the normal tissue and may predispose the tissue to another complication such as infection or erosion (recursive reaction).

Anti-inflammatory agents such as glucocorticosteroids suppress the inflammatory reaction. In general, inflammatory reactions are protective and should not be suppressed. However, in some situations, local application of a glucocorticoid to suppress a low-grade natural reaction is beneficial. For example, steroid-eluting electrodes in most cases eliminate the clinically apparent reaction at the electrode-myocardial interface without causing any adverse consequences.

Pocket Complications

Implant pockets usually heal in an uneventful fashion and mature, reaching an accord with the surrounding tissue. Healing starts with wound healing and encapsulation of the implant device. The tissue is subjected to mechanical stress during both healing and maturation of the pocket. The maturation process continues throughout the duration of the implant. It is a dynamic process with the device-tissue interaction determining the lysis, deposition, and composition of the encapsulating tissue. Normal capsules are made up primarily of fibrous tissue, but with aging some become lined with calcified plaques.

Pocket complications are summarized in Table 28–1 and include pocket hematoma, wound dehiscence, migration, erosion, pain, and infection. Hematoma formation and wound dehiscence are acute events and are usually related to implant technique. A pocket hematoma may form late in anticoagulated patients if the pocket is subjected to trauma. Migration, erosion, and pain are related to device-tissue interaction. Infection is caused by contamination of the pocket and is associated with implant technique and tissue made susceptible by an abnormal device-tissue interaction.

PROPERTIES OF WOUND HEALING AND MATURATION OF THE POCKET

WOUND HEALING

Healing of reapproximated disrupted tissue occurs through an inflammatory reaction called wound healing. The magnitude of this reaction is related to the severity of the injury to the tissue. Sharp dissection using a scalpel, electrosurgical device, or laser causes minimal damage; the tissue heals by a predictable natural reaction called primary union. Tissue disruption resulting from blunt trauma that causes significant tissue injury including tissue necrosis may heal poorly. A large sequestered exudate (unnatural reaction) frequently develops in injuries of this magnitude. Spontaneous drainage of these collections effectively exteriorizes the wound, resulting in an open granulating wound that heals by secondary union. Healing by secondary union is not compatible with a device implant, and the device must be removed. Large wounds with skin loss that are healing by secondary union may not heal and may leave only granulation tissue as the protective barrier. This by definition is a perpetual inflammatory reaction. These wounds must be covered by a skin graft.

MECHANICAL STRESS

Compliant tissues may be compressed and stretched by mechanical stress (exerting positive or negative pressures),

TABLE 28–1. **POCKET COMPLICATIONS**

COMPLICATION	PREDISPOSING FACTORS OR CAUSES	TREATMENT

Pocket hematoma	Tear outside fascial plane
	Arterial bleeding
	Extrusion of venous blood along leads
		If it is large enough to be palpated:
		   Remove clot and debris
		   Obtain hemostasis
		   Reduce pocket size if necessary
		   Use closed drainage system if hemostasis is difficult to
		     achieve
		Avoid repeated needle aspirations

Wound dehiscence	Excessive stress on suture line by hematoma,
	   hemorrhagic effusion, or trauma
	Error in surgical technique
		Immediate:
		   Attempt to salvage site
		Delayed:
		   Treat as infected pocket

Migration	Unknown	No treatment unless another complication exists

Erosion	Device implanted outside correct plane
	Sustained an insult forcing device out of correct plane
	   (compromised blood supply, trauma, sequestered
	   effusion)
		Before pocket sticks to skin:
		   Débride and relocate pocket
		After pocket sticks to skin or skin is broken:
		   Treat as infected (abandon site)

Pain	??	Relocate pocket if necessary

Infection	Perioperative contamination
	Chronic site may have poorer defenses against infection
	Metastatic (seeding from remote infection or procedure
	   such as teeth cleaning)
	Chronic occult infection becomes acute
	Note: pocket infection may present as respiratory distress
	   if infection decompresses into venous system
		Most infections:
		   Antibiotic treatment and abandon site (removing
		     device and leads)
		If no septicemia, no inflammatory build-up around leads
		   near insertion site, and >2.5 cm from pocket to suture
		   sleeve:
		   Antibiotic treatment and abandonment of pocket may
		     be sufficient

directly injuring the tissue. Compliant tissues are compressed at the positive pressure point and stretched some distance away. Negative pressures resulting from pulling on a device stretch and then compress the tissue. The stretching and compression continue until the forces balance. Excessive pressures may compromise the tissue's blood supply, thereby causing additional tissue injury.

The physical properties of the implanted device (size, weight, configuration, and surface texture) determine the amount of pressure applied to the tissue. Weight is a force, and combined with size and configuration, it determines the resultant applied pressure (force/area). Large, heavy, blunt objects and small, light, sharp objects can both cause the same pressures. Motion and other external forces accentuate the force applied to the tissue. Surface texture can also influence pressure. Current devices are smooth, but, if placed within a Dacron mesh pouch (Parsonnet), tissue growth within the interstices of the mesh distribute the forces more uniformly and help negate problems of size, weight, and configuration.

Creation of a pocket of sufficient size will minimize the pressure applied to the surrounding tissues by an implanted device. Forcing a device into too small a pocket stretches the tissue, and the resultant tension (force/length) may injure the tissue. In contrast, too large a pocket will leave disrupted tissue that is not occupied by the device, which will be filled with an exudate and will increase the amount of granulation tissue.

POCKET HEMATOMA

A hematoma developing immediately after implantation of a device is one of the most common complications associated with pacemaker implantation. Although this is a technique-related complication, experienced implanters occasionally have difficulty in obtaining hemostasis. Three conditions pre-

dispose to hematoma formation: a tear outside the fascial plane, arterial bleeding, and extrusion of venous blood back along the leads into the pocket. Electrosurgery is useful for tissue dissection and for coagulation of small venous bleeders but is not recommended for larger venous or arterial structures of any size. Suture ligation is the only sure way of preventing bleeding.

FASCIAL PLANE

The fascial plane between the subcutaneous tissue and the muscle is relatively avascular, but occasional perforating vessels cross the fascial plane. A dissection or tear out of the fascial plane into either the subcutaneous or muscular tissue can, therefore, cause bleeding. In addition, the pectoralis muscle is easily separated in the direction of its muscle fibers, especially in older patients. This leaves the intramural portion of the muscle exposed and frequently bleeding. Hemostasis is best obtained by reapproximating the muscle and fascial tissue using an absorbable running suture.

ARTERIAL BLEEDING

Arterial bleeding within the subcutaneous tissue pocket causes the most dramatic type of hematoma. The hematoma develops rapidly; if not corrected immediately, the pressurized pocket enlarges by dissection into the tissue planes or decompresses by rupturing through the incision. In the pectoral region, a small artery running in the direction of the pectoralis muscle fibers, on or just beneath the surface, is usually involved.

EXTRUSION OF BLOOD

A pocket hematoma can develop from blood forced retrograde out of the implant vein along the leads into the pocket.

Although the pocket may be dry, an elevated venous pressure caused by heart failure, the Valsalva maneuver, or coughing can extrude blood along the leads, filling the pocket with venous blood. If an introducer approach is used, extrusion of blood is prevented by placing a suture around the leads at the muscle entry site. The suture also prevents debris collected within the pocket from being forced back into the venous circulation. If the cephalic vein is used, a suture around the vein and leads at the entry site will suffice.

ORGANIZATION OF CLOT

Once clot forms in the pocket, it is subjected to both lysis and organization. Lysis creates particulate debris, increases the osmotic pressure, and pulls fluid into the pocket, thereby creating a hemorrhagic effusion. As the hemorrhagic effusion increases, the resultant tension on the pocket wall may continue to enlarge the pocket by dissection into the tissue planes or may rupture the incision. Both these complications require surgical intervention for correction.

Organization of a large clot in a pocket may result in excessive granulation tissue and eventually in exuberant fibrous tissue. Granulation tissue may be present years after the organization of a large hematoma. These pockets are not healthy and behave like pockets with exuberant fibrous tissue.

TREATMENT

A pocket hematoma large enough to be palpated should be treated. The most successful treatment is immediate pocket exploration. All clot and tissue debris must be removed and hemostasis obtained. If the pocket has been enlarged, the dissected region should be excluded, leaving an appropriately sized pocket. If adequate hemostasis is difficult to achieve, a closed drainage system (e.g., Jackson-Pratt system) is placed in the excluded pocket to prevent recurrence of the hematoma. Immediate surgical correction of a hematoma and, if necessary, proper placement of a closed drainage system does not adversely affect the healing of the pocket.

Prolonged observation and procrastination must be avoided. This is especially true when the pocket wall is tense. Needle aspiration decompresses the pocket but does not remove the clot. Repeated needle aspirations increase the risk of infection. Other complications of an untreated hematoma include wound dehiscence, migration or erosion, and infection.

WOUND DEHISCENCE

Wound dehiscence is a rare event. It occurs within the first few days or weeks following the implant. During the acute wound healing phase, suture material is required to reapproximate and reinforce the tissue. Most wound dehiscence is caused by excessive stress placed on the suture line by a hematoma, hemorrhagic effusion, or trauma. Traumatic disruption is rare. Dehiscence without a predisposing cause is due to an error in surgical technique.

Treatment consists of attempting to salvage the site by intervening immediately following observation of dehiscence. Treatment is similar to treatment of a hematoma and is usually successful. Delayed intervention allows gross con-

Wound Dehiscence

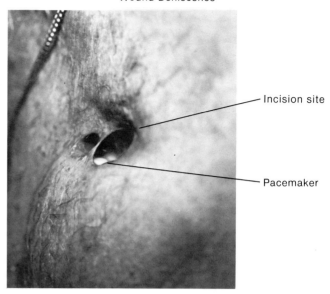

FIGURE 28–3. A wound dehiscence left unattended for more than a week. The pacemaker pocket developed a hematoma, which evacuated spontaneously, rupturing the incision. The incision was not débrided and was reclosed. It became secondarily infected.

tamination, and an infection is likely to develop. When intervention is delayed (Fig. 28–3), dehiscence is treated like an infected pocket with abandonment and reimplantation on the opposite side, if possible. This will be discussed in the section on treatment of infected pockets.

MIGRATION

Migration is the movement of a device through the surrounding tissue. In the past, migration was more common owing to the large size and pointed shape of some devices, even when they were contained in a Dacron (Parsonnet) pouch. Most migrations are slow, occurring over a period of years; they move in an inferior-lateral direction and do not cause complications.

The exact mechanism of migration is not known. One possibility is that the weight of the device interacts with the motion of the musculoskeletal system, creating directed forces that compress or stretch the fibrous capsule and surrounding tissues. A cycle of fibrous tissue lysis and formation associated with a low-grade inflammatory reaction might move the foreign body through the tissue. A migrated device is not treated unless a complication exists.

EROSION

Erosion is the exteriorization of the device following loss of integrity of the skin wall. The pacemaker pocket sticks to the skin prior to erosion (pre-erosion). Before the skin sticks, it can be moved freely over the pocket. At this point, if infection is not present, débridement and relocation of the pocket are usually successful. After the skin sticks, an inflammatory reaction ensues, and bacteria cross the skin, contaminating the pocket. Pockets treated after the skin sticks or following frank erosion are treated like infected pockets.

To erode, the device must migrate outside the normally

enclosing tissue plane. For this to occur, it would have to be implanted outside the correct plane or sustain an insult forcing it out of the plane, such as compromise of the blood supply, trauma, or a sequestered effusion.

IMPLANTS OUTSIDE OF TISSUE PLANES

Flat devices such as pulse generators do well when implanted in a natural tissue plane (fascial plane) between two tissue types (subcutaneous tissue and pectoralis muscle or pectoralis muscle and chest wall). Minimal pressures are exerted by the flat surfaces against the two tissue types. Larger pressures are applied by the device's curved surfaces within the tissue plane. In contrast, poorly positioned implants that have a portion of their curved surfaces extending out into the tissue tend to migrate, and many erode. Erosions occurring within the first few months following an initial implant are not uncommon in these situations.

A pacemaker pulse generator placed under the pectoralis major muscle sometimes protrudes into the axilla when the muscle is flexed. This can lead to migration with pain and possibly erosion. This complication can be avoided by placing the device more medially under both the pectoralis major and minor.

COMPROMISED BLOOD SUPPLY

Compromise of the blood supply causes tissue loss. Blood supply is known to be compromised by mechanical factors and by exuberant fibrous tissue. When the blood supply to a region of subcutaneous tissue and skin is compromised, the resulting dissolution of the subcutaneous tissue (pre-erosion) is caused by lack of nutrition. If this dissolution is severe enough, tissue necrosis occurs, leaving only ischemic or gangrenous skin (Fig. 28–4).

TRAUMA AND SEQUESTERED EFFUSIONS

Traumatic rupture of the fibrous capsule barrier around the device may result in subsequent migration through the rupture site. An effusion in an infected pocket or a hematoma can generate sufficient pressure to erode through the subcutaneous tissue and skin, draining to the outside. Although the mechanism may include ischemia, other contributing factors such as an intense inflammatory reaction or traumatic rupture of the fibrous tissue barrier are usually present.

PAIN

Occasionally patients complain of pain. Pain is usually caused not by the migration per se but by some traumatic event associated with the new anatomic position. For example, trauma to a rib or the costochondral junctions is the most common pain complaint. If pain is persistent, the pocket is relocated to another subcutaneous area or placed beneath the pectoralis major and minor muscles.

INFECTED POCKET

Infections involving implanted devices are challenging not only because of the severity and duration of the inflammatory reaction but also because of the sequelae. The incidence of reported infection of a cardiac pacing system ranges from 0 to 19%.[6-11] Patients with an infection are placed in one group encompassing a spectrum that ranges from contaminated tissue to cellulitis with marked tissue loss. In this classification, a dry pocket erosion with a positive culture is placed in the same group as an acute pocket infection with *Staphylococcus aureus,* cellulitis, marked purulent effusion, and septicemia. The management of these two types of ''infection'' is entirely different. The former is not a tissue infection. This pocket probably had an ischemic erosion with some bacterial contamination but no cellulitis, i.e., the tissue was not invaded by bacteria or their toxins. These examples demonstrate the two extremes encountered in managing ''infected pacing systems.''

Pathogenic organisms cause varying degrees of tissue injury. Mechanisms of injury include direct destructive interaction with the tissue such as intracellular replication, poisoning by toxins, damage by the immunologic defense response, or starvation by passive means such as competitive metabolism.

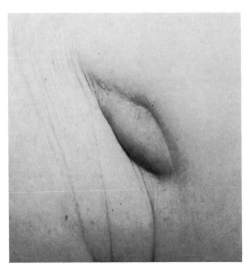

A   Pre-erosion

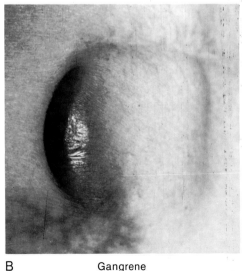

B   Gangrene

FIGURE 28–4. Compromise of the blood supply to the subcutaneous tissue and skin causes a decrease in the supply of nutrients to these cells. *A,* In the early stages (pre-erosion), the fatty tissue begins to lose mass. During the later pre-erosion stages, the tissue becomes ischemic with skin changes. The last stage prior to erosion is adhesion of the skin to the fibrous tissue pocket. Complete loss of blood supply to the skin results in gangrene of the skin prior to erosion *(B).*

Pocket Infections

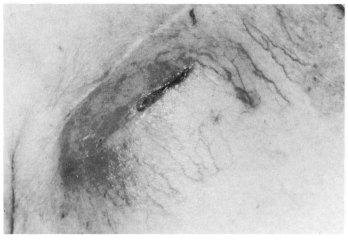

A   Acute infection

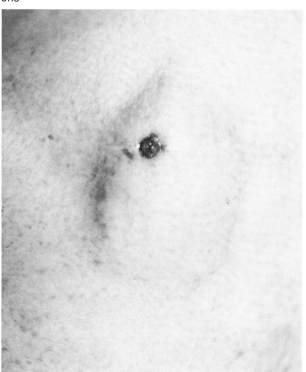

C   Chronic draining sinus

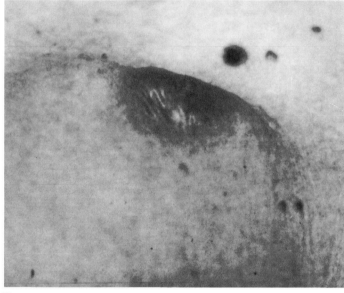

B   Stitch abscess

FIGURE 28–5. An acute pocket infection *(A)* caused by a virulent organism immediately following implantation or reimplantation of a device is rare and is the result of some form of pocket contamination (breach of sterile technique or metastases). These infections are equivalent to an abscess with cellulitis and a sequestered purulent exudate. Treatment consists of antibiotics and incision and drainage, if the exudate is large, or application of pressure to the surrounding tissue.

A chronic draining sinus is a continuously draining infection. In most cases, some part of the implanted device (pulse generator or leads) is infected. As long as drainage continues, the infection is controlled. If drainage stops, the infection is uncontrolled, and an abscess develops.

A local abscess around a suture *(B)* or other isolated implanted object decompresses and forms a chronic draining sinus *(C)*. In these cases, the implanted device may not be infected. However, it is impossible to be sure, and these local infections are treated as if the device was involved.

INFECTION OF AN INITIAL IMPLANT SITE

Acute infections following an initial implant in normal tissue are rare and usually result from some breach of technique, which contaminates the pocket with a virulent form of bacteria (Fig. 28–5). For example, inadvertent contamination of the pocket or device with *S. aureus* will probably cause an acute infection. Most surgical sites are contaminated by mainly nonvirulent bacteria such as *S. epidermidis* and do not become infected. The body's defenses can eradicate a small inoculum of these bacteria. However, a large inoculation or the presence of a culture medium such as devitalized

tissue or hematoma can negate the body's defenses, and an infection will ensue.

An acute infection involving an implanted pulse generator and leads in a subcutaneous tissue pocket causes the most severe tissue reaction. These reactions are characterized by cellulitis, a suppurative effusion within the pocket (abscess), and, in some cases, decompression into the blood causing septicemia or discharge through the skin causing a draining sinus. If septicemia is present, the infection is life threatening and demands immediate treatment. The magnitude of the cellulitis reflects the tissue reaction to the bacteria and their toxins.

INFECTION OF A CHRONIC IMPLANT SITE

An acute infection involving a chronic pocket is more common. Most of the infected pockets that I have seen became infected following an invasive reintervention procedure. They usually occur following replacement of an old device (pulse generator or lead) with a new one inserted into the old pocket. Again, during a surgical procedure, tissue is normally exposed to some degree of contamination such as skin bacteria. Some chronic pacemaker pockets cannot tolerate minimal levels of contamination without developing an infection. For example, pockets with exuberant fibrous tissue that are exposed to a bacteria such as *S. epidermidis* frequently become infected.

METASTATIC INFECTIONS

Another cause of pocket infection is seeding of the pocket by bacteria from a remote infection or from a procedure such as teeth cleaning.[12] The question of whether to give patients prophylactic antibiotics in these situations is still unanswered in the literature.[13–16] I believe that prophylactic antibiotics should be used. Phlebitis and lymphadenitis caused by an infected site of intravenous fluid administration have the potential to infect a new device implant pocket and probably a chronic pocket. Intravenous fluids probably should not be administered on the same side as a new implant.

CHRONIC OCCULT INFECTION

Smoldering or occult infections, causing no signs or symptoms, are defined as chronic infections within the pocket. These low-grade smoldering infections reach some sort of balance between the bacteria and the body's defenses. Such chronic infections are usually caused by *S. epidermidis*. On exploration of the pocket, exuberant fibrous tissue with or without an exudative effusion is found. Granulation tissue may also be present. Bacteria are difficult to culture from small exudates within these pockets. Once the infection has reached a stage at which it cannot be suppressed by the body's defenses, it becomes symptomatic. Chronic infections are reclassified as acute when signs and symptoms become present.

CHRONIC DRAINING SINUS

A chronic draining sinus stabilizes a chronic infection (see Fig. 28–5). An acute infection of a pacemaker pocket behaves like an abscess with a suppurative effusion and cellulitis. The walled-off cavity contains the pulse generator and leads. If the effusion drains through the skin, the abscess cavity is decompressed, the concentration of bacteria and their toxins is decreased, and the cellulitis resolves (usually with the help of antibiotics). With time, a draining sinus develops. The pacemaker pocket is lined with fibrous and granulation tissue. The tissue surrounding the pocket is protected as long as the exudative debris is drained. A balance is achieved, and the infection is tolerated. If the sinus stops draining, the abscess cycle is repeated. Patients with chronic draining sinuses must have lifelong medical management and, in many cases, chronic antibiotic treatment.

In some cases the entire pocket may not be infected. For example, an infected silk suture (stitch abscess) at the suture sleeve causes a localized abscess that drains. This results in a draining sinus from the suture. In these cases, although the lead and pocket may not be directly involved, there is no way to be absolutely sure, and the draining sinus should probably be treated the same way as an infected lead or pocket.

RESPIRATORY DISTRESS

Pocket infections that decompress episodically into the venous system cause fever and pulmonary symptoms. The pulmonary symptoms arise from an interstitial reaction caused by the filtering of bacteria and debris in the pulmonary capillary bed. An interstitial reaction is apparent on chest radiograph. Some patients develop significant respiratory distress, especially when the problem persists for an extensive period of time. Diagnosis is difficult. Patients presenting initially with fever and a persistent cough are sometimes treated for a flulike illness. With antibiotics and time, the symptoms improve but recur following the next episode of bacteremia.

TREATMENT OF AN INFECTED POCKET (AUTHOR'S EXPERIENCE)

Decision making for treatment of an infected intravenous pacing or defibrillator lead causing septicemia is straightforward. The device must be removed, and the pocket abandoned.[17] Decision making for an infection localized to a soft tissue pocket is difficult owing to the confusing plethora of anecdotal information found in the literature. Treatment with antibiotics, local surgery, and combinations of these all have been successful in selected patients. My experiences include antibiotic therapy combined with salvaging the site and abandoning the site (Table 28–2).

ANTIBIOTIC THERAPY

Antibiotic therapy was not tried alone as a curative approach. The negative experience of others, plus our own, was the rationale for combining antibiotics with invasive procedures. All infections were treated with intravenous antibiot-

TABLE 28–2. TREATMENT FOR POCKET INFECTIONS

ANTIBIOTICS AND COMPLETE ABANDONMENT
Abandonment procedure:
  Antibiotic coverage
  Débridement of all inflammatory tissue
  Removal of all foreign material (device and leads)
  Primary closure of site
Reimplantation:
  After patient has been afebrile for 36 hours implant at remote site (opposite side)

ANTIBIOTICS AND PARTIAL ABANDONMENT
Selection criteria:
  No septicemia
  >2.5 cm from pocket to suture sleeve
  No inflammatory build-up around leads
Partial abandonment procedure:
  At incision remote from pocket: cut, seal, and secure leads at pocket; perform abandonment procedure

ics. Vancomycin was used in all patients unless it was medically contraindicated. All staphylococci are sensitive to vancomycin. If gram-negative coverage was needed and sensitivity studies were not available, gentamicin was administered in addition to vancomycin.

The duration of antibiotic therapy prior to the procedure was determined by the magnitude of the infection. For example, patients with an acute *S. aureus* cellulitis and abscess of the pocket may require 2 weeks of antibiotic therapy and incision and drainage of the pocket to resolve the cellulitis. In contrast, a patient with a dry gangrenous erosion without cellulitis needs only the few hours required to reach an appropriate blood level of antibiotic. Regardless of the type of infection present, two clinical conditions must be met prior to performing a surgical procedure. First, the cellulitis must have resolved, and second, the patient must be afebrile.

SALVAGING THE IMPLANT SITE

Salvage procedures are designed to surgically correct a pocket complication, leaving the device at the site. A salvage procedure, at a minimum, includes débridement of all inflammatory tissue and debris, leaving only normal viable tissue (Fig. 28–6). It is followed by reimplantation of the device (decontaminated if necessary) and primary closure of the pocket with or without a closed drainage system.

DÉBRIDEMENT OF INFLAMMATORY TISSUE. All encapsulating and inflammatory tissue must be removed, including the fibrous sheaths tracking the lead or leads into the muscle to near the lead entry site (Fig. 28–7). Successful débridement of encapsulating and inflammatory tissue includes leaving a viable bed of normal tissue and obtaining meticulous hemostasis. Although all tissue dissections are currently performed using an electrosurgical unit, my first successful attempts involved the use of a carbon dioxide laser. The surgical principles that must be followed regardless of the dissecting instrument are the need to minimize the injury to the normal tissue and the need to suture ligate visible veins and all arteries. Care must be taken to reapproximate separated muscle tissue by direct surgical suturing techniques. Reconstitution of this tissue is necessary to achieve hemostasis.

DECONTAMINATION OF DEVICE. The pulse generator in infected cases was decontaminated using Cidex, and the leads were wiped clean with povidone-iodine (Betadine) and saline. Although Cidex has the potential to sterilize the pacemaker, it was applied for only a short time, and sterility was not ensured. The efficacy of lead decontamination by cleaning the surface depended on the integrity of the insulation. Insulation with a rough surface or cracks such as degraded polyurethane could not be cleaned.

REIMPLANTATION USING THE SAME SITE. The pacemaker was reimplanted in the pocket. Most pockets were enlarged following extensive tissue débridement. If necessary, a portion of the débrided pocket was excluded using interrupted sutures, and the pacemaker was replaced in an appropriately sized space. A closed drainage system (e.g., a flat Jackson-Pratt drain) was routinely used to prevent fluid collection prior to the adherence of tissue flaps. An exudative or hemorrhagic effusion jeopardizes the success of the procedure by separating the tissues and acting as a culture medium. The closed drainage system was left in place until the drainage stopped and the tissue flaps were stuck together (2 to 3 days). All incisions were closed primarily.

AUTHOR'S EXPERIENCE. The early salvage procedures involved pacemaker erosions or pocket infections with chronic draining sinuses. Although a few were treated successfully, most failed and the infection immediately recurred. In addition, many patients with early successful treatments suffered

SALVAGING THE IMPLANTATION SITE

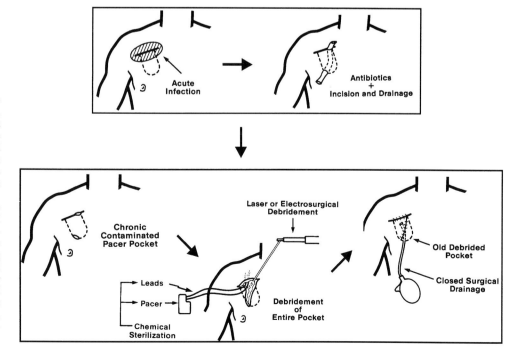

FIGURE 28–6. Acute infections must first be converted into chronic, smoldering infections. The definition of a chronic smoldering infection is absence of cellulitis and a minimal amount of sequestered exudate. In some cases, incision and drainage is performed, and the drain left in place.

Chronic smoldering pockets are débrided of all inflammatory tissue. I use a carbon dioxide laser or an electrosurgical instrument. The pulse generator is decontaminated using Cidex, and the leads are cleaned using Betadine. The pulse generator is reimplanted in the débrided pocket, and the old portion of the débrided pocket is excluded. A closed drainage system (Jackson-Pratt) is used in all cases.

Salvage and Abandonment

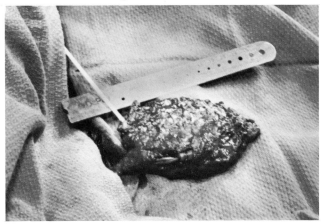

A   Surgical débridement

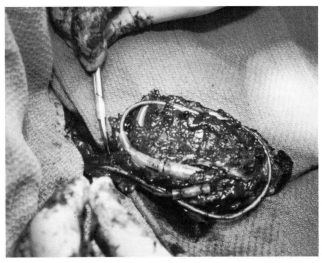

B   Inflammatory tissue

FIGURE 28–7. *A*, Surgical débridement. To attempt to salvage the site, all inflammatory tissue must be removed, including the tissue around the leads near the vein entry site. *B*, Inflammatory tissue. In this case, the inflammatory tissue extended down near the vein entry site, and the pocket was abandoned. To abandon the site, the pulse generator, leads, and any other retained debris (suture material, suture sleeves, insulation boot, etc.) must be removed in addition to the débrided tissue.

a recurrence of the infection 6 months to a year later. I then redefined a success as no recurrence of a complication for at least a year following the salvage procedure.

Patients must be carefully selected to perform successful salvage of an infected pocket (Fig. 28–8). Before patient selection, the percentage of all infected pockets salvaged by me was only 45%. After patients were preselected for the salvage procedure, the success rate in these patients increased to 64%. Preselection criteria were based on experience and included the absence of septicemia, gram-negative sepsis, thin subcutaneous tissue and ischemic skin, and a history of multiple erosions at the site. These preselection criteria excluded 25% of patients, and their pacemaker sites were abandoned without attempting a salvage procedure.

Further selection occurred during the attempted salvage procedure itself, excluding another 9%. In these cases, the débrided pocket was judged not suitable for pacemaker reim-

plantation or the inflammatory tissue could not be completely removed from the leads near the vein entry site (see Fig. 28–8). Exclusion of these patients required a judgment decision based on experience and the ability to recognize inflammatory changes.

During the early and mid 1980s, a salvage rate of 45% was an impressive cure rate. Unfortunately, accurately predicting which patients would have a successful result was not possible. Patients with dry erosions had the highest success rate, and those with acute infections had the lowest. Today, the success rate for lead extraction procedures makes salvage procedures, with their 55% failure rate, an unacceptable alternative for the routine management of pocket infections.

ABANDONMENT OF THE SITE

Abandonment of the implant site includes débridement of all inflammatory tissue and primary closure of the site using the same procedure performed in salvaging a site (Fig. 28–9). In addition, the devices must be removed and reimplanted in another site. Removal of a device such as a pulse generator or defibrillator from an implant pocket is a minor procedure. Formerly, the limitation of abandoning the site was the removal of chronically implanted transvenous leads. Current lead extraction techniques have improved. In my experience, 95% of leads have been successfully extracted using percutaneous transvenous techniques, whereas only 5% required more extensive surgery such as a transatrial or a ventriculotomy procedure. Open heart procedures using cardiopulmonary bypass have not been needed.

All incisions are closed primarily, using a closed drainage system when necessary. Historically, infected abandoned pockets were rarely débrided and were treated by leaving the pocket open to heal by secondary union. Healing by secondary union was slow, caused some morbidity, and required continued antibiotic therapy and medical attention. Also, a transient bacteremia caused by manipulating the wound could infect a remote implantation site (metastatic infection). Unfortunately, this archaic technique still persists today.

ABANDONMENT WITHOUT REMOVING LEADS. In one specific situation, the pocket can be abandoned while removing the proximal portion of the leads and leaving the distal portion intact.[18] The infected chronic pocket must be remote (more than 2.5 cm from the lead insertion site) and free from any visible inflammatory response. Through a separate incision at the lead insertion site, the leads are inspected, and if found free of any inflammatory tissue, they are cut, clipped, and abandoned. Leads should not be allowed to retract into the superior veins. Leads not anchored in the superior veins may migrate, causing another complication. This incision is closed. The pocket is then opened, the proximal portion of the leads removed, all inflammatory tissue débrided, and the pocket closed primarily.

PACEMAKER REIMPLANTATION. Reimplantation of the pacemaker system at a distant site is an integral part of abandoning the site. Pacemakers and leads are reimplanted on the opposite side when possible. If the leads cannot be implanted transvenously on the opposite side, they are implanted using a transatrial, epicardial, or transfemoral approach. The pacemaker is then implanted on the chest wall or in the abdomen. I do not use the transfemoral approach. Although some prac-

Pocket Infections - Attempts to Salvage the Site

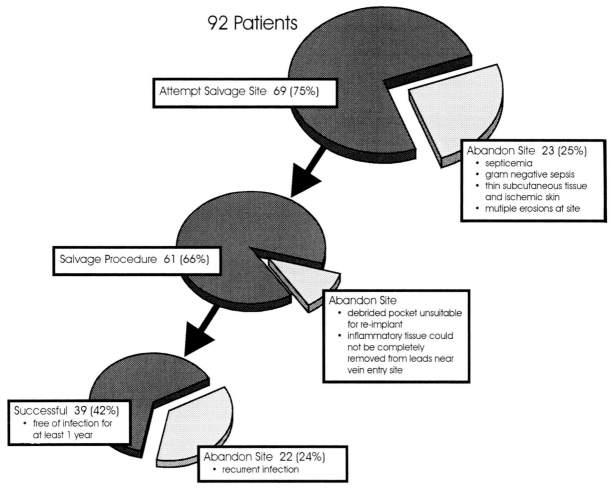

92 Patients

Attempt Salvage Site 69 (75%)

Abandon Site 23 (25%)
- septicemia
- gram negative sepsis
- thin subcutaneous tissue and ischemic skin
- mutiple erosions at site

Salvage Procedure 61 (66%)

Abandon Site
- debrided pocket unsuitable for re-implant
- inflammatory tissue could not be completely removed from leads near vein entry site

Successful 39 (42%)
- free of infection for at least 1 year

Abandon Site 22 (24%)
- recurrent infection

FIGURE 28–8. In this series 92 patients presented with a pocket infection. Only 42% of these patients were successfully treated with the salvage procedure. Of the 69 preselected patients, 57% had a successful result. The salvage procedure was performed on 61 patients and was successful in 39 (64%).

ABANDONING THE IMPLANTATION SITE

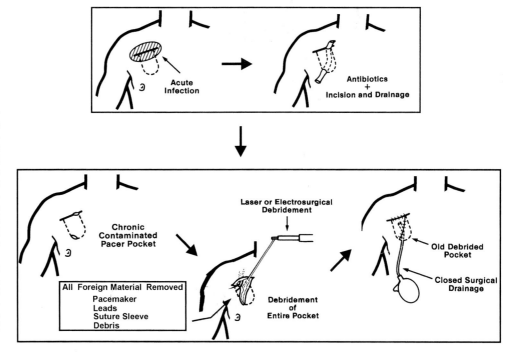

FIGURE 28–9. The initial procedures for abandonment and salvage of an implant site are the same. Acute infections are converted into chronic smoldering infections, and the site is débrided of all inflammatory tissue. The difference lies in the removal of all foreign material, including pacemaker, leads, suture sleeves, permanent suture debris, and plastic terminal caps. The débrided pocket is closed using a closed drainage system if necessary.

This abandonment procedure has a 100% success rate in my experience. This success rate, in combination with current low-morbidity lead extraction techniques, has made abandonment of the site the procedure of choice for treating pocket infections.

titioners promote this approach, it is, in my opinion, potentially dangerous. Transvenous lead implant complications occurring in the superior veins can also occur in the inferior veins. Thrombus formation and venous occlusion occurring in the inferior vena cava, iliac, and femoral veins have life-threatening sequelae.

If no infection is present, a new device is implanted as part of the abandonment procedure. If an infection exists, it is essential for the new system to be implanted without risking a subsequent infection. In these patients, antibiotic therapy is continued, and reimplantation is delayed until the patient has been afebrile for approximately 36 hours. The 36-hour time period was initially an arbitrary choice and has been successful. Most patients are not febrile at the time of abandonment, and the reimplantation is scheduled 36 hours after abandonment of the old site.

CLINICAL RESULTS. Today, following the development of counteraction lead extraction techniques, abandonment of the infected pocket and extraction of transvenous leads is applicable to all patients and has become the preferred treatment. In one of my series, 195 patients were treated by abandonment of the site. In 165 patients, this was the primary modality of therapy; 30 patients had failed salvage procedures with subsequent abandonment of the site. There have been no recurrent infections, and the incisions have healed following a primary closure. Currently, we have treated more than 300 patients using this approach.

Reimplantation of the pacemaker system was performed on the opposite side in most cases. A transatrial implant was performed in 5% of the patients, and two patients received an epicardial implant. In all cases, reimplantation was successful. There were no cases of infection of the new system by cross-contamination or other means.

TYPICAL HOSPITAL STAY. Hospital stay for a typical patient presenting with an infection of a chronic pacemaker pocket without septicemia was 5 days. The patient was admitted on the day of surgery, placed on intravenous antibiotics, and taken to surgery for débridement of the pocket and lead extraction. Intravenous antibiotics were continued, and if the patient was afebrile in 36 hours a new pacemaker was implanted on the opposite side. On the second postimplant day, the intravenous antibiotic was stopped and an oral antibiotic started. The patient was then discharged on the oral antibiotic for a maximum of 10 days. If the lead could not be extracted using transvenous techniques, a cardiac surgical approach added an average of 2 days to the postimplant hospital convalescence.

In my opinion, continued antibiotics are not required. The treatment just outlined is sufficient to treat pacemaker pocket infections. More aggressive chronic antibiotic therapy is reserved for treatment of a concomitant infection such as endocarditis. Endocarditis is rare and was not shown to exist in any of the patients in our series. If endocarditis or some other remote infection does exist, symptoms will recur when the patient is taken off antibiotics, and that infection can then be identified and treated.

Patients with severe infections or other complicating conditions (less than 5%) may have extended hospital stays. For example, patients with an acute infection with marked cellulitis are treated with intravenous antibiotics and, if necessary, incision and drainage until the cellulitis resolves. Hospitalization is usually not required for the entire course of preoperative antibiotics. The interval between corrective surgery and reimplantation may be increased if fever is present. The postimplant interval may be increased by extension of the intravenous antibiotic coverage.

Septic emboli to the lung following débridement and lead extraction is another potential complication that increases hospital stay. A febrile response increases the duration of intravenous antibiotic therapy. In a series of more than 300 patients, 2 with septic emboli superimposed on chronic lung disease developed respiratory insufficiency that required a ventilator postoperatively.

Complications of Permanent Transvenous Leads

The integrity of the electrophysiologic device is dependent on the proper implantation and performance of the permanent transvenous leads. Lead-related complications are associated with both implantation procedure and lead performance. Proper lead implantation includes ensuring that the lead position is uneventful and stable and that the electric parameters are satisfactory. After proper implantation, lead performance includes such issues as lead-tissue interaction and device failure (insulation, conductor coil, adapter, and electrode). Complications related to device failure will not be be discussed in this chapter.

Complications that are primarily implantation related include problems such as dislodgment, perforation, and the presence of poor electric parameters. Performance-related complications (excluding device failure) are associated primarily with lead-tissue interaction. Most chronic complications are performance related. However, sometimes it is difficult to separate implantation from performance complications. For example, a very stiff lead may be associated with both high implantation and high performance complication rates. Currently, the only method of differentiating between the two is statistics and the opinions of experts. Unfortunately, statistics on human implants are not available early in the design process.

Permanent transvenous leads are placed in both extrathoracic and intravascular environments. The extrathoracic lead interaction injures tissue by both disruption and mechanical stress, as previously described for the device pocket. Intravascular interaction also injures tissue owing to endothelial contact and thrombosis.

ENCAPSULATION WITH FIBROUS TISSUE

Depending on the insulation material involved, 30% to 80% of the intravascular portion of the lead may be encapsulated with fibrous tissue initiated by thrombus formation.[19, 20] Fibrous tissue encapsulation ranges from a thin collagenous sheath to thick circumferential bands that bind the lead to the vein or heart wall and to other leads (Fig. 28–10). Leads injure the intima of the veins and cardiac wall by mechanical stress, activating the coagulation mechanism and causing thrombus formation. The slightest touch is sufficient to start the process. Slowing (stasis) or eddying of the blood flow around the lead also has the potential to cause thrombus. In addition, materials such as silicone rubber (Silastic) tend to

Lead Encapsulation

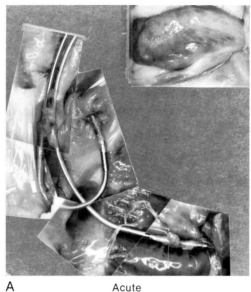

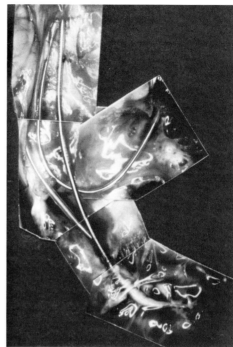

FIGURE 28–10. *A,* Acute thrombus formation 1 week after implantation in a dog. Thrombus forms at each site where the lead touches the wall and in some regions where there is stasis or eddying of blood flow. Most of this early thrombus lyses. It persists and organizes at sites of continued pressure on the wall and in areas with stagnant blood flow. *B,* Organized fibrous tissue encapsulating the lead forms chronically at sites of pressure, motion, and static blood flow. This tissue changes with time from fibrous tissue to cartilaginous tissue and finally to bone.

A   Acute

B   Chronic

be more thrombogenic than polyurethane (Fig. 28–11). The inflammatory reaction associated with organization of thrombus is responsible for encapsulation with fibrous tissue.

Tissue injury resulting from an implanted lead starts at the entry site (tissue disruption) and occurs at each point where the lead body touches the vein and cardiac wall (mechanical stress). At points where the lead does not remain in contact with the wall, the thrombus lyses. At points where the vein remains in contact with the wall, a chronic microthrombus-organization process continues within the encapsulation of the lead at that point. As the vein curves, the lead body contacts the wall. The greater the curvature, the greater the area of contact and the greater the potential for tissue injury.

With time the encapsulating fibrous tissue increases its

Encapsulation at 12 Weeks

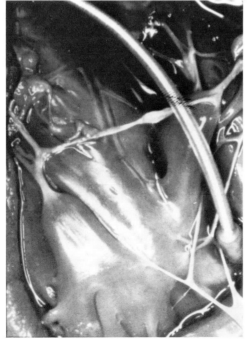

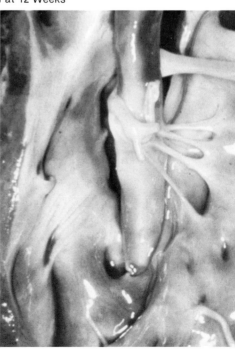

FIGURE 28–11. Polyurethane and silicone rubber leads implanted for 12 weeks. The polyurethane lead *(A)* has minimal encapsulation, and the silicone rubber lead *(B)* is completely encapsulated. This is a surface thrombogenic phenomenon and is not related to the mechanical properties of the lead. The magnitude of the surface encapsulation is probably related to the fact that silicone leads are more difficult to extract than polyurethane in the first 2 to 3 years after implantation.

A   Polyurethane

B   Silicone

tensile strength through maturation of the collagen. Some of the thicker tissue differentiates from dense collagen into cartilage and finally into bone. Mineralized tissue and bone are present in adult humans in 6 to 8 years and in young children in 3 to 4 years.[4, 5] These findings are routinely found in animal models, and human observations are similar.[19–22]

PROPERTIES OF THE ELECTRODE-MYOCARDIAL INTERFACE

The electrode is placed against the myocardial tissue, forming the electrode-myocardial interface. The electrode exerts mechanical stress against the myocardial tissue, causing injury. Electrodes implanted in the ventricular chamber are subjected to more mechanical stress than those in the atrium during contraction. The magnitude and duration of the inflammatory reaction, also known as "electrode maturation," varies. If the inflammatory response is not excessive, steroid-eluting electrodes will suppress the maturation reaction.

PASSIVE FIXATION DEVICES

Passive fixation devices, such as tines or fins, hold the electrode in position by entrapping the fixation device within the trabeculated musculature along the heart wall. The injury caused by the fixation mechanism causes an inflammatory reaction and thrombus formation. Stasis of blood in the trabeculated musculature along the lead body and around the tines also causes thrombus formation. In the ventricle the electrode is acutely secured by the passive fixation device alone. In most cases, in the atrium tension on a J configuration is usually needed to ensure stability (straight flexible leads can be successfully implanted in trabeculated atrial tissue in some cases). Chronically, the electrode is secured by the encapsulating fibrous tissue formed by the inflammatory reaction and organization of thrombus.

Passive fixation devices are separated from the electrode-myocardial interface. The tissue reaction and organization of clot does not seem to influence the maturation reaction at the electrode-myocardial interface. In some cases, the tines or fins absorb some of the mechanical stresses, reducing the pressures at the electrode-myocardial interface.

ACTIVE FIXATION DEVICES

Current active fixation devices are wire helixes screwed into the myocardium. The inflammatory reaction is initiated by the tissue disruption that occurs when the helix is screwed into the myocardium and is continued by mechanical stress. With active fixation devices the wire helix may also serve as the electrode or part of the electrode, or it may be contiguous with but isolated from the electrode. The injury caused by the active fixation device adds in varying degrees to the electrode maturation reaction. Steroid-eluting electrodes are not always successful in eliminating maturation phenomena of this magnitude. All of the acute stability and most of the chronic stability achieved by this type of device depends on the helix. Chronically, fibrous tissue is supportive but may not be sufficiently supportive to stabilize the electrode if the helix is not screwed into the tissue.

LEAD-RELATED COMPLICATIONS

Complications can be grossly divided into lead infections, vein thrombosis, and problems related to the electrode-myocardial interface (Table 28–3). Device failures are not discussed here. Although a new lead must be implanted in many cases, the rationale for abandoning or extracting failed leads is based only on the tissue-related complications described in the following sections.

INDICATIONS FOR REMOVING LEADS

Lead-related complications may require lead removal (lead extraction). Indications for lead extraction have expanded during the last few years. Initially, only patients with life-threatening complications such as septicemia were considered candidates for lead removal. Today, some leads are extracted and replaced for poor performance, to avoid having too many leads passing through the same vein, or even merely because they are abandoned. The risk and morbidity of extracting the leads must be weighed against the medical risk and morbidity of leaving them in place. Based on the risk and morbidity of leaving the leads in place, I have grouped the indications for lead extraction into conditions considered mandatory, necessary, and discretionary.[23–25]

Mandatory indications mean the leads *must* be removed. Mandatory conditions are those in which leaving the leads in place would be life-threatening or disabling. *Necessary* indications mean the leads *should* be removed. Necessary conditions are those in which lead removal would correct a problem or prevent a life-threatening situation from developing, but the existing problem is not considered life-threatening. *Discretionary* indications mean that the leads *could* be removed. Discretionary conditions are those in which it is preferable to remove the leads, but removal is rarely a medical necessity.

TABLE 28–3. TREATMENT OF LEAD-RELATED COMPLICATIONS

Infection
  Remove lead
  Implant new system on opposite side
Vein thrombosis
  Acute venous occlusion
    Anticoagulate (IV heparin, converting to Coumadin)
    Remove lead if abandoned or if clinical events occur (e.g., pulmonary emboli or progressive swelling of the arm)
    May elect to remove lead after fibrous organization occurs
  SVC syndrome
    Administer thrombolytic agents and systemic heparin
    If necessary, perform surgical correction
  Chronic venous occlusion
    Remove abandoned leads
Complications at the electrode-myocardial interface
  Acute dislodgment
    Reposition lead
  Lead migration
    Remove lead
  Acute penetration
    Reposition lead
  Acute perforation
    Immediate pericardiocentesis if there is gradual onset of tamponade
    Immediate cardiac surgery if acute tamponade with low cardiac output occurs

TABLE 28–4. **INDICATIONS AND CONDITIONS FOR LEAD EXTRACTION**

INDICATIONS	BYRD 264 PATIENTS (%)	NATIONAL 856 PATIENTS (%)	CONDITIONS		
			M	N	D
Lead replacement	25.8	38.7		X	X
Infection	24.6	34.7		X	X
Septicemia/ endocarditis	21.6	10.5	X		
Erosion	7.6	5.0		X	
Pain	5.7	1.9			X
Pre-erosion	4.5	2.2		X	
Chronic draining sinus	4.5	2.0		X	
Free-floating or migrating lead	2.6	1.4	X	X	
Thrombosis	0.8	0.5		X	X
Tricuspid regurgitation	0.0	0.5		X	X
Other[a]	2.3	2.6		X	X

[a]Includes isolated presenting conditions such as cancer and trauma and those unknown conditions that could not be classified.
This table combines the Byrd and Cook data bases for indications and conditions for lead extraction. Indications are listed as the presenting condition. M, N, and D refer to the mandatory, necessary, and discretionary conditions for lead extraction (see text). In some cases, the indication group depends on the magnitude of the condition and may be listed in more than one group.

In general, the indications for lead extraction for an individual are directly related to the risk and morbidity of the extraction procedure. If cardiopulmonary bypass is necessary to extract the leads, only patients with mandatory conditions undergo lead extraction. Once proficiency has been gained with the transvenous countertraction techniques, most patients with necessary and some with discretionary conditions have their leads extracted. Experts are now extracting most abandoned leads. Leads not routinely extracted include those in patients with discretionary and noninfected necessary conditions associated with leads that have been implanted longer than 8 to 10 years. Table 28–4 list the indications and conditions for lead extraction in both the Byrd and Cook databases. Table 28–5 lists clinical examples of mandatory, necessary, and discretionary conditions.

TABLE 28–5. **INDICATIONS FOR LEAD EXTRACTION**

Mandatory (life-threatening)
  Septicemia
  Endocarditis
  Lead migration (e.g., perforating, causing arrhythmia, causing emboli)
  Device interference (e.g., abandoned implantable defibrillator lead)
  Obliteration of all usable veins
Necessary (significant morbidity)
  Pocket infection
  Chronic draining sinus
  Erosion
  Vein thrombosis
  Lead migration (not presently causing life-threatening problem)
  Potential device interference
  Lead replacement (e.g., supernumerary, extract and implant thrombosed vein)
Discretionary (optional)
  Pain
  Malignancy
  Lead replacement (e.g., abandoned lead for less than 3 to 4 years)

INFECTED LEADS

The sequelae of infected permanent pacing leads range from an erosion resulting in a draining sinus to a life-threatening systemic infection (septicemia). The mortality associated with persistent infection when infected leads are not removed can be as high as 66%.[17] Because of this statistic, it has been recommended that infected leads be removed, even in the elderly high-risk patient, using open heart surgery if necessary.[26, 27]

An infected pacing system is considered either a mandatory or a necessary condition for lead extraction, depending on the clinical manifestations of the infection.[17, 18, 24, 25, 28] An infection involving only the extravascular portion of the leads with no systemic symptoms may be treated as described earlier for a device pocket infection. However, septicemia may result from a pocket infection with infected tissue along the intravascular portion of the lead or drainage into the bloodstream. Drainage into the bloodstream may occur along the lead, through breaks in the insulation connected by the lead lumen, or by indirect lymphatic or venous drainage. Lead-related septicemia is a mandatory condition for lead extraction. Pockets with negative cultures in the presence of potentially infected leads have only a slightly lower complication rate than those with positive cultures.[29]

An acute infection involving the leads within the vascular space is rare but, if present, causes septicemia. Leads can be infected by vegetation attached to the lead or by actual bacterial growth within the interstices of a degraded insulation polymer or within the lumen if there is a breach in the insulation.[30] If the insulation has failed and bacterial growth occurs in the lumen, it can extend along the entire length of the lead. Treatment is removal of the lead (mandatory condition).

A fresh thrombus may become secondarily infected following lead implantation, causing a suppurative phlebitis or an infected vegetation. These are dangerous infections causing septicemia, septic pulmonary emboli, or, potentially, endocarditis. This problem is best treated by first controlling the infection with systemic antibiotic therapy and then removing the lead. If the infection cannot be controlled, lead removal is mandatory. One of the risks of removing a lead with a fresh infected thrombus is the chance of depositing the infected thrombus at the vein entry site, causing a suppurative phlebitis. Although this infection can be treated successfully, the associated morbidity is great.

Infected vegetations attached to a chronic lead without an insulation fault are usually not a primary lead problem but are probably similar to vegetations on heart valves caused by a systemic infection. Lead removal (mandatory condition) is the treatment of choice, but it is complicated by the vegetation and requires special techniques or open heart surgery.

VEIN THROMBOSIS

Transvenous leads may cause vein thrombosis. The incidence of clinically undetected vein thrombosis has been reported to be as high as 44%.[31]

ACUTE VEIN THROMBOSIS. Acute reactions of the vein wall at or near the lead entry site can cause thrombosis of the subclavian or brachiocephalic veins. These thrombosed veins usually heal without sequelae. If axillary and brachial vein thrombosis occurs, collateral drainage paths are usually not sufficient, and residual swelling of the arm is a frequent complication.

Treatment of acute vein thrombosis consists of anticoagulation therapy with intravenous heparin, converting later to Coumadin. Coumadin is continued for at least 3 months. Clinical data supporting either leaving or removing the lead are not available, although leaving the lead in place does not seem to alter the course. Immediate removal of the lead may extend the clot both proximally and distally. If thrombus on the distal portion of the lead is pulled back toward the subclavian vein, the thrombosis will be extended proximally. Pulling the electrode back through a recently thrombosed subclavian vein may push the thrombus distally into the axillary or brachial veins. Lead removal once the fibrous tissue stage of organization has begun is probably safer.

In my opinion, leads in thrombosed veins should not be removed unless clinical events (acute or chronic) occur, such as pulmonary emboli or progressive swelling of the arm while the patient is on anticoagulant therapy. As mentioned previously, removal may worsen the thrombosis. In addition, a new pacing system must be implanted on the opposite side, and, although unlikely, the new system may have the same problem. Therefore, if clinical events occur or if the leads are abandoned, they should be removed (necessary condition).

An acute thrombosis of the superior vena cava (SVC) does not occur, in my experience, without a preexisting condition that damages the vein. For example, the presence of a chronic pacing lead in the vein or the recent extraction of a lead with thrombus formation along the vein wall predisposes the vein to an acute thrombosis.[32] Treatment of SVC syndrome involves the use of thrombolytic agents, anticoagulation, and a major surgical procedure. Initial treatment consists of administering a thrombolytic agent in an attempt to reopen the lumen. If this is successful, the syndrome resolves. Whether it is successful or not, the patient is placed on systemic heparin and prepared for a surgical procedure. In my experience, débridement of all thrombotic material from the SVC and brachiocephalic veins and a vein patch angioplasty using the saphenous vein have been successful.[33] Construction of a vein conduit (Doty procedure) is an alternative procedure if the remaining surface area of the vein is inadequate.[34]

CHRONIC VENOUS OCCLUSION. Exuberant fibrous tissue forms when transvenous leads cause an exaggerated inflammatory reaction with thrombus formation at sites of contact with the vein or cardiac wall. Mechanical stress is probably the initial cause of this reaction. It is exacerbated by stasis and eddying of blood flow. The consequences of exuberant intravenous fibrous tissue include gradual obliteration of the lumen and acute vein thrombosis as well as the possibility of pulmonary emboli. Obliteration of the subclavian and brachiocephalic veins is common. Occlusion of the SVC is uncommon (Fig. 28–12), but when it occurs, if the lumen is narrowed slowly, development of collateral venous flow prevents the development of the SVC syndrome.

Multiple leads in one vein increase the incidence of venous occlusion.[35] There are additional sites of vein wall contact, and leads bound together apply even greater mechanical stress on the tissue. Mechanical stress is also exacerbated by stasis and eddying of blood flow. In my experience, the incidence of venous occlusion is related to the size and stiffness of the leads and the duration of their implant. The left brachiocephalic vein is occluded more frequently than the right, and small supple leads cause less fibrous tissue reaction than large stiff leads. Abandoned leads in veins compromised by thrombus should be removed (necessary condition).

Exuberant fibrous tissue formation along the heart wall does not cause problems in situ but increases the risk and difficulty of lead removal. Chronic lead extractions from this exuberant fibrous tissue are associated with a high incidence of thrombus formation, and some sites progress to vein thrombosis.

COMPLICATIONS AT THE ELECTRODE-MYOCARDIAL INTERFACE

All complications involving the electrode-myocardial interface present clinically with changes in pacing or inappropriate stimulation of another muscle. These failures are usually due to excessive tissue injury caused by the electrode or to dislodgment of the electrode from its implantation site. Stimulation of other muscles may represent a serious problem such as penetration of the electrode, or it may result from placement of the electrode in close proximity to a nerve.

DISLODGMENT AND MIGRATION. Electrode dislodgment is probably the most common complication encountered. Electrode instability is usually a complication of the implantation procedure and is not a lead-tissue problem (inflammatory reaction). Implantation includes lead performance issues such as stiffness and fixation devices. The great majority of lead dislodgment problems that alter the lead's electric performance are detected and corrected immediately by lead repositioning.

Migration of a dislodged lead out of the heart may be undetected for months in poorly managed patients with an intermittent dysrhythmia. Migration into the pulmonary artery, jugular vein, or an iliac vein can cause complications such as pulmonary emboli and thrombosis of the vein.[36] Once discovered, these leads should be removed (necessary condition) and new leads implanted.

Leads break, and abandoned leads are sometimes cut and left unsecured. Although the incidence of migration is probably low, migration of severed or broken transvenous leads does occur and is potentially dangerous. Fatality secondary to lead migration has been reported to be as high as 66%.[17] For example, if the proximal lead tip is bouncing in the right ventricle causing a ventricular arrhythmia, it is life-threatening. Migrating severed leads have perforated the heart, causing hemorrhage or hemopericardium, and have formed vegetations, causing emboli to the lungs.[37–40] These are mandatory conditions for lead extraction. A severed lead coiled in the right ventricle may not cause acute symptoms, but in my opinion, the scar tissue that forms lead-to-lead and lead-to-heart wall will compromise ventricular function over time. In asymptomatic patients, the potential exists for one of these complications to occur, making lead extraction a necessary condition.

PENETRATION AND PERFORATION. Exaggerated inflammatory reactions, especially those not controlled by steroid-eluting electrodes, represent significant tissue injury. For example, stiff or unstable bouncing leads implanted within the ventricle may apply excessive pressure directly to the electrode-

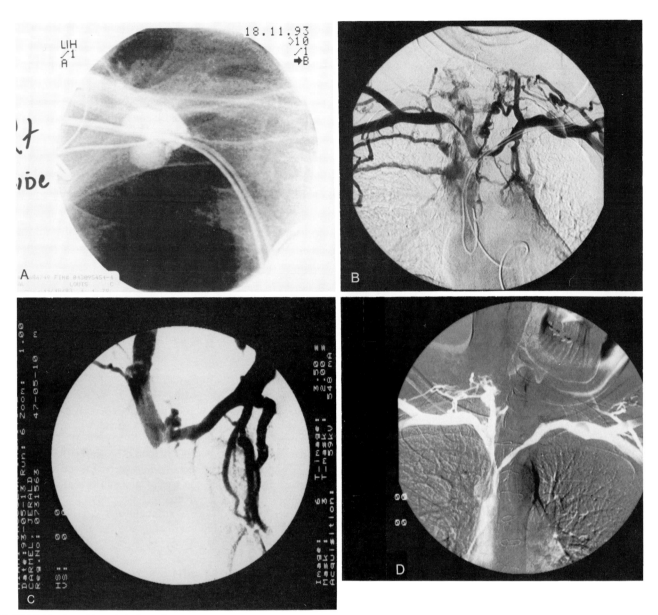

FIGURE 28–12. *A,* The subclavian vein is the most commonly occluded superior vein. Chronic thrombosis and occlusion of the subclavian vein at the lead entry site is shown in this figure. *B,* Chronic thrombosis and occlusion of the superior vena cava (SVC) is unusual. This occlusion is 8 years old, and the collateral venous return is complete. Collateral drainage was inadequate when this young patient exercised, causing swelling of the upper extremities, neck, and head. *C,* The leads were extracted using countertraction through the femoral vein. The postextraction venogram shows the SVC occlusion more clearly. *D,* The brachiocephalic vein and SVC are shown to be patent 6 months after surgical correction. The veins were repaired by débridement of the organized intravenous inflammatory tissue and a vein patch angioplasty. The patient is asymptomatic and has a marked reduction in collateral venous drainage.

myocardial interface. Tissue injury of this magnitude heals with scarring and poor electrode performance, if any. Clinically, exaggerated reactions result in loss of capture (exit block) or loss of sensing.

PENETRATION. The most severe reactions occur when the electrode penetrates the tissue. In these cases, the pressure at the electrode-myocardial interface is great enough to force the electrode into the cardiac muscle. As the electrode works its way through the muscle fibers, the resultant tissue injury causes an intense inflammatory reaction. The intensity of the reaction is sufficient to cause exit block (threshold exceeds the output of the pulse generator). As the electrode nears the epicardial surface, it frequently stimulates the diaphragm.

Patients usually present with threshold elevation and diaphragmatic stimulation. Penetration rarely progresses to perforation of the electrode into the pericardial space. The preferred treatment for acute penetration is to reposition the electrode or replace the lead with a more supple model.

Chronic problems with penetration are not common. Unusually, the clinical manifestations of the acute presentation are so severe that the problem must be corrected. In addition, penetration is slow, and the tissue reaction causes a localized pericarditis that obliterates the pericardial space and prevents perforation. Removal of these leads may be dangerous, and the patient should be prepared for an immediate cardiac procedure prior to the extraction. If the penetration extends to the epicardium and the pericardial reaction is not extensive, extraction by traction or countertraction could avulse the remaining cardiac wall, causing hemorrhage and tamponade.

Limited penetration, however, does occur. For example, an electrode with tines recessed 2 to 3 mm may penetrate to the level of the tines. Although the lead is usable, the resultant chronic reaction causes significant fibrosis and a poor chronic stimulation threshold.

PERFORATION. A perforation is usually an inadvertent misadventure caused by the electrode being pushed through the heart wall. During routine pacemaker implantation, patient monitoring is not adequate to diagnose a perforation unless it is seen on fluoroscopy. It may not be detected until the onset of cardiac tamponade. Unrecognized perforations may present chronically with pericarditis or a hemorrhagic effusion with or without tamponade. Chronic perforation of a pacemaker lead is rare.

Gradual onset of cardiac tamponade is treated differently from marked hemorrhage with tamponade. The treatment for gradual onset is immediate pericardiocentesis, leaving a catheter in the pericardial space and monitoring the blood loss. Preparations for cardiac surgery should be made, although it is usually not required. The lead is pulled back into the heart, and the blood loss is monitored. Treatment for an acute cardiac tamponade with a low cardiac output is more radical. Hemorrhage of this magnitude requires immediate cardiac surgery to ensure a successful result.

Extraction of Chronic Transvenous Leads

The extraction of chronic pacemaker and defibrillator leads has become a challenging endeavor. The goal is to ensure the safe extraction of all transvenous leads. Extraction techniques range from a simple procedure requiring only a few minutes under local anesthesia to a complicated procedure lasting hours under general anesthesia. For example, a simple procedure would consist of unscrewing an active fixation lead implanted for a few months, applying minimal traction. A complicated procedure might be the extraction of multiple leads implanted for 10 years or longer. Some lead extractions may require a more involved surgical procedure to ensure a safe and successful result.

Lead extraction is potentially dangerous. Complications include failure to extract an infected lead, low cardiac output, lead breakage and migration, avulsion of veins and myocardial tissue (e.g., muscle, tricuspid valve), and tears of the veins and heart wall with hemothorax, tamponade, and death. The goal of modern extraction techniques is to devise an approach that is successful in extracting all leads and minimizes, if not eliminates, the complications just listed.

All current lead extraction procedures use some form of traction, a pulling force (Table 28–6). To safely apply the new successful countertraction extraction procedures, it is important to understand the problems associated with direct and indirect traction techniques (Fig. 28–13). Countertraction is applied through the implant vein using an SVC approach and indirectly through the femoral vein using an inferior vena cava (IVC) approach. Occasionally, a more invasive transatrial approach is combined with countertraction. The follow-

ing section provides a detailed discussion of these techniques.

TRACTION

Pulling on the lead was a successful method of extracting the lead during the early years of pacing, when leads lacked efficient fixation devices and were implanted for short periods of time. Traction proved unsafe and had a high incidence of failure when applied to leads with efficient fixation devices and leads implanted for longer periods of time.[41, 42] The amount of traction required increases and becomes more dangerous as the duration of the implant and the tensile strength of the fibrous tissue increase. Leads with efficient passive fixation devices may be difficult to remove 4 to 6 months after implantation. Failure to extract a lead frequently damages the lead, making future extraction attempts more difficult.

Traction must be applied judiciously to minimize the risk to the patient. The pulling force applied to the proximal portion of the lead is distributed to sites where fibrous tissue binds the lead at places where the lead or electrode makes contact with the vein or heart wall. Multiple leads may be bound to the vein or heart wall and to each other. Because the pulling force is not focused, the distribution of force to the binding sites is unknown. It is possible to inadvertently tear a vein or the heart wall.

Accidents are not predictable and frequently happen without warning. This is true in part because it is impossible to accurately judge the force applied to the lead. The applied force varies with lead size, method of grasping the lead, and, most important, the catecholamine (stress) level of the physician. Consequently, the use of procedures such as pulling until you feel the heart contract or applying ''just a little tug'' to see if the lead will come out may not be safe.

Traction can be applied directly (on the proximal lead or a locked stylet) or indirectly.

DIRECT TRACTION ON THE PROXIMAL PORTION OF THE LEAD

Direct traction is applied by pulling on the proximal exposed portion of the lead (Fig. 28–14). Special instrumenta-

TABLE 28–6. **LEAD EXTRACTION APPROACHES***

DIRECT (WITH OR WITHOUT LOCKING STYLET)
Vein entry site
Closed heart (cardiac surgery)
Transatrial
Ventriculotomy
Open heart (cardiopulmonary bypass)
INDIRECT (WITH CATHETER AND SNARE)
Remote vein (usually femoral vein)

*Extraction procedures are separated into those in which the lead is manipulated directly and those in which the lead is manipulated indirectly by snares and catheters. Traction and countertraction techniques are applicable to both approaches. Direct approaches include extraction of the lead through the vein entry site, through a closed heart surgical approach (transatrial and ventriculotomy), and through an open heart surgical approach on cardiopulmonary bypass. Indirect approaches include those made through a vein remote from the entry site, usually the femoral vein. Catheters and snares are used to maneuver and grasp the lead for extraction.

Traction vs. Countertraction

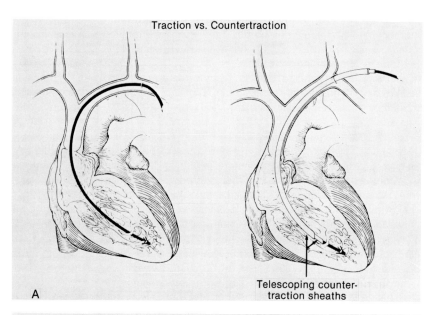

Telescoping counter-
traction sheaths

A

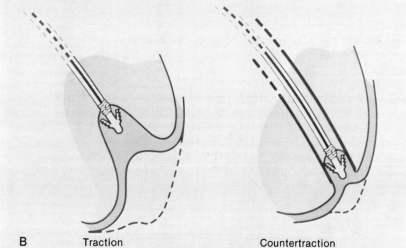

B   Traction   Countertraction

FIGURE 28–13. *A* and *B,* Traction is a pulling force. The lead is grasped at any point and pulled. As the lead is pulled, the right ventricle is everted, and tension is applied to the heart wall. Eversion decreases compliance and compromises the tricuspid valve, both of which cause low cardiac output. The tension is relieved by the tissue tearing. If the scar tissue surrounding the electrode tears, the electrode is freed; if the heart wall tears, a cardiovascular emergency ensues.

Countertraction is the countering of traction force by the countertraction sheaths. Countertraction focuses the traction force at the electrode-myocardial interface; it prevents eversion of the right ventricle and allows only the tissue surrounding the electrode to tear, freeing the electrode.

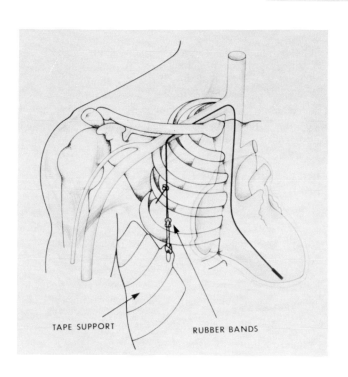

TAPE SUPPORT   RUBBER BANDS

FIGURE 28–14. Direct traction is being applied by pulling on the proximal portion of the lead. Rubber bands are used in this case. Variations include using free weights and weights applied using an orthopedic traction apparatus. If a locking stylet is inserted, the traction point is moved distal to the locking site, usually near the electrode.

tion is not required for this type of direct traction. Traction may be applied for lengths of time ranging from minutes manually to days using various weights or elastic bands.[43–45]

Most direct traction techniques try to apply sufficient force to feel the rhythmic tugging of the heart without producing arrhythmias, hypotension, or chest pain. The force applied is limited by the tensile strength of both the lead and the tissue. Exceeding this force results in a broken lead, a tear of a vein, or an avulsion or tear of the heart wall.

Another danger is the inability to relax the tension placed on a ventricular lead once the traction is removed. If the lead is withdrawn some distance but the electrode is not freed from the myocardium, the lead may become bound so that it cannot return to its original position. If the ventricular wall is pulled toward the tricuspid valve during traction, it causes a decrease in blood flowing into the ventricle and a low cardiac output. If the lead is bound in its withdrawn position, the reduced blood flow causes a cardiovascular emergency.

Successful removal of the lead from the heart wall may terminate with the lead wedged within fibrous tissue in the atrium or in a superior vein. An infected lead must be removed. If a part of the lead protrudes distally, it can be snared and removed. For example, a Dotter basket snare or a loop inserted through the femoral vein is frequently successful. If the snare fails, cardiovascular surgery is the only option.

Applying excessive traction to dislodge a lead wedged in a vein may tear the vein or break the lead. Parts of a broken lead may become dislodged and float freely in the bloodstream. The density of the material influences its behavior. Segments of lead body are usually moved by the blood flow and tend to migrate into the pulmonary artery. Pieces of metal such as the electrodes tend to fall under the influence of gravity and migrate into a dependent position.

DIRECT TRACTION ON A LOCKING STYLET

Recently, locking stylets have become available. The stylet is passed down the lumen of the conductor coil and locked in position, and traction is applied to the locking site. Ideally, the stylet is passed down to the lead tip. If this is not possible, it is locked at the most distal point of passage. Only if the stylet is passed to the electrode is this mode of traction different from pulling on the proximal portion of the lead. Traction on a locking stylet can also be applied for minutes to days.

Traction on a stylet locked at the electrode allows the applied force to be delivered to the electrode. Applying the force at the electrode helps maintain the integrity of the lead but does not by itself eliminate the complications associated with traction. More leads will be removed intact, but the risk of the proximal binding sites absorbing the force or binding a withdrawn lead is still present. Electrodes that are successfully freed from the heart wall may still become impacted in the fibrous tissue within the atrium or a superior vein, and the tensile strength of the heart wall and lead still limit the amount of force that can be applied.

Many companies have tried to develop a locking stylet. Initially attempts were made to develop universal stylets that would fit any size of lead lumen—one size fits all. These attempts failed because of the engineering complexities and cost constraints involved in making such small devices with a tensile strength sufficient to withstand extraction forces. Cook Pacemaker Corporation abandoned this approach and developed the first successful locking stylet, making individually sized stylets for each size of lumen.[46] The technique for using the Cook locking stylet is described later in the section on countertraction. The only limitation of individually sized stylets is the need to maintain an inventory of all sizes for each lead extraction. Although these stylets are reversible, the lumen will probably be damaged with use and is not reusable.

A new universal stylet made by VascoMed (Weil am Rhein, Germany) is being used in Europe.[47] The stylet is reported to have sufficient tensile strength to support lead extractions. I have had no experience with this device. The mechanism for locking consists of two flanges that are forced open and become entrapped within the conductor coil. This locking mechanism is also reported to be removable using a motorized tool.

INDIRECT TRACTION

Indirect traction is traction applied by an instrument such as a snare passed into the heart, usually through a femoral vein. The lead is entrapped in the snare, and traction is applied by pulling or pushing.[48–54] The safety of this technique is enhanced by avoidance of those problems associated with the binding sites in the superior veins and right atrium. Also, it is more successful than direct traction. The difficulty lies in grasping the lead in a fashion that allows sufficient traction to be applied. Only a few snares, such as the Dotter basket snare, have sufficient strength to support extraction forces. Techniques for applying chronic indirect traction safely have not been developed.

The lead must be freed from the superior veins and the heart. One technique is to pull the lead out of the superior veins into the atrium or IVC. The lead is then regrasped and traction is applied to the heart. The techniques used for applying indirect traction are the same as those required for grasping and manipulating the leads used in the countertraction approach and are described in the discussion on countertraction.

Indirect traction has the same potential for breaking the lead or tearing the heart wall as direct traction if their tensile strength is exceeded. However, the risks eliminated by this approach are tearing of the superior veins, wedging the lead in the atrium or in a superior vein, and creating a low cardiac output owing to failure of the lead to return to its original position following traction.

INTRAVASCULAR COUNTERPRESSURE OR COUNTERTRACTION TECHNIQUES

A series of transvenous and thoracic surgical procedures have been developed using countertraction. Countertraction extraction approaches include the SVC, IVC, and transatrial (TA) approaches.[23–25, 55–57] To date, cardiopulmonary bypass has not been necessary. The majority of leads can be removed using the transvenous SVC and IVC approaches individually or in combination. In some situations, both the SVC and IVC approaches fail, and countertraction is applied through a TA approach using a small anterior thoracotomy.[24, 25, 58]

Countertraction is a method of safely extracting an elec-

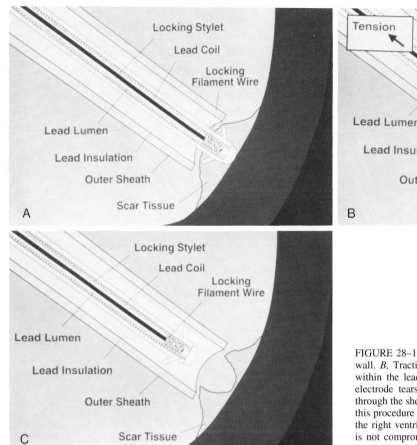

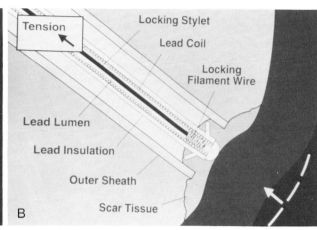

FIGURE 28-15. *A,* The countertraction sheath is placed near the heart wall. *B,* Traction is applied by pulling on the locking stylet anchored within the lead near the electrode. The sheath is not moved. *C,* The electrode tears out of the encapsulating scar tissue and is removed through the sheath. The heart wall returns to its original position. During this procedure tension is not applied to the heart wall, the compliance of the right ventricle is not changed, and the orifice of the tricuspid valve is not compromised. In my experience countertraction is safe and has not damaged the heart.

trode entrapped in fibrous tissue at the electrode-myocardial interface (Fig. 28–15). It is defined as countering the traction on the lead by a sheath. A sheath of slightly larger diameter is passed over the lead to a point approximately 1 cm from the heart wall. Traction is applied on the lead, pulling the myocardial wall to the edge of the sheath, which counters the traction. The edge of the sheath must be blunt; a sharp edge could inadvertently cut myocardial tissue or cut the lead and cause it to break.

Countertraction applied to the heart wall at the electrode-myocardial interface focuses the force perpendicular to the heart wall. Because only scar tissue is present between the sheath and the heart wall, cardiac tissue is not in jeopardy. The amount of traction applied to the lead is limited only by the tensile strength of the lead. Because the traction is countered, the remainder of the heart wall is not subject to this force. Once sufficient traction has been applied, the electrode is torn out of the scar tissue at the electrode-myocardial interface and pulled up into the lumen of the sheath. When the electrode breaks free, the stationary countertraction sheath remains in the ventricular or atrial cavity and is no longer in contact with the heart wall. I do not believe it is possible to tear or perforate the heart wall if countertraction is applied at the myocardium perpendicular to the wall.

PREPARATION FOR PROCEDURE

Patients who are being prepared for a lead extraction are prepared for multiple approaches, including an emergency

cardiac surgical procedure. Although routine lead extractions do not require surgical intervention, a complication such as tearing a large vein or the heart wall may precipitate a cardiovascular emergency. These emergencies must be handled in an expeditious manner to ensure a successful resolution.

Preparations include general endotracheal anesthesia, shave, and preparation of both the chest and groin areas, ECG monitoring, insertion of an arterial line and a Foley catheter, and request for the presence of instruments for pacing and defibrillation, an electrosurgical unit, and a sternal saw for emergencies. Blood is typed and screened but not cross-matched.

TEMPORARY PACING LEAD. A temporary pacing lead is inserted in all patients needing a pacemaker. An exception is made for patients with an implanted permanent pacemaker whose leads are not to be extracted. Because of the maneuvering required to extract some leads, conventional temporary pacing leads are not used. Instead, a permanent unipolar or bipolar active fixation lead is implanted. If a unipolar lead is used, a temporary epicardial lead, the same kind as that used in cardiac surgery, is sutured into the skin over the deltoid muscle and used as an indifferent electrode. I use the less expensive unipolar lead, which fits directly into an external pacemaker without an adapter.

The active fixation lead is placed on the same side as the lead to be extracted, even if the pacemaker site is infected, to avoid contaminating the other side. It is inserted into the subclavian or internal jugular vein using standard introducer techniques. If the lead must be place on the opposite side, the internal jugular vein is used. The lead is secured in a reversible manner for the duration of the procedure.

FLUOROSCOPY. Fluoroscopy should be used to visually monitor all transvenous maneuvers. Most complications involving transvenous insertion and extraction can be avoided if the procedures are performed using fluoroscopy. This is especially true for extraction procedures. If the applied forces are misdirected, the heart or vein wall can be torn. Bleeding into the pleural cavity can be seen with fluoroscopy. The lead being extracted may break and the pieces may float in the bloodstream. If the break is seen immediately, the objects can be retrieved while in a large vein or in the right atrium. They may be difficult to remove if they become lodged in a vein in the head, liver, extremities, or lungs.

SUPERIOR VENA CAVA APPROACH

The SVC approach is the initial approach used by most physicians (Fig. 28–16). The SVC approach combines the pocket abandonment procedure with passage of the dilator sheaths to the electrode. In all cases, the leads are exposed,

débrided of inflammatory tissue, and freed from restraining sutures as part of the abandonment procedure. A locking stylet is passed to the electrode and locked. Stainless steel telescoping sheaths are passed over the lead entering the vein and then exchanged for the plastic sheaths. These sheaths are used to pass through the tissue binding sites to the electrode-myocardial interface. The electrode is extracted by applying countertraction, and the lead is removed through the sheaths. In general, if any difficulty is encountered in advancing the countertraction sheaths, the SVC approach should be abandoned.

The reasons for using the SVC approach are speed, less fluoroscopic exposure, and a high success rate for undamaged leads that have been implanted for less than 6 to 8 years. Almost all undamaged leads implanted for 8 to 10 years are extracted using this approach. The tensile strength at the tissue binding sites for older leads sometimes prohibits passage of the sheaths. In some cases, the amount of scar tissue continues to increase with time, and after 8 to 10 years, it starts to calcify. Consequently, the forces needed to advance the sheaths are greater, and the lead needs greater

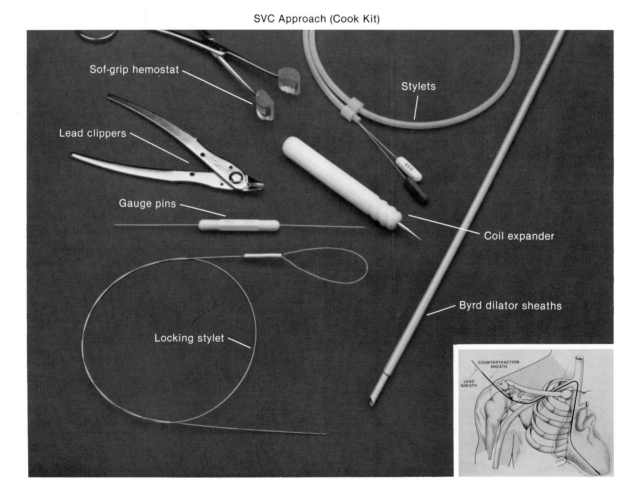

SVC Approach (Cook Kit)

Sof-grip hemostat

Lead clippers

Gauge pins

Locking stylet

Stylets

Coil expander

Byrd dilator sheaths

FIGURE 28–16. The superior vena cava (SVC) approach is currently the most common initial countertraction extraction approach used. The procedure is accomplished by inserting Byrd dilator sheaths over the lead and passing them through the implant site to the electrode. The Cook extraction kit is used for an SVC approach. Tools provided include a wire cutter, lead holder, conductor coil dilator, conductor coil sizing pins, locking stylet, and counterpressure-countertraction sheaths.

The *inset* shows the proximal portion of the lead exposed down to the vein entry site: the vein for a cephalic or external jugular venotomy approach, the pectoralis muscle for an introducer approach, and the tissue near the vein for an internal jugular approach. The counterpressure-countertraction sheaths are passed over the lead, through the vein entry site, and through the veins and heart to a site near the electrode.

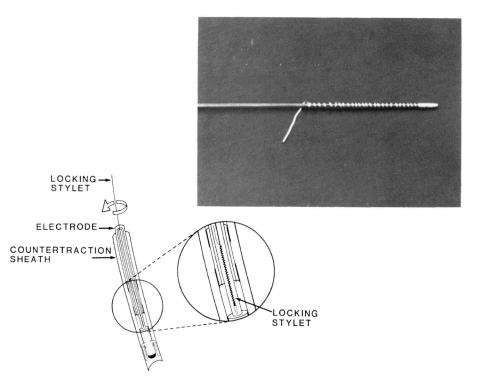

FIGURE 28–17. The locking stylet is passed ideally to the electrode and secured. The locking mechanism is a wire secured to the tip and wrapped around the stylet. When the stylet is turned counterclockwise, the wire bundles together, binding the stylet to the conductor coil. The locking stylet acts primarily as a lead extender for applying traction and secondarily as a means of keeping the lead intact during the extraction. When the stylet is positioned at the electrode, the lead has its best chance of remaining intact. If the stylet is positioned near the proximal end, the fragile leads would be pulled apart when traction is applied.

tensile strength to remain intact during the extraction. Leads implanted for 10 years or more and leads damaged in previous extraction attempts are the most difficult to remove and have the highest failure rate using this approach.

LOCKING STYLET

The development of locking stylets has greatly simplified the methods of applying traction. The locking stylet also functions as a lead extender and as a handle for applying traction, greatly reducing the extraction time and in most cases eliminating the need to improvise. Prior to the development of these stylets, traction was applied by grasping the lead and pulling. The tensile strength of the leads was usually not sufficient, and they broke when subjected to extraction forces. Broken leads were then removed in pieces, complicating the extraction procedure and frequently resulting in an incomplete extraction. Traction applied to a stylet locked within the lumen of the lead near the electrode resulted in extraction of more intact leads.

The Cook locking stylets are successful because of the simplicity and strength of the locking mechanism (Fig. 28–17). The locking mechanism is a small wire attached to the tip of the stylet and wrapped clockwise. To lock the stylet, it is turned counterclockwise, causing the small wire to bundle together, binding the stylet to the conductor coil. The locking does not weaken the conductor coil or reduce the tensile strength of the lead. It is possible to reverse this lock by forcing a clockwise rotation of the stylet, although forced removal of the stylet may damage the conductor coil and prevent insertion of another stylet.

To insert the stylet, the lead is cut, and the insulation is trimmed back to expose the conductor coil. For bipolar leads with coaxial conductors, the inner coil is isolated. The lumen of the conductor coil is measured with the measuring pins provided in the kit. The appropriately sized locking stylet is then advanced down the lumen. While advancing the stylet, if it is bound by a damaged conductor coil, clockwise rotation will sometimes screw the stylet through the area. If the locking wire is uncoiled and stretched, it may not bundle when rotated counterclockwise. To prevent this, the stylet should be advanced a few centimeters and then pulled back to bundle the wire, forming a loose reversible lock. This maneuver is repeated until the electrode is reached.

Failure to lock the stylet is usually caused by improperly measuring the lumen size and inserting too small a stylet. Success in passing the locking stylet depends on the condition of the conductor coil. If it is damaged, the stylet may only be passed to the site of damage. Although it is ideal to pass the stylet to the electrode, passage for any distance down the lumen provides a lead extender and traction handle that are superior to a suture attached to the outside of the lead.

BYRD DILATOR SHEATHS

Passage of the sheaths over the lead and down to the electrode is a prerequisite for applying countertraction. To reach a point near the electrode, the sheaths must pass through the fibrous tissue binding sites along the vein and heart wall. To safely pass the sheaths and prevent problems similar to those associated with direct traction, the proper sheaths and techniques must be used. The same sheaths are used for applying countertraction at the binding sites along the lead and for applying countertraction at the electrode-myocardial interface.

COUNTERPRESSURE AT THE BINDING SITES. Counterpressure is the pressure applied by the sheath to the tissue at a binding site countered by the tissue resistance (Fig. 28–18). The force applied to the fibrous tissue binding sites at the vein entry

Counterpressure

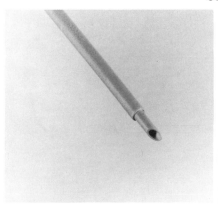

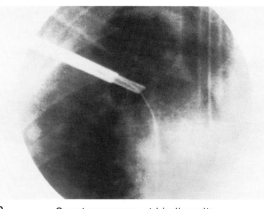

A   Byrd dilator sheaths   B   Counterpressure at binding site

FIGURE 28–18. Counterpressure is defined as the pressure applied (pushing) by the telescoping sheaths countered by tissue. Counterpressure is the opposite of countertraction; the sheath is pushed and the lead is used for support only. The Byrd dilator telescoping sheaths *(A)* are used to apply counterpressure. These sheaths are made of metal (stainless steel) and plastic (Teflon and polypropylene). The metal sheaths are used to pass through the soft tissue and the vein entry site. Once inside, they are replaced by the plastic sheaths.

A radiograph of the sheaths being passed to the right brachiocephalic vein is shown in *B*. The telescoping sheaths apply counterpressure at a binding site when they are manipulated and pushed against the binding site. When the applied pressure exceeds the tensile strength of the binding site, the binding site will dilate, tear, or peel (shear) off the wall.

point and along the veins and heart wall fundamentally differs from the force in countertraction as applied at the electrode-myocardial interface because the sheath is not stationary. It is pushed into the vein against the fibrous tissue at the binding site, creating pressure. The tissue resistance countering this pressure is a combination of the tensile strength of the fibrous tissue binding the lead and the strength of the vein or heart wall.

Counterpressure is applied tangentially as a shearing force. Properly applied, it dilates and tears the fibrous tissue or shears it off the wall. Shearing forces are not as safe as a force applied perpendicular to an electrode at the heart wall. If an excessive shearing force is applied, a misdirected tear may create a false passage that tears the vein or heart wall. Judgment and experience are required for safety.

To focus the pressure, the sheaths must be properly guided and supported. Direct traction on the lead is used to guide the sheaths along the lead, focusing the pushing force to the fibrous tissue binding the lead and not to the vein or heart wall. Direct traction should be limited to the amount needed to supply this support. If too much traction is applied to the lead, the traction has the same attendant risk associated with it as direct traction. If excessive traction is required, this approach should be abandoned. Judgment (common sense) and experience are required to avoid applying excessive force.

In some situations, countertraction may be used in the veins and along the heart wall. If the lead is firmly bound by fibrous tissue that prevents its being pulled through the binding site, countertraction is applied. Traction is applied to the lead and is countered by the sheaths at the bound site. This is a common occurrence when leads pass through chronically occluded veins. It is extremely difficult to pass the sheaths through these areas. If excessive force must be used, this approach should be abandoned.

USING THE COUNTERPRESSURE-COUNTERTRACTION SHEATHS. Sheaths passed over the lead and down to the heart must be strong enough to be forced through the scar tissue and supple enough to make sharp turns. The use of telescoping sheaths allows one sheath to work against the other. Various sizes of plastic sheaths are available; an 11-F inner sheath and a 16-F outer sheath are adequate for most leads. The inner sheath is supple and the outer sheath more rigid. To break through the scar tissue at the vein entry site a telescoping set of rigid

stainless steel sheaths is used. Once inside the vein, the stainless steel sheaths are changed to the flexible plastic sheaths.

STAINLESS STEEL SHEATHS. Telescoping stainless steel sheaths are passed over the lead in the subcutaneous tissue and used to break through the tissue at the vein entry site. The tissue at the vein entry site ranges from fibrous tissue capsule of varying tensile strength to bone. These sheaths were designed to allow a sufficient longitudinal force to be applied to just break into the vein. Both countertraction and counterpressure techniques are applied. We tried a single stainless steel sheath for a period of time, but it was difficult to use and was not as successful as the telescoping sheaths.

Fluoroscopic visualization is essential to follow the lead path and avoid creating a false passage. A false passage will not allow entry into the vein and may damage the lead. Once in the vein, these sheaths are exchanged for the more flexible plastic sheaths. Failure to change to the more flexible sheaths is potentially dangerous.

PLASTIC SHEATHS. The flexible telescoping sheaths are used for maneuvering around curves and forcing a way through the circumferential bands of fibrous tissue. Sufficient traction is applied to support the smaller supple sheath for maneuvering around curves in the vein. The smaller sheath then acts as a guide, supporting the advancement of the larger, more rigid outer sheath. Fluoroscopic visualization is again essential to avoid creating a false passage and tearing the vein or heart wall.

As the sheaths are advanced, fibrous tissue with a low tensile strength is dilated. As the tensile strength increases, the fibrous tissue is torn. After the circumferential bands of fibrous tissue begin to calcify, the sheaths cannot tear through the calcified tissue around the lead, but a larger diameter sheath can be advanced over it (inclusion). It peels the calcified bands off the vein or heart wall.

As previously noted, counterpressure subjects the tissue to a shearing force. The shearing force must be judiciously applied. I use the flexible Teflon sheaths, which are easier to maneuver around curves and limit the applied shearing force. If the counterpressure force is more than can be easily applied with these sheaths, this approach should be abandoned.

Passage of sheaths along the circuitous route down the lead to the heart is successful for most leads that have been implanted for 6 to 8 years or less. Leads implanted for a longer period of time are associated with an increasing incidence of extraction failure because of the tensile strength of the scar tissue. Old, large-diameter leads allow only one large-diameter sheath to be passed over them. The advantages of using telescoping sheaths are lost, and the incidence of failure to extract increases.

INFERIOR VENA CAVA APPROACH

The IVC approach is a more versatile approach (Fig. 28–19). The procedure is performed by inserting a sheath "work station" and extracting the leads through the sheath using snares. The IVC approach is the procedure of choice for extraction of broken or cut leads that are floating free in the veins, heart, or pulmonary artery and for leads passing through occluded veins. A grossly contaminated vein entry site is another indication. The SVC approach, in which sheaths are pushed through this contaminated debris, is unsafe. It has the potential for causing septicemia or showering

pulmonary emboli. The IVC approach is also used to treat the failures of an SVC approach. Physicians who have had extensive training in transfemoral catheter procedures may feel more comfortable in using it as their initial approach.

BYRD WORK STATION

The transvenous approach through a femoral vein requires a special sheath set that functions as an introducer, as a work station for the manipulation of snares, and as countertraction sheaths. The set consists of an introducer needle, guidewire, 16-F work station, 11-F tapered dilator, 11-F telescoping sheath, a Cook deflection snare, and a Dotter basket snare. The work station serves many functions. Initially, it acts as a protective sheath, preventing the insertion, withdrawal, and manipulation of the other sheath and snares from damaging the veins or heart. To prevent clot formation, the work station has a check-flow valve that continuously irrigates the sheath. The work station and snares form a reversible loop that is

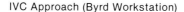

IVC Approach (Byrd Workstation)

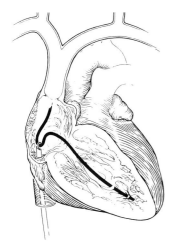

A   IVC approach

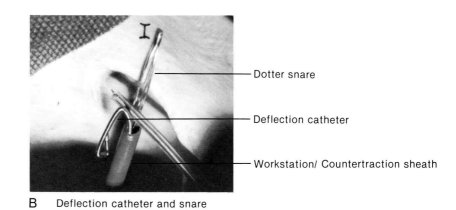

B   Deflection catheter and snare

Dotter snare

Deflection catheter

Workstation/ Countertraction sheath

Cook Deflection Catheter

Check-flow valve

Dotter (basket) snare

C   Byrd workstation

FIGURE 28–19. *A,* IVC approach. The work station is passed through a femoral vein into the heart. The lead is grasped by pulling the proximal end into the heart or IVC. *B* and *C,* Byrd work station. The work station consists of a 16-F Teflon sheath with a check-flow valve and IV site. Components are inserted into the work station as needed. For insertion a tapered dilator is used, and the work station is passed over guidewire (standard introducer approach) into the right atrium. The dilator is replaced by an 11-F sheath through which the Cook deflection catheter and Dotter snare *(B)* are passed. The deflection catheter and snare are used to maneuver the lead, form a reversible loop, and snare the lead for applying countertraction.

used to pull the proximal portion of the lead out of the superior veins; the work station also acts as the outer telescoping countertraction sheath.

INSERTION. The safe insertion and removal of the work station is a prerequisite to extraction of the lead through a femoral vein. The work station is 16 F in size and must be inserted with care. Fluoroscopic monitoring is mandatory. Once the guidewire has been passed into the heart, the work station with its tapered dilator must be maneuvered through the iliac vein, the IVC, and into the right atrium. The route can be circuitous, especially from the left side. In rare cases

the curvature may be too sharp for the stiff dilator to follow the guidewire. Forcing the dilator in this situation is unsafe, and the approach should be abandoned. A torn retroperitoneal iliac vein or IVC is a serious complication. Once the work station has been inserted, irrigation fluids are run continuously through the check-flow valve to prevent clotting.

REVERSIBLE LOOP. A reversible loop is created around the lead body to pull the proximal end of the lead out of the superior veins into the IVC without placing traction on the electrode-myocardial interface (Fig. 28–20). A loop must be created and bound to the lead body. It is mandatory for the

Reversible Loop

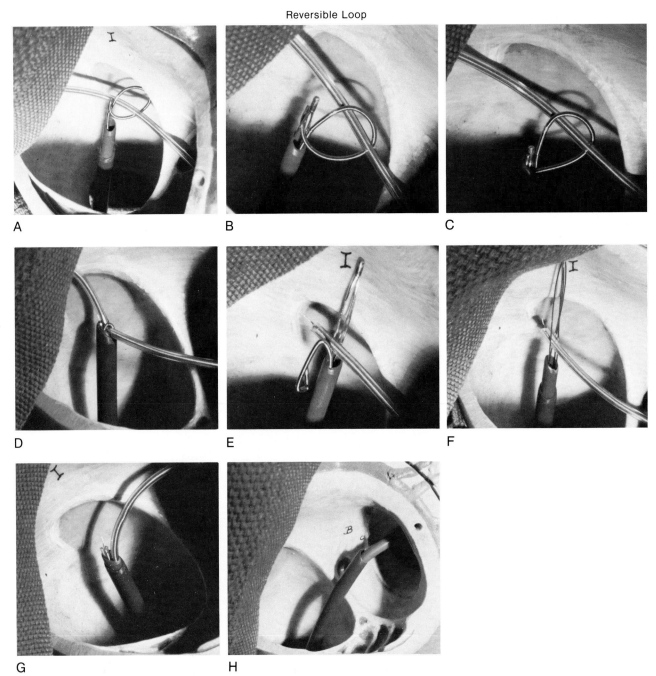

FIGURE 28–20. *A,* The Cook deflection catheter encircles the lead. *B,* The Dotter snare grasps the tip of the deflection catheter, forming a loop. *C,* The loop is pulled into the work station. *D,* The lead is bound and pulled out of the superior vein into the heart or IVC. *E,* The loop is reversed by pushing it out of the work station and separating the catheter and snare. *F,* The catheter is removed, and the proximal portion of the lead is grasped by the snare. *G,* The lead is pulled back into the work station. *H,* The 11-F catheter and work station are advanced into the heart to apply countertraction, extracting the lead.

binding and the loop itself to be reversible. Irreversible binding of the lead or an inability to remove the loop from around the lead may result in dangerous traction maneuvers being performed in desperation in an attempt to extract the lead and the snare. Failure to extract the lead subjects the patient to more invasive procedures to remove both the lead and the snare.

Creating a reversible loop using two snares is a complicated maneuver that requires practice to perfect. One technique is to use a Cook deflecting wire guide and a Dotter basket snare. The Cook deflecting wire guide is wrapped more than 360 degrees around the lead body. Next, the tip of the deflection catheter is passed into the Dotter basket snare. Pulling the basket snare into the work station causes the basket to close, grasping the deflection catheter and completing the loop. The loop is then pulled into the work station, tightly binding the lead body to the work station, and traction is applied. If needed, the loop is relaxed and repositioned on the lead body. This sequence is repeated until the lead is pulled out of the superior veins, through the right atrium, and into the IVC. The reversible loop is then released and the deflection catheter is removed.

PULLING THE LEAD DOWN AND OUT OF THE SUPERIOR VEINS. The removal of leads by pulling them down and out of the superior veins has been remarkably successful. Many leads freed from the heart cannot be pulled up through these same veins. Lead binding by the circumferential bands of fibrous tissue is the same in both directions. The hypothesis for this difference in maneuverability is the free upward mobility of the mediastinal structures. The mediastinum is easily pulled upward, compressing the veins, but is limited in its downward motion. Compression of the fibrous tissue bands around the lead as they bunch together is thought to increase their binding strength.

Failure to extract the proximal lead from the superior veins using this technique is rare and is usually caused by other complicating factors. Examples of such factors are thrombosis of the superior veins and excessive fibrosis around the lead caused by a previous extraction attempt that left the conductor coil exposed or pulled the lead taut against the heart and vein wall. These leads can be removed using approaches such as the transatrial approach, which is reserved for more complicated extractions.

COUNTERTRACTION. To apply countertraction through the work station, the proximal end of the lead must be entangled in the basket snare. This is accomplished by placing the basket snare in close proximity to the lead and rotating it slowly. The lead will flip into the basket. The basket closes by advancing the 11-F sheath over the snare. For most leads, the snare and lead are pulled into the 11-F sheath. The work station and 11-F sheath are then worked in a telescoping fashion to a point near the electrode. At this point, countertraction is applied to extract the electrode as previously described.

REMOVAL. Removal of the work station must be performed carefully. Once the lead has been extracted, clot and debris may be attached to the end of the tubing. If this material dislodges in the femoral vein entry site, it can act as a nidus, forming a thrombus or initiating thrombophlebitis and its sequelae. To prevent this complication, blood is aspirated during the withdrawal of the work station. If the entry site does not bleed freely following withdrawal of the work station, a surgical exploration of the vein is recommended.

Bleeding is controlled by applying slight pressure over the vein entry site. A suture is required to close the skin.

The risk of developing thrombophlebitis and a subsequent pulmonary embolus after an IVC approach was the stimulus for creating the work station. The standard precautions are taken. Patients are given antiembolus stockings (pneumatic, if possible), and subcutaneous heparin (5000 units twice a day) is administered.

PRECISION. The techniques required for grasping the lead in a reversible loop using a Cook deflection catheter and a Dotter snare are more complicated. Once mastered, however, they comprise an effective method of performing a precision extraction. For example, a patient may have six leads in the heart. Two new leads are connected to a pacemaker and are to be saved. Four leads are abandoned and are to be extracted. The abandoned atrial and ventricular leads can be extracted, leaving the newly implanted leads intact. The IVC approach allows this level of precision.

TRANSATRIAL APPROACH

The transatrial approach is a cardiovascular surgical procedure that was first described by our group in 1985.[58] It is a primary approach used for noninfected patients who are candidates for a transatrial lead implantation. In younger patients with occlusion of one brachiocephalic vein or with an SVC syndrome the old leads are extracted through a transatrial approach and new leads are then implanted. The advantage of the TA approach is that it offers the ability to remove leads not accessible or removable by the SVC or IVC approach. Most transatrial extractions are performed in patients in whom the IVC approach has failed. Rarely, a failure with an SVC approach will go directly to a transatrial approach, for example, in situations when the work station cannot be passed through the femoral veins into the heart. In infected patients who are candidates for transatrial lead implants the old leads are extracted using an SVC or IVC approach, and the transatrial implant is performed after the infection has been properly treated.

PROCEDURE

The transatrial approach is performed as originally described, using a limited surgical approach (Fig. 28–21). The right atrium is exposed by removing the third or fourth right costal cartilage. The pericardium is opened and suspended, and a pledgeted pursestring suture is placed in the right atrium. Using fluoroscopy, a pituitary biopsy instrument is inserted through the pursestring, and the lead body is grasped and pulled out of the atrium. The lead is then cut, extracting both the proximal and distal segments separately. The proximal portion can usually be pulled out by traction. On rare occasions the countertraction sheaths are required. The distal segment is extracted by inserting a locking stylet, advancing countertraction sheaths around the lead, and applying countertraction pressure at the electrode-myocardial interface. This procedure is repeated for each lead to be extracted.

THROMBUS OR INFECTED MATERIAL ATTACHED TO LEADS

The presence of large masses of vegetation connected to the leads is a current limitation of all extraction procedures.

Transatrial

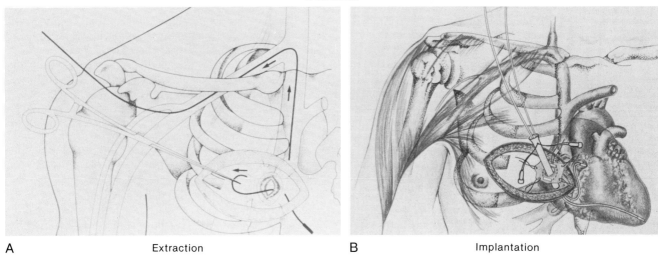

A   Extraction   B   Implantation

FIGURE 28–21. *A,* Extraction. The atrium is exposed through the third or fourth costal cartilage. Through a pursestring suture the lead is grasped using a pituitary biopsy instrument and pulled out of the atrium. The lead is then cut, and the proximal portion is removed using direct traction, and the distal portion using countertraction. *B,* Implantation. An introducer sheath is placed in the atrium, and a pacing or defibrillator lead is implanted as indicated.

Passing sheaths over the lead will shear the vegetation from the lead, causing a pulmonary embolus. This is a dangerous maneuver if the mass is large or if it is infected. Some of these large masses are thrombi that have formed on the lead. Systemic heparin frequently results in dissolution of the thrombus and is tried first if the patient's condition permits. Techniques for extraction of these leads along with the vegetation are being evaluated but have not yet been perfected.

PATIENT MANAGEMENT

Following transatrial extraction, patient management is more involved than that needed with the transvenous extraction techniques. The pericardium must be drained in most cases by a closed drainage system such as a Jackson-Pratt drain. The thoracic cavity is occasionally entered, and a chest tube is inserted to drain both the pericardium and the pleura. These drainage tubes are removed in 2 to 3 days. Although morbidity is not great, the hospital stay is increased by 1 or 2 days.

VENTRICULOTOMY

A lead that must be extracted by this approach is considered a failure of conventional extraction techniques. A ventriculotomy is a cardiovascular surgical procedure (Fig. 28–22). It is reserved for infected broken leads that are not reachable by other means or is used in conjunction with an emergency repair of the heart wall. Some leads are fragile, and if they break near the ventricular wall or within a fibrous tissue tunnel along the ventricular wall, they are impossible to grasp using transvenous or transatrial techniques. If the heart wall tears during an extraction attempt, the lead is extracted through a ventriculotomy following median sternotomy and repair of the tear.

The heart is exposed through a median sternotomy incision. It is then elevated on a pad, exposing the right ventricle. The tip of the electrode is localized by fluoroscopy and by needles used for triangulation of the electrode. A pursestring suture is placed around the electrode, and a ventriculotomy incision is made to the electrode. The electrode is grasped with a clamp and pulled out of the heart.[59] Because the lead segment is being pulled in the direction of the tines, the tines slip out of the embedding scar without resistance.

EMERGENCY SURGERY

Cardiovascular emergencies occur when a vein or the heart wall is torn, resulting in a life-threatening hemorrhage. Bleeding into the pericardium causes tamponade. Marked bleeding with rapid onset of tamponade is treated by an immediate median sternotomy and surgical repair of the torn

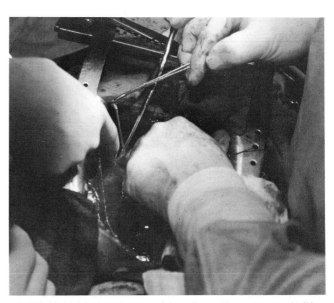

FIGURE 28–22. The heart is exposed through a median sternotomy incision. The electrode is located by palpation and triangulation using fluoroscopy. A pursestring suture is applied, and the electrode is grasped through a small ventriculotomy incision removing the electrode and lead. Cardiopulmonary bypass is not required.

heart or vein wall. To achieve a successful result, contingency plans must be made to treat these complications in an expeditious manner.

Tearing the vein extrapleurally or in the extrapericardial portion of the mediastinum probably will not cause a problem owing to the low venous pressure. Tearing the vein wall and puncturing the pleural cavity is a potential complication of lead extraction procedures and is caused by pushing the sheaths and creating a false passage. Tearing outside the vein and into the pleura can result in a life-threatening hemorrhage into the pleural cavity. Emergency surgery is the treatment. These surgical approaches are generally more difficult, and the approach used depends on the location of the tear. A tear in the subclavian vein is the most difficult to access. The safest approach is probably a median sternotomy. The brachiocephalic veins can be reached through this incision. The subclavian vein is approached by combining this incision with an anterior thoracotomy through the second intercostal space, creating an anterior superior chest wall flap.

BYRD DATA BASE

I have extracted more than 600 leads using countertraction techniques. Analysis of these approaches is based on a consecutive series of 481 leads extracted from 264 patients taken from my own data base. The indications for the procedure are shown in Table 28–4. The average patient age was 66 years and ranged from 10 to 97 years. Of the 481 leads, 63% were ventricular and 37% were atrial. The mean implant time was 62 months ± 46 months and ranged from 5 days to 264 months. Using intravascular countertraction, 476 (99%) leads were removed: 72% using SVC only, 10% using IVC only, and 18% using SVC followed by IVC. The total percentage

of lead extractions using the IVC approach was 28%. In addition, in 9% of extractions the distal tip of the lead, usually just the electrode, remained embedded in the scar tissue at the electrode-myocardial interface. Leads breaking at the tip have not caused a problem to date.

A recent series of 415 leads extracted using countertraction procedures showed that 95% of the leads were removed using intravascular techniques and 5% using the TA approach (Fig. 28–23). The increase in the use of the TA approach reflects the increased number of TA pacemaker implants performed. This percentage will probably increase in the future. The relative percentages of extractions using the SVC and IVC approaches did not change.

SVC APPROACH

The SVC approach was used initially to remove 364 (88%) leads out of a total of 415; 293 (80%) were successfully extracted, and 71 (20%) were failures. Of the 71 failures, 57 (80%) occurred because of excessive scar tissue and 14 (20%) because the lead broke. All of the leads in the failed attempts were successfully extracted using the IVC (67) or the TA (4) approach. There were two complications (0.5%) using this approach. There was one tear of the SVC and one tear of the IVC-atrium.

IVC APPROACH

The IVC approach was the initial approach used for 40 (10%) leads of the total 415. Indications for using the IVC approach were inaccessibility of the leads (96%) and thrombosis of the superior vena cava (4%). Sixty-seven of the failed SVC lead extractions were associated with an IVC

Byrd Database - Extraction Approaches for 415 Leads

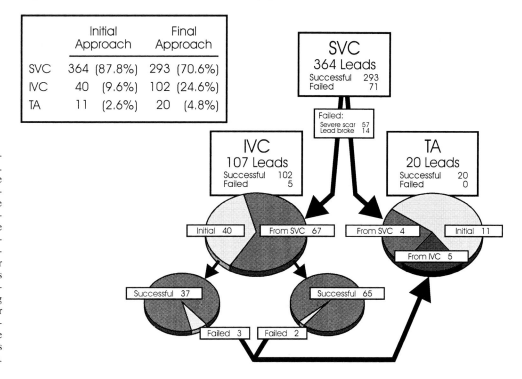

	Initial Approach	Final Approach
SVC	364 (87.8%)	293 (70.6%)
IVC	40 (9.6%)	102 (24.6%)
TA	11 (2.6%)	20 (4.8%)

FIGURE 28–23. Extraction approaches for 415 leads are presented. All leads were extracted using the SVC, IVC, or transatrial (TA) approach. The SVC approach was the initial approach used whenever possible (88%). Leads abandoned in the superior veins and leads in thrombosed superior veins were approached through the IVC (10%) or TA (3%). The initial TA patients plus those in whom the SVC approach failed included mostly young patients with thrombosed superior veins. The remainder of the TA extractions comprised failures of the IVC approach and consisted of leads implanted for longer periods of time.

extraction attempt, bringing the total IVC procedures to 107 (26%). Of these leads, 102 were successfully extracted and 5 were failures. Leads in the 5 failed attempts were extracted using the TA approach. There was one tear of the IVC using this approach.

TRANSATRIAL APPROACH

The TA approach was used as a primary route of extraction for 11 (3%) leads out of 415 in patients who were candidates for a TA lead implant. To this number were added 4 failed SVC extraction leads and 5 failed IVC extraction leads, for a total of 20 (5%) leads extracted using the TA approach. All of the TA extractions were done in patients who had TA implants. If these leads could have been safely extracted by another approach, some of the patients would not have had to undergo a TA implantation. For example, in one patient a broken lead from a previous extraction attempt was pulled taut against the heart and vein walls. The lead was completely encased in fibrous tissue and could not be grasped using a snare. The TA approach was necessary to manually remove the fibrous tissue from a section of the lead so that it could be grasped and removed intact. All lead extractions attempted using this approach were successful, and there were no complications.

VENTRICULOTOMY

To date, three patients with septicemia have had electrodes embedded in the heart; these were removed through a ventriculotomy following attempted lead extraction. Two leads broke, leaving a small segment in the heart. The septicemia recurred, and the lead segments were removed electively. One 20-year-old unipolar lead was removed immediately because the lead pulled apart, and the IVC was lacerated by the conductor coil. All leads were successfully extracted without further complication.

TEAR OF THE HEART OR VEIN WALL

Three patients experienced intrapericardial tears of the heart or vein wall (one of the SVC, one of the IVC, and one of the IVC-atrium). Two tears were inadvertent and progressed dramatically to cardiac tamponade. One patient was prepared for a ventriculotomy, and the IVC lead extraction attempt was pressed beyond known safety limits. All three patients underwent an emergency median sternotomy with surgical repair of the tears and had an uneventful recovery. Extractions of retained ventricular leads were accomplished in two patients during the repair. One lead was removed through an atriotomy and the other through a ventriculotomy as described previously.

DEATHS

Two patients died from pulmonary emboli following an IVC approach. Both patients had histories of thrombophlebitis, and one had documented pulmonary emboli. The latter patient was admitted to the hospital initially in cardiogenic shock following a pulmonary embolus. On recovery, the patient was found to have an infected pacemaker with positive blood cultures. The patient was transferred to our hospi-

tal for removal of the pacing system. Following lead extraction, the patient suffered a fatal pulmonary embolus. An autopsy showed an acute embolus superimposed on chronic emboli as the cause of death. The other patient had a history of thrombophlebitis and was transferred to our hospital a few days after a failed extraction attempt. This patient had positive blood cultures. The patient died a few days following the uneventful lead extraction procedure. A pulmonary embolus was suspected but not proved. An autopsy was not performed.

Except for these two patients, no other patient who underwent an IVC approach developed thrombophlebitis or pulmonary emboli. It is my conclusion that these deaths were caused by a concomitant disease process and were not related directly to the procedure. However, based on this experience, patients with a history of thrombophlebitis should probably have lead extraction performed using another approach.

NATIONAL DATA BASE (COOK)

A growing body of experience at many centers demonstrates the widespread effectiveness of intravascular extraction techniques. Intravascular lead extraction had been attempted for 1441 leads in 856 patients at 147 centers through March 1993.[60] Of the 1441 leads, 86% were completely extracted, 8% were partially extracted, and 6% failed. Success was correlated with shorter implant duration, physician experience, active fixation, and atrial lead placement (Table 28–7). Life-threatening complications occurred in 2.5% (Table 28–8). Five (0.6%) deaths resulted from hemopericardium (2), hemothorax (1), and pulmonary embolus (2). Nonfatal complications included hemopericardium (7), hemothorax (3), bacteremia after failed extraction (1), and migrating lead tip (2).

The SVC approach was used alone for 92% of leads that had been implanted for 1 year or less, 87% of leads implanted 2 to 4 years, 85% of leads implanted 5 to 7 years, and 70% of leads in place for 8 to 22 years. The IVC approach was used alone or following the SVC approach for 8% of the leads implanted for less than 1 year. Use of the IVC approach increased with implant duration, reaching 30%

TABLE 28–7. FACTORS AFFECTING LEAD EXTRACTION OUTCOME FOR 1441 LEADS (NATIONAL DATA BASE)

VARIABLE	EXTRACTION OUTCOME		
	COMPLETE (%)	PARTIAL (%)	FAILED (%)
Implant duration			
1 year	96.5	1.9	1.6
2–4 years	90.7	5.0	4.3
5–7 years	83.0	7.3	9.7
≥8 years	72.0	16.7	11.3
Experience			
First case	78.0	7.5	14.5
>20 cases	89.6	8.8	1.6
Fixation			
Screw	96.8	2.6	0.6
Tines	84.8	8.4	6.8
Placement			
Atrial	94.8	2.2	3.0
Ventricular	81.3	10.5	8.2

TABLE 28–8. POTENTIALLY LIFE-THREATENING COMPLICATIONS FOR 856 PATIENTS (NATIONAL DATA BASE)

NUMBER	PERCENTAGE	DESCRIPTION
9	1.05	Hemopericardium or tamponade (two deaths, one after ventricular perforation by temporary lead)
4	0.47	Hemothorax (one death)
2	0.23	Pulmonary embolism (one immediately after extraction; one 3 days after extraction; both fatal)
3	0.35	Myocardial avulsion (no sequelae)
3	0.35	Migrating lead fragment
1	0.12	Bacteremia followed failed extraction for pocket infection

for leads implanted 8 to 22 years. The TA approach was not performed on a national level.

Summary

Implantable electrophysiologic devices consisting of a pulse generator and leads are designed to be biocompatible. This general term implies that an accord is reached with the implanted tissue for an extended period of time (permanent implant). Unfortunately, these devices are not completely biocompatible. Tissue is injured acutely during the implantation procedure and chronically by device-tissue interactions. When these reactions are excessive, complications may develop. Although some complications continue to remain biocompatible (e.g., excessive inflammatory tissue and migration), others require surgical intervention (e.g., lead dislodgment, pocket hematoma, and wound dehiscence). Many complications are not biocompatible, and the device must be removed and a new device implanted at a remote site.

Management of electrophysiologic device-related complications requires a range of techniques, encompassing both invasive cardiology and cardiovascular surgery procedures. Techniques involving the implantation site include both salvaging and abandoning the site. Techniques involving the leads include repositioning the leads (for those of short implant duration) and extraction of leads (regardless of implant duration).

Some of these procedures can potentially tear the heart or veins, precipitating a life-threatening situation. To minimize the incidence of these complications and to ensure a satisfactory resolution, prior training in these procedures and the availability of appropriate surgical support, should a problem arise, are essential.

The goal of managing complications is to understand the mechanical, biologic, and technical factors responsible for their occurrence to allow design of biocompatible devices and development of complication-free implantation techniques.

REFERENCES

1. Hecker JR, Scandrett LA: Roughness and thrombogenicity of the outer surfaces of intravascular catheters. J Biomed Mater Res 19:381, 1985.
2. Gallin JI, Goldstein IM, Snyderman R (eds): Inflammation. Basic Principles and Clinical Correlates. New York, Raven Press, 1988.
3. Anderson JM: Inflammatory response to implants. ASAIO 11(2):101, 1988.
4. Saab SB, Jung JY, Almond CH: Retention of pacemaker electrode complicated by *Serratia marcescens* septicemia: Removal with total cardiopulmonary bypass. J Thorac Cardiovasc Surg 73:404, 1977.
5. Schoen FJ, Harasaki H, Kim KM, et al: Biomaterial-associated calcification: Pathology, mechanisms, and strategies for prevention. J Biomed Mater Res 22(A1):11, 1988.
6. Jara FM, Toledo-Pereyra L, Lewis JW, et al: The infected pacemaker pocket. J Thorac Cardiovasc Surg 78:298, 1979.
7. Goldman BS, Macgregor DC: Management of infected pacemaker systems. Clin Prog Pacing Electrophysiol 2:220, 1984.
8. Cohen TJ, Pons VG, Schwartz J, et al: *Candida albicans* pacemaker site infection. PACE 14:146, 1991.
9. Hartstein AI, Jackson J, Gilbert DN: Prophylactic antibiotics and the insertion of permanent transvenous cardiac pacemakers. J Thorac Cardiovasc Surg 75:219, 1978.
10. Kennelly BM, Piller LW: Management of infected transvenous permanent pacemakers. Br Heart J 36:1133, 1974.
11. Morgan G, Ginks W, Siddons H, et al: Septicemia in patients with an endocardial pacemaker. Am J Cardiol 44:221, 1979.
12. Firor WB, Lopez JF, Nanson EM, et al: Clinical management of the infected pacemaker. Ann Thorac Surg 6:431, 1968.
13. Muers MF, Arnold AG, Sleight P: Prophylactic antibiotics for cardiac pacemaker implantation: A prospective trial. Br Heart J 46:539, 1981.
14. Ramsdale DR, Charles RG, Rowlands DB, et al: Antibiotic prophylaxis for pacemaker implantation: A prospective randomized trial. PACE 7:844, 1984.
15. Bluhm GL: Pacemaker infections. A 2-year follow-up of antibiotic prophylaxis. Scand J Thorac Cardiovasc Surg 19:231, 1985.
16. De Lalla F, Bonini W, Broffoni T, et al: Prophylactic mezlocillin-netilmicin combination in permanent transvenous cardiac pacemaker implantation: A single-center, prospective, randomized study. J Chemother 2:252, 1990.
17. Rettig G, Doenecke P, Sen S, et al: Complications with retained transvenous pacemaker electrodes. Am Heart J 98:587, 1979.
18. Furman S, Behrens M, Andrews C, et al: Retained pacemaker leads. J Thorac Cardiovasc Surg 94:770, 1987.
19. Robboy SJ, Harthorne JW, Leinbach RC, et al: Autopsy findings with permanent pervenous pacemakers. Circulation 39:495, 1969.
20. Huang TY, Baba N: Cardiac pathology of transvenous pacemakers. Am Heart J 83:469, 1972.
21. Becker AE, Becker MJ, Caludon DG, et al: Surface thrombosis and fibrous encapsulation of intravenous pacemaker catheter electrode. Circulation 46:409, 1972.
22. Fishbein MC, Tan KS, Beazell JW, et al: Cardiac pathology of transvenous pacemakers in dogs. Am Heart J 93:73, 1977.
23. Byrd CL, Schwartz SJ, Hedin N: Intravascular techniques for extraction of permanent pacemaker leads. J Thorac Cardiovasc Surg 101:989, 1991.
24. Byrd CL, Schwartz SJ, Hedin N: Lead extraction: Indications and techniques. Cardiol Clin 10:735, 1992.
25. Byrd CL, Schwartz SJ, Hedin NB: Lead extraction: Techniques and indications. *In* Barold SS, Mugica J (eds): New Perspectives in Cardiac Pacing. Mt Kisco, NY, Futura, 1993, pp 29–55.
26. Choo MH, Holmes DR, Gersh BJ, et al: Permanent pacemaker infections: Characterization and management. Am J Cardiol 48:559, 1981.
27. Brodman R, Frame R, Andrews C, et al: Removal of infected transvenous leads requiring cardiopulmonary bypass or inflow occlusion. J Thorac Cardiovasc Surg 103:649, 1992.
28. Myers MR, Parsonnet V, Bernstein AD: Extraction of implanted transvenous pacing leads: A review of a persistent clinical problem. Am Heart J 121:881, 1991.
29. Parry G, Goudevenos J, Jameson S, et al: Complications associated with retained pacemaker leads. PACE 14:1251, 1991.
30. Marrie TJ, Nelligan J, Costerton JW: A scanning and transmission electron microscopic study of an infected endocardial pacemaker lead. Circulation 66:1339, 1982.
31. Lee ME, Chaux A: Unusual complications of endocardial pacing. J Thorac Cardiovasc Surg 80:934, 1980.
32. Mazzetti H, Dussaut A, Tentori C, et al: Superior vena cava occlusion and/or syndrome related to pacemaker leads. Am Heart J 125:831, 1993.
33. Yakirevich V, Alagem D, Papo J, et al: Fibrotic stenosis of the superior vena cava with widespread thrombotic occlusion of its major tributaries: An unusual complication of transvenous cardiac pacing. J Thorac Cardiovasc Surg 85:632, 1983.

34. Doty DB, Doty JR, Jones KW: Bypass of superior vena cava: Fifteen years' experience with spiral vein graft for obstruction of superior vena cava caused by benign disease. J Thorac Cardiovasc Surg 99:889, 1990.

35. Pauletti M, Di Ricco G, Solfanelli S, et al: Venous obstruction in permanent pacemaker patients: An isotopic study. PACE 4:36, 1981.

36. Toumbouras M, Spanos P, Konstantaras C, et al: Inferior vena cava thrombosis due to migration of retained functionless pacemaker electrode. Chest 82:785, 1982.

37. Dalal JJ, Robinson CJ, Henderson AH: An unusual complication of the unremoved unwanted pacing wire. PACE 4:14, 1981.

38. Dalvi BV, Rajani RM, Lokhandwala YY, et al: Unusual case of pacemaker lead migration. Cathet Cardiovasc Diagn 21:95, 1990.

39. Lassers BW, Pickering D: Removal of an iatrogenic foreign body from the aorta by means of a ureteric stone catcher. Am Heart J 73:375, 1967.

40. Wolfram T, Wirtzfeld A: Pulmonary embolization of retained transvenous pacemaker electrode. Br Heart J 38:326, 1976.

41. Madigan NP, Curtis JJ, Sanfelippo JF, et al: Difficulty of extraction of chronically implanted tined ventricular endocardial leads. J Am Coll Cardiol 3:724, 1984.

42. Jarvinen A, Harjula A, Verkkala K: Intrathoracic surgery for retained endocardial electrodes. J Thorac Cardiovasc Surg 34:94, 1986.

43. Bilgutay AM, Jensen MK, Schmidt WR, et al: Incarceration of transvenous pacemaker electrode: Removal by traction. Am Heart J 77:377, 1969.

44. Imparato AM, Kim GE: The trapped endocardial electrode. Ann Thorac Surg 14:605, 1972.

45. Kaizuka H, Kawamura T, Kasagi Y, et al: An experience of infected catheter removal with continuous traction method and silicon rubber wearing. Kyobu Geka 36:309, 1983.

46. Goode LB, Clarke JM, Fontaine JM, et al: Explanation of chronic transvenous pacemaker leads. PACE 12:677, 1989.

47. Alt E, Theres H, Busch U, et al: Entfernung von drei infizierten Elektro-
den mit Hilfe eines neuen Extraktionsstiletts: Ein Fallbericht. Herzschr Elektrophys 2:29, 1991.

48. Ramo BW, Peter RH, Kong Y, et al: Migration of a severed transvenous pacing catheter and its successful removal. Am J Cardiol 22:880, 1968.

49. Rossi P: "Hook catheter" technique for transfemoral removal of foreign body from right side of the heart. Am J Radiol 109:101, 1970.

50. Taliercio CP, Vlietstra RE, Hayes DL: Pigtail catheter for extraction of pacemaker lead. J Am Coll Cardiol 5:1020, 1985.

51. Foster CJ, Brownlee WC: Percutaneous removal of ventricular pacemaker electrodes using a Dormier basket. Int J Cardiol 21:127, 1988.

52. Zehender M, Buchner C, Geibel A, et al: Diagnosis of hidden pacemaker lead sepsis by transesophageal echocardiography and a new technique for lead extraction. Am Heart J 118:1050, 1989.

53. Kratz JM, Leman R, Gillette PC: Forceps extraction of permanent pacing leads. Ann Thorac Surg 49:676, 1990.

54. Deutsch LS, Dang H, Brandon JC, et al: Percutaneous removal of transvenous pacing lead perforating the heart, pericardium, and pleura. AJR 156:471, 1991.

55. Brodell GK, Castle LW, Maloney JD, et al: Chronic transvenous pacemaker lead removal using a unique, sequential transvenous system. Am J Cardiol 66:964, 1990.

56. Fearnot NE, Smith HJ, Goode LB, et al: Intravascular lead extraction using locking stylets, sheaths, and other techniques. PACE 13:1864, 1990.

57. Byrd CL, Schwartz SJ, Hedin NB, et al: Intravascular lead extraction using locking stylets and sheaths. PACE 13:1871, 1990.

58. Byrd CL, Schwartz SJ, Sivina M, et al: Technique for the surgical extraction of permanent pacing leads and electrodes. J Thorac Cardiovasc Surg 89:142, 1985.

59. Dubernet J, Irarrazaval MJ, Lema G, et al: Surgical removal of entrapped endocardial pacemaker electrodes. Clin Prog Pacing Electrophysiol 4:147, 1986.

60. Sellers TD, Smith HJ, Fearnot NE, et al: Intravascular lead extraction: Technique tips and U.S. database results. PACE 16:1538, 1993.

CHAPTER 29

Approach to Generator Change

Steven P. Kutalek
J. March Maquilan

At some time in the life of any pacemaker patient, replacement of the pulse generator must be considered. Although this is most often the result of the finite life span of the pacemaker battery, replacement of the device may be precipitated by such diverse causes as infection,[1-9] erosion,[10] trauma,[11-13] device malfunction or migration,[14-20] and the need for system upgrade[21, 22] (Table 29-1). Lead replacement or revision may also lead secondarily to generator change.[23-28] Although device or lead replacement includes surgery, the success of the surgery depends on an accurate preoperative evaluation as well as on good surgical technique. Therefore, this chapter addresses the preoperative evaluation of the patient and pacing system and the surgical process of device replacement.

Because of the variety of indications for pacemaker generator replacement, thought about the approach to be used for generator change begins at the initial implantation of the pacemaker system. Meticulous technique in the positioning of endocardial pacing leads to minimize pacing thresholds and maximize sensing capabilities allows optimal programming of the pulse generator to reduce chronic battery drain, thereby prolonging the life of the generator.[29] Careful lead positioning also reduces the likelihood of lead dislodgment that would require reoperation.[26, 27, 30, 31] Cautious venous entry, lead fixation, lead-generator connection, pocket location, and handling of components enhances long-term pacing function. Ensuring that coiled leads in the pacemaker pocket are placed posterior to the pulse generator improves the likelihood of expeditious pulse generator replacement without damage to the lead. Thus, the primary implanting physician prepares the stage for successful reoperation (Table 29-2).

Patient Evaluation

NONINVASIVE EVALUATION

Prior to performing a surgical procedure for pacemaker revision or generator replacement, the need for intervention must be documented. Specific indications are approached with a well-defined plan of evaluation.

DOCUMENTATION OF PULSE GENERATOR BATTERY DEPLETION. Most pulse generators provide direct or indirect indicators of various degrees of battery depletion, documenting the need for enhanced follow-up, elective generator replacement, or

TABLE 29-1. **INDICATONS FOR GENERATOR REPLACEMENT**

PRIMARY
Generator end of service
Unanticipated generator failure
Loss of output
Sensing malfunction
Generator upgrading
Unipolar to bipolar
Single to dual chamber
For rate modulation
Pocket twitch (especially unipolar)
Due to generator insulation break
Due to unipolarity of system
Device recall
SECONDARY[a]
Pocket relocation or generator migration
Pronounced pocket effusion or hematoma
Erosion
Infection of pacing system
Need for lead revision
High thresholds (pacing or sensing)
Lead conductor fracture
Lead insulation break
Trauma
Loose lead-generator connection
Myopotential sensing
Diaphragmatic pacing
Change bifurcated bipolar to unipolar pacemaker due to malfunction of one conductor
Twiddler's syndrome

[a]These are due to factors other than the pulse generator itself. They require reoperation but may or may not require generator replacement.

TABLE 29–2. TECHNICAL FACTORS AT INITIAL DEVICE IMPLANTATION THAT MAY REDUCE THE NEED FOR REOPERATION

> **TISSUES**
> Hemostasis
> Secure closure
> Pocket large enough for generator and leads
> **GENERATOR**
> Integrity of generator insulation
> Active surface toward skin
> Setscrews secure
> **LEADS**
> Meticulous care in positioning for
> Thresholds: pacing and sensing
> Fixation
> Lead selection appropriate for patient
> Integrity of lead insulation
> Gentle handling of stylets
> Secured by anchoring sleeve
> Placement posterior to pulse generator
> Appropriate connections (A, V) to generator
> Adapters secure and not kinked
> Setscrew sealed

TABLE 29–4. GENERAL MAGNET RESPONSES OF PULSE GENERATORS

> Battery depletion indicator
> Mode switch (DOO → VOO)
> Rate change
> Gradual
> Abrupt
> Mode
> AOO, VOO
> Usual asynchronous operation in single-chamber system
> May represent mode switch of battery depletion
> Noise reversion mode
> DOO
> Usual asynchronous operation in dual-chamber system
> AAT, VVT
> P, R synchronous
> OOO
> Inhibited, especially useful with antitachycardia system to avoid initiation of tachyarrhythmia with magnet application
> Rate
> Fixed
> Variable
> First few complexes faster
> Output
> Fixed
> Variable
> Voltage or pulse width decremented in first few complexes for threshold margin test, or pulse width reduced after magnet withdrawal
> Duration
> Continuous as long as magnet applied
> Fixed number of paced complexes

incipient battery failure. Additionally, certain nonspecific indicators may alert the physician to early signs of battery wear (Table 29–3). Since most pacemaker patients are followed via a transtelephonic monitoring system more frequently than by full evaluation in the physician's office, it is not surprising that battery depletion is most often detected through transtelephonic recording.[32–36]

A change in the magnet-activated paced rate remains the most common indicator of reduced battery output voltage (Table 29–4). Some pulse generator models show a gradual reduction in magnet-activated pacing rate; reduced rates indicate the need for enhanced follow-up, with still slower rates suggesting elective or obligatory replacement. Other models demonstrate an abrupt shift in the magnet-activated paced rate at the enhanced follow-up period or at the time of elective replacement. A demand mode switch from DDD to VVI (DOO to VOO in magnet mode) may occur at the elective replacement time or as an obligate replacement indicator for dual-chamber systems prior to complete battery failure (Table 29–5). In the office, other secondary parameters suggest gradual battery depletion. The usual battery impedance in a new pulse generator is less than 1000 ohms. As lithium iodide batteries are depleted, internal battery impedance increases, providing a secondary indicator (Fig. 29–1). With high internal battery impedance, some devices compensate for reduced current output by increasing the pulse width to

maintain adequate energy delivery to the lead tip. The degree of pulse width stretching is measurable and may be precipitated by high-output pacing; it serves as another secondary indicator of battery depletion. Replacement is not required, however, until more definitive indicators appear, such as a change in magnet-activated pacing rate or a mode switch.

Telemetered battery depletion curves (Fig. 29–2) or internal calculations of anticipated device longevity at current programmed settings as well as a general knowledge of the expected performance of various generators assist in anticipating and documenting pacemaker generator end of service. Ultimately, loss of sensing and pacing capabilities occurs with battery exhaustion.[17]

DOCUMENTATION OF LEAD MALFUNCTION. Various causes of

TABLE 29–3. BATTERY DEPLETION INDICATORS

> **PRIMARY**
> Abrupt decrease in magnet paced rate
> Gradual decrease in magnet paced rate
> Mode switch (especially DDD to VVI or DOO to VOO magnet mode)
> Abrupt loss of pacing or sensing capability
> **SECONDARY**
> Rise in internal battery impedance
> Fall in battery voltage
> Pulse width stretch
> Battery depletion curve

PACING RATE	60	PPM
PACING INTERVAL	1003	MSEC
CELL VOLTAGE	2.61	VOLTS
CELL IMPEDANCE	6.75	KOHMS
CELL CURRENT	20.9	UA

	ATRIAL (Uni)	VENTRICULAR (Uni)	
SENSITIVITY	1.6	1.5	MV
LEAD IMPEDANCE	613	504	OHMS
PULSE AMPLITUDE	2.49	4.97	VOLTS
PULSE WIDTH	0.50	0.50	MSEC
OUTPUT CURRENT	3.8	9.3	MA
ENERGY DELIVERED	4.4	20.8	UJ
CHARGE DELIVERED	1.94	4.66	UC

FIGURE 29–1. Acquired telemetry data from Intermedics Cosmos II 284-05 dual-chamber (DDD) pacemaker programmed to the unipolar mode. Cell impedance has increased to 6750 ohms, a secondary indicator of battery depletion. Pulse amplitude and pulse width are maintained. Lead impedances in both chambers are acceptable.

TABLE 29–5. **EXAMPLES OF SPECIFIC MAGNET RESPONSES**

MANUFACTURER	MODEL	MODE			RATE (ppm)			OUTPUT (≤ERI)	DURATION OF MAGNET RESPONSE
		BOL	ERI	EOL	BOL	ERI	EOL		
Biotronik	178	DOO	VDD	VOO	PR	PR minus 11%(AD)	PR 11%	PO	Cx
Cardiac Control Systems	505	DOO	DOO	VOO	80[a]	80–70(AD) (alternate cycles)	50	PO	Cx
Cook	500	VOO	VOO	[d]	100	90(AD)	[d]	PO	Cx
Cordis	233GL	DOO	DOO	VOO	70	62.5(AD)	52.5[b]	PO	Cx
CPI	936	DOO	DOO	[d]	100	85(GD)	[d]	PO	Cx
ELA	6034	DOO	DOO	DOO	96	80(GD)	69.8	PO[e]	Cx
Intermedics	294–03	DOO	VOO	[d]	4C @ 90, then PR	90–80[f](AD)	[d]	PW ↓ 50% on 4th C	Fx (60 C)
Medtronic	7086	DOO	VOO	[d]	3C @ 100, then 85	3C @ 100, then 65(AD)	[d]	PO; PW ↓ 25% on 3rd C	Cx
Pacesetter	2028L	DOO	DOO	[d]	PR	PRI plus 100 msec(AD)	[d]	PO	Cx
Telectronics	1250H	VOO	VOO	VOO	91.1[c]	≤78(GD)	63.3	PO	Cx

[a] 80 ppm × 16C, then PR for 16C, then 80 ppm.

[b] 62.5 ppm for serial numbers ≥4000.

[c] Magnet response in rate-responsive mode is valid after 18 seconds of magnet application. Magnet rate of 91.1 valid for DDD and DDDR programmed modes.

[d] No specific additional EOL indicator before battery failure.

[e] Output is increased to 5.0 V and 0.49 msec (if programmed less than these values) during magnet application, then is reduced to PO for 6 complexes at the magnet rate after magnet removal with shortening of the AV interval.

[f] Intensified follow-up indicator is 90 ppm, ERI is 80 ppm.

AD, abrupt decrease; BOL, beginning of life; C, complexes; Cx, continuous; EOL, end of life; ERI, elective replacement indication; Fx, fixed; GD, gradual decrease—indicated rate defines ERI; PO, programmed output; ppm, pulses per minute; PR, programmed rate; PRI, programmed rate interval; PW, pulse width.

lead malfunction may require reoperation[29, 37] owing to primary lead dysfunction or secondarily to premature battery depletion due to excessive battery drain (see Table 29–1). Primary lead malfunction may be due to outer insulation break,[38–44] inner insulation break in a bipolar lead,[45, 46] lead conductor fracture,[11, 13, 47] or lead dislodgment.[26, 27, 30, 31, 48] High pacing thresholds that increase current drain[23, 25, 49] or failure to optimize generator output for chronic pacing after lead maturation (about 3 months after implantation) can result in premature battery depletion. Before reoperation for lead malfunction is performed, consideration should be given to upgrading or replacing the pulse generator, especially if the battery is old.

Lead malfunction can usually be documented by noninvasive telemetric evaluation.[21, 50] A measured lead impedance below 200 ohms suggests an insulation break. An outer insulation break may be the result of lead wear or may have been inadvertently produced during surgery; an inner insulation break between the two coils of a bipolar system occurs most commonly at the subclavian insertion site as the result of crush injury to the lead, especially with leads inserted into the subclavian vein in a far medial position in patients with a tight clavicular–first rib space. Lead telemetry may demonstrate markedly low impedance in bipolar pacing in patients with an inner insulation break. The impedance varies with manipulation of the pacemaker, which causes intermittent shorting of the two lead conductors (Fig. 29–3).

High lead impedance (>1200 ohms) may be the result of lead conductor fracture or an incomplete circuit caused by a loose lead–pulse generator connection. The introduction of high-impedance leads makes it essential to compare the impedance at implantation with the follow-up impedances. Depending on the point of discontinuity, lead impedance may vary with manipulation of the pulse generator or with respiration. Lead conductor fractures may be evident on chest radiographs or fluoroscopy; however, absence of visual evidence does not exclude lead fracture. A break in the connection of the lead to the generator, or within the lead itself, can produce intermittent loss of energy delivery to the heart. This results in absence of pacemaker spikes. Undersensing, or oversensing due to chatter, may also occur with lead conductor fracture.

Lead dislodgment produces intermittent noncapture or failure to sense that may be related to respiration. Pacing thresholds needed to achieve consistent capture may increase significantly. Lead impedance increases or remains unchanged. Fluoroscopy may demonstrate a loose or displaced lead tip.

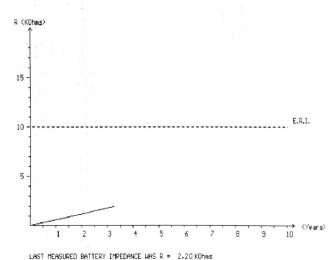

LAST MEASURED BATTERY IMPEDANCE WAS R = 2.20 KOhms

FIGURE 29–2. Example of a battery depletion curve from an Ela Chorus 6034 DDD pacemaker. The curve graphically presents the true increase in internal battery impedance (R) over time with an indication of the anticipated impedance at elective replacement time (ERI). Changes in programming that affect battery current drain alter the slope of the battery depletion curve.

PACING RATE	68	PPM
PACING INTERVAL	876	MSEC
AVERAGE CELL VOLTAGE	2.63	VOLTS
CELL IMPEDANCE	<1.00	KOHMS
SENSITIVITY	.8	MV
LEAD IMPEDANCE	41	OHMS
PULSE AMPLITUDE	7.42	VOLTS
PULSE WIDTH	0.45	MSEC
OUTPUT CURRENT	96.5	MA
ENERGY DELIVERED	173.2	UJ
CHARGE DELIVERED	42.85	UC
TACHYCARDIA DETECTED	NO	

FIGURE 29–3. Acquired telemetry data from an Intermedics Intertach 264-14 VVICP antitachycardia pacemaker connected through a bipolar coaxial lead to the right ventricular apex. Battery voltage and cell impedance are normal. Measured lead impedance of 41 ohms is, however, extremely low. In this patient, measured lead impedance was normal in the supine position but decreased with sitting or when the device was pulled inferiorly. This indicates a break in the inner insulator between the coaxial conductor strands in the area of the clavicle. With movement, the conductors contact one another, resulting in low impedance and preventing delivery of electric current to the heart. Because output voltage is fixed, the low lead impedance results in a high delivered current (96.5 mA) and energy.

DETERMINATION OF PULSE GENERATOR–LEAD INTERFACE MALFUNCTION. Pulse generator–lead interface problems can be grouped into three categories, as follows: (1) loose or improper connection, (2) reversal of atrial and ventricular leads in the pulse generator connector block, and (3) improper pulse generator–to-lead match.

A loose lead connection should become apparent by noninvasive testing. The device may fail to deliver pacemaker spikes when appropriate, it may intermittently fail to sense, or both of these can occur. Capture or sensing problems can be exacerbated by manipulating the device. A loose connection most commonly produces current leakage (an electric short circuit in the system) that inhibits pacing or sensing. This can occur if a setscrew is not properly insulated or tightened, or if sealing rings do not prevent body fluid from oozing into the pulse generator connector block around a loosely fitting lead. Leakage around sealing rings may result from a loose lead connection or lead–pulse generator mismatch. Lead impedance in pulse generator–lead interface problems varies, depending on the specific situation. A loose lead that remains in the pulse generator connector block, so that sealing rings prevent fluid from entering, causes a break in the electric circuit and thus a very high impedance. If fluid enters the pulse generator connector block around a loose lead, however, the resultant electric short circuit can produce a very low measured impedance. As with lead fractures, impedance can vary with manipulation of the device.

Reversed lead connections (i.e., atrial lead in the ventricular port, and vice versa) should be readily evident prior to leaving the implantation laboratory, allowing immediate correction. Some atrial and ventricular leads are marked to allow easy identification; however, it is not uncommon to place ''generic'' leads into both chambers, especially straight screw-in leads, which may not be so marked. It is also possible, in patients in whom the pacemaker remains inhibited because of intrinsic electric activity, to see no pacemaker spikes initially after implantation. To be certain that the pulse generator–lead system functions appropriately immediately after implantation, one should program the device to an atrioventricular (AV) delay shorter than the intrinsic PR interval, or place a magnet over the device after the leads are attached, to document appropriate function before the pocket is closed. Caution exercised at implantation should avoid reversed leads.

Beyond ensuring the presence of adequate and appropriate lead connections to the pulse generator, the battery connector block and leads must be compatible[51–53] (see later section). Incompatibility can result in fluid leakage or loose connections, with resultant loss of pacing or sensing capabilities, requiring reoperation.

DETECTION OF NEED FOR REOPERATION FOR OTHER REASONS. Other indications for generator replacement or lead revision (see Table 29–1) are generally apparent through careful patient evaluation. Abrupt pulse generator failure with no antecedent signs of battery depletion is rare but can occur, producing symptoms in pacemaker-dependent patients. In others, abnormal pacing output or rate, lack of pacing output, or inappropriate sensing due to generator malfunction may be detected transtelephonically or in the office.[17]

Development of pacemaker syndrome in patients with implanted ventricular demand (VVI), ventricular rate-responsive (VVIR), or atrial rate-responsive (AAIR)[22] pacemakers should be apparent through the history and physical examination, although confirmatory blood pressure or cardiac output measurements may be required. Documentation of hemodynamic improvement with dual-chamber synchronization may require placement of a temporary atrial lead prior to reoperation for upgrading to a dual-chamber system. Pacemaker syndrome occurring with an implanted functioning dual-chamber pacemaker must be managed by reprogramming.[54, 55]

Reoperation may be required for complications resulting from the initial implantation procedure.[10, 15, 16, 56–63] Decisions about surgery in patients with large unresolving pocket hematomas or effusions, cardiac chamber perforation by a pacing lead, or a need for repositioning of the pulse generator

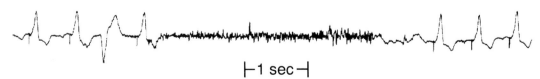

⊢1 sec ⊣

FIGURE 29–4. Myopotential inhibition in a unipolar dual-chamber pacing system induced by pectoral muscle contraction in a patient who noted recurrent lightheadedness with activity. Atrial sensitivity is programmed to 0.5 mV and ventricular sensitivity to 2.5 mV. Two atrially tracked complexes are followed by a ventricular premature depolarization. The fourth QRS complex occurs early owing to atrial myopotential tracking. Thereafter, ventricular pacing output is inhibited for nearly 6 seconds, after which normal DDD function resumes. Intrinsic QRS complexes occurring during the period of inhibition may be obscured by myopotential activity.

Programming the ventricular sensitivity to 5 mV avoided myopotential inhibition and the need for lead revision. Although atrial sensitivity could not be adjusted owing to the low intrinsic P-wave amplitude, atrial myopotential tracking remained asymptomatic.

must be made on an individual basis. Most small to moderate hematomas resolve; the risk of secondarily introducing infection through reoperation or aspiration can thus be avoided. Large hematomas or effusions that do not resolve and that compromise the blood supply through pressure on the overlying skin of the pacemaker pocket may require evacuation; however, primary closure should be attempted because the pocket cannot be left open with a device in place.

Pocket twitch (due to lead insulation break, loose lead-generator connection, exposed setscrew, battery insulation break, inverted unipolar pulse generator, or the need for high-output pacing in a unipolar system), diaphragmatic pacing, or myopotential pacing or inhibition[64] (Fig. 29–4) may also require repeat surgical intervention.

IDENTIFICATION OF PULSE GENERATOR MAKE AND MODEL (Table 29–6)

The most straightforward means of identifying a pulse generator showing signs of malfunction or operating in a mode suggestive of end of service is to obtain information directly from the patient. An identification card is provided by the manufacturer for each pacemaker patient, specifying the type of device, the model and serial number, implantation date, implanting or following physician, and often the lead model and serial numbers. This information may also be obtained from records kept by the implanting physician, following physician, transtelephonic service that follows the patient, or the institution at which the device was placed. If none of these sources of information is available, alternative methods must be used to identify the pulse generator. Identification of the make and model of the existing pulse generator is crucial to (1) determine its true functional status and (2) have the necessary information to select a replacement or upgraded device and/or compatible lead. In the rare situation in which a pulse generator cannot be identified before surgery, the implanting physician must have available a full array of leads, generators, and adaptors at the time of reoperation.

MAGNET RESPONSE. The response of a pulse generator to placement of a magnet adjacent to the device can assist in the identification of its manufacturer (see Table 29–5; Fig. 29–5). Most pulse generators respond to magnet application by entering a fixed-rate single- or dual-chamber pacing mode corresponding to the type of generator and the programmed mode. Magnet rates vary among manufacturers and may provide a clue as to the origin of the device. To properly perform a magnet-activated test, the patient must be connected to an electrocardiographic recorder *before* the magnet is applied and remain connected after the magnet is removed. The first few paced complexes after magnet application may occur at a rate or an output other than that seen later in the recording, providing critical identification data as well as information regarding the integrity of the pulse generator and lead system (e.g., the delivered pulse width may be reduced during the first few paced complexes). Furthermore, with constant magnet application over the pacemaker, some devices continue to pace at a fixed rate, while pacing ceases after a programmed number of intervals in others. Devices temporarily reprogrammed to a backup mode by electric interference (e.g., electrocautery during surgery) may exhibit magnet responses that vary from the standard for devices that are not in a backup mode.

X-RAY OR FLUOROSCOPIC IDENTIFICATION OF THE PULSE GENERATOR. Most pulse generators can be identified by their appearance under radiography. The shape and size of the generator may characterize a particular manufacturer (e.g., square, oval, elongated ellipse, round). Pulse generator shape can vary significantly from one device model to another, however, even when they are produced by the same manufacturer. Considering that the life span of some devices may exceed 10 or 12 years, various shapes and sizes will be encountered.

More specific to identification of the pulse generator are radiopaque markings placed near the connector block that code for manufacturer and device model. These markings appear under fluoroscopic or x-ray examination when the device is positioned perpendicular to the radiographic beam (Fig. 29–6).

The shape and orientation of internal components, which can often be identified, provide further clues as to the device type, manufacturer, and model. Comparison of these radiographic features (size and shape, identification markings, internal components) to compiled x-ray photographs available from manufacturers facilitates identification of the pulse generator.

X-RAY OR FLUOROSCOPIC IDENTIFICATION OF LEADS.[65] Radiographic examination of leads serves two purposes. First, it allows one to ascertain the presence of unipolar versus bipolar distal electrodes and, frequently, the fixation mechanism. Distal active fixation screws may be quite evident by their radiographic appearance, whereas passive fixation leads often demonstrate a bulbous tip. Second, radiographic examination identifies evident lead conductor fractures where the conductor has clearly separated, leaving a gap. Lead information of this sort is important for programming (bipolar vs. unipolar), for selecting an appropriate generator, and for lead extraction.

Radiography of leads must involve an examination of the

TABLE 29–6. IDENTIFICATION OF THE PULSE GENERATOR

IMPLANT DATA
ID card
Transtelephonic monitoring records
Implant or following physician's records

NONINVASIVE TESTING
Size, shape, thickness
Magnet response
Interrogation (if manufacturer identified)

FLUOROSCOPY
Size, shape
Connector block
Unipolar or bipolar
Single or dual chamber
Identifying markings/codes
Lead
Unipolar or bipolar
Active or passive fixation

INVASIVE
Direct identification of pulse generator
Lead
Manufacturer code
Type of connector

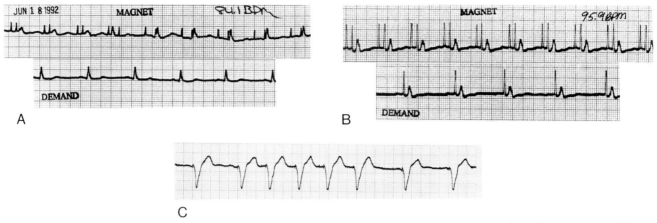

A

B

C

FIGURE 29–5. Examples of normal pacemaker generator magnet response. Tracings *A* and *B* were recorded transtelephonically during routine follow-up. Upper tracings in both *A* and *B* show magnet response (DOO), and lower tracings show demand mode with the magnet off. Tracing *C* was recorded by real-time surface electrocardiography at follow-up in the office.

A, Representative tracings from Medtronic dual-chamber pacing systems, here from a model 7070 Synergyst II device programmed DDD. The first three AV sequentially paced complexes are delivered at a rate 10% higher than the magnet rate; the AV interval is shortened to ensure both atrial and ventricular capture. The first two AV complexes are delivered at programmed atrial and ventricular outputs, whereas the delivered pulse width of the third complex is reduced by 25% ("threshold margin test"). Thereafter, the device delivers AV sequentially paced complexes at a fixed rate of approximately 85 bpm at programmed output. The device in this example remains entirely inhibited in the demand mode.

B, Representative tracings from Ela dual-chamber pacing systems, here from a model 6034 Chorus device programmed DDD. Magnet application results in fixed-rate DOO pacing at a rate of 96 bpm at the programmed AV interval. The AV interval in this example is short owing to activation of the rate-adaptive AV delay. Output during magnet application may be increased but reverts to programmed levels for six complexes after magnet withdrawal (see Table 29–6). The pacemaker appropriately tracks in the demand mode.

C, Representative electrocardiographic recording from Intermedics dual-chamber pacing systems, here from a model 294-03 Relay device programmed DDD. The first four complexes are delivered at 90 bpm with a shortened AV delay. Programmed pulse width for the fourth complex is reduced by 50%. Thereafter, the device delivers AV sequential paced complexes in a fixed mode (DOO) at the programmed rate while the magnet remains in place for a total of 60 AV complexes in the DOO mode.

insertion site (e.g., subclavian, cephalic, jugular) for acute bends or fractures in the lead, the location of lead coils beneath the pulse generator in the event they need to be freed for lead repositioning or extraction, the position of the pulse generator connector block, and a general preview of the character of the connector block–lead interface (see Fig. 29–6). Fluoroscopically, the lead should be examined throughout its course for kinking, fracture, or excessive tension as well as for fixation at the distal tip. A thorough x-ray examination

of lead integrity and pulse generator–lead interface prior to reoperation in pacemaker patients saves much distress when the pocket is opened.

INVASIVE EVALUATION

After as much information as possible has been gathered noninvasively regarding the hardware of the pacing system and functional status of all its components, further invasive

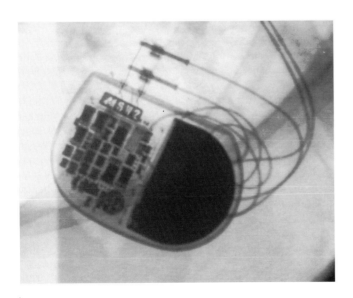

FIGURE 29–6. X-ray identification of a pulse generator. The unit is clearly connected to two leads, and each lead has only a single electrically active pole, i.e., unipolar. Although the shape and arrangement of electronic components assist in identification, the specific radiopaque code block inside the pulse generator provides the primary means of identifying the device. Here, a Medtronic logo, followed by *S W 2* indicates that the pulse generator is a Synergyst II model 7071 DDDR unit with a connector block that will accept two (atrial and ventricular) 5-mm or 6-mm unipolar leads.

evaluation may proceed at the time of reoperation. Invasive evaluation does not supplant noninvasive analysis but adds to it. Invasive evaluation involves (1) measuring the functional capacity of implanted leads, (2) examining the structural integrity of leads and the lead-generator interface, and (3) venography.

MEASURING THE FUNCTIONAL CAPACITY OF IMPLANTED LEADS. By far one of the most critical parts of invasive analysis during reoperation involves measurement of pacing and sensing thresholds in existing chronic leads. Vigorous noninvasive evaluation should provide the operator with a significant amount of information regarding lead viability and functional status as well as a determination of pulse generator end of life.[28, 29, 34, 42, 50] Verification of lead integrity and precise threshold determination must, however, be performed at reoperation. If surgery is undertaken for pulse generator replacement, demonstrating viability of existing leads is critical to the appropriate long-term performance of the new battery. Surgery for lead repair or revision itself involves extensive testing of chronic leads to (1) confirm the lead as the source of malfunction, (2) ensure normal operation of other leads, and (3) evaluate new leads for optimal positioning inside the heart.

After the pacemaker pocket is opened, the pulse generator is disconnected from the leads to enable testing of lead sensing and pacing functional capacity.[66] Disconnecting the lead from the pulse generator must be done cautiously in pacemaker-dependent patients; to avoid prolonged ventricular asystole, the operator must be prepared to immediately connect the lead to a cable attached to a functioning external pacing system. The external device should be activated and should be delivering pacing impulses before the ventricular lead is disconnected from the pulse generator in a pacemaker-dependent patient. Alternatively, although not usually necessary, a temporary pacing wire may be placed before disconnecting the lead in a pacemaker-dependent patient; such additional instrumentation, however, may increase the risk of infection.

The most important aspect of invasive testing involves measurement of pacing and sensing thresholds in chronically implanted leads. Chronic lead thresholds rarely remain as low as those at initial lead implantation. Most leads show some deterioration in thresholds over the first 4 to 8 weeks after implantation, then reach a relatively stable level for the long term.[23, 49] It is possible, however, for chronic thresholds to continue to increase over time, a change that may not be recognized by transtelephonic monitoring alone. The change in chronic threshold from baseline appears greatest with active fixation leads; threshold increases are reduced with passive fixation and steroid-eluting leads. Noninvasive testing should give the operator some clue as to the usefulness of chronic leads, but invasive testing confirms their functional utility.

Both atrial and ventricular leads must be tested. If bipolar, they should be evaluated in both unipolar and bipolar configurations. The external pacing analyzer is connected to the lead; pacing and sensing thresholds as well as lead impedance are determined. The voltage pacing threshold at a fixed pulse width is recorded as that which produces reliable capture. Delivered current can then be measured. Lead impedance is best determined at a high output voltage (e.g., 5.0 V) to ensure accuracy.

Low voltage pacing thresholds are desirable for chronic leads. This allows programming of the pulse generator output to a reduced level, ensuring battery longevity. For leads that have been in place for several years, the operator may decide to accept a pacing threshold (at 0.5 msec pulse width) of up to 2.5 V, since this provides a two-times pacing safety margin for most pulse generators and since chronic leads generally show little additional increase in threshold over time. However, a pacing threshold of 2.5 V that occurs early after implantation (e.g., within 6 months) may not be acceptable. This situation suggests excessive early fibrosis around the lead tip and the possibility of developing exit block and noncapture in the future if the pacing threshold continues to increase. Care at initial implantation helps ensure lower chronic pacing thresholds and improved sensing capabilities.

Thresholds for sensing likewise tend to increase after lead implantation. Acceptable measurable intracardiac electrogram amplitudes depend on the maximum programmable sensitivity of the new pulse generator. For most systems, P-wave amplitude of 1.0 mV or more and R-wave amplitude of 3.0 mV or more constitute minimally acceptable chronic values. Such low amplitudes, however, leave little room for further deterioration in lead function. Values of 1.5 mV or more and of 4.0 mV or more for P and R sensing, respectively, provide an additional safety margin. If atrial or ventricular ectopy is present, the operator should determine electrogram amplitude of ectopic complexes to ensure that they will be sensed by the pacemaker. In patients with paroxysmal atrial fibrillation, excellent atrial sensing may be required to reliably detect atrial fibrillation when it occurs. Larger amplitude electrograms are required for unipolar (vs. bipolar) leads to allow programming of lower sensitivities in order to avoid myopotential interference.

Inadequate sensing or pacing thresholds at the time of generator replacement are indications for placement of a new lead in the affected chamber. This may entail capping an old lead while leaving it in place or removing it. The new lead can usually be placed through the same subclavian vein, although it is preferable to avoid having too many leads (especially more than three) pass through the same vessel, to reduce the chance for venous occlusion and thrombosis. A single new lead may also be placed via the internal jugular vein, external jugular vein, or the contralateral subclavian vein. The proximal tip can be tunneled to the original pocket to meet a second, functional chronic lead for a dual-chamber system if required. Alternatively, an entirely new generator or lead system may be placed on the contralateral side.[67]

EXAMINING THE STRUCTURAL INTEGRITY OF LEADS AND THE LEAD-GENERATOR INTERFACE. Visual inspection provides some clue as to lead integrity. Fluid inside the lead body suggests an insulation break. Undue tension on the lead near the fixation site may cause kinking, conductor uncoiling, conductor fracture, or thinning of the electric insulator. A hazy appearance of the insulator surrounding an area of tension or repeated stress is common in older leads. This represents surface erosion of the lead insulator and does not itself imply lead malfunction. It should, however, alert the operator to the possibility of lead damage in areas of stress to the insulation. An examination of the suture location ensures that the ligature remains around the suture sleeve, and gentle tension on the lead body ensures its fixation at the venous entry site. Visual inspection of the specific course of a coiled lead in the pocket may be hampered by a significant thickness of overlying capsule scar; fluoroscopy can assist in this regard.[38–41]

Direct examination of the lead connector can assist in the identification of lead model if not previously known.[51–53] This is particularly important for lead models that have been found to have excessive premature failure rates; such leads in the ventricular position should be replaced in pacemaker-dependent patients.

VENOGRAPHY. Venography is not commonly required as part of the device replacement procedure. It does, however, play an important role when insertion of replacement leads into the subclavian vein is rendered difficult, since it can (1) ensure patency of the subclavian and superior vena cava systems or (2) demonstrate the point of venous occlusion.

Venography is indicated (1) when the subclavian vein cannot be accessed, in order to demonstrate its location, and (2) when the vein is accessed but a guide wire cannot be passed into the superior vena cava. Inability to access the subclavian vein that carries a chronically implanted lead suggests either an incorrect needle insertion angle or an occluded subclavian or innominate venous system.[68–72] Finding an appropriate location to insert the access needle can be facilitated by advancing the needle fluoroscopically in the direction of the chronic electrode site under the clavicle, taking care not to damage the chronic lead. The vein should be approached with the bevel of the needle facing the chronic lead. If access is not possible, venography may provide better definition of the course of the subclavian vein. In this situation, radiopaque dye must be injected distal to the subclavian vein, that is, into the basilic or median cubital vein.

Occasionally, access to the subclavian vein is possible, but the guide wire will not pass freely to the superior vena cava. Assuming adequate needle placement in the vessel, this suggests proximal venous occlusion.[73–77] Venography demonstrates (1) whether occlusion is indeed present and (2) the site of occlusion. Chronic venous occlusion may occur asymptomatically through the development of collateral venous circulation around the shoulder. Delineation of the location and length of occlusion indicates to the operator an appropriate needle insertion site for placement of a new lead. It also ensures patency of the superior vena cava. Dye is injected directly into the subclavian vein. Occlusion of the subclavian system proximal to the junction of the internal jugular vein excludes the ipsilateral jugular system as an alternative site for a new lead. Alternatively, if the subclavian vein is occluded and the internal jugular vein remains patent, a new lead may still be placed via the jugular approach.

Occlusion of the superior vena cava precludes the use of any new endocardial lead placed from a superior site.

Anomalous left superior vena cava (that may enter the coronary sinus) makes placement of right ventricular endocardial leads difficult or impossible.[78, 79] Venography defines the anatomy of the venous system in such a situation, which may be suggested by an unusual intravascular guide wire course. Finally, leakage of venography dye into perivascular tissues or into the pericardial space suggests vessel or cardiac chamber perforation, respectively.

The technique is performed by injecting 10 to 20 mL of radiopaque dye (a 50% dilution generally suffices) into a vein distal to the occlusion site. The dye may be injected directly into the subclavian vein if accessed, or into the antecubital or brachial vein if subclavian access is not possible. Fluoroscopy and permanent storage of images is necessary to properly evaluate flow.

GENERATOR-LEAD ADAPTABILITY

LEAD CONNECTORS. Replacing a pulse generator onto one or more chronic leads requires that the generator connector block be compatible with the proximal lead tip.[51–53] Through years of development by multiple manufacturers, pacemaker leads have evolved to an International Standard (IS-1) proximal lead connector configuration, which involves the following: (1) a 3.2-mm lead connector with a short pin that is electrically connected to the distal electrode tip, (2) a lead connector ring wired to the proximal pacing pole (the ring is electrically active in a bipolar lead), and (3) sealing rings. The proximal lead connector configuration is the same for unipolar or bipolar leads, except that the ring is inactive in unipolar leads. Modern pulse generators have connector block specifications that conform to IS-1 leads and that also fit the prior Voluntary Standard (VS-1) lead type. Thus, generator replacement onto implanted leads of either of these two types poses no difficulty because of the wide array of compatible pulse generators from multiple manufacturers.

A variety of other lead connector configurations had previously been developed, however (Table 29–7; Fig. 29–7). Because implanted leads may remain useful for many years, a number of these older lead connector configurations remain implanted. If sensing and pacing thresholds are adequate, old leads with such configurations may be used, but a pulse generator with a compatible connector block should be selected. An alternative, but less desirable approach involves using an adapter. Most very old leads are unipolar; upgrading to a bipolar system should be considered but is not always necessary.

TABLE 29–7. COMMON ENDOCARDIAL LEAD CONNECTOR CONFIGURATIONS

DESIGNATION	UNIPOLAR/ BIPOLAR	LINEAR/ BIFURCATED (Bipolar)	PIN: LONG/ SHORT	CONNECTOR DIAMETER (mm)	SEALING RINGS	FIXATION ACTIVE/PASSIVE	ATRIAL J AVAILABLE
IS-1	U or B	L	S	3.2	Yes	A or P	Yes
VS-1	U or B	L	S or L[a]	3.2	Yes	A or P	Yes
3.2-mm low profile	U or B	L	L	3.2	Yes or no	A or P	Yes
5-mm	U	—	L	5	Yes	A or P	Yes
5-mm	B	B	L	6	Yes	A or P	Yes
6-mm	U or B	L or B	S or L	6	Yes	A or P	Yes

[a]Long pin on VS-1 A or VS-1 B configurations.

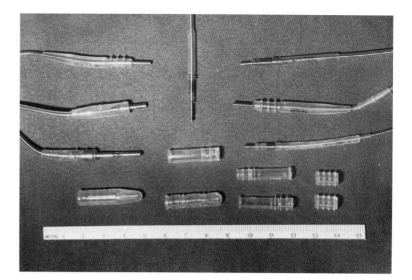

FIGURE 29–7. A variety of lead connectors *(top)*, nonconducting adapters *(bottom right, five)*, and lead caps *(bottom left, two)*. Lead connectors shown are *(clockwise from bottom left)*: Intermedics 6-mm linear bipolar, 6-mm unipolar, Medtronic 5-mm unipolar, Cordis 3.2-mm linear bipolar, Pacesetter IS-1, Medtronic atrial 5-mm unipolar, Medtronic IS-1.

Lead caps include 5-mm cap *(bottom left)* and 3.2-mm low-profile or IS-1/VS-1 *(bottom left, center)*. Upsizing sleeves include 5- to 6-mm *(top left, center)*, 3.2- to 5-mm *(top right, center)*, 3.2- to 6-mm *(bottom right, center)*. Unipolarizing sleeves for 6-mm bipolar leads are shown on bottom right. (Photography by Andrew C. Floyd, Chief CVT, Hahnemann University Hospital, Philadelphia.)

Prior to IS-1 and VS-1 lead connector configurations,[51, 52] the most commonly used pacing leads included 3.2-mm low-profile leads (unipolar or linear bipolar), 5-mm or 6-mm unipolar or linear bipolar leads, or bifurcated bipolar systems. Pulse generators available from some manufacturers remain compatible with each of these lead models, especially 3.2-mm and 5- to 6-mm linear bipolar or unipolar leads. Precise compatibility, however, is essential to ensuring that no fluid leaks into the pulse generator connector block and that electric continuity to proximal and distal poles remains intact. One must be particularly cautious to ensure that sealing rings are located either on the lead connector or in the pulse generator connector block, since not all older lead models had sealing rings placed on the lead connector itself.

Review of manufacturers' specifications of devices should provide the necessary details regarding lead–pulse generator compatibility. Since the lead model may not always be known before reoperation and since it may not be determined even with visual inspection, careful evaluation of the lead connector configuration may be required in the laboratory after the old pulse generator has been removed. Although the lead and pulse generator should have been compatible at the initial implantation, one cannot make this assumption without visual inspection of the type of lead connector at reoperation.

Bifurcated bipolar leads were implanted primarily with ventricular demand pacing systems with 5- to 6-mm lead connectors that plugged side by side into the pulse generator connector block. Some of these leads continue to function. Replacement of the pulse generator entails (1) selection of a new battery with a compatible connector block to maintain bipolar capability, (2) use of an adapter to convert the bifurcated bipolar lead to a linear bipolar system, or (3) conversion to unipolar by using only one pole of the bifurcated lead, capping the other. The third option is particularly useful in the event that only one pole of a bifurcated bipolar lead functions well. This also allows conversion to a unipolar dual-chamber pacing system, if desired, by placing a new atrial unipolar lead with a 5- to 6-mm connector, or by placing an IS-1 atrial lead and adapting the functional pole of the old lead in a unipolar configuration to an IS-1 connector. If the bifurcated bipolar lead is adapted to linear bipolar,

placing a linear bipolar atrial lead can convert the system to bipolar DDD.

Other lead types may be used only with particular pulse generators that have specific rate-responsive sensors, including the following: (1) temperature sensors having a thermistor within the lead body, (2) oxygen saturation sensor systems that measure by photometry, (3) respiratory (minute ventilation) sensors that require a particular (bipolar) lead configuration, and (4) intracavitary pressure recording leads. Each of these sensor systems requires specific lead types that may be compatible with pulse generators available only from a particular manufacturer. Most such leads require additional connections into the pulse generator. This information must be available preoperatively.

ADAPTERS. Two general categories of adapters are available, (1) electrically conducting units that change the size or configuration of lead connectors to fit specific pulse generators, and (2) upsizing sleeves to allow IS-1 or 3.2-mm low-profile leads to fit into 5- to 6-mm pulse generator connector blocks while maintaining a fluid seal (Table 29–8; Fig. 29–8).

Electrically conducting adapters necessarily contain wires attached on one end to a lead pin to enter the new pulse generator and a socket on the other to accept the old lead, as well as a mechanism to connect to the old lead, generally a setscrew. Produced by most manufacturers, an array of adapter types exists (see Table 29–8). The most common downsize 5- to 6-mm leads to IS-1 unipolar or bipolar configurations or adapt 3.2-mm low-profile connectors to the IS-1 variety. Adapters are also available to convert bifurcated bipolar leads to the linear IS-1 bipolar configuration. This may be particularly useful for a patient who requires upgrading from VVI to DDD pacing when maintenance of bipolar pacing is important, such as with an implanted defibrillator or to avoid myopotential sensing.

Despite the available variety of electrically conducting adapters, these units prove bulky in the pacemaker pocket. Furthermore, they provide another weak link, that is, one additional set of connections in the pacing circuit for delivery of current to the patient and for sensing, increasing the chance for malfunction as compared with direct attachment of a lead into a pulse generator connector block. Some

TABLE 29–8. **COMMON ADAPTER CONFIGURATIONS**

FROM (LEAD)	TO (GENERATOR)
CONDUCTING ADAPTERS	
6-mm UNI	5-mm UNI
6-mm BIF	3.2-mm LP BI
6-mm BI	3.2-mm LP BI
5-mm BIF	3.2-mm LP BI
5-mm BIF	IS-1 BI
5-mm UNI	IS-1 UNI
3.2-mm LP BI	5-mm BIF
3.2-mm LP BI	IS-1 BI
NONCONDUCTING UPSIZING SLEEVE ADAPTERS	
3.2-mm LP BI	5-mm or 6-mm UNI (± pin extender)
IS-1 UNI or BI	5-mm or 6-mm UNI
5-mm UNI	6-mm UNI

BI, linear bipolar; BIF, bifurcated bipolar; LP, low profile; UNI, unipolar.

TABLE 29–9. **COMMONLY USED TOOLS FOR GENERATOR OR LEAD REPLACEMENT OR REVISION OR FOR LEAD REPAIR**

Allen wrenches[a]
   0.035 inch (No. 2)
   0.050 inch (No. 4)
   0.062 inch (No. 6)
   0.093 inch (No. 10)
Screwdrivers
   0.100 inch
   0.200 inch
Setscrews
Probes (to unlock lead connector block in some devices)
Anchoring sleeves
Lead repair kit
   Conductor with crimp ends
   Crimping tool
   Insulating sleeve
Medical adhesive
Lead end caps
   6.5-mm
   5-mm
   3.2-mm LP
   IS-1

[a]Specific torque wrenches may be available from some manufacturers; these are especially important for tightening setscrews with appropriate force. Wrench numbers are standardized for ease in identification.

adapter setscrews need to be sealed with medical adhesive after being fastened to the lead; a poor seal can result in a short circuit in the system. Because of internal connections, not all adapters have the reliability inherent in most pacemaker leads.

TOOLS. Several specially designed tools assist the operator in replacing pulse generators and repairing leads (Table 29–9; Fig. 29–9). Most important are wrenches to loosen setscrews in the pulse generator connector block to allow the old lead to be withdrawn. If the old generator manufacturer and model are known, a specific wrench may be obtained. If these are not known, it is best to have available an array of small Allen wrenches to remove the hexagonal setscrew. Some pulse generators must be removed from the lead by using a small flat screwdriver. The new battery can be attached using wrenches available in the sterile packet housing the new device. Some pulse generators are connected to the lead without setscrews by pressing an attachment unit into place; to loosen this unit requires that a small probe be inserted into the side of the connector block to push open the locking mechanism. It is unusual to lose setscrews because they are generally held in place by a seal. It is advisable, however, to have additional setscrews available in a busy pacing laboratory.

Occasionally, repair can salvage an old lead, as long as the conductor fracture or insulation break is accessible several centimeters from the point at which the lead enters the vas-

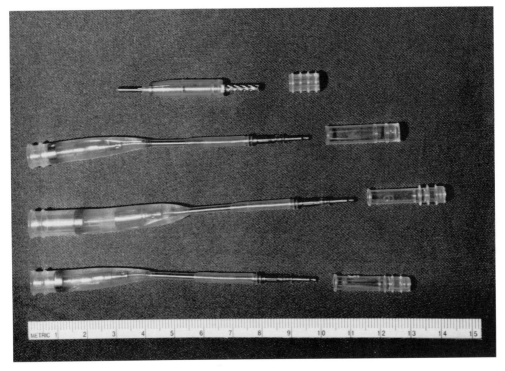

FIGURE 29–8. Eight lead adapters, four conducting *(left)*, and four nonconducting *(right)*. Conducting adapters shown include *(top to bottom)*: 6-mm lead pin replacement, 3.2-mm low-profile linear bipolar (to accept a lead connector without sealing rings) to VS-1 linear bipolar, 6-mm linear bipolar to 3.2-mm linear bipolar, and 3.2-mm low-profile linear bipolar to VS-1 linear bipolar. Nonconducting adapters shown are *(top to bottom)*: unipolarizing sleeve for 6-mm bipolar lead, upsizing sleeve from 5- to 6-mm, upsizing unipolarizing sleeve from 3.2- to 6-mm, upsizing unipolarizing sleeve from 3.2- to 5-mm. (Photography by Andrew C. Floyd, Chief CVT, Hahnemann University Hospital, Philadelphia.)

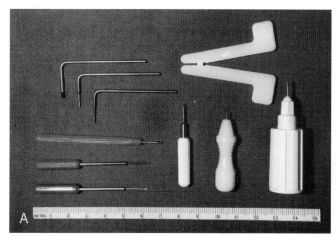 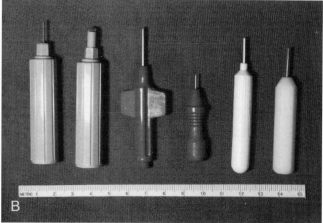

FIGURE 29–9. Tools commonly required for reoperation. *A,* Three nondeformable Allen wrenches *(top left)* of various sizes; a pinch-on tool (Medtronic) *(top right)* to extend and retract the distal screw of an active fixation lead; three wrenches *(bottom left)*; two torque wrenches (Medtronic and CPI) *(bottom right)* on either side of a probe (Intermedics) used to unlock a pacemaker connector block. Some wrenches are deformable to avoid placing excess torque on the setscrew, whereas others are not; caution is required in using the various systems (see text).

B, Left to right, Intermedics ratchet torque wrench; Intermedics flat-bladed ratchet torque screwdriver; Cordis No. 6 Allen wrench; unlocking probe; two Allen wrenches with handles (not deformable). (Photography by Andrew C. Floyd, Chief CVT, Hahnemann University Hospital, Philadelphia.)

cular system. Lead insulation breaks can be repaired by gluing over a Silastic sleeve with medical adhesive. Conductor fracture can be repaired by (1) severing the lead; (2) placing the two cut conductor ends into an electrically conducting sleeve, which is crimped down onto both ends of the lead conductor; and (3) gluing a Silastic sleeve over the insulator with medical adhesive. This procedure is recommended only for a lead on which the patient is not entirely dependent, since recurrent conductor fracture may occur. Repair of polyurethane leads can prove functionally inadequate, since adhesive may not bond properly with the lead insulator.

Surgical Considerations

Device replacement and/or revision in a tertiary care institution with an active electrophysiology service and long-term follow-up may constitute more than a quarter of all pacemaker procedures (Table 29–10). The timing of intervention depends on the specific indication. The majority of patients require reoperation for elective battery replacement or battery or lead revision, whereas 1 to 6% of patients may return to the laboratory for other problems, such as pocket hematoma, pocket twitch, diaphragmatic pacing, and pocket relocation (Table 29–11).

TABLE 29–10. **PULSE GENERATOR IMPLANTS AND REVISIONS OR REPLACEMENTS** (**July 1986–December 1992**)

DDD implants	51%
VVI implants	23%
Revisions or replacement	26%

The frequency of dual-chamber (DDD) and single-chamber (VVI) pulse generator implantations and battery or lead revisions or replacements over 5½-year period at the Likoff Cardiovascular Institute of Hahnemann University.

CHRONIC OR ELECTIVE INTERVENTION

Most reoperative implants fall into this category. Preoperative blood work is performed, aspirin is stopped for at least 5 days, and other anticoagulants are discontinued. The patient fasts from midnight and receives preoperative antibiotics, most commonly being admitted on the day of the procedure. Elevated coagulation times may be corrected with fresh-frozen plasma if necessary. Procedures are routinely performed with local anesthetic, with supplemental intravenous anxiolytics. Precordial electrocardiographic lead monitoring and sterile preparation and draping are standard procedure.

TABLE 29–11. **DEVICE REOPERATIONS: FREQUENCY OF VARIOUS INDICATIONS**

GENERATOR INDICATIONS	
Battery end of service	53%
DVI → DDD conversion	2.2%
Battery insulation break	1.1%
DDD → VVIR conversion	1.1%
LEAD INDICATIONS	
Lead revision	17%
Exit block	
Lead injury	
Diaphragmatic pacing	2.2%
Lead fracture	1.1%
Lead insulation break	1.1%
BATTERY OR LEAD INDICATIONS	
Battery end of service and lead replacement	6.8%
VVI → DDD conversion	4.4%
Unipolar DDD → bipolar DDD	1.1%
Pocket twitch	1.1%
SURGICAL	
Pocket relocation	5.6%
Pocket effusion	2.2%

The frequency of indications for device reoperation over a 5½-year period at the Likoff Cardiovascular Institute of Hahnemann University (July 1986–December 1992).

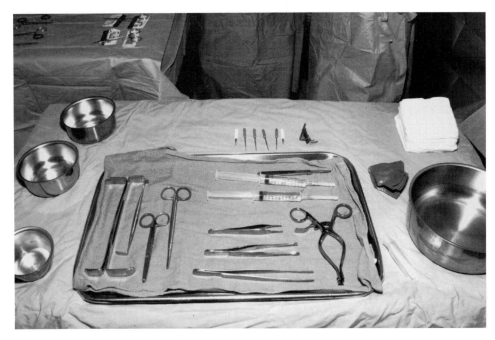

FIGURE 29–10. Preparation for surgery. A typical array of instruments required for reoperation. *Foreground,* Retractors, scissors, forceps, scalpel, syringes filled with Xylocaine anesthetic, sterile saline solution, sponges, and a variety of wrenches. *Background,* Hemostats and absorbable and nonabsorbable sutures. (Photography by Andrew C. Floyd, Chief CVT, Hahnemann University Hospital, Philadelphia.)

GENERAL GUIDELINES AND TECHNIQUES. There is no substitute for (1) careful surgical planning in approaching the chronic pacemaker pocket and (2) gentleness to the tissues. Perfect hemostasis, avoidance of a tight-fitting pacemaker pocket, and multilayered incisional closure are basic principles that will help prevent future difficulties. These principles are similar to those required at initial implantation (see Table 29–2). Electrocautery must not be used directly over an implanted pulse generator to avoid (1) induction of ventricular fibrillation, (2) development of fibrosis at the lead tip, or (3) damage to the generator itself. Electrocautery must also not be used during battery changes with the generator disconnected when pacemaker leads are grounded to the patient for testing, as current may be shunted directly to the heart. Hemostasis at reoperation can usually be secured by direct ligature. Use of surgical absorbable cellulose or topical thrombin assists in treating persistently "oozy" pockets. Clinical judgment should be used in the application of various technical approaches (Fig. 29–10).

SPECIFIC TECHNIQUES. Local anesthesia is administered most commonly as 1% xylocaine infiltrated into the scar line from the previous procedure; additional xylocaine may be given under direct vision once the capsule of the pacemaker pocket has been defined. The skin and subcutaneous tissues are opened with sharp dissection over the prior scar. Deeper dissection with Metzenbaum scissors is carried out to clearly delineate the pacemaker capsule. The capsule is sharply incised with a blade to make a small opening, which is then extended with direct visualization of the implanted pulse generator and leads (Fig. 29–11). The capsule must be opened far enough to allow extraction of the pulse generator and lead connector assembly without undue force. The posterior capsule may need to be carefully dissected away from the leads to allow mobility. Access to leads and generator may be facilitated through the use of retractors. Extreme care is required throughout the procedure to preserve the integrity of the leads and lead connectors; they must not be punctured with anesthetic needles or cut with blades or scissors.

Once the generator is delivered out of the pocket, the leads are disconnected and analyzed, as described earlier. Leads from pacemaker-dependent patients will need to be expeditiously reconnected to an external pacemaker (Fig. 29–12). Unipolar leads require direct grounding to subcutaneous tissue; the active part of the unipolar generator must remain in contact with the patient before the lead is disconnected. Grounding can best be accomplished through a large surface area ground electrode placed directly into the open pocket. Making contact with this electrode onto the active surface of a unipolar pulse generator allows the generator to be safely removed from the pocket before the lead is disconnected, even in a pacemaker-dependent patient.

After being secured to temporary pacing cables, leads can be completely freed from adhesions up to their entry point into the subclavian vein, if necessary, to examine lead integ-

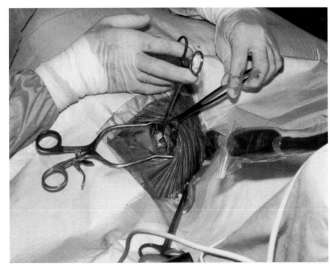

FIGURE 29–11. Opening the capsule of the chronic generator pocket to expose the pulse generator. (Photography by Andrew C. Floyd, Chief CVT, Hahnemann University Hospital, Philadelphia.)

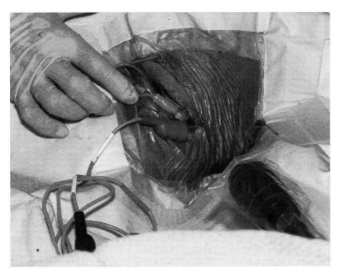

FIGURE 29–12. Disconnecting the chronic lead. The active surface of the unipolar pulse generator remains in contact with the open pocket to maintain pacing output until the lead is withdrawn from the connector block. The surgeon has adequately mobilized the proximal portion of the 5-mm lead to allow rapid connection to an external pacing cable, one end of which has already been securely grounded to the patient. A ligature previously placed around the lead connector block entry post has been removed. After the external pacemaker has been activated, the surgeon will loosen the setscrew (here covered by a seal on the top right side of the connector block) and withdraw the lead from the pulse generator, immediately connecting it to the negative pole of the external pacing cable. (Photography by Andrew C. Floyd, Chief CVT, Hahnemann University Hospital, Philadelphia.)

rity or for extraction. If lead replacement or repair is not necessary, and if chronic lead function is adequate, dissection of the complete course of each lead may not be necessary. One must ascertain, however, lead connector mobility sufficient to attach it to a new pulse generator without tension.

Inadequate chronic lead pacing or sensing thresholds may require placement of one or two new leads. Upgrading from a single-chamber to a DDD system may require placement of one additional lead. If a chronic lead is extracted through a dilating sheath, the new lead or a guide wire can usually be inserted into the vascular system through the extraction sheath. In other cases, repeated subclavian puncture, brachiocephalic cutdown, or an internal jugular approach provide alternative means of inserting a new lead. If new leads are placed via the same subclavian system by direct puncture, the operator must be cautious to avoid lead damage.

After the old pulse generator has been detached from leads, and lead integrity and functional status have been ascertained, a new pulse generator can be attached. The principles of generator-lead adaptability must be maintained. Redundant lead coils are placed posterior to the pulse generator, and the pocket is closed with three layers of absorbable suture, two subcutaneous and one subcuticular.

Generator replacement most commonly uses the chronic pacemaker pocket location, usually opposite the patient's dominant side. Since the majority of pacemakers are placed infraclavicularly in a subcutaneous location anterior to the pectoralis fascia, the location of replacement devices is similar. Various modifications suit individual patient needs. In very thin patients, subpectoral or axillary locations may be required. Abdominal wall, subcostal, or intrathoracic positions represent other alternatives for positioning of a replacement pulse generator.

APPROACH TO THE ERODING DEVICE. Although relatively uncommon, chronic erosion through the skin of the pulse generator or lead can occur.[1, 10, 60] Incipient erosion manifests as localized erythema in an area of thinned skin that is adherent to the underlying device. The area gradually becomes necrotic and may drain serosanguineous fluid. Outright erosion and drainage necessarily imply that the pacemaker pocket is no longer sterile;[1, 80] in such instances, the system (generator and leads) should be removed if possible.[5, 8] Occasionally, the pocket will heal with removal of the pulse generator alone, but only when skin integrity has not been breeched. After removal of the pulse generator and leads, eroded pockets are packed for secondary closure. Administration of intravenous antibiotics proceeds for 1 to 6 weeks (the longer duration if bacteremia has occurred). A new device should be implanted on the contralateral side only (1) after all signs of infection have resolved at the old pacemaker site, (2) if the patient has not developed recurrent fever after antibiotics have been stopped, and (3) if there is no elevation of white blood cell count. Replacement of the pulse generator on the original side is not recommended but may be possible if (1) complete erosion did not occur, (2) the pocket could be closed after primary generator removal, and (3) there are no signs of active infection after antibiotics have been discontinued. Alternative approaches are discussed in Chapter 28.

ACUTE INTERVENTION

Indications for acute intervention involve primary complications of pacemaker implantation (e.g., pocket hematoma, infection,[1–3] or cardiac perforation[56–60]), as well as other less critical indications, such as iatrogenic lead damage and lead dislodgment.

Pacemaker pocket hematoma occurs most frequently in patients receiving anticoagulants, including aspirin, or in those with platelet dysfunction, commonly in patients undergoing chronic hemodialysis. The range in hematoma size varies from a contained, small amount of fluctuance and ecchymosis to a large hematoma that may drain through the skin. A minor hematoma requires only observation, whereas a breech of skin integrity after operation may require complete removal of the entire pacemaker and lead system. If the patient remains pacemaker dependent, a temporary wire must be placed when the original system is removed, and after an appropriate course of intravenous antibiotic therapy the old pocket can be closed, and a new pacemaker placed on the contralateral side. Prolonged antibiotic therapy may be required in some cases. Antibiotic therapy alone and conservative surgical approaches other than complete removal of the eroded or infected generator and leads prove unsatisfactory.[5–8]

Acute reoperation may also be required for cardiac perforation.[56–60, 62] Perforation is suggested by curvature of the lead beyond the confines of the right ventricular apex, an abrupt rise in pacing threshold or deterioration of sensing, precordial discomfort, hypotension, or hemodynamic collapse. Although most perforations close spontaneously, development of a large pericardial bleed or tamponade requires immediate intervention.[62] Pericardiocentesis usually suffices, but occasionally a subxiphoid approach to pericardial drainage is necessary. Proper lead selection to match the patient's anatomy and gentle technique are vital to avoiding acute perforation. Subcostal placement of epicardial screw-in leads has been associated with a high incidence of serious or fatal ventricular perforations; chronic perforation of endocardial leads is distinctly rare.[24]

Early surgical exploration is indicated to confirm the diagnosis of iatrogenic lead insulation damage. This is an uncommon complication and manifests early in the form of pocket twitch,[64] failure to capture, or failure to sense, with associated low measured lead impedance.[50] Chronic implantation lead damage has been associated with excessively tight anchoring sutures, especially if they are placed around the lead and not the anchoring sleeve. The damaged lead, be it a passive or an active fixation variety, should be removed and replaced, if possible; alternatively, it may be repaired, although this is difficult if damage has occurred near the venous insertion site.

Lead dislodgment occurs most commonly during the first 24 to 48 hours following system implantation.[26, 27] It can, however, occur later, the result of a loose anchoring sleeve, excessive diaphragmatic motion, or patient manipulation of the device (i.e., the twiddler's syndrome).[48] Before the development of leads with active fixation or a fin-like mechanism at the distal tip, the incidence of lead dislodgment remained as high as 5 to 18%. With careful technique and selection among a variety of active and passive fixation leads, the incidence should range no higher than 1 to 2%.[30, 31, 81] Most spontaneous dislodgments occur with atrial passive fixation leads. The diagnosis may be facilitated by chest radiograph or fluoroscopy; pacing analysis reveals an increased pacing threshold with, usually, normal lead impedance. The operator has the option of repositioning or lead replacement. If a distinct cause cannot be identified, placement of an active fixation lead may avoid a second dislodgment. To prevent recurrent lead dislodgment in the twiddler's syndrome, leads must be sutured to prepectoral fascia or firm pacemaker pocket fibrous tissue using nonabsorbable suture around anchoring sleeves at more than two points; the pacemaker connector block may also be anchored to the pectoralis fascia. The use of a polyester (Dacron) pouch can improve device stability in this syndrome and in patients with very loose subcutaneous tissue.[82]

INTERVAL OR UNSCHEDULED INTERVENTION

In the course of pacemaker follow-up and before the patient requires elective replacement, interval intervention may be required to correct other complications. These include pulse generator migration,[15] lead dislodgment,[16, 23, 26, 27, 31, 48] high pacing thresholds,[23, 49] pocket twitch or diaphragmatic pacing,[24, 64] lead insulation break or lead fracture,[11, 13, 26] and premature pacemaker generator failure (which could be due to intrinsic component failure or the result of externally induced failure, such as that caused by electrocautery, radiation, or cardioversion).[19, 20] The pacemaker clinic may prove particularly useful in recognizing early surgical or functional problems.[36] Evaluation and technique are approached using the principles described earlier.

Summary

Successful pacemaker replacement is the result of an accurate preoperative evaluation and careful surgical interven-

tion. The preoperative status of the pulse generator battery and lead pacing and sensing function, and the appropriateness of both to the future pacing system, need to be determined in order to plan the surgery. There should be no surgical surprises, and all the tools, adapters, leads, and generators need to be ready for the intervention. The goal should be to avoid reoperation for as long as possible with careful initial implantation and programming. However, when properly planned, the surgery is likely to proceed smoothly.

REFERENCES

1. Bonchek LI: New methods in the management of extruded and infected cardiac pacemakers. Ann Surg 176(5):686, 1972.
2. Corman LC, Levison ME: Sustained bacteremia and transvenous cardiac pacemakers. JAMA 233(3):264, 1975.
3. Morgan G, Ginks W, Siddons H, Leatham A: Septicemia in patients with an endocardial pacemaker. Am J Cardiol 44(2):221, 1979.
4. Wohl B, Peters RW, Carliner N, et al: Late unheralded pacemaker pocket infection due to *Staphylococcus epidermidis*: A new clinical entity. PACE 5(2):190, 1982.
5. Praeger PI, Kay RH, Somberg E, et al: Pacemaker remnants—another source of infections. PACE 7(4):763, 1984.
6. Mansour KA, Kauten JR, Hatcher CR Jr: Management of the infected pacemaker: Explantation, sterilization, and reimplantation. Ann Thorac Surg 40(6):617, 1985.
7. Buch J, Mortensen SA: Late infections of pacemaker units due to silicone rubber insulation boots. PACE 8(4):494, 1985.
8. Ruiter JH, Degener JE, Van Mechelen R, Bos R: Late purulent pacemaker pocket infection caused by *Staphylococcus epidermidis*: Serious complications of in situ management. PACE 8(6):903, 1985.
9. Vilacosta I, Zamorano J, Camino A, et al: Infected transvenous permanent pacemakers: Role of transesophageal echocardiography. Am Heart J 125(3):904, 1993.
10. Garcia-Rinaldi R, Revuelta JM, Bonnington L, Soltero-Harrington L: The exposed cardiac pacemaker: Treatment by subfascial pocket relocation. J Thorac Cardiovasc Surg 89(1):136, 1985.
11. Kronzon I, Mehta SS: Broken pacemaker wire in multiple trauma: A case report. J Trauma 14(1):82, 1974.
12. Tegtmeyer CJ, Bezirdjian DR, Irani FA, Landis JD: Cardiac pacemaker failure: A complication of trauma. Southern Med J 74(3):378, 1981.
13. Grieco JG, Scanlon PJ, Pifarre R: Pacing lead fracture after a deceleration injury. Ann Thorac Surg 47(3):453, 1989.
14. Wallace WA, Abelmann WH, Norman JC: Runaway demand pacemaker: Report, in vitro reproduction, and review. Ann Thorac Surg 9(3):209, 1970.
15. Bello A, Yepez CG, Barcelo JE: Retroperitoneal migration of a pacemaker generator: An unusual complication. J Cardiovasc Surg 15(2):256, 1974.
16. Kim GE, Haveson S, Imparato AM: Late displacement of cardiac pacemaker electrode due to heavyweight pulse generator. JAMA 228(1):74, 1974.
17. Austin SM, Kim CS, Solis A: Electrical alternans of pacemaker spike amplitude: An unusual manifestation of permanent pacemaker generator malfunction. PACE 4(3):313, 1981.
18. Campo A, Nowak R, Magilligan D, Tomlanovich M: Runaway pacemaker. Ann Emerg Med 12(1):32, 1983.
19. Venselaar JL, Van Kerkeorle HL, Vet AJ: Radiation damage to pacemakers from radiotherapy. PACE 10(3,pt1):538, 1987.
20. Lewinn AA, Serago CF, Schwade JG, et al: Radiation-induced failures of complementary metal oxide semiconductor containing pacemakers: A potentially lethal complication. Int J Radiol Oncol Biol Phys 10(10):1967, 1984.
21. Halperin JL, Camunas JL, Stern EH, et al: Myopotential interference with DDD pacemakers: Endocardial electrographic telemetry in the diagnosis of pacemaker-related arrhythmias. Am J Cardiol 54(1):97, 1984.
22. den Dulk K, Lindemans FW, Brugada P, et al: Pacemaker syndrome with AAI rate-variable pacing: Importance of atrioventricular conduction properties, medication, and pacemaker programmability. PACE 11(8):1226, 1988.
23. Aris A, Shebairo RA, Lepley D Jr: Increasing myocardial thresholds to pacing after cardiac surgery. Surg Forum 24:167, 1973.
24. Gaidula JJ, Barold SS: Elimination of diaphragmatic contractions from

chronic pacing catheter perforation of the heart by conversion to a unipolar system. Chest 66(1):86, 1974.

25. Contini C, Papi L, Pesola A, et al: Tissue reaction to intracavitary electrodes: Effect on duration and efficiency of unipolar pacing in patients with A-V block. J Cardiovasc Surg 14(3):282, 1973.

26. Holmes DR Jr, Nissen RG, Maloney JD, et al: Transvenous tined electrode systems: An approach to acute dislodgement. Mayo Clin Proc 54(4):219, 1979.

27. Snow N: Elimination of lead dislodgement by the use of tined transvenous electrodes. PACE 5(4):571, 1982.

28. Alt E, Volker R, Blomer H: Lead fracture in pacemaker patients. Thorac Cardiovasc Surg 35(2):101, 1987.

29. Woscoboinik JR, Maloney JD, Helguera ME, et al: Pacing lead survival: Performance of different models. PACE 15(11,pt2):1991, 1992.

30. Morse D, Yankaskas M, Johnson B, et al: Transvenous pacemaker insertion with a zero dislodgement rate. PACE 6(2,pt1):283, 1983.

31. Hakki AH, Horowitz LN, Reiser J, Mundth ED: Improved pacemaker fixation and performance using a modified finned porous surfaced tip lead. Int Surg 69(4):291, 1984.

32. Mond H, Twentyman R, Smith D, Sloman G: The pacemaker clinic. Cardiology 57(5):262, 1972.

33. Starr A, Dobbs J, Dabolt L, Pierie W: Ventricular tracking pacemaker and teletransmitter follow-up system. Am J Cardiol 32(7):956, 1973.

34. Janosik DL, Redd RM, Buckingham TA, et al: Utility of ambulatory electrocardiography in detecting pacemaker dysfunction in the early postimplantation period. Am J Cardiol 60(13):1030, 1987.

35. Mugica J, Henry L, Rollet M, et al: The clinical utility of pacemaker follow-up visits. PACE 9(6,pt2):1249, 1986.

36. Byrd CL, Schwartz SJ, Gonzales M, et al: Pacemaker clinic evaluations: Key to early identification of surgical problems. PACE 9(6,pt2):1259, 1986.

37. Kertes P, Mond H, Sloman G, et al: Comparison of lead complications with polyurethane tined, silicone rubber tined, and wedge tip leads: Clinical experience with 822 ventricular endocardial leads. PACE 6(5,pt1):957, 1983.

38. van Gelder LM, El Gamal MI: False inhibition of an atrial demand pacemaker caused by an insulation defect in a polyurethane lead. PACE 6(5,pt1):834, 1983.

39. Sanford CF: Self-inhibition of an AV sequential demand (DVI) pulse generator due to polyurethane lead insulation disruption. PACE 6(5,pt1):840, 1983.

40. Timmis GC, Westveer DC, Martin R, Gordon S: The significance of surface changes on explanted polyurethane pacemaker leads. PACE 6(5,pt1):845, 1983.

41. Chawla AS, Blais P, Hinberg I, Johnson D: Degradation of explanted polyurethane cardiac pacing leads and of polyurethane. Biomater, Artif Cells Artif Organs 16(4):785, 1988.

42. Van Beek GJ, den Dulk K, Lindemans FW, Wellens HJ: Detection of insulation failure by gradual reduction in noninvasively measured electrogram amplitudes. PACE 9(5):772, 1986.

43. Stokes KB, Church T: Ten-year experience with implanted polyurethane lead insulation. PACE 9(6,pt2):1160, 1986.

44. Phillips R, Frey M, Martin RO: Long-term performance of polyurethane pacing leads: Mechanisms of design-related failures. PACE 9(6,pt2):1166, 1986.

45. Barold SS, Gaidula JJ: Demand pacemaker arrhythmias from intermittent internal short circuit in bipolar electrode. Chest 63(2):165, 1973.

46. Adler SC, Foster AJ, Sanders RS, Wuu E: Thin bipolar leads: A solution to problems with coaxial bipolar designs. PACE 15(11,pt2):1986, 1992.

47. Barold SS, Scovil J, Ong LS, Heinle RA: Periodic pacemaker spike attenuation with preservation of capture: An unusual electrocardiographic manifestation of partial pacing electrode fracture. PACE 1(3):375, 1978.

48. Bayliss CE, Beanlands DS, Baird RJ: The pacemaker-twiddler's syndrome: A new complication of implantable transvenous pacemakers. Can Med Assoc J 99(8):371, 1968.

49. Starr DS, Lawrie GM, Morris GC Jr: Acute and chronic stimulation thresholds of intramyocardial screw-in pacemaker electrodes. Ann Thorac Surg 31(4):334, 1981.

50. Ferek B, Pasini M, Pustisek S, et al: Noninvasive detection of insulation break. PACE 7(6,pt1):1063, 1984.

51. Calfee RV, Saulson SH: A voluntary standard for 3.2-mm unipolar and bipolar pacemaker leads and connectors. PACE 9(6,pt2):1181, 1986.

52. Doring J, Flink R: The impact of pending technologies on a universal connector standard. PACE 9(6,pt2):1186, 1986.

53. Tyers GF, Sanders R, Mills P, Clark J: Analysis of setscrew and sidelock connector reliability. PACE 15(11,pt2):2000, 1992.

54. Torresani J, Ebagosti A, Allard-Latour G: Pacemaker syndrome with DDD pacing. PACE 7(6,pt2):1183, 1984.

55. Cunningham TM: Pacemaker syndrome due to retrograde conduction in DDI pacemaker. Am Heart J 115(2):478, 1988.

56. Peters RW, Scheinman MM, Raskin S, Thomas AN: Unusual complications of epicardial pacemakers: Recurrent pericarditis, cardiac tamponade and pericardial constriction. Am J Cardiol 45(5):1088, 1980.

57. Foster CJ: Constrictive pericarditis complicating an endocardial pacemaker. Br Heart J 47(5):497, 1982.

58. Phibbs B, Marriott HJ: Complications of permanent transvenous pacing. N Engl J Med 312(22):1428, 1985.

59. Villanueva FS, Heinsiner JA, Burkman MH, et al: Echocardiographic detection of perforation of the cardiac ventricular septum by a permanent pacemaker lead. Am J Cardiol 59(4):370, 1987.

60. Hill PE: Complications of permanent transvenous cardiac pacing: A 14-year review of all transvenous pacemakers inserted at one community hospital. PACE 10(3,pt1):564, 1987.

61. Pizzarelli G, Dernevik L: Inadvertent transarterial pacemaker insertion: An unusual complication. PACE 10(4,pt1):951, 1987.

62. Sandler MA, Wertheimer JH, Kotler MN: Pericardial tamponade associated with pacemaker catheter manipulation. PACE 12(7,pt1):1085, 1989.

63. Mueller X, Sadeghi H, Kappenberger L: Complications after single-versus dual-chamber pacemaker implantation. PACE 13(6):711, 1990.

64. Ekbom K, Nilsson BY, Edhag O, Olin C: Rhythmic shoulder girdle muscle contractions as a complication in pacemaker treatment. Chest 66(5):599, 1974.

65. Chun PK: Characteristics of commonly utilized permanent endocardial and epicardial pacemaker electrode systems: Method of radiologic identification. Am Heart J 102(3,pt1):404, 1981.

66. Angello DA: Principles of electrical testing for analysis of ventricular endocardial pacing leads. Prog Cardiovasc Dis 27(1):57, 1984.

67. Kemler RL: A simple method for exposing the external jugular vein for placement of a permanent transvenous pacing catheter electrode. Ann Thorac Surg 26(3):266, 1978.

68. Sethi GK, Bhayana JN, Scott SM: Innominate venous thrombosis: A rare complication of transvenous pacemaker electrodes. Am Heart J 87(6):770, 1974.

69. Fritz T, Richeson JF, Fitzpatrick P, Wilson G: Venous obstruction: A potential complication of transvenous pacemaker electrodes. Chest 83(3):534, 1983.

70. Sharma S, Kaul U, Rajani M: Digital subtraction venography for assessment of deep venous thrombosis in the arms following pacemaker implantation. Int J Cardiol 23(1):135, 1989.

71. Antonelli D, Turgeman Y, Kaveh Z, et al: Short-term thrombosis after transvenous permanent pacemaker insertion. PACE 12(2):280, 1989.

72. Spittell PC, Vlietstra RE, Hayes DL, Higano ST: Venous obstruction due to permanent transvenous pacemaker electrodes: Treatment with percutaneous transluminal balloon venoplasty. PACE 13(3):271, 1990.

73. Wertheimer M, Hughes RK, Castle CH: Superior vena cava syndrome: Complication of permanent transvenous endocardial cardiac pacing. JAMA 224(8):1172, 1973.

74. Toumbouras M, Spanos P, Konstantaras C, Lazarides DP: Inferior vena cava thrombosis due to migration of retained functionless pacemaker electrode. Chest 82(6):785, 1982.

75. Blackburn T, Dunn M: Pacemaker-induced superior vena cava syndrome: Consideration of management. Am Heart J 116(3):893, 1988.

76. Goudevenos JA, Reid PG, Adams PC, et al: Pacemaker-induced superior vena cava syndrome: Report of four cases and review of the literature. PACE 12(12):1890, 1989.

77. Mazzetti H, Dussaut A, Tentori C, et al: Superior vena cava occlusion and/or syndrome related to pacemaker leads. Am Heart J 125(3):831, 1993.

78. Chaithiraphan S, Goldberg E, Wolff W, et al: Massive thrombosis of the coronary sinus as an unusual complication of transvenous pacemaker insertion in a patient with persistent left, and no right superior vena cava. J Am Geriatr Soc 22(2):79, 1974.

79. Kennelly BM: Permanent pacemaker implantation in the absence of a right superior vena cava: A case report. South Afr Med J 55(25):1043, 1979.

80. Wade JS, Cobbs CG: Infections in cardiac pacemakers. Curr Clin Topics Infec Dis 9:44, 1988.

81. Boake WC, Kroncke GM: Pacemaker Complications. Cardiac Pacing. Philadelphia, Lea & Febiger, 1979.

82. Parsonnet V: A stretch fabric pouch for implanted pacemakers. Arch Surg 105:654, 1972.

CHAPTER 30

PACEMAKER RADIOGRAPHY

Lon W. Castle
Sebastian Cook

Both posteroanterior and left lateral chest roentgenograms are essential in evaluating a pacing system. As in any radiologic series, a deliberate systematic approach lends itself to the best diagnostic interpretation. It is imperative to be knowledgeable of the components of the pacing systems, especially the various pulse generators and various lead types. A fundamental knowledge of the location and relationships of the various vascular structures and compartments that the leads traverse in their course is also important. Therefore, a brief review of the soft tissue and osseous anatomy pertinent to pacing devices is described.

The pacing system consists of an energy source, the pulse generator, wires connecting the source to the leads, and electrodes that are located either in the cardiac chambers along the endocardial surface (transvenous) or in the myocardium itself (epicardial leads).

For transvenous systems, the generator is typically situated in the subcutaneous pectoralis major region, away from the axilla or heart. For epicardial systems, the source is usually in the left upper quadrant of the abdomen, in the epigastrium, or, occasionally, in the chest wall.

Practical Radiographic Anatomy

Although the subclavian vein is most commonly used in the placement of the electrodes, cephalic and jugular vein approaches can also be employed. The cephalic vein is located along the radial aspect of the forearm. After coursing lateral to the biceps, it continues in a groove between the deltoid and pectoralis major, penetrating the clavipectoral fascia and emptying into either the axillary or proximal subclavian vein. A cut-down procedure is required to visualize the cephalic vein adequately. The axillary vein, which anatomically originates at the lower border of the teres major,

drains the basilic and brachial veins. The axillary vein then continues medially to become the subclavian vein at the lateral margin of the first rib.[1] Radiographically, this marks the typical site for insertion of the pacemaker's wires (Fig. 30–1).

The brachiocephalic vein is formed by the internal jugular vein and the subclavian vein behind the clavicular head near the sternoclavicular joint. The right brachiocephalic artery is posterior and medial to the vein. The right brachiocephalic vein receives the vertebral and internal mammary veins; its length is typically about 2 cm. Together with the left brachiocephalic vein, it forms the superior vena cava. A wire in the right brachiocephalic vein on a lateral view enters the superior vena cava in an almost straight line (Fig. 30–2).

The left brachiocephalic vein forms behind the medial aspect of the left clavicle and, for a distance of approximately 7 cm, runs obliquely behind the sternum to join its counterpart from the right to form the superior vena cava.[1] On a lateral view, it has a bend, touching or coming close to the sternum as it courses posteriorly over the arch vessels to join the right (Fig. 30–3). A skeletal landmark for the origin of the superior vena cava is the inferior aspect of the first costochondral junction. The superior vena cava and inferior vena cava drain into the right atrium. The right atrium can be identified as a slightly convex soft tissue bulge along the right side of the cardiac silhouette on the PA view. In a small percentage of cases, a persistent left superior vena cava is present, which typically drains into a coronary sinus (Fig. 30–4).

Venous cardiac anatomy must also be familiar to the physician interpreting the plain chest roentgenogram. The coronary sinus, which enters the inferior aspect of the right atrium just in front of the opening of the inferior vena cava, receives most of the venous drainage from the heart. This major venous compartment is approximately 3 cm long and is situ-

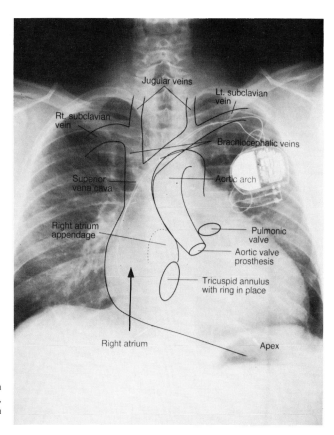

FIGURE 30–1. Overlay of diagram on a posteroanterior chest roentgenogram demonstrating the typical location for the formation of the subclavian veins, brachiocephalic veins, the superior vena cava, and the right atrium along with their associated osseous landmarks. Rt., right; Lt., left.

ated posteriorly in the atrioventricular (AV) groove. It drains the great, small, and middle cardiac veins, the posterior vein of the left ventricle, and the oblique vein of the left atrium.[2]

The great cardiac vein is situated anteriorly in the interventricular sulcus, beginning at the apex and ending in the cor-

onary sinus. The small cardiac vein drains part of the right atrium and ventricle. The middle cardiac vein begins in the apex and runs in the posterior interventricular sulcus. Occasionally, the pacemaker wires can have their tips either in the coronary sinus or in the middle cardiac vein (Fig. 30–5). The

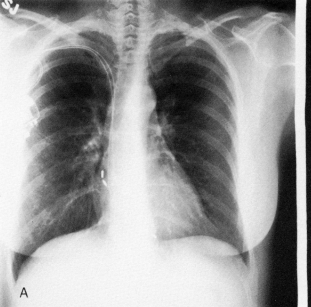

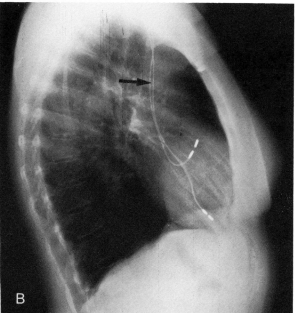

FIGURE 30–2. Posteroanterior *(A)* and lateral *(B)* views of a patient who has had a dual-chamber unipolar passively fixed system installed. Note on the lateral view the vertical course of the wires located by the arrow, indicating that it has been inserted from the right and is directed down the right brachiocephalic vein into the superior vena cava.

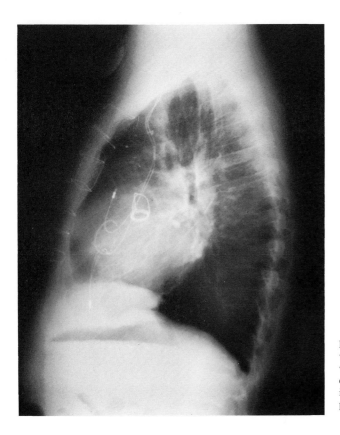

FIGURE 30–3. The pacing system has been inserted from the left subclavian vein. Note on the lateral view the bend toward the sternum, indicating that the wires are coursing around the arch vessels before entering the superior vena cava. The patient has an annuloplasty ring in the tricuspid position, which identifies the right atrioventricular valve; there is also a high-profile mechanical prosthetic valve in place in the aortic position.

AV node is situated close to the coronary sinus foramen (Fig. 30–6).

The tricuspid valve, which overlies the vertebral bodies on the posteroanterior view, forms the left border of the right atrium. It extends from its superior margin where it is incorporated into the central fibrinous tendon, adjacent to the mitral and aortic valves of the heart to the diaphragmatic surface of the heart inferiorly. The posterior medial wall of the atrium is formed by the atrial septum. The fossa ovalis, a thin fibrous area in the middle portion of the septum, represents the closed embryologic foramen ovale.

An important structure to remember is the right atrial appendage, which frequently houses the atrial wire of a dual-chamber system. This structure curves around the right side of the heart; it is triangular with a rather broad base as opposed to the left atrial appendage, which has a narrower base and is more elongated. The tip of the right atrial appendage usually overlies the root of the aorta (Fig. 30–7).

The right ventricle (into which blood from the right atrium) flows can be divided into an inflow tract adjacent to the tricuspid valve and an outflow tract (infundibulum) related to the pulmonic valve. A muscular ring (formed by the crista supraventricularis, the septal band, the moderator band, and the parietal band) separates the two tracts. The crista supraventricularis is a muscular segment that extends from the upper part of the membranous portion of the interventricular septum and the tricuspid valve to the pulmonic valve and forms the right posterior wall of the outflow tract. The right aortic sinus of Valsalva lies against the other side of the crista. Because of the obliquity of the aortic valve, the crista lies inferior to the pulmonic valve on the right side of the heart and is part of the outflow tract; however, on the left

Persistent Left Superior Vena Cava

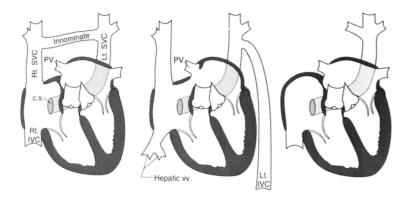

FIGURE 30–4. Schematic representation of the three different types of persistent left SVC with various insertions of the left SVC into the right heart system. SVC, superior vena cava; IVC, inferior vena cava; PV, pulmonary vein; Rt., right; Lt., left; c.s., coronary sinus; VV., veins.

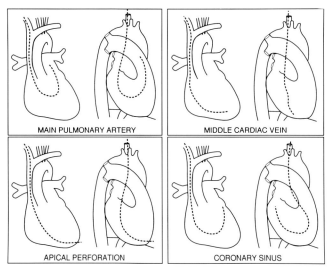

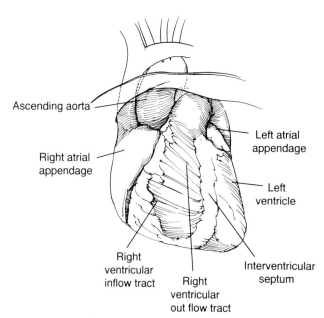

FIGURE 30–5. Diagram demonstrating the course of various improperly placed ventricular leads and the location of the electrode with respect to the cardiac structures. (Modified and redrawn from Steiner RM, Tegtmeyer CJ, Morse D, et al: The radiology of cardiac pacemakers. Radiographics 6:381, 1986.)

FIGURE 30–7. Anatomy of the right atrial appendage and its relationship to the root of the ascending aorta.

side, it reinforces the root of the aorta, being situated mostly above the aortic valve. The septal, parietal, and moderator bands anteriorly primarily end along the free wall of the right ventricle. There are many trabeculations in the wall of the right ventricle.[3]

Flow returns from the lungs to the left atrium, which is an ovoid chamber that is the most posteriorly situated of the four cardiac chambers. There are four pulmonary veins: two superior and two inferior. The left atrium is located partly to the left, partly above, and partly posteriorly to the right atrium because of the oblique orientation of the septum. An elongated fingerlike projection, with a relatively narrow base, extending anteriorly from the upper corner of the atrium and curving around the right ventricular outflow tract and main pulmonary artery, is the left atrial appendage.[4] The mitral valve is situated anteroinferiorly in the left atrial chamber. Blood drains through the mitral valve into the left ventricle,

which is an ellipsoid chamber with fewer and finer trabeculations along with a thicker wall than the right ventricle. No muscular structure separates the mitral and aortic valves in the left ventricle, as there is the crista supraventricularis on the right.[3]

Because the interventricular septum has an undulating course, similar to that of an airplane's propeller, it is impossible to visualize the septum in any single projection. The membranous portion is situated just below the commissure between the right and noncoronary cusps. On the right side, the septal leaflet of the tricuspid valve attaches to the membranous septum, almost bisecting it. The portion of the septum behind the tricuspid valve lies between the right atrium and the left ventricle; the portion in front of the valve attachment is interposed between the right and left ventricles.[3] Except for complications or congenital anomalies, the pacing wires are situated in the right heart; therefore, the primary focus of this chapter is right-sided anatomy.

Atrial Lead Positioning and Malpositioning

In the placement of the right atrial lead, the approach can be from the right or left side of the body, depending on the anatomy and the patient's or physician's preference. Typically, the approach is made from the left side. Generally, it is percutaneous through the subclavian vein, using a modified Seldinger approach. The wire traverses the subclavian vein, the brachiocephalic vein, the superior vena cava, and the body of the right atrium before typically being fixed in the right atrial appendage.[5] A cut-down procedure can also be used in the cephalic vein or external or internal jugular veins. If the patient has not had previous open heart surgery, the atrial appendage (which is an anteromedial cardiac structure) is the typical site where the lead is positioned.

If the patient, however, has had previous open heart sur-

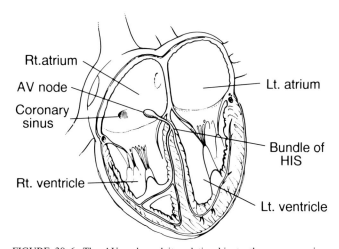

FIGURE 30–6. The AV node and its relationship to the coronary sinus foramen. AV, atrioventricular; Rt., right; Lt., left.

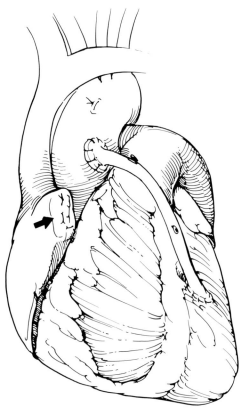

FIGURE 30–8. Diagram depicting a heart that has undergone previous revascularization. Note the saphenous vein graft to the left anterior descending (LAD) and the transected right atrial appendage *(arrow)*.

gery, the atrial appendage has generally been truncated at the time of the procedure (Fig. 30–8). Positioning in these patients is more likely to be in the anterior wall of the right atrium. The lead can be unipolar, the one electrode being the tip of the pacing lead (cathode) and the ground portion of the electrical system being the pulse generator (anode), or a bipolar lead system can be used. In the latter, the two electrodes are situated near the end of the lead, with the most distal being the cathode and the more proximal, the anode. The leads can be passive or active; the former have fine tines that mesh in the trabeculation of the right atrium that are not apparent on the standard roentgenogram and require several weeks for fibrosis to occur; the latter have screws that have the appearance of tiny coils that may be either retractable or fixed. There are some active fixed leads that have a ''stab'' fixation apparatus.[6]

On occasion, leads have been placed in the coronary sinus rather than the atrial appendage or the body of the right atrium. If the body of the right atrium is used, the position of the electrode can be either in the septum or anteriorly, either high or low but usually not laterally because of the presence of the phrenic nerve and the possibility of diaphragmatic stimulation (Fig. 30–9).

The atrial lead can be the primary lead for pacing, as part of an atrial pacemaking system (AAI), or it can be part of a dual-chambered system, such as DVI or DDD. In positioning the atrial lead, if there is either an atrial septal defect or patent foramen ovale, the lead can cross over and be inadvertently positioned in the left atrium. It is identified on routine chest roentgenograms as being situated posteriorly in the region of the left atrium. In certain patients with congenital heart disease, such positioning can be seen after a Senning operation with a baffle (Fig. 30–10). Patients with dextrocardia can also present challenges in the optimal placement of the electrodes.

If the lead that is placed in the right atrium is dislodged, it can migrate to either a new atrial position, the inferior vena cava, the tricuspid valve area, the right ventricle, or occasionally, the superior vena cava. Perforation by the atrial lead can lead to pericarditis or pericardial tamponade and produce a lack of either sensing or pacing.[7] Both ultrasonography[8] and computed tomography[9] have been reported to be diagnostic in patients who have had atrial perforation. Magnetic resonance imaging has not been used in patients with pacing devices because of the possible electrical and thermal complications produced by exposure to the high radiofrequency signals. Presently, research is being performed on the development of devices that may not respond unfavorably when exposed to magnetic resonance imaging.

Ventricular Lead Positioning and Malpositioning

The approach for a ventricular lead system is the same as that for the atrial lead. Again, the leads may be either active, fixed, or passive or unipolar or bipolar. The ventricular lead traverses the same venous structures, the right atrium, and finally, the right ventricular chamber. Typically, the electrode is situated near the right ventricular apex. This structure is generally to the left of the spine on the posteroanterior view and is situated slightly inferiorly. The wire should have a gentle curve. There should not be a redundant amount of wire, nor should it be too taut. The placement of pacing systems in the pediatric population poses certain problems related to growth. A sufficient amount of wire must be inserted to allow for the normal increase in the dimensions of the torso.

On the lateral view, the wire of the ventricular lead is directed anteriorly, with its tip in the distal inflow tract behind the sternum. Other locations in the right ventricle can be the proximal inflow tract, the septal area, or the outflow tract. The ventricular pacing lead may inadvertently be placed in the coronary sinus, which would demonstrate a more posterior course on the lateral view, or occasionally, in one of its tributaries, such as the middle cardiac vein (Fig. 30–11).

If malfunction occurs, such as an exit block with excessive fibrosis (Fig. 30–12), a second lead must be placed in the ventricle or a new lead from a completely different system must be used. Ventricular leads may exist as part of an implantable cardioverter-defibrillator (ICD). The original ICD systems consisted of a myocardial patch with a spring electrode in the superior vena cava–right atrial area and a transvenous lead in the right ventricle for sensing purposes. Subsequent devices used two myocardial patches and two myocardial sensing and pacing leads. However, with the recent development of transvenous defibrillators, right ventricular paced and sensed leads are used.[10] On occasion, with older-generation ICDs, new sensing leads can be positioned

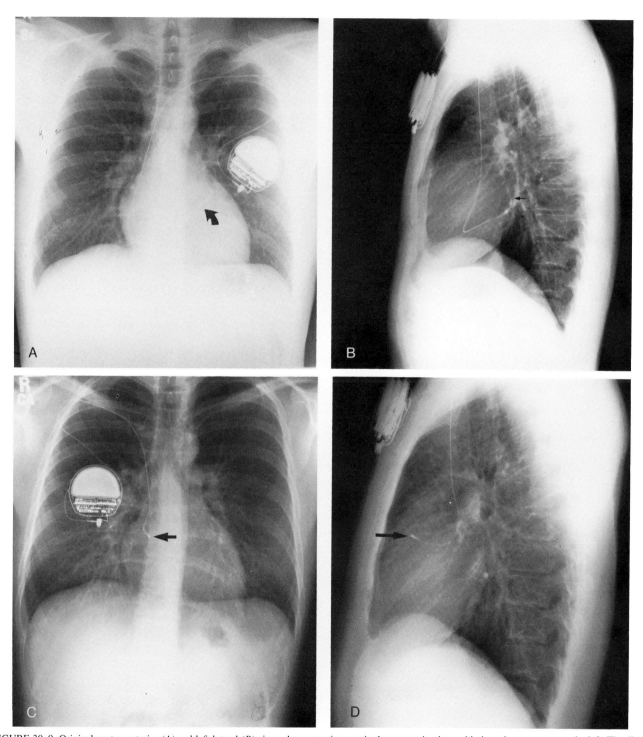

FIGURE 30–9. Original posteroanterior (A) and left lateral (B) views demonstrating a unipolar system in place with the pulse generator on the left. The distal aspect of the wire is in the coronary sinus on the posteroanterior view (curved arrow). On the lateral view, the wire is directed posteriorly. This is an AAI system. On posteroanterior (C) and left lateral (D) views obtained 4 years later, the original system has been removed, and now a unipolar right-sided system has been inserted whose tip (arrow) is in the anterior wall of the right atrium. This also is an AAI system.

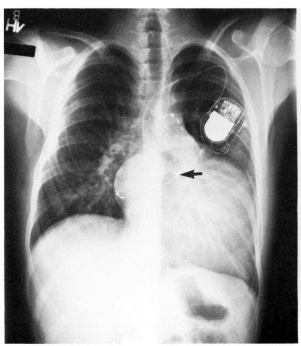
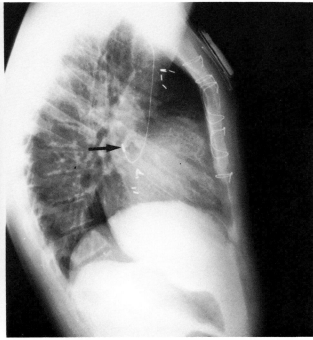

FIGURE 30–10. Sternotomy wires are in place. There is a unipolar, single-chamber AAI pacing system in place with the generator on the left. The active fixed wire is located in an unusual position, traversing the midline and being located in the left atrium *(arrow)*. The patient has a diagnosis of transposition of the great vessels and has undergone previous multiple surgeries to correct his congenital heart defect.

in the right ventricle using a transvenous approach. Although there are right ventricular leads with antitachycardia pacing devices, these pacemakers are no longer implanted since the availability of tiered-therapy cardioverter defibrillator systems.[11] ICD devices may exist with single- or dual-chambered bradycardia pacemakers.

Occasionally, the right ventricular wire can perforate the ventricle; this is diagnosed by showing its tip extending beyond the cardiac silhouette. If the right ventricular lead perforates the septum or the wall of the ventricle, it paces externally on the left ventricle; therefore, there will be electrocardiographic evidence of right bundle branch block while pacing. This would require repositioning of the pacing lead. The pacing lead may also be placed inadvertently into the left ventricle by a patent ventricular septal defect, a patent foramen ovale, or perforation through the septum (Fig. 30–13). One of the major complications from left ventricular placement is systemic embolic disease. The most catastrophic

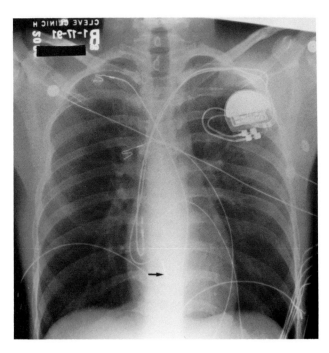

FIGURE 30–11. A portable chest roentgenogram demonstrating a pacing system that has been inserted from a left-sided approach. Note the rather abrupt angulation of the ventricular lead in its distal course *(arrow)*, which descends in an almost vertical direction. It is located in the middle cardiac vein.

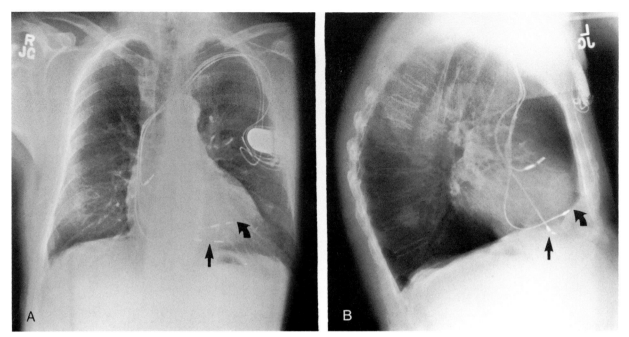

FIGURE 30–12. Posteroanterior *(A)* and left lateral *(B)* chest views demonstrating a dual-chamber pacing system in place with a bipolar passive fixed electrode in the right atrial appendage, a bipolar active fixed electrode just above the right ventricular apex *(curved arrow)*, and an unused (capped) passively fixed electrode in the right ventricular apex *(straight arrow)*. The capped ventricular lead was replaced because of high pacing thresholds.

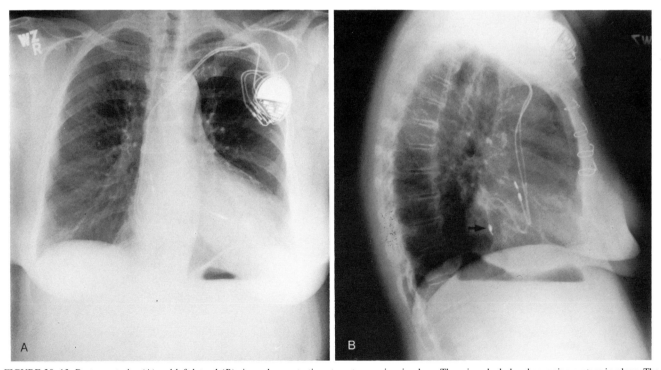

FIGURE 30–13. Posteroanterior *(A)* and left lateral *(B)* views demonstrating sternotomy wires in place. There is a dual-chamber pacing system in place. The ventricular wire has a peculiar curve on the posteroanterior view, and on the lateral view it is noted to extend in a posterocranial direction, only then to curve back on itself with the tip of the wire in the wall of the left ventricle *(arrow)*. This is an example of improper placement, with the wire traversing the foramen ovale and extending through the body of the left atrium through the mitral valve and into the left ventricle. Of note is the fact that the patient did develop incomplete right bundle branch block in the interim between the placement of the system and the first electrocardiogram that was obtained during clinical follow-up. (From Trohman RG, Wilkoff BL, Byrne T, Cook S: Successful percutaneous extraction of a chronic left ventricular pacing lead. PACE Pacing Clin Electrophysiol 14:1448, 1991.)

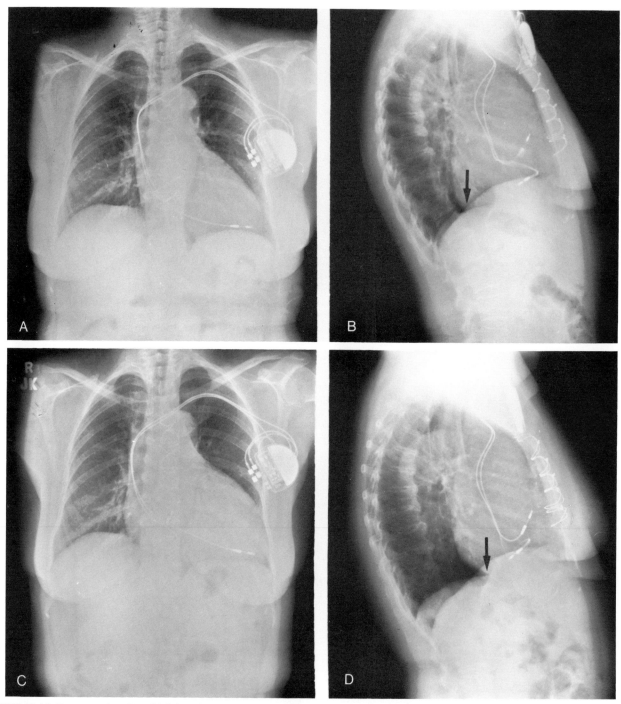

FIGURE 30–14. Posteroanterior *(A)* and left lateral *(B)* views demonstrating sternotomy wires in place with a bipolar DDD pacemaker with active fixed leads. There is evidence of cardiomegaly with straightening of the posterior heart border near its interface with the left hemidiaphragm *(arrow)*. The pulmonary vasculature is not congested. The findings suggest a pericardial effusion. *C* and *D*, Follow-up chest roentgenograms obtained several months later demonstrating a decrease in heart size with now a sharp angle at the ventricular diaphragmatic interface *(arrow)*. This is an example of perforation of the myocardium secondary to pacemaker placement, with the development of hemorrhage into the pericardium and subsequent resolution.

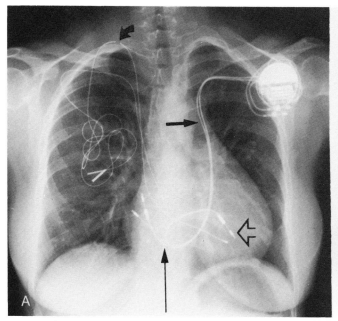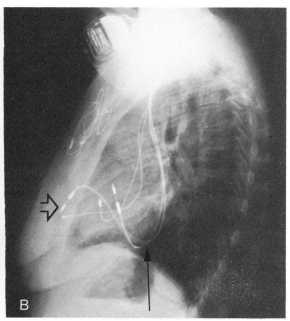

FIGURE 30–15. Posteroanterior *(A)* and left lateral *(B)* views demonstrating an abandoned system on the right, which is of the dual-chamber variety with a passive fixed electrode in the right ventricle and an active fixed electrode in the right ventricle. Note disruption of the ventricular wire near the right lung apex *(curved arrow)*, indicating a fracture. A new system had been placed on the left side, which is situated near the axilla, having two active fixed electrodes. Note the unusual course of the wires to the left of midline *(straight arrow)*, indicating that it descends down a persistent left superior vena cava and into the coronary sinus *(narrow arrow)*. The wires loop around and ultimately reach their final destination in the right atrial appendage and the outflow tract of the right ventricle *(open arrow)*, respectively.

is related to neurologic complications.[12–14] On occasion, there may be perforation of the right ventricular wall because of its thickness, being typically only 2 to 3 mm. This can lead to a lack of sensing and/or pacing and is often associated with pericardial effusion (Fig. 30–14).

Although computed tomography has been used in diagnosing malplacement and perforation,[9] cardiac echography is helpful in noninvasively assessing the course of wires that are suspected of being aberrant and also in diagnosing pericardial effusions.[15, 16]

On occasion, the ventricular lead can extend into the coronary sinus and appear to be in the region of the right ventricular apex on the posteroanterior view; on the lateral view, however, a more posterior position is appreciated. A persistent left superior vena cava may be present, which makes access to the right atrium and right ventricle difficult. However, this can be accomplished by active-fixed atrial and ventricular leads (Fig. 30–15).[17] Rarely, the ventricular lead is located in the pulmonary artery.

Lead Positioning in Children and Adults with Congenital Heart Disease

Generally, in small children, especially those younger than 5 years of age, epicardial leads of the screw-in variety are used. These can be placed either in the right and/or left ventricle or the right and/or left atrium. Epicardial leads are only unipolar; therefore, to create a bipolar system, two electrodes connected to an adapter are necessary to produce a

complete system. If a dual-chambered bipolar epicardial system is used, four electrodes are required, two in the atria and two in the ventricle with two sets of adapters connected to the pulse generator. These leads usually are tunneled into the abdominal cavity because of the small chest size of the child. In older children, transvenous pacing systems can be used. In growing children, however, it is important to determine the appropriate length of the wires so that frequent replacement is not necessary and dislodgement of the lead does not occur because of a short wire.[18] Lead fractures of epicardial systems are easy to identify, and multiple leads are often required in the long-term management of a child requiring a pacing system (Fig. 30–16).[19]

Epicardial leads may also be used in patients undergoing valve replacement to obviate the need of transvenous electrodes, which on occasion, cannot be manipulated across the tricuspid valve. Other congenital anomalies, such as Ebstein's, may also prevent the transvenous placement of an electrode in the right ventricle.

Epicardial systems in children, if there are no contraindications, can be changed to transvenous systems as the child grows. Dextrocardia may present another challenge for the placement of a lead system (Fig. 30–17). Corrected transposition of the great vessels is another congenital anomaly that poses problems. In this condition, the great vessels are transposed in the setting of a discordant AV connection.[4] The anatomic left ventricle becomes the functional right, and the anatomic right ventricle becomes the functional left ventricle. The morphologic left ventricle, which is the functioning right ventricle, has fewer trabeculations, and it is therefore more difficult to place a passive ventricular lead in such a ventricle.

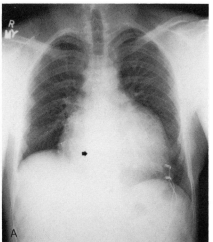

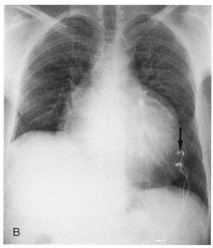

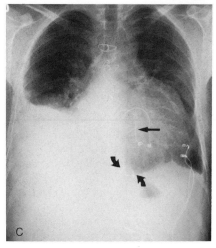

FIGURE 30–16. This patient is a young male adult with complex congenital heart disease. *A*, Posteroanterior roentgenogram dated 9/88 demonstrating a Hancock valve in the tricuspid position *(arrow)* and a St. Jude's valve in the mitral position. The patient initially had two sets of epicardial wires, which were attached to an energy source on the left side of the abdomen. Note the intact screw-in electrodes near the apex. *B*, Roentgenogram obtained approximately 4 years later demonstrating disruption of one of the screw-in electrodes, which is situated near the apex of the heart *(arrow)*. *C*, Final roentgenogram obtained approximately 1 month later demonstrating insertion of a new set of epicardial wires *(curved arrows)*, which are situated adjacent to the left cardiophrenic angle. The new system was installed at the same time that the patient underwent a surgical procedure to replace his mitral valve *(straight arrow)* and also his annuloplasty ring with a prosthetic tricuspid valve. Note the large right-sided effusion secondary to recent surgery.

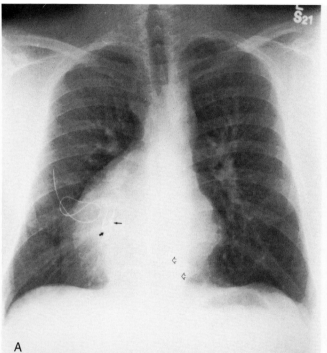
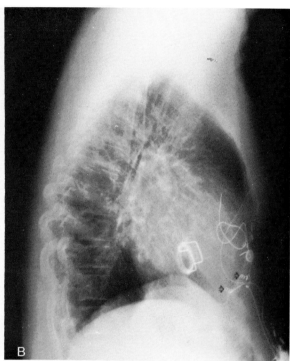

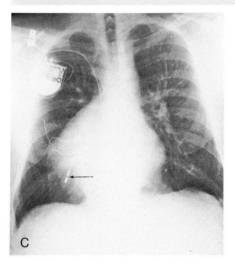

FIGURE 30–17. Posteroanterior *(A)* and left lateral *(B)* views obtained 8/85 demonstrating dextrocardia, with a prosthetic mitral valve in place. There are remnant stab electrodes identified overlying the right precordium *(small curved and straight black arrows)*. The energy source for a single-chamber pacing system, which has two screw-in electrodes near the subxiphoid area *(open arrows)*, is identified at the margin of the lateral view. *C*, Single posteroanterior view dated 7/89 demonstrates abandonment of the previously placed generator. A single-chamber bipolar system has now been installed with the pulse generator on the right. The position of the new lead is near the right ventricular apex *(narrow arrow)*.

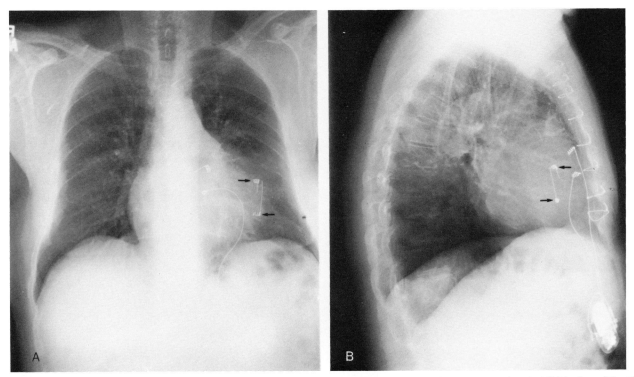

FIGURE 30–18. Posteroanterior *(A)* and left lateral *(B)* views demonstrating sternotomy wires in place. Remnant screw-in epicardial leads are identified along the lateral aspect of the cardiac silhouette, which are identified approximately 3 cm posterior to the sternum on the lateral view. There is a functioning set of epicardial screw-in leads *(arrows)*, which are attached to the myocardium in the region of the right ventricular outflow tract. These are situated more anteriorly on the lateral view.

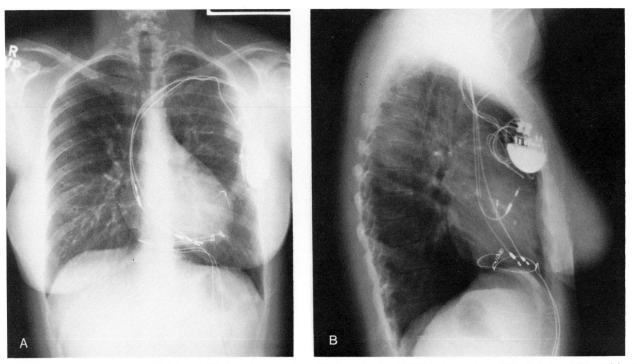

FIGURE 30–19. Posteroanterior *(A)* and left lateral *(B)* views demonstrating a bipolar active fixed DDD pacing system with leads in the right ventricle and right atrial appendage. The pacemaker is buried in the left axillary region. There is also a passive right ventricular bipolar lead that is capped. Two unipolar screw-in epicardial leads have been capped and can be traced down into the left side of the abdomen. There is an abandoned unipolar stab-type epicardial lead that has been fractured, which is situated along the lateral wall of the cardiac silhouette near the junction of the mid and distal thirds.

Unusual Lead Location: Epicardial Tunneling

Although epicardial lead systems generally are tunneled to the abdomen, on occasion, they can be placed in the chest wall (Fig. 30–18). Because of impending erosion, it may be necessary to bury a pulse generator beneath a muscle, move it to a different area, or revise the pocket (Fig. 30–19).[20] In patients who have had a temporary pacing system installed at the time of open heart surgery, it is important to be aware that retained fragments of wires may migrate years later and cause complications.[21] Transvenous and myocardial lead systems can be tunneled into the axillary area, particularly in a thin patient in whom the axillary fat pad tends to decrease the likelihood of erosion.

Lead Problems: Fractures, Dislodgements, Abandonments, and Connector Pins

Plain roentgenograms provide a simple valuable method of diagnosing complications secondary to insertion of the pacemaker's wire. During the introduction of the lead system, using the modified Seldinger approach, the needle can puncture the pleura and lung, leading to a pneumothorax[22, 23] (Fig. 30–20), or profuse bleeding into the pleural space can occur if the subclavian artery is inadvertently entered. Arterial bleeding obviously occurs acutely, and the chest roent-

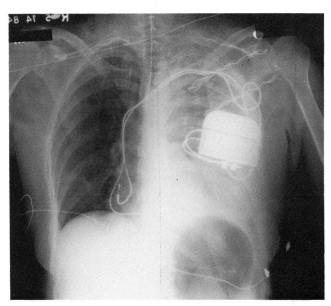

FIGURE 30–21. Anteroposterior portable chest roentgenogram obtained immediately after pacemaker insertion demonstrates a large hemothorax on the left secondary to perforation of the left subclavian artery. There is almost complete opacification of the left hemithorax.

genogram show a large amount of fluid on the side that has been entered (Fig. 30–21). Large pneumothoraces are usually relatively easy to diagnose. If the clinician is concerned, however, about a small pneumothorax, a roentgenogram obtained during expiration in the upright position has a greater likelihood of documenting such a small collection. If bleeding occurs from the subclavian vein, the bleeding is less profuse and may not require aggressive therapy. With arterial bleeding, however, a more aggressive approach with occasional surgical intervention may result.

Although infection can occur at the site of the implantation and the clinician would be suspicious of such a complication by identifying gas in the subcutaneous tissue adjacent to the pulse generator, we have not found this to be a common radiographic manifestation of infection. Sequential roentgenograms of an individual patient that demonstrate placement changes can imply removal secondary to infection (Fig. 30–22).[17]

The patient can also develop partial venous thrombosis secondary to the wires being in various venous channels (Fig. 30–23). Thrombosis may occur in the subclavian vein or in the smaller tributaries of the subclavian vein;[24] however, superior vena caval thrombosis is a relatively unusual but significant complication that can produce serious clinical sequelae.[26] Typically, when thrombosis and occlusion of the superior vena cava occur secondary to insertion of the pacemaker, there is a long latency period of more than 10 months (Fig. 30–24).[25]

Mitrovic and associates,[27] in studying 100 patients, demonstrated occlusion at the site of wire insertion in 39 of these patients. In 15, complete occlusion of the venous segment was identified; collateral vessels varied, depending on the site and extent of the occlusion. In the remaining 24 patients, there was only partial occlusion, without evidence of collateralization. In 12 of the 39 patients, impairment of venous flow was indicated by clinical signs and symptoms, and in 10, impairment was suggested by the medical history. Con-

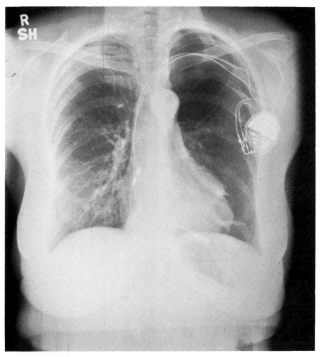

FIGURE 30–20. Posteroanterior chest roentgenogram demonstrating a dual-chamber pacing system in place with fixed electrodes in both the right atrial appendage and the right ventricular apex. Note the relative radiolucency over the left chest compared with the right. There is a moderate-sized pneumothorax on the left, with evidence of subsegmental atelectasis in the lingula and in the left lower lobe. Note absence of lung markings superiorly.

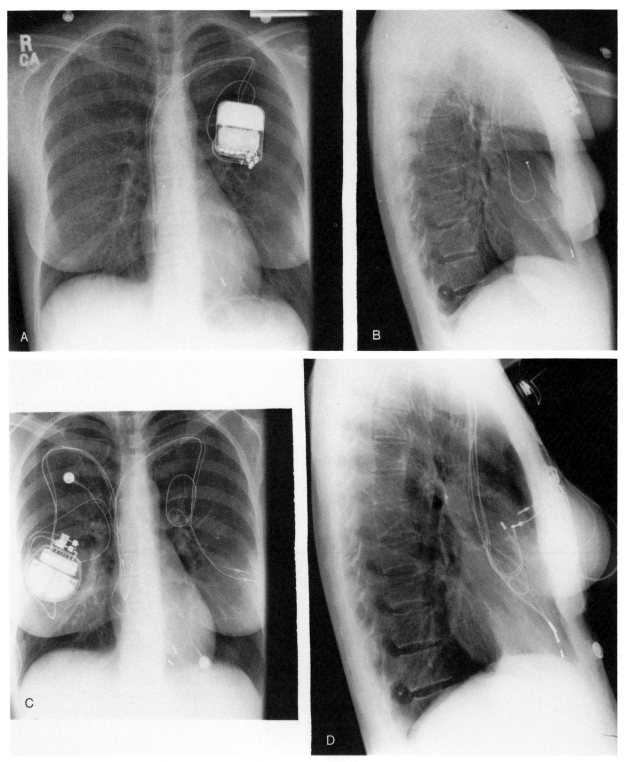

FIGURE 30–22. Original posteroanterior *(A)* and left lateral *(B)* chest roentgenograms demonstrating a dual-chamber passive lead system in place with the generator on the left. Note the position of the generator superior to the breast parenchyma, which is easily identifiable on both views. Posteroanterior *(C)* and left lateral *(D)* views obtained 3 years later demonstrating abandonment of the wires on the left side. A new system has been inserted from the right. The patient simultaneously requested that an augmentation mammoplasty procedure be performed, and therefore the new generator was placed in the right retromammary region.

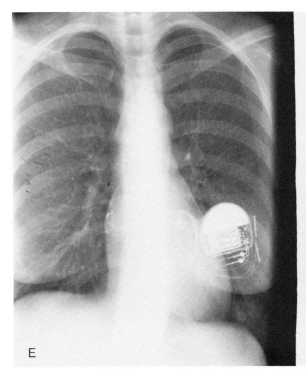 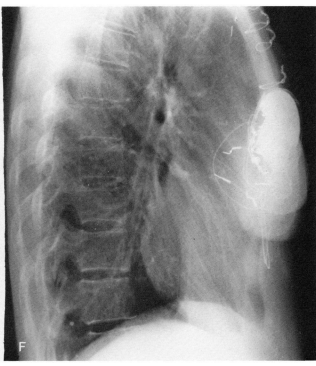

FIGURE 30–22 *Continued* Final posteroanterior *(E)* and left lateral *(F)* views demonstrating a completely new system installed with epicardial stab leads being placed anteriorly in the right atrium and right ventricle. The patient developed an infection after the augmentation procedure, and both breast implants were removed. The four epicardial leads are situated anteriorly in the right atrium and ventricle. Note the sternotomy wires that are now in place.

ventional analog venography can sometimes be misleading in diagnosing thrombosis of the subclavian vein. A digital subtraction technique provides improved contrast and also enables the clinician to use a smaller volume of contrast to provide exquisite detail in diagnosing thrombotic complications.[28] Lytic therapy has been effective in treating patients who develop superior vena cava syndrome secondary to acute thrombosis.

Narrowing of the superior vena cava, because of fibrosis secondary to remnant pacemaker wires, is a relatively unusual complication.[29] This complication frequently responds to intravascular balloon dilatation.[29] In one of our patients, unfortunately, we were unsuccessful in satisfactorily dilating the narrowing (Fig. 30–25).

Serial roentgenograms visually demonstrate the advancements in technology in this ever-changing field (Fig. 30–26). By being aware of the appearance of various pacemaking systems, the clinician appreciates the developing complexity of various devices and the importance of being familiar with the various components and their potential complications.[30, 31]

Roentgenograms of pacing systems show abnormalities of lead systems with obvious lead fractures[32] (Figs. 30–27 and 30–28) or leads that have been previously fractured and spliced with subsequent refracturing near the splice (Fig. 30–29). Few fractures tend to occur in the pacing pocket where the lead changes from a large to a smaller diameter near the connector pin. Fractures tend to occur at the point of entrance into the venous system and also where the stabilizing sutures have been used to fix the lead to prevent movement. Also, if leads are used in the jugular system and are looped over the clavicle, they have a higher likelihood of fracture, particularly if they are positioned laterally across the clavicle, be-

cause of the motion of the shoulder and clavicular area. Leads that have tight coils or excessive angulation also are at greater risk. Occasionally, lead fractures occur in the intravascular space secondary to metallic fatigue, which is produced by the motion of the heart and vascular system.

At times, there may be abnormalities on the roentgenogram that have the appearance of fractures without an actual fracture of the lead system. These are called "pseudofractures." The term pseudofracture has been used to refer to two different roentgenographic observations.

One type occurs when tight ligatures (Fig. 30–30) are placed around the pacemaker's lead, which is generally coated by polyurethane, with the ligature compressing the insulation and producing the appearance of a fracture.[33] The wire coil is often opened by this external pressure. Although it does not represent an actual fracture, this can lead to a subsequent true fracture with time. Tight ligatures can also lead to insulation fractures, which can cause pacing systems to malfunction (generally manifested by low impedances). This can occur also at the time of surgery if the lead is partially bisected.

A second type of pseudofracture is associated with a particular system's construction in which the appearance of the bifurcated bipolar lead changes at the transition of the lead from a coaxial to a linear configuration, giving the appearance on the roentgenogram of a wire fracture, although actually there is continuity of the lead system (Fig. 30–31).[34, 35] The actual integrity of the lead can be determined by checking the pacing system through programming.

Although pin reversal is not common and is usually a diagnosis made by an evaluation of the pacemaker and electrocardiographic findings, careful attention to the pace-

Text continued on page 558

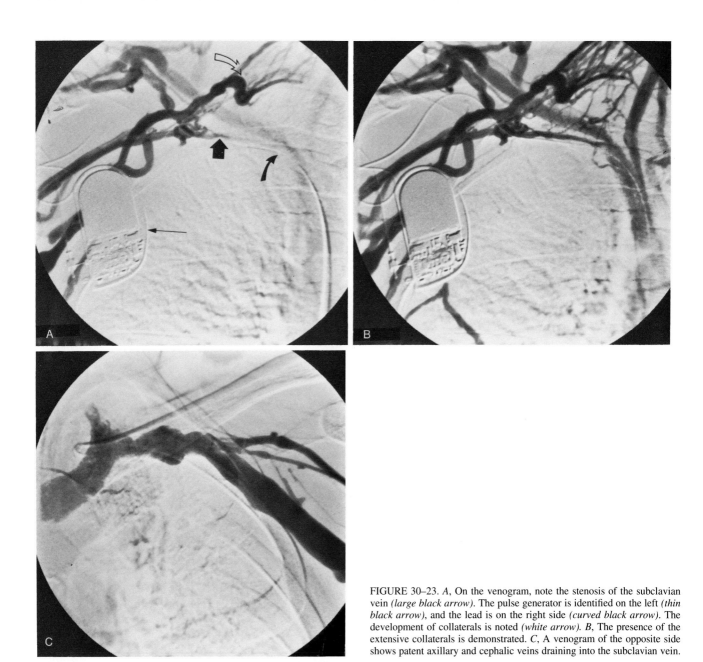

FIGURE 30–23. *A*, On the venogram, note the stenosis of the subclavian vein *(large black arrow)*. The pulse generator is identified on the left *(thin black arrow)*, and the lead is on the right side *(curved black arrow)*. The development of collaterals is noted *(white arrow)*. *B*, The presence of the extensive collaterals is demonstrated. *C*, A venogram of the opposite side shows patent axillary and cephalic veins draining into the subclavian vein.

FIGURE 30–24. *A*, Posteroanterior view demonstrating abandoned wires *(arrow)*, which previously had been connected to a pulse generator over the right chest. A functioning dual-chamber unipolar system has been inserted on the left. Note the normal-appearing superior mediastinum *(open arrows)*. *B*, Subsequent film obtained 3 weeks later demonstrating removal of the left-sided pacing system. There is also evidence of a sternotomy. Only parts of the previously described bipolar system, which had been previously inserted on the right, are identified. The tips of two other wires are identified in the superior vena cava. Wires from an energy source that has been placed in the left side of the abdomen, are identified with four screw-in electrodes overlying the cardiac silhouette, two near the left cardiophrenic angle and two overlying the right atrium. There is a left-sided pleural effusion. Note the significant increase in the width of the superior mediastinum *(open arrows)*. The patient at this time had signs and symptoms of superior vena cava syndrome. *C*, Sternotomy wires remain in place, as do the remnant pacing wires from the previously placed right-sided system. There has been a definite decrease in the width of the mediastinum *(open arrows)*. The patient responded well to thrombolytic therapy.

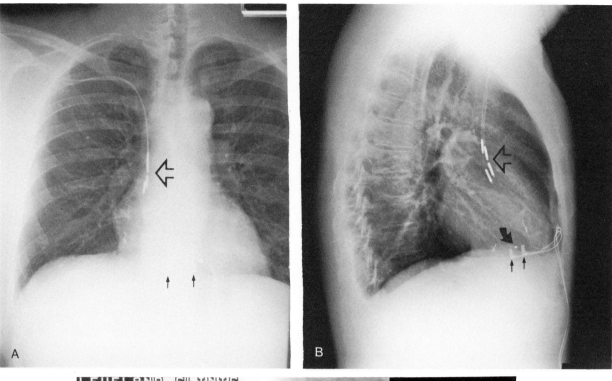

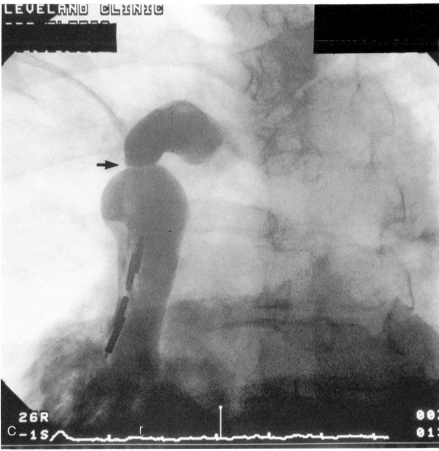

FIGURE 30–25. Posteroanterior *(A)* and left lateral *(B)* chest roentgenograms demonstrating remnants of previously placed pacing system, which had been inserted through a right subclavian vein with wires extending from the axillary vein and the electrode tips into the distal superior vena cava *(open arrows).* An epicardial system is identified in place, with two screw-in *(tiny arrows)* and two stab electrodes identified along the inferior aspect of the cardiac silhouette. There is also a tiny metallic density identified on the lateral view between the two screw-in electrodes, which represents a remnant passively fixed electrode *(curved arrow).* Despite multiple attempts, the transvenously placed remnant wires could not be extracted. *C,* Single anteroposterior venogram of the superior vena cava demonstrates a stenotic lesion at the origin of the superior vena cava adjacent to the inferior aspect of the first right rib *(arrow).* Several attempts to dilate the narrowing were unsuccessful.

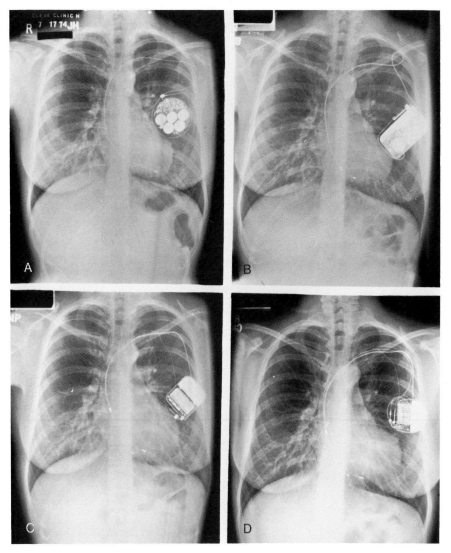

FIGURE 30–26. Natural history of pacemakers in a single patient. *A,* Posteroanterior chest roentgenograms demonstrating a unipolar VVI mercury cell pacemaker in place with the battery on the left. *B,* Posteroanterior chest roentgenogram obtained 7 years later demonstrating the insertion of a bipolar nickel-cadmium rechargeable pacemaker. *C,* Posteroanterior chest roentgenogram obtained approximately 3 years later demonstrating a unipolar VVI lithium-powered pacemaker with a retained ventricular bipolar lead, which has been capped. This is an increase in distance between the bipolar electrodes, secondary to attempted but failed extraction. *D,* Posteroanterior chest roentgenogram obtained 4 years later demonstrating the insertion of a lithium-powered DDD unit. A new atrial appendage electrode has been inserted. The retained wire described in *C* is again visualized.

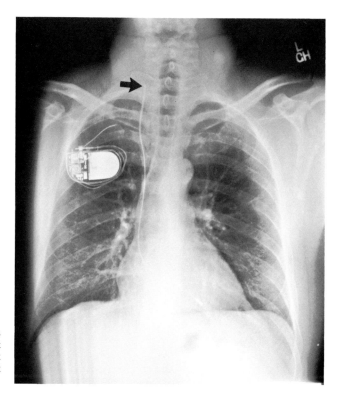

FIGURE 30–27. Posteroanterior chest roentgenogram demonstrating an obvious fracture of the pacing wire with the proximal end of the long distal component in the jugular vein *(arrow)*. The generator is in place on the right, and a short segment of wire is attached to it, which ends in the proximal portion of the right subclavian vein. The pacemaker is a VVI bipolar model.

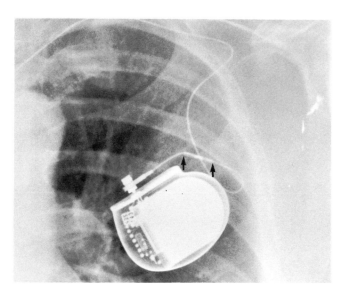

FIGURE 30–28. A close-up view of a single-chamber unipolar pacing system demonstrating the appearance of a splice *(small arrows)* overlying the right fifth rib near the posterior axillary line, which is part of the right ventricular wire.

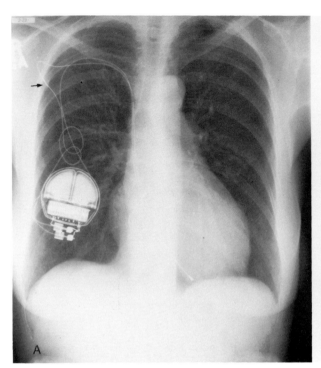

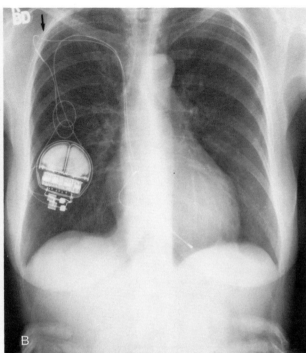

FIGURE 30–29. *A,* Posteroanterior chest roentgenogram after pacemaker insertion demonstrating a spliced wire *(arrow),* which is situated a few centimeters from the pulse generator. The wire is connected to a passively fixed unipolar electrode, which is located in the inflow tract of the right ventricle. *B,* Follow-up roentgenogram demonstrating a new fracture *(arrow)* a few centimeters above the splice.

maker's header and lead positioning can diagnose a lead reversal (Fig. 30–32). Leads should always leave the pulse generator in a clockwise fashion when viewed on the posteroanterior roentgenogram. Otherwise, the pacemaker is upside down toward the underlying muscle, which may cause

skeletal muscle stimulation or myopotential sensing during unipolar pacing and sensing.

The twiddler syndrome (Fig. 30–33) was described in the literature more than 25 years ago and generally implies an intentional rotation of the pulse generator in the pocket by the patient.[36] However, pacemakers can flip in the pocket because of physical activity, and this can be a source of discomfort to the patient. This can frequently be diagnosed by sequential roentgenograms that provide the opportunity to

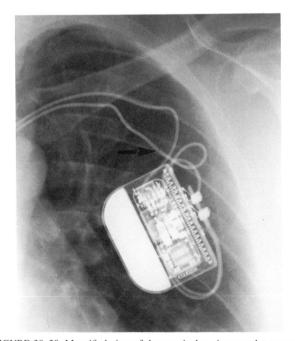

FIGURE 30–30. Magnified view of the ventricular wire near the generator showing a localized indentation *(arrow)* superior to the generator. This does not represent disruption of the wire but merely too tight a placement of the ligature.

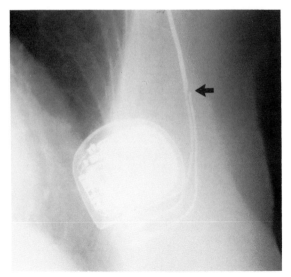

FIGURE 30–31. Example of a pseudofracture *(arrow).* This appearance is related to the design and construction of the coaxial system and not to a disruption of the wire (see text).

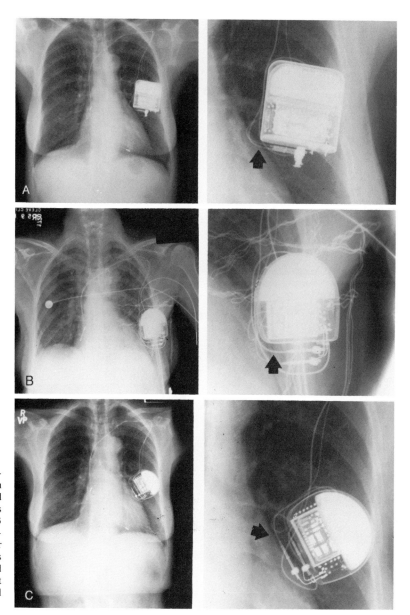

FIGURE 30–32. Sequential roentgenograms showing pin reversal. *A*, Original roentgenogram after pacemaker insertion shows the wire that has the wider diameter *(arrow)* connected to the channel that is situated further from the battery, which is the atrial channel. *B*, Roentgenogram obtained approximately 3 weeks later demonstrates pin reversal with the now wider diameter wire *(arrow)* being situated closer to the pacemaker battery, which is the ventricular channel. The pacemaker was malfunctioning at this time. *C*, Final roentgenogram obtained approximately 1 month later demonstrates normal placement with the thicker wire *(arrow)* now being situated in the atrial channel (more distant to the battery), which is normal.

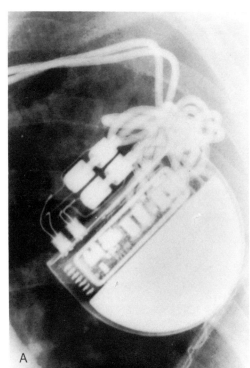
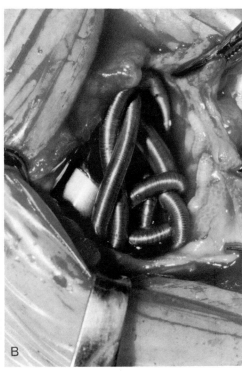

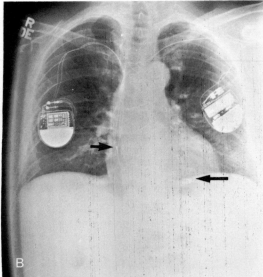

FIGURE 30–33. *A*, Magnified view of a roentgenogram of a patient with "twiddler's syndrome." *B*, During surgical exploration, the pacer had to be twisted 18 revolutions to uncoil the leads. Note the wormlike characteristic of the multiple loops of the electrode wires, which are coiled on themselves.

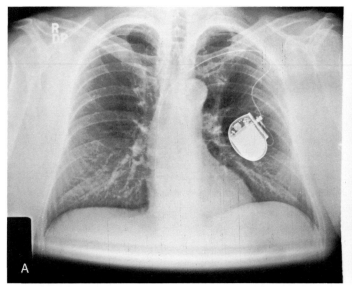

FIGURE 30–34. *A*, Posteroanterior chest view demonstrating a unipolar VVI pacemaker system. The tip of the electrode is in the inflow tract of the right ventricle. *B*, The sternotomy wires are now noted. There are now two pacemakers, one over the right and the other over the left chest. The battery on the left has been changed. This continues to be a unipolar VVI system. On the right side, however, a unipolar DDD pacing system has been inserted. This pacemaker has two wires: one in the right atrial appendage *(short arrow)* and the other in the right ventricular apex *(long arrow)*.

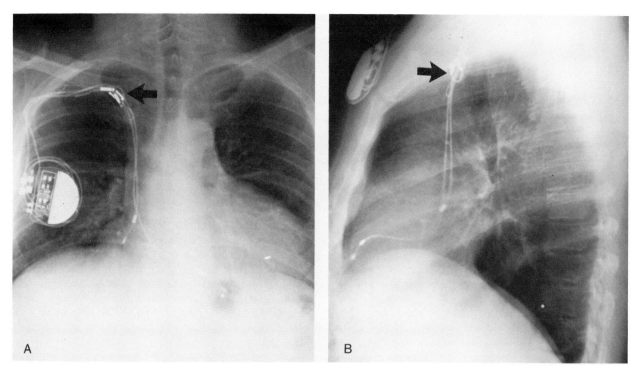

FIGURE 30–35. Posteroanterior *(A)* and left lateral *(B)* views demonstrate a DDD bipolar pacemaker with the atrial lead situated lower in the body of the atrium than is typical. There is evidence of retained fragmented wires in the right subclavian vein *(arrow)*. This makes the patient more liable to develop thrombosis in the left subclavian vein. Of incidental note, is the presence of a tiny metallic foreign body in the posterior medial basilar segment of the left lower lobe.

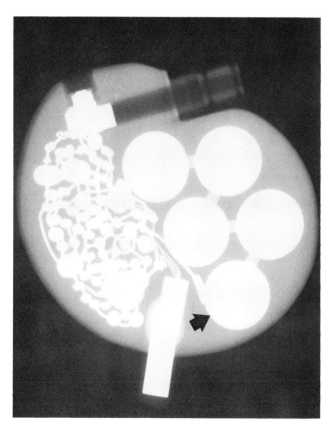

FIGURE 30–36. Early-generation mercury-zinc–powered pulse generator with five batteries and early circuitry. The arrow points to one of the mercury-zinc batteries.

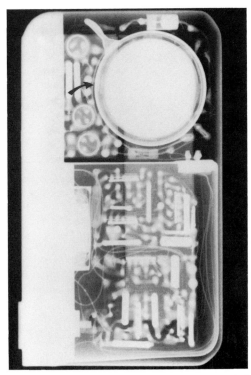

FIGURE 30–37. Rechargeable pulse generator with an arrow pointing to the power source of a nickel-cadmium rechargeable battery. Note the multiple circuitry boards.

appreciate a change in the orientation of the pacemaker's battery.[37]

Rarely, there are unusual situations in which a previous pacing system is not removed when an upgraded pacer sys-

tem is installed, and two completely functioning separate pacemakers can be identified in one patient (Fig. 30–34).

When certain pacing systems malfunction or no longer satisfactorily treat the patient's arrhythmia, it becomes necessary to remove the previous pacing system and to install a new one. Although the pulse generator is technically easy to exchange or remove, the pacing leads are often difficult to remove, and roentgenographic evidence may demonstrate retained lead systems with pacemakers. These can provide a nidus for subsequent thrombosis and possibly for pulmonary embolization.[38] At other times, retained leads in the superior vena cava can also be the nidus of thrombosis, which can propagate and cause evidence of clinical thrombosis[27] (Fig. 30–35).

Numerous companies manufacture various pulse generators, which appear roentgenographically as different units. Although virtually all pacing power sources in the modern era use lithium, roentgenograms can identify other power sources, such as mercury cells and rechargeable batteries. In the past, a few nuclear energy sources were implanted.[39] Manufacturers provide charts of their systems with identification numbers and identification clues that enable clinicians to identify the manufacturer and model number of a pacing system by roentgenography (Figs. 30–36 to 30–40). How-

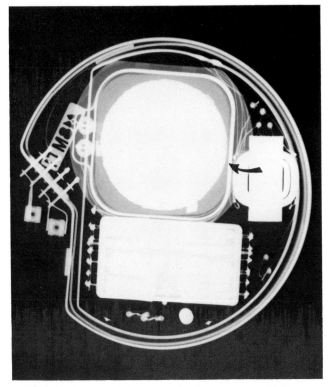

FIGURE 30–38. Early lithium-powered pulse generator, with the arrow pointing to the lithium battery.

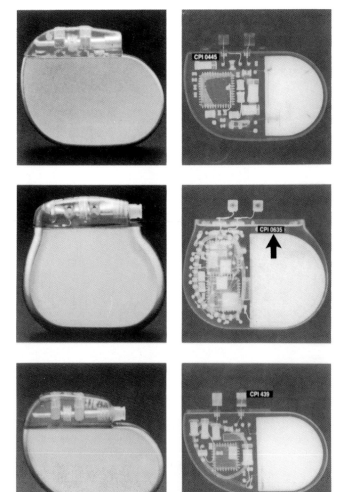

FIGURE 30–39. Series of lithium-powered pacemakers of various model types. Note the manufacturer's identification code, with an arrow pointing to the code in the middle figure.

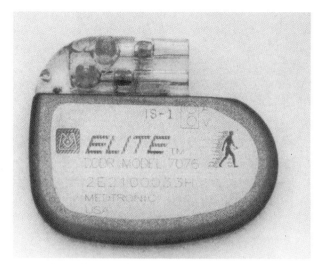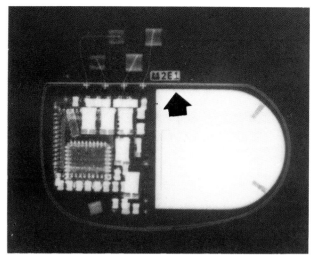

FIGURE 30–40. Modern dual-chambered rate-responsive pacemaker, with an arrow pointing to the manufacturer's identification number.

ever, it is more difficult to identify a specific type of lead system, unless the clinician is relatively familiar with the various leads that a manufacturer produces.

Summary

In approaching the roentgenogram of a patient with a pacing system, it is important to evaluate not only the system, but also the normal thoracic anatomic structures. The roentgenograms, which typically include a posteroanterior and left lateral chest view, provide information related to the pulse generator that should be identified both in terms of its location and, if possible, its model type. Notation of the device's polarity and connector blocks should also be made. The connection of the lead system to the pulse generator should be evaluated, and a determination should be made of whether the electrodes are of the transvenous or epimyocardial variety. The clinician should also describe whether the leads are atrial, ventricular, or both. Brief mention should be made of the type of fixation, the polarity, and the lead's integrity. If other remnant lead systems have been abandoned, a description of such should be included in the report. Any unusual observation or abnormality should be noted.

By using a systematic approach in the evaluation of the roentgenograms of patients who have undergone insertions of pacing systems, the clinician can make more accurate and appropriate interpretations, with subsequently better care for the patient.

REFERENCES

1. Wechsler RJ, Steiner RM, Kinori I: Monitoring the monitors: The radiology of thoracic catheters, wires, and tubes. Semin Roentgenol 23:61, 1988.
2. Netter FH: The CIBA Collection of Medical Illustration, Vol. 5. New York, CIBA Pharmaceutical Company, 1969.
3. Baron MG: Anatomy of the heart. In Taveras JM, Ferrucci JT (eds): Radiology. Philadelphia, JB Lippincott, 1987, pp 1–13.
4. Hurst JW, Anderson RH, Wilcox BR, et al: Atlas of the Heart. New York, Gower Medical Publishing, 1988, pp 1.1–1.20.
5. Hertzberg BS, Chiles C, Ravin CE: Right atrial appendage pacing: Radiographic considerations. AJR Roentgenol 145:31, 1985.
6. Filice R, Hutton L, Klein G: Cardiac pacemaker leads: A radiographic perspective. Can Assoc Radiol J 35:20, 1984.
7. Van Nooten G, Verbeet T, Deuvaert FE: Atrial perforation by a screw-in electrode via a left superior vena cava. Am Heart J 119:1439, 1990.
8. Iliceto S, Antonelli G, Sorino M, et al: Two-dimensional echocardiographic recognition of complications of cardiac invasive procedures. Am J Cardiol 53:846, 1984.
9. Sussman SK, Chiles C, Cooper C, Lowe JR: CT demonstration of myocardial perforation by a pacemaker lead. J Comput Assist Tomogr 10:670, 1986.
10. Brady GH, Troutman C, Poole JE, et al: Clinical experience with a tiered-therapy, multiprogrammable antiarrhythmia device. Circulation 85:1689, 1992.
11. Rosenthal ME, Marchlinski FE, Josephson ME: Complications of implantable antitachycardia devices: Diagnosis and management. In Saksena S, Goldschlager N (eds): Electrical Therapy for Cardiac Arrhythmias. Philadelphia, WB Saunders, 1990, pp 574–588.
12. Ross WB, Mohiuddin SM, Pagano T, Hughes D: Malposition of a transvenous cardiac electrode associated with amaurosis fugax. PACE Pacing Clin Electrophysiol 6:119, 1983.
13. Schiavone WA, Castle LW, Salcedo E, Graor R: Amaurosis fugax in a patient with a left ventricular endocardial pacemaker. PACE Pacing Clin Electrophysiol 7:288, 1984.
14. Winner SJ, Boon NA: Transvenous pacemaker electrodes placed unintentionally in the left ventricle: Three cases. Postgrad Med J 65:98, 1989.
15. Villanueva FS, Heinsmer JA, Burman MH, et al: Echocardiographic detection of perforation of the cardiac ventricular septum by a permanent pacemaker lead. Am J Cardiol 59:370, 1987.
16. Brenner JI, Gaines S, Cordier J, et al: Cardiac strangulation: Two-dimensional echo recognition of a rare complication of epicardial pacemaker therapy. Am J Cardiol 61:654, 1988.
17. Steiner RM, Tegtmeyer CJ, Morse D, et al: The radiology of cardiac pacemakers. Radiographics 6:373, 1986.
18. Gheissari A, Hordof AJ, Spotnitz HM: Transvenous pacemakers in children: Relation of lead length to anticipated growth. Ann Thorac Surg 52:118, 1991.
19. El-Sherif N, Samet P: Cardiac Pacing and Electrophysiology, 3rd ed. Philadelphia, WB Saunders, 1991.
20. Siclari F, Uhlschmid G, Zwicky P, Turina M: Intracolonic migration of a pacemaker generator. Thorac Cardiovasc Surg 34:338, 1986.
21. Korompai FL, Hayward RH, Knight WL: Migration of temporary epicardial pace wire fragment retained after a cardiac operation. J Thorac Cardiovasc Surg 94:446, 1987.
22. Grier D, Cook PG, Hartnell GG: Chest radiographs after permanent pacing: Are they really necessary? Clin Radiol 42:244, 1990.
23. Kattan KR, Gutman E, Pantoja E, Makkar JC: Tubes, wires, and rods seen in chest roentgenograms. Crit Rev Diagn Imaging 21:257, 1984.
24. Knudsen F, Ring T, Nielsen ST: Thrombosis of the subclavian vein: A rare complication of transvenous cardiac pacing. Scand J Thorac Cardiovasc Surg 17:125, 1983.

25. Angeli SJ: Superior vena cava syndrome following pacemaker insertion post atrial septal defect repair. Am Heart J 120:433, 1990.

26. Murakami Y, Matsuno T, Izumi S, et al: Superior vena cava syndrome as a complication of DDD pacemaker implantation. Clin Cardiol 13:298, 1990.

27. Mitrovic V, Thormann J, Schlepper M, Neuss H: Thrombotic complications with pacemakers. Int J Cardiol 2:363, 1983.

28. Sharma S, Kaul U, Rajani M: Digital subtraction venography for assessment of deep venous thrombosis in the arms following pacemaker implantation. Int J Cardiol 23:135, 1989.

29. Walpole HT, Lovett KE, Chuang VP, et al: Superior vena cava syndrome treated by percutaneous transluminal balloon angioplasty. Am Heart J 115:1303, 1988.

30. Cope C, Larrieu AJ, Isaacson CS, et al: Transfemoral removal of a chronically implanted pacemaker lead: Report of a case. Ann Thorac Surg 42:329, 1986.

31. Trohman RG, Wilkoff BL, Byrne T, Cook S: Successful percutaneous extraction of a chronic left ventricular pacing lead. PACE Pacing Clin Electrophysiol 14:1448, 1991.

32. Dunbar RD: Radiologic appearance of compromised thoracic catheters, tubes, and wires. Radiol Clin North Am 22:699, 1984.

33. Hayes DL: Pacemaker complications. *In* Furman S, Hayes DL, Holmes DR (eds): A Practice of Cardiac Pacing. New York, Futura Publishing, 1993, pp 361–400.

34. Hecht S, Berdoff R, Van Tosh A, Goldberg E: Radiographic pseudofracture of bipolar pacemaker wire. Chest 88:302, 1985.

35. Dunlap TE, Popat KD, Sorkin RP: Radiographic pseudofracture of the Medtronic bipolar polyurethane pacing lead. Am Heart J 106:167, 1983.

36. Roberts JS, Wagner NK: Pacemaker twiddler's syndrome. Am J Cardiol 63:1013, 1989.

37. Kallinen LM, Hauser RG, Warren J: Complications of permanent pacing systems: Diagnosis and management. *In* Saksena S, Goldschlager N (eds): Electrical Therapy for Cardiac Arrhythmias. Philadelphia, WB Saunders, 1990, pp 320–334.

38. Neuwirth J, Bohutova J, Kolar J, et al: DSA diagnosis of pulmonary embolization from intracardial thrombus in a patient with permanent pacing catheter. PACE Pacing Clin Electrophysiol 13:7, 1990.

39. Smyth N, Millett ML: Complications of pacemaker implantation. *In* Barold SS (ed): Modern Cardiac Pacing. New York, Futura Publishing, 1985, pp 257–304.

PACEMAKER ELECTRO-CARDIOGRAPHY

CHAPTER 31

Timing Cycles and Operational Characteristics of Pacemakers

S. Serge Barold

Understanding the timing cycles of pacemakers is important because "all comprehension of pacemaker electrocardiography depends on the interpretation of pacemaker timing cycles," as emphasized by Furman.[1] Characterization of the various timing cycles that control pacemaker function must be clear and unambiguous to reflect the mathematical behavior of the timing circuits.[2] The increasing complexity of pacemakers and their timing cycles has led to the pacemaker code[3] that has become the essential language of pacing.

Pacemaker Code

Pacemakers are categorized according to the site of pacing electrodes and the mode of pacing[3] (Table 31–1). The letters in the identification code are few and easy to remember: V = ventricle, A = atrium, D = double (A and V), I = inhibited, T = triggered, and 0 = none. The first position denotes the chamber or chambers paced. The second position indicates the chamber or chambers sensed. The third position describes the response to sensing, if any, with I response indicating an inhibited response (output suppressed by a sensed signal), T indicating a triggered response (output discharged by a sensed signal, either P or QRS), and D indicating both inhibited and triggered functions. Both I and T responses reset the timing circuit. In the third position, 0 indicates that the pulse generator is not influenced by cardiac events because it does not sense. Therefore, when the first position is set to pace and the third position is 0, the second one must always be 0, and vice versa. Occasionally the letter

TABLE 31–1. **THE NASPE-BPEG GENERIC PACEMAKER CODE**

POSITION	I	II	III	IV	V
CATEGORY	CHAMBERS PACED	CHAMBERS SENSED	RESPONSE TO SENSING	PROGRAMMABILITY, RATE MODULATION	ANTITACHYARRHYTHMIA FUNCTIONS
	0 = none	0 = none	0 = none	0 = none	0 = none
	A = atrium	A = atrium	T = triggered	P = simple programmable	P = pacing (anti-tachyarrhythmias)
	V = ventricle	V = ventricle	I = inhibited	M = multi-programmable	S = shock
	D = dual (A + V)	D = dual (A + V)	D = dual (T + I)	C = communicating R = rate modulation	D = dual (P + S)
Manufacturer's designation only	S = single (A or V)	S = single (A or V)			

Abbreviations: BPEG, British Pacing and Electrophysiology Group; NASPE, North American Society of Pacing and Electrophysiology.

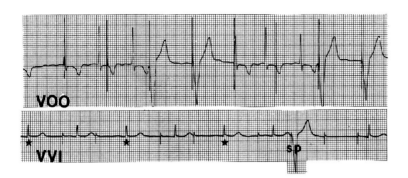

FIGURE 31–1. *Top*, VOO pacing. The pacemaker competes with the spontaneous rhythm. Pacemaker stimuli capture the ventricle only beyond the myocardial refractory period. *Bottom*, Supernormal phase (sp). The recording shows a ventricular demand (VVI) pacemaker with ineffectual pacemaker stimuli. The high pacing threshold was close to the output of the pulse generator. The third last stimulus captures the ventricle in the supernormal phase when the excitability threshold attains its lowest value. Spontaneous QRS complexes falling within the pacemaker refractory period (350 msec after the stimulus) are not sensed; those beyond the pacemaker refractory period are sensed and recycle the pacemaker. (From Barold SS, Zipes DP: Cardiac pacemakers and antiarrhythmic devices. *In* Braunwald E [ed]: Heart Disease: A Textbook of Cardiovascular Medicine. Philadelphia, WB Saunders, 1991, pp 726–755.)

S is used in the first and second positions to indicate that a single-chamber unit is suitable for either atrial or ventricular pacing, depending on how its parameters are programmed. For most pacemakers, the first three positions contain all the information of practical importance. The fourth and fifth positions describe additional functions, but the letters are infrequently stated in practice except for R, which indicates a rate-adaptive, sensor-driven pulse generator.

Operational Characteristics of Single-Chamber Pacemakers

ASYNCHRONOUS AOO AND VOO MODES

In the AOO and VOO modes, pacemaker stimuli are generated asynchronously at a ''fixed-rate'' with no relationship to the spontaneous rhythm. During VOO pacing, stimuli capture the ventricle only when they fall outside the ventricular myocardial refractory period that follows spontaneous ventricular beats (Fig. 31–1). The VOO and AOO modes require only one timing interval (automatic interval). Dedicated VOO or other asynchronous pacemakers that cannot sense are now obsolete. However, asynchronous modes are often used temporarily during testing, when a special magnet is applied over the pacemaker, or by programming the asyn-

chronous mode with an external programmer. The asynchronous mode can occasionally be used for competitive pacing for the treatment of reentrant tachycardia. Rarely, a multiprogrammable pacemaker is permanently programmed to the asynchronous mode to prevent undesirable oversensing.

VVI MODE

In the early 1970s, sensing circuits were added to ventricular pacemakers to allow stimulation only when required or on demand whenever the sensing circuit detects no underlying ventricular activity. A VVI, or ventricular demand pacemaker, senses the intracardiac ventricular depolarization or electrogram, that is, the potential difference between the two electrodes (anode and cathode) also used for pacing (Fig. 31–2). A VVI pacemaker programmed to a predetermined rate of 70 pulses per minute (ppm) will pace with a cycle length of 857 msec whenever the spontaneous rate falls below 70 ppm or the R-R-interval lengthens beyond 857 msec. The timing cycle (or internal clock) of a VVI pulse generator begins with either a sensed or paced ventricular event. The initial portion of the cycle consists of a refractory period (usually 200 to 350 msec), during which the pulse generator cannot sense any signals. The refractory period prevents the pulse generator from sensing its own stimulus waveform, the paced or spontaneous QRS complex, T waves, and the decaying residual voltage (polarization or afterpotential) at the

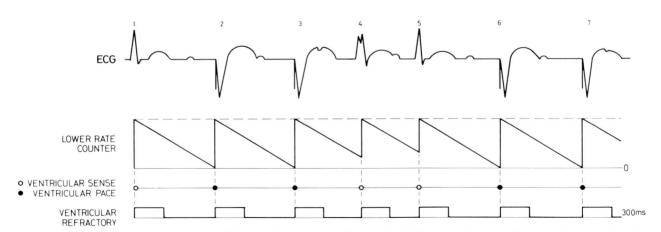

FIGURE 31–2. Diagrammatic representation of the VVI mode of pacing (rate = 80 ppm). The QRS marked 1 is sensed. Beats 2 and 3 are paced complexes. A ventricular extrasystole (4) and a normal QRS (5) are then sensed. The sixth and seventh beats are paced. The pacemaker ventricular refractory period (300 msec) is shown by a rectangle. Complexes 4 and 5 reset and start the lower rate counter before the zero level has been reached, that is, before completion of the escape or automatic interval. The pacemaker emits its stimulus only from the zero level. (From Lindemans FW: Diagrammatic representation of pacemaker function. *In* Barold SS [ed]: Modern Cardiac Pacing. Mt Kisco, NY, Futura Publishing, 1985, pp 323–353.)

electrode-myocardial interface because of an electrochemical process.[4–6] Beyond the pacemaker refractory period, a sensed ventricular event inhibits and resets the pacemaker so that its timing clock returns to the baseline; a new pacing cycle is initiated and the output circuit therefore remains inhibited for a period equal to the programmed pacemaker (or lower rate) interval. Any ventricular event within the ventricular pacemaker refractory period cannot reset the timer responsible for the lower rate interval (LRI). If no signal is sensed, the timing cycle ends with the delivery of a ventricular stimulus, and a new cycle is started. The sensing function prevents competition between pacemaker and intrinsic rhythm and conserves battery capacity.

SINGLE-CHAMBER PACEMAKERS: INTERVALS AND RATES

There are several basic intervals or rates in single-chamber pacemakers. The *automatic interval* is the period between two consecutive stimuli during continuous pacing and corresponds to the programmed free-running or lower rate. For the sake of simplicity, the *escape interval* is measured in the electrocardiogram (ECG) from the onset of the sensed QRS complex (or other signal) to the succeeding pacemaker stimulus. In the case of a VVI pulse generator, sensing ventricular activity, the exact time when the ventricular electrogram activates the sensing circuit (when the timing clock returns to the baseline as in Fig. 31–2) and initiates a new (electronic) escape interval cannot be determined precisely from the surface ECG.[7] Consequently, in pacemakers with identical automatic and "electronic" escape intervals, the escape interval determined from the surface ECG must of necessity be slightly longer than the automatic interval by a value ranging from a few milliseconds to almost the entire duration of the QRS complex, depending on the time of intracardiac sensing according to the temporal relationship of the intracardiac electrogram and the surface ECG. It is evident that a VVI pacemaker requires only two timing intervals: an LRI (automatic interval, usually equal to the electronic escape interval) and the pacemaker refractory period.

Application of a special magnet over a pulse generator closes a magnetic reed switch that inactivates the sensing function with conversion to the asynchronous mode.[8] The *magnet rate* (interval) varies according to the manufacturer and is generally faster (shorter interval) than the programmed rate to override the spontaneous rhythm. The magnet interval is often used for assessment of battery status; it lengthens with impending battery depletion. The *interference rate* is the rate (often equal to the lower rate) at which a pulse generator will revert automatically in the presence of continually sensed extraneous interference.

RATE OR INTERVAL?

The pulse generator and the pacemaker physician both "think" in terms of interval rather than rate.[1, 9] Yet for ease of programming, manufacturers have expressed parameters in terms of rate rather than interval. The terms lower rate and upper rate should be deemphasized but not completely discarded because the traditional rate terminology can be useful under certain circumstances. For example, programmed rates may provide useful information when communicating with the patient or the referring physician with little or no knowledge of cardiac pacing who simply want to know the upper and lower rates (in the case of rate-adaptive single-chamber or dual-chamber devices) without having to understand the complexity and timing cycles of contemporary pacemakers.[9]

AAI MODE

AAI pacing may be used for patients with sick sinus syndrome and intact atrioventricular (AV) conduction. The AAI mode is identical to the VVI mode except that it paces the atrium and senses atrial electric activity (Fig. 31–3). AAI pacemakers differ from VVI pacemakers in two respects: (1) they need a higher sensitivity because the atrial electrogram is considerably smaller than the ventricular one and (2) the pacemaker refractory period should be longer ($\geq$400 msec) to prevent sensing of the conducted QRS complex or the "far-field" ventricular electrogram (registered by the atrial lead), which may cause inappropriate inhibition of the pacemaker.[10] Ideally an AAI pacemaker should not sense ventricular activity. Oversensing of ventricular activity is more common with unipolar systems than with bipolar systems[11] and can often be corrected by lengthening the pacemaker atrial refractory period or decreasing atrial sensitivity.

VVT MODE

In the VVT mode, a sensed ventricular event causes immediate release or triggering of a pacemaker stimulus. The VVT mode therefore requires at least three timing intervals: (1) an LRI, (2) an upper rate interval (URI), and (3) a refractory period. In a simple VVT design, the pacemaker refractory period determines the maximal pacing rate according to the formula:

$$\text{upper rate (ppm)} = \frac{60}{\text{refractory period (sec)}}$$

On sensing a QRS complex, a VVT pacemaker discharges its stimulus during the absolute refractory period of the ventricular myocardium (Figs. 31–4 and 31–5). Such ineffectual stimulation wastes battery capacity and distorts the ECG. As

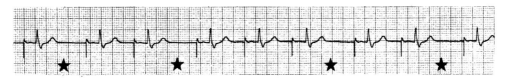

FIGURE 31–3. AAI pacemaker rate = 70 ppm (automatic interval = 857 msec), and refractory period = 250 msec. There is intermittent prolongation of the interstimulus interval because the atrial lead senses the far-field QRS complex just beyond the 250-msec pacemaker refractory period. When the refractory period was programmed to 400 msec, the irregularity disappeared, with restoration of regular atrial pacing at a rate of 70 ppm. (From Barold SS, Zipes DP: Cardiac pacemakers and antiarrhythmic devices. *In* Braunwald E [ed]: Heart Disease: A Textbook of Cardiovascular Medicine. Philadelphia, WB Saunders, 1992, pp 726–755.)

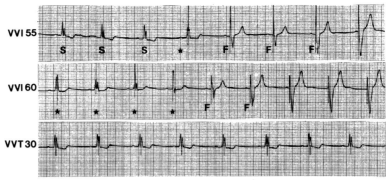

FIGURE 31–4. *Top*, VVI pacemaker at a rate of 55 ppm. The first three beats are sensed, and the fourth beat (*star*) is a pseudofusion beat (i.e., superimposition of a pacemaker stimulus on the surface QRS complex because the intracardiac ventricular electrogram registered by the pacing lead has not yet developed sufficient amplitude to inhibit the pacemaker output). The fifth, sixth, and seventh complexes are ventricular fusion beats (F). *Middle*, VVI pacemaker at a rate of 60 ppm. The first three beats (*stars*) are pseudofusion beats. The fourth beat (*star*) appears to be a pseudofusion beat because the initial QRS vector occurs just before the stimulus. Note that in beat 4 the T wave is identical to that of the previous beats, suggesting that depolarization was also identical. The fifth and sixth complexes are fusion beats (F), while the last three beats are pure ventricular paced beats. *Bottom*, Same patient as above. The pacemaker was programmed to the VVT mode, rate = 30 ppm. The pacemaker emits a stimulus immediately on sensing each QRS complex. Thus, a stimulus marks the precise time of sensing in the VVT mode. This may be correlated with the pseudofusion beats in the middle tracing in which the first pseudofusion beat is deformed by a stimulus just before the R wave returns to the baseline, that is, just before sensing would have occurred as determined from the VVT mode in the lower tracing. (From Barold SS, Zipes DP: Cardiac pacemakers and antiarrhythmic devices. *In* Braunwald E [ed]: Heart Disease: A Textbook of Cardiovascular Medicine. Philadelphia, WB Saunders, 1992, pp 726–755.)

in the VVI mode, if no QRS is sensed during the LRI, the pacemaker delivers its impulse at the completion of the LRI. Dedicated single-mode VVT (AAT) pulse generators are now obsolete, but in the early days of pacing they constituted important systems because they prevented prolonged inhibition (exhibited by unsophisticated VVI pacing systems) secondary to detection of extraneous or electromagnetic interference (EMT). The triggered VVT mode therefore ensures stimulation (i.e., prevents inhibition) whenever the pulse generator senses signals other than the QRS complex.

The triggered function is generally available in contemporary single- and dual-chamber pacemakers as a programmable mode for either temporary or permanent use. The VVT (AAT) mode of some pulse generators possesses a short inhibitory window beyond the pacemaker refractory period in which sensed signals can inhibit rather than trigger the output circuit.[12] As a rule, this occurs when the URI is longer than the programmed refractory period.[12] In the temporary VVT (AAT) mode, the capability of triggering an implanted pacemaker by the application of chest wall stimuli (generating signals for sensing) from an external pacemaker provides a way of performing noninvasive electrophysiologic studies or terminating reentrant tachycardias by appropriately timed stimuli or burst pacing[13–15] (see Fig. 31–5). The temporary VVT or AAT mode may also delineate the presence and exact time of sensing by "marking" the sensed signals with a stimulus, a function useful in the diagnosis of oversensing spurious signals (invisible on the surface ECG) generated by a fractured or defective lead.[10] Rarely, the VVT (AAT) mode is used to prevent inhibition of a unipolar pulse generator by

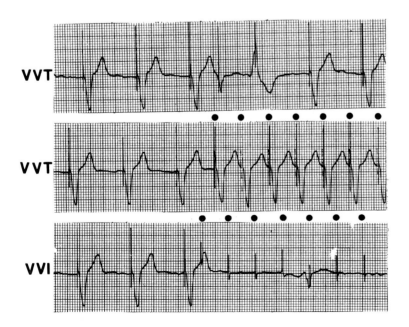

FIGURE 31–5. VVI pacemaker programmed to the VVT mode, rate = 70 ppm. *Top*, There are two sensed ventricular extrasystoles, both deformed by ventricular stimuli. *Middle*, VVT mode. Chest wall stimulation (*solid black circles*) delivered from an external pacemaker (to electrodes on the chest) provides signals detected by the implanted VVT pacemaker, which therefore discharges its stimuli in synchrony with the sensed signals. This leads to an increase in the rate of ventricular pacing equal to the rate of chest wall stimulation. *Bottom*, Same patient. The pacemaker was reprogrammed back to the VVI mode, rate = 70 ppm. Chest wall stimulation at the same rate and amplitude as in the *middle tracing* now causes inhibition, with the emergence of a slow spontaneous rhythm. (From Barold SS: Single- and dual-chamber pacemakers: Electrophysiology, pacing modes, and multiprogrammability. *In* Singer I, Kupersmith J [eds]: Clinical Manual of Electrophysiology. Baltimore, Williams & Wilkins, 1993, pp 231–273.)

myopotentials (musculoskeletal electric activity originating near the anodal electrode on the pacemaker case) when programming of sensitivity in the VVI (AAI) mode cannot correct the problem without compromising QRS (or P) sensing.[12] In the VVT mode, a unipolar pulse generator will increase its pacing rate on sensing myopotentials, which is a better tradeoff than ventricular inhibition.

HYSTERESIS

When the escape interval is significantly longer than the automatic interval, the pacemaker is said to operate in the hysteresis mode[16] (Fig. 31–6). The purpose of hysteresis is to maintain sinus rhythm (i.e., AV synchrony) for as long as possible at a spontaneous rate lower (e.g., 50 ppm) than the automatic rate of the pacemaker (e.g., 70 ppm). Thus when the spontaneous rate drops below 50 bpm, the pacemaker will take over and pace at a rate of 70 ppm. The pacemaker will continue to pace at a rate of 70 ppm until the spontaneous rate exceeds the automatic rate, that is, when the spontaneous QRS complex occurs before the 857 msec automatic interval has timed out. Thus, if the spontaneous rate never exceeds 70 bpm, ventricular pacing will continue indefinitely at a rate of 70 ppm.

In some advanced systems, a device with hysteresis (e.g., 50 ppm/70 ppm) lengthens one or more pacing cycles automatically (to 1200 msec) after a given number of paced cycles at the programmed value (857 msec) to allow the return of a slower spontaneous rhythm (search hysteresis).[17] The length of the extended interval (or "search" interval) corresponds to the programmed hysteresis rate, that is, 50 ppm. If no event is sensed during a search interval (1200 msec), the pulse generator delivers a stimulus at the end of that interval or intervals (depending on the number of search intervals programmed for the search function) and resumes pacing at the programmed rate of 70 ppm. Periodic activation of the search hysteresis function eventually promotes the return of the spontaneous rhythm.

Hysteresis is a frequent source of confusion in electrocardiographic interpretation of pacemaker function. Although hysteresis is available as a programmable option in many contemporary pacemakers, it is probably used infrequently because its advantages are more theoretical than real and it may predispose the patient to undesirable arrhythmias.[18, 19] Indeed, hysteresis appears to have no advantage over simply decreasing the pacing rate in patients with symptoms due to loss of AV synchrony.[20] When pacing is required for carotid sinus syndrome or malignant vasovagal syndrome (neurally mediated syncope), however, a dual-chamber pulse generator with search hysteresis is often recommended.[21, 22]

FUSION AND PSEUDOFUSION BEATS

Ventricular fusion beats occur when the ventricles are depolarized simultaneously by spontaneous and pacemaker-induced activity. A ventricular fusion beat is often narrower

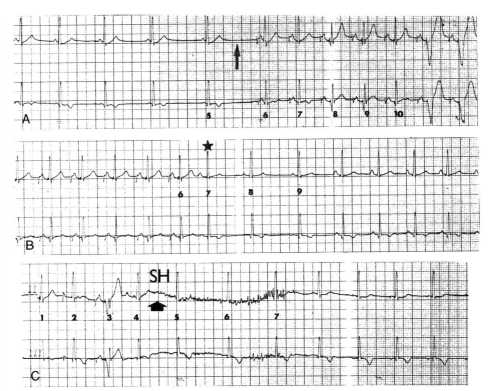

FIGURE 31–6. Two-lead ECG of a patient with cardioneurogenic syncope who received an Intermedics Relay DDDR pacemaker programmed to the DDD mode with hysteresis (50/85 ppm). The pacemaker is programmed to pace in the (AV sequential) DDD mode at 85 ppm (AV interval = 200 msec) whenever the spontaneous rate falls below 50 ppm (R-R interval > 1200 msec) as shown in A (arrow) where the R-R interval initiated by the fifth QRS complex is longer than 1200 msec. With standard 50/85 ppm hysteresis, the pacemaker should continue pacing at 85 ppm indefinitely unless the spontaneous rate exceeds 85 ppm to inhibit the device. In B the pacemaker senses a relatively early spontaneous beat (star) with an R-R interval of 600 msec (6–7), shorter than the 705-msec interval corresponding to the pacing rate of 85 ppm. Consequently, pacing is inhibited, and the device remains inhibited by sensing of a spontaneous rate faster than 50 ppm. In C, the search hysteresis function was programmed. After 255 paced beats, the search hysteresis (SH) option is activated, and the pacemaker automatically extends the pacing interval (in this case it was programmed for three intervals). The length of the extended or search intervals corresponds to a programmed hysteresis rate of 50 ppm, that

is, 1200 msec. Sensed events in the search intervals inhibit the pacemaker and allow resumption of a spontaneous rhythm of less than 85 ppm. If no event is sensed during a search interval, the pacemaker will deliver a stimulus at the end of the interval and resume pacing at the programmed rate after the last search interval. In C, the three intervals (4–5, 5–6, 6–7) during the search intervals all are shorter than 1200 msec. Consequently, the pacemaker is inhibited. Note that when search option is selected (C), the patient's intrinsic rate need not exceed the programmed pacing rate (as in B) to inhibit the pulse generator with hysteresis function.

In A, beat 6 shows ventricular inhibition from a conducted QRS complex (see Fig. 31–10). Beat 7 is a ventricular pseudofusion beat. Beats 8, 9, and 10 are ventricular fusion beats, as are all the paced beats in B. In C, beat 1 is a ventricular fusion beat, beat 2 is a ventricular pseudofusion beat, and beat 3 is a ventricular fusion beat. Beat 4 may be a ventricular fusion beat.

than a pure paced beat and can exhibit various morphologic features depending on the relative contribution of the two foci to ventricular depolarization. Ventricular fusion can mimic lack of capture if it produces an isoelectric complex in a single ECG lead: ventricular depolarization should be obvious in other leads, and the presence of a T wave (repolarization) indicates that preceding depolarization has taken place.

Pseudofusion beats consist of the superimposition of an ineffectual pacemaker stimulus on the surface QRS complex originating from a single focus; they represent a normal manifestation of VVI pacing.[7, 23] A substantial portion of the *surface* QRS complex can be inscribed before *intracardiac* electric activity or the electrogram monitored by the pacing lead generates the required voltage or signal to inhibit the output circuit of a VVI pacemaker (Fig. 31–7). Therefore, a VVI pacemaker functioning normally according to its programmed timing mechanism can deliver its impulse within a spontaneous surface QRS complex (mimicking undersensing) before the pulse generator has the opportunity to sense the "delayed" *intracardiac* signal or electrogram at the right ventricular apex. In a pseudofusion beat, the pacemaker stimulus falls within the absolute refractory period of the myocardium. In the presence of normal ventricular sensing, striking examples of ventricular pseudofusion beats with pacemaker stimuli released late within the surface QRS complex can occur in right bundle branch block, left ventricular extrasystoles, and deranged intraventricular conduction (such as hyperkalemia) because of delayed arrival of activation at the sensing electrode or electrodes at the right ventricular apex.[24] Whenever pseudofusion beats are observed, true sensing failure must be excluded with long electrocardiographic recordings. Pacemaker stimuli falling clearly beyond the surface QRS complex indicate undersensing. Fusion and pseudofusion atrial beats can also occur with atrial pacing but are more difficult to recognize in view of the smaller size of the P wave in the ECG.

Operational Characteristics of a Simple DDD Pulse Generator

The function and timing intervals of the various modes of dual-chamber pacing are best understood by focusing first on the DDD mode, in which pacing and sensing occur in the atrial and ventricular "electric" chambers.

VENTRICULAR CHANNEL (LOWER RATE INTERVAL AND VENTRICULAR REFRACTORY PERIOD)

As in a standard VVI pacemaker, the ventricular channel of a DDD device requires two basic timing cycles. The first is the LRI that corresponds to the programmed lower rate. In most dual-chamber pacemakers, lower rate timing (LRT) is ventricular-based (V-V timing) in that the LRI is controlled and initiated only by a paced or sensed ventricular event.[25] In this situation, the LRI is the longest interval from a paced or sensed ventricular event to the succeeding ventricular stimulus (without any intervening atrial or ventricular sensing events). The second timing cycle is the period when the pacemaker cannot sense (ventricular refractory period), traditionally defined as the time when the pulse generator is insensitive to incoming signals.[6] Yet many contemporary

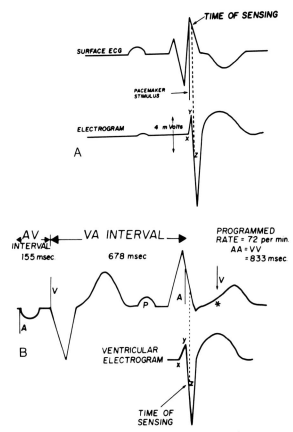

FIGURE 31–7. *A,* Diagrammatic representation of the mechanism of pseudofusion. The surface electrocardiogram (ECG) and ventricular electrogram are recorded simultaneously. The electrogram generates the necessary intracardiac voltage to inhibit the pacemaker (yz, assumed at 4 mV) at a point corresponding to the descending limb of the surface QRS complex in its second half (*at dotted line*). Consequently, it is possible for a pacemaker stimulus to occur at the apex of the R just before the dotted line (or point of sensing) because the ventricular electrogram has not yet generated the voltage required to inhibit the pulse generator. *B,* Diagrammatic representation of the mechanism of pseudopseudofusion. Assume a DVI pulse generator with an AV interval of 155 msec and an atrial escape (pacemaker VA) interval of 678 msec. The atrial channel cannot sense in the DVI mode. The first beat shows atrial and ventricular capture by the atrial and ventricular stimuli. The relatively early occurrence of a spontaneous P wave and the ensuing conducted QRS complex allows the atrial stimulus to fall within the surface QRS complex according to the programmed atrial escape interval (AEI) of 678 msec. The ventricular electrogram generates the necessary voltage for sensing (yz) relatively late in relation to the surface QRS complex (corresponding to the dotted line). Consequently, the pulse generator delivers its atrial stimulus within the surface QRS complex (before the point of sensing at the dotted line) according to its programmed VA interval because the electrogram has not yet generated sufficient intracardiac voltage to suppress the pulse generator. In a DVI (or DDD) pulse generator, release of the atrial stimulus initiates a short ventricular refractory period (known as the blanking period) to prevent the ventricular channel from sensing the atrial stimulus as crosstalk. If a substantial portion of the ventricular electrogram falls within the ventricular blanking period, the ventricular channel will not sense the QRS complex, leading the pacemaker to deliver its ventricular stimulus on the ascending limb of the T wave at the completion of the programmed AV delay (*asterisk*). The atrial stimulus within the QRS may be called pseudopseudofusion because two chambers are involved. The same mechanism can occur during DDD pacing with ventricular extrasystoles or atrial undersensing (see Figs. 31–12 and 31–13). (In ventricular pseudofusion, the ventricular stimulus deforms the QRS complex.) (From Barold SS, Falkoff MD, Ong LS, et al: Electrocardiographic analysis of normal and abnormal pacemaker function. Cardiovasc Clin 14[2]:97, 1983.)

pulse generators can sense during part of the refractory period (as discussed later) and use such signals to initiate or reset certain timing cycles with the exception of the inviolable LRI.[25]

VVI PACING WITH AN ATRIAL CHANNEL (ATRIOVENTRICULAR INTERVAL AND UPPER RATE INTERVAL)

The addition of an atrial channel to a VVI system (the latter supplying the LRI and ventricular refractory period) creates a simple DDD pulse generator.[3] Two new intervals are required: an AV interval (the electronic analog of the PR interval) and a URI (the speed limit) to control the response of the ventricular channel to sensed atrial activity. The AV interval is initiated either by an atrial paced or sensed event. If the pulse generator does not detect ventricular activity during the AV interval, it emits a ventricular stimulus at the end of the programmed AV delay (Fig. 31–8).

If the upper rate interval (URI) of a DDD pacemaker is 500 msec (upper rate = 120 ppm), a P wave occurring earlier than 500 msec from the previous atrial event will not be followed by a ventricular stimulus. Such an arrangement allows atrial sensing with 1:1 AV synchrony between the LRI and URI. In such a simple DDD pulse generator with only four intervals, the URI is equal to the refractory period of the atrial channel or total atrial refractory period (TARP), which is initiated by a paced or sensed atrial event. As before, if the TARP is equal to 500 msec, the pacemaker will maintain 1:1 AV synchrony up to an atrial rate of 120 ppm, corresponding to a P-P interval of 500 msec. When the atrial rate exceeds 120 ppm, P waves will fall within the TARP, and 1:1 AV synchrony can no longer occur. The TARP actually provides the URI.

The atrial escape (pacemaker VA) interval is a *derived* timing interval obtained by subtracting the programmed AV delay from the LRI (Fig. 31–8). In a pacemaker with ventricular-based (V-V) lower rate timing, the atrial escape (pacemaker VA) interval always remains constant and starts with a sensed or paced ventricular event and terminates (in the absence of sensed atrial or ventricular activity) with the release of an atrial stimulus[26–28] (see Fig. 31–8). The behavior of the atrial escape interval (AEI) of pacemakers with atrial-based (A-A) lower rate timing is discussed later.

INFLUENCE OF EVENTS OF ONE CHAMBER ON THE OTHER

The functions of the two channels of a DDD pacemaker are intimately linked, and an event detected by one channel generally influences the other.[26–28] A sensed atrial event alters pacemaker response in two ways: (1) it triggers a ventricular stimulus after the completion of the programmed AV interval provided that the ventricular channel senses no signal during the AV interval and (2) it inhibits the release of the atrial stimulus expected at the completion of the atrial escape (pacemaker VA) interval because there is no need for atrial stimulation. Thus the atrial channel functions simultaneously in the triggered mode by delivering ventricular stimulation (it triggers a ventricular output after a sensed P wave) and in the inhibited mode by preventing competitive release of an atrial stimulus when a P wave is sensed, that is, the AEI does not time out in its entirety. When the ventricular channel senses a signal, both atrial and ventricular channels are inhibited simultaneously. A sensed ventricular event inhibits release of the atrial stimulus (the AEI does not time out) and initiates a new AEI and LRI.

If a sensed ventricular event occurs during the AV interval, there is obviously no need for a ventricular stimulus at the completion of the programmed AV interval. The AV interval is therefore terminated (i.e., abbreviated) and the pacemaker initiates a new AEI and LRI. The ventricular channel of a DDD pulse generator functions in the inhibited mode under all circumstances. The code DD TI/I was originally proposed

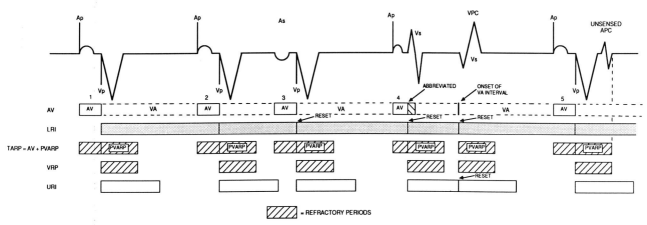

FIGURE 31–8. Diagram showing the function of a simple DDD pacemaker with only four basic intervals. Lower rate timing is ventricular based and controlled by ventricular events (paced or sensed). Ap = atrial paced beat; As = atrial sensed event; Vp = ventricular paced beat; Vs = ventricular sensed event. The four fundamental intervals: LRI = lower rate interval; VRP = ventricular refractory period; AV = atrioventricular delay; PVARP = postventricular atrial refractory period. The two derived intervals: atrial escape (pacemaker VA) interval = LRI – AV; total atrial refractory period (TARP) = AV + PVARP. Reset refers to the termination and reinitiation of a timing cycle before it has timed out to its completion according to its programmed duration. Premature termination of the programmed AV delay by Vs is indicated by its abbreviation. The upper rate interval (URI) is equal to TARP. As (third beat) initiates an AV interval terminating with Vp; As also aborts the atrial escape interval initiated by the second Vp. The third Vp resets the LRI and starts the PVARP, VRP, and URI. The fourth beat consists of Ap, which terminates the AEI initiated by the third Vp, followed by a sensed conducted QRS (Vs). The AV interval is therefore abbreviated. Vs initiates the AEI, LRI, PVARP, VRP, and URI. The fifth beat is a ventricular extrasystole (ventricular premature contraction [VPC]) that initiates an AEI, PVARP, and VRP and resets the LRI and URI. The last beat is followed by an unsensed atrial extrasystole because it occurs within the PVARP. (From Barold SS, Zipes DP: Cardiac pacemakers and antiarrhythmic devices. *In* Braunwald E [ed]): Heart Disease: A Textbook of Cardiovascular Medicine. Philadelphia, WB Saunders, 1992, pp 726–755.)

for the DDD mode because the atrial channel functions both in the triggered and inhibited modes, whereas the ventricular channel is restricted to the inhibited mode. This designation, although correct, was considered unwieldy and was eventually replaced by a simpler but less descriptive DDD mode requiring that the last position be labeled D (double) if both T and I responses occur, regardless of other considerations.

REFRACTORY PERIODS

In a DDD pulse generator, an atrial sensed or paced event initiates the AV interval and atrial refractory period. The atrial channel of a DDD pulse generator must remain refractory during the entire AV interval to prevent initiation of a new AV interval while one is already in progress.[29] Thus the first part of the atrial refractory period lasts for the duration of the AV interval in the form of Ap-Vs, Ap-Vp, As-Vp, As-Vs (Ap = atrial paced event, As = atrial sensed event, Vp = ventricular paced event, Vs = ventricular sensed event). The AV interval terminates with a ventricular event (Vp or Vs), which immediately restarts (or continues) the atrial refractory period. The part of the atrial refractory period initiated by a ventricular event is called the postventricular atrial refractory period (PVARP). The PVARP is designed to prevent the atrial channel from sensing a variety of signals such as retrograde P waves related to retrograde ventriculoatrial (VA) conduction, very early atrial extrasystoles, and far-field ventricular signals registered in the atrial electrogram.[30, 31] The TARP is equal to the sum of the AV delay and the PVARP. Thus programming a long PVARP limits the upper rate of the pacemaker by lengthening the TARP.

In a DDD pulse generator, does a paced or sensed event in one channel initiate a refractory period in both atrial and ventricular channels to ensure that a given paced or sensed event in one (electric) chamber or channel does not interfere with the function of the other? Four possible events may be considered, that is, Ap, As, Vs, and Vp.

1. Vs or Vp initiates the ventricular refractory period and the PVARP simultaneously.
2. Ap initiates the AV interval and the atrial refractory period and simultaneously initiates a short ventricular refractory period (ventricular blanking period) to avoid sensing of the atrial stimulus by the ventricular channel (interference known as crosstalk).[26, 32, 33] Thus, the ventricular channel can sense throughout most of the AV interval because the ventricular blanking period is relatively short. This allows intrinsic ventricular activity to inhibit the ventricular output if sensed before the AV interval times out.
3. As is the only one of the four possible events (As, Ap, Vs, Vp) that generates a refractory period only in the atrial channel. No ventricular refractory period is needed after As because ordinarily it cannot be sensed by the ventricular electrode and therefore cannot directly disturb the function of the ventricular channel.

CONTROL OF UPPER RATE INTERVAL IN A SIMPLE DDD DEVICE

In a simple DDD pulse generator (without a separately programmable URI), the URI is equal to the TARP. The TARP (AV delay + PVARP) and URI are interrelated according to the formula:

$$\text{upper rate (ppm)} = \frac{60,000}{\text{TARP (msec)}}$$

In the previously discussed example, if TARP is equal to 500 msec (AV delay = 200 msec and PVARP = 300 msec), the pulse generator will sense atrial signals (P waves) 500 msec or longer apart up to a repetition rate of 120 ppm. An atrial signal occurring earlier than 500 msec (the URI) from the previous atrial event will fall in the atrial refractory period and will not be sensed.[26, 27, 29]

BASIC AND DERIVED TIMING CYCLES OF DDD PULSE GENERATORS

Although the URI was previously considered a basic timing cycle, it is preferable at this stage to use the PVARP as a fundamental interval and relegate the URI and TARP to derived functions. At this point in the discussion, a simple DDD pulse generator can be built with only four basic intervals—LRI, AV interval, ventricular refractory period, and PVARP—and three derived intervals—AEI, TARP (AV delay + PVARP), and URI (equal to the TARP). Theoretically, a DDD pulse generator equipped with these timing cycles should function well provided that the ventricular channel does not sense the atrial stimulus (crosstalk).[32, 33] Prevention of crosstalk is mandatory and requires the addition of a fifth fundamental timing interval in the form of a brief ventricular refractory (blanking) period starting with the release of the atrial stimulus. Indeed, a DDD device with only these five basic intervals was successfully used clinically in early DDD pulse generators manufactured by the Cordis Corporation (now part of Telectronics, Inc., Englewood, CO). Further refinements related to crosstalk and the upper rate response created the need for two other basic intervals—the ventricular safety pacing (VSP) period (to complement the ventricular blanking period in dealing with crosstalk) and a URI that is programmable independently of the TARP for an upper rate response smoother than the sudden mechanism provided only by the TARP[26–29, 34, 35] (Fig. 31–9).

CROSSTALK INTERVALS

Crosstalk with self-inhibition refers to the inappropriate detection of the atrial stimulus by the ventricular channel. It occurs more commonly in unipolar than in bipolar dual-chamber pacemakers. In patients without an underlying ventricular rhythm, inhibition of the ventricular channel by crosstalk could be catastrophic by causing ventricular asystole.

VENTRICULAR BLANKING PERIOD

The prevention of crosstalk requires a basic timing cycle called the ventricular blanking period that consists of a brief absolute ventricular refractory period starting coincidentally with the release of the atrial stimulus (Fig. 31–10). The duration of the ventricular blanking period varies from 10 to

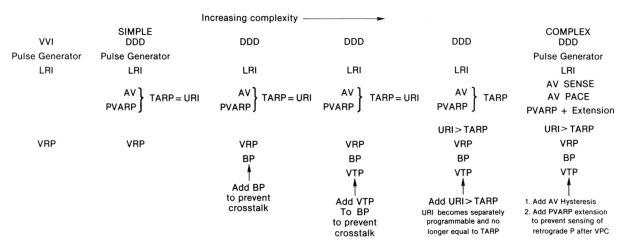

FIGURE 31–9. The progressive addition of new timing cycles to a simple DDD pacemaker (*left*) creates a more complex device (*right*) (see text for details). Abbreviations as in Figure 31–8: AV pace = AV interval initiated by Ap; AV sense = AV interval initiated by As; BP = blanking period; VTP = ventricular triggering period or ventricular safety pacing period. (From Barold SS, Falkoff MD, Ong LS, et al: Timing cycles of DDD pacemakers. *In* Barold SS, Mugica J [eds]: New Perspectives in Cardiac Pacing. Mt Kisco, NY: Futura Publishing Co., 1988, pp 69–119.)

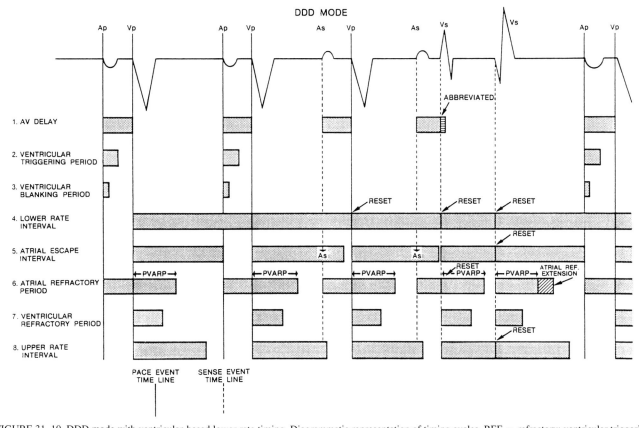

FIGURE 31–10. DDD mode with ventricular-based lower rate timing. Diagrammatic representation of timing cycles. REF = refractory; ventricular triggering period = ventricular safety period. The second Vs event is a sensed ventricular extrasystole. The fourth AV interval initiated by As is abbreviated because Vs occurs before the AV interval has timed out. The PVARP generated by the ventricular extrasystole is automatically extended by the atrial refractory period extension. This design is based on the concept that most episodes of endless loop tachycardia (pacemaker macroreentrant tachycardia due to repetitive sensing of retrograde atrial depolarization) are initiated by ventricular extrasystoles with retrograde ventriculoatrial conduction. Whenever possible, the AV interval and atrial escape (pacemaker VA) interval are depicted in their entirety for the sake of clarity. The arrow pointing down within the atrial escape (pacemaker VA) interval indicates that As has taken place; As inhibits the release of the atrial stimulus expected at the completion of the AEI. The abbreviations and format used in this illustration are the same as those for Figures 31–17, 31–19, 31–25, 31–29, 31–30, and 31–43. (From Barold SS, Falkoff MD, Ong LS, et al: All dual-chamber pacemakers function in the DDD mode. Am Heart J 115:1353, 1988.)

60 msec according to the manufacturer and is programmable in some pulse generators.[33] A QRS occurring soon after Ap within the ventricular blanking period will be unsensed, whereupon the pulse generator will emit a competitive ventricular stimulus. Thus if the programmed AV interval is relatively long, this particular ventricular stimulus could fall on the T wave of the unsensed ventricular beat (whose QRS falls within the ventricular blanking period). There is no need for ventricular blanking after atrial sensing. Sensing of a ventricular stimulus or QRS complex by the atrial channel, which is the reverse of crosstalk, is also prevented by appropriate blanking of the atrial channel provided automatically by the PVARP.

VENTRICULAR SAFETY PACING

In many dual-chamber pulse generators, the AV interval initiated by an atrial stimulus contains an additional safety mechanism to prevent the potentially serious consequences of crosstalk. The AV delay initiated by an atrial stimulus is divided into two parts (see Fig. 31–10). The first part is the ventricular safety pacing (VSP) period (also known as the nonphysiologic AV delay, ventricular triggering period, or crosstalk sensing window).[33, 36, 37] Traditionally, the VSP period encompasses the first 100 to 110 msec of the AV interval and is programmable in some devices. During the VSP period, a signal (crosstalk, QRS, and so forth) sensed by the ventricular channel does not inhibit the pulse generator. Rather the signal initiates or triggers a ventricular stimulus delivered prematurely only at the completion of the VSP period, producing a characteristic abbreviation of the paced

AV (Ap–Vp) interval (usually 100 to 110 msec)[36] (Fig. 31–11). In this way, if the ventricular channel detects crosstalk beyond the ventricular blanking period, activation of the VSP mechanism prevents ventricular asystole by delivering an early Vp. Consequently, during continual crosstalk in pacemakers with ventricular (V-V) lower rate timing, because the atrial escape (pacemaker VA) interval remains constant and the AV interval shortens, the AV sequential pacing rate becomes faster than the programmed lower rate.[25] When a QRS complex is sensed during the VSP period, the early triggered ventricular stimulus is supposed to fall harmlessly during the absolute refractory period of the myocardium because of the abbreviated AV interval (Fig. 31–12).

Although the duration of the VSP is generally described as beginning from the atrial stimulus, obviously ventricular sensing cannot occur until termination of the initial ventricular blanking period. A sensed ventricular signal beyond the VSP period in the second part of the AV interval inhibits rather than triggers the ventricular output. Pulse generators without a VSP period generally require a relatively long ventricular blanking period to prevent crosstalk. A long ventricular blanking period (being an absolute refractory period) predisposes to undersensing by the ventricular channel (Fig. 31–13). Consequently VSP provides a "backup" mechanism to deal with crosstalk and allows the use of relatively short ventricular blanking periods to optimize ventricular sensing. Figure 31–14 shows further refinements of the VSP response of contemporary dual-chamber pacemakers.[38]

In pulse generators (ventricular-based lower rate timing) without a VSP mechanism, crosstalk produces distinctive electrocardiographic manifestations.[39, 40]

COSMOS DDD
LOWER RATE = 80 ppm (750 ms)
AV INTERVAL = 300 ms
ATRIAL ESCAPE INTERVAL = 450 ms
VTP = 100 ms

VENTRICULAR SENSITIVITY = 2 mV   VENTRICULAR SENSITIVITY = 5 mV
CROSSTALK VV = 550 ms (109 ppm)   VV = 750 ms (80 ppm)

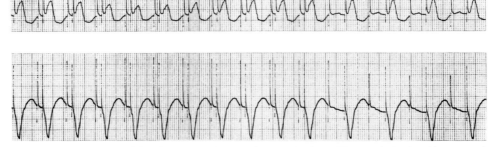

FIGURE 31–11. Cosmos I Intermedics unipolar DDD pulse generator (Intermedics, Inc., Angleton, TX) (ventricular-based lower rate timing) with ventricular safety pacing mechanism (VTP = ventricular triggering period) showing on the *left* crosstalk characterized by abbreviation of the AV interval to 100 msec. The LRI is controlled by ventricular events. Consequently, the AEI remains constant at 450 msec. The interval between two consecutive ventricular stimuli (Vp-Vp) therefore shortens from 750 to 450 + 100 = 550 msec, increasing the AV sequential pacing rate from 80 to 109 ppm during continual crosstalk. On the right, crosstalk disappears when the ventricular sensitivity is reduced from 2 to 5 mV (less sensitive setting). Two ECG leads were recorded simultaneously. (From Barold SS: Single- and dual-chamber pacemakers: Electrophysiology, pacing modes, and multiprogrammability. *In* Singer I, Kupersmith J [eds]: Clinical Manual of Electrophysiology. Baltimore, Williams & Wilkins, 1993, pp 231–273.)

FIGURE 31–12. Activation of the VSP function during DDD pacing (ventricular-based lower rate timing) (LRI = 857 msec; AV interval = 200 msec). The second last QRS complex is a ventricular extrasystole sensed by the ventricular channel during the VSP period, whereupon the pulse generator triggers a ventricular stimulus at the termination of the VSP period, producing characteristic abbreviation of the AV interval (100 msec). An atrial stimulus falls within the QRS complex because the ventricular electrogram at that point has not yet generated sufficient voltage to inhibit the pulse generator, in effect producing a pseudofusion beat, which in this situation has been called a pseudopseudofusion beat because an atrial and not a ventricular stimulus falls within the QRS complex (see Figure 31–7 for description of pseudopseudofusion beats).

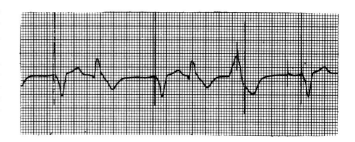

1. There is unexpected prolongation of the interval between the atrial stimulus and the succeeding conducted (spontaneous) QRS complex to a value greater than the programmed AV interval. If there is no AV conduction, ventricular asystole will occur. Myopotential interference sensed during the AV interval of unipolar DDD pulse generators can superficially resemble crosstalk (Fig. 31–15).

2. The rate of atrial pacing increases compared with the programmed free-running AV sequential (lower) rate. There is no paced QRS complex. The atrial stimulus (sensed by the ventricular channel) initiates a new atrial escape (pacemaker VA) interval. Consequently, the interval between two consecutive atrial stimuli (A-A interval) becomes equal to the atrial escape (pacemaker VA) inter-

val (ignoring the negligible duration of the blanking period).

PREVENTION OF CROSSTALK

Crosstalk is best prevented by using bipolar dual-chamber devices. The presence of crosstalk and effective (ventricular) blanking is tested by reprogramming the atrial output to its maximal value and the ventricular sensitivity to its most sensitive setting.[40] To avoid competition, the lower rate is set above the patient's own spontaneous rate, and the AV delay is shortened to less than the spontaneous PR interval. If crosstalk is observed, the atrial voltage output should be decreased before decreasing the atrial pulse width and the ventricular sensitivity. If these maneuvers are unsuccessful or undesirable, the blanking period should be prolonged, but

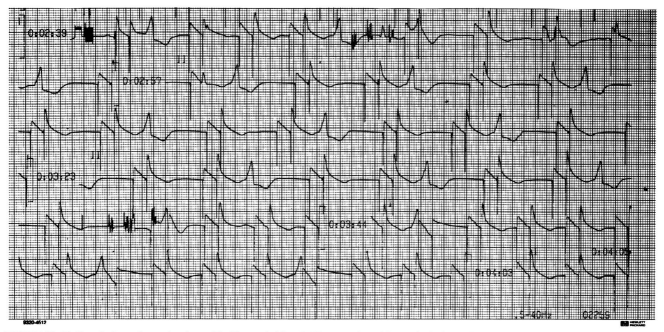

FIGURE 31–13. Ventricular undersensing due to blanking period in a DDD pacemaker with ventricular-based lower rate timing. The ECG shows a normally functioning Cordis Gemini DDD pulse generator (Telectronics, Inc., Englewood, CO) programmed to a relatively slow lower rate. There are frequent ventricular extrasystoles with a varying coupling interval. The ventricular extrasystoles all are sensed by the pulse generator. At the beginning of the fifth strip, the pacemaker was reprogrammed to a faster lower rate. Atrial stimuli now fall within the QRS complexes of the ventricular extrasystoles because of "late sensing" of these beats by the ventricular channel (pseudopseudofusion beats) (see Fig. 31–7). The ventricular channel does not sense the ventricular extrasystoles because their ventricular electrogram falls within the ventricular blanking period (39–47 msec). The pulse generator therefore emits a ventricular stimulus on the apex of the T wave at the completion of the full AV interval of 250 msec. (From Barold SS, Ong LS, Falkoff MD, et al: Crosstalk or self-inhibition in dual-chambered pacemakers. *In* Barold SS [ed]: Modern Cardiac Pacing. Mt Kisco, NY, Futura Publishing Co., 1985, pp 615–623.)

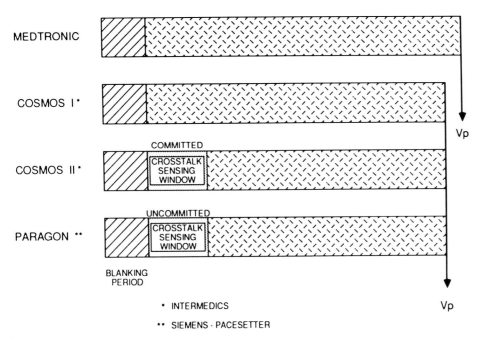

MEDTRONIC

COSMOS I*

COSMOS II*

PARAGON **

COMMITTED

UNCOMMITTED

CROSSTALK SENSING WINDOW

BLANKING PERIOD

Vp

Vp

• INTERMEDICS

•• SIEMENS - PACESETTER

FIGURE 13–14. Behavior of the ventricular safety pacing (VSP) mechanism of DDD pacemakers. The VSP period actually begins at the completion of the ventricular blanking period, but its total duration is generally expressed as starting from the atrial stimulus with the onset of the ventricular blanking period. Medtronic dual-chamber pulse generators (Medtronic Inc., Minneapolis, MN) possess a VSP period of 110 msec, while other pulse generators have a VSP period with a nominal value of 100 msec. In the Medtronic and Intermedics Cosmos I pulse generators, a signal sensed at any time during the VSP period (beyond the blanking period) by the ventricular channel of these pulse generators triggers an obligatory (committed) ventricular stimulus at the termination of the VSP period. In the Intermedics Cosmos II and Relay DDDR pulse generator, the VSP period contains an initial crosstalk sensing window. When the ventricular channel senses a signal during the crosstalk window, the pulse generator triggers a committed ventricular stimulus at the termination of the VSP period regardless of any other sensed ventricular events sensed during the VSP period beyond the crosstalk sensing window. In contrast, an isolated ventricular signal sensed in the VSP beyond the crosstalk sensing window inhibits the ventricular output. In the Pacesetter Siemens Paragon DDD and Synchrony DDDR pulse generators, the crosstalk sensing window functions as in the Cosmos II pulse generator. A signal sensed by the ventricular channel during the crosstalk sensing window triggers a ventricular stimulus at the termination of the VSP period. In contrast to the Cosmos II pulse generator, the ventricular output triggered by sensing in the VSP is uncommitted. Thus another ventricular event sensed in the VSP (beyond the crosstalk sensing window) will inhibit the triggered ventricular response initiated by ventricular sensing within the crosstalk sensing window. (From Barold SS: Single- and dual-chamber pacemakers: Electrophysiology, pacing modes, and multiprogrammability. *In* Singer I, Kupersmith J [eds]: Clinical Manual of Electrophysiology. Baltimore, Williams & Wilkins, 1993, pp 231–274.)

FIGURE 31–15. Crosstalk during DDD pacing without a VSP mechanism (ventricular-based lower rate timing). *Top strip*, The lower rate was increased to test for crosstalk (LRI = 580 msec; AV = 170 msec). During crosstalk the interval between atrial stimuli on the right becomes shorter than the LRI because the ventricular channel initiates a new AEI on sensing the atrial stimulus. Crosstalk therefore causes an increase in the atrial pacing rate faster than the free-running AV sequential LRI on the *left*. Continual crosstalk causes prolonged ventricular asystole. *Bottom strip*, Crosstalk with AV conduction (LRI = 857 msec; AV interval = 200 msec). Crosstalk occurs with the third atrial stimulus and produces characteristic prolongation of the interval between the atrial stimulus and the succeeding conducted QRS complex to a value longer than the programmed AV interval. The rate of atrial pacing increases because the sensed atrial stimulus by the ventricular channel

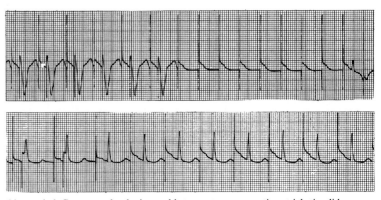

initiates a new AEI just beyond the termination of the ventricular blanking period. Consequently, the interval between two consecutive atrial stimuli becomes equal to the atrial escape interval of 657 msec (857 − 200) plus the duration of the ventricular blanking period (50 msec), providing a total of about 700 msec. (From Barold SS, Zipes CP: Cardiac pacemakers and antiarrhythmic devices. *In* Braunwald E [ed]: Heart Disease: A Textbook of Cardiovascular Medicine. Philadelphia, WB Saunders, 1992, pp 726–755.)

it is not programmable in some pulse generators, which automatically adjust the duration of the blanking period according to the programmed atrial output (volts and pulse width), ventricular sensitivity, and polarity (unipolar vs. bipolar).

Upper Rate Response of DDD Pacemakers

In the DDD mode, the *atrial*-driven URI refers to the shortest Vs-Vp or Vp-Vp, in which the second Vp is triggered by a sensed *atrial* event. The URI always refers to the shortest *ventricular* paced interval. The second Vp can be released only at the completion of the atrial-driven *ventricular* URI initiated by a preceding Vs or Vp. In the DDD mode, URI always refers to the *atrial*-driven (ventricular) URI because there are no sensor-driven intervals (SDI) in a device without a nonatrial sensor.

NO SEPARATELY PROGRAMMABLE UPPER RATE INTERVAL

In a DDD pacemaker without a separately programmable URI, the TARP is equal to the (ventricular) URI and provides a simple way of controlling the paced ventricular response to a fast atrial rate. This upper rate response is often called fixed-ratio AV block (Fig. 31–16). The TARP defines the fastest atrial rate associated with 1:1 AV pacemaker response or the fastest paced ventricular rate associated with 1:1 AV synchrony.[27, 29, 30, 34] As the atrial rate increases, any P wave falling within the PVARP is unsensed. The degree of block depends on the atrial rate and where the P waves occur in the pacemaker cycle. The AV interval (As-Vp) always remains constant and equal to its programmed value. As the atrial rate increases, more P waves fall within the TARP and the degree of block increases. If the upper rate is 120 ppm, (TARP = 500 msec) and the lower rate is 70 ppm, the rate will not drop by half to 60 ppm (i.e., 2:1) when atrial tachy-

cardia occurs because the paced ventricular rate cannot fall below the lower rate. This response is often called 2:1 block, although it is really a misnomer. Actually the paced ventricular rate will be exactly half the atrial rate or equal to the lower rate of the pacemaker, whichever is higher. When half the atrial rate is slower than the programmed lower rate, the pulse generator must pace AV sequentially according to the LRI, that is, an atrial stimulus rather than a sensed P wave initiates the AV interval. An upper rate response using fixed-ratio AV block can be inappropriate in young or physically active individuals because the sudden reduction of the ventricular rate with activity may be poorly tolerated.

WENCKEBACH UPPER RATE RESPONSE

Only DDD pulse generators with an independently programmable upper rate (interval) produce a Wenckebach (or pseudo-Wenckebach) response to faster atrial rates. In order for a Wenckebach response to occur with *prolongation* of the AV interval (As-Vp), the URI must be *longer* than the TARP[27, 28, 30, 34, 35, 37, 41–44] (Fig. 31–17). The maximal prolongation of the AV interval during a Wenckebach sequence represents the difference between these two intervals (Fig. 31–18). If As-Vp as programmed is less than Ap-Vp as programmed, the maximum extension of the basic As-Vp interval will be equal to

[(Ap-Vp) − (As-Vp)] + [URI − TARP] where TARP = PVARP + Ap-Vp as programmed—that is, maximal AV extension = URI − (PVARP + As-Vp).

When the separately programmable URI becomes equal to the TARP, a Wenckebach response cannot occur, and the URI becomes a function of the programmed TARP, thereby creating fixed-ratio AV block. With a progressive increase in the atrial rate, the Wenckebach response of a pacemaker with a URI longer than the TARP eventually switches to (2:1) fixed-ratio AV block when the P-P interval becomes shorter than the TARP (Fig. 31–19).

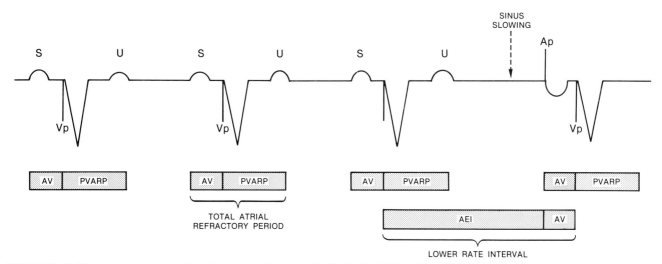

FIGURE 31–16. Diagrammatic representation of pacemaker fixed-ratio AV block. The TARP (AV + PVARP) controls the URI. Every second P wave is unsensed because it falls within the PVARP (2:1 block). When sinus slowing occurs on the right, the pacemaker functions according to the programmed LRI, thereby delivering an atrial stimulus that terminates the pause. AEI = atrial escape interval; Ap = atrial paced event; S = sensed P wave; U = unsensed P wave; Vp = ventricular paced event. (From Barold SS, Falkoff MD, Ong LS, et al: Electrocardiography of contemporary DDD pacemakers. A. Basic concepts, upper rate response, retrograde ventriculoatrial conduction, and differential diagnosis of pacemaker tachycardias. *In* Saksena S, Goldschlager N [eds]. Electrical Therapy for Cardiac Arrhythmias: Pacing, Antitachycardia Devices, Catheter Ablation. Philadelphia, WB Saunders, 1990, pp 225–264.)

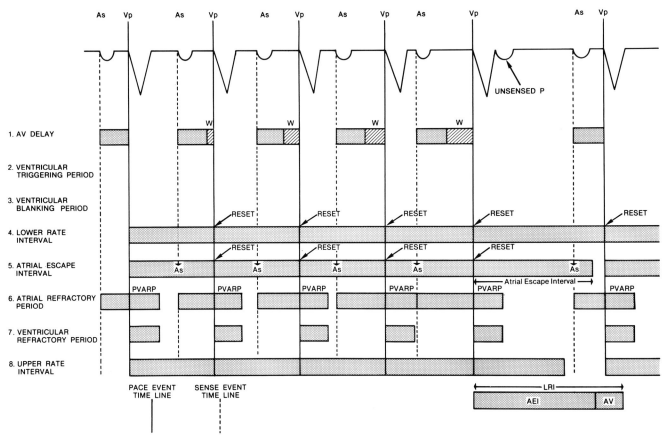

FIGURE 31–17. DDD mode (ventricular-based lower rate timing). Upper rate response with pacemaker Wenckebach AV block. AEI = atrial escape interval. The URI is longer than the programmed TARP. The P-P interval (As-As) is shorter than the URI, but longer than the programmed TARP. The As-Vp interval lengthens by a varying period (w) to conform to the URI. During the Wenckebach response, the pacemaker synchronizes Vp to As, and because the pacemaker cannot violate its (ventricular) URI, Vp can be released only at the completion of the URI. The AV delay (As-Vp) becomes progressively longer as the ventricular channel waits to deliver its Vp until the URI has timed out. The maximum prolongation of the AV interval represents the difference between the URI and the TARP (see Fig. 31–18). The As-Vp interval lengthens as long as the As-As interval (P-P) is longer than the TARP. The sixth P wave falls within the PVARP and is unsensed and not followed by Vp. A pause occurs, and the cycle restarts. In the first four pacing cycles, the intervals between ventricular stimuli (Vp-Vp) are constant and equal to the URI. When the P-P interval becomes shorter than the programmed TARP, Wenckebach pacemaker AV block cannot occur, and fixed-ratio pacemaker AV block (e.g., 2:1) supervenes. Same format as Figure 31–10. (From Barold SS, Falkoff MD, Ong LS, et al: All dual-chamber pacemakers function in the DDD mode. Am Heart J 115:1353, 1988.)

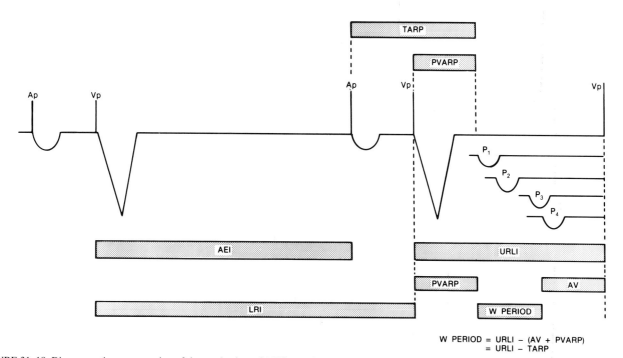

W PERIOD = URLI − (AV + PVARP)
= URLI − TARP

FIGURE 31–18. Diagrammatic representation of the mechanism of AV interval prolongation in a pulse generator with a separately programmable TARP and upper rate limit interval (URLI). Lower rate timing is ventricular based. The maximum AV extension, or waiting, period (W) = URLI − (AV + PVARP) = URLI − TARP. A P wave (P₁) occurring immediately after the termination of the PVARP exhibits the longest AV interval, that is, AV + W. A P wave just beyond the W period (P₄) initiates an AV interval equal to the programmed value. P waves occurring during the W period (P₂ and P₃) exhibit varying degrees of AV prolongation to conform to the URLI depicted as the shortest interval between two consecutive ventricular paced beats. If the pacemaker is programmed with As-Vp shorter than Ap-Vp, W becomes URLI − (As-Vp) − PVARP, that is, AV extension becomes longer if basic As-Vp is shorter than Ap-Vp. However, the maximum As-Vp duration is (URLI − PVARP) regardless of programmed AV interval. AEI = atrial escape interval; LRI = lower rate interval; Ap = atrial paced beat; Vp = ventricular pacing beat. (From Barold SS, Falkoff MD, Ong LS, et al: Electrocardiography of contemporary DDD pacemakers. A. Basic concepts, upper rate response, retrograde ventriculoatrial conduction, and differential diagnosis of pacemaker tachycardias. *In* Saksena S, Goldschlager N [eds]: Electrical Therapy for Cardiac Arrhythmias: Pacing, Antitachycardia Devices, Catheter Ablation. Philadelphia, WB Saunders, 1990, pp 225–264.)

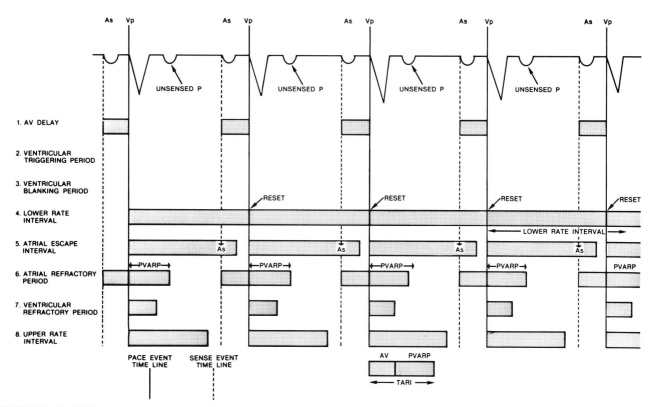

FIGURE 31–19. DDD mode with ventricular-based lower rate timing. *Top,* Upper rate response with fixed-ratio pacemaker AV block. The URI is longer than the TARP (AV + PVARP), and the P-P interval (As-As) is shorter than the TARP. Thus, a Wenckebach upper rate response cannot occur. Every second P wave falls within the PVARP and is unsensed. The AV interval remains constant. Same format as Figure 31–10. (Reprinted with permission from Barold SS: Management of patients with dual-chamber pulse generators: Central role of pacemaker atrial refractory period. Learning Center *Highlights* (Heart House, American College of Cardiology) 5[4]:10, 1990.)

During the Wenckebach response, the pacemaker synchronizes its ventricular stimulus to sensed atrial activity. The ventricular stimulus can be released only at the completion of the URI because the pacemaker cannot violate its (ventricular) URI. The AV delay (initiated by a sensed P wave) becomes progressively longer as the ventricular channel waits to deliver its stimulus until the URI has timed out (see Fig. 31–17). The atrial channel remains refractory and therefore insensitive to incoming signals through the entire duration of the AV interval, regardless of its duration. Eventually a P wave falling within the PVARP is not followed by a ventricular output, and a pause occurs. In other words, Wenckebach behavior limits the paced ventricular rate by extending the AV interval. The Wenckebach upper rate response provides a smoother transition rather than a sudden decrease in the ventricular rate as the pacemaker shifts from a 1:1 ventricular response to fixed-ratio AV block. The Wenckebach upper rate response also allows some degree of AV synchrony.

The pacemaker Wenckebach upper rate response exhibits variability of the AV (As-Vp) interval, a sustained fast paced-ventricular rate (the programmed upper rate), and an occasional abrupt change in the ventricular beat-to-beat interval. Basically a pacemaker Wenckebach sequence contains only two ventricular intervals: (1) Vp-Vp pacing at the URI and (2) Vp-Vp longer than the URI following the undetected P wave in the PVARP. The actual duration of the pause can be calculated with a formula published by Higano and Hayes[45] by knowing the P-P interval, TARP, and URI. The *maximal* duration of the pause terminating the Wenckebach cycle measured between two consecutive ventricular stimuli (after a blocked or unsensed P wave) is equal to the sum of the PVARP, P-P interval, and programmed AV interval provided that the pulse generator senses the P wave that follows the unsensed one in the PVARP at the end of the Wenckebach sequence.[46] Should a P wave not occur before the end of the atrial escape (pacemaker VA) interval, the pause will be equal to the LRI, and the pacemaker will release Ap.

ARTIFICIAL VERSUS NATURAL WENCKEBACH PHENOMENON

There are important differences between the artificial and the natural Wenckebach phenomena:

1. Although a spontaneous, atypical AV nodal Wenckebach phenomenon may occasionally cause some regularization of the R-R intervals, it is never associated with absolutely constant R-R intervals as seen with the pacemaker response to a rapid atrial rate. The intervals between the pacemaker stimuli are constant because they are locked at the URI.
2. There appears to be AV dissociation during the pacemaker Wenckebach period because the P waves march through the ventricular cycle. In contrast to spontaneous AV dissociation, in which atrial and ventricular events are unrelated, in pacemaker Wenckebach periods there is a definite link between each P wave and its triggered ventricular stimulus.
3. The blocked P wave is not really blocked but is unsensed when it falls within the PVARP. The pacemaker then synchronizes its ventricular output to the next P wave.

DISADVANTAGES OF THE WENCKEBACH UPPER RATE RESPONSE

1. In patients with retrograde VA conduction, progressive lengthening of the AV delay to conform to the URI during the Wenckebach response may result in the atria being "ready" to accept a retrograde impulse generated by the ventricular paced beat. Critical prolongation of the AV interval during a pacemaker Wenckebach sequence may therefore initiate endless loop tachycardia (discussed later). Rarely, the same mechanism may also initiate endless loop tachycardia during exercise in predisposed individuals.[47, 48]
2. The hemodynamic benefit of AV synchrony is attenuated or even lost because of the wide variability of the As-Vp intervals.
3. The pause at the end of a Wenckebach sequence may not be tolerated during exercise in some active individuals. (the pause can be reduced or eliminated by sensor-driven rate smoothing during DDDR pacing as discussed later).

MATHEMATICS OF THE WENCKEBACH UPPER RATE RESPONSE

If w is equal to the increment of the AV interval per cycle during the Wenckebach upper rate response w = URI − (P-P interval). If W is equal to the maximal increment of the AV (As-Vp) interval, W is equal to the URI minus the TARP. Thus the AV interval will vary from the basic value of As-Vp (as programmed) to a value equal to (As-Vp) + (URI − TARP). For example, if the URI = 600 msec, the AV interval = 200 msec, the PVARP = 200 msec, and the P-P interval = 550 msec, the increment per cycle w = URI − (P-P interval) = 50 msec. The maximal increment of the AV interval, W = URI − TARP = 600 − 400 = 200 msec. Thus the As-Vp interval will vary from 200 to 400 msec. The Wenckebach ratio can be calculated according to the formula of Higano and Hayes[45] as follows: n = W/w = 4. If N is the next integer above n, N = 5, Wenckebach ratio = N + 1/N = 6/5. Thus, with the preceding parameters, a DDD pulse generator will exhibit 6:5 Wenckebach pacemaker AV block. The pacemaker will respond to an atrial rate faster than 100 ppm and less than 150 ppm with a Wenckebach upper rate response. When the atrial rate reaches 150 ppm, the Wenckebach upper rate response gives way to fixed-ratio AV block.

In contrast, if a DDD pulse generator were programmed with an AV interval equal to 200 msec, a PVARP equal to 250 msec, and an upper rate equal to 125 ppm (URI = 480 msec), it would be difficult to produce an actual pacemaker Wenckebach effect. Maximal prolongation of the AV interval during Wenckebach behavior (W interval) would be only 30 msec (480 − 450). The maximal duration of the AV interval would therefore be 230 msec. In the preceding situation in which the TARP is equal to 450 msec (corresponding to a rate of 133 ppm), the pulse generator will respond with a Wenckebach response to an atrial rate higher than 125 ppm but less than 133 ppm. When the atrial rate exceeds 133 ppm, fixed-ratio AV block will occur without a Wenckebach response. A short W period means that the pulse generator will respond basically with fixed-ratio AV block.

RELATIONSHIP OF UPPER RATE INTERVAL AND TOTAL ATRIAL REFRACTORY PERIOD: AN OVERVIEW

UPPER RATE INTERVAL SHORTER THAN TOTAL ATRIAL REFRACTORY PERIOD

When the URI is programmed to a shorter value than the TARP (despite the fact that the programmer and the pulse generators may seem to have accepted the command), the pacemaker obviously cannot exhibit Wenckebach pacemaker AV block. The URI will be the longer of the two intervals—that is, equal to the TARP. The programmer should alert the operator that such values are not acceptable in the DDD mode. However, this paradoxical relationship (TARP > URI) may actually be programmable and clinically useful in some DDDR pacemakers, as discussed later.

UPPER RATE INTERVAL EQUAL TO THE TOTAL ATRIAL REFRACTORY PERIOD

If a separately programmable URI is equal to the TARP, a Wenckebach upper rate response cannot occur and the pulse generator will respond to fast atrial rates with only a fixed-ratio pacemaker AV block.

UPPER RATE INTERVAL LONGER THAN TOTAL ATRIAL REFRACTORY PERIOD

When the URI is longer than the TARP, the upper rate response of a DDD pulse generator depends on the duration of three variables: TARP, URI, and P-P interval (corresponding to the atrial rate) and three situations can occur.

1. *P-P interval* is longer than the *URI*. The pulse generator maintains 1:1 AV synchrony because the atrial rate is slower than the programmed upper rate.
2. *P-P interval* is shorter than the *URI*. When the P-P interval becomes shorter than the URI but remains longer than the TARP—that is, the URI is longer than the P-P interval, which is longer than the TARP, the pulse generator responds with a Wenckebach pacemaker AV block.
3. *P-P interval* is shorter than the *TARP*. When the P-P interval is shorter than the TARP (and therefore also shorter than the URI), a Wenckebach upper rate response cannot occur, and the upper rate response consists of only a fixed-ratio pacemaker AV block regardless of the duration of the separately programmable URI (see Fig. 31–19). Therefore, when the URI is longer than the TARP, a progressive increase in the atrial rate (shortening of the P-P interval) causes first a pacemaker Wenckebach upper rate response (when P-P < URI), and when the P-P interval becomes equal to or shorter than the TARP, the upper rate response switches from pacemaker Wenckebach AV block to fixed-ratio pacemaker AV block.

UPPER RATE AND DURATION OF THE ATRIOVENTRICULAR INTERVAL

The AV interval initiated by atrial sensing As (i.e., As-Vp) and not the one initiated by Ap (i.e., Ap-Vp) (either equal to or longer than the As-Vp interval) determines the point at which fixed-ratio pacemaker AV block occurs, that is, when the P-P interval becomes equal to or shorter than the TARP, where TARP = (As-Vp) + PVARP. In many pacemakers, As-Vp can be programmed to a value shorter than the Ap-Vp interval, thereby shortening the TARP during atrial sensing. In some pulse generators, the TARP can shorten further on exercise by one of three mechanisms: (1) the As-Vp decreases with an increase of the sensed atrial rate or sensor activity, or both, (adaptive AV interval); (2) the PVARP shortens on exercise (adaptive PVARP); or (3) both the As-Vp interval and PVARP shorten on exercise. In terms of the upper rate response, abbreviation of the TARP, especially in relation to the AV interval initiated by atrial sensing (As-Vp < Ap-Vp) provides important advantages.

1. There is a shorter TARP duration (As-Vp + PVARP) compared with the situation in which As-Vp is equal to Ap-Vp. The shorter TARP induces fixed-ratio pacemaker AV block only at faster sensed atrial rates whenever the P-P interval becomes equal to or shorter than the TARP.
2. With a constant separately programmable URI, a shorter TARP widens the range of atrial rates associated with pacemaker Wenckebach AV block, that is, the Wenckebach upper rate response begins at the same atrial rate (determined by URI), but fixed-ratio pacemaker AV block begins at a faster atrial rate (determined by TARP).
3. A shorter TARP allows programming of a shorter (separately programmable) URI (keeping URI > TARP) with preservation of the Wenckebach pacemaker AV block response at faster atrial rates.

SO-CALLED WENCKEBACH UPPER RATE RESPONSE IN SINGLE CYCLES

The response of a DDD pacemaker (with URI > TARP) to a sensed atrial extrasystole may at first appear complicated (Fig. 31–20). The AV interval engendered by a sensed premature atrial depolarization depends on its timing within the pacing cycle, bearing in mind that the release of a triggered ventricular stimulus must wait until the URI has timed out. Thus, an atrial extrasystole prolongs the As-Vp for a single cycle to conform to the URI. The URI can be identified on the ECG by moving calipers from a premature ventricular stimulus back to the previous ventricular event. If this interval corresponds to the URI, it provides presumptive proof that an atrial sensed event occurred between the two ventricular events bracketing the URI.

Some workers have called this response a manifestation of Wenckebach upper rate behavior, creating potential confusion because a Wenckebach sequence does not actually occur. Rather, a single-cycle response is best described as an ''AV extension'' upper rate response (to conform to the relationship URI > TARP).[29]

ABORTED WENCKEBACH UPPER RATE RESPONSE

In a traditional Wenckebach sequence, a dual-chamber pulse generator (e.g., DDD mode) extends the AV (As-Vp) interval so that Vp occurs at the completion of the (atrial-driven) URI. An aborted Wenckebach sequence is defined as repetitive partial extension of the AV interval, which, however, never attains its expected value in any given cycle according to the programmed URI because an earlier Vp or

APC   APC   URLI = 600 ms

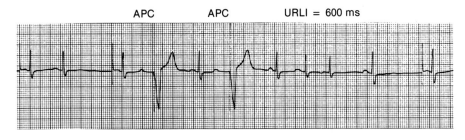

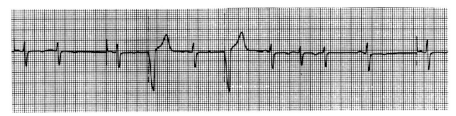

FIGURE 31–20. Two-lead ECG showing DDD pacing (ventricular-based lower rate timing) with sensed atrial premature contractions (APC) (LRI = 1000 msec; AV = 200 msec; URI = 600 msec; PVARP = 155 msec). Note the extended AV interval generated by the APCs to conform to the URI. This response with single beats should not be called a Wenckebach upper rate response. Rather it is best called an AV extension upper rate response.

Vs event continually usurps control of the ventricular channel away from the atrial-driven URI.[40, 49] In other words, a premature Vp or Vs event prevents timing out of the atrial-driven URI, which is therefore reset by an earlier Vp or Vs event. Consequently, the AV (As-Vp) interval never completes its full extension according to the programmed atrial-driven URI. Repetitive aborted Wenckebach upper rate sequences can be classified either as ventricular sensed or ventricular paced responses.

VENTRICULAR SENSED REPETITIVE ABORTED WENCKEBACH UPPER RATE RESPONSE

A DDD pacemaker with a URI longer than the TARP can produce a repetitive aborted Wenckebach upper rate response in the presence of sinus tachycardia, with preserved AV conduction when the spontaneous ventricular rate is faster than the programmed upper rate. A ventricular sensed repetitive aborted Wenckebach upper rate response is characterized by an R-R or Vs-Vs interval shorter than the URI and a PR interval (As-Vs) longer than the programmed As-Vp interval. Should TARP be less than P-P and P-P be less than the URI, sinus tachycardia with complete AV block would produce a classic pacemaker Wenckebach upper rate response. However, the same sinus tachycardia now associated with normal AV conduction forces the pulse generator to sense the conducted QRS (Vs) before the URI has timed out: Vs resets the URI, initiates a new URI, and the process repeats itself creating a self-perpetuating mechanism, with Vs always preempting the expected ventricular stimulus Vp (Fig. 31–21). The aborted Wenckebach response simulates atrial undersensing (lack of atrial tracking) because the partially extended As-Vs interval (to conform to the URI) is longer than the programmed As-Vp interval (without extension). The pulse generator actually senses As beyond the PVARP but cannot emit Vp until completion of the URI. With slowing of the sinus rate, the R-R interval lengthens so that it becomes longer than the URI, whereupon the pacemaker immediately emits Vp after the "correct" programmed (As-Vp) AV interval (now shorter than the partially extended AV interval seen during the aborted Wenckebach sequence) (Fig. 31–22). A single cycle with an extended As-Vs interval should not qualify as an aborted Wenckebach

sequence, as previously argued; it is best described as an AV extension upper rate response (to conform to the relationship URI > TARP).

The concept of ventricular sensed repetitive aborted Wenckebach upper rate response has assumed greater importance in view of the increasing use of DDDR pulse generators and exercise testing (or other forms of activity) necessary to program these complex devices appropriately.[50]

VENTRICULAR-PACED ABORTED-WENCKEBACH UPPER RATE RESPONSE

A ventricular-paced aborted-Wenckebach upper rate response can occur only in the DDDR mode under certain circumstances when delivery of Vp occurs before termination of the atrial-driven URI (discussed later).[49] In this context, shortening or obliteration of the pause at the end of a Wenckebach sequence during DDDR pacing (discussed later) should not be called an aborted-Wenckebach upper rate response. Rather it could be called an "aborted Wenckebach pause."

WENCKEBACH UPPER RATE RESPONSE AND TACHYCARDIA TERMINATION ALGORITHM

When the sinus rate produces a P-P interval essentially equal to the URI but longer than the TARP (URI > TARP), the pacemaker continues to function with an extended As-Vp interval (longer than the programmed As-Vp) to conform to the URI. In this situation, Wenckebach progression can occur for a long time without discernible prolongation of the AV (As-Vp) delay. In the absence of the characteristic pause at the end of the pacemaker Wenckebach block upper rate response, this type of upper rate behavior can resemble a ventricular-paced repetitive aborted-Wenckebach upper rate response. The latter diagnosis is untenable because the As-Vp interval and the URI both time out in their entirety.

Some pulse generators possess a tachycardia-terminating algorithm to abolish endless loop tachycardia automatically (discussed later). In the Intermedics Relay DDDR pacemaker (Intermedics, Inc., Angleton, TX),[17] after 15 paced ventricular beats (triggered by sensed P waves) at the URI, the 16th paced ventricular beat is blocked by inhibiting the delivery

FIGURE 31–21. ECG showing a ventricular sensed repetitive aborted Wenckebach upper rate response during DDDR pacing on exercise (ventricular-based lower rate timing). The PR interval (As-Vs) measures 160 to 180 msec. For this particular level of sensor activity, the rate-adaptive AV interval should be close to 100 msec (see Fig. 31–22). Therefore, the ECG shows apparent lack of atrial tracking (sensing). The sinus rate is faster than the atrial-driven upper rate, that is, R-R interval is shorter than the atrial-driven URI (atrial D − URI = 600 msec). The DDDR pacemaker senses the P waves beyond the PVARP and initiates an extended AV interval to conform to the atrial-driven URI. The spontaneous QRS complex (Vs) occurs before completion of the atrial-driven URI. Vs repeatedly resets the atrial-driven URI. The latter never times out in its entirety. Two ECG leads were recorded simultaneously (paper speed = 50 mm/sec). (From Barold SS: Electrocardiography of rate-adaptive (DDDR) pacemakers. 2. Upper rate behavior. *In* Alt E, Barold SS, Stangl K [eds]: Rate-Adaptive Cardiac Pacing. Berlin, Springer-Verlag, 1993, pp 195–221.)

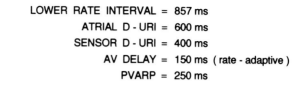

LOWER RATE INTERVAL = 857 ms
ATRIAL D - URI = 600 ms
SENSOR D - URI = 400 ms
AV DELAY = 150 ms (rate - adaptive)
PVARP = 250 ms

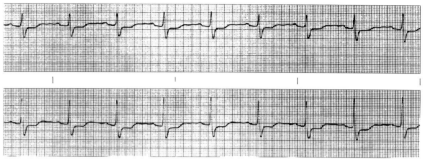

of the 16th ventricular stimulus. This pause terminates endless loop tachycardia by reestablishing AV synchrony with the next pacing cycle. This algorithm is based on the concept that endless loop tachycardia occurs at the programmed upper rate. Although this is frequently the case, it is not always true. An algorithm linked to the URI does not come into play when the cycle length of the endless loop tachycardia is longer than the URI—that is, the sum of the retrograde VA conduction time and the programmed AV interval is longer than the URI. Occasionally the tachycardia termination algorithm comes into play during sinus tachycardia, particularly when the programmed upper rate is relatively slow. Sinus tachycardia with a P-P interval slightly shorter than the URI can cause a Wenckebach progression without discernible prolongation of the AV delay, especially if the programmed AV interval is relatively long and the P wave is concealed within the T wave of the previous beat. This Wenckebach sequence does not terminate in the usual fashion with a P wave ultimately falling within the PVARP (Fig. 31–23). Rather, after 15 cycles at the URI, the pulse generator activates the tachycardia termination algorithm and omits the 16th ventricular stimulus. The P wave never falls in the PVARP, but a pause occurs, although its mechanism differs from that seen in the classic pacemaker Wenckebach block upper rate response (see Fig. 31–23).

Rate-Adaptive Pacemakers

SINGLE-CHAMBER PACEMAKERS: LOWER RATE INTERVAL

In the VVIR (AAIR) mode, the LRI is variable and changes according to the activity of the sensor (which monitors activity in terms of body vibration, minute ventilation volume, temperature, and so forth) designed to increase the pacing rate with effort. At any given time, the duration of the LRI can be either its basic programmed value or the constantly changing sensor-controlled LRI, whichever is shorter (Fig. 31–24). The shortest sensor-driven LRI is equal to the programmed sensor-driven URI.

FIGURE 31–22. Same patient as in Figure 31–21. With slowing of the sinus rate, ventricular stimuli (Vp) begin to appear when the R-R interval is longer than the atrial-driven URI. Initially Vp falls within the QRS complex, producing pseudofusion beats (PF). Then as the ventricular stimulus falls earlier in relation to the spontaneous QRS complex, Vp produces ventricular fusion beats (F). The PR interval (As-Vp) preceding the first two fusion beats is shorter than the PR intervals associated with pseudofusion beats and those in Figure 31–21. The second last beat (labeled F) could be a pseudofusion beat rather than a fusion beat. The pulse generator senses the last P wave (*arrow*) and initiates a short AV interval that represents the prevailing rate-adaptive AV interval at this particular level of exercise. Two ECG leads were recorded simultaneously at a paper speed equal to 50 mm/sec. (From Barold SS: Electrocardiography of rate-adaptive (DDDR) pacemakers. 2. Upper rate behavior. *In* Alt E, Barold SS, Stangl K [eds]: Rate-Adaptive Cardiac Pacing. Berlin, Springer-Verlag, 1993, pp 195–221.)

LOWER RATE INTERVAL = 857 ms
ATRIAL D - URI = 600 ms
SENSOR D - URI = 400 ms
AV DELAY = 150 ms (rate - adaptive)
PVARP = 250 ms

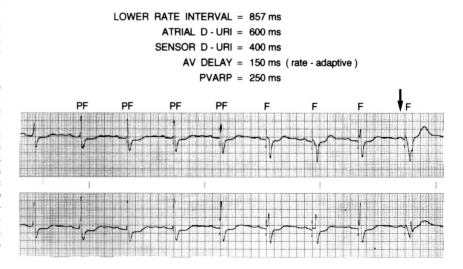

LOWER RATE = 70 ppm (857 ms)
UPPER RATE = 94 ppm (638 ms)
AV INTERVAL = 200 ms
PVARP = 270 ms

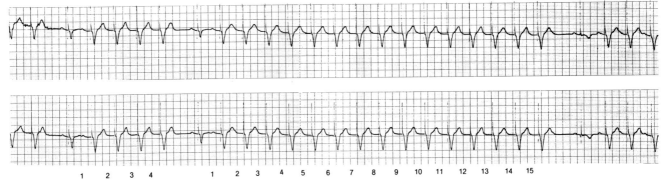

FIGURE 31–23. Operation of the tachycardia termination algorithm of the Intermedics Cosmos I DDD pulse generator (Intermedics, Inc., Angleton, TX) during sinus rhythm (AEI = 657 msec). The sinus rate is close to the programmed upper rate of 94 ppm. On the left there is a pacemaker Wenckebach sequence with four cycles (indicated by the numbers 1–4). The P wave following cycle 4 falls in the PVARP and is unsensed. The subsequent AEI is equal to 657 plus the VA extension (300 msec for this particular pulse generator after a preceding cycle at the URI). This is equal to 957 msec. The extended AEI or VA interval terminates prematurely because of P wave sensing. The next sequence is another pacemaker Wenckebach response with very small increments of the AV (As-Vp) interval, so all the cycles occur at the URI and no P waves fall in the PVARP. The pulse generator activates the tachycardia-terminating algorithm after detecting 15 cycles at the URI. The pause at the end of the tachycardia-terminating algorithm is equal to the URI (638) + AEI (657) = 1295 msec. This interval is aborted by sensing of a P wave about 1000 msec after the previous ventricular stimulus. Note that the pause (Vp-As) after the tachycardia termination algorithm is longer than the maximum extended AEI or VA interval, that is, 1000 msec is longer than 957 msec, the maximum duration of the extended AEI from the previous 6:5 Wenckebach sequence. Note that the sinus P wave that follows the 15th ventricular paced beat does not fall in the PVARP. (From Barold SS, Falkoff MD, Ong LS, et al: Upper rate response of DDD pacemakers. *In* Barold SS, Mugica J [eds]: New Perspectives in Cardiac Pacing. Mt Kisco, NY, Futura Publishing Co., 1988, pp 121–172.)

DUAL-CHAMBER PACEMAKERS: LOWER RATE INTERVAL

In the DDDR mode (as in the VVIR mode), the LRI is variable and varies as the sensor-driven rate varies. At any given time, the duration of the LRI can be either the programmed LRI or the constantly changing sensor-driven LRI, whichever is shorter (see Fig. 31–24). The shortest sensor-driven LRI is equal to the programmed sensor-driven URI.

DDDR PACEMAKERS: UPPER RATE RESPONSE

Control of the upper rate involves (1) only two intervals (TARP and P-P intervals) with a simple DDD pacemaker;

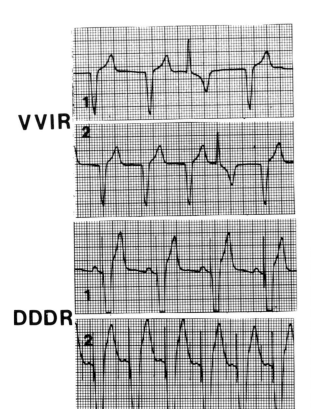

FIGURE 31–24. Response of rate-adaptive VVIR and DDDR pacemakers to exercise. *Top*, VVIR. The tiny bipolar stimuli cannot be discerned. *Panel 1* shows pacing at the programmed lower rate interval (LRI) − 857 msec (corresponding to a rate of 70 ppm). The third beat is a ventricular extrasystole sensed by the pacemaker. The escape interval is essentially equal to the automatic interval. *Panel 2* shows the response on exercise when the ventricular rate increases to about 88 ppm (sensor-driven interval = 680 msec), so the sensed ventricular extrasystole now recycles the pacemaker with an escape interval of about 680 msec. *Bottom Panels*, DDDR. *Panel 1* shows DDD pacing with sensing of P waves (LRI = 1000 msec). In *panel 2* during exercise the AV sequential pacing rate increases to 107 ppm (cycle length 560 msec). (From Barold SS, Falkoff MD, Ong LS, et al: Cardiac pacing in the nineties: Technologic, hemodynamic, and electrophysiologic considerations in the selection of the optimal mode of pacing. *In* Rackley CE [ed]: Challenges in Cardiology I. Mt Kisco, NY, Futura Publishing Co., 1992, pp 39–83.)

(2) three intervals (TARP, P-P interval, and URI) with a more complex DDD pacemaker with a separately programmable URI that is longer than the TARP; and (3) four intervals (TARP, P-P interval, atrial-driven URI, and sensor-driven URI) in DDDR devices.[49]

A DDDR device may function with either a common ventricular URI or two separate ventricular URIs as follows: (1) atrial-driven URI (sometimes known as the maximum tracking rate) and (2) sensor-driven URI. The *atrial-driven* URI refers to the shortest Vs-Vp or Vp-Vp interval in which the last Vp is triggered by an atrial sensed event (As). The pacemaker releases the terminal Vp output only at the completion of the atrial-driven URI initiated by the preceding Vs or Vp. The *sensor-driven* URI refers to the shortest Vs-Vp or Vp-Vp interval in which the last Vp is controlled by *sensor* activity. The pacemaker releases the last Vp output only at the completion of the sensor-driven URI initiated by the preceding Vs or Vp. Note that both the sensor-driven URI and the atrial-driven URI begin with either Vs or Vp and are therefore ventricular intervals.

The relationship between the sensor-driven URI and atrial driven URI can take one of three forms:[49] (1) a sensor-driven URI that is longer than the atrial-driven URI—that is, the sensor-driven upper rate is slower than the atrial-driven upper rate; (2) a sensor-driven URI that is equal to the atrial-driven URI (common upper rates); and (3) a sensor-driven URI that is shorter than the atrial-driven URI—that is, the sensor-driven upper rate is faster than the atrial-driven upper rate. The upper rate behavior of DDDR pacemakers is described in detail later in the text.

Types of Dual-Chamber Pacemakers

Simpler pacing modes can be derived by the removal of "building blocks" from the DDD mode and equalizing certain timing intervals.[41] A DDD pacemaker may have to be downgraded to a simpler mode for the treatment of certain complications. In contrast, a DDDR pacemaker consists of a DDD system upgraded with the addition of a non–P-wave sensor to provide an increase in the pacing rate in patients with abnormal atrial chronotropic function on exercise.

DVI MODE

Dedicated permanent DVI pacemakers (but not the DVI mode) are now obsolete. The DVI mode may be considered as the DDD mode with the PVARP extending through the entire AEI[41] (Fig. 31–25). Thus, in the DVI mode, the TARP in effect lasts through the entire LRI because during the AV interval, the atrial channel of a DDD pacemaker always remains refractory. The URI cannot exist because a DVI pacemaker cannot sense atrial activity. In the DVI mode, therefore, the LRI, TARP, and URI are equal. Asynchronous atrial pacing may precipitate atrial fibrillation.[51]

In the uncommitted DVI mode,[52] the ventricular channel can sense through the entire duration of the AV interval (no ventricular blanking period), whereas in the partially committed DVI mode, the ventricular channel can sense only during part of the AV interval beyond the initial ventricular blanking period (see Fig. 31–25).[53] In contrast, a committed DVI pacemaker may be regarded as having a ventricular

blanking period that encompasses the entire AV interval, rendering crosstalk impossible.[54] In the committed DVI mode, AV sequential stimulation therefore occurs in an all-or-none fashion, that is, no stimuli occur during inhibition and two sequential stimuli always occur during pacing because the ventricular channel cannot sense during the AV interval (Vp is committed after Ap).[54]

DDI MODE

The DDI mode was first mentioned by Levine and Seltzer[55] in 1983 and subsequently described in detail by Floro and associates[56] in 1984. The functional characteristics, limitations, adverse effects, and indications for the DDI mode and the relatively new DDIR mode are still not fully appreciated.[57] The lack of understanding of the DDI mode stems in part from its widely divergent characterizations by various workers as follows: AAI mode with ventricular back-up,[58] AAI plus VVI modes,[38, 56, 59] DVI mode without the potential for atrial competition by virtue of atrial sensing,[60] improved or upgraded DVI with atrial sensing,[61, 62] upgrade of DVI noncommitted pacing,[60] intermediate pacemaker between DVI and DDD modes[63] (a hybrid of DVI and DDD modes),[64] DDD mode without P wave tracking capability,[61, 62, 65] non–P-synchronous DDD mode,[62] AV sequential non–P-synchronous pacing with dual-chamber sensing,[60] and DDD mode with identical upper rate (interval) and lower rate (interval).[66]

Atrial sensing prevents competitive atrial pacing characteristic of the DVI mode in which atrial sensing does not occur. In the DDI mode, atrial sensing occurs beyond the PVARP as in the DDD mode (Fig. 31–26). Atrial sensing inhibits release of the atrial stimulus at the end of the AEI. The subsequent Vp can occur only at the completion of the LRI. Constancy of the paced ventricular rate in the DDI mode requires a ventricular-based (V-V) LRT after a paced or sensed ventricular event, that is, the LRI starts with Vp or Vs. With this arrangement, the DDI mode can be considered as the DDD mode with identical upper and lower intervals.[65] Like the DDD mode, the DDI mode requires an LRI, AV delay, PVARP, ventricular refractory period, and crosstalk intervals (ventricular blanking and safety pacing), but no URI because the LRI equals the URI. A sensor-driven "URI" is obviously required for the DDIR mode (i.e., shortest rate-adaptive LRI).

In the DDI mode with V-V lower rate timing, an atrial extrasystole or sinus P wave (As) sensed beyond the PVARP will initiate an AV interval (as in the DDD mode) so that the pulse generator will release its ventricular stimulus (Vp) only at the completion of the (ventricular) URI (equal to the ventricular LRI). Thus a very early atrial extrasystole (As) can produce an extremely long As-Vp interval. A shorter AV interval after atrial sensing than atrial pacing, an important feature of contemporary DDD (DDDR) systems, is incompatible with the DDI mode in which the As-Ap interval by definition must be longer than the programmed Ap-Vp interval. Despite atrial sensing, a DDI pacemaker cannot increase its ventricular pacing rate in response to a faster atrial rate (unlike the DDD or VDD mode), and ventricular pacing always occurs at the programmed lower rate. This response is sometimes described as an inability to track the atrial rate, that is, no atrial tracking means that the ventricular paced rate cannot increase beyond the programmed rate (except in

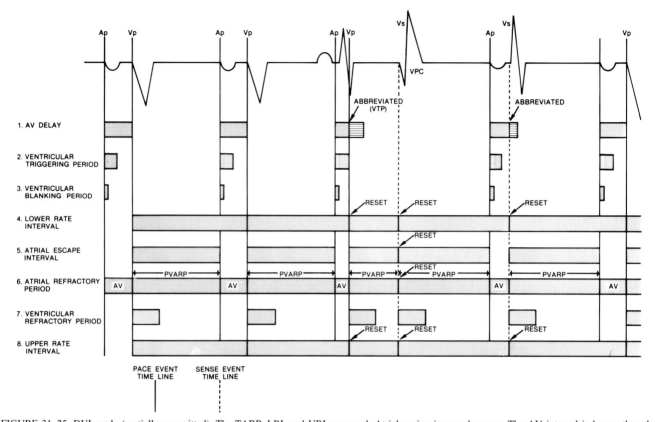

FIGURE 31–25. DVI mode (partially committed). The TARP, LRI, and URI are equal. Atrial pacing is asynchronous. The AV interval is longer than the VSP (triggering) period, and the latter is in turn longer than the ventricular blanking period. The third P wave is unsensed because the atrial channel functions asynchronously. The first spontaneous QRS complex (between the third Ap and the third Vp) is sensed within the VSP period (or VTP), so the ventricular channel delivers Vp at the completion of the VSP period. Therefore, the third AV interval (Ap-Vp) is abbreviated by premature delivery of Vp. The fourth Ap initiates an AV interval that is terminated prematurely because Vs occurs before the AV interval has timed out; premature emission of Vp does not occur because Vs is sensed beyond the VSP period. The fourth beat is a ventricular extrasystole (VPC) sensed by the ventricular channel. In an uncommitted DVI device, the ventricular blanking period and VTP are absent. In a committed DVI device, the ventricular blanking period is equal to the AV interval. Same format as Figure 31–10. (From Barold SS, Falkoff MD, Ong LS, et al: All dual-chamber pacemakers function in the DDD mode. Am Heart J 115:1353, 1988.)

FIGURE 31–26. DDI mode. With ventricular-based (V-V) lower rate timing, the DDI mode is equivalent to the DDD mode, with LRI equal to URI. However, the URI (equal to LRI) is longer than the programmed TARP (AV + PVARP). As in the DDD mode, P waves outside the 250-msec PVARP are sensed and initiate an AV interval (i.e., atrial stimulus is inhibited). With atrial sensing the As-Vp interval lengthens by a varying period to conform to the URI (equal to the LRI). As in the DDD mode (see Figs. 31–17 and 31–18), the maximum prolongation of the AV interval during Wenckebach pacemaker AV block represents the difference between the URI and the programmed TARP. When the P wave is unsensed during the PVARP, the pulse generator emits an atrial stimulus at the end of its programmed AEI. Three ECG leads were recorded simultaneously. (From Barold SS, Falkoff MD, Ong LS, et al: Electrocardiography of contemporary DDD pacemakers. A. Basic concepts, upper rate response, retrograde ventriculoatrial conduction, and differential diagnosis of pacemaker tachycardias. *In* Saksena S, Goldschlager N [eds]: Electrical Therapy for Cardiac Arrhythmias: Pacing, Antitachycardia Devices, Catheter Ablation. Philadelphia, WB Saunders, 1990, pp 225–264.)

PACESETTER AFP 283 DDI MODE
LOWER RATE = 70 ppm, AV = 165 ms, PVARP = VRP = 250 ms

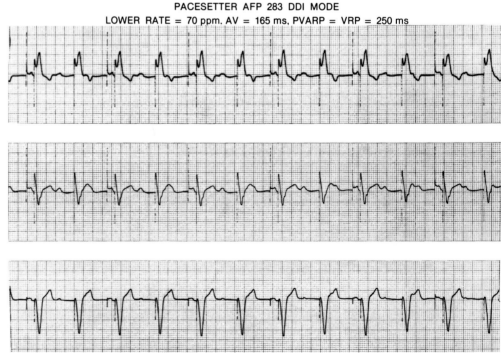

devices with ventricular-based V-V LRT during VSP when the AV sequential pacing rate increases as it does in the DDD mode).[25] In the DDIR mode, the paced ventricular rate becomes equal to the sensor-driven rate.[67]

ATRIAL AND VENTRICULAR STIMULI. The DDI mode provides AV synchrony when the programmed rate exceeds the spontaneous atrial rate and AV conduction is slower than the programmed AV delay so that both channels pace sequentially, a situation that provides no advantage over DDD pacing.

NO STIMULI WITH RELATIVELY NORMAL AV CONDUCTION. If the spontaneous atrial rate exceeds the programmed lower rate (P-P interval < LRI), the P waves and conducted QRS complexes inhibit the pulse generator, a situation that provides no advantage over DDD pacing.

NORMAL ATRIAL CHRONOTROPIC FUNCTION WITH AV BLOCK. When the sinus rate exceeds the programmed lower rate in patients with AV block and normal atrial chronotropic function, AV synchrony (at the programmed AV interval) does *not* occur in the DDI mode (Fig. 31–27). P waves sensed by the atrial channel gradually march through the pacing cycles, moving closer and closer to the preceding paced ventricular beat, which produces constantly changing AV intervals, mostly unphysiologic in duration regardless of the programmed AV interval. More obvious AV dissociation occurs with faster atrial rates. The pacemaker therefore functions like the VVI mode (with AV dissociation) except when the P wave falls in the PVARP (and is unsensed), whereupon the pulse generator delivers an atrial stimulus at the termination of the AEI (ventricular stimuli with occasional atrial stimuli). During episodes of rapid atrial tachyarrhythmias with constant inhibition of the atrial channel, a DDIR pacemaker merely paces at the programmed lower ventricular rate or at the sensor-driven ventricular rate during DDI pacing. For example, during atrial fibrillation, when the pacemaker continually senses atrial activity, the DDI mode looks exactly like VVI pacing without any atrial stimuli whatsoever (ventricular stimuli only) (Fig. 31–28).

ATRIAL COMPETITION. No atrial competition occurs except with a substantial increase in the ventricular pacing rate in the DDI or DDIR mode when the pacemaker can discharge

its atrial stimulus relatively close to a preceding P wave unsensed in the PVARP. Atrial stimulation may then fall in the atrial vulnerable period or may be ineffectual if delivered in the myocardial atrial refractory period generated by the preceding atrial depolarization.

VENTRICULOATRIAL SYNCHRONY. In the DDI mode, sensing of retrograde P waves due to VA conduction (beyond the PVARP) produces a pacemaker endless loop arrangement (obviously at the programmed lower rate) similar to its counterpart (endless loop tachycardia) in the DDD mode, an arrangement capable of causing the pacemaker syndrome as in the VVI mode with retrograde VA conduction (Fig. 31–29).[68]

ATRIAL STIMULI ONLY (VENTRICULAR INHIBITION). In the DDI as in the DDD mode with ventricular-based LRT, when Ap-Vs is shorter than Ap-Vp, the sequence Ap-Vs-Ap-Vs causes an increase in the atrial pacing rate and an increase in the ventricular rate (the Vs-Vs interval shortens), but the ventricular *paced* rate cannot increase by definition.

Despite their limitations,[69] the DDI mode and its rate-adaptive counterpart the DDIR mode have become popular for the treatment of patients with alternating bradycardia and tachycardia as in the sick sinus syndrome.[70–74] In the latter, the DDI mode provides atrial pacing and AV synchrony (in the absence of atrial tachyarrhythmias), with the potential of preventing atrial tachyarrhythmias by overdrive suppression. During episodes of atrial tachyarrhythmias, a DDI (DDIR) pacemaker simply paces at the constant programmed (lower) ventricular rate (or sensor-driven rate). In patients with paroxysmal supraventricular tachyarrhythmias with a normal sinus mechanism and AV block, the DDI (DDIR) mode produces almost continual AV dissociation with possible intolerance of pacing (pacemaker syndrome). AV dissociation can be prevented by implanting a DDD or DDDR unit (that maintains AV synchrony) with the capability of recognizing pathologic supraventricular tachycardia and designed with a protective fallback mechanism to a lower pacing rate (with or without automatic conversion of the pacing mode) to avoid rapid ventricular pacing from tracking rapid atrial rates (discussed later). Reversion to the original DDD or DDDR mode of pacing subsequently occurs when the atrial rate drops below the programmed upper rate or the tachycardia

FIGURE 31–27. Electrocardiograms of a patient who developed the pacemaker syndrome with the DDIR mode. A dual-chamber pulse generator was implanted after His bundle ablation for intractable paroxysmal atrial fibrillation. *Top,* The DDIR mode at rest functions at the programmed lower rate of 60 ppm, slower than the prevailing sinus rate. Note that sinus P waves march through the cardiac cycle, producing AV dissociation. The P wave following the first ventricular paced beat falls in the 300-msec PVARP and is unsensed, thereby allowing the release of an atrial stimulus at the end of the AEI initiated by the first ventricular paced complex. *Bottom,* On exercise, when the sinus rate is slightly faster than the sensor-driven rate, sinus P waves march through the cardiac cycle, producing AV dissociation. The pulse generator does not sense the P wave following the first ventricular paced beat because it falls in the PVARP. This allows emission of an atrial stimulus at the termination of the sensor-driven AEI initiated by the first ventricular paced beat. (From Barold SS, Ong LS, Falkoff MD, et al: Cardiac pacing update: Guidelines in choosing pacemakers and optimal pacing m modes. *In* Zipes DP, Rowlands DJ [eds]: Progress in Cardiology. Philadelphia, Lea & Febiger, 1992, pp 171–196.)

DDIR

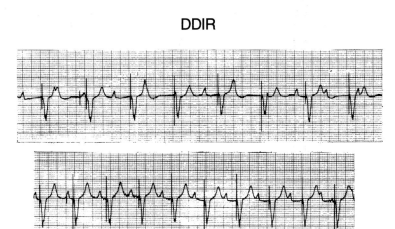

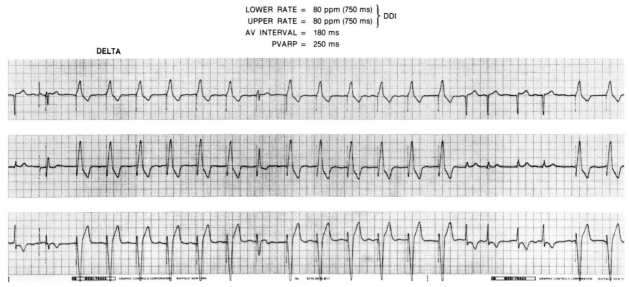

FIGURE 31–28. DDI mode in CPI Delta DDD pacemaker (Cardiac Pacemakers, Inc., St. Paul, MN) with ventricular-based lower rate timing. Although the pulse generator was left programmed to the DDD mode, it functions as in the DDI mode because the upper rate was programmed to a value equal to the lower rate (80 ppm). The underlying rhythm is atrial fibrillation. Barring the first beat, the DDI mode resembles VVI pacing at 80 ppm with normal ventricular pacing and sensing. The presence of atrial and ventricular stimuli in relation to the first beat provides the only clue that the pulse generator functions in the DDI mode. The atrial fibrillatory waves generate sufficient voltage to inhibit the atrial channel continually except on the left before the first QRS complex. Three ECG leads were recorded simultaneously. (From Barold SS, Falkoff MD, Ong LS, et al: Timing cycles of DDD pacemakers. *In* Barold SS, Mugica J [eds]: New Perspectives in Cardiac Pacing. Mt Kisco, NY, Futura Publishing Co., 1988, pp 69–119.)

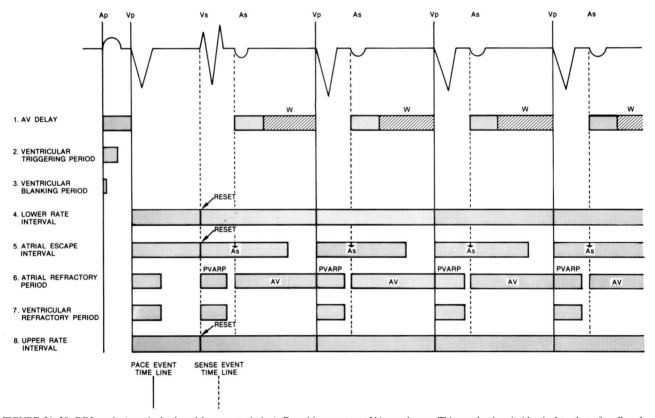

FIGURE 31–29. DDI mode (ventricular-based lower rate timing). Repetitive reentrant VA synchrony. This mechanism is identical to that of endless loop tachycardia (see Fig. 31–43), but no tachycardia occurs in the DDI mode because URI equals LRI. A sensed ventricular extrasystole (Vs) generates retrograde VA conduction (As). The pacemaker senses As and initiates an extended AV interval lengthened by W to conform to the URI (Vp-Vp) also equal to the lower rate interval. Same format as Figure 31–10. (From Barold SS, Falkoff MD, Ong LS, et al: All dual-chamber pacemakers function in the DDI mode. Am Heart J 115:1353, 1988.)

detection rate. The DDI mode will probably become obsolete as a primary pacing mode when fallback mechanisms and automatic mode conversion (which prevent rapid ventricular pacing during paroxysmal supraventricular tachyarrhythmias) become more refined and commonplace.

VDD MODE

The VDD mode functions like the DDD mode except that the atrial output is turned off [41] (Fig. 31–30). The VDD mode is a programmable option in many dual-chamber pacemakers. If not, it can be obtained by programming the atrial output to zero. If the design does not allow the latter, the lowest pulse width and atrial voltage usually do not capture the atrium, so the pulse generator functions essentially in the VDD mode. In the case of bipolar atrial pacing, the stimuli often become invisible and the VDD mode is mimicked. In the VDD mode, failure to deliver an atrial stimulus precludes initiation of crosstalk intervals (ventricular blanking and safety pacing periods). The required timing cycles of the VDD mode include LRI, URI, AV interval, ventricular refractory period, and PVARP.[41] As far as the timing cycles are concerned, the omitted atrial stimulus begins an implied AV interval during which the atrial channel must be refractory as in the DDD mode. This behavior explains why in most contemporary VDD designs, a P wave occurring during the implied AV interval (after an aborted atrial stimulus) cannot initiate a new AV interval. However, in some DDD pulse generators programmed to the VDD mode, a P wave during the implied AV interval can be sensed and can actually reinitiate an entirely new AV interval so that the Vs-Vp or Vp-Vp interval becomes longer (maximum extension equal to As-Vp interval) than the programmed (ventricular-based) LRI, producing a form of hysteresis.[1, 38]

In the absence of sensed atrial activity, the VDD mode will continue to pace effectively in the VVI mode (at the LRI of the DDD mode) because the VDD mode preserves all the other timing cycles of the DDD mode despite the missing atrial output. Dedicated VDD devices became obsolete with the introduction of DDD pacemakers. However, single-lead AV systems with floating atrial electrodes on the intra-atrial portion of the ventricular lead can provide reliable VDD pacing and will almost certainly lead to a renaissance of dedicated VDD devices.[75, 76]

Automatic Mode Conversion

Conventional or specially designed pacemakers can convert automatically to another pacing mode in a variety of

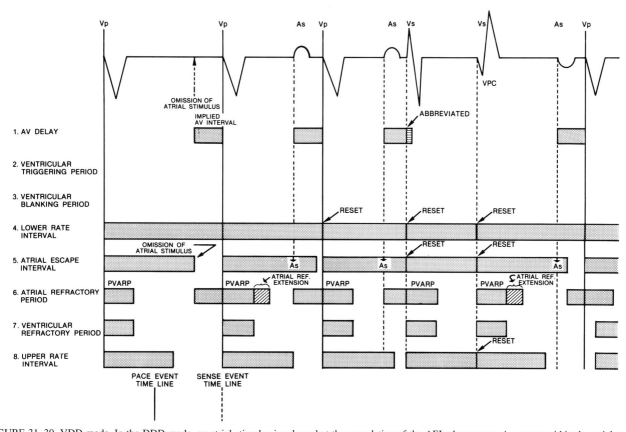

FIGURE 31–30. VDD mode. In the DDD mode, an atrial stimulus is released at the completion of the AEI whenever no As occurs within the atrial escape interval. In the VDD mode (equivalent to the DDD mode without an atrial output), the atrial stimulus is omitted. Nevertheless, the pulse generator initiates an implied AV interval with the same characteristics as in the DDD mode. Most pacemakers do not sense (or track) a P wave falling in the implied AV interval. In the first Vp-Vp cycle, the pacemaker extends its PVARP automatically, as after a sensed ventricular extrasystole (see Fig. 31–10), because Vp terminating the implied AV interval is not preceded by Ap or As. No ventricular blanking and VSP (triggering) periods are needed because there are no atrial stimuli in the VDD mode. With the omission of Ap at the end of the implied AV interval and the absence of As, the pulse generator effectively paces in the VVI mode at the programmed DDD lower rate interval (first cycle). Same format as in Figure 31–10. (From Barold SS, Falkoff MD, Ong LS, et al: All dual-chamber pacemakers function in the DDD mode. Am Heart J 115:1353, 1988.)

circumstances.[77-79] Automatic conversion of the pacing mode of single- and dual-chamber devices may be classified as follows:

1. *Apparent*: A VDD pulse generator effectively paces in the VVI mode in the presence of sinus bradycardia slower than the programmed lower rate, whereas a DDI pacemaker appears to function in the VVI mode in the presence of an atrial tachyarrhythmia when the atrial channel consistently senses P or f waves beyond the PVARP.

2. *Temporary*: When the mechanism causing the automatic change of pacing mode no longer exists, the pulse generator reverts immediately to its original pacing mode. In this way, a VVI pacemaker can revert to the VOO mode and a DDD pacemaker to the VOO or DOO mode as a temporary response to sensed electromagnetic interference (EMI) or other extraneous signals (interference mode). Additionally, a pacemaker in the DDD mode may respond to an atrial rate faster than the programmed upper rate by automatic conversion to a fallback mode (such as VVI) with a gradual or sudden reduction of the pacing rate to a predetermined level; reversion to the DDD mode subsequently occurs when the atrial rate drops below the programmed upper rate[80] (see later discussion of fallback response). Tachycardia-terminating pacemakers also belong to this group.

3. *Permanent until reprogrammed* (pacemaker reset): The DDD mode can be converted to the VVI or VOO mode, and the VVIR mode to the VVI mode as a permanent (unless reprogrammed) response to sensed EMI or as an indicator of the elective replacement time.[81]

4. *Permanent and unresponsive to reprogramming*: Conversion to the reset mode with an inability to reprogram the pulse generator to its original mode may occur with advanced battery depletion (end of life) or component malfunction (including damage from defibrillation, therapeutic radiation, and electrocautery).

Types of Lower Rate Timing

Traditional and many contemporary dual-chamber pacemakers are designed with ventricular-based LRT or simply V-V timing (see Fig. 31–8). With ventricular-based LRT, the LRI is initiated (and therefore controlled) by a ventricular event (Vp or Vs) and is the longest Vp-Vp or Vs-Vp interval (without intervening atrial and ventricular sensed events.)[25] Similarly the AEI (Vp-Ap or Vs-Ap) always remains constant provided that there are no intervening atrial or ventricular sensed events. A ventricular sensed event either in the AV interval or during the AEI resets both the LRI and the AEI so that both start again. Constancy of the AEI is the cardinal feature of ventricular-based LRT. Hence the term V-V timing is often used interchangeably with VA timing to emphasize constancy of the AEI in ventricular-based LRT.[25, 82] Despite the well-established performance of dual-chamber pacemakers with ventricular-based LRT, recently a number of manufacturers introduced dual-chamber pulse generators with atrial-based LRT (A-A timing) designed to avoid cycle-to-cycle fluctuations or beat-to-beat oscillations.[25, 83] With atrial-based LRT, the LRI is initiated and therefore controlled by atrial (As or Ap) rather than ventricular events (Fig. 31–31). In A-A LRT, the LRI is the longest Ap-Ap or As-Ap interval (without an intervening atrial sensed event or ventricular premature contraction [VPC]). Other forms of lower rate control include a variety of hybrids with either atrial or ventricular LRT, according to the circumstances. These new designs have introduced great complexity in the understanding of timing cycles related to lower rate function of dual-chamber pacemakers.[60, 61, 82-89] Nevertheless, the definition of the AEI as the interval from Vp or Vs to the succeeding Ap remains identical for all LRT mechanisms. In the subsequent discussion, AV delay as programmed refers only to the paced AV interval, that is, Ap-Vp.

V-V and A-A Responses

For descriptive purposes, the behavior of a *single* pacemaker cycle initiated by any combination of atrial and ventricular events (As-Vs, As-Vp, Ap-Vs, Ap-Vp, or isolated Vs) can be considered in terms of one of the two basic LRT mechanisms. The characterization of single cycles is important because some manufacturers have designed pacemakers with hybrid timing systems for LRT, using either A-A or V-

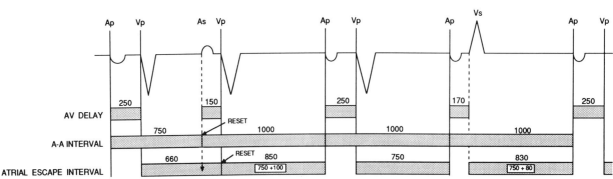

A-A TIMING (As - Vp < Ap - Vp)

FIGURE 31–31. Diagrammatic representation of the timing cycles of a DDD pulse generator with pure atrial-based (A-A) lower rate timing showing the effect of differential AV delays (LRI = 1000 msec; basic AEI = 750 msec during free-running AV sequential pacing; As-Vp = 150 msec; and Ap-Vp = 250 msec). The second Vp terminates the As-Vp interval that is equal to 150 msec and initiates an AEI of 750 + (250 − 150) = 850 msec to maintain constancy of the A-A or Ap-Ap interval. On the *right*, the third Ap initiates an Ap-Vs interval equal to 170 msec. The corresponding AEI becomes 750 + (250 − 170) = 830 msec to maintain constancy of the A-A or Ap-Ap interval. The last interventricular interval (Vs-Vp) = 830 + 250 = 1080 msec and longer than the atrial-based LRI (1000 msec). (From Barold SS, Falkoff MD, Ong LS, et al: A-A and V-V lower rate timing of DDD and DDDR pulse generators. *In* Barold SS, Mugica J [eds]: New Perspectives in Cardiac Pacing 2. Mt Kisco, NY, Futura Publishing Co., 1991, pp 203–247.)

TABLE 31–2. **TYPES OF AV INTERVALS**

	SHORTER	BASIC	LONGER
Ap-Vp	+	+	–
Ap-Vs	+	+	–
As-Vp	+	+	+
As-Vs	+	+	+

Abbreviations: AV, atrioventricular.
From Barold SS: Electrocardiography of rate-adaptive dual-chamber (DDDR) pacemakers: Lower rate behavior. *In* Alt E, Barold SS, Stangl K (eds): Rate-Adaptive Pacing. Heidelberg, Berlin, Springer-Verlag, 1993, pp 173–194. Copyright 1993 Springer-Verlag.

V LRT according to the relationship of atrial and ventricular events (Table 31–2).

V-V RESPONSE. A ventricular paced or sensed event determines the duration of the succeeding pacing cycle, that is, Vp or Vs initiates a *constant* AEI (Vs-Ap or Vp-Ap) equal to its basic value in the free-running mode. If Ap terminating the AEI is followed by Vp, the Vs-Ap-Vp or Vp-Ap-Vp intervals will be constant and equal to the programmed ventricular-based LRI (see Figs. 31–8 and 31–10). An isolated Vs (e.g., a VPC not preceded by an atrial event) initiates a V-V response (constant AEI) in all dual-chamber pulse generators with V-V timing. All DDD and DDDR pacemakers from the following manufacturers exhibit ventricular-based (V-V) lower rate timing: Siemens-Pacesetter, Inc. (Sylmar, CA), Telectronics, Inc. (Englewood, CO), and Cardiac Pacemakers, Inc. (CPI) (St. Paul, MN). The timing behaviors of the dual-chamber pacemakers manufactured by Intermedics, Inc. (Angleton, TX), and Medtronic Inc. (Minneapolis, MN) and those CPI pacemakers manufactured by Medtronic Inc. are expressed in Tables 31–3, 31–4 and 31–5. In most dual-chamber devices with either a pure atrial-based or a hybrid LRT mechanism, a VPC also initiates a V-V cycle, as discussed later.

A-A RESPONSE. An atrial paced or sensed event determines the duration of the succeeding pacing cycle, that is, As or Ap initiates a constant LRI (As-Ap or Ap-Ap) disregarding any Vs or Vp following the atrial event (As or Ap) that initiates the pacing cycle. Consequently, the AEI adapts its duration (longer, shorter, or unchanged) to maintain a constant Ap-Ap or As-Ap relationship equal to the atrial-based LRI (see Fig. 31–31). In some designs, a VPC initiates an A-A rather than a V-V response (as previously emphasized), that is, (Vs-Ap) interval = atrial-based LRI.[82, 84]

Lower Rate Timing Versus Upper Rate Timing

Control of the LRI by either an A-A or V-V response should not be confused with behavior of the URI. All DDD and DDDR pacemakers possess a URI controlled by and therefore initiated by a ventricular (paced or sensed) event regardless of the LRT mechanism.

The term atrial-driven ventricular URI is not contradictory because, as already emphasized, it refers to the shortest Vs-Vp or Vp-Vp in which an *atrial* sensed event (As) triggers or drives the terminal Vp output. The pacemaker can release the last Vp output only at the completion of the *ventricular* URI initiated by the preceding Vs or Vp. An atrial-based LRT does not mean that the URI is also atrial-based because no DDD or DDDR pacemakers can function with URI solely controlled by atrial events. (Some DDD pacemakers[25, 40] [Medtronic Symbios; Medtronic, Inc., Minneapolis, MN] and DDDR pacemakers[25, 89, 90] [Medtronic Synergyst II] occasionally function with separate but linked atrial and ventricular URIs [i.e., each URI is initiated by a paced or sensed event in its respective chamber and terminated by a *paced* event in the same chamber], which may become evident only under special circumstances.)

Ventricular-Based Lower Rate Timing

ANALYSIS OF PACEMAKER FUNCTION ON A CYCLE-TO-CYCLE BASIS

The behavior of a DDD pulse generator can be analyzed on a cycle-to-cycle basis (Fig. 31–32). In any given cycle, a DDD pulse generator with ventricular-based LRT can be considered to function in one of the following modes: AAI, DVI, VDD, or inhibited mode. Under exceptional circumstances, a DDD pulse generator can also function in the VVI, VOO, DOO, or DDT mode.

NO PACEMAKER STIMULI

If there are no stimuli, the pacemaker could be operating in any one of its three modes for any given cycle (AAI, VDD, or DVI) or all of them together. In this situation, the R-R interval is shorter than the LRI, and the PR interval is

TABLE 31–3. **LOWER RATE BEHAVIOR OF INTERMEDICS DDD AND DDDR PULSE GENERATORS**

AV INTERVAL	COSMOS I DDD	COSMOS II DDD	RELAY DDDR	RELAY DDD
Ap-Vs	V-V	A-A	A-A	A-A
Abbreviated Ap-Vp (VSP)	V-V	A-A	A-A	A-A
As-Vp is shorter than programmed Ap-Vp	V-V	A-A	A-A	A-A
As-Vp is longer than programmed Ap-Vp (prolongation in Wenckebach upper rate response)	V-V	A-A	V-V	V-V
As-Vs is shorter than programmed Ap-Vp	V-V	A-A	A-A	A-A
As-Vs is longer than programmed Ap-Vp (as in Wenckebach upper rate response)	V-V	A-A	V-V	V-V
VPC not preceded by As	V-V	V-V	V-V	V-V

Abbreviations: VSP, ventricular safety pacing; VPC, ventricular premature contraction.
From Barold SS: Electrocardiography of rate-adaptive dual-chamber (DDDR) pacemakers: Lower rate behavior. *In* Alt E, Barold SS, Stangl K (eds): Rate-Adaptive Pacing. Heidelberg, Berlin, Springer-Verlag, 1993, pp 173–194. Copyright 1993 Springer-Verlag.

TABLE 31–4. **LOWER RATE BEHAVIOR OF MEDTRONIC DDD AND DDDR PULSE GENERATORS**

AV INTERVAL	SYMBIOS DDD MODE	SYNERGYST I AND II[a] DDD MODE	SYNERGYST II[a] DDDR MODE	ELITE I AND II[a] DDDR MODE	ELITE I AND II[a] DDD MODE MINUET DDD
Ap-Vs	V-V	A-A	A-A	A-A	V-V
Abbreviated Ap-Vp (VSP)	V-V	V-V	V-V	A-A	V-V
As-Vp shorter than programmed Ap-Vp	NA	NA	NA	V-V	V-V
As-Vp longer than programmed Ap-Vp (as in Wenckebach response)	V-V	V-V	V-V	V-V	V-V
As-Vs shorter than programmed Ap-Vp	V-V	A-A	A-A	V-V	V-V
As-Vs longer than programmed Ap-Vp (as in Wenckebach upper rate response)	V-V	V-V	V-V	V-V	V-V
VPC not preceded by As	V-V	V-V	V-V	V-V	V-V

Abbreviations: VSP, ventricular safety pacing; VPC, ventricular premature contraction or extrasystole; NA, not applicable.
[a]The CPI Triumph DR DDDR pacemaker and the Medtronic Synergyst II pacemaker share the same circuit and therefore these devices have identical timing cycles. The CPI Prelude DR DDDR pacemaker and the Medtronic Elite I share the same circuit and have identical timing cycles.
From Barold SS: Electrocardiography of rate-adaptive dual-chamber (DDDR) pacemakers: Lower rate behavior. *In* Alt E, Barold SS, Stangl K (eds): Rate-Adaptive Pacing. Heidelberg, Berlin, Springer-Verlag, 1993, pp 173–194. Copyright 1993 Springer-Verlag.

shorter than the AV interval. However, pacemaker inhibition does not always mean that the device senses both ventricular and atrial signals. Thus, during total inhibition, a DDD pulse generator may actually be working continuously in the DVI mode, for example, if the atrial signal is too small to be sensed and if the R-R interval is shorter than the AEI, atrial undersensing can be masked.[40]

ONE PACEMAKER STIMULUS

If there is only one stimulus, the pacemaker could be operating in any one of three modes:

TABLE 31–5. **COMMITTED AV INTERVALS**

PACEMAKER MODEL	CIRCUMSTANCES ASSOCIATED WITH COMMITTED AV INTERVAL (OR A-A INTERVALS)
Medtronic Elite I and II[a]	After Ap only
Intermedics Relay	After all AV intervals (initiated by Ap or As)[b] *shorter* than the programmed Ap-Vp interval
Medtronic Synergyst I and II[c]	After all AV intervals (initiated by Ap or As)[b] *shorter* than the programmed Ap-Vp interval *except* when Ap-Vp is abbreviated because of ventricular safety pacing
Intermedics Cosmos II and ELA Chorus	After *all* AV intervals (initiated by Ap or As)[b]

The following AV combinations do not occur during normal function: (1) Ap-Vs longer than programmed Ap-Vp; (2) Ap-Vp longer than programmed Ap-Vp.
[a]CPI Prelude DR DDDR pacemakers have identical timing cycles to the Medtronic Elite I devices.
[b]As-Vs may be shorter than, equal to, or longer than the programmed Ap-Vp during normal function. When URI is longer than total atrial refractory period, As-Vs can be longer than the programmed Ap-Vp during Wenckebach block upper rate response.
[c]CPI Triumph DR DDDR pacemakers have identical timing cycles to the Medtronic Synergyst II devices.
Modified from Barold SS: Electrocardiography of rate-adaptive dual-chamber (DDDR) pacemakers: Lower rate behavior. *In* Alt E, Barold SS, Stangl K (eds): Rate-Adaptive Pacing. Heidelberg, Berlin, Springer-Verlag, 1993, pp 173–194. Copyright 1993 Springer-Verlag.

AAI MODE. If there is an atrial stimulus only, the pacemaker functions in the AAI mode. This occurs if the atrial rate is slow, with intact AV conduction. The conducted QRS causes ventricular inhibition.

VDD (VAT) MODE. If there is a ventricular stimulus only, the pacemaker functions in the VDD (VAT) mode. This occurs with a normal atrial rate but abnormal AV conduction.

VVI (VOO) MODE. If there is a single ventricular stimulus, the pacemaker may also be functioning in the VVI or VOO mode rather than the VDD mode. Automatic conversion of a DDD or DDDR pulse generator to the VVI (or VOO) mode (pacemaker reset) can occur as a result of sensing extraneous interference or battery depletion.[81] In the latter situation, the reset mode (VVI or VOO) functions as the elective replacement indicator. The VVI (VOO) mode can usually be ignored in the routine electrocardiographic analysis of pacemaker function because it occurs only under unusual circumstances. Some DDD pulse generators convert to the VOO mode on application of the magnet.

TWO PACEMAKER STIMULI

If there are two pacemaker stimuli, three possibilities exist:

DVI MODE. This is the most likely mode, and it occurs with a slow atrial rate and abnormal AV conduction. In this context, the DVI mode refers to a partially committed system, that is, the pulse generator is capable of sensing ventricular activity during part of the AV interval (after termination of the ventricular blanking period to prevent detection of the atrial stimulus or crosstalk).

DOO MODE. This may occur in the presence of excessive noise or interference or on application of the test magnet.

DDT (TRIGGERED) MODE. Under certain circumstances, a DDD pulse generator may be considered to be working in the DDT mode, a code suggested by Garson and colleagues[91] to denote VSP.

The duration of a DVI cycle (initiated by Vs or Vp and terminating with Ap-Vp) is equal to the (ventricular) LRI and always remains constant. AAI and VDD cycles are variable and produce interventricular intervals shorter than the LRI. In the case of VDD cycles, shortening of the ventricular

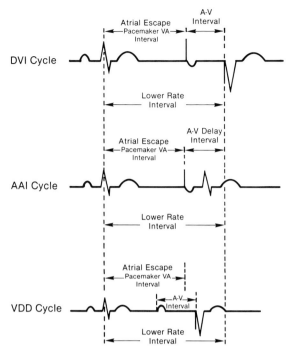

FIGURE 31–32. Behavior of a DDD pacemaker with ventricular-based (V-V) lower rate timing based on examination of a single cycle at a time in a continuous ECG. The DDD mode incorporates the essentials of three simpler modes: DVI, AAI, and VDD. In any one pacemaker cycle, starting with either a sensed or a paced ventricular event (Vs or Vp), one of these three modes may be seen. The descriptive mode for a single pacemaker cycle is determined only by the way the cycle terminates: (a) DVI mode if there are two stimuli. The DVI mode occurs with a slow atrial rate and abnormal AV conduction. (In this context, the DVI mode refers to a partially committed system.) (b) AAI mode. If there is only an atrial stimulus, the pacemaker functions in the AAI mode. The AAI mode occurs if the atrial rate is slow, with intact AV conduction. (c) VDD mode. If there is only a ventricular stimulus, the pacemaker functions in the VDD mode. The VDD mode occurs with a normal atrial rate, but abnormal AV conduction. If there are no stimuli, the pacemaker is fully inhibited, and the mode for a given cycle cannot be determined. Thus, if there are no stimuli, the pacemaker could be operating in any one of its three modes for any given cycle (AAI, VDD, or DVI). In this situation the R-R interval (Vs-Vs) is shorter than the LRI, and the PR interval is shorter than the programmed AV interval. However, inhibition does not always mean that the pulse generator senses both ventricular and atrial signals. Thus, during total inhibition a DDD pulse generator may actually be working continuously in the DVI mode with atrial undersensing (if the atrial signal is too small to be sensed), if the RR interval is shorter than the AEI. (From Barold SS, Falkoff MD, Ong LS, et al: Electrocardiography of contemporary DDD pacemakers. A. Basic concepts, upper rate response, retrograde ventriculoatrial conduction, and differential diagnosis of pacemaker tachycardias. *In* Saksena S, Goldschlager N [eds]: Electrical Therapy for Cardiac Arrhythmias: Pacing, Antitachycardia Devices, Catheter Ablation. Philadelphia, WB Saunders, 1990, pp 225–264.)

cycles is due to early P wave sensing (i.e., Vp-As-Vp or Vs-As-Vp) and with AAI cycles it is due to early sensing of the conducted QRS by the ventricular lead (Vp-Ap-Vs, Vs-Ap-Vs). In *dual*-chamber devices, the AAI cycles are shorter than the LRI, in contrast to *single*-chamber AAI pacing in which the pacing cycles remain constant (Ap-Ap is equal to the LRI) because the far-field QRS should be unsensed (by the atrial lead) with appropriate programming of the refractory period, sensitivity, and the use of a bipolar lead.

RATE FLUCTUATION DUE TO VENTRICULAR INHIBITION DURING PROGRAMMED AV DELAY

During traditional DDD, DVI, and DDI pacing with ventricular-based LRT, when AV conduction is relatively nor-

mal, atrial capture (Ap) may give rise to a normally conducted QRS complex that may, in turn, inhibit the ventricular channel (Vs). In this situation, the QRS complex must occur before the completion of the programmed AV interval (Ap-Vp). Because the sensed QRS complex also starts a new LRI and AEI, this situation causes a faster atrial pacing rate (i.e., faster than the constant programmed lower rate for ventricular pacing) either on a beat-to-beat basis or continually when atrial pacing is followed by ventricular inhibition (Ap-Vs-Ap-Vs, and so on).[25, 61, 83, 84, 88, 89] Ventricular intervals such as Vp-Ap-Vs or Vs-Ap-Vs become shorter than the programmed lower rate for ventricular pacing (Vs-Ap-Vp or Vp-Ap-Vp). With atrial-based LRT, the atrial pacing rate remains constant and independent of ventricular inhibition (discussed later).

In pulse generators with a ventricular-based LRT, an increase in the paced atrial rate (and therefore the conducted ventricular rate) due to ventricular inhibition is slight when pacing occurs according to the LRI interval (Fig. 31–33). An increase in the atrial pacing rate (and therefore the conducted ventricular rate) becomes more pronounced at faster basic pacing rates, an important consideration in the design of rate-adaptive DDDR pulse generators with ventricular-based LRTs. Figure 31–33 shows how a programmed DDDR pulse generator with a common upper rate of 120 ppm (equal sensor- and atrial-driven upper rates) can actually result in a faster atrial pacing rate of 150 ppm with exercise because of ventricular inhibition (in the absence of Ap-Vp adaptation on exercise). Rate-adaptive shortening of the Ap-Vp interval during DDDR pacing on exercise diminishes or eliminates this discrepancy and allows the maximum ventricular rate (during a sequence of Ap-Vs-Ap-Vs) to remain close to the programmed upper rate for ventricular pacing[84] (Fig. 31–34).

MODIFIED VENTRICULAR-BASED LOWER RATE TIMING

The new CPI Vigor DDDR pacemaker (Cardiac Pacemakers, Inc., St. Paul, MN) was designed with modified ventricular-based LRT. This modification eliminates the potential for the atrial pacing rate to exceed the programmed sensor-driven upper rate in the presence of intact AV conduction at high rates. The AEI is automatically extended by the difference between the programmed AV delay and the Ap-Vs interval.[88] This results in sensor-driven pacing that cannot exceed the maximum sensor-driven rate regardless of AV conduction.

RATE FLUCTUATION DUE TO VENTRICULAR SAFETY PACING

In ventricular-based LRT pulse generators with a VSP mechanism, activation of VSP (by ventricular sensing of signals such as crosstalk) also causes an increase in the atrial pacing rate because of abbreviation of the Ap-Vp interval, with the AEI (Vp-Ap) remaining constant (see Fig. 31–11).

A-A Lower Rate Timing

Some DDD pulse generators are designed with a pure atrial-based LRT (see Table 31–3).[25] When the LRI of a DDD pacemaker with atrial-based LRT is equal to the LRI

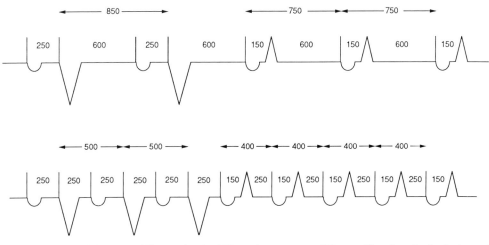

FIGURE 31–33. Diagrammatic representation of the function of a DDDR pacemaker with ventricular-based (V-V) lower rate timing showing the effect of ventricular inhibition. *A*, DDD mode: LRI = 850 msec; AV = 250 msec; AEI = 600 msec. On the *right*, when Ap is followed by a conducted QRS complex, the PR (Ap-Vs) interval shortens to 150 msec, but the AEI remains constant at 600 msec. Therefore, the Ap-Ap interval decreases to 750 msec, that is, the atrial pacing rate increases from 70 to 80 ppm. *B*, DDDR mode: the programmed maximum sensor-driven rate is 120 ppm (500 msec). The AV interval remains at 250 msec, so the AEI shortens to 250 msec. On the *right*, when Ap is followed by a conducted QRS complex, the PR (Ap-Vs) interval shortens to 150 msec, but the AEI remains constant at 250 msec. Therefore, the Ap-Ap interval decreases to 400 msec, that is, the atrial pacing rate increases from 120 to 150 ppm. (From Barold SS, Falkoff MD, Ong LS, et al: A-A and V-V lower rate timing of DDD and DDDR pulse generators. *In* Barold SS, Mugica J [eds]: New Perspectives in Cardiac Pacing 2. Mt Kisco, NY, Futura Publishing Co., 1991, pp 203–247.)

of a DDD pacemaker with ventricular-based LRT, the basic AEI of both types of devices is identical during the free-running state with continuous atrial and ventricular pacing, that is, DVI cycles terminate with an atrial stimulus (Ap) when there is no spontaneous ventricular activity. In a DDD pulse generator with atrial-based LRT, the duration of the AEI must adapt to preserve constancy of the atrial-based LRI or A-A interval (As-Ap, Ap-Ap) (Figs. 31–35 and 31–36; see also Fig. 31–31). The actual AEI of a given pacing cycle becomes equal to the sum of the basic AEI (as defined previously) plus an extension equal to the difference of the programmed AV delay (Ap-Vp) and the actual PR interval (Ap-Vs, As-Vs, As-Vp, or Ap-Vp) that immediately precedes the AEI. Alternatively, the duration of the AEI can be calculated as the LRI less the AV interval immediately preceding the particular AEI. The AEI may therefore change by a

positive value, zero, or even a negative value. This response assures that the atrial-based LRI or A-A interval (As-Ap or Ap-Ap) remains constant under all circumstances, even when the sensed AV interval (As-Vp) and the paced AV interval (Ap-Vp) are different. During A-A timing in pacing sequences consisting of As-Vs-Ap-Vp or Ap-Vs-Ap-Vp, the interventricular (or V-V) interval (Vs-Vp or Vp-Vp) can be longer than the programmed atrial-based LRI (see Figs. 31–31 and 31–36). When a pulse generator with atrial-based LRT senses a late VPC preceded by a (nonconducted) P wave, it actually detects a short AV interval (i.e., Ap-Vs or As-Vs). In this situation, constancy of the atrial-based LRI mandates delay of the subsequent Ap. The AEI initiated by the VPC therefore lengthens and produces a form of hysteresis with regard to the interval between the VPC and the subsequent Vp output. Such slowing of the ventricular rate

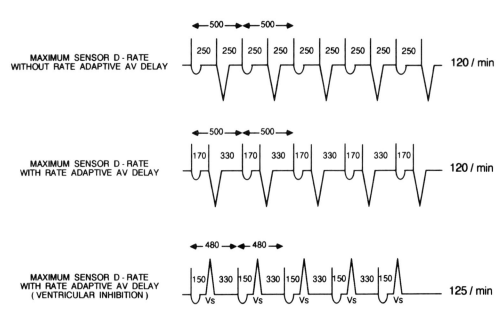

FIGURE 31–34. Diagrammatic representation of the function of a DDDR pacemaker with ventricular-based (V-V) lower rate timing showing the effect of a rate-adaptive AV delay that shortens on exercise. The maximum sensor-driven rate is 120 ppm (500 msec). The basic AV interval is 250 msec. *Top*, Maximum sensor-driven rate without rate-adaptive AV delay. *Middle*, Maximum sensor-driven rate with rate-adaptive AV delay. Note that the AV delay has shortened from 250 to 170 msec, and the sensor-driven AEI has lengthened from 250 msec (*top*) to 330 msec. *Bottom*, The maximum sensor-driven rate is 120 ppm (500 msec). The AV interval shortens to 150 msec because a conducted QRS complex (Vs) is sensed before termination of the rate-adaptive AV interval. As in the *middle example*, the sensor-driven AEI remains at 330 msec, so the atrial pacing rate increases to only 125 ppm (compare with the atrial pacing rate of 150 ppm) in Figure 31–33*B*. (From Barold SS: Single- and dual-chamber pacemakers: Electrophysiology, pacing modes, and multiprogrammability. *In* Single I, Kupersmith J [eds]: Clinical Manual of Electrophysiology. Baltimore, Williams & Wilkins, 1993, pp 231–273.)

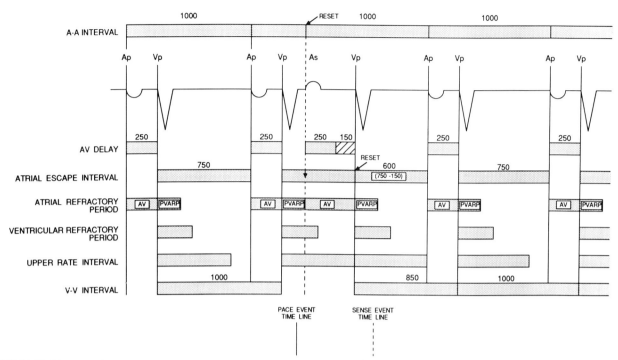

FIGURE 31–35. Diagrammatic representation of timing cycles of a DDD pulse generator with pure atrial-based (A-A) lower rate timing (LRI = 1000 msec; basic AEI = 750 msec during free-running AV sequential pacing). An atrial extrasystole (As) initiates an AV interval of 400 msec (As-Vp) to conform to the ventricular URI. Therefore the pulse generator emits Vp at the completion of the URI. Vp initiates an AEI of 750 + (250 − 400) = 750 − 150 = 600 msec. The A-A interval (As-Ap) remains constant at 1000 msec and equal to the LRI. However, the Vp-Vp interval from the third Vp to the fourth Vp is equal to 850 msec, a value shorter than the programmed LRI. The PVARP (200 msec) was deliberately shortened to demonstrate the effect of AV extension upper rate response (URI > TARP) on the timing of Vp. (From Barold SS, Falkoff MD, Ong LS, et al: A-A and V-V lower rate timing of DDD and DDDR pulse generators. *In* Barold SS, Mugica J [eds]: New Perspectives in Cardiac Pacing 2. Mt Kisco, NY, Futura Publishing Co., 1991, pp 203–247.)

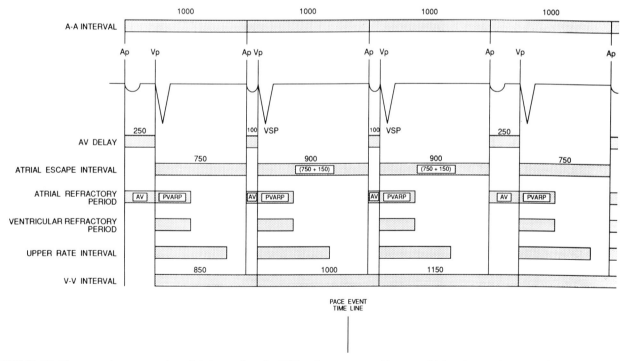

FIGURE 31–36. Diagrammatic representation of timing cycles of a DDD pulse generator with pure atrial-based (A-A) lower rate timing (LRT). (LRI = 1000 msec; AEI = 750 msec during free-running AV sequential pacing.) Crosstalk induces ventricular safety pacing (VSP) with abbreviation of the Ap-Vp interval to 100 msec. The Ap-Ap interval remains constant so that the AEI lengthens to 750 + (250 − 100) = 900 msec. During VSP, the pacing rate of a pulse generator with A-A LRT remains constant, in contrast to an increase in the pacing rate in a DDD pulse generator with V-V LRT (see Fig. 31–11). At the termination of crosstalk, the Vp-Vp interval lengthens to 1150 msec, longer than atrial LRI. (From Barold SS, Falkoff MD, Ong LS, et al: A-A and V-V lower rate timing of DDD and DDDR pulse generators. *In* Barold SS, Mugica J [eds]: New Perspectives in Cardiac Pacing 2. Mt Kisco, NY, Futura Publishing Co., 1991, pp 203–247.)

predisposes to ventricular bigeminy and may be undesirable in some patients.

ANALYSIS OF PACEMAKER FUNCTION ON A CYCLE-TO-CYCLE BASIS

During atrial-based LRT, in the pacing sequence Ap-Vs-Ap-Vs, the atrial pacing rate remains constant at the programmed lower rate and independent of ventricular inhibition, in contrast to ventricular-based LRT in which the atrial pacing rate increases. Any given cycle may be considered to start with an atrial paced or sensed event and terminate either with As or Ap (see Figs. 31–31, 31–35, and 31–36). A DVI cycle begins with Ap-Vp, a VDD cycle begins with As-Vp (even if As-Vp is shorter than Ap-Vp), and an AAI cycle begins with Ap-Vs. To qualify as AAI, DVI, or VDD cycles, the cycle must terminate with Ap. In cases terminating with As, the cycle is considered to be an inhibited or aborted AAI, DVI, or VDD cycle. All three cycles (AAI, DVI, and VDD) terminating with Ap will exhibit constant A-A intervals equal to the atrial LRI regardless of As-Vp being programmed to be shorter than Ap-Vp. In this respect, the timing behavior of an AAI cycle resembles that of a single-chamber AAI system that ignores the far-field QRS complex. In circumstances already described, DDD pacemakers with an atrial-based LRT, like those with a ventricular-based LRT, can function in the VVI, VOO, DOO, or DDT modes.

VENTRICULAR PREMATURE BEATS AND ATRIAL-BASED LOWER RATE TIMING

In defining atrial-based LRT, Hayes and colleagues and other workers[60, 61, 82, 84, 87, 88] stated categorically that "when a ventricular premature beat (defined as Vs without a preceding As) is sensed during the VA interval (atrial escape interval) the timers are also reset but now it is the A-A interval rather than the VA interval that is reset." This statement actually violates the concept that A-A timing is based on atrial rather than ventricular events. The definition of Hayes and coworkers[60, 61, 82] is probably based on the behavior of the original and now defunct Siemens 674 and 740 DDD pulse generators designed with an atrial-based LRT.[25, 92] In these pulse generators, when Ap or As started an LRI, the latter timed out to the next Ap as follows: (1) When Ap or As was followed by Vs, A-A timing of the LRI initiated by Ap or As was uninterrupted by Vs. (2) The LRI (A-A interval) was reset by As sensed outside the atrial refractory period. (3) The A-A or LRI timer was also reset by a VPC interpreted as a ventricular sensed event without any preceding atrial event. The now obsolete Intermedics Cyberlith committed DVI pulse generator (Intermedics, Inc., Angleton, TX) also exhibited A-A timing because Vs initiated an AEI equal to the sum of the basic (as programmed) AEI (Vp-Ap) and the AV (Ap-Vp) interval.[25] These original designs created the notion that in a pure atrial-based LRT system, the AEI initiated by a VPC should be equal to the LRI.

In an atrial-based LRT system, a VPC-initiated AEI equal to the LRI constitutes a form of obligatory hysteresis. Yet, the atrial-based LRT of contemporary pacemakers was designed primarily to avoid rate fluctuation, especially during ventricular inhibition. Furthermore, many contemporary pulse generators with a pure atrial-based LRT or a hybrid

LRT system (atrial- or ventricular-based according to circumstances) exhibit mostly V-V or VA timing in response to a VPC (Fig. 31–37). For these reasons, the definition of atrial-based LRT should not include the requirement that a VPC-initiated AEI be equal to the LRI. Devices with a pure atrial-based LRT can therefore be classified into two groups in terms of their VPC response:[85] (1) pure A-A timing with a VPC-induced V-V or VA response (by far the commonest type) and (2) pure A-A timing with a VPC-induced A-A or hysteresis response (AEI = LRI).

Lower Rate Timing Cycles: Ventricular-Based, Ventricular-Based With Committed AV Intervals, Atrial-Based, Modified Atrial-Based, Pseudoatrial-Based, and Hybrids

A few years ago, Medtronic (Minneapolis, MN) introduced pacemakers (Synergyst I and II) with two different mechanisms for LRT consisting of either A-A or V-V response according to circumstances (hybrid system)[25] (see Table 31–4). Some workers described this LRT as modified atrial LRT.[60, 84] At the time, I explained the function of the Medtronic Synergyst dual-chamber pulse generators in terms of pseudo A-A timing because the device could be considered as having ventricular-based LRT with a "committed" AV interval under specific circumstances.[25, 89] All LRT mechanisms can be conceptualized as being ventricular-based with a committed AV interval (in terms of timing cycles) under specific circumstances (Fig. 31–38).[2, 89] In such a system, under specific circumstances the full Ap-Vp interval times out, but the pacemaker does not necessarily release the actual ventricular stimulus (Vp) at the completion of the Ap-Vp interval. For example, when Ap-Vs (shorter than Ap-Vp) initiates a pacing cycle, Vs inhibits the release of Vp. Yet the Ap-Vp interval times out in its entirety so that Vp is implied (Vpi). The manufacturer has called Vpi the "impending or scheduled V-pace."[2] Vpi controls initiation of the AEI and the LRI precisely as if Vp had actually been released. This behavior gave rise to the term committed AV interval during ventricular-based LRT (see Table 31–5). In such a response, when Ap-Vs is shorter than Ap-Vp, Vs initiates the PVARP and the ventricular refractory period. In contrast, the implied Vp (Vpi) initiates the LRI and AEI, both constant in duration, characteristic of ventricular-based LRT.[2]

The concept of a committed AV interval during ventricular-based LRT can be somewhat confusing with VSP. In the Medtronic Elite I and II pacemakers (Medtronic, Inc., Minneapolis, MN), VSP causes premature delivery of Vp (abbreviated Ap-Vp). Yet the LRI, AEI, and sensor-driven interval (SDI) cannot begin with the release of the premature Vp. Consequently, the pacemaker waits until the entire programmed Ap-Vp interval has timed out to initiate these intervals coincidentally with Vpi or the scheduled Vp.[2, 93–95] Obviously the pacemaker cannot issue two Vp (Vp and Vpi) outputs in quick succession.

In the published literature concerning the Medtronic Synergyst series and the Elite I DDDR pacemakers, Medtronic

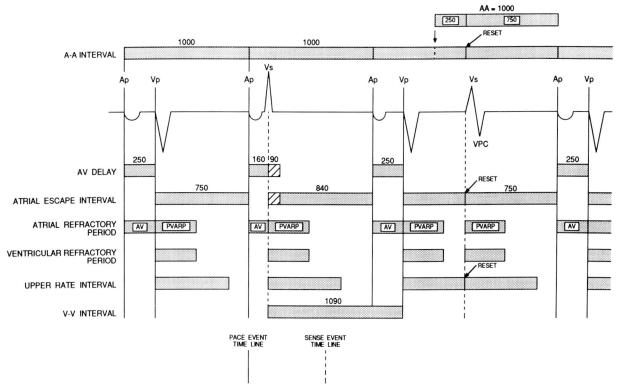

FIGURE 31–37. Diagrammatic representation of timing cycles of a DDD pulse generator with pure atrial-based (A-A) lower rate timing (LRT). LRI = 1000 msec; AV = 250 msec (As-Vp = Ap-Vp); basic AEI = 750 msec (during free-running pacing). The second Ap is followed by a conducted QRS complex Vs, and Ap-Vs = 160 msec. Ap initiates an A-A (Ap-Ap) interval of 1000 msec. Consequently, the AEI is equal to 750 + (250 − 160) = 840 msec. Note that the Vs-Vp interval is equal to 1090 msec and longer than atrial LRI. A ventricular extrasystole (VPC) beyond the AV interval initiates an AEI of 750 msec, equal to the basic value. The VPC response is similar to that seen in devices with a ventricular-based (V-V) LRT. (From Barold SS, Falkoff MD, Ong LS, et al: A-A and V-V lower rate timing of DDD and DDDR pulse generators. *In* Barold SS, Mugica J [eds]: New Perspectives in Cardiac Pacing 2. Mt Kisco, NY, Futura Publishing Co., 1991, pp 203–247.)

describes a lower rate response based on A-A timing under certain circumstances, establishing the devices as having a hybrid system for LRT[2, 90, 96, 97] (see Table 31–4). The same literature also mentions the concept of a committed AV interval in the control of ventricular-based LRT. With regard to the Elite II DDDR pulse generator, Medtronic no longer uses the concept of A-A timing to describe the behavior of its hybrid LRT mechanism:[94, 95] the technical manual states only that "the PAV interval (P = paced) always times out to its programmed duration in case of ventricular inhibition." Also, "scheduled V-pace (Vpi) starts the lower rate VA interval and sensor-driven VA interval"[95] (see Table 31–5).

Each of the pacing cycles initiated by one of the eight possible A-V combinations shown in Figure 31–39 can be translated into a V-V cycle with or without a committed AV interval.[2, 89] In this way, A-A cycles automatically become V-V cycles with a committed AV interval, whereas V-V cycles without a committed AV interval remain V-V cycles (see Table 31–5). However, with better understanding of LRT, much of the preceding terminology, including pseudo A-A timing[25, 87] and modified atrial lower timing, becomes of little value because all cycles in hybrid systems can be characterized simply in terms of A-A or V-V cycles. Thus, for the understanding of lower rate behavior, one only needs to know which combinations of atrial and ventricular events initiate A-A cycles. Similarly, if one assumes that all pacemakers have ventricular-based LRT, one only needs to know

which cycles are associated with a committed AV interval as described earlier.

FEASIBILITY OF DDI, DDIR, DDD, AND DDDR MODES WITH ATRIAL-BASED LOWER RATE TIMING

Pure atrial-based LRT is compatible with normal pacemaker function in the DVI and VDD modes but is incompatible with normal function in the DDI mode.[25] A conventional DDI pulse generator is really a DDD pulse generator with ventricular-based LRT in which the ventricular URI and LRI (rates) are identical. The ventricular pacing rate cannot exceed the programmed LRI. The DDI mode with atrial-based LRT (controlling the LRI) creates a paradoxical situation in which the LRI is an atrial interval controlled by atrial events, whereas the URI (which should be equal to the LRI) is a ventricular interval. A DDI pacemaker with atrial-based LRT must, however, retain constancy of the atrial LRI (As-Ap or Ap-Ap) (Fig. 31–40). Preservation of the atrial LRI takes hierarchical precedence over any other intervals including the ventricular URI (equal to the atrial LRI), a situation that can produce violation of the LRI (whenever Ap-Vp never exceeds its programmed value) as shown in Figure 31–44. For this reason, a dual-chamber pulse generator functioning in the DDI or DDIR mode requires ventricular-based LRT in most circumstances. Actually the DDI (DDIR) mode can

PSEUDO A-A TIMING

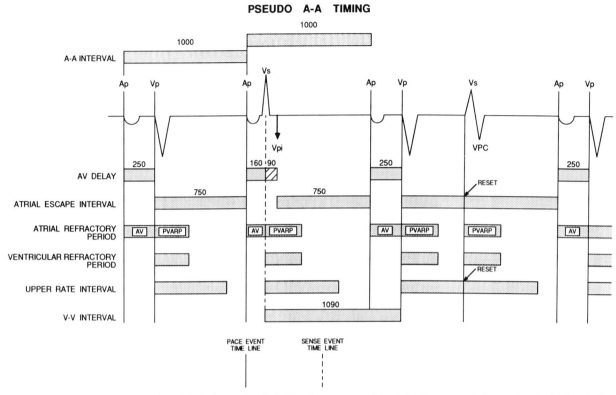

FIGURE 31–38. Diagrammatic representation of the timing cycles of a DDD pulse generator with a hybrid lower rate timing, such as the Medtronic Synergyst II DDDR pacemaker (Medtronic Inc., Minneapolis, MN), showing the concept of "committed" AV interval. (LRI = 1000 msec; Ap-Vp = 250 msec [equal to As-Vp], AEI = 750 msec during free-running AV sequential pacing). Note that the second AV interval Ap-Vs (160 msec) initiates an A-A response, so Ap-Ap (interval between the second and third Ap) remains constant at the LRI equal to 1000 msec. Alternatively, the pacemaker can be considered as having ventricular-based LRT with a "committed" AV interval. In this way, the second Ap is followed by a conducted QRS complex Vs; Ap-Vs = 160 msec. Ap initiates a "committed" AV interval of 250 msec, at the end of which an implied ventricular stimulus (Vpi) occurs. Vs initiates the PVARP, ventricular refractory period, but not the AEI. Vpi initiates the AEI of 750 msec (and therefore the LRI). Note that the Vs-Vp interval = 1090 msec, longer than LRI (typical of an A-A response). A VPC beyond the AV interval initiates an AEI of 750 msec, as in devices with ventricular-based LRT. (From Barold SS, Falkoff MD, Ong LS, et al: A-A and V-V lower rate timing of DDD and DDDR pulse generators. *In* Barold SS, Mugica J [eds]: New Perspectives in Cardiac Pacing 2. Mt. Kisco, NY, Futura Publishing Co., 1991, pp 203–247.)

function with a hybrid LRT in which short AV intervals (shorter than programmed Ap-Vp) initiate A-A cycles, whereas AV intervals longer than programmed Ap-Vp or VPCs initiate V-V cycles (as in the Intermedics Relay DDD or DDDR pacemakers [Intermedics, Inc., Angleton, TX] in the DDI and DDIR modes). With this arrangement in the DDI mode, Ap-Vs-Ap-Vs sequences (ventricular inhibition) will show an atrial pacing rate equal to the programmed lower rate, in contrast to the DDI mode with ventricular-based LRT in which Ap-Vs-Ap-Vs sequences will show an atrial pacing rate faster than the programmed lower ventricular pacing rate.

As with the DDI and DDIR modes, pure atrial-based LRT does not lend itself to smooth functioning of DDD or DDDR pulse generators.[89] Indeed, at present there are no DDDR pacemakers with pure atrial-based LRT.[98] It seems that all DDDR pulse generators with atrial-based LRT consist of hybrid forms.

In the DDD mode with pure atrial-based LRT, the greater the separation of LRI and URI, the less the likelihood of violation of the atrial-driven URI as seen in the DDI mode. The closer the LRI and URI, the greater the likelihood of violation of the atrial-driven URI. Violation of the URI can occur only with AV interval extension as a response to

Wenckebach upper rate limitation. Mathematically, violation of the atrial-driven URI will occur when

2 (atrial-driven URI) > LRI − TARP.
The largest degree of violation Δ msec = (URI − LRI) + W, where
W = URI − TARP as previously defined.

For example, in the case of a DDD pulse generator with pure atrial-based LRT and the following indices, violation of the upper rate interval can be calculated mathematically: LRI = 750 msec (80 ppm), URI = 600 msec (100 ppm), AV delay = 200 msec, PVARP = 200 msec.

2 URI > LRI + TARP
1200 > 1150

Therefore, a 50-msec violation of the atrial-driven URI can occur.

Δ = (URI − LRI) + W
= (600 − 750) + 200 = +50 msec

If Δ = 0 or negative value, no violation of the atrial-driven URI can occur.

The same argument applies to DDDR pulse generators with pure atrial-based LRI. In the DDDR mode, the LRI

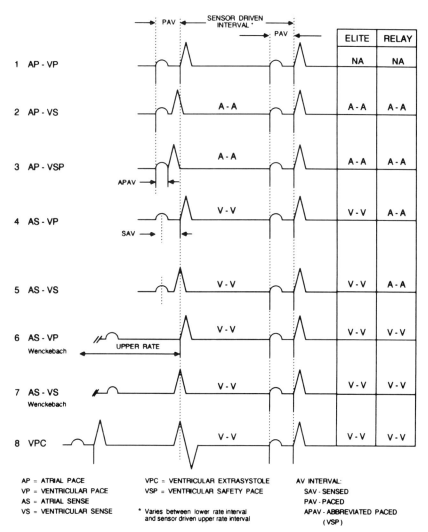

FIGURE 31–39. Comparison of timing cycles of the Medtronic Elite I and II (Medtronic Inc., Minneapolis, MN) and Intermedics Relay DDDR pulse generators (Intermedics, Inc., Angleton, TX) (when programmed to the DDDR mode). The diagrams show the behavior of only the Medtronic Elite I and II pulse generators. Ap = atrial pace; VP = ventricular pace; AS = atrial sense; VS = ventricular sense; VPC = ventricular premature contraction; VSP = ventricular safety pace. AV interval: SAV sensed, PAV paced, APAV abbreviated paced (ventricular safety pacing); NA not applicable. Note that in 4, the SAV is shorter than the PAV in 1. In 6, upper rate refers to the upper rate interval. The first dotted vertical lines on the left indicate the response of the atrial channel to either AP or AS. The dotted vertical line beyond AP or AS represents the beginning of the LRI of the Elite I and II pulse generators, assuming that the lower rate timing of all the cycles is ventricular based with a "committed" AV interval (that times out the entire duration of the PAV or Ap-Vp interval, as in 1 on top). Note that the two cycles with a committed AV interval (2 and 3) can also be described in terms of A-A timing. *Asterisk*: sensor-driven interval varies between lower rate interval and sensor-driven upper rate interval. (From Barold SS: Electrocardiography of rate-adaptive dual-chamber (DDDR) pacemakers: Lower rate behavior. *In* Alt E, Barold SS, Stangl K [eds]: Rate-Adaptive Cardiac Pacing. Berlin, Springer-Verlag, 1993, pp 173–194.)

obviously gets closer and closer to the URI with increasing sensor activity, and violation of the atrial-driven URI can occur as in the DDD mode. This is illustrated in Figure 31–41, in which the sensor-driven URI is equal to the atrial-driven URI, which equals 500 msec. The sensor-driven interval (SDI) equals 600 msec, the AV interval equals 150 msec, and the PVARP equals 200 msec. Violation of the common URI will occur if

2 (atrial-driven URI) > LRI + TARP. 1000 > 600 + 350, + 50 msec. This represents a violation of 50 msec. Alternatively, Δ = (URI − LRI) + W, = (500 − 600) + 150 = 50 msec. This represents the maximum violation of the common URI.

In some DDDR pulse generators the situation is more complex when the atrial-driven URI is longer than the sensor-driven URI. When the atrial-driven URI is longer than the sensor-driven URI, which is greater than the SDI minus W, violation of both the atrial-driven URI and the sensor-driven URI will occur. In this situation, the sensor-driven URI is only slightly shorter than the atrial-driven URI. When the sensor-driven URI becomes substantially shorter than the atrial-driven URI, only the atrial-driven URI can be violated. If the sensor-driven URI is shorter than the SDI minus W, violation of the sensor-driven URI cannot occur.

Endless Loop Tachycardia

Endless loop tachycardia (sometimes called pacemaker-mediated tachycardia) is a well-known complication of DDD (DDDR, VDD) pacing and represents a form of VA synchrony or the reverse of AV synchrony.[27, 28, 35, 43, 47, 99–101] Any circumstance causing AV dissociation with separation of the P wave away from the paced or spontaneous QRS complex, coupled with the capability of retrograde VA conduction, can initiate endless loop tachycardia (Fig. 31–42, Table 31–6). The most common initiating mechanism is a ventricular extrasystole with retrograde VA conduction (Figs. 31–43 and 31–44). Other initiating mechanisms are outlined in Table 31–6 (Fig. 31–45). The atrial channel of a dual-chamber pacemaker can sense retrograde atrial activation only when it falls beyond the PVARP. Therefore, a short PVARP and a long AV interval predispose to endless loop tachycardia. A relatively long AV interval allows recovery of the AV conduction system to permit retrograde VA conduction (Fig. 31–46). The following terminology best describes the mechanism of endless loop tachycardia: repetitive pacemaker reentrant VA synchrony, pacemaker VA reentrant tachycardia,[102] or antidromic reentrant dual-chamber pacemaker tachycardia (the pacemaker acting as an electronic accessory pathway).

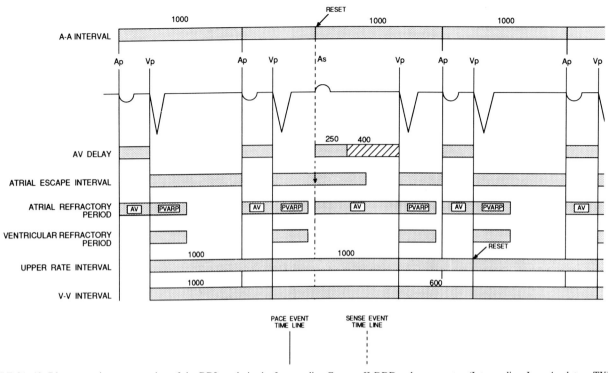

FIGURE 31–40. Diagrammatic representation of the DDI mode in the Intermedics Cosmos II DDD pulse generator (Intermedics, Inc., Angleton, TX) with pure atrial-based (A-A) LRT. For this generator, the lowest programmable upper rate is 80 ppm, and the closest programmable lower rate is 78 ppm. For the sake of discussion, it was assumed that both the upper rate and the lower rate were programmable to 60 ppm, in an attempt to obtain the DDI mode (LRI = 1000 msec; AV = 250 msec). In the DDI mode, the ventricular URI should be equal to the LRI, which in this case is atrial based (as opposed to ventricular based in Figures 31–26 through 31–29). An early As initiates a long As-Vp interval of 650 msec, as in any DDD pulse generator (regardless of LRT), simply to conform to the ventricular URI (1000 msec and equal to LRI). With A-A LRT, because Vp terminates the As-Vp interval, Vp initiates an AEI equal to 750 + (250 − 650) = 350 msec, as shown. The As-Ap interval, however, is maintained at 1000 msec. The Vp-Ap-Vp = 350 + 250 = 600 msec, in violation of the ventricular URI. This illustration demonstrates the incompatibility of A-A LRT with the DDI mode of pacing. (From Barold SS, Falkoff MD, Ong LS, et al: A-A and V-V lower rate timing of DDD and DDDR pulse generators. *In* Barold SS, Mugica J [eds]: New Perspectives in Cardiac Pacing 2. Mt Kisco, NY, Futura Publishing Co., 1991, pp 203–247.)

FIGURE 31–41. Timing cycles of a hypothetical DDDR pulse generator with pure atrial-based lower rate timing. The sensor-driven URI is equal to the atrial-driven URI (500 msec). In the DDDR mode with the sensor-driven interval (SDI) of 600 msec (effective sensor-driven LRI = 600 msec), a spontaneous P (As) initiates an AV interval, As-Vp, that is extended to conform to the atrial-driven ventricular URI (500 msec) initiated by the second Vp. The interval from the second Vp to the third Vp is equal to the atrial-driven ventricular URI. The sensed P wave, As, initiates a sensor-driven (atrial-based) LRI of 600 msec, which by definition must terminate with Ap (i.e., last Ap). Since the programmed Ap-Vp interval is not allowed to lengthen, the last Vp is delivered according to the programmed Ap-Vp interval of 150 msec. Delivery of the last Vp violates the sensor-driven ventricular

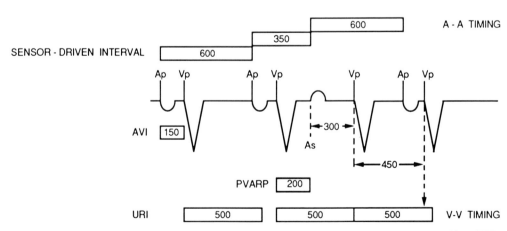

URI and the atrial-driven ventricular URI because the last Vp-Vp interval is 450 msec, less than 500 msec (duration of the common or sensor-driven URI). This example illustrates the two conditions required for violation of the URI by an atrial-based DDDR system: (a) atrial-driven URI is longer than total atrial refractory period (TARP). This allows a Wenckebach upper rate response with extension of the As-Vp interval; W = maximal increment of the As-Vp interval (atrial-driven URI − TARP). In this case the W interval = 500 − 350 = 150 msec. (b) Violation of the URI occurs because Δ = W − (SDI − URI), which is equal to 150 − (600 − 500) = 50 msec, that is, the value of Δ is greater than zero and represents the maximum degree of shortening or violation of the common URI, as shown in the diagram. Violation of the URI could be avoided by prolonging the last Ap-Vp, so the last Vp-Vp interval is equal to 500 msec, which is equal to URI. (See text for details.) (From Barold SS: Electrocardiography of rate-adaptive dual-chamber (DDDR) pacemakers: Lower rate behavior. *In* Alt E, Barold SS, Stangl K [eds]: Rate-Adaptive Cardiac Pacing. Berlin, Springer-Verlag, 1993, pp 173–194.)

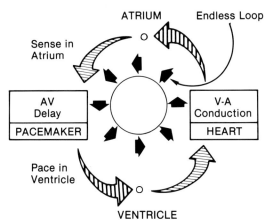

FIGURE 31–42. Diagrammatic representation of the mechanism of endless loop tachycardia. When the atrial channel senses a retrograde P wave, a ventricular pacing stimulus is issued at the completion of the programmed AV interval. The pulse generator itself provides the anterograde limb of the macroreentrant loop because it functions as an artificial AV junction. Retrograde VA conduction following ventricular pacing provides the retrograde limb of the reentrant loop. The pulse generator again senses the retrograde P wave, and the process perpetuates itself. Termination of endless loop tachycardia can be accomplished by disrupting either the anterograde limb (by eliminating atrial sensing) or the retrograde limb (by eliminating retrograde VA conduction). (Reprinted from Barold SS, Falkoff MD, Ong LS, et al: Pacemaker endless loop tachycardia: Termination by simple techniques other than magnet application. The American Journal of Medicine 85:817, 1988.)

Endless loop tachycardia may terminate spontaneously because of VA conduction block either from a fatigue phenomenon in the conduction system or the occurrence of a ventricular extrasystole sufficiently premature to cause retrograde VA conduction block:

I. Elimination of atrial sensing terminates endless loop tachycardia by affecting the anterograde limb of the reentrant process in a variety of circumstances:
   A. Magnet application when the pulse generator converts to the DOO or VOO mode. Rarely, the tachycardia recurs on magnet removal
   B. PVARP prolongation
   C. Decrease of atrial sensitivity
   D. Programming to a nonatrial tracking mode such as the DVI or VVI mode
II. Disruption of the retrograde limb of the reentrant process can also terminate endless loop tachycardia by one of two mechanisms:
   A. Direct effect on VA conduction with carotid sinus massage (rarely successful unless VA conduction is already quite prolonged)[103] or the administration of drugs such as verapamil or beta blockers[104] or
   B. Uncoupling of VA synchrony by
      1. Any ventricular sensed event unaccompanied by retrograde VA conduction block, such as a sufficiently premature ventricular extrasystole with retrograde VA conduction block, myopotentials (in unipolar pulse generators) or chest wall stimulation[105]
      2. Omission of a single ventricular stimulus as in the automatic tachycardia-terminating algorithm of some DDD pacemakers after the detection of a given number of pacing cycles at the programmed upper rate or other predetermined rate[106]

Uncoupling of VA synchrony allows restoration of AV synchrony by promoting either a paced or sensed atrial event (other than retrograde P waves).

Approximately 80% of patients with sick sinus syndrome and 35% of patients with AV block exhibit retrograde VA conduction.[107, 108] Consequently, more than 50% of patients receiving dual-chamber pacemakers are susceptible to endless loop tachycardia. The VA conduction time ranges from 100 to 400 msec, rarely longer. All patients should be considered capable of retrograde VA conduction until proved otherwise, with particular emphasis on its unpredictable behavior. Retrograde VA conduction is influenced by various circumstances, including the resting heart rate, level of activity, and changes in autonomic tone, pacing rate, catecholamines, and concurrent drug therapy.[101, 104, 109–111] In some patients, measurements made at the time of pacemaker implantation may have little bearing on future VA conduction patterns because improvement in VA conduction may occur with ambulation and may indeed return when it was absent at the time of implantation. However, only a minority of patients (5% to 10%) with no VA conduction at the time of implantation will subsequently acquire VA conduction.[112]

With appropriate programming of sophisticated contemporary pulse generators, endless loop tachycardia can now be prevented in most cases.[113–115] Even with appropriate programming, endless loop tachycardia may still occur because of unpredictable variation of VA conduction that is either

TABLE 31–6. INITIATING MECHANISMS OF ENDLESS LOOP TACHYCARDIA

1. Ventricular extrasystoles
2. Subthreshold atrial stimulation
3. Chest wall stimulation selectively sensed by the atrial channel
4. Atrial extrasystoles with prolongation of the AV interval (to conform to the programmed URI > TARP)
5. Decrease in atrial sensitivity; undersensing of anterograde P waves with preserved sensing of retrograde P waves
6. Application and withdrawal of the magnet
7. (a) Myopotential oversensing by the atrial channel only
   (b) Myopotential inhibition of the ventricular channel can also initiate endless loop tachycardia by allowing ventricular escape beats without preceding atrial depolarization, thereby favoring retrograde VA conduction
8. Programmer-generated EMI sensed by the atrial channel only
9. Excessively long programmed AV interval
10. Paradoxical induction with excessively long PVARP, also with automatic PVARP extension
11. Programming to the VDD mode when the sinus rate is slower than the programmed lower rate
12. Omission of the atrial stimulus in certain circumstances during normal function of some DDD pulse generators
13. Exercise treadmill stress testing with development of pacemaker Wenckebach upper rate response with lengthening of the AV interval initiated by a sensed P wave
14. Sensing of a far-field QRS signal by the atrial lead—that is, far-field endless loop tachycardia without atrial participation (only with inappropriate abbreviation of the PVARP)

Abbreviations: URI, upper rate interval; TARP, total atrial refractory period; AV, atrioventricular; EMI, electromagnetic interference; PVARP, postventricular atrial refractory period.

Adapted from a table that appeared in Barold SS: Repetitive reentrant and nonreentrant ventriculoatrial synchrony in dual-chamber pacing. Clin Cardiol 14(9):754, 1991. Copyrighted and reprinted with the permission of Clinical Cardiology Publishing Company, Inc., P.O. Box 832, Mahwah, NJ 07430.

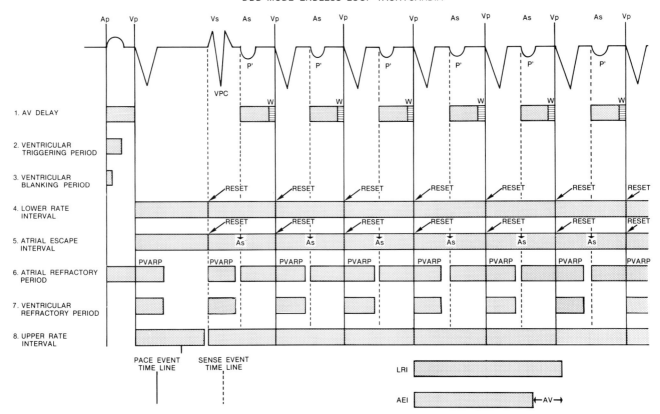

FIGURE 31–43. DDD mode with ventricular-based lower rate timing. Endless loop tachycardia initiated by a ventricular extrasystole (VPC, second beat) with retrograde VA conduction (As). The atrial channel senses the retrograde P wave (P'), and a ventricular pacing stimulus (Vp) is issued after extension of the AV interval to conform to the URI. Vp generates another retrograde P wave, again sensed by the pulse generator, and the process perpetuates itself. The pulse generator itself provides the anterograde limb of the macroreentrant loop because it functions as an artificial AV junction. Retrograde VA conduction following ventricular pacing provides the retrograde limb of the reentrant loop. The cycle length of the endless loop tachycardia may occasionally be longer than the URI if retrograde VA conduction is prolonged (see Figs. 31–44 and 31–47B). Same format as in Figure 31–10. (From Barold SS, Falkoff MD, Ong LS, et al: All dual-chamber pacemakers function in the DDD mode. Am Heart J 115:1353, 1988.)

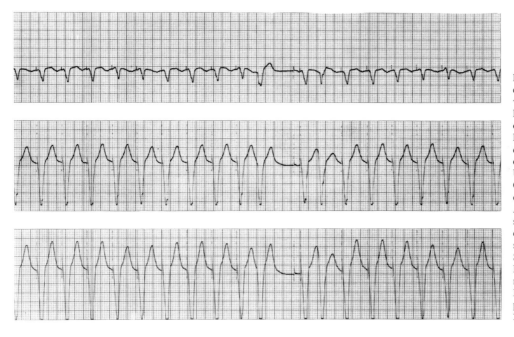

FIGURE 31–44. Endless loop tachycardia terminated and reinitiated by a ventricular extrasystole. The three ECG leads were recorded simultaneously. URI = 500 msec (120 ppm); LRI = 857 msec (70 ppm); and AV delay = 150 msec. The cycle length of the tachycardia is longer than the URI. (From Barold SS, Falkoff MD, Ong LS, et al: Electrocardiography of contemporary DDD pacemakers. A. Basic concepts, upper rate response, retrograde ventriculoatrial conduction, and differential diagnosis of pacemaker tachycardias. In Saksena S, Goldschlager N [eds]: Electrical Therapy for Cardiac Arrhythmias: Pacing, Antitachycardia Devices, Catheter Ablation. Philadelphia, WB Saunders, 1990, pp 225–264.)

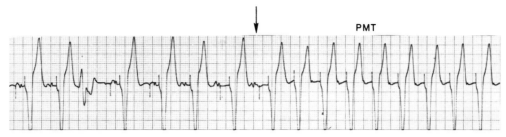

FIGURE 31–45. Initiation of endless loop tachycardia (PMT) due to undersensing of sinus P waves and normal sensing of retrograde P waves. The arrow points to the unsensed P wave responsible for initiation of PMT. (From Barold SS, Falkoff MD, Ong LS, et al: Electrocardiography of contemporary DDD pacemakers. A. Basic concepts, upper rate response, retrograde ventriculoatrial conduction, and differential diagnosis of pacemaker tachycardias. *In* Saksena S, Goldschlager N [eds]: Electrical Therapy for Cardiac Arrhythmias: Pacing, Antitachycardia Devices, Catheter Ablation. Philadelphia, WB Saunders, 1990, pp 225–264.)

spontaneous or secondary to the administration of cardiac drugs.

EVALUATION OF RETROGRADE VENTRICULOATRIAL CONDUCTION AND PROPENSITY FOR ENDLESS LOOP TACHYCARDIA

Although the presence and duration of retrograde VA conduction can be determined in the VVI mode (with or without telemetry of the atrial channel), or even automatically by telemetry connected to the programmer of advanced pacemakers, the propensity for endless loop tachycardia is best tested by programming the parameters of the pulse generator as follows: (1) DDD mode, (2) lower rate faster than the spontaneous rate, (3) highest atrial sensitivity, (4) shortest PVARP, (5) lowest possible atrial output (pulse width and voltage) to produce subthreshold atrial stimulation.[28, 47, 116] An ineffectual atrial stimulus preceding a paced ventricular beat favors retrograde VA conduction by separating the spontaneous P wave from the paced QRS complex. Endless loop tachycardia will occur if retrograde VA conduction is sustained and the retrograde P wave falls beyond the PVARP (Figs. 31–47 and 31–48). As an alternative, a pulse generator may be programmed to the VDD mode with the preceding parameters, the VDD mode being equivalent to the DDD mode with zero atrial output. However, the VDD mode is not universally available as a programmable option. Furthermore, in the presence of a relatively fast sinus rate, programming to the VDD mode with a lower rate faster than the sinus rate makes evaluation difficult. Occasionally, in the DDD mode, the threshold for atrial pacing is so low that

FIGURE 31–46. "Spontaneous" endless loop tachycardia in a patient with a Symbios 7006 DDD pulse generator (Medtronic Inc., Minneapolis, MN). The programmed parameters are shown above the ECG of three leads recorded simultaneously. The paced AV (Ap-Vp) interval is not associated with retrograde VA conduction. When the AV interval is initiated by a sensed sinus P wave (As-Vp), retrograde VA conduction occurs and initiates an endless loop tachycardia. This initiating mechanism was repeatedly documented in long ECG recordings. Endless loop tachycardia was prevented (on a short-term basis) by programming the AV interval to 150 msec without changing the PVARP. No atrial extrasystoles were observed. The sequence of events suggests that a sinus impulse reaches the AV junction earlier than a paced atrial depolarization. Earlier recovery of the AV junction permits retrograde VA conduction only after a sinus P wave. The relatively late recovery of the AV junction after a paced atrial depolarization prevents retrograde VA conduction. (From Barold SS, Falkoff MD, Ong LS, et al: Electrocardiography of contemporary DDD

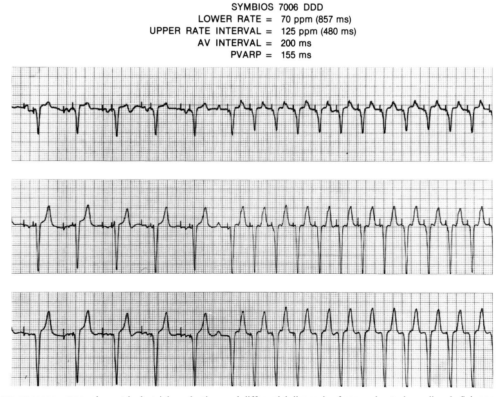

SYMBIOS 7006 DDD
LOWER RATE = 70 ppm (857 ms)
UPPER RATE INTERVAL = 125 ppm (480 ms)
AV INTERVAL = 200 ms
PVARP = 155 ms

pacemakers. A. Basic concepts, upper rate response, retrograde ventriculoatrial conduction, and differential diagnosis of pacemaker tachycardias. *In* Saksena S, Goldschlager N [eds]: Electrical Therapy for Cardiac Arrhythmias: Pacing, Antitachycardia Devices, Catheter Ablation. Philadelphia, WB Saunders, 1990, pp 225–264.)

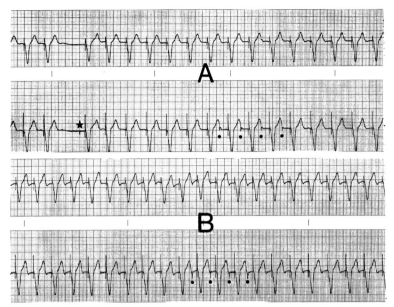

FIGURE 31–47. Endless loop tachycardia initiated by subthreshold atrial stimulation in a patient with an Intermedics Cosmos DDD pulse generator (Intermedics, Inc., Angleton, TX). In *A* (two ECG leads recorded simultaneously), the pulse generator was programmed as follows: URI = 600 msec (100 ppm); AV interval = 150 msec; PVARP = 200 msec. The atrial pacing output was programmed to a value less than the pacing threshold (*star* in the second strip). When the sensed atrial event marker functions is activated, special markers are delivered for four consecutively sensed P waves (*solid black circles*). The retrograde VA conduction time is approximately 360 msec, and the consequent AV interval measures approximately 240 msec, thereby yielding the URI of approximately 600 msec. This time value is the cycle length of the endless loop tachycardia precipitated by subthreshold atrial stimulation (*star*). In *B* (two ECG leads recorded simultaneously), the pacemaker parameters were identical except that the upper rate was programmed to 125 ppm. Note the presence of endless loop tachycardia at a rate less than 125 ppm (480 msec). The cycle length measured 520 msec because of delayed retrograde VA conduction. The marker channels (*solid black circles*) demonstrate a VA conduction interval of approximately 370 to 380 msec. This interval plus the AV interval of 150 msec gives approximately 520 msec, the cycle length of the endless loop tachycardia. (From Barold SS, Falkoff MD, Ong LS, et al: Electrocardiography of contemporary DDD pacemakers. A. Basic concepts, upper rate response, retrograde ventriculoatrial conduction, and differential diagnosis of pacemaker tachycardias. *In* Saksena S, Goldschlager N [eds]: Electrical Therapy for Cardiac Arrhythmias: Pacing, Antitachycardia Devices, Catheter Ablation. Philadelphia, WB Saunders, 1990, pp 225–264.)

subthreshold stimulation cannot be achieved by programming the lowest atrial output. In this situation, chest wall stimulation (with an external pacemaker providing signals sensed selectively by the atrial channel) can easily precipitate endless loop tachycardia in susceptible individuals by separating the P wave from the paced QRS complex[15, 105, 117, 118]

(Fig. 31–49). Other techniques such as application and withdrawal of the magnet, isometric muscle exercise (unipolar devices), maximum prolongation of the AV interval, treadmill exercise, and chest thumping (to produce ventricular extrasystoles) are inconsistently effective and are not recommended.[28]

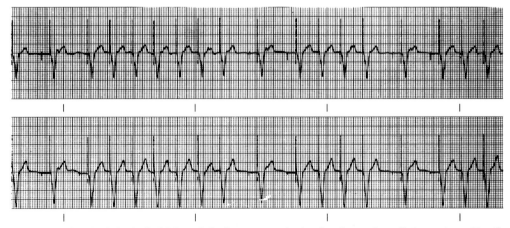

FIGURE 31–48. Subthreshold atrial stimulation in the DDD mode leading to unsustained endless loop tachycardia in a patient with a Cosmos (Intermedics) DDD pulse generator (two-lead ECG). The programmed parameters were as follows: LRI = 880 msec; URI = 480 msec; PVARP = 200 msec; AV interval = 180 msec. The retrograde VA conduction time is just over 200 msec, so the retrograde P wave is sensed by the atrial channel, thereby initiating runs of nonsustained endless loop tachycardia. Two ECG leads were recorded simultaneously. (From Barold SS, Falkoff MD, Ong LS, et al: Function and electrocardiography of DDD pacemakers. *In* Barold SS [ed]: Modern Cardiac Pacing. Mt Kisco, NY, Futura Publishing Co., 1985, pp 645–675.)

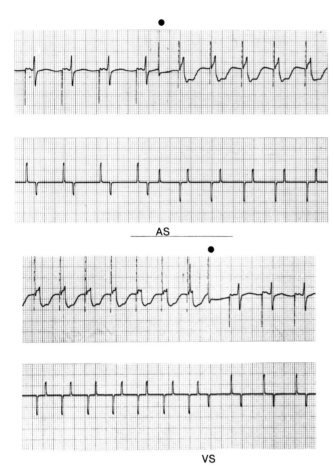

FIGURE 31–49. Effect of chest wall stimulation (CWS) on Medtronic Symbios 7005 unipolar DDD pulse generator (Medtronic Inc., Minneapolis, MN). Real-time event markers are shown below the ECG, with atrial events on top and ventricular events at the bottom. The markers depicting sensed events are smaller than those related to paced events. *Top*, Chest wall stimulation (*solid black circle*) sensed only by the atrial channel initiates endless loop tachycardia. *Bottom*, Endless loop tachycardia terminated by the second chest wall stimulation (*solid black circle*) sensed by the ventricular channel. The first chest wall stimulation falls within the refractory period of the ventricular channel (As = atrial sensed event; Vs = ventricular sensed event). (From Barold SS, Falkoff MD, Ong LS, et al: Electrocardiography of contemporary DDD pacemakers. A. Basic concepts, upper rate response, retrograde ventriculoatrial conduction, and differential diagnosis of pacemaker tachycardias. *In* Saksena S, Goldschlager N [eds]: Electrical Therapy for Cardiac Arrhythmias: Pacing, Antitachycardia Devices, Catheter Ablation. Philadelphia, WB Saunders, 1990, pp 225–264.)

PREVENTION OF ENDLESS LOOP TACHYCARDIA

Maneuvers to initiate endless loop tachycardia are repeated until appropriate programming of the pacemaker prevents induction of tachycardia. The rate of the tachycardia is often equal to the programmed upper rate. When the rate of endless loop tachycardia is slower than the programmed upper rate, the retrograde VA conduction time is equal to the difference between the tachycardia cycle length and the AV interval, which in this case is equal to the programmed value.[119] Telemetry by means of event markers or transmission of the atrial electrogram facilitates measurement of the retrograde VA conduction time. Programmability of the PVARP constitutes the most effective way of preventing endless loop tachycardia at present. In general, the PVARP should be programmed at 50 to 75 msec beyond the duration of the retrograde VA conduction time determined noninvasively. A PVARP of 300 msec offers protection against endless loop tachycardia in most patients with retrograde VA conduction. If possible, patients without demonstrable retrograde VA conduction at the time of the implantation should have a PVARP programmed to 300 msec, provided that there is no compromise of the upper rate. A long PVARP limits the upper rate of the pacemaker, but this may be partially circumvented in some pacemakers with automatic shortening of the As-Vp interval as the sinus rate increases (rate-adaptive AV delay). Such devices allow programming of a faster upper rate because the shorter AV delay shortens the TARP despite the relatively long PVARP. A long PVARP can also cause atrial undersensing and the induction of repetitive non-reentrant VA synchrony (discussed later).

Other measures to prevent endless loop tachycardia (Table 31–7) include (1) a shorter AV interval; (2) differential discrimination of the larger anterograde P wave from the smaller retrograde atrial depolarization, a theoretical option in 60% to 75% of patients;[120, 121] and (3) response to ventricular extrasystoles. A sensed ventricular event (outside the AV delay) that the pacemaker interprets as a ventricular extrasystole activates a special mechanism consisting of either (1) automatic extension of the PVARP for one cycle to ensure containment of retrograde atrial depolarization[26, 28, 37, 122] (discussed later in the section on Atrial Refractory Period) or (2) delivery of synchronous atrial stimulation (to preempt retrograde atrial depolarization).[122, 123]

The measures listed in Table 31–7 can be useful in minimizing or eliminating endless loop tachycardia, but they may also create new problems, as shown in Figure 31–50. A contemporary DDD pacemaker should rarely if ever be downgraded to a simpler mode (e.g., DVI or VVI) to prevent endless loop tachycardia.

AUTOMATIC TERMINATION AND PREVENTION OF ENDLESS LOOP TACHYCARDIA

Some pulse generators can terminate endless loop tachycardia automatically almost as soon as it starts with diagnostic algorithms using rate recognition[106, 124, 125] or AV interval modulation regardless of the rate[126, 127] (automatic shortening of a single AV interval by advancing ventricular activation may occasionally terminate tachycardia by causing retrograde VA conduction block). In one algorithm (ELA Chorus [ELA, Montrouge, France]) the pacemaker automatically shortens one As-Vp interval (As being a retrograde P wave in case of endless loop tachycardia). The pacemaker identifies endless loop tachycardia if the same Vp gives rise to a Vp-As interval that remains constant, that is, retrograde VA conduction remains constant. In a supraventricular tachycardia, the Vp-As will lengthen by the amount the As-Vp interval is shortened by the pacemaker algorithm. The pacemaker identifies endless loop tachycardia if the Vp-As remains constant after previous shortening of the AV interval. A pacemaker can reliably terminate endless loop tachycardia automatically either by omitting a single ventricular stimulus (uncoupling of VA synchrony) or by substantial PVARP prolongation for one cycle.[124–127] A smart pacemaker should know when the automatic tachycardia-terminating algorithm is being activated too frequently, whereupon it could automatically increase the PVARP permanently, a change that

TABLE 31–7. **PROGRAMMABILITY FOR THE PREVENTION OF ENDLESS LOOP TACHYCARDIA**

PARAMETERS	ADVANTAGES	DISADVANTAGES
Programmable PVARP	Applicable to all patients unless VACT is excessively long	Limits programmable upper rate. Long TARP precludes pacemaker Wenckebach upper rate response and may cause sudden undesirable 2:1 pacemaker AV block at relatively low levels of exercise
Automatic PVARP extension for one cycle after a ventricular premature event, i.e., ventricular extrasystole[a]	Standard PVARP remains unchanged. Upper rate not compromised. Useful with long VACT or if short PVARP is required	(a) Not operative with ventricular paced beat (b) Cannot be programmed off in some units[b] (c) Long PVARP may cause atrial undersensing with perpetuation of PVARP extension if the pacemaker senses only ventricular events (d) Long PVARP may paradoxically induce ELT (e) Delivery of atrial stimulus close to the preceding unsensed P wave may theoretically induce supraventricular arrhythmias
DDX mode after a ventricular premature event (DVI cycle)	As above	As above except for (b). The DVI mode is not necessarily restricted to one cycle. The pacemaker will remain in the DVI mode until emission of an atrial stimulus
Synchronous atrial pacing on sensing a ventricular premature event	As above Preempts atrial depolarization so that retrograde impulse encounters refractory atrium	(a) Not operative following a ventricular paced beat (b) May cause pacemaker orthodromic tachycardia
Programmable atrial sensitivity	Upper rate not compromised. Allows shorter PVARP. 60%–75% of anterograde P waves are at least 0.5 mV larger than retrograde P waves	Requires device with extensive selection of atrial sensitivity to allow fine-tuning. This approach never became popular, probably because of technical reasons.
Shortening of AV interval	Allows a faster programmable upper rate by shortening TARP. If the atrial-sensed ventricular-paced AV interval is shorter than the atrial-paced ventricular-paced AV interval and further decreases on exercise, a faster upper rate can be programmed.	Limited value
Faster upper rate to induce VA conduction block at faster ventricular rates	ELT either unsustainable or of shorter duration and better tolerated	Limited application. Sustained rapid ELT may occur with improvement of VA conduction
Adaptive TARP (either AV or PVARP or both can shorten on exercise)	Longer TARP at rest limits upper rate often with fixed-ratio block if TARP = URI. Shortening of PVARP on exercise allows a high programmed upper rate. ELT much less likely on exercise.	More complex pacemaker behavior. Rarely prolonged VA conduction may be absent at rest or may occur only on exercise
Elimination of effective atrial tracking by programming to another mode—e.g., VVI (VVIR), DVI (DVIR), DDI (DDIR)	Ventricular pacing rate always remains at the programmed lower rate	(a) VVI (VVIR) and DVI (DVIR) are unphysiologic paced modes (b) DDI (DDIR) mode may not prevent repetitive reentrant VA synchrony at lower rate (ELT without tachycardia)

Abbreviations: TARP, total atrial refractory period; PVARP, postventricular atrial refractory period; VACT, ventriculoatrial conduction time; ELT, endless loop tachycardia.

[a]Interpreted by a pacemaker as two ventricular events without an intervening sensed atrial event.

[b]Automatic PVARP extension may also come into effect with magnet removal, VDD mode without a preceding atrial event, inhibition of atrial output in the DDI mode, and noise sensed by atrial channel.

In some pulse generators, automatic PVARP extension is accompanied by a longer atrial escape interval to favor AV synchrony and prevent ELT (see Fig. 31–72).

Adapted from a table that appeared in Barold SS: Repetitive reentrant and nonreentrant ventriculoatrial synchrony in dual-chamber pacing. Clin Cardiol 14(9):754, 1991. Copyrighted and reprinted with the permission of Clinical Cardiology Publishing Company, Inc., P.O. Box 832, Mahwah, NJ 07430.

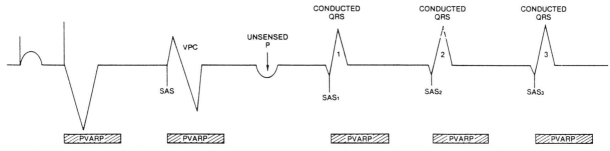

FIGURE 31–50. Diagram illustrating the mechanism of orthodromic pacemaker tachycardia during DDD pacing with a synchronous atrial stimulation (SAS) algorithm to prevent endless loop tachycardia. SAS delivers an atrial stimulus on detection of a VPC. In this way, retrograde VA conduction engendered by a VPC cannot cause atrial depolarization because it is preempted by SAS that renders the atrium refractory. A ventricular extrasystole (VPC) is sensed by the ventricular electrode, thereby triggering SAS. This is followed by an unsensed P wave outside the PVARP. The unsensed P wave is conducted and gives rise to the first conducted QRS complex that is sensed beyond the ventricular refractory period of the pacemaker. The pulse generator interprets this conducted QRS complex as a VPC and delivers SAS. This again leads to a conducted QRS complex (2) with a very long PR interval. The second QRS complex causes SAS 2, and SAS 2 causes QRS 3, and so forth, and the process perpetuates itself. The reentrant loop is composed of an anterograde limb in the heart (AV junction), and the retrograde limb occurs in the pacemaker (sensing by the ventricular channel). Such an orthodromic pacemaker tachycardia could also be initiated by a sensed VPC (without retrograde conduction) or any other signal sensed by the ventricular channel and interpreted as a VPC (e.g., myopotentials in a unipolar system), provided SAS causes prolonged but successful AV conduction. A related pacemaker tachycardia can occur during single-chamber AAT pacing. In this particular case, the far-field QRS complex is sensed in the atrium, and the pacemaker delivers an atrial stimulus synchronously with sensing of the QRS complex. (From Barold SS: Repetitive reentrant and nonreentrant ventriculoatrial synchrony in dual-chamber pacing. Clin Cardiol 14:754, 1991. Copyrighted and reprinted with the permission of Clinical Cardiology Publishing Company, Inc., P.O. Box 832, Mahwah, NJ 07430.)

would be telemetered at the time of the next follow-up interrogation of the device.[128] Obviously algorithms for the detection of endless loop tachycardia should not be based solely on the detection of the programmed upper rate because some tachycardias are slower than the upper rate in the presence of relatively prolonged VA conduction. Furthermore, the pulse generator should recognize the nature of tachycardia because pacing at the upper rate obviously does not discriminate endless loop tachycardia from tracking of a normal sinus tachycardia.

A smart DDDR pacemaker can differentiate physiologic from nonphysiologic rate variations.[128, 129] This discrimination can be achieved in the passive sensor mode, with the pulse generator itself not necessarily functioning in the rate-adaptive mode. During endless loop tachycardia, the atrial channel senses a rapid rate, but the input to the nonatrial sensor indicates physical inactivity and therefore no need to increase the pacing rate. The pulse generator can use this information to increase its PVARP for one cycle to terminate endless loop tachycardia immediately. If tachycardia persists, the pulse generator would then identify it as a supraventricular tachycardia other than endless loop tachycardia, whereupon it might switch its pacing mode automatically to avoid rapid ventricular pacing. A smart pacemaker will also analyze the relationship between atrial and ventricular events. The smart pacemaker will then automatically lengthen the PVARP or omit the Vp related to an atrial sensed event in situations favoring retrograde VA conduction, for example, lack of atrial capture (detected by evoked response recognition) or detection of early atrial events such as retrograde P waves[130] with prolongation of AV conduction. A smart pacemaker may eventually be capable of differentiating anterograde from retrograde P waves in all cases, and it should also detect atrial signals other than the P wave by improved electronics for better signal discrimination. Further refinements of these designs may eliminate the need to compromise the upper rate of the pacemaker by programming a long PVARP to contain relatively slow retrograde VA conduction.

REPETITIVE NONREENTRANT VENTRICULOATRIAL SYNCHRONY

VA synchrony can occur without endless loop tachycardia when a paced ventricular beat engenders an *unsensed* retrograde P wave falling within the PVARP of a DDD (DDDR, DDI, DDIR) pacemaker. Under certain circumstances this form of VA synchrony may become self-perpetuating because the pacemaker continually delivers an *ineffectual* atrial stimulus during the atrial *myocardial* refractory period generated by the preceding retrograde atrial depolarization[102, 131–135] (Fig. 31–51). By definition, the amplitude of the atrial stimulus must exceed the atrial pacing threshold tested during atrial pacing with a normal relationship of atrial and ventricular events. This form of VA synchrony has been called "AV desynchronization arrhythmia,"[133] repetitive nonreentrant VA synchrony, or VA synchrony nonreentrant arrhythmia.[102] Schüller and Brandt have called this situation "pseudoatrial exit block."[136]

During repetitive nonreentrant VA synchrony, the pacemaker provides an anterograde pathway (atrial stimulus followed by ventricular stimulus) whereas the conduction system provides a retrograde pathway back to the atrium (Fig. 31–52). In contrast to endless loop tachycardia, the potential reentrant circuit does not close because the pacemaker does not sense the retrograde P wave. The process repeats itself with each cardiac cycle and release of the ventricular stimulus does not depend on the timing of the retrograde P wave.

A long AV interval or a relatively fast lower rate (or sensor-driven rate with DDDR pacing), or both, favor the development of repetitive nonreentrant VA synchrony, usually in the setting of relatively long retrograde VA conduction with retrograde P waves in the PVARP. A retrograde P wave beyond the PVARP, but unsensed because of low amplitude or low sensitivity of the atrial channel, can also initiate the same form of VA synchrony. Rarely AV synchrony (with atrial capture) and VA synchrony (retrograde P waves) coexist in the same cardiac cycle whenever a relatively long

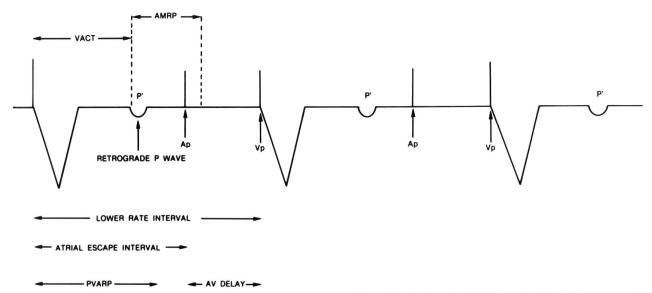

FIGURE 31–51. Diagrammatic representation of nonreentrant VA synchrony or AV desynchronization arrhythmia. There is relatively slow retrograde VA conduction. The first ventricular paced beat causes retrograde VA conduction. The retrograde P wave (P′) is unsensed either because it falls within the PVARP or because the magnet causes asynchronous DOO pacing. At the completion of the AEI, the pacemaker delivers an atrial stimulus (Ap) falling too close to the preceding P wave and therefore still within the atrial myocardial refractory period (AMRP) engendered by the preceding retrograde atrial depolarization. Ap is therefore ineffectual. Barring any pertubations, this process becomes self-perpetuating. VACT = retrograde VA conduction time; Vp = ventricular stimulus. (From Barold SS, Falkoff MD, Ong LS, et al: Magnet unresponsive pacemaker endless loop tachycardia. Am Heart J 116:726, 1988.)

AV interval (e.g., 250 msec) favors retrograde VA conduction. Both endless loop tachycardia and repetitive nonreentrant VA synchrony depend on retrograde VA conduction and are physiologically similar (Figs. 31–53 through 31–55). Both share similar initiating and terminating mechanisms, and under certain circumstances one arrhythmia may convert spontaneously to the other.[102] Repetitive nonreentrant VA synchrony rarely terminates spontaneously because of VA conduction block or improved VA conduction, situations that

can displace the subsequent atrial stimulus beyond the atrial myocardial refractory period with resultant atrial capture.

Once initiated, two scenarios are possible during repetitive nonreentrant VA synchrony: (1) The atrial stimulus continually falls in the absolute atrial myocardial refractory period and is always ineffectual even if the atrial output of the pacemaker is increased to its maximal value. (2) The atrial stimulus falls within the relative refractory period of the atrial myocardium so that the threshold for atrial pacing is in-

LOWER RATE INTERVAL = 750 ms

AV DELAY = 250 ms

PVARP = 400 ms

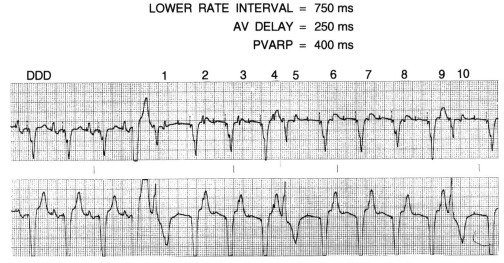

FIGURE 31–52. Initiation of nonreentrant VA synchrony by ventricular extrasystole (VPC) during DDD pacing (parameters shown above the ECG). The numbers indicate retrograde P waves. The fourth and fifth complexes are VPCs. The second VPC initiates retrograde VA conduction (1). The succeeding atrial stimulus is ineffectual because it falls within the myocardial atrial refractory period related to retrograde P wave no. 1. The accompanying ventricular paced beat perpetuates retrograde VA conduction (2), thereby starting nonreentrant VA synchrony. VPCs with retrograde VA conduction (5 and 10) during nonreentrant VA synchrony do not disturb the basic mechanism. Two electrocardiographic leads were recorded simultaneously. (From Barold SS: Repetitive reentrant and nonreentrant ventriculoatrial synchrony in dual-chamber pacing. Clin Cardiol 14:754, 1991. Copyrighted and reprinted with the permission of Clinical Cardiology Publishing Company, Inc., P.O. Box 832, Mahwah, NJ 07430.)

FIGURE 31–53. Initiation of nonreentrant VA synchrony or AV desynchronization arrhythmia (AVDA) by chest wall stimulation adjusted to be selectively sensed by the atrial channel. Chest wall stimuli are depicted by solid black circles. The first chest wall stimulus sensed by the atrial channel triggers a ventricular paced beat followed by retrograde VA conduction. The retrograde P wave falls within the long PVARP (400 msec) and deforms the apex of the T wave. The succeeding atrial stimulus falls within the atrial myocardial refractory period. The second and third chest wall stimuli fall within the atrial refractory period and are unsensed by the atrial channel. Two ECG leads were recorded simultaneously. (From Barold SS: Nonreentrant ventriculoatrial synchrony in dual-chamber pacing. *In* Santini M, Pistolese M, Alliegro A [eds]: Progress in Clinical Pacing 1990. Amsterdam, Excerpta Medica, 1990, pp 451–471.)

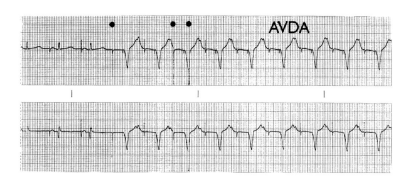

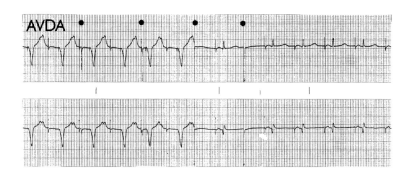

FIGURE 31–54. Termination of nonreentrant VA synchrony or AV desynchronization arrhythmia (AVDA) by chest wall stimulation. Same patient and parameters as in Figure 31–53. Chest wall stimuli are depicted by solid black circles. The first chest wall stimulus is unsensed. The amplitude of chest wall stimulation was increased, so the second chest wall stimulus is sensed by the ventricular channel activating the ventricular safety pacing mechanism, with resultant abbreviation of the AV interval. The ventricular channel of the DDD pulse generator senses the third chest wall stimulus, and nonreentrant VA synchrony terminates immediately. Two ECG leads were recorded simultaneously. (From Barold SS: Repetitive nonreentrant ventriculoatrial synchrony in dual-chamber pacing. *In* Santini M, Pistolese M, Alliegro A [eds]: Progress in Clinical Pacing 1990. Amsterdam, Excerpta Medica, 1990, pp 451–471.)

FIGURE 31–55. Two-lead ECG showing termination of nonreentrant VA synchrony or AV desynchronization arrhythmia at 80 ppm by ventricular extrasystole (VPC). On the left, the atrial stimuli are ineffectual because they fall in the atrial myocardial refractory period generated by the preceding retrograde atrial depolarization. The VPC restores AV synchrony (*on the right*). It is impossible to determine from the ECG whether the VPC is associated with retrograde VA conduction block (because of prematurity) or retrograde conduction that is sufficiently removed from the subsequent atrial stimulus to allow it to capture the atrium.

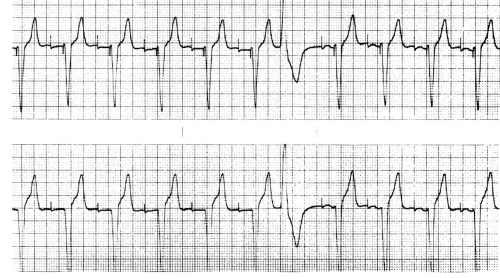

creased. After the induction of repetitive nonreentrant VA synchrony, the higher atrial pacing threshold seems to decrease gradually and then stabilize (all other parameters remaining unchanged) over a period of less than 1 minute to a value greater than the one tested during atrial pacing with a normal relationship of atrial and ventricular events.[135] The mechanism of such threshold behavior is unknown. One of two situations can then occur: (1) Spontaneous return of atrial capture without altering any of the pacemaker parameters when the diminishing atrial pacing threshold attains a value equal to the atrial output of the pacemaker. Indeed, repetitive nonreentrant VA synchrony is often unsustained for this reason. (2) Repetitive nonreentrant VA synchrony persists until a deliberate increase in the atrial output of the pacemaker promotes atrial capture with all other parameters remaining constant.

When sustained, repetitive nonreentrant VA synchrony can cause unfavorable hemodynamics similar to the pacemaker syndrome during normal function of a DDD/DDI (DDDR/DDIR) pulse generator.[137] Because the duration of the atrial escape (pacemaker VA) and AV intervals can be easily controlled, repetitive nonreentrant VA synchrony should not be an important problem with conventional DDD or DDI pulse generators. However, DDDR or DDIR pulse generators could induce repetitive nonreentrant VA synchrony on exercise when the sensor-driven increase in pacing rate shortens the atrial escape (pacemaker VA) interval. Conceivably, during exercise a ventricular extrasystole could precipitate repetitive nonreentrant VA synchrony with perpetuation of retrograde VA conduction, thereby negating the beneficial effect of AV synchrony by producing a VVIR-like pacemaker syndrome.

A pacemaker can be easily designed with an algorithm to terminate repetitive nonreentrant VA synchrony by automatic prolongation of the AEI for one cycle whenever the pacemaker detects a predetermined number of P waves within the PVARP. Repetitive nonreentrant VA synchrony that starts with a ventricular extrasystole and associated retrograde VA conduction can be prevented by lengthening the AEI after a ventricular extrasystole during DDD and especially DDDR pacing to ensure AV synchrony initiated either by As or (delayed) Ap.[89]

MAGNET-UNRESPONSIVE ENDLESS LOOP TACHYCARDIA

When magnet application causes relatively fast DOO pacing, endless loop tachycardia may convert to a slower repetitive nonreentrant VA synchrony without disturbing VA conduction. On withdrawal of the magnet and restoration of atrial sensing, repetitive nonreentrant VA synchrony is immediately converted to an endless loop tachycardia that cannot be terminated by magnet application[134] (Fig. 31–56A and

FIGURE 31–56. A, Inability to terminate endless loop tachycardia (ELT) by magnet application in a patient with a Medtronic 7000 DDD pulse generator (Medtronic Inc., Minneapolis, MN). Application of the magnet converts endless loop tachycardia to nonreentrant VA synchrony or AV desynchronization arrhythmia. Two ECG leads were recorded simultaneously. The pulse generator was programmed to the following settings: LRI = 750 msec (rate 80 ppm); URI = 480 msec (rate = 125 ppm); AV interval = 250 msec; PVARP = 155 msec (nonprogrammable); atrial output = 5.0 V at 0.3 msec (threshold for atrial pacing was less than 5.0 V at 0.05 msec). The rate of the endless loop tachycardia is approximately 107 ppm (cycle length = 560 msec). Retrograde P waves are not discernible, but the retrograde VA conduction time (VACT) can be calculated because the endless loop tachycardia is slower than the programmed upper rate. Therefore the cycle length of the endless loop tachycardia (560 msec) must be equal to the sum of the VACT and the AV interval. Consequently, the VA conduction time is approximately 560 − 250 = 310 msec. In the top tracing, application of the magnet converts the DDD pulse generator to the DOO mode for

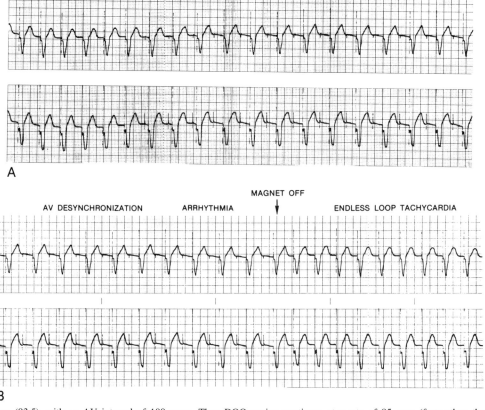

three cycles at a rate 10% above 85 ppm (93.5), with an AV interval of 100 msec. Then DOO pacing continues at a rate of 85 ppm (faster than the programmed rate) at the programmed AV interval (250 msec). During magnet application, all atrial stimuli appear ineffectual. Retrograde VA conduction continues because the atrial stimuli fall within the atrial myocardial refractory period initiated by the preceding retrograde atrial depolarization. This results in nonreentrant VA synchrony (AV desynchronization arrhythmia). Endless loop tachycardia recurs on magnet removal in B. B, Same patient as in A. Nonreentrant VA synchrony or AV desynchronization arrhythmia continues as long as the magnet remains in place. Magnet removal (arrow) causes immediate return of endless loop tachycardia. Identical responses were observed with repeated application and removal of the magnet. Two ECG leads were recorded simultaneously. (A and B from Barold SS, Falkoff MD, Ong LS, et al: Magnet-unresponsive pacemaker endless loop tachycardia. Am Heart J 116:726, 1988.)

B). Other causes of magnet-unresponsive endless loop tachycardia include inadvertent programming of the "magnet off" operation and insufficient magnetic field when a magnet is applied over the pulse generator of an obese patient. In the absence of an appropriate programmer, magnet-unresponsive endless loop tachycardia can be terminated in a variety of ways. Carotid sinus massage may occasionally be successful by causing block of retrograde VA conduction.[103] Pharmacologic therapy to block retrograde VA conduction is not recommended. Uncoupling of VA synchrony with immediate termination of endless loop tachycardia can be accomplished easily by chest wall stimulation sensed by the ventricular channel.[105] Without special equipment, chest wall stimulation can be easily and reliably delivered by transcutaneous external pacing (pulse width 20–40 msec) with the large pad electrodes separated by 10 to 15 cm and an output invariably less than 20 mA (well below the external pacing threshold).[105]

COEXISTENCE OF REPETITIVE REENTRANT AND NONREENTRANT VENTRICULOATRIAL SYNCHRONY

Manipulation, such as application or removal of the magnet, may convert an endless loop tachycardia to nonreentrant VA synchrony and vice versa. Occasionally conversion of nonreentrant VA synchrony to endless loop tachycardia and back to nonreentrant VA synchrony can occur spontaneously. The predisposing factors for spontaneous conversion include (1) PVARP close to the retrograde VA conduction time; minor variations of P wave timing may cause periods of P wave sensing alternating with undersensing. (2) Progressive prolongation of the retrograde VA conduction time with eventual stabilization; repetitive nonreentrant VA synchrony converts to sustained endless loop tachycardia when the retrograde P wave falls beyond the PVARP. (3) Borderline voltage for atrial sensing provided by the retrograde P wave. Endless loop tachycardia occurs with P wave sensing, but when the P wave is unsensed, the subsequent atrial stimulus falls within the refractory period of the atrial myocardium and creates a situation akin to repetitive nonreentrant VA synchrony. A situation like repetitive nonreentrant VA synchrony will continue until the pulse generator resumes sensing the P wave.

Upper Rate Response of DDDR Pulse Generators

In DDDR pulse generators, the sensor-driven URI can be longer or shorter than or equal to the atrial-driven URI.[49, 67, 98, 138] There appears to be no clinical use for a sensor-driven upper rate slower than the atrial-driven upper rate except perhaps to attenuate the effect of sudden deceleration of the sinus rate after effort. As a rule, a sensor-driven URI greater than an atrial-driven URI should not be programmed, and this combination will not be discussed further.

SENSOR-DRIVEN UPPER RATE EQUAL TO ATRIAL-DRIVEN UPPER RATE

When the sensor-driven URI is equal to the atrial-driven URI, three responses can occur: (1) Wenckebach pacemaker AV block if the TARP is shorter than the P-P interval, which is shorter than the atrial-driven URI, which is shorter than the SDI; (2) fixed-ratio pacemaker AV block if the P-P interval is shorter than the TARP, which is shorter than the SDI; (3) AV sequential pacing if the SDI is shorter than the P-P interval, with the AV sequential (Ap-Vp-Ap-Vp) pacing rate faster than the one that could be provided by atrial sensing with 1:1 AV synchrony (Table 31–8). The maximal AV sequential pacing rate is equal to both the sensor-driven URI and the atrial-driven URI.

PACEMAKER WENCKEBACH AV BLOCK

A Wenckebach pacemaker upper rate response occurs only when the TARP is shorter than the P-P interval, which is shorter than the atrial-driven URI, which is shorter than the SDI. During the Wenckebach block upper rate response in the DDD mode, the atrial-driven URI times out with each constant Vp-Vp cycle (equal to URI) until a pause occurs, that is, Vp-Vp lengthens only when a P wave falls in the PVARP. Thus the atrial-driven URI controls Vp release ex-

TABLE 31–8. **DDDR UPPER RATE RESPONSE: ATRIAL-DRIVEN UPPER RATE INTERVAL EQUAL TO SENSOR-DRIVEN UPPER RATE INTERVAL**

PARAMETERS	RESPONSE	COMMENTS
P-P < TARP = atrial-driven URI < SDI	Fixed-ratio (2:1) AV block with sensor-induced rate smoothing	
P-P < TARP < atrial-driven URI < SDI	As above	
P-P < TARP ≥ SDI	Atrial sensing cannot occur	Functions in DVIR mode
TARP < P-P < atrial-driven URI = sensor-driven URI < SDI	Wenckebach block upper rate response with sensor-driven rate smoothing and shorter pause at end of sequence	Atrial-driven URI times out. The pause at the end of Wenckebach sequence is equal to SDI
TARP < P-P < atrial-driven URI = sensor driven URI = SDI	Wenckebach block upper rate response *without* a pause at the end of sequence. Vp-Vp remains constant	Identical to DDIR mode and therefore functionally equivalent to VVIR mode; atrial-driven URI times out

Abbreviations: TARP, total atrial refractory period; URI, upper rate interval; SDI, sensor-driven interval; P-P, interval between two consecutive P waves; Vp-Vp, interval between two consecutive ventricular paced beats.

Modified from Barold SS: Electrocardiography of rate-adaptive dual-chamber (DDDR) pacemakers: Upper rate behavior. *In* Alt E, Barold SS, Stangl K (eds): Rate-Adaptive Cardiac Pacing. Heidelberg, Berlin, Springer-Verlag, 1993, pp 195–221. Copyright 1993 Springer-Verlag.

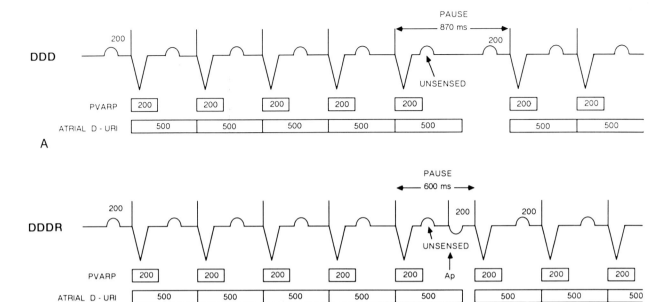

A

B

FIGURE 31–57. DDD (*A*) and DDDR (*B*) pacing with pacemaker Wenckebach block upper rate response. LRI = 1000 msec; atrial-driven URI (ATRIAL D-URI) = 500 msec; PVARP = 200 msec; AV interval = 200 msec (As-Vp = Ap-Vp in both the DDD and the DDDR modes). A Wenckebach upper rate response occurs because the atrial-driven URI is longer than the TARP. *A*, DDD pacing with typical Wenckebach upper rate response. The pulse generator does not sense the sixth P wave in the PVARP but senses the succeeding P wave, so the pause at the end of the Wenckebach cycle measures approximately 870 msec. *B*, In the DDDR mode with the same basic parameters as in the DDD mode above, the SDI is equal to 600 msec and is longer than the atrial-driven URI. The pulse generator does not sense the sixth P wave in the PVARP. The pause at the end of the Wenckebach sequence is shorter than that in the DDD mode above because the SDI equals 600 msec, and the sensor-driven AEI equals 400 msec. Thus, Ap occurs earlier (and closer to the preceding P wave in the PVARP) because its release is sensor controlled. The pause at the end of the Wenckebach sequence therefore shortens to the 600-msec SDI. (From Barold SS: Electrocardiography of rate-adaptive (DDDR) pacemakers. 2. Upper rate behavior. *In* Alt E, Barold SS, Stangl K [eds]: Rate-Adaptive Cardiac Pacing. Berlin, Springer-Verlag, 1993, pp 195–221.)

cept in the pause terminating the Wenckebach sequence. In contrast to the DDD mode, DDDR pacing shortens the pause, terminating the Wenckebach sequence to a value equal to the SDI (Fig. 31–57). Higano and coworkers[139] have called this effect "sensor-driven rate smoothing." Unlike true rate smoothing, sensor-driven rate smoothing occurs only at atrial rates faster than the atrial-driven upper rate (P-P < atrial-driven URI).[34, 140] In the DDDR mode, the duration of the pause terminating the Wenckebach cycle depends on sensor activity, and it becomes progressively shorter as the SDI shortens or as the sensor-driven rate increases.

A DDDR pulse generator working with a shorter sensor-

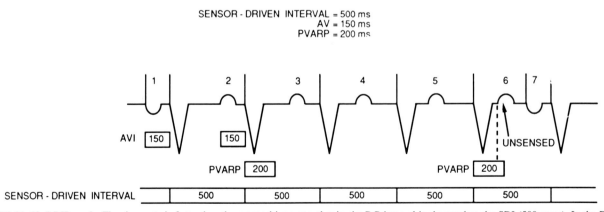

FIGURE 31–58. DDIR mode. The sinus rate is faster than the sensor-driven rate, that is, the P-P interval is shorter than the SDI (500 msec). In the DDI or DDIR mode, the ventricular paced rate (or the Vp-Vp interval) always remains constant and equal to the programmed LRI or sensor-driven (lower rate) interval. The first atrial stimulus captures the atrium. The pulse generator senses the subsequent P waves (2 to 5). The P waves march through the pacing cycle with progressive prolongation of the AV interval. The sixth P wave falls in the 200-msec PVARP and is therefore unsensed. The pacemaker delivers its next atrial stimulus (which captures the atrium and generates the seventh P wave) at the end of the sensor-driven AEI (500 − 150 = 350 msec). Because the ventricular pacing rate (or Vp-Vp interval) remains constant, the DDIR mode is functionally equivalent to the VVIR mode (with AV dissociation) with the occasional occurrence of atrial extrasystoles (premature beats) when the pulse generator delivers Ap relatively close to the preceding (unsensed) P wave in the PVARP. (From Barold SS: Electrocardiography of rate-adaptive (DDDR) pacemakers. 2. Upper rate behavior. *In* Alt E, Barold SS, Stangl K [eds]: Rate-Adaptive Cardiac Pacing. Berlin, Springer-Verlag, 1993, pp 195–221.)

driven AEI delivers Ap earlier in relation to the preceding ventricular event (Vs or Vp) than in the conventional DDD mode. The consequences of sensor-controlled earlier release of the atrial stimuli (when the preceding P wave falls in the PVARP) is discussed later. The pause at the end of the Wenckebach cycle disappears when the SDI eventually becomes equal to the sensor-driven URI. At that point, the pulse generator will continue to pace the ventricle regularly with constant Vp-Vp intervals at the sensor-driven URI (equal to the atrial-driven URI) and function as if it were in the DDIR mode (with a constant ventricular pacing rate and P waves marching through the cardiac cycle) (Fig. 31–58). In the DDD mode, some otherwise healthy young patients do not tolerate the beat-to-beat variations in cycle length due to the pause at the end of a Wenckebach block upper rate response. In these individuals without atrial chronotropic incompetence, an appropriately programmed DDDR pacemaker will shorten the pause, with its minimum value being equal to the sensor-driven URI. At that point the pacemaker functions basically in the DDIR mode (see Fig. 31–58).

PACEMAKER FIXED-RATIO AV BLOCK

When the P-P interval is shorter than the TARP, which is shorter than the SDI, fixed-ratio pacemaker AV block occurs. During DDD pacing, rapid acceleration of sinus rate may cause shortening of the P-P interval to a value less than the TARP, whereupon sudden fixed-ratio pacemaker AV block will occur. The abrupt fall in the paced ventricular rate seen in the DDD mode is attenuated in a DDDR system in the same way as the SDI abbreviates the pause at the end of Wenckebach cycles during DDDR pacing[141] (Fig. 31–59).

SENSOR-CONTROLLED RATE SMOOTHING AND ATRIAL COMPETITION

During DDDR pacing, the shorter SDI and sensor-driven AEI generates an Ap earlier than in the DDD mode (Ap can be relatively close to a preceding unsensed P wave in the PVARP). Ap occurs earlier in abbreviated pauses related to (1) fixed-ratio pacemaker AV block and (2) the cycle terminating Wenckebach pacemaker AV block.

Sensor-controlled rate smoothing[139] can be useful in active patients who require a long PVARP for the prevention of endless loop tachycardia. For example, in the DDD mode in a pulse generator with the following parameters—lower rate equal to 70 ppm, PVARP equal to 350 msec—if As-Vp shortens to 100 msec at the programmed (common) upper rate, a TARP of 450 msec will produce fixed-ratio pacemaker AV block when the atrial rate exceeds 140 pm. In this circumstance, as already emphasized, in a DDDR device the sensor-driven rate and its corresponding SDI can reduce or

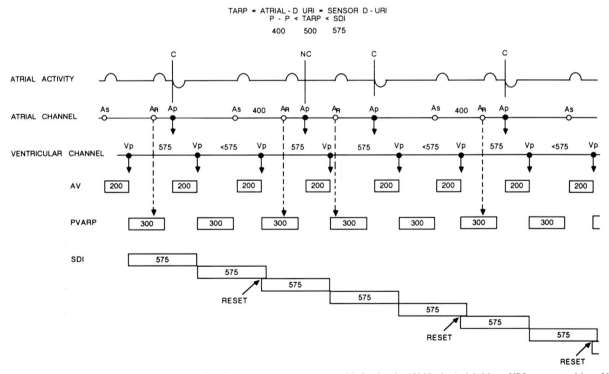

FIGURE 31–59. Pacing by a DDDR pulse generator showing an upper rate response with fixed-ratio AV block. Atrial-driven URI = sensor-driven URI = TARP. Fixed-ratio pacemaker AV block occurs because P-P interval (400 msec) is shorter than the TARP (500 msec). The Vp-Vp remains constant and equal to the SDI (575 msec). The second P (A_R) falls in the PVARP and is therefore unsensed. The succeeding Ap is delivered at the end of the sensor-driven atrial escape interval (AEI) and captures the atrium (C) very close to the preceding spontaneous P (A_R). The fourth (As) P wave falls beyond the PVARP and initiates an AV interval of 200 msec. The Vp-Vp interval between the second Vp and the third Vp is shorter than 575-msec SDI (sensor-driven Vp-Vp interval) because the third Vp is controlled by As and not the sensor. The fifth P wave (A_R) falls in the PVARP. The pulse generator fires Ap at the end of the sensor-driven AEI, but Ap falls too close to the previous P wave (in the PVARP). Ap delivery within the atrial myocardial refractory period produces no capture (NC). Note that the SDI is reset whenever Vp occurs prematurely (earlier than the SDI of 575 msec) when triggered by As. Competitive atrial pacing produces complex electrocardiographic patterns. (From Barold SS: Electrocardiography of rate-adaptive (DDDR) pacemakers. 2. Upper rate behavior. *In* Alt E, Barold SS, Stangl K [eds]: Rate-Adaptive Cardiac Pacing. Berlin, Springer-Verlag, 1993, pp 195–221.)

even eliminate the abrupt drop in the paced ventricular rate produced by fixed-ratio pacemaker AV block in the DDD mode.

On the basis of the preceding considerations, in the DDDR mode, fixed-ratio and Wenckebach pacemaker AV block can create complex electrocardiographic patterns[50, 141] with various combinations of (1) ineffectual Ap (no capture) when an early sensor-controlled Ap (delivered at the completion of sensor-driven AEI) falls in the atrial *myocardial* refractory period generated by the preceding unsensed P wave in the PVARP and (2) effectual with atrial capture but close to the previous P wave—that is, atrial competition. Stimulation in the atrial vulnerable period (with the risk of inducing an atrial arrhythmia) represents at this time only a theoretical concern until more experience is obtained with these devices.[142] Thus at any one time in the DDDR mode, Vp can be preceded by one of the following: (1) ineffectual Ap, (2) effectual Ap sometimes close to the previous P wave, (3) sensed P wave (As) triggering Vp, or (4) sensed P wave (As) with Vp controlled by the SDI and not triggered by atrial activity (discussed later). Furthermore, a DDDR pulse generator can release Ap either in the PVARP or beyond the PVARP (discussed later). Atrial competition during Wenckebach or fixed-ratio pacemaker AV block can be reduced or minimized with correct selection of the pacing mode (is the DDDR mode really indicated?) and programmable settings.

TOTAL ATRIAL REFRACTORY PERIOD LONGER THAN THE UPPER RATE INTERVAL

Patients with atrial chronotropic incompetence and paroxysmal supraventricular tachyarrhythmias may benefit from a DDDR pulse generator programmed with (1) a relatively slow atrial-driven upper rate to avoid tracking of fast unphysiologic atrial rates at rest and (2) a faster sensor-driven upper rate to provide an increase in the pacing rate on exercise. However, in some DDDR pulse generators with equal atrial-driven and sensor-driven upper rates, the two upper rates (intervals) cannot be dissociated.

Obviously in the DDD mode, a TARP longer than the atrial-driven URI cannot exist because the atrial-driven URI becomes equal to the TARP. Consequently one could easily conclude that the two upper rates (atrial-driven and sensor-driven) in a DDDR device with a common upper rate are inextricably linked and cannot be dissociated. Indeed, as in the conventional DDD mode, some DDDR pulse generators with a common URI (e.g., Intermedics Relay, Intermedics, Angleton, TX) permit programming of the TARP to a value equal to or shorter than, but not longer than, the atrial-driven URI (equal to the sensor-driven URI). Yet, in any DDD or DDDR pulse generator it should be theoretically possible to program the TARP to a value longer than the atrial-driven URI or common URI. Indeed, in the Medtronic DDDR devices (Synergyst II and Elite I and II, Medtronic, Inc., Minneapolis, MN), the TARP can actually be programmed to a value longer than the common URI. Obviously if the TARP is longer than or equal to the common URI, no Wenckebach upper rate response can occur. When the TARP is longer than the common URI, the TARP actually becomes equal to the atrial-driven URI. This manipulation allows programming of a sensor-driven upper rate faster than the atrial-driven upper rate in pacemakers without a separately pro-

TABLE 31–9. DDDR UPPER RATE RESPONSE: SENSOR-DRIVEN UPPER RATE INTERVAL EQUAL TO SENSOR-DRIVEN UPPER RATE INTERVAL.
RELATIONSHIP OF TOTAL ATRIAL REFRACTORY PERIOD AND SENSOR-DRIVEN INTERVALS

PARAMETERS	RESPONSE	COMMENTS
P-P < sensor-driven URI < TARP < SDI	Fixed ratio AV block with sensor-driven rate smoothing	Ap beyond PVARP
P-P[a] < sensor-driven URI < SDI < TARP[b]	DVIR pacing	Ap in PVARP
P-P[a] < TARP = SDI	DVIR pacing	Ap at end of PVARP
P-P[a] > TARP = SDI	As above	As above

Abbreviations: TARP, total atrial refractory period; PVARP, postventricular atrial refractory period; URI, upper rate interval; P-P, interval between two consecutive P waves; SDI, sensor-driven interval.

[a]Duration of P-P interval is immaterial as pacer functions in DVIR mode, atrial sensing cannot occur because SDI is ≤ TARP.

[b]Capability of programming TARP > common URI is required (see Table 31–11). In this way, sensor-driven URI < TARP—i.e., sensor-driven URI < SDI < TARP is possible in devices that allow programming of TARP > common URI.

Modified from Barold SS: Electrocardiography of rate-adaptive dual-chamber (DDDR) pacemakers: Upper rate behavior. *In* Alt E, Barold SS, Stangl K (eds): Rate-Adaptive Cardiac Pacing. Heidelberg, Berlin, Springer-Verlag, 1993, pp 195–221. Copyright 1993 Springer-Verlag.

grammable atrial-driven URI and sensor-driven URI. The atrial-driven URI becomes equal to the TARP and corresponds to the rate at which fixed-ratio pacemaker AV block supervenes. Thus, the atrial-driven URI can be *functionally* separated from the sensor-driven URI by programming a TARP longer than the common URI—that is, the atrial-driven URI is equal to the TARP, which is longer than the sensor-driven URI. In this way, fixed-ratio pacemaker AV block will occur at atrial rates slower than the programmed sensor-driven upper rate. This approach may be useful in limiting the atrial-driven upper rate in patients with paroxysmal supraventricular tachyarrhythmias (Table 31–9). It is not really useful with the Medtronic Elite II pacemaker because the device also allows programming of a separate atrial-driven URI and sensor-driven URI without the aforementioned manipulation of the TARP.

ATRIAL PACING IN THE POSTVENTRICULAR ATRIAL REFRACTORY PERIOD

During DDD pacing, the delivery of Ap cannot occur in the PVARP because Ap can be released only at the completion of the LRI, that is, after the completion of the PVARP. In the DDDR mode, atrial pacing can occur in the PVARP only when the sensor-driven URI is shorter than the TARP, allowing an SDI that is shorter than the TARP (Figs. 31–60 and 31–61). When the P-P interval shortens to a value shorter than the TARP, P waves fall in the terminal portion of the PVARP and are therefore unsensed. The DDDR pulse generator then takes over control of the atrial rhythm. Sensor-driven release of Ap may occur either in the PVARP or beyond it, according to the SDI at any given time. As previously stated, an earlier Ap may result in lack of capture (i.e., Ap in atrial *myocardial* refractory period generated by previous atrial depolarization) or atrial capture with competition.

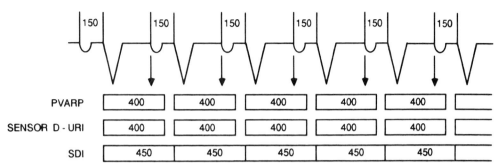

FIGURE 31–60. Pacing by a DDDR pacemaker with a TARP longer than the common URI. Ap-Vp = 150 msec. The atrial-driven URI and sensor-driven URI should be equal (400 msec) according to pacemaker specifications when a 400-msec URI is programmed. However, TARP (AV + PVARP) = 550 msec (TARP > URI is allowed only in certain DDDR pulse generators). A 550-msec TARP actually represents an atrial-driven URI of the same duration, and a Wenckebach upper rate response cannot occur. At that particular level of activity with an SDI of 450 msec, the sensor-driven AEI (300 msec) is shorter than the 400-msec PVARP. Therefore, the atrial stimulus is continually delivered with the PVARP. (From Barold SS: Electrocardiography of rate-adaptive (DDDR) pacemakers. 2. Upper rate behavior. *In* Alt E, Barold SS, Stangl K [eds]: Rate-Adaptive Cardiac Pacing. Berlin, Springer-Verlag, 1993, pp 195–221.)

Note that it is possible for Ap to fall in the *myocardial* atrial refractory period generated by a preceding unsensed P wave and also within the *pacemaker* atrial refractory period (or PVARP).

SENSOR-DRIVEN UPPER RATE FASTER THAN ATRIAL-DRIVEN UPPER RATE

When sensor-driven URI is shorter than atrial-driven URI, the upper rate response of a DDDR pulse generator depends on the interplay of four variables: P-P interval, TARP, atrial-driven URI, and sensor-driven URI.[84, 143–145] The Siemens-Pacesetter Synchrony I, II, and III DDDR devices (Siemens-Pacesetter, Sylmar, CA) and the Medtronic Elite II DDDR devices (Medtronic, Inc., Minneapolis, MN) allow programming of separate atrial-driven URIs and sensor-driven URIs (Table 31–10). A sensor-driven upper rate faster than an atrial-driven upper rate can be useful in patients with paroxysmal supraventricular tachyarrhythmias and in patients requiring a very long PVARP to prevent endless loop tachycardia.[145] When the TARP is shorter than the atrial-driven URI, a Wenckebach block upper rate response can occur (with extension of the As-Vp interval) only when the TARP is shorter than the P-P interval. When the SDI is shorter than or equal to the atrial-driven URI, no pause occurs at the end of a Wenckebach block upper rate sequence. This contrasts

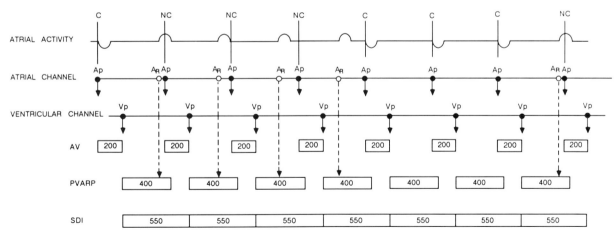

FIGURE 31–61. Pacing in the DDDR mode with a common URI of 450 msec, an AV of 200 msec, a PVARP of 400 msec, a TARP of 600 msec, and an SDI of 550 msec. Provided that the pulse generator allows programming a TARP longer than the common URI, these parameters indicate that the atrial-driven URI (600 msec = TARP) is longer than the sensor-driven URI (450 msec = programmed common URI). There is an atrial sensing window beyond the PVARP, but it closes when SDI is shorter than or equal to the TARP. In this example, because the SDI is shorter than the TARP, the pulse generator cannot sense spontaneous atrial activity (A$_R$). Atrial pacing is asynchronous, and Ap competes with A, producing a response functionally equivalent to the DVIR mode. Therefore, both Ap-Ap and Vp-Vp intervals remain constant. C = capture; NC = no capture (when Ap in atrial myocardial refractory period). (From Barold SS: Electrocardiography of rate-adaptive (DDDR) pacemakers. 2. Upper rate behavior. *In* Alt E, Barold SS, Stangl K [eds]: Rate-Adaptive Cardiac Pacing. Berlin, Springer-Verlag, 1993, pp 195–221.)

TABLE 31–10. **DDDR UPPER RATE RESPONSE: SENSOR-DRIVEN UPPER RATE INTERVAL IS SHORTER THAN THE ATRIAL-DRIVEN UPPER RATE INTERVAL.**
TOTAL ATRIAL REFRACTORY PERIOD IS SHORTER THAN THE ATRIAL-DRIVEN UPPER RATE INTERVAL

PARAMETERS	ATRIAL-DRIVEN UPPER RATE INTERVAL TIMES OUT	PAUSE AT END OF WENCKEBACH SEQUENCE	VENTRICULAR PACED REPETITIVE ABORTED WENCKEBACH UPPER RATE RESPONSE	VP-VP INTERVAL SOLELY CONTROLLED BY SENSOR OR SENSOR-DRIVEN INTERVAL	COMMENTS
1. P-P < SDI < ATRIAL-DRIVEN URI Sensor-driven URI < TARP[a] < P-P < SDI < atrial-driven URI	No	No	Yes	Yes	Functionally equivalent to DDIR
TARP[a] < sensor-driven URI < P-P < SDI < atrial-driven URI	As above	As above	As above	As above	As above
2. P-P < SDI = ATRIAL-DRIVEN URI Sensor-driven URI < TARP[a] < P-P < SDI = atrial-driven URI	Yes	No	No	No because Vp-Vp = atrial-driven URI = SDI	Functionally equivalent to DDIR
TARP[a] < sensor-driven URI < P-P < SDI = atrial-driven URI	As above	As above	As above	As above	As above
3. P-P = SDI < ATRIAL-DRIVEN URI Sensor driven URI < TARP[a] < P-P = SDI < atrial-driven URI	No	No	Yes	Yes; Vp-Vp controlled by SDI < atrial-driven URI	Apparent P wave tracking above atrial-driven upper rate, i.e., at the sensor indicated rate. Extended As-Vp interval
TARP[a] < sensor-driven URI < P-P = SDI < atrial-driven URI	As above	As above	As above	As above	

Abbreviations: URI, upper rate interval; TARP, total atrial refractory period; P-P, interval between two consecutive P waves; SDI, sensor-driven interval; Vp-Vp, interval between two consecutive ventricular paced beats.
[a]TARP < atrial-driven URI permits Wenckebach block upper rate response with extension of As-Vp longer than programmed value.
Modifed from Barold SS: Electrocardiography of rate-adaptive dual-chamber (DDDR) pacemakers: Upper rate behavior. *In* Alt E, Barold SS, Stangl K (eds): Rate-Adaptive Cardiac Pacing. Heidelberg, Berlin, Springer-Verlag, 1993, pp 195–221. Copyright 1993 Springer-Verlag.

with the occurrence of pauses during DDDR pacing when the atrial-driven URI is equal to the sensor-driven URI and the SDI is longer than the atrial-driven URI.

ATRIAL-DRIVEN UPPER RATE INTERVAL LONGER THAN TOTAL ATRIAL REFRACTORY PERIOD

1. *P-P interval longer than sensor-driven interval.* Obviously when the P-P interval is longer than the SDI, the pulse generator paces AV sequentially. Complexity occurs when the P-P interval is equal to or shorter than the SDI and sensor-driven URI.
2. *P-P interval shorter than sensor-driven interval.* When the atrial rate exceeds the sensor-driven rate (P-P interval < SDI), the SDI may also become shorter than the atrial-driven URI (i.e., P-P interval < SDI < atrial-driven URI), a relationship that cannot occur when the sensor-driven URI and atrial-driven URI are common and cannot be dissociated.

SENSOR-DRIVEN INTERVAL SHORTER THAN THE ATRIAL-DRIVEN UPPER RATE INTERVAL

In the absence of atrial activity, when the SDI is shorter than the atrial-driven URI, a pulse generator delivers an atrial stimulus (Ap) at the termination of the sensor-driven AEI and an accompanying ventricular stimulus (Vp) at the completion of the Ap-Vp interval. Vp occurs at the end of the SDI initiated by the preceding ventricular event, but before completion of the atrial-driven URI, also initiated by the same preceding ventricular event (Fig. 31–62). If a sensed P wave (As) occurs before the expected emission of Ap (controlled by the SDI), the pulse generator inhibits the subsequent release of the sensor-controlled Ap. Although the pulse generator omits Ap, it delivers Vp on time according to the SDI. Consequently the As-Vp interval extends beyond its programmed value, a response analogous to the classic Wenckebach block upper rate behavior (possible only if the atrial-driven URI > TARP). In this response, when the P-P interval is shorter than the SDI, which is shorter than the atrial-driven URI, P waves march through the pacing cycles and initiate As-Vp intervals of progressively longer duration until a P wave falls in the PVARP and is unsensed, a behavior resembling the typical pacemaker Wenckebach block upper rate response. There is no pause when the P wave falls in the PVARP because release of the subsequent Ap and Vp is sensor controlled according to the SDI and the sensor-driven AEI. Thus, in this type of pacing either As or Ap can occur, but the Vp-Vp interval remains constant and equal to the prevailing SDI (either longer than the sensor-driven URI or equal to it) but shorter than the atrial-driven URI. The constant sensor-driven Vp-Vp interval with the occasional release of Ap (when P is unsensed in the PVARP) resembles DDIR pacing (see Table 31–10). In other words, when P-P

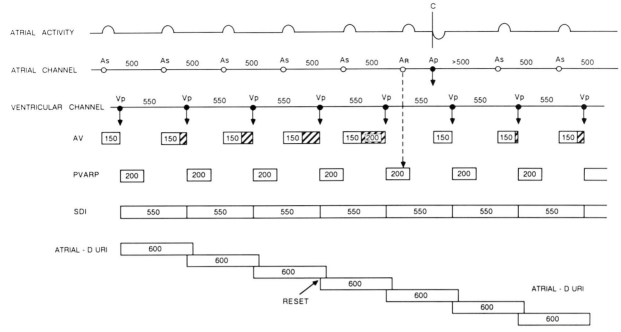

FIGURE 31–62. Pacing by a DDDR pulse generator with the sensor-driven URI (400 msec) shorter than the atrial-driven URI (600 msec). Sensor-driven URI (400 msec) is shorter than the P-P interval (500 msec), which is shorter than the SDI (550 msec), which is shorter than the atrial-driven URI (600 msec). As-Vp = Ap-Vp = 150 msec; PVARP = 200 msec; TARP = 350 msec. The TARP is shorter than the P-P, which is shorter than the atrial-driven URI. The maximal increment of the AV interval during the Wenckebach upper rate response is 600 − 350 = 250 msec. The first P wave initiates an AV interval of 150 msec. The second P wave initiates an AV interval extended beyond 150 msec to conform to the atrial-driven URI, which does not time out because the SDI is shorter than the atrial-driven URI. Thus, the delivery of Vp is sensor controlled, and the Vp-Vp interval is controlled by the sensor or the SDI. The AV interval cannot fully extend to the completion of the atrial-driven URI because an earlier Vp (sensor-controlled) terminates the AV interval. This response may be called a ventricular paced repetitive aborted Wenckebach upper rate response. The sixth P wave falls in the PVARP and is therefore unsensed (A_R). The next Ap released at the end of the sensor-driven escape interval (550 − 150 = 400 msec) occurs 400 msec from the previous Vp, close to the sixth P wave, but capable of atrial capture. There is no pause at the end of the Wenckebach sequence because the Vp-Vp interval is reset by the earlier Vp. On the *right*, the process repeats itself. (From Barold SS: Electrocardiography of rate-adaptive (DDDR) pacemakers. 2. Upper rate behavior. *In* Alt E, Barold SS, Stangl K [eds]: Rate-Adaptive Cardiac Pacing. Berlin, Springer-Verlag, 1993, pp 195–221.)

is shorter than the sensor-driven URI, which is shorter than the atrial-driven URI, the atrial-driven URI does not time out because the SDI or the sensor-driven URI usurp control of the paced ventricular rate. This modified form of pacemaker Wenckebach block upper rate response can therefore be called a ventricular paced repetitive aborted Wenckebach upper rate response because the atrial-driven URI never times out. (Compare this response with the previously described ventricular sensed repetitive aborted Wenckebach upper rate behavior.) In this response, SDI obviously times out, and when SDI becomes equal to the sensor-driven URI, the latter also times out.

SENSOR-DRIVEN INTERVAL EQUAL TO THE ATRIAL-DRIVEN UPPER RATE RESPONSE

When P-P is shorter than the atrial-driven URI, which is equal to the SDI, a Wenckebach upper rate response will also occur with no pause at the end of the sequence in the cycle containing the unsensed P wave within the PVARP (see Table 31–10). The Vp-Vp interval remains equal to the SDI and to the atrial-driven URI. Therefore, both the SDI and the atrial-driven URI time out, but the sensor-driven URI does not. The effect is therefore identical to the situation in which the atrial-driven URI is equal to the sensor-driven URI, which is equal to the SDI; this also creates a classic Wenckebach upper rate response without a pause at the end of the

sequence provided that the TARP is shorter than the P-P, which is shorter than the SDI. In the latter situation, all three intervals (atrial-driven URI, sensor-driven URI, and SDI) time out at the end of every Vp-Vp cycle.

P-P INTERVAL EQUAL TO THE SENSOR-DRIVEN INTERVAL

If atrial sensing produces sustained inhibition of Ap, pacemaker behavior resembles P wave tracking seen in DDD pulse generators, a situation called "apparent tracking" by Higano and Hayes.[143] When the TARP is shorter than the P-P, which is equal to the SDI, which is shorter than the atrial-driven URI, sustained apparent P wave tracking occurs with an extended As-Vp interval that remains constant (Fig. 31–63).[67] In this situation, the Vp-Vp interval is shorter than the atrial-driven URI (see Table 31–10). P waves followed by Vp give the appearance of P wave tracking at a rate faster than the programmed atrial-driven upper rate. Such P waves actually inhibit the sensor-controlled atrial output Ap, but obviously not the succeeding sensor-controlled Vp. The same behavior can occur during DDIR pacing.

OVERVIEW

When the sensor-driven URI is shorter than the atrial-driven URI, the response of a DDDR pacemaker depends on

FIGURE 31–63. Pacing with a DDDR pulse generator showing apparent P wave tracking. Atrial-driven URI is longer than sensor-driven URI. As-Vp = Ap-Vp = 150 msec. The sinus rate is equal to the sensor-driven rate (P-P interval = SDI = 450 msec). The pulse generator senses the last three spontaneous P waves (As). A sensed P wave initiates an AV interval of 150 msec, but at the completion of the 150-msec AV interval, the atrial-driven URI (600 msec) has not yet timed out. Consequently, the pacemaker extends the AV interval to conform to the atrial-driven URI (600 msec). The latter does not time out because the pulse generator emits Vp at the termination of the 450-msec SDI initiated by the preceding ventricular event. The As-Vp interval is stretched to 250 msec. (In the absence of sensor activity or SDI, the As-Vp interval would have stretched to 400 msec to conform to the atrial-driven URI.) Delivery of the last three ventricular stimuli is sensor controlled. The atrial-driven URI is repeatedly reset by the early delivery of sensor-controlled Vp, producing apparent P wave tracking at a rate faster than the programmed atrial-driven upper rate. (From Barold SS: Electrocardiography of rate-adaptive (DDDR) pacemakers. 2. Upper rate behavior. *In* Alt E, Barold SS, Stangl K [eds]: Rate-Adaptive Cardiac Pacing. Berlin, Springer-Verlag, 1993, pp 195–221.)

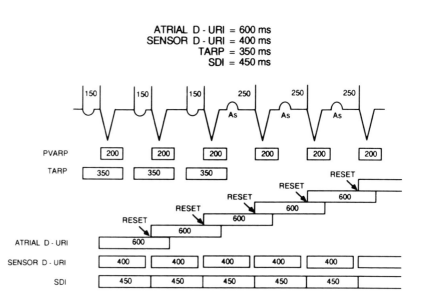

the relationship of the P-P interval to the SDI, and there are four possibilities provided that the P-P is longer than the TARP, making AV extension possible. (1) P-P is longer than the SDI: AV sequential pacing. (2) P-P is shorter than the SDI, which is shorter than the atrial-driven URI: modified Wenckebach upper rate response with P waves marching through the pacing cycle and no pauses. When the SDI is shorter than the atrial-driven URI, the P waves start an AV interval, but unlike the Wenckebach response in the DDD mode, the pulse generator never completes the expected AV interval (although it is extended to some extent) because the pulse generator emits Vp at the completion of the SDI, causing continual reset of the atrial-driven URI by the sensor-controlled Vp. The Vp-Vp interval is sensor driven and the atrial-driven URI does not time out. (3) P-P is equal to the SDI, which is shorter than the atrial-driven URI: sustained apparent P wave tracking with a fixed but extended As-Vp interval. (4) Fluctuation of the P-P interval to a value equal to, longer, or shorter than the SDI leads to irregular patterns with intermittent inhibition of Ap creating complex ECGs. In all these situations, apparent P wave tracking should not be misinterpreted as pacemaker malfunction. Interpretation of DDDR pacemaker function requires knowledge of device specifications as shown in Table 31–11.

DDDR Pacing: Functional Mode Versus Programmed Mode

During DDDR pacing, a particular programmed pacing mode may effectively function in another mode according to

TABLE 31–11. **CHARACTERISTICS OF DDD AND DDDR PULSE GENERATORS**

MODE	MANUFACTURER	URI > TARP WENCKEBACH UPPER RATE RESPONSE	FIXED-RATIO AV BLOCK	SENSOR-DRIVEN URI < ATRIAL-DRIVEN URI	SENSOR-DRIVEN URI INDEPENDENT OF TARP; TARP > URI	ATRIAL PACING IN PVARP	ADAPTIVE PVARP WITH EXERCISE
DDD	Cordis DDD	No	Yes	NA	NA	No	No
DDD	Standard DDD	Yes	Yes	NA	NA	No	No
DDDR	Medtronic Synergyst I and II, Elite I[a]	Yes	Yes	No	Yes	Yes	No
DDDR	Medtronic Elite II	Yes	Yes	Yes	Yes	Yes	No
DDDR	Siemens-Pacesetter Synchrony I, II, and III	Yes	Yes	Yes	Yes	Yes	No
DDDR	Intermedics Relay	Yes	Yes	No	No	No (as TARP never > SDI)	No
DDDR	Telectronics Meta DDDR (1250)	Yes[b]	No because of AMS[c]	At rest	NA	No	Yes
DDDR	Telectronics Meta DDDR (1254)	Yes[d]	Yes	At rest	NA	No	Yes

Abbreviations: NA, not applicable; TARP, total atrial refractory period; URI, upper rate interval; PVARP, postventricular atrial refractory period; AMS, automatic mode switching.

[a]CPI Prelude DR DDDR pacemakers and Medtronic Elite I devices have identical characteristics. CPI Triumph DR DDDR pacemakers and Medtronic Synergyst II devices have identical characteristics.

[b]Only with software unavailable in the United States.

[c]Atrial activity sensed in PVARP causes AMS whereby the succeeding Ap is inhibited—i.e., VVIR mode.

[d]Atrial Protection Interval (PI) is equivalent to Wenckebach window. An atrial event in API inhibits an atrial output and initiates an AV delay. API is a minimum of 30% of the pacing interval at maximum rate to prevent competitive atrial pacing.

circumstances. A DDDR pacemaker can switch its functional pacing mode in the following situations.

DDDR TO DVIR MODE

When the SDI is shorter than or equal to the TARP, the atrial channel paces asynchronously and the DDDR mode functions as a DVIR mode. For example, if AV is equal to 200 msec, the PVARP is equal to 400 msec, and the TARP is equal to 600 msec. When the SDI reaches 600 msec or less, the pacemaker functions in the DVIR mode because these parameters obliterate the atrial sensing window.

DDIR TO DVIR MODE

In the DDIR mode with an AV equal to 150 msec, the PVARP is equal to 350 msec, and the LRI is equal to 1000 msec, the atrial sensing window is equal to the LRI minus the TARP, which equals 500 msec. As the sensor-driven LRI shortens with exercise, the atrial sensing window also shortens. Eventually when the SDI reaches 500 msec (corresponding to a rate of 120 ppm), the programmed indices obliterate the atrial sensing window and the pacemaker then functions in the DVIR mode.

DDDR TO DDIR MODE

1. Any Wenckebach upper rate response without a pause at the termination of the cycle (when the P wave falls within the PVARP) is functionally equivalent to the DDIR mode. In a pulse generator with equal atrial-driven URI and sensor-driven URI, shortening of the SDI (i.e., sensor-driven LRI) on exercise brings it closer to the atrial-driven or common URI. The pacing mode begins to resemble the DDIR mode. When the difference between the URI and the SDI diminishes, the pause at the end of a Wenckebach cycle becomes inconspicuous so that the pacing mode looks like the DDIR mode (constant rate of ventricular pacing) with an occasional, hardly discernible, slight prolongation of the Vp-Vp interval at the end of the Wenckebach sequence. When the SDI is equal to the atrial-driven URI, which is equal to the sensor-driven URI, no pauses occur at the end of the Wenckebach cycle and the pacing mode becomes effectively DDIR. In this situation, the Vp-Vp interval becomes equal to the common URI.
2. A Wenckebach upper rate response without pauses (functionally equivalent to the DDIR mode) can also occur when P-P is shorter than the SDI, which is shorter than the atrial-driven URI provided that the TARP is shorter than the atrial-driven URI. The SDI becomes the Vp-Vp interval when the SDI is shorter than the atrial-driven URI. The atrial-drive URI times out only when the SDI is equal to the atrial-driven URI, the Vp-Vp interval being equal to the SDI.

Other Upper Rate Responses of Dual-Chamber Pacemakers: Fallback and Automatic Mode Conversion

The response of antibradycardia pacemakers to rapid unphysiologic atrial rates has become important now that dual-chamber pacemakers are recommended for patients with alternating bradycardia and tachycardia, as in the sick sinus syndrome.[78–80]

Traditional fallback mechanisms introduced about 10 years ago in certain (VDD) DDD pacemakers provided a reasonably satisfactory degree of protection against sustained rapid ventricular pacing rates during supraventricular tachycardia. In traditional fallback, when the atrial rate exceeds the programmed upper rate or tachycardia detection rate (for a given duration that may be programmable), the pulse generator activates a mechanism that produces a slower ventricular pacing rate with or without maintaining the same pacing mode. During traditional fallback, a DDD pulse generator functions either in the VVI mode with uncoupling of atrial activity from the ventricular paced complexes (actually the VDI mode because atrial sensing is maintained) (Fig. 31–64) or it stays in the DDD (VDD) mode.[34, 146, 147] The ventricular pacing rate drops *gradually* to a programmed fallback rate anywhere between the upper and lower rates according to design or programmability. The pulse generator automatically returns to its previous DDD (VDD) mode with 1:1 AV synchrony when the sensed atrial rate drops below the programmed upper rate or tachycardia detection rate.

Many DDD and DDDR devices are now available with a more refined "atrial tachy response" specific to each manufacturer,[78–80, 148–151] and the field has become quite complex. Figures 31–65 and 31–66 show some of the shortcomings of present algorithms. A detailed analysis of the various forms of fallback from a growing number of manufacturers is beyond the scope of this discussion, and only the general principles are emphasized.

Contemporary pulse generators with a fallback mechanism should have programmability of the following:

1. Fallback rate—the slowest ventricular paced rate that will be maintained as long as the spontaneous atrial rate exceeds the programmed upper rate or tachycardia detection rate.
2. Parameters such as the number of atrial events at the upper rate or tachycardia detection rate required to initiate the fallback mechanism.
3. Deceleration of the fallback response in terms of prolongation of the pacing cycles in milliseconds per cycle until attainment of the programmed fallback mechanism. The capability of rapid or immediate conversion to the fallback rate or mode should be available as a programmable option.
4. Fallback response. Dual-chamber pulse generators can respond to supraventricular tachycardia by (1) maintaining the same pacing mode but slowing the paced ventricular rate, for example, a DDD mode with gradual lengthening of the URI (slowing of upper rate) or (2) converting to another pacing mode with control of the ventricular pacing rate by virtue of a new pacing mode without atrial tracking capability, with or without rate-adaptive fallback response, for example, VVI, VVIR, DDI, DDIR modes (automatic mode conversion) (Figs. 31–67 and 31–68). Although some DDD pulse generators are designed to maintain some semblance of AV synchrony during the fallback mechanism by using the DDD (by continually reducing the URI) or DDI (DDIR) mode, the constantly changing AV intervals during this process probably provide little or no hemodynamic benefit. Indeed, with con-

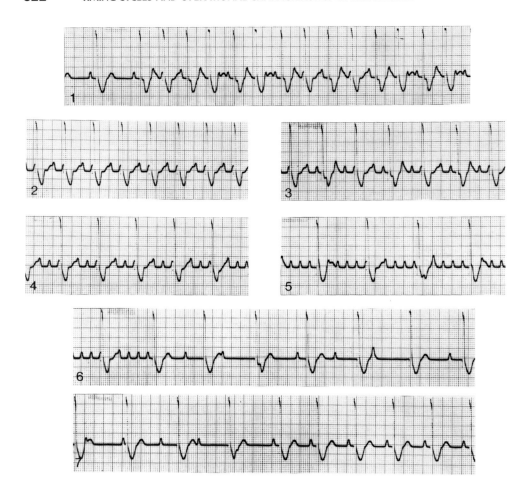

FIGURE 31–64. Traditional fallback mechanism of the CPI 925 Delta DDD pulse generator (Cardiac Pacemakers, Inc., St. Paul, MN) to the VVI mode. Eight cycle onset and 4 msec/cycle. 1 = onset of supraventricular tachycardia (SVT); 2 = 20 seconds after onset of SVT; 3 = 40 seconds after onset of SVT; 4 = 1 minute after onset of SVT; 5 = 2 minutes after onset of SVT; 6 = SVT stops; 7 = pacemaker resynchronization. (From Barold SS, Falkoff MD, Ong LS, et al: Upper rate response of DDD pacemakers. *In* Barold SS, Mugica J [eds]: New Perspectives in Cardiac Pacing. Mt Kisco, NY, Futura Publishing Co., 1988, pp 121–172.)

LOWER RATE INTERVAL = 1000 ms
UPPER RATE INTERVAL = 414 ms (145 / min)
PVARP (BASE) = 400 ms
ATRIAL SENSITIVITY = 0.5 mV

VVIR

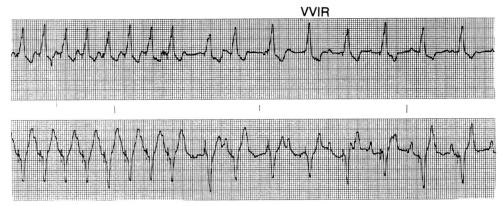

FIGURE 31–65. Two-lead ECG showing pacing with the Telectronics Meta DDDR (1250) pacemaker (Telectronics, Inc., Englewood, CO) during treadmill exercise. On the left there is 1:1 AV synchrony. When the sinus rate generates a P-P interval shorter than the prevailing TARP at that given point in time (adaptive atrial refractory period shortens with exercise), the pulse generator automatically reverts the VVIR mode (automatic mode switching) at a relatively slow rate controlled by sensor activity. When the pacemaker senses a P wave in the PVARP, it omits the succeeding atrial stimulus, thereby effectively switching to the VVIR mode as long as P waves fall within the PVARP (beyond the initial blanking period). The sudden slowing of the paced ventricular rate and loss of AV synchrony may not be tolerated in some individuals. Appropriate programming (upper rate or sensor response, or both) and testing should prevent or minimize such a nonphysiologic response. (From Barold SS: Repetitive reentrant and nonreentrant ventriculoatrial synchrony in dual-chamber pacing. Clin Cardiol 14:754, 1991. Copyrighted and reprinted with the permission of Clinical Cardiology Publishing Co., Inc., P.O. Box 832, Mahwah, NJ 07430 USA.)

FIGURE 31–66. *A*, Meta DDDR (1250) pace-maker (Telectronics, Inc., Englewood, CO) showing automatic mode switching (AMS) initiated by a ventricular extrasystole (V) with retrograde VA activity sensed in the PVARP. Subsequent ventricular paced beats in the VVIR mode perpetuate retrograde VA conduction and AMS. After sensing eight consecutive retrograde P waves within the PVARP, the pacemaker alters its function as follows: (a) automatic prolongation of the next pacing interval (actually the sensor-driven AEI) by 240 msec; (b) automatic uncoupling of the AMS function, thereby allowing successful atrial pacing with immediate termination of retrograde VA conduction. The original 1250 Meta DDDR device activates AMS by sensing a single atrial event (sinus, single APC, or retrograde P wave) in the PVARP. The recently released second-generation 1254 Meta DDDR pulse generator was redesigned to avoid the problem shown in *A* and

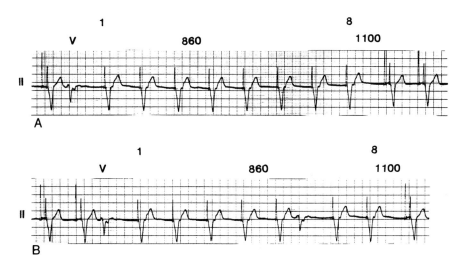

B. In the new device, AMS occurs after the pacemaker detects 5 or 11 atrial intervals (programmable) faster than the automatic mode switching rate (programmable to 150, 175, or 200 bpm). Automatic mode switching is now independent of the PVARP. *B*, Same patient as in *A*. The ECG shows that automatic prolongation of the pacing cycle (sensor-driven AEI) during AMS depends on sensing eight consecutive atrial events within the PVARP rather than the occurrence of eight consecutive ventricular paced cycles. (*A* and *B* from Barold SS, Mond HG: Optimal antibradycardia pacing in patients with paroxysmal supraventricular tachyarrhythmias: Role of fallback and automatic mode switching mechanisms. *In* Barold SS, Mugica J [eds]: New Perspectives in Cardiac Pacing 3. Mt Kisco, NY, Futura Publishing Co., 1993, pp 483–518.)

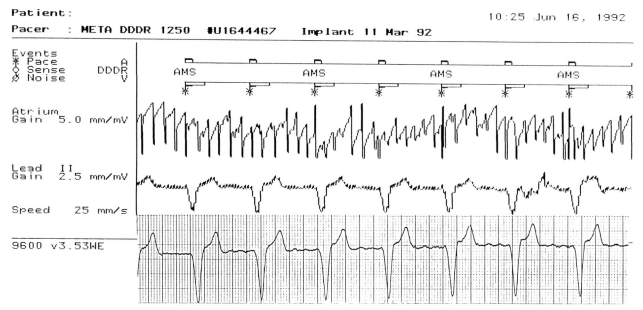

FIGURE 31–67. Meta DDDR 1250 pulse generator (Telectronics, Inc., Englewood, CO) showing automatic mode switching (AMS) with atrial fibrillation in a patient at rest. A high-quality ECG below the printout was recorded simultaneously. Sensing of f waves in the postventricular atrial refractory period perpetuates AMS. (From Barold SS, Mond HG: Optimal antibradycardia pacing in patients with paroxysmal supraventricular tachyarrhythmias: Role of fallback and automatic mode switching mechanisms. *In* Barold SS, Mugica J [eds]: New Perspectives in Cardiac Pacing 3. Mt. Kisco, NY, Futura Publishing Co., 1993, pp 483–518.)

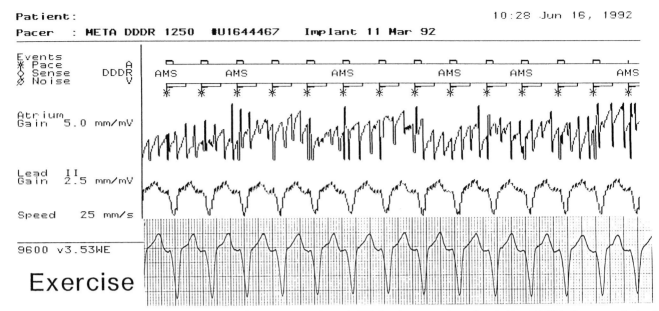

FIGURE 31–68. Meta DDDR 1250 pulse generator (Telectronics, Inc., Englewood, CO) showing automatic mode switching (AMS) in the same patient as in Figure 31–67, but now on exercise. A high-quality ECG below the printout was recorded simultaneously. During AMS in the VVIR mode, the pacemaker increases its rate. (From Barold SS, Mond HG: Optimal antibradycardia pacing in patients with paroxysmal supraventricular tachyarrhythmias: Role of fallback and automatic mode switching mechanisms. *In* Barold SS, Mugica J [eds]: New Perspectives in Cardiac Pacing 3. Mt Kisco, NY, Futura Publishing Co., 1993, pp 483–518.)

tinual atrial sensing during rapid supraventricular tachycardia, the DDI mode effectively paces in the VVI mode, and the DDIR mode functions like the VVIR mode.

5. Relative contribution of nonatrial sensor and atrial inputs for the diagnosis of pathologic supraventricular tachycardia in DDDR devices that use more than simply the atrial sensor for diagnosis of supraventricular tachycardia.[149, 151]

The spontaneous atrial rate versus the sensor-driven (or indicated) rate to initiate fallback should be programmable. In other words, the level of nonatrial sensor activity required to initiate fallback should be variable to deal with patients who experience supraventricular tachycardia on exercise.

6. Restoration of AV synchrony. When fallback is no longer

FIGURE 31–69. Rate smoothing with the CPI Delta 925 DDD pulse generator (Cardiac Pacemakers, Inc., St. Paul, MN). The programmed parameters were as follows: lower rate = 65 ppm; upper rate = 150 ppm; AV interval = 150 msec; and PVARP = 250 msec. The top tracing shows 1:1 P wave tracking during supraventricular tachycardia without rate-smoothing operation. The bottom strip shows the same supraventricular tachycardia with rate-smoothing operation (smoothing factor of 6%). The pulse generator stores in its memory the most recent R-R interval, either paced or sensed. It then calculates "rate control windows" for the next cycle based on the R-R interval and the programmed rate-smoothing value (6% in this ex-

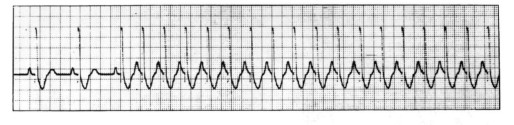

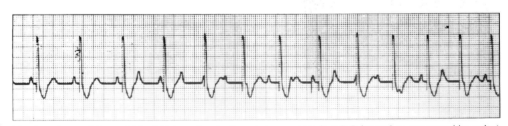

ample). A separate window is calculated for the atrium and the ventricle. Atrial synchronization window = (previous R-R interval ± rate-smoothing value) − AV delay. Ventricular synchronization window = previous R-R interval ± rate-smoothing value. The timing for both windows is initiated at the end of a ventricular event. For example, if the previous R-R interval is 800 msec with a 6% rate-smoothing factor, the ventricular window would be 800 ± 6% = 800 ± 48 msec. The window would therefore extend from 752 to 848 msec. Paced activity (atrial or ventricular), if it is to occur, must occur during these rate control windows. When an atrial event occurs before the atrial synchronization window, the ventricle is paced after an interval that equals the previous R-R interval less the rate-smoothing value. When an atrial event occurs within the synchronization window, the programmed AV delay is initiated, and the ventricle is paced at the end of the AV delay period. When no atrial event occurs during the synchronization window, the interval becomes equal to (previous R-R interval + rate-smoothing value) − AV delay, so the atrium is paced at the end of this interval, followed by ventricular pacing at the end of the programmed AV delay. (Courtesy of Cardiac Pacemakers, Inc., St. Paul, MN.)

needed, restoration of AV synchrony could be either abrupt or gradual with a progressive increase in the paced ventricular rate until AV synchronization occurs.

RATE SMOOTHING

Rate smoothing is a programmable option that is not specifically an upper rate response because it is designed to eliminate pronounced variations in cycle length and therefore functions over all rate ranges. At the upper rate, rate smoothing prevents marked change in cycle length.[152] This mode of operation is complex and its clinical advantages and disadvantages are not fully known, especially in the DDDR mode. Rate smoothing can provide an effective ventricular response to pathologic atrial rates (Fig. 31–69). Rate smoothing is an attempt to replace abrupt changes in rate with gradual transition by limiting the maximal change in the pacing rate from cycle to cycle to some percentage of the previous R-R interval (smoothing factor). Rate smoothing controls the response of a pulse generator because of increases and decreases in the intrinsic rate. Rate smoothing may be useful in patients who cannot tolerate marked fluctuations of paced rate during fixed-ratio or Wenckebach block response during the upper rate response of a DDD pulse generator.[140, 153] Rate smoothing may prevent the sudden deceleration of the ventricular rate during exercise, as with the development of 2:1 or 3:1 fixed-ratio block. During rate smoothing, the pulse generator loses effective AV synchrony and thus sacrifices optimal AV relationships to maintain pacing rates. For increasing atrial rates, rate smoothing will look similar to a Wenckebach

response with prolonged AV delays and occasional unsensed P waves falling in the PVARP.

Rate smoothing modifies the onset of endless loop tachycardia by preventing abrupt variations in the paced rhythm. Actually rate smoothing may itself precipitate endless loop tachycardia because of its propensity to induce AV dissociation.

Atrial Refractory Period

The TARP (AV interval + PVARP) is the most important timing cycle of dual-chamber pacemakers, and many factors influence its duration[26, 30, 31, 37] (Fig. 31–70). The various factors determining the duration of the AV interval are discussed later in the section on the Atrioventricular Interval and the factors determining PVARP duration are described in the discussion herein.

The shortest possible TARP (AV + PVARP) occurs when the AV interval is zero, that is, the TARP is equal to the PVARP. When the URI is longer than the TARP, the longest possible TARP (excluding PVARP extension) is equal to the separately programmable URI. The PVARP was originally designed as an absolute refractory period during which the pulse generator cannot sense. However, a number of contemporary designs permit atrial sensing during the PVARP to fulfill a number of functions (by definition a sensed atrial event within the PVARP cannot be tracked, so it cannot initiate an AV interval). The first part of the PVARP (sometimes programmable) now becomes the atrial blanking period

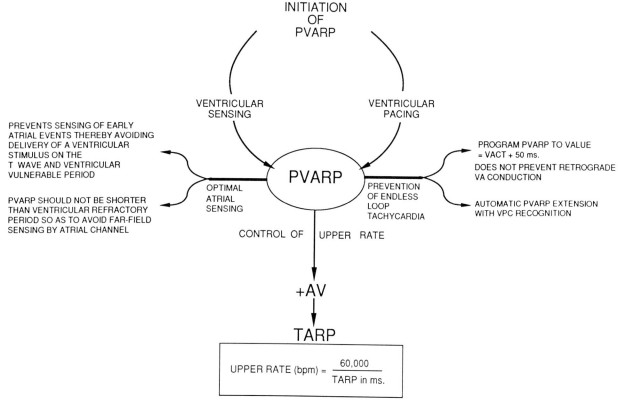

FIGURE 31–70. Central role of the PVARP in dual-chamber pacing (see text for details). (Reprinted with permission from Barold SS: Management of patients with dual-chamber pulse generators: Central role of pacemaker atrial refractory period. Learning Center *Highlights* (Heart House, American College of Cardiology) 5[4]:8, 1990.)

or an absolute refractory period. Published pacemaker specifications by manufacturers are somewhat confusing because some refer to the atrial refractory period as the TARP, whereas others refer only to the PVARP.

UPPER RATE LIMITATION

As previously discussed, the TARP defines the longest P-P interval (corresponding to the slowest atrial rate) that will produce an upper rate response characterized by pacemaker fixed-ratio AV block (e.g., 2:1) whether or not the pacemaker can respond to a longer P-P interval with Wenckebach block upper rate behavior.

POSTVENTRICULAR ATRIAL REFRACTORY PERIOD

AUTOMATIC EXTENSION

Many DDD pulse generators incorporate an automatic extension of the PVARP (for one cycle only) after a sensed ventricular event (outside the AV delay) that the pacemaker interprets as a VPC. In some pulse generators, PVARP extension after a VPC is programmable and in others it is automatic and nonprogrammable. PVARP extension is based on the concept that most episodes of endless loop tachycardia are initiated by VPCs with retrograde VA conduction. Another design related to PVARP extension, the so-called DDX mode, consists of conversion to the DVI mode (i.e., asynchronous atrial channel)[26] (Fig. 31–71). The DDX mode in effect functions like an automatic PVARP extension after a VPC, with the atrial channel remaining refractory for a complete cycle (corresponding to the programmed lower rate). The pacemaker may continue to function in the DVI mode indefinitely as long as the R-R interval between two consecutive sensed ventricular events remains shorter than the pacemaker AEI (Vs-Ap or Vp-Ap).[154] Termination of the DVI

mode requires delivery of an atrial stimulus either spontaneously or by application and removal of the magnet (see Fig. 31–71).

The advantage of an automatic PVARP extension or the DDX mode is that it may play a role in the prevention of endless loop tachycardia. Automatic PVARP extension does not sacrifice the atrial tracking capability (upper rate) because the standard PVARP remains unchanged. Its *limitation* is that the PVARP extension does not provide protection when the first retrograde P wave is engendered by a ventricular *paced* event. The *disadvantage* of this design is that under certain circumstances both the DDX and excessive extension of the PVARP may themselves paradoxically increase susceptibility to endless loop tachycardia[155] (Fig. 31–72). Automatic PVARP extension can also cause atrial undersensing despite a large intracardiac signal[156] (discussed later).

APPARENT OR FUNCTIONAL UNDERSENSING

The differential diagnosis of atrial undersensing, not an uncommon problem in dual-chamber pacing, requires knowledge of atrial refractory period behavior under a variety of circumstances to avoid unnecessary surgical intervention to correct an apparent problem when the amplitude of the atrial signal is actually sufficiently large for sensing by the atrial channel. Apparent or functional atrial undersensing (or lack of P wave tracking in the presence of an adequate atrial signal) originates from two main sources: (1) an atrial signal in the PVARP and (2) upper rate limitation (Fig. 31–73, Table 31–12).

ATRIAL UNDERSENSING RELATED TO THE REFRACTORY PERIOD. P wave undersensing can occur in the presence of an adequate atrial electrogram if the PVARP is excessively prolonged, especially when the atrial rate is relatively fast. This form of undersensing is more likely with prolongation of

DDX MODE, LOWER RATE = 45 ppm, AV = 165 ms, UPPER RATE = 145 ppm

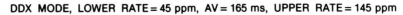
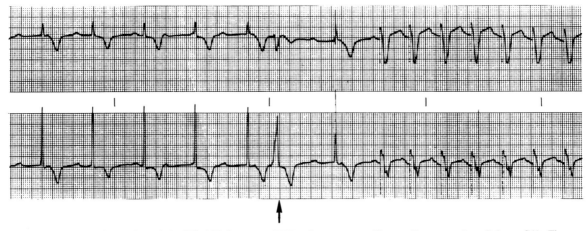

FIGURE 31–71. DDX mode of operation of the 283 AFP Pacesetter DDD pulse generator (Siemens-Pacesetter, Inc., Sylmar, CA). The programmed parameters are shown above the ECG with two leads recorded simultaneously. The DDX mode of operation initiated the DVI mode after sensing of a ventricular extrasystole. The DVI mode can terminate only with the emission of an atrial stimulus. This stimulus does not occur because the R-R interval of the AV junctional escape rhythm (approximately 1000 msec) is shorter than the AEI (1333 − 165 = 1168 msec). A ventricular extrasystole (*arrow*) induces a longer pause, thereby allowing the release of an atrial stimulus at the termination of the AEI. The atrial stimulus produces a pseudopseudofusion beat. This atrial stimulus terminates the DVI mode, with the return of P wave tracking in the DDX (or DDD) mode. (From Barold SS, Falkoff MD, Ong LS, et al: Electrocardiography of contemporary DDD pacemakers. A. Basic concepts, upper rate response, retrograde ventriculoatrial conduction, and differential diagnosis of pacemaker tachycardias. *In* Saksena S, Goldschlager N [eds]: Electrical Therapy for Cardiac Arrhythmias: Pacing, Antitachycardia Devices, Catheter Ablation. Philadelphia, WB Saunders, 1990, pp 225–264.)

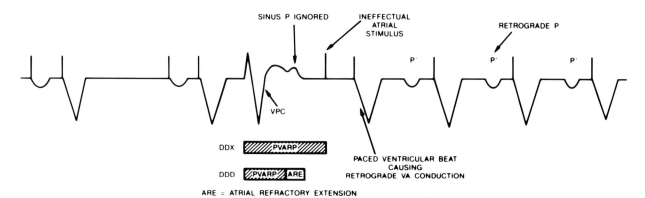

FIGURE 31–72. Diagrammatic representation of the mechanism of paradoxical induction of endless loop tachycardia by excessive prolongation of the PVARP with either atrial refractory period extension (ARE) or the DDX mode, in which the PVARP extends for the entire duration of the pacemaker cycle. An unsensed sinus P wave renders the succeeding atrial stimulus ineffectual because the stimulus falls within the atrial myocardial refractory period. This ineffectiveness of the atrial stimulus causes AV dissociation followed by retrograde VA conduction and initiation of endless loop tachycardia. (From Barold SS, Falkoff MD, Ong LS, et al: Electrocardiography of contemporary DDD pacemakers. A. Basic concepts, upper rate response, retrograde ventriculoatrial conduction, and differential diagnosis of pacemaker tachycardias. *In* Saksena S, Goldschlager N [eds]: Electrical Therapy for Cardiac Arrhythmias: Pacing, Antitachycardia Devices, Catheter Ablation. Philadelphia, WB Saunders, 1990, pp 225–264.)

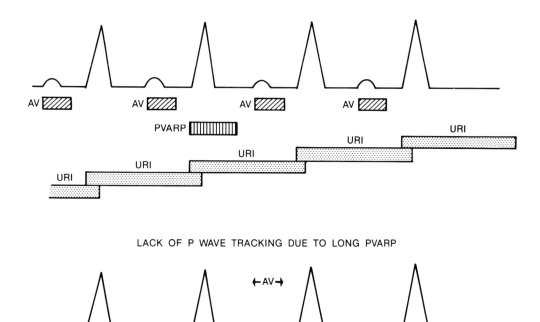

LACK OF P WAVE TRACKING DUE TO LONG PVARP

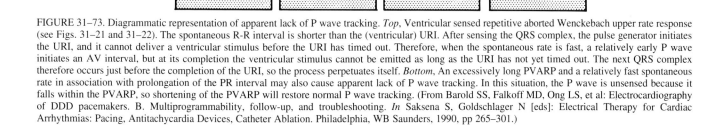

FIGURE 31–73. Diagrammatic representation of apparent lack of P wave tracking. *Top*, Ventricular sensed repetitive aborted Wenckebach upper rate response (see Figs. 31–21 and 31–22). The spontaneous R-R interval is shorter than the (ventricular) URI. After sensing the QRS complex, the pulse generator initiates the URI, and it cannot deliver a ventricular stimulus before the URI has timed out. Therefore, when the spontaneous rate is fast, a relatively early P wave initiates an AV interval, but at its completion the ventricular stimulus cannot be emitted as long as the URI has not yet timed out. The next QRS complex therefore occurs just before the completion of the URI, so the process perpetuates itself. *Bottom*, An excessively long PVARP and a relatively fast spontaneous rate in association with prolongation of the PR interval may also cause apparent lack of P wave tracking. In this situation, the P wave is unsensed because it falls within the PVARP, so shortening of the PVARP will restore normal P wave tracking. (From Barold SS, Falkoff MD, Ong LS, et al: Electrocardiography of DDD pacemakers. B. Multiprogrammability, follow-up, and troubleshooting. *In* Saksena S, Goldschlager N [eds]: Electrical Therapy for Cardiac Arrhythmias: Pacing, Antitachycardia Devices, Catheter Ablation. Philadelphia, WB Saunders, 1990, pp 265–301.)

TABLE 31–12. POSTVENTRICULAR ATRIAL REFRACTORY PERIOD AND ATRIAL UNDERSENSING

NORMAL PVARP DURATION
Relatively fast sinus rate with long PR interval (P wave falls close to the preceding QRS—i.e., within PVARP)
LONG PVARP
As programmed, or DDX mode
AUTOMATIC PVARP EXTENSION
(Secondary to two ventricular events without an intervening P wave, interpreted by pacemaker as a ventricular extrasystole.) P-wave undersensing may be perpetuated from cycle to cycle if the pulse generator continually interprets the spontaneous supraventricular QRS complex (i.e., preceded by a P wave) as a ventricular extrasystole or premature ventricular event and P waves occur consistently within the extended PVARP and remain undetected.
Some contemporary devices allow atrial sensing in the PVARP. If pacemaker detects a P wave in the PVARP, it prevents VPC status for any subsequent intrinsic ventricular event, i.e., PVARP does not lengthen automatically.
PVARP REINITIATION BY INAPPARENT VENTRICULAR SIGNALS
Oversensing by ventricular channel, e.g., T wave, myopotentials. With relatively low voltage signals, decrease in ventricular sensitivity may restore atrial sensing.
RETRIGGERABLE ATRIAL REFRACTORY PERIOD
Atrial sensing occurs in the PVARP during the noise-sampling period. This mechanism creates overlapping atrial refractory periods and asynchronous atrial pacing when the P-P interval < TARP.
Oversensing of far-field QRS initiates a new TARP that can cause atrial undersensing. A decrease in atrial sensitivity often eliminates atrial sensing of far-field QRS complex with correction of atrial undersensing.

Abbreviations: PVARP, postventricular atrial refractory period; VPC, ventricular premature contraction; TARP, total atrial refractory period.

spontaneous AV conduction (long PR interval) pushing the P wave closer to the preceding PVARP (Fig. 31–74). Occasionally P wave undersensing can occur when the programmed PVARP is quite short, for example, 155 msec. This paradox is explained by the onset of P wave undersensing within an automatically extended PVARP (e.g., 400 msec) initiated by a VPC or any other signal, for example, a sinus conducted QRS complex, false signal, not preceded by a detected P wave, and interpreted as a VPC by the pacemaker. The unsensed P wave in the PVARP gives rise to a spontaneous conducted QRS complex that is then interpreted by the pacemaker as a VPC (no preceding sensed P wave), thereby generating another automatically extended PVARP (Fig. 31–75). This excessively long PVARP is perpetuated from cycle to cycle (the pacemaker continually interprets the spontaneous conducted QRS as a VPC) especially if the atrial rate remains relatively fast and AV conduction is delayed so that P waves consistently occur within the extended PVARP. The

relatively long PR interval suggests lack of atrial tracking.[156–159] This self-perpetuating mechanism can be unlocked by slowing of the atrial rate, improvement of AV conduction, or by a VPC (without retrograde VA conduction), circumstances that create a new and premature PVARP. By starting earlier, the new, premature PVARP finishes earlier, thereby giving the succeeding P wave an opening for being sensed outside the PVARP, whereupon AV synchrony is immediately restored. A similar situation can occur on exercise following the last unsensed P wave (in the PVARP) of a Wenckebach block upper rate response (see Fig. 31–75). If the unsensed P wave is conducted to the ventricle, the pacemaker can interpret the QRS as a VPC because it ignores the preceding P wave. Such a situation leads to automatic PVARP extension, perpetuated by each succeeding QRS complex as the P wave continually falls within the extended PVARP. The ECG therefore suggests lack of atrial tracking. After exercise, as the sinus rate decreases, P wave sensing is restored only

LOWER RATE = 70 ppm (857 ms)
UPPER RATE INTERVAL = 135 ppm
AV INTERVAL = 150 ms
PVARP = 400 ms
VRP = 250 ms

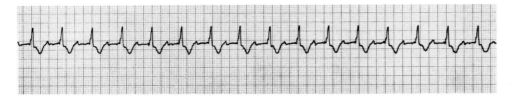

FIGURE 31–74. Lack of P wave tracking due to long PVARP (PVARP = 400 msec). The sinus rate is about 85 ppm, and there is first-degree AV block. The P waves fall within the PVARP initiated by the preceding sensed QRS complex. Shortening the PVARP to 375 msec (*bottom*) restores 1:1 atrial tracking with the programmed AV interval (150 msec). VRP = ventricular refractory period. (From Barold SS, Falkoff MD, Ong LS, et al: Timing cycles of DDD pacemakers. *In* Barold SS, Mugica J [eds]: New Perspectives in Cardiac Pacing. Mt Kisco, NY, Futura Publishing Co., 1988, pp 69–119.)

PVARP = 400 ms   PVARP = 375 ms

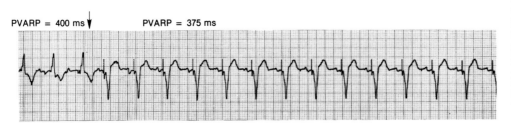

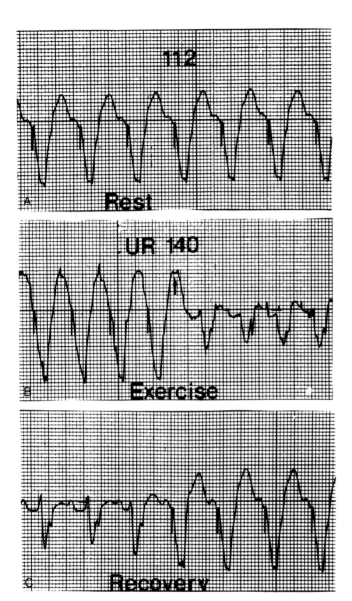

FIGURE 31–75. Apparent P wave undersensing in an Intermedics Cosmos II DDD pacemaker (Intermedics, Inc., Angleton, TX) on exercise in a patient with intermittent AV block. Lower rate = 60 ppm; upper rate = 140 ppm; AV delay after P wave sensing = 135 msec (adaptive AV delay with minimum AV delay of 75 msec); PVARP = 320 msec; automatic PVARP extension = 100 msec. *A*, At rest the atrial rate is 112 bpm, causing atrial sensing and ventricular pacing with AV interval of approximately 100 msec. *B*, After 1 minute of exercise, Wenckebach block upper rate response occurs, and the pacemaker does not sense a P wave (*arrow*) in the PVARP. The P wave in the PVARP allows spontaneous AV conduction with a PR interval of approximately 260 msec. The pacemaker interprets the spontaneous QRS as a VPC and therefore automatically lengthens the PVARP to 320 + 100 = 420 msec. Subsequent events all are spontaneous, that is, P wave and conducted QRS complex with PR interval longer than programmed As-Vp interval at that particular atrial rate (apparent lack of atrial tracking). The spontaneous QRS complex continually activates the PVARP extension as the P waves continually fall within the extended PVARP. *C*, In the recovery phase, the ECG shows sinus rhythm (PR = 200 msec) and conversion to an atrial synchronous ventricular paced rhythm with an AV interval of 100 msec. The PR interval preceding ventricular pacing shows an abrupt shortening of approximately 40 msec without a change in the P-P interval. This results in earlier detection of the conducted QRS complex, and subsequently the next P wave falls outside the extended PVARP of 420 msec. (From vanGelder BM, vanMechelen R, denDulk K, et al: Apparent P wave undersensing in a DDD pacemaker postexercise. PACE 15:1651, 1992.)

when the P-P interval is longer than or equal to the PR interval plus the PVARP as programmed plus the PVARP extension.

Ventricular oversensing (T wave, false signals, and so forth) causes reinitiation of the PVARP as occurs with any ventricular sensed event. The new PVARP can, in turn, cause atrial undersensing. This diagnosis is confirmed if a decrease in ventricular sensitivity restores atrial sensing.[26]

APPARENT ATRIAL UNDERSENSING AND UPPER RATE LIMITATION. In this situation, as previously discussed, P waves are sensed outside the PVARP, but the pacemaker does not emit its ventricular stimulus at the end of the programmed AV interval (ventricular sensed repetitive aborted Wenckebach upper rate response) (see Figs. 31–21, 31–22, and 31–73). Apparent atrial undersensing occurs during continual AV conduction when the P-P and R-R intervals are shorter than the URI.[49] P waves are actually sensed beyond the PVARP and give rise to a conducted QRS complex, but the PR interval is longer than the programmed value of the AV interval. The pulse generator cannot emit a ventricular stimulus at the end of the programmed AV interval (As-Vp) because it cannot violate the URI. This relationship represents another cause of lack of P wave tracking or sensing. When the P-P and the R-R intervals exceed the URI, normal P-wave tracking returns.

PREVENTION OF UNDESIRABLE ATRIAL SENSING

EARLY SENSING

If the PVARP is too short, very premature atrial extrasystoles can be sensed and cause triggering of a ventricular pacing beat very close to the apex of the T wave linked to the previous beat; a short URI and long AV interval favor ventricular capture beyond the myocardial ventricular refractory period. Such a situation could lead to repetitive ventricular responses and potentially serious unsustained or sustained ventricular tachyarrhythmias.[30, 160, 161]

FAR-FIELD SENSING

A ventricular event (Vs or Vp) may generate a substantial QRS deflection in the atrial electrogram registered by the atrial lead. Obviously when the ventricular channel senses the tail end of the near-field QRS complex before the atrial channel can sense its far-field counterpart, the pulse generator responds only to Vs because the far-field QRS signal (delivered to the atrial electrode) then falls in the PVARP initiated by ventricular sensing (Vs). If sufficiently large, the far-field QRS complex (paced or spontaneous) picked up via the atrial electrogram can be sensed by the atrial channel under certain circumstances:[162–164] (1) relatively short PVARP, (2) low ventricular sensitivity preventing or delaying ventricular sensing, or (3) atrial channel sensing the far-field QRS signal before the ventricular channel senses the near-field QRS signal. Atrial sensing of the far-field QRS complex is far more common in unipolar than in bipolar sensing systems. With far-field atrial sensing, the signal delivered to the atrial channel initiates an AV interval. At the completion of the programmed AV delay, the pulse generator releases a ventricular stimulus that falls within the ST segment or the T

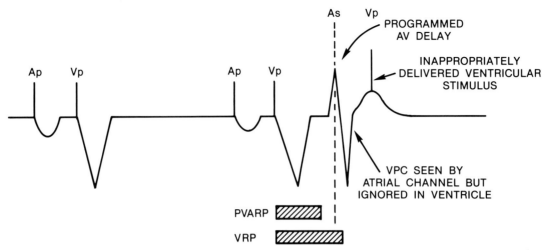

FIGURE 31–76. Diagrammatic representation of far-field sensing by the atrial electrode of a DDD pulse generator. When the VRP is substantially longer than the PVARP, it creates a window within which a ventricular signal can be sensed by the atrial channel and ignored by the ventricular channel. On sensing the VPC, the atrial channel initiates an AV interval with the ultimate delivery of the ventricular stimulus on the T wave of the VPC. The likelihood of delivering a ventricular stimulus at the apex of the T wave is increased by programming a relatively long AV interval. Ap = atrial paced event; As = atrial sensed event; Vp = ventricular paced event; PVARP = postventricular atrial refractory period; VRP = ventricular refractory period; VPC = ventricular premature contraction. (From Barold SS, Falkoff MD, Ong LS, et al: Electrocardiography of DDD pacemakers. B. Multiprogrammability, follow-up, and troubleshooting. *In* Saksena S, Goldschlager N [eds]: Electrical Therapy for Cardiac Arrhythmias: Pacing, Antitachycardia Devices, Catheter Ablation. Philadelphia, WB Saunders, 1990, pp 265–301.)

wave (Fig. 31–76). A long programmed AV delay favors early ventricular capture. Repetitive atrial sensing of the far-field tail end of the QRS complex may also cause a sustained endless loop tachycardia in the absence of regular retrograde VA conduction (Figs. 31–77 and 31–78). During normal DDD pacing (in the absence of lead displacement), far-field sensing of the QRS complex generally occurs only when the PVARP is relatively short and the ventricular refractory period is substantially longer than the PVARP, a situation favoring selective atrial sensing of far-field events. Thus, the PVARP should not be less than 200 msec and should always be equal to or longer than the ventricular refractory period to avoid far-field sensing by the atrial channel.

OPTIMAL DURATION OF ATRIAL AND VENTRICULAR REFRACTORY PERIODS

As mentioned previously, the duration of the ventricular refractory period should not exceed the value of the PVARP to avoid far-field sensing by the atrial channel. A relatively

LOWER RATE =	70 ppm
UPPER RATE INTERVAL =	180 ms
AV INTERVAL =	130 ms
PVARP =	125 ms

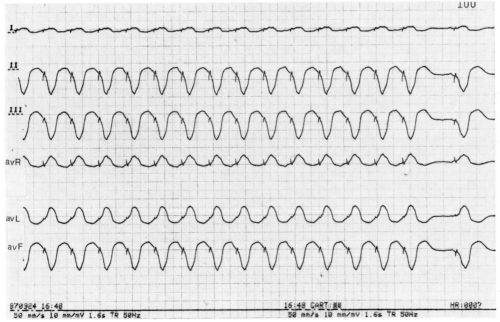

FIGURE 31–77. Far-field endless loop tachycardia with a CPI 925 Delta DDD pulse generator (Cardiac Pacemakers, Inc., St. Paul, MN). The programmed parameters are shown above the ECG with six leads recorded simultaneously. The atrial channel senses far-field ventricular depolarization and not retrograde P waves. This diagnosis cannot be made from the surface ECG because there was no clear-cut evidence of AV dissociation during the tachycardia. (From Barold SS, Falkoff MD, Ong LS, et al: Electrocardiography of contemporary DDD pacemakers. A. Basic concepts, upper rate response, retrograde ventriculoatrial conduction, and differential diagnosis of pacemaker tachycardias. *In* Saksena S, Goldschlager N [eds]: Electrical Therapy for Cardiac Arrhythmias: Pacing, Antitachycardia Devices, Catheter Ablation. Philadelphia, WB Saunders, 1990, pp 225–264.)

LOWER RATE = 70 ppm (750 ms)
UPPER RATE INTERVAL = 180 ms
AV = 130 ms
PVARP = 125 ms

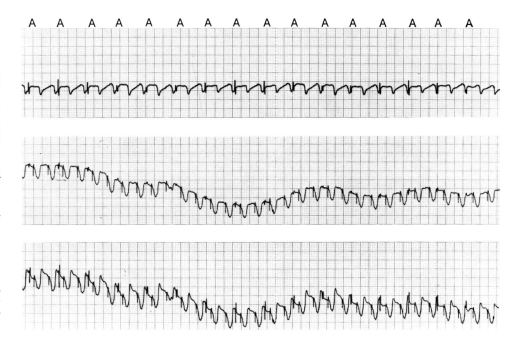

FIGURE 31–78. Same patient as in Figure 31–77. Three-lead ECG with bipolar esophageal recording in the upper strip and compound leads below. A = atrial depolarization. AV dissociation excludes the usual type of near-field endless loop tachycardia related to sensing of retrograde P waves. The tachycardia was terminated and prevented by lengthing the PVARP. (From Barold SS, Falkoff MD, Ong LS, et al: Electrocardiography of contemporary DDD pacemakers. A. Basic concepts, upper rate response, retrograde ventriculo-atrial conduction, and differential diagnosis of pacemaker tachycardias. *In* Saksena S, Goldschlager N [eds]: Electrical Therapy for Cardiac Arrhythmias: Pacing, Antitachycardia Devices, Catheter Ablation. Philadelphia, WB Saunders, 1990, pp 225–264.)

long ventricular refractory period that is longer than or equal to 300 msec predisposes to undersensing of early ventricular events. A VPC may be unsensed when it falls within a relatively long VRP. However, if the VPC engenders retrograde VA conduction, the atrial channel can sense the retrograde P wave if it falls beyond the PVARP. In this situation, the retrograde P wave can trigger an undesirable ventricular stimulus falling within the T wave of the unsensed VPC.

ADAPTIVE POSTVENTRICULAR ATRIAL REFRACTORY PERIOD

AUTOMATIC REFRACTORY PERIOD ABBREVIATION WITH EXERCISE

Wittkampf and Boute[165] suggested that a DDD pulse generator could be designed with shortening of the PVARP on exercise whenever the atrial channel interprets atrial activity as being physiologic according to the actual rate and rate of change of atrial sensed events. PVARP abbreviation during exercise coupled with adaptive shortening of the AV interval (As-Vp) on exercise would therefore produce substantial shortening of the TARP. A long PVARP and TARP at rest provide protection against atrial arrhythmias (by limiting the upper ventricular paced rate) in patients with bradycardia-tachycardia syndrome. A shorter PVARP on exercise allows programming of a faster upper rate.

Mathematically, the timing of pacemaker and spontaneous events make initiation of endless loop tachycardia by retrograde VA conduction (from a VPC) highly unlikely at fast ventricular pacing rates because the retrograde P wave cannot arrive at the atrium before the occurrence of the next spontaneous P wave. In most cases, therefore, there is no need for the PVARP on exercise to equal the required duration at rest to prevent endless loop tachycardia. Thus under normal cir-

cumstances, at rest the URI could be equal to the TARP, as there is no need for a Wenckebach upper rate response at rest. With this arrangement at rest, an early atrial extrasystole would not prolong the AV interval (As-Vp) with the potential of inducing endless loop tachycardia as it does when the URI is longer than the TARP. With a constant URI, TARP shortening on exercise would establish a Wenckebach upper rate response only on exercise.

The Telectronics Meta DDDR Model 1250, and especially the recently released Model 1254 (Telectronics, Inc., Englewood, CO) incorporate many of the preceding concepts.[79, 150, 151, 166] The Meta DDDR pacemakers are minute ventilation rate-adaptive devices that exhibit automatic AV delay shortening dependent on a metabolic indicated rate (MIR) interval (calculated pacing rate interval determined by the algorithm during both atrial pacing and sensing). The MIR interval is dependent on the programmed rate-response factor, the upper and lower pacing rates, and the measured transthoracic impedance changes. Shortening of the PVARP (adaptive PVARP) on exercise is also dependent on the MIR interval and the programmable indices. The longer TARP at rest limits the maximum tracking rate of the pacemaker and promotes mostly fixed-ratio AV block in response to supraventricular tachycardia at rest, a situation clinically preferable to a Wenckebach upper rate response. A long TARP at rest will not limit the upper rate of an appropriately programmed Meta DDDR device, as the AV interval and PVARP (i.e., TARP) shorten with exercise.

AUTOMATIC PVARP PROLONGATION WITH ATRIAL TACHYARRHYTHMIAS

Some DDD pulse generators are designed with an automatic PVARP extension (and therefore longer TARP if the

AV interval does not shorten) on sensing a nonphysiologic atrial rate, with consequent reduction in the maximum ventricular pacing rate.[34] This response avoids an unnecessary fast ventricular paced response to unphysiologic atrial tachyarrhythmias and represents a form of fallback.

RETRIGGERABLE ATRIAL REFRACTORY PERIOD

In some DDD pulse generators, the first part of the PVARP consists of the absolute refractory period during which atrial sensing cannot occur. However, atrial sensing may take place in the second and terminal portion of the PVARP, sometimes known as the noise sampling period. A sensed P wave within the noise sampling period does not initiate a new AV interval as ordinarily occurs in all DDD pulse generators by a P wave outside the TARP. Rather a sensed P wave in the noise sampling period retriggers a complete TARP (i.e., AV + PVARP)[78, 80] (Fig. 31–79). In a pulse generator with a retriggerable TARP of 500 msec, when the P-P interval becomes slightly shorter than 500 msec, every alternate P wave will fall within the noise sampling period generated by the preceding P wave. Sensing of the P wave within the noise sampling period restarts another full TARP of 500 msec (not just the AV interval). As long as the P-P interval remains shorter than the 500-msec TARP, the atrial refractory periods will overlap. In effect, the pulse generator reverts to the DVI mode (asynchronous atrial pacing) and provides an effective way of avoiding a faster paced ventricular rate in response to atrial tachyarrhythmias by automatic mode conversion to the DVI mode (Biotronik Diplos 06 and Physios 01-Gemnos 04, Biotronic, Lake Oswego, OR). When the P-P interval becomes shorter than the TARP, a pulse generator with a retriggerable atrial refractory period cannot exhibit a fixed-ratio AV block upper rate response because the P waves never occur beyond the TARP. Conceptually this design is similar to that of automatic tachycardia-terminating dual-demand pacemakers with overlapping refractory periods and activation of the pulse generator

to pace at the same lower rate automatically in response to both bradycardia and tachycardia.[168]

In pulse generators with a retriggerable atrial refractory period, atrial sensing of a far-field QRS signal may cause reinitiation of the TARP and loss of atrial sensing. In this situation, decreasing *atrial* sensitivity may paradoxically restore atrial sensing, whereas decreasing ventricular sensitivity produces no effect. Decrease of atrial sensitivity abolishes atrial sensing of the far-field QRS complex so that the additional TARP initiated by the previously sensed far-field QRS complex cannot occur. This response is in sharp contrast to loss of atrial sensing secondary to PVARP (not TARP) reinitiation by ventricular oversensing. The diagnosis of PVARP reinitiation is certain if a decrease in the ventricular sensitivity restores atrial tracking, as previously described, whereas reduction of atrial sensitivity alone produces no effect.

ADVANTAGES OF ATRIAL SENSING DURING THE POSTVENTRICULAR ATRIAL REFRACTORY PERIOD

1. Atrial sensing can be used to make the diagnosis of physiologic or pathologic atrial rates to provide an appropriate pacemaker response. In advanced DDDR devices, the pulse generator compares the spontaneous atrial rate with the sensor-driven rate. These responses are reviewed in the discussion on fallback and automatic conversion of the pacing mode.
2. Repetitive nonreentrant VA synchrony can be diagnosed with atrial sensing.
3. Atrial sensing can avoid atrial competition during DDDR pacing. In this mode, an unsensed P wave in the PVARP can be followed by an atrial stimulus either in the PVARP (according to design) or beyond it according to the sensor-driven interval. The sensor-driven atrial output may thus occur within the vulnerable period of atrial depolarization and carries the potential of inducing atrial arrhythmias. Therefore, an intelligent pacemaker should provide a programmable option that permits omission or delay of the

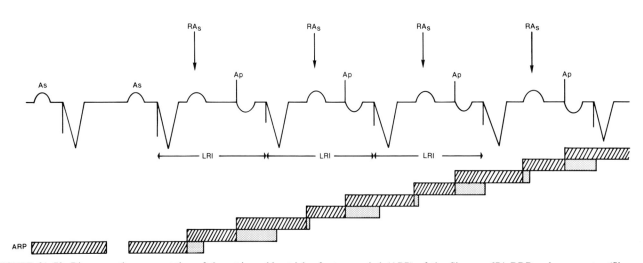

FIGURE 31–79. Diagrammatic representation of the retriggerable atrial refractory period (ARP) of the Siemens 674 DDD pulse generator (Siemens-Pacesetter, Inc., Sylmar, CA). As = atrial sensed event outside ARP; RAs = atrial sensed event within ARP; Ap = atrial paced event. The first 125 msec of the PVARP represents the absolute refractory period during which signals cannot be sensed. The second part of the PVARP (and AV interval) consists of the noise sampling period. P waves falling within the noise sampling period may be sensed, and although they do not initiate a new AV interval, they retrigger a full ARP. Continual retriggering of the ARP causes the DDD pulse generator to operate in the atrial asynchronous mode at the lower rate, that is, DVI mode when the P-P interval is shorter than the ARP. (From Barold SS, Falkoff MD, Ong LS, et al: Upper rate response of DDD pacemakers. *In* Barold SS, Mugica J [eds]: New Perspectives in Cardiac Pacing. Mt Kisco, NY, Futura Publishing Co., 1988, pp 121–172.)

atrial stimulus after sensing one or a programmable number of P waves within a particular portion of the PVARP. Prevention of atrial competition may become desirable when more becomes known about this potential problem.

4. Atrial sensing can prevent inappropriate automatic PVARP extension by a conducted atrial extrasystole or sinus beat (P wave unsensed in the PVARP followed by a sensed conducted QRS falling beyond the ventricular refractory period) when the pulse generator interprets the ventricular signal as a ventricular extrasystole. Sensing of a preceding P wave in the PVARP would eliminate the PVARP extension applied to the succeeding conducted and sensed QRS complex (a feature incorporated in some contemporary pacemakers). This arrangement would therefore avoid atrial undersensing perpetuated by P waves continually falling within an automatically extended (and long) PVARP, for example, as in relatively fast sinus rhythm associated with first-degree AV block.

5. Extension of the AEI can be provided by atrial sensing. A number of Intermedics dual-chamber pulse generators are designed with an extension of the AEI interval to prevent atrial pacing in the pause of a Wenckebach block upper rate response most likely when the lower rate is faster than 80 ppm as required by pediatric pacing. The extension allows sensing of spontaneous activity whenever the preceding cycle or cycles occur at the URI or when an atrial event is sensed within the terminal portion of the PVARP (relative refractory period).

6. Automatic detection of retrograde VA conduction by the pulse generator during follow-up evaluation obviously requires sensing of P waves within the PVARP.

Atrial sensing during the PVARP constitutes an important characteristic of contemporary pacemakers. Other advantages of this function will undoubtedly come to light when it becomes better understood.

Ventricular Refractory Period

With the advent of sophisticated pulse generators, the definition of the ventricular refractory period has changed and is now known as the period during which the lower rate timer cannot be reset or restarted. Therefore, a pulse generator can actually recognize ventricular signals during the second part of the ventricular refractory period (also known as the relative refractory period or noise sampling period) beyond the first part or the absolute refractory period. The detected signals can only reset timing intervals other than the inviolable LRI.[169] In most cases, the duration of the ventricular refractory period initiated by a ventricular stimulus is equal to the ventricular refractory period initiated by ventricular sensing (with or without a preceding P wave).

The noise sampling (or noise interrogation) period may be considered as a relative refractory period (usually in the terminal portion of the ventricular refractory period) with design, function, and duration varying from manufacturer to manufacturer. Single- and dual-chamber pacemakers (sometimes both the atrial and ventricular channels) can be designed with a noise sampling period. There are at least three types of responses when a signal is sensed within the noise sampling period.[169] (1) The sensed signal may reset the entire

refractory period (retriggerable refractory period). (2) The sensed signal resets only the noise sampling period rather than the entire refractory period. Repetitive retriggering of the noise sampling period eventually leads to asynchronous pacing. (3) The sensed signal may cause reversion to asynchronous pacing for one full cycle, that is, the refractory period is extended for the duration of one pacing cycle only.

The ventricular refractory period of Medtronic dual-chamber pulse generators (Medtronic, Inc., Minneapolis, MN) provides a good example of a retriggerable design.[167] The ventricular refractory period is composed of an initial 125-msec absolute refractory period (also called the ventricular blanking period by Medtronic) followed by the noise sampling period, which occupies the terminal part of the ventricular refractory period. Sensing cannot occur during the "ventricular blanking period." Such terminology is potentially misleading because this particular blanking period could be confused with the brief ventricular blanking period occurring coincidentally with the atrial stimulus and designed to prevent crosstalk. When Medtronic DDD pulse generators (Medtronic, Inc., Minneapolis, MN) sense a VPC in the noise sampling period (defined as two successive ventricular events without any sensed intervening atrial activity), an entirely new ventricular refractory period is reinitiated. (In the case of Medtronic pulse generators 7001, 7005, and 7006, reinitiation of a new ventricular refractory period occurs with automatic prolongation of the noise sampling period) (Fig. 31–80, Table 31–13). A signal sensed during the noise sampling period of Medtronic pulse generators is represented by a telemetered marker pulse indicating a ventricular "sense refractory" (SR or VR event). Such a signal does not reset the lower rate timer, but it resets (restarts) other intervals as follows:

1. Initiation of a complete ventricular refractory period, with the blanking period occupying the first 125 msec takes place. The duration of the ventricular refractory period remains unchanged and nonprogrammable except in older models (7001, 7005, 7006) in which the ventricular refractory period extends to 345 msec, as after a VPC (see Table 31–13).

2. A new PVARP is started, together with nonprogrammable automatic extension to 400 msec, because the pacemaker interprets the sensed signal (in the refractory period) as a VPC.

3. A new URI is set. By design the upper rate circuit governs only the rate of atrial-triggered ventricular pacing.

These considerations have important implications. When a ventricular signal is detected during a noise sampling period, it retriggers another complete ventricular refractory period. With continual retriggering, the pulse generator will eventually time out at the LRI and appear to be pacing asynchronously. Such ventricular refractory period design is particularly effective in preventing inhibition of the pacing output by electromagnetic or skeletal muscle interference.[12]

Atrioventricular Interval

Variability of the AV interval is common during DDD and DDDR pacing, and its interpretation requires a thorough understanding of pacemaker timing cycles. One must consider

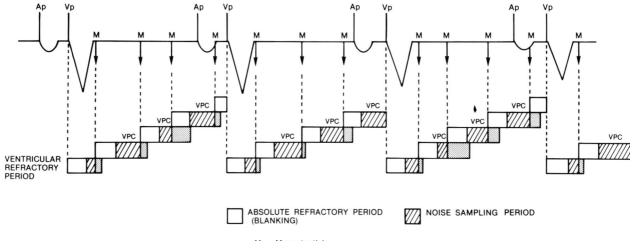

FIGURE 31–80. Conversion of the Medtronic Symbios dual-chamber pacemaker (Medtronic Inc., Minneapolis, MN) from the DDD to the DOO mode from repetitive myopotential (M) oversensing by the ventricular channel. When M signals are sensed by the ventricular channel in the noise sampling period (beyond the absolute refractory period), a new and complete ventricular refractory period (VRP) is initiated. The VRP is automatically extended when the pulse generator detects two ventricular events without an intervening P wave (VPC extension). This VRP extension occurs only with Models 7001, 7005, and 7006 DDD pulse generators. Subsequent generations of devices function in the same way except that a sensed event in the noise sampling period reinitiates the VRP without any extension. The overlapping VRPs cause the pulse generator to pace asynchronously at the lower rate. The stippled parts indicate where the VRP would have terminated had sensing not occurred in the noise sampling period. (From Barold SS, Falkoff MD, Ong LS, et al: Timing cycles of DDD pacemakers. *In* Barold SS, Mugica J [eds]: New Perspectives in Cardiac Pacing. Mt Kisco, NY, Futura Publishing Co., 1988, pp 69–119.)

the following events that constitute the AV interval: As, Ap, Vs, Vp, as already defined, as well as P waves and QRS complexes not necessarily sensed at the correct time.

DIFFERENTIAL DIAGNOSIS OF VARIABLE ATRIOVENTRICULAR INTERVALS DURING DUAL-CHAMBER PACING

Obviously, during normal function, As-Vs is shorter than As-Vp, and Ap-Vs is shorter than Ap-Vp according to the status of AV conduction. Application of the magnet produces changes in the AV interval specific to a particular device.

1. *Spontaneous activity*
   (a) As-Vs < As-Vp normal situation
   (b) As-Vs > As-Vp as programmed
            > Ap-Vp as programmed

Repetitive aborted Wenckebach sequence. The P wave is sensed. URI has not timed out when Vs occurs.
   (c) P-Vs (P = P wave) > As-Vp
   The P wave falls in the PVARP and is therefore unsensed despite an adequate atrial electrogram. Possible PVARP automatic extension or PVARP reinitiation.
   (d) As-R (R = QRS complex) > As-Vp
   Ventricular oversensing during the AV interval.
2. *Atrial stimulation followed by spontaneous ventricular activity*
   (a) Ap-Vs < Ap-Vp normal situation
   (b) Ap-R > Ap-Vs or Ap-Vp as programmed
   Oversensing during AV interval, including crosstalk.
3. *Paced AV interval*
   (a) Ap-Vp < Ap-Vp as programmed
   Ventricular safety pacing

TABLE 31–13. **MEDTRONIC RETRIGGERABLE VENTRICULAR REFRACTORY PERIODS**

MODEL	VENTRICULAR BLANKING PERIOD (msec)	VENTRICULAR REFRACTORY PERIOD (msec)	VENTRICULAR REFRACTORY PERIOD EXTENSION AFTER VENTRICULAR REFRACTORY PERIOD (msec)[a]	POSTVENTRICULAR ATRIAL REFRACTORY PERIOD EXTENSION	EFFECT OF SENSING P WAVE IN POSTVENTRICULAR ATRIAL REFRACTORY PERIOD (msec)
7001		225	345	400	No effect
7005		225	345	400	No effect
7006		225	345	400	No effect
Synergyst I	125	230	No	400	No effect
Synergyst II	125	230	No	400	No effect
Elite I	125	230	No	400	Prevents VPC status (no PVARP extension)
Elite II	125	230	No	400	As above
Minuet	125	230	No	400	As above

Abbreviations: VPC, ventricular premature contraction; PVARP, postventricular atrial refractory period.
[a]The total value of the ventricular refractory period = 345 msec. The actual extension is 120 msec.

Rate-adaptive (sensor-controlled shortening)

(b) Ap-Vp > Ap-Vp as programmed

During DDD pacing in devices with pure atrial-based lower rate timing, some pacemakers deliver Ap on time but delay Vp to avoid violation of the URI.[170]

4. *Spontaneous atrial activity followed by ventricular stimulation*

(a) As-Vp > As-Vp as programmed
> Ap-Vp as programmed

Wenckebach block upper rate upper rate limitation. AV extension can occur with a single atrial premature depolarization.

(b) As-Vp < As-Vp as programmed

A rate-adaptive AV delay mimics the physiologic shortening of the PR interval during physiologic increase in the atrial rate. The pacemaker AV interval can shorten progressively secondary to an increase in the atrial rate (duration of previous cycle) or an increase in the sensor-controlled rate related to increase in sensor activity, or both.

(c) P-Vp < As-Vp as programmed

This occurs during VDD pacing when the P wave is late and falls in the implied AV interval that has already started. The pacemaker therefore does not sense the P wave. The pacemaker releases Vp at the end of the LRI. The P wave does not trigger Vp.

(d) P-Vp < As-Vp (P = P wave)

Atrial oversensing before the P wave initiates the AV interval. The P wave is unsensed as it falls in the already initiated and refractory AV interval.

REFERENCES

1. Furman S: Comprehension of pacemaker timing cycles. *In* Furman S, Hayes DL, Holmes DR Jr: A Practice of Cardiac Pacing, 3rd ed. Mt Kisco, NY, Futura Publishing, 1993, pp 135–194.
2. Barold SS: Lower rate and related timing cycles of dual-chamber pacemakers: The need for precise definitions and language. Eur J Cardiac Pacing Electrophysiol 3:278, 1993.
3. Bernstein AD, Camm AJ, Fletcher R, et al: The NASPE/BPEG generic pacemaker code for antibradyarrhythmia and adaptive-rate pacing and antitachy-arrhythmia devices. PACE 10:794, 1987.
4. Barold SS, Carrol M: ''Double reset'' of demand pacemakers. Am Heart J 84:276, 1972.
5. Barold SS, Falkoff MD, Ong LS, et al: Oversensing by single-chamber pacemakers: Mechanisms, diagnosis, and treatment. Cardiol Clin 3:565, 1985.
6. Barold SS: Clinical significance of pacemaker refractory periods. Am J Cardiol 28:237, 1971.
7. Barold SS, Gaidula JJ: Evaluation of normal and abnormal sensing functions of demand pacemakers. Am J Cardiol 28:201, 1971.
8. Driller J, Barold SS, Parsonnet V: Normal and abnormal function of the pacemaker magnetic switch. J Electrocardiol 6:1, 1973.
9. Barold SS: Upper rate of DDD pacemakers: The view from the atrial side. PACE 11:2149, 1989.
10. Barold S, Mugica J, Falkoff MD, et al: Multiprogrammability in cardiac pacing: *In* Barold SS (ed): Modern Cardiac Pacing. Mt Kisco, NY, Futura Publishing, 1985, pp 377–409.
11. Brandt J, Fahraeus T, Schüller H: Far-field QRS complex sensing in the atrial pacemaker lead. II. Prevalence, clinical significance, and possibility of intraoperative prediction in DDD pacing. PACE 11:1540, 1988.
12. Barold SS, Falkoff MD, Ong LS: Interference in cardiac pacemakers: Endogenous sources. *In* El-Sherif N, Samet P (eds): Cardiac Pacing and Electrophysiology, 3rd ed. Philadelphia, WB Saunders, 1991, pp 634–651.
13. Barold SS, Falkoff MD, Ong LS, et al: Cardiac pacing for the treatment of tachycardia. *In* Barold SS (ed): Modern Cardiac Pacing. Mt Kisco, NY, Futura Publishing, 1985, pp 693–725.
14. Barold SS, Falkoff MD, Ong LS, et al: Termination of ventricular tachycardia by chest wall stimulation during DDD pacing. Am J Med 84:549, 1988.
15. Barold SS: Clinical uses of chest wall stimulation in patients with DDD pulse generators. Intel Rep Cardiac Pacing Electrophysiol 7:2, 1988.
16. Friedberg HD, Barold SS: On hysteresis in pacing. J Electrocardiol 6:1, 1973.
17. Technical Manual, Relay Models 293-03 and 294-03. Angleton, TX, Intermedics, Inc., 1992.
18. Rosenqvist M, Vallin HO, Edhag KO: Rate hysteresis pacing: How valuable is it? A comparison of the stimulation rates of 70 and 50 beats per minute and rate hysteresis in patients with sinus node disease. PACE 7:332, 1984.
19. Thompson ME, Shaver JA: Undesirable cardiac arrhythmias associated with rate hysteresis pacemakers. Am J Cardiol 38:685, 1976.
20. Hollins WJ, Leman RB, Kratz JM, et al: Limitations of the long-term clinical application of rate hysteresis. PACE 10:302, 1987.
21. Morgan JM, Amer AS, Ingram A, et al: Diagnosis and treatment of vasovagal syndrome. PACE 14:667, 1991.
22. Katritsis D, Ward DE, Camm AJ: Can we treat carotid sinus syndrome? PACE 14:1367, 1991.
23. Spritzer RC, Donoso E, Gadboys HI, et al: Arrhythmias induced by pacemaking on demand. Am Heart J 77:619, 1969.
24. Vera Z, Mason DT, Awan NA, et al: Lack of sensing by demand pacemakers due to intraventricular conduction defects. Circulation 815:51, 1975.
25. Barold SS, Falkoff MD, Ong LS, et al: A-A and V-V lower rate timing of DDD and DDDR pulse generators. *In* Barold SS, Mugica J (eds): New Perspectives in Cardiac Pacing. Mt Kisco, NY, Futura Publishing, 1991, pp 203–247.
26. Barold SS, Falkoff MD, Ong LS, et al: Timing cycles of DDD pacemakers. *In* Barold SS, Mugica J (eds): New Perspectives in Cardiac Pacing. Mt Kisco, NY, Futura Publishing, 1988, pp 69–119.
27. Barold SS, Falkoff MD, Ong LS, et al: Function and electrocardiography of DDD pacemakers. *In* Barold SS (ed): Modern Cardiac Pacing. Mt Kisco, NY, Futura Publishing, 1985, pp 645–676.
28. Barold SS, Falkoff MD, Ong LS et al: Electrocardiography of contemporary DDD pacemakers. A. Basic concepts, upper rate response, retrograde ventriculoatrial conduction, and differential diagnosis of pacemaker tachycardias. *In* Saksena S, Goldschlager N (eds): Electric Therapy for Cardiac Arrhythmias: Pacing, Antitachycardia Devices, Catheter Ablation. Philadelphia, WB Saunders, 1990, pp 225–264.
29. Furman S: Comprehension of pacemaker cycles. *In* Furman S, Hayes DL, Holmes DR (eds): A Practice of Cardiac Pacing, 2nd ed. Mt Kisco, NY, Futura Publishing, 1989, pp 115–166.
30. Barold SS: Management of patients with dual-chamber pacemakers: Central role of the pacemaker atrial refractory period. Learning Center Highlights (Heart House). Am Coll Cardiol 5:8, 1990.
31. Levine PA: Postventricular atrial refractory periods and pacemaker-mediated tachycardias. Clin Prog Pacing Electrophysiol 1:394, 1983.
32. Furman S, Reicher-Reiss H, Escher DJW: Atrio-ventricular sequential pacing and pacemakers. Chest 63:783, 1973.
33. Barold SS, Ong LS, Falkoff MD, et al: Crosstalk or self-inhibition in dual-chamber pacemakers. *In* Barold SS (eds): Modern Cardiac Pacing. Mt Kisco, NY, Futura Publishing, 1985, pp 615–623.
34. Barold SS, Falkoff MD, Ong LS, et al: Upper rate response of DDD pacemakers. *In* Barold SS, Mugica J (eds): New Perspectives in Cardiac Pacing. Mt Kisco, NY, Futura Publishing, 1988, pp 121–172.
35. Furman S, Gross J: Dual-chamber pacing and pacemakers. Curr Prob Cardiol 15:119, 1990.
36. Barold SS, Belott PH: Behavior of the ventricular triggering period of DDD pacemakers. PACE 10:1237, 1987.
37. Levine PA: Normal and abnormal rhythm associated with dual-chamber pacemakers. Cardiol Clin 3:595, 1985.
38. Levine PA: Base rate behavior of dual-chamber pacing systems. *In* Barold SS, Mugica J (eds): New Perspectives in Cardiac Pacing 3. Mt Kisco, NY, Futura Publishing, 1993, pp 215–232.
39. Barold SS, Falkoff MD, Ong LS, et al: Arrhythmias caused by dual-chambered pacing. *In* Steinbach K (ed): Proceedings of the 7th World Symposium on Cardiac Pacing. Darmstadt, Steinkopff Verlag, 1983, pp 505–510.
40. Barold SS, Falkoff MD, Ong LS, et al: Electrocardiography of DDD pacemakers. B. Multiprogrammability, follow-up, and troubleshooting. *In* Saksena S, Goldschlager N (eds): Electrical Therapy for Cardiac Arrhythmias. Pacing, Antitachycardia Devices, Catheter Ablation. Philadelphia, WB Saunders, 1990, pp 265–301.

41. Barold SS, Falkoff MD, Ong LS, et al: All dual-chamber pacemakers function in the DDD mode. Am Heart J 115:1353, 1988.

42. Furman S: Dual-chamber pacemakers: Upper rate behavior. PACE 8:197, 1985.

43. Luceri RM, Castellanos A, Zaman L, et al: The arrhythmia of dual-chamber cardiac pacemakers and their management. Ann Intern Med 99:354, 1983.

44. Stoobrandt R, Willems R, Holvoet G, et al: Prediction of Wenckebach behavior and block response in DDD pacemakers. PACE 9:1040, 1986.

45. Higano ST, Hayes DL: Quantitative analysis of Wenckebach behavior in DDD pacemakers. PACE 13:1456, 1990.

46. Fearnot NE, Smith HJ, Geddes LA: A review of pacemakers that physiologically increase rate: The DDD and rate-responsive pacemakers. Prog Cardiovasc Dis 29:145, 1986.

47. DenDulk K, Lindemans FW, Wellens HJJ: Noninvasive evaluation of pacemaker circus movement tachycardia. Am J Cardiol 53:537, 1984.

48. Warren J, Falkenberg E: Wenckebach type upper rate behavior: A mixed blessing. (Abstract.) PACE 8:A-37, 1985.

49. Barold SS: Electrocardiography of rate-adaptive dual-chamber (DDDR) pacemakers: Upper rate behavior. In Alt E, Barold SS, Stangl K (eds): Rate-Adaptive Pacing. Heidelberg, Berlin, Springer-Verlag, 1993, pp 195–221.

50. Ritter P: La stimulation DDDR définitive: Aspects techniques. Stimucoeur 18:29, 1990.

51. Furman S, Cooper A: Atrial fibrillation during AV sequential pacing. PACE 5:133, 1982.

52. Barold SS, Falkoff MD, Ong LS, et al: Characterization of pacemaker arrhythmias due to normally functioning AV demand (DVI) pulse generators. PACE 3:712, 1980.

53. Barold SS, Falkoff MD, Ong LS, et al: Function and electrocardiography of DVI pacing systems. In Barold SS (eds): Modern Cardiac Pacing. Mt Kisco, NY, Futura Publishing, 1985, p 625.

54. Barold SS, Falkoff MD, Ong LS, et al: Interpretation of electrocardiograms produced by a new unipolar multiprogrammable ''committed'' AV sequential (DVI) pulse generator. PACE 4:692, 1981.

55. Levine PA, Seltzer JP: AV universal (DDD) pacing and atrial fibrillation. Clin Prog Pacing Electrophysiol 1:275, 1983.

56. Floro J, Castellanet M, Florio J, et al: DDI: A new mode for cardiac pacing. Clin Prog Pacing Electrophysiol 2:255, 1984.

57. Barold SS: The DDI and DDIR modes of cardiac pacing. Characteristics and indications. Cardiostimolazione 11:317, 1993.

58. Sutton R, Ingram A, Kenny RA, et al: Clinical experience of DDI pacing. In Belhassen B, Feldman S, Copperman Y (eds): Cardiac Pacing and Electrophysiology. Proceedings of the VIIIth World Symposium on Cardiac Pacing and Electrophysiology. Jerusalem, Keterpress Enterprises, 1987, pp 161–163.

59. Guzy P, Goldschlager N: Considerations in the selection of cardiac pacing systems. In Saksena S, Goldschlager N (eds): Electrical Therapy for Cardiac Arrhythmias: Pacing, Antitachycardia Devices, Catheter Ablation. Philadelphia, WB Saunders, 1990, pp 154–162.

60. Hayes DL, Levine PA: Pacemaker timing cycles. In Ellenbogen KA (ed): Cardiac Pacing. Boston, Blackwell Scientific Publication, 1992, pp 263–308.

61. Hayes DL: Timing cycles of permanent pacemakers. Cardiol Clin 10:593, 1992.

62. Hayes DL, Osborn MJ: Pacing. A. Antibradycardia devices. In Giuliani ER, Fuster V, Gersh BJ, et al (eds): Cardiology: Fundamentals and Practice. St. Louis, Mosby-Year Book, 1991, pp 1014–1079.

63. Dodinot B, BarrosCosta A: Intérêts et limites du mode DDI. Stimucoeur 20:205, 1992.

64. Brinker JA, Platia EV: Bradyarrhythmias and pacemaker therapy. In Platia EV (ed): Management of Cardiac Arhythmias: The Nonpharmacologic Approach. Philadelphia, JB Lippincott, 1987, pp 156–200.

65. Clarke M, Sutton R, Ward D, et al: Recommendations for pacemaker prescription for symptomatic bradycardia. Br Heart J 66:185, 1991.

66. Barold SS: The DDI mode of cardiac pacing. PACE 9:480, 1987.

67. Lau CP: DDDR pacing. Lower and upper rate behaviors. In Lau CP: Rate-adaptive Cardiac Pacing: Single and Dual Chamber. Mt Kisco, NY, Futura Publishing, 1993, pp 271–290.

68. Cunningham TM: Pacemaker syndrome due to retrograde conduction in a DDI pacemaker. Am Heart J 115:478, 1988.

69. Markowitz HT: DDI and DDIR: Unforeseen Limitations: Technical Concept. Minneapolis, Medtronic, 1989.

70. Markewitz A, Schad N, Hemmer W, et al: What is the most appropri-

ate simulation mode in patients with sinus node dysfunction? PACE 9:1115, 1986.

71. Sutton R: Pacing in atrial arrhythmias. PACE 13:1823, 1990.

72. Vanerio G, Maloney JD, Pinski SL, et al: DDIR versus VVIR pacing in patients with paroxysmal atrial tachyarrhythmias. PACE 14:1630, 1991.

73. Bana G, Locatelli V, Piatti L, et al: DDI pacing in the bradycardia-tachycardia syndrome. PACE 13:264, 1990.

74. Dreifus LS, Fisch C, Griffin JC, et al: Guidelines for implantation of cardiac pacemakers and antiarrhythmia devices. A report of the American College of Cardiology (American College of Cardiology/American Heart Association Task Force on Assessment of Diagnostic and Therapeutic Cardiovascular Procedures, Committee on Pacemaker Implantation). J Am Coll Cardiol 18:1, 1991.

75. Varriale P, Pilla AG, Tekriwal M: Single-lead VDD pacing system. PACE 13:757, 1990.

76. Antonioli GE, Ansani L, Barbieri D, et al: Single-lead VDD pacing. In Barold SS, Mugica J (eds): New Perspectives in Cardiac Pacing 3. Mt Kisco, NY, Futura Publishing, 1993, pp 359–381.

77. Barold SS: Automatic mode switching during antibradycardia pacing in patients without supraventricular tachycardia. In Barold SS, Mugica J (eds): New Perspectives in Cardiac Pacing 3. Mt Kisco, NY, Futura Publishing, 1993, pp 455–481.

78. Barold SS, Mond HG: Optimal antibradycardia pacing in patients with paroxysmal supraventricular tachyarrhythmias; Role of fallback and automatic mode switching mechanisms. In Barold SS, Mugica J (eds): New Perspectives in Cardiac Pacing 3. Mt Kisco, NY, Futura Publishing, 1993, pp 483–518.

79. Mond HG, Barold SS: Dual-chamber rate-adaptive pacing in patients with paroxysmal supraventricular tachyarrhythmias: Protective measures for rate control. PACE 16:2168, 1993.

80. Barold SS, Mond HG: Fallback responses of dual chamber (DDD and DDDR) pacemakers. A proposed classification. PACE (in press.)

81. Sanders R, Barold SS: Understanding elective replacement indicators and automatic parameter conversion mechanisms in DDD pacemakers. In Barold SS, Mugica J (eds): New Perspectives in Cardiac Pacing. Mt Kisco, NY, Futura Publishing, 1991, pp 203–227.

82. Hayes DL, Ketelson A, Levine P, et al: Understanding timing systems of current DDDR pacemakers. Eur J Cardiac Pacing Electrophysiol 3:70, 1993.

83. Markowitz T, Prest-Berg K, Betzold R, et al: Clinical implications of dual-chamber responsive rate pacing. In Belhassen B, Feldman S, Copperman Y (eds): Cardiac Pacing and Electrophysiology. Proceedings of the VIIIth World Symposium on Cardiac Pacing and Electrophysiology. Jerusalem, Keterpress, 1987, pp 165–170.

84. Levine PA, Hayes DL, Wilkoff BL, et al: Electrocardiography of rate-modulated pacemaker rhythms. Sylmar, CA, Siemens-Pacemaker, 1990, pp 1–90.

85. Stroobandt R, Willems R, Sinnaeve A: Dual-chamber rate-responsive (DDDR) pacing: Ventricular versus atrial timing. In Andries E, Brugada P, Stroobandt R (eds): How to Face ''The Faces'' of Cardiac Pacing. Dordrecht, The Netherlands, Kluwer Academic Publishers, 1992, pp 127–137.

86. Stroobandt R, Willems R, Vandenbulcke F, et al: DDDR pacemakers: A framework for the understanding of atrial and ventricular based device timing. Eur J Cardiac Pacing Electrophysiol 2:151, 1992.

87. Lau CP: DDDR pacing: Lower and upper rate behaviors. In Lau CP: Rate-Adaptive Cardiac Pacing: Single and Dual Chamber. Mt Kisco, NY, Futura Publishing, 1993, pp 271–

88. Merillat JC: Understanding and assessing DDDR pacing systems in adaptive rate pacing: Perspectives in cardiac rhythm management. St. Paul, MN, Cardiac Pacemakers, 1993, pp 53–85.

89. Barold SS: Electrocardiography of rate-adaptive dual-chamber (DDDR) pacemakers. 1. Lower rate behavior. In Alt E, Barold SS, Stangl K (eds): Rate-Adaptive Pacing. Heidelberg, Berlin, Springer-Verlag 1993, pp 173–194.

90. Medtronic Synergystics: Synergyst II Guidelines to Operation and Patient Management. Minneapolis, Medtronic, 1989.

91. Garson A Jr, Coyner T, Shannon CE, et al: A systematic approach to the fully automatic (DDD) pacemaker electrocardiogram. In Gillette PC, Griffin JC (eds): Practical Cardiac Pacing. Baltimore, Williams & Wilkins, 1986, pp 181–270.

92. Siemens 674 DDD Pulse Generator, Technical Manual. Solna, Sweden, Siemens, 1984.

93. Technical Manual, Elite 7074/75/76/77. Activity-responsive dual-chamber pacer with telemetry. Minneapolis, Medtronic, 1991.

94. User's Guide for the Medtronic Elite II Pacemaker. Minneapolis, MN, Medtronic, 1992.

95. Technical Manual, Elite II 7084/85/86. Activity-responsive dual-chamber pacemaker with telemetry. Minneapolis, Medtronic, 1992.

96. Technical Manual, Synergyst 7026/7027 Dual-Chamber Pacer with VVI Activity Response and Telemetry. Minneapolis, Medtronic, 1989.

97. Technical Manual, Synergyst II 7070/7071 Activity Responsive Dual-Chamber Pacer with Telemetry. Minneapolis, Medtronic, 1989.

98. Hayes DL: DDDR timing cycles: Upper rate behavior. *In* Barold SS, Mugica J (eds): New Perspectives in Cardiac Pacing 3. Mt Kisco, NY, Futura Publishing, 1993, pp 233–257.

99. Tolentino AO, Javier RP, Byrd C, et al: Paced-induced tachycardia associated with an atrial synchronous ventricular inhibited (ASVIP) pulse generator. PACE 5:251, 1982.

100. Furman S, Fisher JD: Endless loop tachycardia in an AV universal (DDD) pacemaker. PACE 5:476, 1982.

101. Akhtar M, Gilbert C, Mahmud R, et al: Pacemaker-mediated tachycardia: Underlying mechanism, relationship to ventriculoatrial conduction, characteristics, and management. Clin Prog Pacing Electrophysiol 3:90, 1985.

102. Barold SS: Repetitive reentrant and nonreentrant ventriculoatrial synchrony in dual-chamber pacing. Clin Cardiol 14:754, 1991.

103. Friart A: Termination of magnet-unresponsive pacemaker endless loop tachycardia by carotid sinus massage. Am J Med 87:1, 1989.

104. Perrins EJ, Morley CA, Dixy J, et al: The pharmacologic blockade of retrograde atrioventricular conduction in paced patients. (Abstract.) PACE 6:A-112, 1983.

105. Barold SS, Falkoff MD, Ong LS, et al: Pacemaker endless loop tachycardia: Termination by simple techniques other than magnet application. Am J Med 85:817, 1988.

106. Fontaine JW, Maloney JD, Castle LW, et al: Noninvasive assessment of ventriculoatrial conduction and early experience with the tachycardia termination algorithm in pacemaker-mediated tachycardia. PACE 9:212, 1986.

107. Hayes DL, Furman S: Atrioventricular and ventriculoatrial conduction times in patients undergoing pacemaker implant. PACE 6:38, 1983.

108. Westveer DC, Stewart JR, Goodfleish R, et al: Prevalence and significance of ventriculoatrial conduction. PACE 7:784, 1984.

109. Altamura G, Boccadamo R, Toscano S, et al: Incidence of and drug effect on ventriculoatrial conduction in patients with bradyarrhythmias. *In* Pérez Gómez F (ed): Cardiac Pacing: Electrophysiology: Tachyarrhythmias. Mt Kisco, NY, Futura Media Services, 1985, pp 735–742.

110. Harriman RJ, Pasquariello JL, Gomes JAC, et al: Autonomic dependence of ventriculoatrial conduction. Am J Cardiol 56:285, 1985.

111. Cazeau S, Daubert C, Mabo P, et al: Dynamic electrophysiology of ventriculoatrial conduction: Implications for DDD and DDDR pacing. PACE 13:1649, 1990.

112. VanMechelen RV, Ruiter J, Vanderkerckhove Y, et al: Prevalence of retrograde conduction in heart block after DDD pacemaker implantation. Am J Cardiol 57:797, 1986.

113. Hayes DL, Holmes DR, Vliestra RE, et al: Changing experience with dual-chamber (DDD) pacemakers. J Am Coll Cardiol 4:556, 1984.

114. Calfee RV: Pacemaker-mediated tachycardia: Engineering solutions. *In* Barold SS, Mugica J (eds): New Perspectives in Cardiac Pacing. Mt Kisco, NY, Futura Publishing, 1988, pp 357–373.

115. Hayes DL: Endless loop tachycardia: The problem has been solved? *In* Barold SS, Mugica J (eds): New Perspectives in Cardiac Pacing. Mt Kisco, NY, Futura Publishing, 1988, pp 375–386.

116. Barold SS, Falkoff MD, Ong LS, et al: Programmability in DDD pacing. PACE 7:1159, 1984.

117. Littleford P, Curry RC Jr, Schwartz KM, et al: Pacemaker-mediated tachycardia: A rapid bedside technique for induction and observation. Am J Cardiol 52:287, 1983.

118. Greenspon AJ, Greenberg RM: Noninvasive evaluation of retrograde conduction times to avoid pacemaker tachycardia. J Am Coll Cardiol 5:1403, 1985.

119. Gabry MD, Klementowicz P, Furman S: Balanced endless loop tachycardia. PACE 9:294, 1986.

120. Klementowicz PT, Furman S: Selective atrial sensing in dual-chamber pacemakers eliminates endless loop tachycardia. J Am Coll Cardiol 7:590, 1986.

121. Bernheim C, Markewitz A, Kemkes BM: Can reprogramming of atrial sensitivity avoid an endless loop tachycardia? (Abstract.) PACE 9:293, 1986.

122. DenDulk K, Lindeman FW, Wellens HJJ: Merits of various antipacemaker circus movement tachycardia features. PACE 9:1055, 1986.

123. DenHeijer P, Grinjns HJGM, VanBinsbergen EJ, et al: Orthodromic pacemaker circus movement tachycardia. PACE 10:955, 1987.

124. Duncan JL, Clark MF: Prevention and termination of pacemaker-mediated tachycardia in a new DDD pacing system (Siemens-Pacesetter Model 2010T). PACE 11:1679, 1988.

125. Goldschlager N: Advances in avoidance and termination of pacemaker-mediated tachycardia. *In* Barold SS, Mugica J (eds): New Perspectives in Cardiac Pacing. Mt Kisco, NY, Futura Publishing, 1991, pp 459–471.

126. Bonnet JL, Limousin M: A new algorithm to solve endless loop tachycardia (ELT): A multicenter study of 1816 ELTs. PACE 13:555, 1990.

127. Nitzsché R, Gueunoun M, Lamaison D, et al: Endless loop tachycardia: Description and first clinical results of a new fully automatic protection algorithm. PACE 13:1711, 1990.

128. Mugica J, Barold SS, Ripart A: The smart pacemaker. *In* Barold SS, Mugica J (eds): New Perspectives in Cardiac Pacing. 2. Mt Kisco, NY, Futura Publishing, 1991, pp 545–577.

129. Goy J, Vogt P, Kappenberger L: Activity sensing for prevention of pacemaker-mediated tachycardia in DDD pacing. PACE 11:531, 1988.

130. Nitzsché R, Girodo S, Limousin M, et al: Use of a new fallback function to prevent endless loop tachycardia: First clinical results. PACE 15:1851, 1993.

131. VanGelder LM, El Gamal MIH: Ventriculoatrial conduction: A cause of atrial malpacing in AV universal pacemakers. A report of two cases. PACE 8:140, 1985.

132. Sudduth B, Goldschlager N: Retrograde ventriculoatrial conduction in atrial refractoriness: Cause of apparent failure of atrial capture. Clin Prog Electrophysiol Pacing 4:56, 1986.

133. Barold SS, Falkoff MD, Ong LS, et al: AV desynchronization arrhythmia during DDD pacing. *In* Belhassen S, Feldman S, Cooperman Y (eds): Cardiac Pacing and Electrophysiology. Jerusalem, Keterpress Enterprises, 1987, pp 177–184.

134. Barold SS, Falkoff MD, Ong LS, et al: Magnet-unresponsive pacemaker endless loop tachycardia. Am Heart J 116:726, 1988.

135. Barold SS: Repetitive non-reentrant ventriculoatrial synchrony in dual-chamber pacing. *In* Santini M, Pistolese M, Alliegro A (eds): Progress in Clinical Pacing 1990. Amsterdam, Excerpta Medica, 1990, pp 451–471.

136. Schüller H, Brandt J: The pacemaker syndrome: Old and new causes. Clin Cardiol 14:336, 1991.

137. Chien WW, Foster E, Phillips B, et al: Pacemaker syndrome in a patient with DDD pacemaker for long QT interval. PACE 14:1209, 1991.

138. Hayes DL: Pacemaker electrocardiography. *In* Furman S, Hayes DL, Holmes DR (eds): A Practice of Cardiac Pacing, 3rd ed. Mt Kisco, NY, Futura Publishing, 1993, pp 309–359.

139. Higano ST, Hayes DL, Eisinger G: Sensor-driven rate smoothing in a DDDR pacemaker. PACE 12:922, 1989.

140. VanMechelen R, Ruiter J, DeBoer H, et al: Pacemaker electrocardiography of rate smoothing during DDD pacing. PACE 8:684, 1985.

141. Hanich RF, Midei MG, McElroy BP, et al: Circumvention of maximum tracking limitations with a rate-modulated dual-chamber pacemaker. PACE 12:392, 1989.

142. Feuer JM, Shandling AH, Ellstad MH: Sensor-modulated dual-chamber cardiac pacing: Too much of a good thing too fast? PACE 13:816, 1990.

143. Higano ST, Hayes DL: P-wave tracking above the maximum tracking rate in a DDDR pacemaker. PACE 12:1044, 1989.

144. Hayes DL, Higano ST, Eisinger G: Electrocardiographic manifestations of a dual-chamber rate-modulated (DDDR) pacemaker. PACE 12:555, 1989.

145. Higano ST, Hayes DL, Eisinger G: Advantages of discrepant upper rate limits in a DDDR pacemaker. Mayo Clin Proc 64:932, 1989.

146. Lescault G, Frank G, Girodo S, et al: Tachycardias atriales et stimulation double chambre. Utilité potentielle de l'algorithme de repli. Stimucoeur 18:8, 1990.

147. Van Wyhe G, Sra J, Rovang K, et al: Maintenance of atrioventricular sequence after His bundle ablation for paroxysmal supraventricular rhythm disorders: A unique use of the fallback mode in dual-chamber pacemakers. PACE 14:410, 1991.

148. Vaneiro G, Patel S, Ching E, et al: Early clinical experience with a minute ventilation sensor DDDR pacemaker. PACE 14:1815, 1991.

149. Lee MT, Adkins A, Woodson D, et al: A new feature for control of inappropriate high rate tracking in DDDR pacemaker. PACE 13:1852, 1990.

150. Lau CP, Tai YI, Fong PC, et al: Atrial arrhythmia management with sensor controlled atrial refractory period and automatic mode switching in patients with minute ventilation sensing dual-chamber rate-adaptive pacemakers. PACE 15:1504, 1992.

151. Lau CP, Tai YT, Fong PC, et al: The use of implantable sensors for the control of pacemaker-mediated tachycardias: A comparative evaluation between minute ventilation sensing and acceleration sensing dual-chamber rate-adaptive pacemakers. PACE 15:34, 1992.

152. Azara D, Girardi C, Ruffa H, et al: Assessment of rate smoothing in dual-chamber pacemakers. Am J Cardiol 70:548, 1992.

153. Papp MA, Mason T, Gallastegni J: Use of rate smoothing to treat pacemaker-mediated tachycardias and symptoms due to upper rate response of a DDD pacemaker. Clin Prog Pacing Electrophysiol 2:547, 1984.

154. Satler LF, Rackley CE, Pearle DL, et al: Inhibition of a physiologic pacing system due to its antipacemaker-mediated tachycardia mode. PACE 8:806, 1985.

155. DenDulk K, Wellens HJ: Failure of the postventricular premature beat DVI mode in preventing pacemaker circus movement tachycardia. Am J Cardiol 54:1371, 1984.

156. Greenspon AJ, Volasin KJ: "Pseudo" loss of atrial sensing by a DDD pacemaker. PACE 10:943, 1987.

157. Wilson JH, Lattner S: Undersensing of P waves in the presence of adequate P wave due to automatic postventricular atrial refractory period extension. PACE 12:1729, 1989.

158. vanGelder BM, vanMechelen R, denDulk K, et al: Apparent P wave undersensing in a DDD pacemaker post exercise. PACE 15:1651, 1992.

159. Dodinot B, Beurrier D, Simon JP, et al: "Functional" loss of atrial sensing causing sustained first to high-degree AV block in patients treated with dual-chamber pacemakers. (Abstract.) PACE 16:1189, 1993.

160. Freedman RA, Rothman MT, Jason JW: Recurrent ventricular tachycardia induced by an atrial synchronous ventricular inhibited pacemaker. PACE 5:490, 1982.

161. Furman S, Fisher JD: Repetitive ventricular firing caused by AV universal (DDD) pacing. Chest 83:586, 1983.

162. Dodinot BP, Medeiros P, Galvão SS, et al: Endless loop dual-chamber pacemaker tachycardias related to R-wave sensing by the atrial circuit. PACE 8:301, 1985.

163. Dodinot B, Medeiros P, Galvão S, et al: Dual-chamber pacemaker sustained tachycardias related to "cross ventricular sensing." Stimucoeur Med 14:15, 1986.

164. Pimenta J, Soldá R, Britto Pereiva C: Tachycardia mediated by an AV universal (DDD) pacemaker triggered by a ventricular depolarization. PACE 9:105, 1986.

165. Wittkampf FHM, Boute W: Return to Wenckebach. Improved timing cycles for dual-chamber pacemakers. In Barold SS, Mugica J (eds): New Perspectives in Cardiac Pacing. Mt Kisco, NY, Futura Publishing, 1988, pp 173–186.

166. User's Guide Meta DDDR 1254 Telectronics Pacing System. Englewood, CO, Telectronics, 1993.

167. Ahmed R, Worzewski W, Ingram A, et al: A new pacemaker algorithm preventing atrial tracking during atrial flutter/fibrillation in DDD pacing. (Abstract.) Eur Heart J 12:414, 1991.

168. Curry PVL, Rowland E, Krikler DM: Dual demand pacing for refractory atrioventricular reentry tachycardias. PACE 2:137, 1979.

169. Barold SS, Falkoff MD, Ong LS, et al: Interference in cardiac pacemakers: Exogenous sources. In El-Sherif N, Samet P (eds): Cardiac Pacing and Electrophysiology, 3rd ed. Philadelphia, WB Saunders, 1991, pp 608–633.

170. Fredman CS, Bjerregaard P, Janosik DL, et al: Unusual Wenckebach upper rate response of an atrial-based DDD pacemaker. PACE 15:975, 1992.

CHAPTER 32

PACEMAKER DIAGNOSTICS: MEASURED DATA, EVENT MARKER, ELECTROGRAM, AND EVENT COUNTER TELEMETRY

Paul A. Levine
Richard Sanders
H. Toby Markowitz

Over the years, pacemakers have advanced from nonprogrammable single-chamber asynchronous devices (VOO) to dual-chamber systems with extensive programmability, including the ability to automatically adjust the pacing rate based on signals that are independent of the intrinsic heart rhythm (DDDR). The analysis of a pacing system was comparatively easy during the early days of pacing, but the difficulty in evaluating the modern pacemaker has increased to the degree that is concordant with the sophistication of the current devices. To facilitate these evaluations, manufacturers have incorporated a multiplicity of diagnostic tools into the pacemaker. These features can be accessed by the programmer and are the subject of this chapter. The various capabilities commonly complement one another and either eliminate the need for ancillary testing or focus the direction for additional tests. Occasionally, a given feature provides absolutely unique information that is not readily available by any other technique.

Bidirectional Telemetry

Telemetry is the ability to transmit information or data from one device to another. The development of telemetry was essential to the introduction of programmability, which is the ability to noninvasively change the functional parameters of the pacing system by coded commands transmitted to the pacemaker from a programmer.[1-4] In the early days of programmability, it was often suggested that if the clinician was changing a parameter, such as sensitivity or refractory period, that could not be independently confirmed on the electrocardiogram (ECG), a parameter, such as rate, should also be programmed. The change in the rate would confirm that the pacemaker received the programming command and responded appropriately. The first generation of programmable pacemakers used unidirectional telemetry from the programmer to the pacemaker. These systems were not able to transmit data from the pacemaker to the programmer.

Bidirectional telemetry is communication in two directions. With respect to pacing systems, the pacemaker and programmer can communicate with each other. Bidirectional telemetry was essential for the development of the multiple diagnostic capabilities that are the subject of this chapter.[5, 6] Bidirectional telemetry in pacing was first implemented in rechargeable pacemakers. It was used to confirm the proper alignment of the recharging head with the implanted pacemaker. When the recharging wand was not aligned properly with the pacemaker, there was an audible beep from the charging unit to notify the patient and whomever was in attendance of this condition. When the two were correctly aligned, the system was silent.

Bidirectional telemetry was next applied to confirmation of programming. This was particularly valuable for those parameters that did not result in an obvious change in pacing system performance or which could not be independently identified on an ECG recording. This capability is essential for the DDDR pacemaker and third-generation implantable cardioverter-defibrillators, which may have 20, 30, or even more independently programmable parameters, most of which are invisible on the ECG (Fig. 32–1). Bidirectional telemetry not only confirms the pacemaker's correct response to a program command but also allows the unit to be interrogated as to its programmed parameters when the patient is seen during follow-up or is evaluated for a suspected pacing system malfunction.

Measured Data

Complementing the interrogation of programmed data is the provision of measured data. This includes data obtained from the pacemaker, which detail lead and battery function at the time of evaluation and demand and asynchronous rates (see Fig. 32–1).

BATTERY STATUS

Although not all systems provide the same information, data concerning battery function often include a measure of battery voltage, current drain, and/or impedance.[7–9] All three parameters are interrelated. The battery current drain is a measure of the average current being drained from the battery at 100% pacing at the programmed rate and output settings. Lead or stimulation impedance is a nonprogrammable parameter that may dramatically affect the current drain of the battery. The current drain provides a worst-case assessment of system function because if the pacemaker is inhibited in one or both chambers for some part of the day, the actual current drain is less than that reported and the projected longevity calculations based on the reported current drain understate the effective longevity of the system.

The current drain of the battery can be used to qualitatively assess the effect of programming changes on the longevity of the system. After the rate and/or output is changed, the measured data can be interrogated. Most manufacturers provide the usable battery capacity reported in Ampere-hours. If the battery's capacity is converted to microampere-hours and then divided by the current drain of the battery, this results in the anticipated number of hours of normal function at the programmed rate and output. This number, when divided by 8760, the number of hours in 1 year, yields an estimate of the longevity of the system in years.

Although virtually every pacemaker incorporates a change in the magnet and demand rates and sometimes mode or

Pacesetter® Systems, Inc. A Siemens Company ©1991
APS: Version 3039a – 2013M

Synchrony® II

Feb 25 1993 3:40 pm
MODEL: 2022   SERIAL: 14209

PATIENT: _____

PHYSICIAN: _____

PROGRAMMED PARAMETERS

	INITIAL	PRESENT
Mode	DDDR	DDDR
Sensor	ON	ON
Rate	50	50 ppm
A-V Delay	150	150 msec
Max Track	175	175 ppm
Vent. Pulse Config.	BIPOLAR	BIPOLAR
V. Pulse Width	.4	.4 msec
V. Pulse Amplitude	2.5	2.5 Volts
V. Sense Config.	BIPOLAR	BIPOLAR
V. Sensitivity	2.0	2.0 mVolts
V. Refractory	250	250 msec
Atr. Pulse Config.	BIPOLAR	BIPOLAR
A. Pulse Width	.4	.4 msec
A. Pulse Amplitude	2.5	2.5 Volts
A. Sense Config.	BIPOLAR	BIPOLAR
A. Sensitivity	1.0	1.0 mVolts
A. Refractory	275	275 msec
Blanking	38	38 msec
V. Safety Option	ENABLE	ENABLE
PVC Options	NORMAL DDD	NORMAL DDD
PMT Options	10 BEATS >175	10 BEATS >175
Rate Resp. A-V Delay	ENABLE	ENABLE
Magnet	TEMPORARY OFF	TEMPORARY OFF
Threshold	AUTO (+0.0)	AUTO (+0.0)
Measured Average Sensor	2.9	2.9
Slope	8 (Normal)	8 (Normal)
Maximum Sensor Rate	150	150 ppm
Reaction Time	FAST	FAST
Recovery Time	MEDIUM	MEDIUM

MEASURED DATA

Pacer Rate	49.7	ppm

Ventricular:
Pulse Amplitude	2.4	Volts
Pulse Current	4.6	mAmperes
Pulse Energy	4	μJoules
Pulse Charge	2	μCoulombs
Lead Impedance	511	Ohms

Atrial:
Pulse Amplitude	2.4	Volts
Pulse Current	4.6	mAmperes
Pulse Energy	4	μJoules
Pulse Charge	2	μCoulombs
Lead Impedance	519	Ohms

Battery Data: (W.G. 8077 – NOM. 1.8 AHR)
Voltage	2.74	Volts
Current	16	μAmperes
Impedance	2	KOhms

FIGURE 32–1. Initial interrogation of a Synchrony II rate-modulated dual-chamber pacemaker (Siemens-Pacesetter, Sylmar, CA) with the programmed parameters, measured data telemetry, model, serial number, date, and time. AV, atrioventricular; A, atrial; V, ventricular.

other functions to signal a depletion of the battery that warrants pulse generator replacement, most of these changes occur when the battery's voltage reaches a predefined level, which is specific for each manufacturer and, sometimes, for each model pacemaker. These changes are termed elective or recommended replacement time indicators (ERT, ERI, or

$$\frac{\text{Number of Ampere-hours}}{\text{Battery}} \times \frac{1 \times 10^6 \text{ Microampere-hours}}{1.0 \text{ Ampere-hours}} \times \frac{1 \text{ year}}{8760 \text{ hours}} = \text{Longevity}$$

RRT). Although they are often abrupt, there is commonly a 3- to 6-month period between activation of the ERT indicator and erratic behavior caused by the depletion of the battery. A marker to determine when to increase the frequency of pacing system surveillance, either transtelephonically or in the office, included in some systems and called an intensified follow-up indicator, provides an indication of the battery status, even before reaching the ERT.

Given the degree of programmability of most pacemakers today, a dual-chamber pacemaker programmed to a rapid base rate with a maximal output on each channel may last only 2 years; the identical model programmed to a low base rate, with outputs of 2.5 V or even lower on each channel and inhibited a significant portion of the time, may be anticipated to function properly for 10 years or longer. It would be inappropriate to follow the second unit on a monthly basis, beginning 1 year after implantation; it would be equally inappropriate to plan annual checks on a pacing system programmed with high outputs and rapid rates. By being able to follow some measure of the status of the battery, the clinician can achieve a qualitative assessment as to when to increase the frequency of pacing system follow-up.[10]

There are two primary indicators of battery status. One is the battery voltage itself, which progressively decreases over time (see Chapter 4). At the present time, virtually all pulse generators are powered by a lithium-iodine power cell. The nominal unloaded output voltage is 2.8 V, with each manufacturer triggering the RRT indicator at a specified battery voltage. The battery voltage and programmed output voltage are not identical. The programmed output voltage is achieved with either voltage multipliers or charge pumps to provide a higher voltage, or a voltage can be divided to deliver a voltage lower than 2.8 V. As energy is consumed, the battery voltage progressively decreases, even when the manufacturer has included circuitry to maintain the stability of the delivered programmed voltage to the patient. The ability to track the progressive decrease in battery voltage provides a guideline to the physician to prescribe the frequency with which the pacing system is routinely checked for signs of battery depletion.

Inversely related to battery voltage is battery impedance. In the lithium-iodine power cell, the release of electrons occurs by the combination of the lithium ion with two iodine atoms. The result of this chemical reaction is the release of two electrons (negatively charged particles) and the formation of lithium iodide. As the lithium iodide accumulates, it forms a resistive barrier between the anode and the cathode. Thus, as progressive cell depletion occurs, the increasing amount of lithium iodide results in a rise in the internal impedance of the battery. Some pacemakers report battery impedance in the telemetered measured data. The higher the battery impedance, the lower the cell voltage is.

Either or both of these parameters, battery voltage and impedance, may be tracked, and if these measurements are provided to the manufacturer's technical service engineers along with the programmed parameters, an estimate of the percentage of time during which the pacemaker is inhibited, and the measured current drain of the battery, the remaining longevity of that pacing system can be estimated, assuming that these parameters remain stable. These calculations have also been incorporated into the programmer to provide an online estimate of longevity based on the assumption of 100% pacing. The accuracy of this prediction is dependent on the tolerances and accuracy of the measurements of battery status and is, at best, an approximation because projections of a battery's function are based on accelerated testing and not battery monitoring under normal conditions. Thus, the understanding of actual battery function may be modified based on normal battery depletion experience with implanted units.

LEAD STATUS

Although many systems provide data concerning lead function, including pulse voltage, current, charge, and energy, the measurement that is used most frequently is that of lead impedance. Changes in lead impedance affect the other measures of lead function. The terms resistance and impedance, while different, are used interchangeably in pacing. Impedance is a complex concept in which changes in various factors result in varying resistance. The resistance to electron flow in a pacing system progressively rises during the delivery of the stimulation pulse as a result of polarization at the electrode-myocardial interface and, thus, is appropriately termed impedance. However, many systems, whether it be the pulse generator or pacing system analyzer, usually make this measurement at a specific point within the pacing stimulus; other devices report an average resistance throughout the pulse. Furthermore, the actual resistance to current flow imparted by the conductor coil is fixed and represents only a portion of the total lead resistance. The progressive polarization at the electrode-myocardial interface and the conduction through the body's tissues play a larger role in the overall resistance of the system. All this is loosely incorporated in the measurement termed either lead or stimulation impedance.

Stimulation impedance is affected by many factors, not the least of which are electrode size, configuration, and materials. Manufacturers are attempting to design electrodes with a low capture threshold but a high impedance to reduce the overall current drain of the battery and effectively increase the unit's longevity. For any given lead model, there is a range of normal impedances, and for a specific lead within that model series, the impedance should fall within a relatively narrow range.

The clinician can use knowledge of the lead impedance to follow and identify a developing lead problem, but only if the baseline data are available. In addition, it is essential to know what device is being used to make these measurements because different devices, particularly pacing system analyzers, may obtain these data at different points in the pacing stimulus. Furthermore, the impedance measurement obtained with a pacing system analyzer at the time of implantation may be significantly different from that obtained by telemetry from the implanted pacemaker. This difference does not imply a problem. Impedances may evolve over time, with a fall in impedance occurring in the days to weeks after implantation followed by a gradual rise toward the initial measurements on a chronic basis. Multiple factors may affect impedance, particularly in a unipolar system, such that measurements obtained during deep inspiration may significantly differ from those obtained during maximal exhalation. In the same patient, impedance measurements obtained that are based on a single output pulse may normally vary by 100 ohms or even more during the same follow-up evaluation.

If a marked change in lead impedance (>200 ohms) is encountered during a routine follow-up evaluation and the patient is clinically asymptomatic with stable capture and sensing thresholds, increased follow-up is appropriate, but operative intervention would be premature. However, a dramatic change in telemetered lead impedance in the presence of a clinical problem directs the physician toward the likely source of the difficulty (Fig. 32–2).

A dramatic fall in impedance usually reflects a break in the insulation.[11–13] This effectively increases the surface area of the electrode, resulting in a lower impedance. In a unipolar system, an insulation problem provides an alternative pathway for current flow, starting closer to the pulse generator and resulting in less energy reaching the heart, possibly causing a loss of capture. The amplitude of the stimulus artifact determined by the distance from the point at which the current exits the lead to the housing of the pulse generator may also decrease, particularly if it is recorded with an analog ECG machine, giving the appearance of bipolar pacing.

In a bipolar pacing system, an insulation defect between the proximal conductor and the tissues of the body is not likely to affect capture thresholds, but it results in a larger stimulus artifact, making it appear unipolar. Depending on the actual location of the insulation failure in either the bipolar or unipolar lead, stimulation of the extracardiac muscle contiguous to the insulation defect may occur. Insulation failures may also attenuate the electrical signal reaching the pacemaker, possibly resulting in sensing failure.

In a coaxial bipolar lead, an insulation defect developing between the proximal and distal conductors can present with a number of clinical manifestations. As the two conductors make contact, a voltage transient is generated, which the pacemaker can sense, resulting in inhibition or triggering, depending on the programmed sensing mode. This signal is not seen on the surface ECG and, thus, is appropriately termed oversensing. If the two conductors remain in contact,

current flowing down the distal conductor is short-circuited to the proximal conductor and never reaches the electrodes. This may result in a loss of capture and a further reduction in the amplitude of the normally diminutive bipolar stimulus artifact. Here too, loss of appropriate sensing may occur.

Although programming the output configuration to unipolar in those systems that have this capability prevents the loss of capture and possibly undersensing from a total short circuit, it does not prevent the oversensing behavior from make-break electrical transients generated by intermittent contact between the two conductors. When programmed to the unipolar output configuration, the telemetered lead impedance rises. This, however, is not a cure and should only be considered a temporary measure. The malfunctioning lead should be replaced expeditiously.

An increase in lead impedance may be the result of a conductor fracture or a connection problem.[14] When this occurs, the lead impedance often rises to high levels. If the impedance is high, there is no current flow and, hence, no output, with loss of capture. The reduced current flow also results in a fall in the measured current drain of the battery.

Prior to the availability of telemetry for lead impedance measurements, physicians could obtain similar information by oscilloscopic analysis of the pacemaker stimulus. In the 1970s, some manufacturers included a photograph of the pulse wave contour at various impedances with the technical manual accompanying each pacemaker. More recently, some computer-based ECG systems can record and display the pacemaker pulse at an expanded scale so that its waveform can be recorded and tracked as a routine part of the periodic pacing system evaluation.

Unfortunately, lead impedance measurements have an indeterminate incidence of false-negative results when the lead problem is only intermittently manifested. The system forces the pacemaker to function asynchronously to make these measurements. However, the measurements are made over only a few cycles. If there is a true lead problem but it is intermittent and was not present when the measurements were being made, the telemetered lead impedance may be normal. Thus, if a problem is suspected, repeated measurements are required. In addition, stressing the lead by placing manual pressure on it or having the patient raise or in other ways manipulate the ipsilateral arm may be required to unmask a problem. It is often awkward to obtain measurements during these maneuvers.

There are some pacemakers that can report lead impedance measurements on a beat-by-beat basis, allowing the physician to observe the digital read-out of lead impedance on the programmer screen over a protracted number of cycles to look for an intermittent unexpected fluctuation. Like the oscilloscopic monitoring of the pulse wave morphology, this reduces the incidence of false-negative studies but does not totally exclude this limitation.

Event Marker Telemetry

Interpretation of the paced ECG has challenged the medical profession since the early days of pacing. This reflects a learning curve on the part of medical personnel from the time when single-chamber rhythms with a limited number of timing cycles were relatively easy to interpret. However, even

294-03-001024		APR 13 '93	11:46 AM	*
RELAY	TELEMETRY DATA			I
PACING RATE			70 PPM	N
PACING INTERVAL	860 MSec			T
CELL VOLTAGE			2.48 VOLTS	E
CELL IMPEDANCE			< 2.5 KOHMS	R
CELL CURRENT			40.1 UA	M
	ATRIAL (Bi)		VENTRICULAR (Bi)	E
SENSITIVITY	1.3		3.0 MV	D
LEAD IMPEDANCE	501		Low OHMS	I
PULSE AMPLITUDE	3.43		3.13 VOLTS	C
PULSE WIDTH	0.45		0.45 MSEC	S
OUTPUT CURRENT	6.5		HIGH MA	
ENERGY DELIVERED	9.1		HIGH UJ	I
CHARGE DELIVERED	2.94		HIGH UC	N
				C
			RETURN	*

FIGURE 32–2. Measured data telemetry from a Relay rate-modulated dual-chamber pacemaker (Intermedics, Angleton, TX) reporting a low impedance on the ventricular lead as a result of an insulation failure. This also results in an increase in the battery or cell current caused by a higher output current, charge, and energy being delivered by the pacemaker, whether or not it reaches the heart.

then, multiple assumptions had to be made; the clinician evaluated a surface ECG composed of P waves, representing native atrial depolarizations, and QRS complexes or R waves, representing native ventricular depolarizations. The pacemaker responds to the intrinsic deflection, the electrical potential inside the heart that occurs when the wave of depolarization passes by the pacing electrode. Although the events inside the heart frequently correspond to events recorded by the ECG, there may be events inside the heart that are not visible on the ECG. In addition, the pacemaker may sense and, hence, respond to events occurring outside the heart when detected by the sense amplifier. These same electrical events may not be easily observed by the standard ECG recordings.

The development of dual-chamber pacing increased the level of complexity of the paced rhythm. The interaction between the two channels of the pacing system, with the spontaneous rhythms occurring in either the atria or ventricles, added to the potential for confusion. The addition of rate-modulated pacing (i.e., allowing the pacemaker to also respond to one or more sensor signals that are invisible on the ECG) further contributes to the challenge of interpreting the paced ECG.

In the modern pacemaker, an interpretation of the paced rhythm requires a knowledge of the basic timing intervals, a variety of refractory periods (postventricular atrial refractory periods, ventricular refractory periods, ventricular blanking periods, and atrioventricular [AV] intervals), and the intervals that may change depending on the rate (AV intervals, atrial escape intervals when under sensor drive, and postventricular atrial refractory periods). The clinician also needs to be aware of a number of device-specific responses to protect the system from a variety of known but undesirable behaviors, including crosstalk, a premature ventricular beat initiating a pacemaker-mediated tachycardia (PMT), and multiblock upper rate behavior.

To facilitate interpretation of the paced rhythm, many pacing systems incorporate the ability of the pacemaker to trans-

mit information to the programmer continuously, detailing its beat-by-beat behavior. Both pacing stimulus events and sensing events are communicated to the programmer. This information is displayed as a series of positive or negative marks, with or without alphanumeric annotation, that are generically termed event markers. These have the greatest diagnostic value when superimposed above or below a simultaneously recorded surface ECG (Fig. 32–3). Some systems also display the duration of the atrial and ventricular refractory periods; others show events that are sensed during the refractory period but do not play a role in altering the system timing (sensed but not used). Many systems have the ability to provide interval measurements, either online or after the tracing has been frozen on the programmer screen by using cursors to identify the interval that should be measured. If a monitor-type screen is used to show the rhythm and event markers, the frozen tracing can often be printed for inclusion in the medical record (Fig. 32–4).

Event markers, also called marker channel, annotated event markers, and main timing events, are most effectively used when displayed with a simultaneously recorded ECG rhythm.[15-18] Without the ECG, the event marker simply reports the behavior of the pacemaker. This information is valuable, implying that energy has been released or that sensing has occurred. What it does not confirm is that the stimulus effectively depolarized the heart. It also does not confirm that the stimulus reached the heart. An open circuit, for example, a severe breach in the insulation, may preclude the output pulse from reaching the heart, or there may have been a native depolarization, which was not sensed, allowing the stimulus to be released at a time when the myocardium was physiologically refractory. If the markers reported that an event was sensed on the atrial channel followed by a ventricular output pulse after a preset delay (P-wave synchronous ventricular pacing), the clinician would know that the pacemaker was capable of sensing in the atria and pacing in the ventricle. However, without a simultaneously recorded ECG, it would be impossible to determine whether the pacemaker

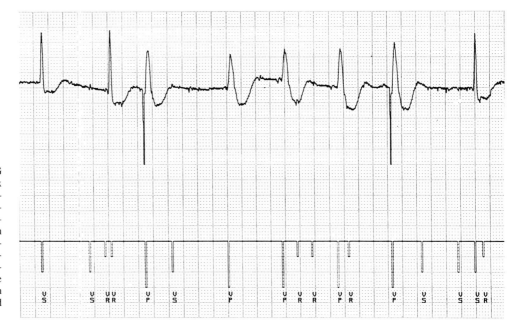

FIGURE 32–3. Simultaneous ECG and event markers from an Activitrax bipolar rate-modulated single-chamber pacemaker (Medtronic, Minneapolis, MN) with an internal insulation failure of the lead. There is both oversensing (VS and VR) and functional undersensing when the true native complex coincides with the refractory period initiated by the oversensing. During the intervention for lead replacement, the measured lead impedance was 125 ohms.

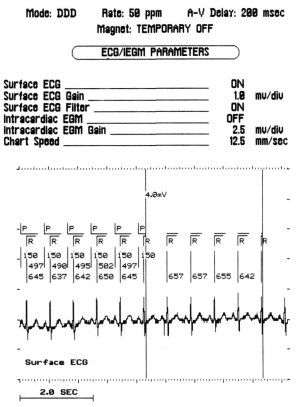

FIGURE 32–4. Event markers were recorded during an atrial sensing threshold test with a Synchrony II pulse generator (Siemens-Pacesetter). The horizontal line following each letter symbol identifies the length of the refractory period on the respective channel. Loss of atrial sensing occurs at a sensitivity setting of 4 mV, with normal sensing at 3 mV. The numbers are the millisecond durations for the PR, RP, and RR intervals, respectively. The tracing sweep speed was compressed to 12.5 mm/sec. ECG, electrocardiograph; EGM, electrogram; IEGM, intracardiac EGM; A-V, atrioventricular.

was responding to inappropriate signals on the atrial channel or, as mentioned earlier, the ventricular stimulus was effective.

EVENT MARKER DISPLAYS

A variety of different displays have been used over the years. Although not intended for this purpose, the simplest event marker for sensed events was achieved with single-chamber triggered mode pacing, particularly if the output configuration was unipolar. A sensed event would now be marked by the simultaneous release of a pacing stimulus coincident with sensing. This was easily recorded on an ECG. The next evolutionary step in this technology involved the pacemaker emitting a series of varying amplitude subthreshold stimuli to represent the release of an output pulse, a sensed event, and the end of the refractory period. Both of these systems, the triggered mode and the series of markers, were limited by the fact that the signals were emitted by the pacemaker through the intact lead system. If the output pulse were bipolar, the diminutive signal might not be readily visible, particularly in the triggered mode, because it could be obscured by the native complexes. In addition, if there were an open circuit, most commonly a conductor fracture, no marker would be visible.

The next improvement was to transmit coded signals that represented pacing and sensing from the pacemaker to the programmer. The programmer then reconstituted these signals into a series of varying amplitude pulses, reflecting paced or sensed events and displaying these either on a monitor screen or recorded by a printer, which was an integral part of the programming system. These systems all allowed for the simultaneous recording of a surface ECG acquired by way of a separate set of cables so that the clinician could directly correlate the behavior of the pacemaker with the patient's rhythm to determine whether the system was functioning properly. A calibration signal composed of a series of different amplitude pulses allowed the clinician to interpret the various markers. The largest reflected a pacing output, the midsized one indicated a sensed event, and the smallest represented either the end of the refractory period or a sensed complex that occurred during the refractory period itself. With the advent of dual-chamber pacing systems, atrial events were identified by a marker pulse extending above the baseline; ventricular events were labeled with a pulse extending below the baseline.

A further refinement to this system was the addition of alphanumeric annotations. Two common sets of notations have been used and are summarized later. These are not the only possibilities because some manufacturers use a unique set of symbols to identify paced and sensed events, with the location of the symbol on the recording identifying whether it represented atrial or ventricular events.

Many of the single-chamber pacing systems with event marker telemetry used the letters P to reflect a paced event and S to represent a sensed event. This has the potential for causing confusion with the output of some dual-chamber systems in which the letter P reflects a sensed atrial event indicating a native P wave (with which most medical personnel are familiar, based on their knowledge of the standard ECG). The interpretation of the alphanumeric event markers is often product specific, and this must be taken into account by the clinical personnel who evaluate the pacing system.

In the case of dual-chamber pacing or when the pacemaker knows that it is providing atrial pacing and sensing, a native atrial depolarization may be identified as either the letter P or the combination As. P is taken from the standard ECG identifier for an atrial depolarization. As is the abbreviation for an atrial sensed event. An atrial stimulus is identified by either the letter A or the combination Ap for atrial paced.

Analogous lettering is used on the ventricular channel. Again, single-chamber pacing in some systems might still use the letters P to represent a paced event and S to refer to a sensed event. Other systems use R to refer to a native ventricular depolarization, which is generically called an R wave on the standard ECG. This may also be identified by the letter combination Vs for a ventricular sensed event. The letter V in one system might be used to represent a ventricular pacing stimulus, which may also be shown as Vp for ventricular pacing.

Other symbols may be used for a paced or sensed event, and when this is done, these symbols are commonly displayed with an identifying key on the resultant printout. Each paced or sensed event may also be identified by a vertical line, going up in the case of atrial events and down for ventricular events. In some cases, a difference in the amplitude of these lines has been retained in conjunction with the alphanumeric lettering.

Medtronic (Minneapolis, MN) uses the letter R in conjunction with an A for atrium or V for ventricle to identify and mark events that are sensed during the refractory period but are not used to alter the basic timing of the pacemaker. This is termed ''sensed but not used.'' Other manufacturers incorporate a horizontal line beginning at the onset of either sensing or pacing to indicate the duration of the refractory period. Events coinciding with the refractory period are not otherwise displayed, although an extension of the refractory period marker would signal an event sensed during the terminal portion of the refractory period and, thus, extending it, an integral component of the noise mode response of some pacemakers.

In many systems, interval measurements between the various events are either automatically calculated and displayed or can be measured after cursors are aligned with specific events. There may be a time delay between the actual sensed or paced event and the release of the event marker because a finite period is required for the pacemaker to recognize the event and then transmit this information to the programmer through the telemetry channel. In most cases, priority is given to the normal function of the pacemaker, with the diagnostic marker feature being delayed. Misalignments of up to 40 msec have been noted.

LADDERGRAMMING

Laddergramming, a standard adjunct to the interpretation of clinical arrhythmias, is now being incorporated in some programming systems by using the known programmed parameters of the pacemaker combined with the event marker information telemetered from the implanted pacemaker (Fig. 32–5).[16, 19] For all the elegance of these graphic interpretations of the pacemaker's behavior, they still require the simultaneously recorded ECG rhythms. Although the pacemaker may be functioning normally, in that it is behaving properly with respect to its programmed parameters, failure to capture, undersensing, or oversensing would not be diagnosed from the laddergrams without the surface ECG.

EVENT MARKER LIMITATIONS

There are a number of limitations associated with event marker telemetry. The first is that, by itself, it reports the behavior of the pacemaker but does not allow the clinician to determine whether this behavior is appropriate for the patient.[20] In this regard, it is analogous to the small hand-held digital counters that report pacing rates and intervals. The counters only detect and report the pacing stimuli, not whether these output pulses are effective in causing a cardiac depolarization, whether a long interval between consecutive pacing stimuli reflects normal function because the pacemaker responded appropriately to a native complex, or whether it represents a system malfunction, with oversensing or no output (e.g., from an intermittent lead fracture). Neither event marker telemetry nor the digital counters should be used independent of a simultaneously monitored ECG rhythm.

The second limitation is that the report of a stimulus output does not mean that there is capture. Confirmation of capture requires ECG or concomitant pulse monitoring. In addition, if the markers report that the pacemaker is sensing a signal but this signal is not visible on the surface ECG, is it an appropriate signal that the pacemaker should sense (sometimes intrinsic atrial rhythms may not be visible on the specific lead that is being monitored), or is the system responding to an inappropriate or nonphysiologic signal, such as the make-break potentials associated with a breach of the internal insulation in a coaxial bipolar lead?

In addition, event marker telemetry is limited to real-time recordings. The markers must be telemetered from the pacemaker to the programmer or another display system while the rhythm is being evaluated. The pacemaker or programmer cannot retrospectively provide markers for a previously recorded rhythm. If the pacemaker is responding to events that are not visible on the surface ECG, the event marker simply confirms this fact but does not identify the specific signal. An evaluation of sensed but invisible events requires electrogram (EGM) telemetry or an invasive procedure to record the signal from the implanted lead.

Electrogram Telemetry

The clinician evaluates a pacing system based on an analysis of the ECG, but the pacemaker does not respond to P waves or QRS complexes, which are surface manifestations of the atrial and ventricular depolarization. The recorded signal that enters the pacemaker's sense amplifier by way of the electrode located within or on the heart is termed an EGM or intracardiac EGM. The EGM is composed of a number of components. The portion that is sensed by the

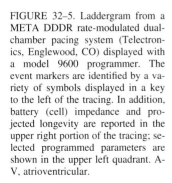

FIGURE 32–5. Laddergram from a META DDDR rate-modulated dual-chamber pacing system (Telectronics, Englewood, CO) displayed with a model 9600 programmer. The event markers are identified by a variety of symbols displayed in a key to the left of the tracing. In addition, battery (cell) impedance and projected longevity are reported in the upper right portion of the tracing; selected programmed parameters are shown in the upper left quadrant. A-V, atrioventricular.

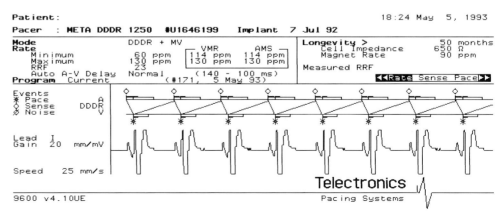

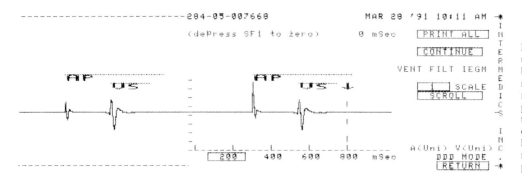

FIGURE 32–6. Telemetered ventricular electrograms are shown after being processed by the pacemaker's sense amplifier and annotated event markers from a Cosmos II dual-bipolar dual-chamber pacemaker (Intermedics) with functional single-chamber atrial pacing (ApVs). The horizontal bar in the event markers represents the length of the refractory period.

pacemaker is termed the intrinsic deflection and reflects the rapid deflection that occurs when the wave of cardiac depolarization passes by the electrode. The intrinsic deflection can be characterized by both the amplitude and slew rate. The derivative of the voltage or the change in voltage amplitude divided by the time duration of this portion of the signal is the slew rate. The unit of measurement is volts per second or millivolts per milliseconds. Most implanted pacemakers require a slew rate of more than 0.5 V/sec for proper sensing. The other portions of the cardiac depolarization, as reflected by the EGM, are termed the extrinsic deflection, and although they may have an adequate amplitude, the slew rate is usually too low, precluding this portion of the cardiac signal from being sensed by the pacemaker (see Chapter 2).

At the time of implantation, the amplitude of the EGM is commonly measured with a pacing system analyzer that reports a millivolt amplitude. The pacing system analyzer uses its own unique set of amplifiers, which may not be identical to that of the pacemaker's sense amplifier. Thus, the analyzer's reported signal, at best, provides an approximation of what the pacemaker effectively sees. The morphology of the EGM observed on a high-fidelity monitor is not identical to the signal as seen by the pacemaker because the filters in the pacemaker's sense amplifier usually have a narrower bandpass and therefore block out some of the frequencies (Fig. 32–6). However, examining the recorded EGM by using a physiologic recorder or telemetry with a wide bandpass can provide valuable information as to the slew rate, splintering of the intrinsic deflection, and other morphologic abnormalities.

Although measuring the peak-to-peak amplitude of the EGM, as recorded at the time of implantation or telemetered from the already implanted pacemaker, is commonly used to determine the "sensing threshold," this may be inappropriate when the frequency content of the signal is outside the constraints of the bandpass filter of the sense amplifier. If the clinician wants to determine the sensing threshold for a given patient, the sensitivity of the system should be progressively reduced until the system no longer consistently senses the native signal. The highest number of the sensitivity settings, usually identified by a millivolt amplitude, at which there is consistent sensing is the sensing threshold (Fig. 32–7). The precision of this measurement is limited by the number and range of the programmable sensitivity options in the specific model of pacemaker.[21–23]

Although the telemetered EGM should not be used to determine the sensing threshold, it has many other roles.[24, 25] A primary value is identifying signals that are being sensed but are not visible on the surface ECG. Another is to facili-

tate an analysis of the timing of the pacing system because a sensed intrinsic deflection resets one or more timers. The intrinsic deflection at which sensing occurs can be best identified from the EGM and only indirectly measured from the surface ECG. Under unique circumstances, the telemetered EGM has been used to confirm capture, particularly atrial, when the evoked complex is not visible in any lead of the surface ECG.[26, 27] This requires a unique output pulse configuration either to cancel the residual polarization artifact or to record the signal through electrodes that are not directly involved with the output pulse. The output pulse has a tendency to overload the telemetry or sense amplifier, driving the signal off scale. This is then followed by a refractory period before anything can again be recognized (Fig. 32–8). The telemetered EGM has been effectively used to diagnose native arrhythmias in which the pacemaker is simply an innocent bystander or to identify retrograde P waves not visible on the surface ECG, facilitating programming of the postventricular atrial refractory period (PVARP) to prevent pacemaker-mediated tachycardias.[27–35] In the case of episodes of undersensing, the telemetered EGM provides clues as to why this may be occurring, including splintering of the EGM or low slew rates that may place the signal outside the tight constraints of the pacemaker's sense amplifier despite an appropriate peak-to-peak amplitude (Fig. 32–9).[36]

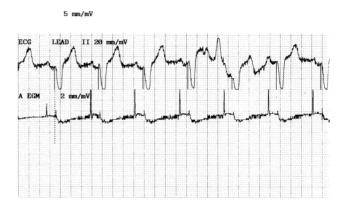

FIGURE 32–7. Simultaneously displayed atrial electrogram and surface electrocardiogram were obtained from an Elite rate-modulated dual-chamber pacemaker (Medtronic) as recorded with the Medtronic 9760 programmer. The peak-to-peak amplitude of atrial electrogram measures 6 mV. Assessing the amplitude of the signal by adjusting the sensitivity settings of the pacemaker, normal sensing was present at 3.5 mV, with loss of sensing occurring at 4.0 mV.

```
PROGRAMMING SELECTED VALUES  13:18:21
** PROGRAMMING CONFIRMED **
VALUES JUST PROGRAMMED:

                         TEMP  PERM

MODE:                          DDD
LOWER RATE:                     50  PPM
UPPER TRACKING RATE:           160  PPM
A-V PACE INTERVAL:             190  MS
A-V SENSE INTERVAL:            120  MS
```

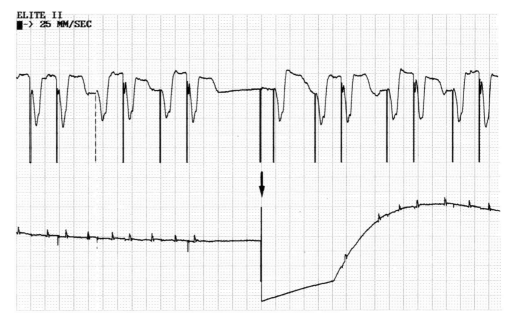

FIGURE 32–8. Atrial-tracking ventricular pacing occurring with an Elite II pacing system (Medtronic) and displayed with simultaneously telemetered atrial electrograms recorded with a Medtronic 9710 programmer. The patient has bradycardia-tachycardia syndrome with an unstable atrial mechanism. With abrupt termination of the endogenous atrial rhythm, the pacemaker escapes with atrial and ventricular pacing. The atrial stimulus *(arrow)* drives the telemetered electrogram off the scale, and in this case, it required 1000 msec before there was a return of an identifiable signal. A-V, atrioventricular.

The telemetered EGM can also be followed on a periodic basis to monitor the progression of the patient's intrinsic disease process. A decrease in the amplitude of the telemetered EGM was reported to effectively identify early rejection in cardiac transplanted patients, with a return to the baseline amplitude correlating with a resolution of the rejection process.[37] Preliminary work on the signal-averaged EGM, either atrial or ventricular, suggests that this may be effective in identifying disease in the respective chamber that may be beyond the resolution of the signal-averaged ECG.[38]

LIMITATIONS OF ELECTROGRAM TELEMETRY

That the telemetered EGM appears to be adequate for sensing does not mean that this is the case. Often, the telemetry amplifier uses different filters from the sensing circuit, providing qualitative rather than quantitative data concerning the EGM. Telemetered EGMs also suffer from limitations that are similar to those of event markers. They are real-time recordings and cannot be retrospectively provided by the programmer to facilitate the interpretation of an earlier ECG.

Real-time telemetry allows the physician to analyze the behavior of the pacing system when the patient is in the physician's office or clinic and these diagnostics are being accessed with the programmer. This is impractical over a long period. In addition, it does not allow the patient to move around much while these recordings are being obtained. Recordings of pacing system behavior require either a Holter monitor, which is expensive and cumbersome, or event counter telemetry, depending on the degree of precision that is desired.

Event Counter Telemetry

Simplistically, the pacemaker "knows" when it has released an output pulse or responded to a sensed event. The availability of high-density, low-power RAM and ROM that can be incorporated in the pacemaker has given pacemakers the ability to store information as to system performance for retrieval at a later date. The objective of the event counters is to facilitate the clinician's ability to analyze and manage the patient's pacing therapy more effectively. Although this may add to the time required for the evaluation, namely to retrieve and interpret these data, the additional time is usually only a few minutes. This technology can provide the clinician with information that is critical to understanding the performance of the system over time, which in turn guides the programming of the system to achieve optimal performance. Other techniques, such as standard Holter recordings or repeated exercise tolerance tests, while valuable, are impractical and arduous to acquire on a routine basis.

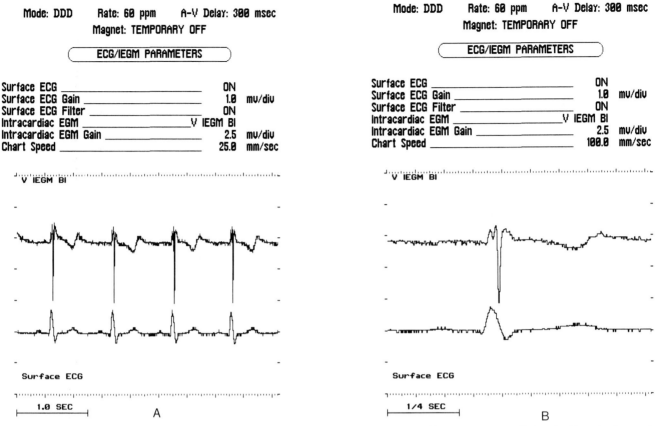

FIGURE 32–9. *A,* Ventricular electrogram telemetered from a Paragon dual-chamber pacemaker (Siemens-Pacesetter) displayed with a simultaneously recorded surface at a chart speed of 25 mm/sec. Although the peak-to-peak amplitude can be measured, additional details regarding the signal are not visible. *B,* The same signal displayed at a chart speed of 100 mm/sec revealing an initial splintering of the early part of the complex with the intrinsic deflection of the EGM occurring late within the QRS. ECG, electrocardiogram; EGM, electrogram; A-V, atrioventricular; IEGM, intracardiac EGM.

The first use of stored diagnostic data in cardiac pacemakers was associated with the introduction of multiparameter programmability. Programmable modes, rates, outputs, sensitivities, and refractory periods made it necessary to keep track of the programmed parameters or know the programmed parameters at the time of the system's evaluation. There was also concern regarding the potential for phantom programming, which is the unexpected uncontrolled alteration of various pacing parameters by exposure to electromagnetic fields in the environment. Although there were infrequent but well-documented cases of phantom programming, the most common cause was poor record keeping. It did not take long before manufacturers included the ability to report the programmed values on command in their pacemakers.

An adjunct to this ability allowed the clinician to enter specific information concerning the patient and pacing system into the pacemaker for retrieval at subsequent evaluations. The date of implant, lead model numbers, pharmacologic regimens, and even acute implant measurements, including capture and sensing thresholds and lead impedances, usually within ranges rather than specific numbers, could be entered into the memory of the implanted pacemaker (Fig. 32–10). This information was printed with the programmed parameters each time the pacemaker was interrogated.

STORAGE OF SYSTEM PERFORMANCE PARAMETERS

Some systems keep track of the number of times a pacing stimulus is released or a native complex is sensed. This allows for an assessment of the degree to which the pacemaker was used. A refinement of this ability allows the pacemaker to diagnose bradycardias and, in the dual-chamber modes, to tell whether the bradycardia was the result of sinus node dysfunction or AV block. Event counters with this ability have been variably called diagnostic data, implanted Holter systems, and event histograms.[39–45]

With the introduction of dual-chamber pacing and specifically the DDD mode, the potential interactions between the pacemaker and the patient increased from two (pacing or sensing in one chamber) to five (pacing or sensing in the atria or ventricles and sensing ventricular activity without preexisting atrial activity). Knowing how the pacing system behaves over time, combined with the clinician's knowledge of the patient, provides invaluable information toward assessing the system's performance.

The various annotations described in the event marker section were combined to provide a cryptic description of the different operational states of the DDD mode, which is often similar to that used for the event markers. These include an atrial sensed event followed by a ventricular sensed event

MAR   4, 1993
12:16 PM

1603 5.5BUE/2.51

PACER STATUS

PHYSICIAN:

PATIENT:

META II 1204H
5N U00064046
IMPLANT DATE
MAY 8, 1992
PROG. NO. 027
ON MAR 4, 1993
LEAD TYPE
VENT. BIPOLAR
MODE
VVIR + MV
RRF
18

FIGURE 32–10. Initial portion of the interrogation printout from a META II single-chamber rate-modulated pacemaker (Telectronics) reporting a variety of administrative data, including the date of implantation, number of times the pacemaker has been programmed, and the lead type. Vent., ventricular; Prog. No., program number.

(AsVs or PR). This indicates that the pacemaker is inhibited on both channels. Atrial sensing followed by a ventricular paced event (AsVp or PV) refers to P wave synchronous ventricular pacing. Atrial pacing with intact AV nodal conduction or functional single-chamber atrial pacing would be indicated by ApVs or AR. Base rate pacing in both chambers would be represented by ApVp or AV. A ventricular sensed event not preceded by atrial activity, either paced or sensed, is a PVE, which refers to a premature sensed ventricular event identified by the letter R or combination Vs.

Additional data that have been collected include the percentage of pacing in the atrium and ventricle, the amount of time at the maximum tracking rate, and the number of episodes in which the pacing system reached the programmed upper rate limit. Another counter reports the number of times special features were activated, such as the pacemaker-mediated tachycardia termination algorithm.

The counters are able to continue to accumulate data until one of the pacing state bins is full and cannot accept one additional bit of information; at this point, all the counters are frozen (Fig. 32–11). The volume of data that can be stored depends on the memory capacity of the pacemaker that is dedicated to this feature.

The following example provides a general idea as to the amount of data that can be stored or the quantity of memory. All data are stored in a binary code, represented by a series of 1s and 0s. A binary unit of memory is called a bit. Eight bits is also called a byte and results in 256 combinations of 1s and 0s. If each series of combinations represents a single item of data, a total of 256 pieces of information can be stored in a system with eight bits of memory. As the number of bits increases, the amount of data that can be stored in-

creases geometrically. If each pacing state is represented by a single combination of bits and there are 24 bits in the RAM devoted to these counters, upward of 17 million events can be counted and stored in memory for retrieval at the time of routine pacing system follow-up. Reading the counters requires access to the memory banks in the pacemaker by using specific coded commands from the programmer. One DDD system introduced in the mid-1980s had this ability, which provided a summary of the pacing system behavior over approximately a 6-month period. As the memory capacity is increased, systems will be able to store more data for longer periods (Fig. 32–12).

Storing a simple marker as to the pacing state and rate requires relatively little memory compared with that required to store waveform data representing the rhythm, as depicted by a consecutive series of EGMs. A theoretical 100-Hz bandwidth with 200 samples per cardiac cycle at eight bits of resolution per sample and recording the entire rhythm during a 24-hour period would require 140,000,000 bits per day and, then, only if the rate was a steady 60 beats per minute. One implantable defibrillator system stores a series of EGMs preceding and following the delivery of antitachycardia therapy. A second manufacturer provides "snapshots" of representative complexes with the trigger to store these data being the delivery of antitachycardia therapy. Extensive storage of cardiac rhythm data, even with the most sophisticated compression algorithms, is going to require more memory than is currently available but is the active goal of many manufacturers.

Furthermore, even if RAM chips with sufficient memory were small enough to be incorporated into a pacemaker, other problems also need to be solved before extensive EGM storage becomes a reality. First, the microprocessors in a pacemaker, unlike those in desk-top or even lap-top computers, must operate in an undernourished power environment. The transmission of data to and from the programmer cannot require great surges of power, which would place a heavy load on the pacemaker's battery. In addition, because such transmission is basically wireless, sophisticated error detection and correction algorithms are needed, which further slow

283-01-017021   MAR 10 '88   11:15 AM   *
               Diagnostic Data (Cardiac Cycles)   I
                                                                       N
EVENT COUNTERS LAST CLEARED......FEB 25, 06:00 pm   T
NO. OF PREMATURE VENTRICULAR EVENTS......10,830   E
NO. OF ATRIAL SENSE EVENTS FOLLOWED   R
        BY VENTRICULAR SENSE EVENT...........15,088,068 M
NO. OF ATRIAL SENSE EVENTS FOLLOWED   E
        BY VENTRICULAR PACE EVENT.................3,122,267 D
NO. OF ATRIAL PACE EVENTS FOLLOWED   I
        BY VENTRICULAR SENSE EVENT................627,336   C
NO. OF ATRIAL PACE EVENTS FOLLOWED   S
        BY VENTRICULAR PACE EVENT................3,417,647
PERCENT PACED – ATRIUM..18%   I
PERCENT PACED – VENTRICLE...................................29%   N
        DISPLAY MISCELLANEOUS EVENTS   C

PRINT   CLEAR EVENT COUNTERS   RETURN   *

FIGURE 32–11. Event counter data from a Cosmos pacemaker (Intermedics) showing the number of counts in each of the pacing states. On a second page, the number of times the system reached its upper rate limit is listed, and the number of times the tachycardia termination algorithm was used is not shown.

Pacesetter® Systems, Inc.
A Siemens Company ©1990
APS: Version 3037a - 4647

Synchrony®II

7 Apr 1993 1:34 pm
MODEL: 2022   SERIAL: 55866

PATIENT: _____

PHYSICIAN: _____

```
┌────────── EVENT HISTOGRAM ──────────┐
```

Total Time Sampled: 413d 10h 22m 60s
Sampling Rate: EVERY EVENT

```
Mode _____ DDD
Sensor _____ PASSIVE
Rate _____ 60  ppm
Max Track _____ 120  ppm
Maximum Sensor Rate _____ 130  ppm
A-V Delay _____ 175  msec
Rate Resp. A-V Delay _____ DISABLE
```

Note: The above values were obtained
when the histogram was interrogated.

Rate	Event Counts				
ppm	PV	PR	AV	AR	PVE
0-60	157,186	145	2,444,581	6,262	0
61-67	4,928,327	3,847	51	423	0
68-75	8,898,433	4,960	0	0	191
76-85	13,038,331	19,694	0	0	1,229
86-100	12,945,813	38,751	0	0	28,291
101-119	4,066,127	13,878	0	0	81,692
120-149	0	14,843	0	0	36,672
> 149	0	1,207	0	0	14,218
Total:	44,034,217	97,325	2,444,632	6,685	162,293

Total Event Count: 46,745,152

```
Percent Paced in Atrium _____ 5%
Percent Paced in Ventricle _____ 99%
Total Time at Max Track Rate _____ 0d 22h 36m 31s
```

Percent of Total Time

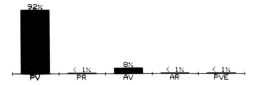

FIGURE 32–12. Event counter data from a Synchrony II (Siemens-Pacesetter) showing the cumulative counts and rate distributions of the various pacing states over a monitoring period of 413 days with every event being sampled. These data are simultaneously displayed as a histogram representing the percentages of use of each of the pacing states. A-V, atrioventricular.

the information exchange. Higher bandwidth data transmission channels are required for data storage, particularly long series of rhythms, so that transmission can be accomplished efficiently and almost instantaneously.

Although an implanted Holter monitor complete with stored rhythms is a laudable goal, the current practicality is limited to data reflecting the total number of times a pacing state was encountered and, in some systems, the distribution of rates or intervals, rate ranges, or mean rates within these pacing states. This information provides the physician with an overview as to the function of the system in the patient. Predominant base rate pacing is expected in a patient with marked sinus node dysfunction or the patient receiving antianginal medications. On the other hand, predominant base

rate pacing, ApVp, in the patient whose primary indication for pacing was complete heart block suggests either the development of sinus node dysfunction or primary atrial undersensing. In this same patient with high-grade AV block, frequent counts of AsVs and PVEs, particularly in the absence of known ventricular ectopy, suggests episodes of ventricular oversensing or the resolution of the AV block. Large numbers of counts regarding PMTs warrant a reassessment of retrograde conduction and the optimal PVARP or PMT programming; a large number of counts at the maximum tracking rate suggests that the upper rate limit should be reassessed. Event counter telemetry can provide an insight into the overall function of the pacing system, and if it varies from the clinician's knowledge of the patient, it might suggest a direction for reevaluation.

When the additional ability to monitor a series of rates and pacing states is added, chronotropic function can be assessed by the distribution of atrial sensed rates (AsVs or PR and AsVp or PV; see Fig. 32–12). Furthermore, atrial pacing at rates above the programmed base rate reflect sensor drive in the DDDR pacing systems. When there is the ability to report rates and pacing state, the clinician can obtain a better insight into the cause of the PVEs. True premature ventricular contractions tend to occur at short coupling intervals, which is equivalent to a rapid rate, and large numbers might suggest recurrent ventricular arrhythmias. If there are large numbers of PVE counts at relatively low rates, the clinician should consider episodes of atrial undersensing or accelerated junctional rhythms, which would also fulfill the pacemaker's criteria for a PVE (i.e., a sensed R wave not preceded by an atrial event).

STORAGE OF SENSOR DATA

Other sources of event counter data are the sensor signal and the theoretical rates that would have been achieved had the sensor been controlling the pacing system. Thus, these have been called sensor-indicated rates and can be displayed as either a histogram of various rates or a table reflecting the actual counts and total accumulated time in each rate bin. This feature allows the clinician to assess sensor performance, even when the pacemaker is being inhibited by a faster native rhythm. As such, it enables the clinical staff caring for the patient to set the sensor parameters while the patient performs activities of daily living in an unmonitored environment. If the monitoring period is short, the sensor-indicated rate counter reflects the system's response to a specific activity.[46, 47] If the period of data collection extends over weeks to months, the sensor-indicated rate counter provides an overview of the sensor performance during this period, although specific activities cannot be identified within the mass of data (Fig. 32–13).

The sensor-indicated rate counters complement the system performance counters. If the patient has severe chronotropic incompetence, then any rate increase is the result of the sensor, and the data in the two counters should be similar. However, if the pacing system either is inhibited by a faster native rhythm or predominantly tracks sensed atrial activity, the system performance counter reflects the actual behavior of the pacemaker with respect to pacing and sensing; the sensor-indicated rate counter provides data as to the distribution of rates that would have occurred had there been chronotropic incompetence.

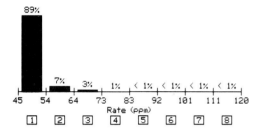

SENSOR INDICATED RATE HISTOGRAM

Total Time Sampled: 28d 1h 37m 52s
Sampling Rate: 1.6 seconds

Sensor	PASSIVE
Rate	50 ppm
Maximum Sensor Rate	120 ppm
Slope	8 (Normal)
Threshold	4.0
Reaction Time	FAST
Recovery Time	MEDIUM
Measured Average Sensor	3.3

Note: The above values were obtained
when the histogram was interrogated.

Bin Number	Range (ppm)	Time	Sample Counts
1	45 – 54	25d 0h 13m 41s	1,329,736
2	54 – 64	1d 20h 51m 16s	99,370
3	64 – 73	0d 19h 23m 6s	42,945
4	73 – 83	0d 6h 37m 16s	14,668
5	83 – 92	0d 1h 29m 55s	3,320
6	92 – 101	0d 0h 47m 21s	1,748
7	101 – 111	0d 0h 12m 2s	444
8	111 – 120	0d 0h 3m 17s	121
		Total:	1,492,352

Percent of Total Time

FIGURE 32–13. The event counter data from a Synchrony II (Siemens-Pacesetter) pulse generator showing the distribution of rates that would have occurred over a period of 28 days had the sensor been driving the pacemaker. The sensor parameter data are displayed above the sensor indicated rate count table and histogram.

The principal limitation associated with the two types of counters described to this point is that counts are placed in a bin, either the pacing state alone or the pacing state and rate, which provides a one-dimensional view of the system's behavior. If the period of monitoring is short, as during a casual or brisk walk, the clinician can reasonably assess the behavior of the pacing system. Longer periods of monitoring overlap the results of many activities, precluding an assessment of the pacing system's behavior during a specific activity or symptomatic episode occurring at an earlier time. The ability of the system to store pacing state and rate data with respect to time (identified as time-based event counters) has been variably termed event record or Holter systems. Technically, this is not yet a true Holter monitor because continuous rhythm recordings are not retained in memory, even though rate data may be available.

TIME-BASED EVENT COUNTERS

Time-based event counters require an extensive amount of memory. Not only is the pacing state and rate stored, it must be stored with respect to the preceding and subsequent events. Thus, the data cannot be simply dumped into a rate or pacing state bin. Each piece of data (i.e., every cardiac

event) must have a time reference. Therefore, it takes significantly more memory to achieve time-referenced data storage.

There are two techniques available for storing real-time data. One is to continue to accumulate the data until the memory is full and then freeze the counter(s). Freezing all the counters maintains the ratios between the events. A clearing function is usually provided to reset the counters; however, sometimes reprogramming of either any parameter or specific parameters, such as the rate or pacing mode, can result in the automatic clearing of these data. This technique is especially useful for short-term monitoring, as in office-based exercise evaluations. This also allows the system's response to exercise to be evaluated, often without the need for simultaneous ECG monitoring.

The other option is to continuously collect the data. As the counters fill, new data are added at the expense of the oldest data (Fig. 32–14). This has been called a rolling trend or

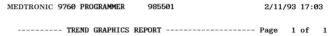

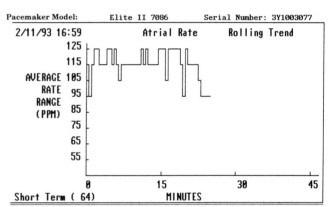

```
MEDTRONIC 9760 PROGRAMMER      985501           2/11/93 17:03

---------- TREND GRAPHICS REPORT -------------------- Page  1 of  1

Pacemaker Model:      Elite II 7086      Serial Number: 3Y1003077
```

| 2/11/93 16:59 | Atrial Rate | Rolling Trend |

```
MEDTRONIC 9760 PROGRAMMER      985501           2/11/93 17:03

---------- TREND TABLE REPORT --------------------- Page  1 of  4

Pacemaker Model:      Elite II 7086    Serial Number: 3Y1003077
Format:      Rolling Trend            Collected:  2/11/93 16:59
Source:      Atrial Rate
Term:        Short

Trend Values:
```

Data Point	Average Rate	Accumulated Time Range	Average % Paced
1	115	.56	0–<25
2	95	1.23	0–<25
3	115	1.79	0–<25
4	125	2.30	0–<25
5	125	2.81	0–<25
6	115	3.37	0–<25
7	115	3.93	0–<25
8	115	4.49	0–<25
9	125	5.00	0–<25
10	125	5.51	0–<25
11	115	6.07	0–<25
12	125	6.58	0–<25

FIGURE 32–14. *A*, Time-dependent event counter (rolling trend) display reporting atrial rates, both paced and sensed, obtained from an Elite II dual-chamber rate-modulated pacing system (Medtronic). In this case, slightly less than 30 minutes of data is displayed because of the relatively rapid rates, which fill the available memory. *B*, The first page of a tabular display of the average rates at each data point is also shown, along with the percentage of complexes that were paced.

continuous data storage. Thus, when the patient is seen in follow-up, the data acquired over the time immediately preceding the interrogation of the system are available for review. The patient can often recall symptoms and activities during this period. These can be correlated with the behavior of the pacing system (Fig. 32–15). In this manner, the clinical staff caring for the patient may further assess chronotropic function, the behavior of the pacemaker during a variety of special or usual activities, and whether the sensor is behaving appropriately and gain insight into the cause of palpitations and other symptoms that may have occurred during this time.[41, 48, 49]

Combining sensor-input data with the actual rates that have been achieved has been used to facilitate programming of the sensor parameters. The data, once acquired, are retained in the memory of the programmer; the rates achieved over time are displayed on a screen. Because the system's performance occurred at a given set of sensor parameters and the system has the actual sensor-signal data, it knows how the unit should perform in response to a different set of sensor parameters. If these other sensor parameters are entered into the programmer, the curves that are based on the original input data are redrawn to display the system's behavior in response to the new set of parameters. The clinical staff can then determine which are the best set of sensor parameters for the individual patient without having the pa-

tient perform repeated activities (Fig. 32–16). This feature has been termed "redraw."[50]

LIMITATIONS OF EVENT COUNTER TELEMETRY

The major value of event counters are that they provide a review of system performance over time. This is not available from the real-time diagnostic features of measured data and event counter and EGM telemetry. However, the data are only interpretable after a detailed assessment as to the capture and sensing thresholds in a manner analogous to event marker telemetry. The pacemaker can only store information that it knows about, namely output or sensed events. If there is a problem with undersensing, the pacemaker releases a pacing pulse, and the counters report a predominant paced rhythm. Similarly, a large number of sensed events cause the pacemaker to be inhibited on the respective channel. The counter simply reports a large percentage of sensed events, but this may be clinically inappropriate if the cause is oversensing.

With respect to pacing, if the rhythm is predominantly composed of AV or PV paced complexes, this does not necessarily indicate complete heart block. It might result from a programmed AV delay that was not sufficiently long to allow for full conduction through the AV node. Although the ventricular complex could have been fully paced, it could

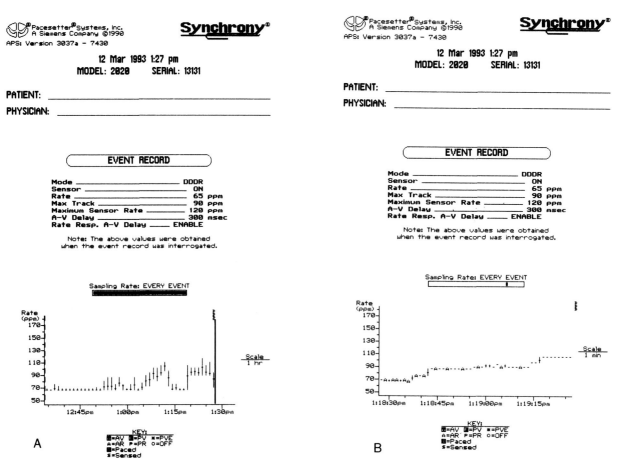

FIGURE 32–15. *A,* Real-time event counter display (event record) from a Synchrony II dual-chamber rate-modulated pacing system (Siemens-Pacesetter) reporting data over the previous 1 hour. The vertical bars reflect maximum and minimum rates; the crossbar identifies the mean rate. *B,* An expansion of the time scale from the middle of the event record display taken from one of the periods of rate increase. The steady rise in rate is associated with functional single-chamber atrial pacing (the AR pacing state identified by the letter A), indicative of sensor drive increasing the paced rate.

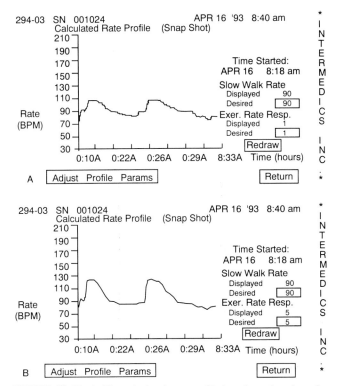

A

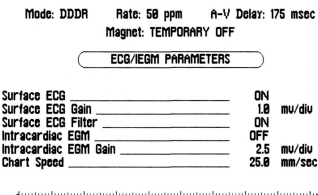

B

FIGURE 32–16. *A*, The calculated rate profile based on time-dependent sensor input data obtained from a Relay dual-chamber rate-modulated pacing system (Intermedics) following a couple of slow walks over a period of 15 minutes. These rates would have been achieved for a rate-response setting of 1. *B*, The calculated rate profile based on these data is shown with the rate-response setting of 5. The clinician can observe the potential system's behavior associated with the various rate-response settings to decide which would be best for the particular patient.

the programmed parameters for pacing and sensing have been determined and the status of the native rhythm is known. If the pacemaker is programmed to provide a good margin of safety for both pacing and sensing, the event counters are likely to be an accurate reflection of the patient's clinical rhythms. This also provides insight as to the degree to which the patient requires pacing support at the current programmed parameters, chronotropic function of the sinus node, and responsiveness of the sensor function. Evidence of oversensing or lead dysfunction renders the event counter data suspect with regard to these findings. The event counter data cannot be adequately interpreted without a knowledge of them and the clinical status of the patient.

Summary

As pacing systems increase in complexity (including both the ability to deliver antitachycardia and bradycardia therapy), use multiple sensors, incorporate a variety of automatic

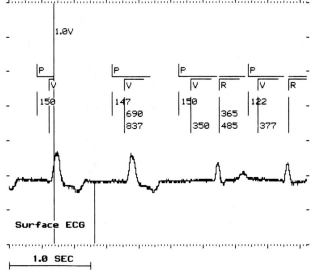

FIGURE 32–17. Although obtained during a ventricular capture threshold test in a Synchrony II pacing system (Siemens-Pacesetter), this printout demonstrates the limitations of some of the telemetry data in the absence of a simultaneously recorded ECG. The last two ventricular output pulses were subthreshold, resulting in a loss of capture. The endogenous P wave conducts with a marked first-degree AV block, placing the R wave outside the ventricular refractory period and allowing it to be sensed. Based on event marker and event counter data, this patient would be interpreted as having frequent "PVEs" interspersed in a stable atrial-sensed ventricular-paced rhythm; in actuality, there was a loss of ventricular capture and intact AV conduction. AV, atrioventricular; ECG, electrocardiogram; EGM, electrogram.

also have been a fusion or pseudofusion beat, and the counters cannot differentiate between these complexes. In addition, there could have been a total loss of ventricular capture with intact AV nodal conduction (Fig. 32–17). The conducted R wave would not have been sensed because it occurred during the refractory period that followed the ventricular output pulse.

The clinician must also be aware of how the pacemaker defines PVEs. Although most true premature ventricular contractions are counted as PVEs, late-cycle PVEs occurring after a sensed P wave (PR or AsVs) or an atrial output pulse (AR or ApVs) are counted as either inhibited or effective single-chamber atrial paced beats with intact AV nodal conduction. In some devices, an atrial premature beat that falls within the PVARP but is conducted is counted as a PVE. This may also be true for accelerated junctional rhythms and very fast supraventricular arrhythmias in which the P wave is not sensed because it falls into an atrial refractory period. Further refinements in some current and future pacemakers enable the system to recognize a P wave during the relative refractory period and to classify a subsequent conducted and sensed R wave as a PR or an AsVs rather than a PVE. True atrial undersensing and episodes of ventricular oversensing are also called PVEs by the pacemaker with event counter capability.

The event counters simply report the system's performance without making any statement as to the appropriateness of this behavior. The information provided by the event counters can be interpreted only after the appropriateness of features (such as rate and possibly AV interval modulation based on sensor input), and increase the adjustment of output and sensitivity, the need for event counters and other diagnostic features increases. The roles of programmed parameter, battery, and lead measured data and event marker and EGM telemetry along with event counters were reviewed as to their utility and some of their limitations. Many products available today include at least some of these abilities with varying levels of sophistication. It was not the purpose of this chapter to review the individual abilities of each model pacemaker that is currently on the market or under investigation. The illustrations, of necessity, reflect the features of a given manufacturer's product, but they are intended to be illustrative only and not an endorsement of one product over another. Space did not allow for comparable examples of a given technology from each of the manufacturers whose products incorporate this ability.

Furthermore, it should be recognized that, although the diagnostic features incorporated in an implanted pulse generator often facilitate the evaluation of the patient and a suspected system malfunction, the same final results can usually be obtained without these features. In addition, the various abilities complement one another and often achieve their greatest value when used together.

The clinical staff caring for a patient who has a pacemaker that incorporates one or more of the diagnostic features discussed in this chapter should be familiar with each of these features and routinely use them during each evaluation of the patient. This not only facilitates the evaluation, but may also uncover subclinical problems that might not be otherwise suspected, allowing them to be corrected before the patient is symptomatic. This is the major value of both the real-time and event counter diagnostic abilities incorporated in the modern pacemaker.

REFERENCES

1. Furman S: Pacemaker programmability. PACE Pacing Clin Electrophysiol 1:161, 1978.
2. Furman S, Escher DJW, Fisher JD: Seven-year experience with programmable pulse generators. *In* Meere C (ed): Cardiac Pacing. Montreal, Pacesymp Publications, 1979, Chap. 19–1.
3. Levine PA: Why Programmability? Indications for and Clinical Utility of Multiparameter Programmability. Sylmar, CA, Pacesetter Systems, 1981.
4. Gold RD, Saulson SH, MacGregor DC: Programmable pacing systems: The medium and the message. PACE Pacing Clin Electrophysiol 5:777, 1982.
5. Sholder J, Levine PA, Mann BM, Mace RC: Bidirectional telemetry and interrogation in cardiac pacing. *In* Barold SS, Mugica J (eds): The Third Decade of Cardiac Pacing: Advances in Technology and Clinical Applications. Mt Kisco, NY, Futura Publishing, 1982, pp 145–166.
6. Levine PA (ed): Proceedings of the Policy Conference of the North American Society of Pacing and Electrophysiology on Programmability and Pacemaker Follow-up Programs. Clin Prog Pacing Electrophysiol 2:145, 1984.
7. Del Marco CJ, Tyers GFO, Brownlee RR: Lithium pacers with self-contained multiparameter telemetry: First-year follow-up. *In* Meere C (ed): Cardiac Pacing. Montreal, Pacesymp Publications, 1979, Chap. 28–1.
8. Tanaka S, Nanba T, Harada A, et al: Clinical experience with telemetry pacing systems and long-term follow-up: Clinical aspects of lead impedance and battery life. PACE Pacing Clin Electrophysiol 6:A-30, 1983.
9. Castellanet MJ, Garza J, Shaner SP, Messenger JC: Telemetry of programmed and measured data in pacing system evaluation and follow-up. J Electrophysiol 1:360, 1987.
10. Markewitz A, Kronski D, Kammeyer A, et al: Adequate pulse generator selection increases cost-effectiveness in pacemaker therapy (abstract). PACE Pacing Clin Electrophysiol 16:882, 1993.
11. Levine PA: Clinical manifestations of lead insulation defects. J Electrophysiol 1:144, 1987.
12. Clarke M, Allen A: Early detection of lead insulation breakdown. PACE Pacing Clin Electrophysiol 8:775, 1985.
13. Winoker P, Falkenberg E, Gerard G: Lead resistance telemetry: Insulation failure prognosticator. PACE Pacing Clin Electrophysiol 8:A-85, 1985.
14. Schmidinger H, Mayer H, Kaliman J, et al: Early detection of lead complications by telemetric measurement of lead impedance. PACE Pacing Clin Electrophysiol 8:A-23, 1985.
15. Kruse I, Markowitz T, Ryden L: Timing markers showing pacemaker behavior to aid in the follow-up of a physiologic pacemaker. PACE Pacing Clin Electrophysiol 6:801, 1983.
16. Olson W, McConnell M, Sah R, et al: Pacemaker diagnostic diagrams. PACE Pacing Clin Electrophysiol 8:691, 1985.
17. Levine PA, Schuller H, Lindgren A: Pacemaker ECG: Utilization of Pulse Generator Telemetry. Solna, Sweden, Siemens Elema AB, 1988.
18. Furman S: The ECG interpretation channel (editorial). PACE Pacing Clin Electrophysiol 13:225, 1990.
19. Olson WH, Goldreyer BA, Goldreyer BN: Computer-generated diagnostic diagrams for pacemaker rhythm analysis and pacing system evaluation. J Electrocardiol 1:376, 1987.
20. Levine PA: Pacemaker diagnostic diagrams (letter). PACE Pacing Clin Electrophysiol 9:250, 1986.
21. Furman S, Hurzeler P, DeCaprio V: Cardiac pacing and pacemakers III. Sensing the cardiac electrogram. Am Heart J 93:794, 1977.
22. Levine PA, Klein MD: Discrepant electrocardiographic and pulse analyzer endocardial potentials, a possible source of pacemaker sensing failure. *In* Meere C (ed): Cardiac Pacing. Montreal, Pacesymp Publications 1979, Chap. 18–1.
23. Levine PA, Podrid PJ, Klein MD, et al: Pacemaker sensing: Comparison of signal amplitudes determined by electrogram telemetry and noninvasively measured sensing thresholds (abstract). PACE Pacing Clin Electrophysiol 12:1294, 1989.
24. Levine PA, Sholder J, Duncan JL: Clinical benefits of telemetered electrograms in the assessment of DDD function. PACE Pacing Clin Electrophysiol 7:1170, 1984.
25. Clarke M, Allen A: Use of telemetered electrograms in the assessment of normal pacemaker function. J Electrophysiol 1:388, 1987.
26. Edery T: Clinical applications of pacemaker-telemetered intracardiac electrograms: Technical concept paper. Minneapolis, MN, Medtronic Inc., 1991.
27. Hughes HC, Furman S, Brownlee RR, Del Marco C: Simultaneous atrial and ventricular electrogram transmission via a specialized single-lead system. PACE Pacing Clin Electrophysiol 7:1195, 1984.
28. Feuer J, Florio J, Shandling AH: Alternate methods for the determination of atrial capture thresholds utilizing the telemetered intracardiac electrogram. PACE Pacing Clin Electrophysiol 13:1254, 1990.
29. Sarmiento JJ: Clinical utility of telemetered intracardiac electrograms in diagnosing a design dependent lead malfunction. PACE Pacing Clin Electrophysiol 13:188, 1990.
30. Marco DD, Gallagher D: Noninvasive measurements of retrograde conduction times in pacemaker patients. J Electrophysiol 1:388, 1987.
31. Nalos PC, Nyitray W: Benefits of intracardiac electrograms and programmable sensing polarity in preventing pacemaker inhibition due to spurious screw-in lead signals. PACE Pacing Clin Electrophysiol 13:1101, 1990.
32. Halperin JL, Camunas JL, Stern EH, et al: Myopotential interference with DDD pacemakers: Endocardial electrographic telemetry in the diagnosis of pacemaker-related arrhythmias. Am J Cardiol 54:97, 1984.
33. Gladstone PJ, Duxbury GB, Berman ND: Arrhythmia diagnosis by electrogram telemetry: Involvement of dual-chamber pacemaker. Chest 91:115, 1987.
34. Hassett JA, Elrod PA, Arciniegas JG, et al: Noninvasive diagnosis and treatment of atrial flutter utilizing previously implanted dual-chamber pacemaker. PACE Pacing Clin Electrophysiol 11:1662, 1988.
35. Luceri RM, Castellanos A, Thurer RJ: Telemetry of intracardiac electrograms: Applications in spontaneous and induced arrhythmias. J Electrophysiol 1:417, 1987.
36. Levine PA: The complementary role of electrogram, event marker, and measured data telemetry in the assessment of pacing system function. J Electrophysiol 1:404, 1987.
37. Pirolo JS, Tweddel JS, Brunt EM, et al: Influence of activation origin, lead number, and lead configuration on the noninvasive electrophysio-

logic detection of cardiac allograft rejection. Circulation 84(Suppl III):III-344, 1991.

38. Berbari EJ, Lander P, Geselowitz DB, et al: Correlating late potentials from the body surface with epicardial electrograms. Eur J Cardiac Pacing Electrophysiol 2:A-156, 1992.

39. Sanders R, Martin R, Frumin H, et al: Data storage and retrieval by implantable pacemakers for diagnostic purposes. PACE Pacing Clin Electrophysiol 7:1228, 1984.

40. Levine PA, Lindenberg BS: Diagnostic data: An aid to the follow-up and assessment of the pacing system. J Electrocardiol 1:396, 1987.

41. Levine PA: Utility and clinical benefits of extensive event counter telemetry in the follow-up and management of the rate-modulated pacemaker patient. Sylmar, CA, Siemens-Pacesetter, January 1992.

42. Newman D, Dorian P, Downar E, et al: Use of telemetry functions in the assessment of implanted antitachycardia device efficiency. Am J Cardiol 70:616, 1992.

43. Wang PJ, Manolis A, Clyne C, et al: Accuracy of classification using a data log system in implantable cardioverter defibrillators. PACE Pacing Clin Electrophysiol 14:1911, 1991.

44. Luceri RM, Puchferran RL, Brownstein SL, et al: Improved patient surveillance and data acquisition with a third-generation implantable cardioverter defibrillator. PACE Pacing Clin Electrophysiol 14:1870, 1991.

45. Stangl K, Sichart U, Wirtsfeld A, et al: Holter Functions for the Enhancement of the Diagnostic and Therapeutic Capabilities of Implantable Pacemakers, Vitatext. Dieren, The Netherlands, Vitatron Medical, 1987, pp 1–6.

46. Hayes DL, Higano ST, Eisinger G: Utility of rate histograms in programming and follow-up of a DDDR pacemaker. Mayo Clin Proc 64:495, 1989.

47. Levine PA, Sholder JA, Florio J: Obtaining maximal benefit from a DDDR pacing system: A reliable yet simple method for programming the sensor parameters of Synchrony. Sylmar, CA, Siemens-Pacesetter, 1990.

48. Lascault GR, Frank R, Fontaine G, et al: Ventricular tachycardia using the Holter function of a dual-chamber pacemaker (abstract). PACE Pacing Clin Electrophysiol 16:918, 1993.

49. Lascault GR, Frank R, Barnay C, et al: Clinical usefulness of a "diagnostic" dual-chamber pacemaker (abstract). PACE Pacing Clin Electrophysiol 16:918, 1993.

50. Intermedics Technical Manual. Relay DDDR Pacing System. Angleton, TX, Intermedics, 1992.

CHAPTER 33

EVALUATION OF PACEMAKER MALFUNCTION

Charles J. Love
David L. Hayes

The evaluation of the patient with a pacemaker has been transformed from the relatively simple job of evaluating single-chamber asynchronous devices to the monumental task of trouble-shooting dual-chamber, modulated-rate, dual-sensor devices.[1] It is no longer possible to simply look at an electrocardiographic (ECG) strip to determine the operating characteristics of a modern pulse generator. The clinician must have an in-depth knowledge of pacing systems. This includes, not only the pulse generator, but also the lead(s), sensor(s), connector(s), other implanted devices, and patient's physiology. It is critical that the clinician understand the importance of evaluating the entire system, rather than isolating the individual components.

Before attempting to determine the cause of a pacing system malfunction, it is important to determine whether or not an actual problem is present. Many devices have special programming features and idiosyncrasies that may appear to be malfunctions to those not completely familiar with the particular system under scrutiny. It is not unusual to hear about devices being explanted and returned to the manufacturer for failure to pace at the programmed rate, only to find that hysteresis had been enabled. The latter is but one of many examples of "pseudomalfunctions" that are discussed in greater detail.[2–5] This discussion is divided into six sections: Historical Clues, Physical Examination and Telemetry, Failure of Output, Failure to Capture, Failure to Sense, and Special Dual-Chamber Pacemaker Issues.

Historical Clues

The first step in the evaluation of the patient with a suspected pacing system problem is to gather as much informa-

tion about the patient as is possible (Table 33–1). This includes the indications for the pacemaker implantation, the operative record of the implant, the model numbers of all portions of the implanted pacing system, and the pro-

TABLE 33–1. EVALUATION OF THE PATIENT WITH A POTENTIALLY MALFUNCTIONING PACEMAKER

KNOW THE PATIENT
Cardiac and noncardiac diagnosis
Exposure to environmental extremes
Programming changes performed by others
Trauma to device or leads
Electromagnetic interference
Therapeutic radiation
Surgery using electrocautery
Defibrillation or cardioversion

KNOW THE PACEMAKER
Manufacturer
Model
Serial number
Alerts or recalls
Current programming (as interrogated by a programmer)
Device idiosyncrasies
Mode idiosyncrasies (DVI-C, Hysteresis, etc.)

KNOW THE LEAD(S) AND ADAPTERS
Manufacturer
Model
Serial number
Alerts or recalls
Connector type
Polarity
Insulation material
Fixation mechanism
Idiosyncrasies
Normal radiographic appearance

656

TABLE 33–2. NONINVASIVE TESTING

```
12-Lead surface ECG
24-Hour continuous ECG recording (Holter)
ECG loop memory recorders
Real-time transtelephonic transmission
ECG event recorders
Chest radiography
Fluoroscopy
Echocardiography
Magnet application
Telemetric analysis
    Current programming
    Measured lead data
        Lead impedance
        Pulse charge
        Pulse current
        Pulse energy
    Measured battery data
        Voltage
        Impedance
        Mean current drain
    Intracardiac electrograms
        Amplitude
        Frequency (slew rate)
        Artifacts
        Arrhythmias
        PVCs/PACs
        Atrial fibrillation
        Atrial flutter
    Pacemaker marker annotations
```

Abbreviations: ECG, electrocardiogram; PVC, premature ventricular contraction; PAC, premature atrial contraction.

grammed parameters. The latter data all are absolutely critical to the correct evaluation of the device.

Even in the current "high-tech" environment of cardiac pacing, the history and physical examination still play important roles. The patient should be asked about symptoms relating to potential device malfunction. These include presyncope, syncope, palpitations, slow or fast pulse rates, pain or erythema around the implanted devices, fevers, chills, night sweats, and extracardiac stimulation. It is also important to obtain any history of trauma to the device, exposure to intense electromagnetic or therapeutic radiation, use of electrocautery or defibrillation (internal or external), programming changes, or exposure to environmental extremes.

Information related to the actual implant procedure can be important when making clinical decisions. If the implanting physician was unable to obtain an adequate electrogram in the atrium for sensing, then atrial undersensing of P waves by the device would be expected. Knowledge of such a situation might prevent a second futile operation for the patient. Another common situation occurs with unusual roentgenographic findings. What may appear to be a dislodgement of an atrial lead into the low atrium might actually be the site of placement because of poor sensing or capture thresholds in the high atrium. Thus, a stable situation might lead an uninformed evaluator to an invalid conclusion regarding an apparent malfunction or problem.

The analysis of a potentially malfunctioning pacemaker system may require telemetry and programming information and noninvasive or invasive evaluation (Tables 33–2 and 33–3). The correct information with regard to the pacemaker system model numbers should be determined before any attempt at the evaluation of the system begins. Without this information, a serious error may occur because a safe and

rational assessment of the system cannot proceed without knowledge of these data. In many cases, the patient has an identification card that records at least the pulse generator's model and serial number. If the patient has had more than one device implanted, be sure that the card is the most recent one. Many patients like to keep their old and invalid identification cards as mementos of their previous pacemaker(s). Unfortunately, the data relating to the leads may or may not be on this card. This is often the case when the lead(s) and pacemaker are supplied by different manufacturers. It is also necessary to track down the lead information because many "pacemaker problems" are the result of a malfunction of the lead. Certain leads are less reliable than others, and there have been multiple recalls and alerts regarding leads; thus, such information is vital.

If the patient does not have an identification card, the information may be obtained from the operative report or from adhesive labels (provided with each pulse generator and lead) that may have been charted at the time of the implant. Finally, if none of these are available, a roentgenogram of the patient, including the area of the pulse generator, allows the clinician to match the identification label inside the pulse generator to those in a reference source (Fig. 33–1).[6–8] Although not all pulse generators have these labels, many have a distinct roentgenographic skeleton from which the clinician can determine the name of the manufacturer if not the model. All manufacturers provide toll-free numbers that the clinician may call to obtain further information regarding the pulse generator and the leads that are implanted.

Some manufacturers' programmers and devices are capable of automatically identifying the model and even the serial number of the pacemaker. Certain pulse generators are also capable of storing data concerning the patient, implant date, and lead model(s). If the pacemaker and programmer have this function, the programmer provides much of the data necessary for tracking down additional patient data. It may be possible to obtain further information from the manufacturer's patient tracking data base. Finally, pulse generators often have a characteristic magnet response signature on an ECG strip. However, the clinician should never "blindly" interrogate a device without knowing at least the name of the manufacturer. Unexpected and possibly disastrous reprogramming results may occur when using one manufacturer's programmer on another's pacemaker.

As previously stressed, knowing the specifics about the implanted pacing system's components is a critical first step. However, once known, it is also important to know what, if any, special considerations apply to the device. These might include recalls, alerts, known idiosyncrasies, and the functions of specialized programmable features and rate-modulation sensors.[9–15] Any of these items may have an impact and guide a further evaluation of the system or affect a decision to modify the system. For example, a pulse generator that is

TABLE 33–3. INVASIVE ANALYSIS

Visual inspection	Capture threshold
Connector	Voltage
Setscrews	Current
Grommets	Sensing threshold
Insulation	Intracardiac electrogram
Conductor	Impedance
Suturing sleeve	

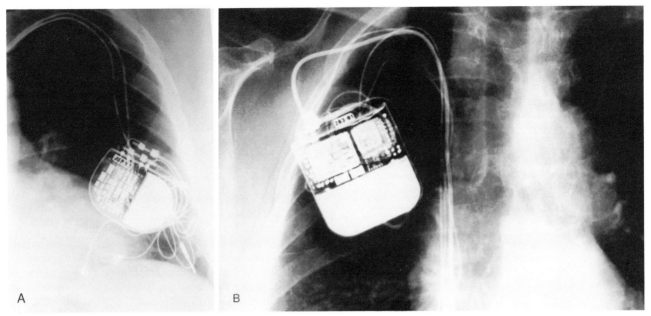

FIGURE 33–1. Roentgenograms of two pulse generators showing radiopaque identification tags. Some units may not have this helpful feature, but they can still be identified by the appearance of their unique radiographic ''skeletons.'' *A*, Medtronic (Minneapolis, MN) and *B*, Intermedics (Angleton, TX).

exhibiting its elective replacement parameters would typically be replaced using the same lead system if the latter had a good capture threshold, a good sensing threshold, and a normal impedance. However, if it was known that the lead was under a safety alert or recall, the clinician should follow recommended guidelines and, if appropriate, replace the vulnerable lead system at the time of generator replacement. Unfortunately, some patients must undergo a subsequent operation to revise another element of the pacing system because the implanter was unaware of known product deficiencies.

Many devices may exhibit idiosyncrasies that may be mistaken for malfunctions. Functional undersensing as a result of blanking periods, hysteresis, automatic mode switching, and endless loop tachycardia (ELT) prevention and termination algorithms are but a few examples of features that may cause confusion.

Physical Examination and Telemetry

After the history has been obtained and the pacemaker system's specifics are known, the patient should be examined. The implant site is examined for proper healing, erosion of suture material, erosion of leads or the generator, erythema, hematoma, seroma, excessive pain to palpation, evidence of trauma, pocket stimulation, and generator displacement.

The precordium is inspected for chest wall or diaphragmatic stimulation. The presence of the latter may indicate a number of possible problems (Table 33–4). If the system is unipolar, the pacemaker may have the noninsulated side facing posteriorly. This may have been done inadvertently at implant or have occurred spontaneously, or the patient may be a ''twiddler.''[16–20] Alternatively, the insulation coating may have been damaged or may have degraded over time. In some situations, pocket stimulation may occur, even with the

generator in the correct position and the insulation intact.[21] High-output settings, placement in or below the pectoral musculature, or high-current delivery as a result of low lead impedance may be at fault. Outer lead insulation failure may also allow problematic current leakage.

The neck veins should be evaluated for distention or the presence of cannon ''A'' waves. The latter might indicate an atrial lead problem or malprogramming in a dual-chamber system or the pacemaker syndrome in a single-chamber system. Auscultation of the heart for variable heart sounds, rubs, or gallops may also give clues as to the physiology related to the patient-device interaction.[22–23]

Physical maneuvers may be useful to manifest an intermittent symptom or malfunction during an examination. Carotid sinus massage and other vagal maneuvers may slow the intrinsic rhythm so that device function or malfunction becomes evident. Positional changes (sitting or standing up) or having the patient do in-place exercise or isometric maneuvers may accelerate the heart rate to observe for sensing (proper tracking and inhibition). Manipulation of the device and lead may make an intermittent lead fracture, loose connection, or insulation failure evident. Other helpful maneuvers include movement of the patient's ipsilateral arm (reach-

TABLE 33–4. CAUSES OF EXTRACARDIAC STIMULATION

Improper lead position
  Gastric vein
  Cardiac vein
Proximity of electrode to diaphragm
Lead perforation of heart
Phrenic nerve stimulation
Lead insulation failure
Device coating failure
Device movement (twiddler's syndrome)
Device placed upside down
Unipolar device at high output
Low chest wall muscle capture threshold

ing overhead or reaching behind the back), isometric exercise (pressing hands together in front of the chest), and sitting up (for an abdominal implant).[24]

A 12-lead ECG is required to document the function of the device at baseline. The use of a 12-lead or a multiple-lead ECG, instead of a single-lead rhythm strip, is mandatory when trouble-shooting. A myocardial infarction may have occurred, resulting in a change of capture and/or sensing thresholds. A change in the paced QRS axis might be a clue to lead dislodgement, whereas a change in the intrinsic axis (a new bundle branch block) may be associated with sensing problems. Multiple leads are frequently necessary to recognize the relatively low-amplitude atrial depolarization. In addition, the pacing artifact may not be visible in any given lead, especially if the pacing system is bipolar (Figs. 33–2 and 33–3). Care should be taken in the interpretation of the ECG tracing with regard to the type of recording system used. The older style analog systems have been generally replaced with digital recording systems. The digital systems can cause many types of artifacts and have several idiosyncrasies that can lead easily to misinterpretation (Fig. 33–4).[25–27]

After the baseline ECG is obtained, it should be inspected closely for any abnormalities of rate, sensing, loss of capture, or change in paced axis. A tracing with the magnet applied should then be performed. This gives information about the status of the battery and the pacemaker's function. If the pacemaker was inhibited during the baseline tracing, the magnet tracing allows a confirmation of the device's output and of the output into the appropriate chamber(s). If no output is seen during application of the magnet, several possibilities should be considered. The battery may be depleted, the device may be nonfunctional, or an open circuit (such as a lead fracture) may be present. The magnet response is programmable (enabled or disabled) on some models and may have been disabled. Alternatively, the magnet may not have been positioned properly, the reed switch may be stuck open, or an improper magnet may have been used.

The magnet function of each device is unique with regard to the rate and mode of response. This may differ by manufacturer, model, and programmed mode of the pacemaker. The clinician cannot assume that a DDD device exhibits a DOO response to application of the magnet. Some DDD devices respond with DVI and even VOO modes. Thus, the physician's manual that is supplied with the pacemaker, another reference source, or the manufacturer should be consulted to determine the appropriateness of the response obtained.

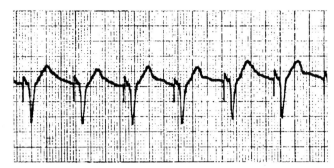

FIGURE 33–3. Electrocardiographic rhythm strip of a patient with 100% ventricular pacing. The pace artifact is easily identified because of the large electrical potential generated by the unipolar pacing polarity.

If the pacemaker is capable of telemetry or communication, it should be interrogated and the programmed settings printed.[28, 29] The latter is important because it provides documentation of the initial settings and serves as a reference should the clinician wish to restore the device to these settings when the evaluation is complete. If measured telemetry is available, all data should be requested and printed. Some models have extensive histograms, trend data, or other counters that are useful. These may keep track of many events, including the number of noise detections, high-rate episodes, and times the patient achieved the upper rate limit. A significant time spent at the upper rate in a patient with complaints related to exertion may be an indication of a pseudo-Wenckebach or 2:1 block. Data relating to the sensor's function are now available in many devices that are capable of rate modulation. These data provide useful information to confirm appropriate sensor's function. If any of this information is available, it should be obtained and printed, and the counters should be cleared so that they will reflect any changes made to the device.

When reviewing the results of the interrogation, an evaluation of the programmed setting data is always the first step. What are the mode and base rate? Many suspected device "malfunctions" have occurred because the programming has been changed by someone since the last evaluation. This has been referred to as "phantom reprogramming." It is often caused by another physician who did not notify the physician responsible for following the patient of the changes made to the pacemaker. Depletion of the battery may also cause a change in the mode or rate. Some dual-chamber devices change to a single-chamber mode to conserve power when the battery's voltage drops below a certain value. Likewise, the sensor may be disabled in modulated-rate devices to save

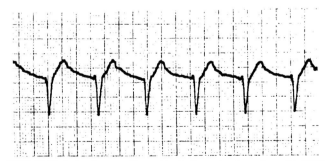

FIGURE 33–2. An electrocardiographic rhythm strip of a patient with 100% ventricular pacing. The pace artifact is not readily identified as a result of the small electrical potential generated by the bipolar pacing polarity.

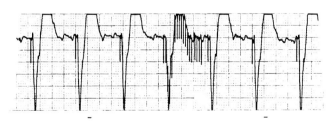

FIGURE 33–4. This electrocardiographic rhythm has a recording artifact that appears to be a pace artifact. Many recording and monitoring systems place an artificial "spike" on the recording when any high-frequency electrical transient is noted. This artifact was caused by interference during a programming session.

TABLE 33–5. **CAUSES OF MODE AND SETTING CHANGES**

Programming
Automatic mode switching
Battery depletion
Sticking reed switch (VOO, AOO, DOO, DVI)
Electrocautery
Internal defibrillation
External defibrillation
Airport security metal detectors
Magnetic resonance imaging scanners
Pacemaker-mediated tachycardia prevention/termination
   algorithms
Electronic article surveillance
Reset caused by cold (prior to implant)
Search hysteresis

power. Other causes of mode changes are listed in Table 33–5.

In colder climates and high altitudes, new devices that are shipped or transported may get cold enough to allow the battery's voltage to drop. If the battery gets cold enough, this may trigger the elective replacement behavior to occur, even though the device is new. The programmer must then be used to reset the pacemaker so that normal function may resume. Electrocautery and defibrillation can cause mode and/or polarity changes to occur on some models. The latter may also trigger the elective replacement indicator of the pacemaker. Pacing rate changes may also occur for many other reasons (Table 33–6). Thus, any assumption as to the expected operating characteristics of a device cannot be made without the most basic data, that is, the current programmed mode and rate.

After the mode and rate have been verified, an evaluation of the remaining programmed data is necessary. The output, pulse width, sensitivity, and refractory period(s) should be reviewed for each channel. The presence and status of any special programmable features should be checked. The latter includes rate-modulation settings, ELT prevention and termination algorithms, hysteresis, search hysteresis, time of day dependent rate changes (circadian function), rate-adap-

TABLE 33–6. **CAUSES OF RATE CHANGE**

Normal device-to-device variation
Fever
Circuitry failure
Battery failure
Battery depletion
Rate response
Magnet mode (sticking reed switch)
Crosstalk
Phantom programming
Sensor-driven rate changes
Atrial tracking
Triggered mode
Oversensing
Myopotentials
Intrinsic rhythm
Pseudomalfunction
   Holter/monitor recorder/electrocardiographic recorder speed changes
   Pulse enhancement artifact
   Rate smoothing
   Hysteresis
Runaway
Mode or rate reset as a result of cold

tive atrioventricular (AV) delay, differential AV delay, rate smoothing, and others. An evaluation of the device's function in relation to all programmed data is then performed by comparing the programmed data with ECG and Holter data obtained at these settings.

The measured data are then reviewed.[30–32] Impedance of the lead is one of the most important elements of the measured data. However, proper interpretation of the lead's impedance is dependent on the manufacturer and model of the lead used and the historical values of an individual lead's impedance. Very high impedance measurements may indicate an open circuit. This may be caused by a failure of the conductor, a loose setscrew, or failure of the connector or adaptor. The range of "normal" varies tremendously. Some older unipolar leads may have nominal impedance values of only 290 ohms; some newer leads are being designed with impedance values of more than 2000 ohms. Impedance values of less than 250 ohms are highly suggestive of an insulation failure. Although many lead models have a normal range, the data suggest that a marked change in the lead's impedance from the implant ($\pm 30\%$) or from the last visit is more important than any single value. Thus, a steady trend or an abrupt change may be more meaningful than any single value (Fig. 33–5).[33]

Not only should the impedance be evaluated but also other parameters of the lead's performance should be correlated with the measured impedance. These include pulse voltage, pulse charge, pulse energy, and current. If the impedance is very high, the charge, energy, and current should be very low or zero (Fig. 33–6). The voltage remains at or near the programmed voltage for "constant-voltage" devices. This is because no energy is being delivered as a result of the open circuit. Conversely, a low impedance should be associated with higher than normal values for charge, energy, and current measurements. If the impedance and the other data do not support each other, then a telemetry or calculation error may be present. This does not necessarily mean that the generator is defective, although the latter must be considered

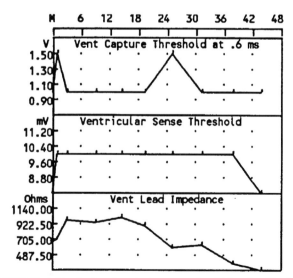

FIGURE 33–5. Graph of noninvasively measured and telemetered lead impedance versus time showing a progressive decay. Also note the drop in sensing threshold. This coaxial lead model was on alert for a high level of polyurethane insulation failure between the anodal and the cathodal conducting coils. Vent, ventricular.

A

```
╭─────────── MEASURED DATA ───────────╮
```

Pacer Rate _____ 59.8 ppm

Ventricular:
Pulse Amplitude _____ 4.1 Volts
Pulse Current _____ .0 mAmperes
Pulse Energy _____ 0 µJoules
Pulse Charge _____ 0 µCoulombs
Lead Impedance _____ > 1990 Ohms

Atrial:
Pulse Amplitude _____ 4.1 Volts
Pulse Current _____ .0 mAmperes
Pulse Energy _____ 0 µJoules
Pulse Charge _____ 0 µCoulombs
Lead Impedance _____ > 1990 Ohms

Battery Data: (W.G. 8077 – NOM. 1.8 AHR)
Voltage _____ 2.82 Volts
Current _____ 11 µAmperes
Impedance _____ < 1 KOhms

B

```
╭─────────── MEASURED DATA ───────────╮
```

Pacer Rate _____ 70.5 ppm

Ventricular:
Pulse Amplitude _____ 2.3 Volts
Pulse Current _____ 8.4 mAmperes
Pulse Energy _____ 8 µJoules
Pulse Charge _____ 4 µCoulombs
Lead Impedance _____ 276 Ohms

Atrial:
Pulse Amplitude _____ 3.0 Volts
Pulse Current _____ 5.6 mAmperes
Pulse Energy _____ 8 µJoules
Pulse Charge _____ 3 µCoulombs
Lead Impedance _____ 528 Ohms

Battery Data: (W.G. 8074 – NOM. 2.3 AHR)
Voltage _____ 2.78 Volts
Current _____ 33 µAmperes
Impedance _____ < 1 KOhms

C

```
╭─────────── MEASURED DATA ───────────╮
```

Pacer Rate _____ 70.5 ppm

Ventricular:
Pulse Amplitude _____ 2.5 Volts
Pulse Current _____ 3.6 mAmperes
Pulse Energy _____ 5 µJoules
Pulse Charge _____ 2 µCoulombs
Lead Impedance _____ 684 Ohms

Atrial:
Pulse Amplitude _____ 3.0 Volts
Pulse Current _____ 4.9 mAmperes
Pulse Energy _____ 7 µJoules
Pulse Charge _____ 3 µCoulombs
Lead Impedance _____ 598 Ohms

Battery Data: (W.G. 8074 – NOM. 2.3 AHR)
Voltage _____ 2.81 Volts
Current _____ 29 µAmperes
Impedance _____ < 1 KOhms

FIGURE 33–6. *A,* Measured data from a pulse generator not connected to the leads. These readings reflect an open circuit. The potential voltage remains as programmed; however, there is no current, energy, or charge flow. *B,* Measured data from a pulse generator connected to a coaxial lead with failing inner insulation. Note the high current, energy, and charge drain associated with the markedly low lead impedance on the ventricular lead. *C,* Measured data from a pulse generator connected to a properly functioning lead system.

in the differential diagnosis. It is prudent to repeat the measurements several times if such a conflict is noted.[34]

Be aware that some lead problems may be intermittent. Thus, a single measurement of lead-related parameters may not provide the diagnosis in all cases. At least one manufacturer provides real-time, pulse-by-pulse measurements of the lead's impedance. This is useful in cases of intermittent pacing system problems. Some devices take several measurements (the number varies by manufacturer and/or device model) and average them to give a single number. Thus, it may be important to obtain the measured data several times to reduce the chance of missing an intermittent problem (Fig. 33–7).

Another important data set that may be available measures the battery's status. This can include a measured magnet rate; measured base pacing rate; projected longevity; elective replacement indicator or status message; and the voltage, impedance, and mean current drain of the battery. The latter measurement may be useful to corroborate the measured data from the lead. If the mean current drain remains unchanged, despite a major change in the lead's impedance or current, then a telemetry or measurement error should be suspected.

Normal mean current drains vary greatly for each generator model, the lead system implanted, and the programmed settings. Once again, the importance of tracking these data over time allows a more accurate interpretation. The mean current drain may also be used to calculate the expected longevity of the device (Fig. 33–8). Rises in the battery's impedance result in decreasing voltage. This signals progressive depletion of the battery in a manner that is usually predictable and may be apparent long before any change in the magnet's rate occurs (Fig. 33–9).

After all the telemetry and measured data are obtained and reviewed, the next step should be an evaluation of the pacing and sensing thresholds. A complete threshold evaluation should be performed for each lead present. Marked changes in capture or sensing thresholds may imply a malfunction of a lead. There are other causes of both permanent and transient increases in threshold that are discussed subsequently.

An oscilloscopic evaluation of the pulse's waveform may be useful. This is true especially in older devices that lack the ability to measure lead performance parameters or telemeter intracardiac electrograms or provide pulse identification markers. The presence of noise in the pulse's waveform may

A

Jan. 13, 1992 1:50 pm MODEL: 2011 SERIAL: 14440
MEASURED DATA

Pacer Rate ———————————————— 70.5 ppm

Ventricular:
Pulse Amplitude ———————————— 2.9 Volts
Pulse Current ——————————————— 6.0 mAmperes
Pulse Energy ———————————————— 9 µJoules
Pulse Charge ———————————————— 3 µCoulombs
Lead Impedance ——————————————— 492 Ohms

Atrial:
Pulse Amplitude ———————————— 2.4 Volts
Pulse Current ——————————————— 5.6 mAmperes
Pulse Energy ———————————————— 6 µJoules
Pulse Charge ———————————————— 3 µCoulombs
Lead Impedance ——————————————— 422 Ohms

Battery Data: (W.G. 8077 – NOM. 1.8 AHR)
Voltage ——————————————————— 2.83 Volts
Current ——————————————————— 14 µAmperes
Impedance ————————————————— < 1 KOhms

B

Jan. 13, 1992 1:50 pm MODEL: 2011 SERIAL: 14440
MEASURED DATA

Pacer Rate ———————————————— 70.5 ppm

Ventricular:
Pulse Amplitude ———————————— 3.1 Volts
Pulse Current ——————————————— 2.2 mAmperes
Pulse Energy ———————————————— 4 µJoules
Pulse Charge ———————————————— 1 µCoulombs
Lead Impedance ——————————————— 1413 Ohms

Atrial:
Pulse Amplitude ———————————— 2.3 Volts
Pulse Current ——————————————— 5.3 mAmperes
Pulse Energy ———————————————— 6 µJoules
Pulse Charge ———————————————— 3 µCoulombs
Lead Impedance ——————————————— 438 Ohms

Battery Data: (W.G. 8077 – NOM. 1.8 AHR)
Voltage ——————————————————— 2.83 Volts
Current ——————————————————— 14 µAmperes
Impedance ————————————————— < 1 KOhms

FIGURE 33–7. *A,* Measured data from a pacing system exhibit normal values. *B,* Measured data from the same pacing system taken immediately after the first measurements. Note the lead impedance value is markedly different. This demonstrates the intermittent nature of many lead problems.

indicate a conductor coil fracture, a failure of insulation between the conductors of a bipolar lead, a loose setscrew, or a loose fixation screw. For constant-voltage devices, a square wave is indicative of a low current drain on the output capacitor, which is consistent with a fracture of the lead or an open circuit. Conversely, a very steep slope is seen with large current drains on the output capacitor because of low impedance (Fig. 33–10). This technique is an adjunct to other methods of diagnosing problems and should probably not be used to make a diagnosis without additional evidence of a malfunction.

If a pacemaker system's problem is suspected, posteroanterior and lateral chest roentgenograms should be obtained. It is usually best to request a slightly overpenetrated exposure. The film should be inspected for evidence of conductor disruption, insulation failure, proper lead placement in the generator connector block, proper slack in the lead system, electrode perforation, dislodgement or malposition of a lead, generator movement, and proper orientation of the coated side of the can posteriorly (i.e., leads exiting in a "clockwise" direction).[35] The latter is especially important when evaluating pocket stimulation in unipolar systems. Close attention should be paid to the infraclavicular area where pressure from the clavicle and first rib may cause lead failure (see Chapter 30).[36–46]

On occasion, a fluoroscopic evaluation of the patient may

be useful. This shows many of the problems and defects listed earlier. It also provides a dynamic view of the lead system. The clinician may therefore demonstrate excessive electrode movement (indicating unstable fixation) or insufficient slack with respiratory movement. Either of these would provide an explanation of intermittent capture and sensing.

Differential Diagnosis of Pacing System Malfunction

Although many pacing system malfunctions are common to single- and dual-chamber devices, the latter present a greater challenge. The section that follows deals with problems seen in both single- and dual-chamber devices. The subsequent section deals with problems unique to dual-chamber devices.

Battery Data: (W.G. 8077 – NOM. 1.8 AHR)
Voltage ——————————————————— 2.80 Volts
Current ——————————————————— 22 µAmperes
Impedance ————————————————— < 1 KOhms

FIGURE 33–8. The telemetered mean battery current drain may be used to calculate the expected longevity of the pulse generator:

Usable battery capacity = 90% of rating
0.9 × 1.8 Ah = 1.62 Ah
= 1,620,000 µAh

Mean current drain = 22 µA

Capacity/drain = 73,636 hr
24 hr/day = 3068 days
365 days/year = 8.4 years estimated longevity

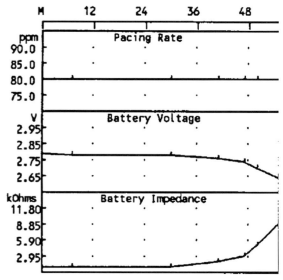

FIGURE 33–9. Graph of magnet rate, battery voltage, and battery impedance versus time. Note the drop in voltage relative to the rise in impedance. Also note that although the battery is showing significant wear, there has been no indication of this by the magnet rate.

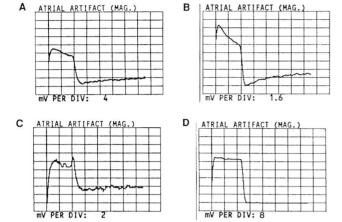

FIGURE 33–10. Oscilloscopic analysis of pacing impulses. *A,* A normal lead on a constant voltage pacemaker. Note that there is a gradual decay of the waveform. *B,* A lead with a low impedance caused by an insulation failure. Note the voltage decay as a result of the high current drain off the capacitors. *C,* A lead with a high impedance because of a conductor coil failure. Note the lower voltage decay as there is reduced current drain off the capacitors. Also note the noise at the end of the waveform, which is common with lead fractures. *D,* A normal lead on a constant current pacemaker. Note that the waveform is more squared with this type of output circuit.

TABLE 33–7. **FAILURE TO PACE (NO OUTPUT)**

Battery failure
Circuit failure
Lead fracture
Internal insulation failure (bipolar lead) with ''dead short''
Oversensing
    Electromagnetic interference
    Myopotentials
    Make-break signals (lead fracture or insulation failure)
    Polarization currents
Improper positioning of lead in header
Incompatible lead or header
Lack of anodal connector contact during implantation
    Unipolar lead in bipolar device
    Bipolar lead in device programmed unipolar
    Air in pacemaker pocket (unipolar device)
    Pacemaker not in pocket (unipolar device)
Crosstalk (dual-chamber device)
Pseudomalfunction
    Bipolar spike not seen
    Hysteresis (single- and dual-chamber devices)
    Search hysteresis
    Automatic mode switching
    Unrecognized intrinsic activity
    Pacemaker-mediated tachycardia prevention and termination
       algorithms

FAILURE OF OUTPUT (NO ARTIFACT PRESENT)

When it occurs, failure to pace represents a potentially catastrophic and lethal situation. The ECG appearance in a single-chamber system is that of no pacing artifact, with an intrinsic rate below the lower rate limit of the device. This may be intermittent or continuous. In a dual-chamber device, the clinician may see an atrial pace alone, ventricular pace alone, or no pacing artifacts at all. The latter may be entirely normal, depending on the patient's sinus rate, AV nodal conduction, AV interval settings, enabling of hysteresis, and sensor settings. The causes of a no-output condition are listed in Table 33–7. In evaluating this situation, the clinician must be certain that a malfunction truly exists before taking any corrective action. Remember that the ECG (especially in a single surface lead) may not display the pacing artifact because of technical factors (Fig. 33–11). This is common in bipolar systems and systems programmed to a lower-than-nominal voltage output. Thus, the problem may be failure to capture rather than failure to output. Another common source of misinterpretation is the presence of hysteresis. As previously noted, many pacemakers have been returned to their manufacturers as defective when this feature was enabled. In these cases, the physician was either not aware of the programming or did not understand this feature. Other causes of intermittent prolongation of the pacing interval are listed in Table 33–8.

Another source of evaluation error is failure to recognize intrinsic complexes that are causing appropriate inhibition of the device. This problem is not uncommon in the hospital's telemetry unit in which only a single lead is monitored. Premature beats may be present, with the ectopic complexes appearing nearly isoelectric (Fig. 33–12). Although the observer may not recognize the premature ventricular (PVC) or atrial contraction (PAC) on casual observation, the pacemaker senses these events and is appropriately inhibited. The

use of multiple leads or a 12-lead ECG recording virtually eliminates this cause of pseudomalfunction.

The lack of an output pulse is frequently caused by oversensing. The pacemaker, for all of its complexity, operates from a relatively simple set of rules. Any event that generates an electrical signal of adequate strength and frequency content is sensed and resets the timing cycle. Oversensing can come from cardiac, extracardiac, and nonphysiologic sources. A common intracardiac cause of oversensing in AAI systems is the sensing of the far-field QRS complex (Fig. 33–13). This is most common in unipolar systems when the lead is placed in close proximity to the tricuspid valve, with high sensitivity settings, and with short atrial refractory periods. Far-field sensing is uncommon in VVI systems because of the diminutive size of the P wave, as seen electrically from the ventricle. Sensing of the intracardiac T wave may occur in VVI systems with similar results (Fig. 33–14). The other intracardiac source that may be oversensed is postpace polarization (Fig. 33–15). Chapter 1 provides a description of polarization and the evoked response. Oversensing of this

TABLE 33–8. **INTERMITTENT PROLONGATION OF THE PACING INTERVAL**

Far-field sensing
T-wave sensing
After potential sensing
Myopotential sensing
Lead fracture
Loose connection
Inner or outer insulation failure
Electromagnetic or radiofrequency interference
Hysteresis
Search hysteresis
Electrocardiogram or Holter recorder speed
Inadvertent or intermittent magnet application
Pacemaker-mediated tachycardia prevention or termination algorithms
Automatic mode switching

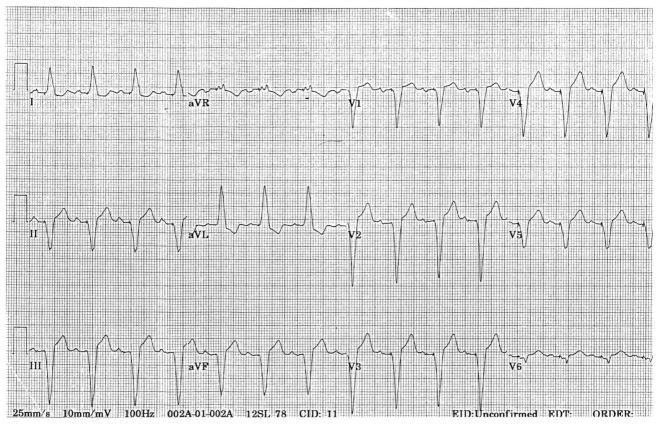

FIGURE 33–11. A 12-lead electrocardiogram of a patient with a normally functioning bipolar pacing system. Note that lead V4 shows the pace artifact, whereas others do not show it at all.

event may occur with short refractory periods combined with high outputs on certain lead systems.

The most frequent source of a physiologic extracardiac signal that causes oversensing is myopotentials. The pacemaker is capable of sensing muscle depolarizations of not only the heart but also noncardiac structures, such as the pectoralis and rectus abdominis muscles. Myopotential inhibition of pacemaker output can be seen during arm movements (prepectoral implant) or when the patient sits up (abdominal implant, Fig. 33–16). This is primarily a problem of unipolar systems because the anode is the pacemaker's case, which remains in close proximity to these muscular structures.[47–56] Nonphysiologic signals may also cause oversensing. Formerly, electromagnetic interference (EMI) from mi-

crowave ovens was a significant problem when pacemakers were encased in plastic or epoxy. The newer devices are shielded from EMI by their metal cases, although strong EMI sources can still cause oversensing (Table 33–9).[57–74]

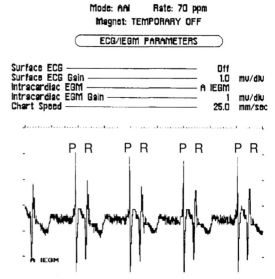

FIGURE 33–13. An IEGM recorded from a unipolar atrial lead. Note the large size of the "far-field" ventricular EGM (R). If the near-field atrial EGM (P) was not as large, the device could undersense the atrium, sensing the ventricular EGM in error. ECG, electrocardiogram; EGM, electrogram; IEGM, intracardiac EGM.

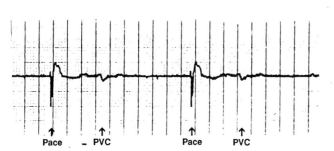

FIGURE 33–12. An electrocardiographic rhythm strip of a pacemaker programmed to VVI with a demand rate of 50 bpm. This seems to show an inappropriate bradycardia. Note the low-amplitude waves that map out to the escape interval. These are PVCs that appeared almost isoelectric in this lead. PVC, premature ventricular contraction.

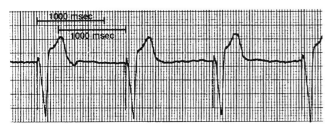

FIGURE 33–14. Electrocardiographic rhythm strip of a device programmed VVI at 60 bpm. T-wave oversensing is present. The last sensed event can always be determined by mapping back by the escape interval.

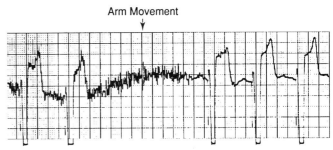

FIGURE 33–16. An electrocardiographic rhythm strip showing an obvious somatic artifact associated with and in the absence of pacemaker output. This is oversensing caused by myopotentials.

It has been well documented that intermittent metal-to-metal contact can create electrical signals. These "make-break" signals may be of sufficient amplitude to be detected by pacing systems. Signals exceeding 25 mV have been recorded in some cases (Fig. 33–17). The latter presents a major problem because this false signal can be greatly in excess of the physiologic signal, which causes an oversensing situation with inhibition of the output pulse. As a result of the large size of these artifacts, decreasing the pacemaker's sensitivity is frequently not an effective option. The sources of these electrical signals include a loose setscrew, fracture of the conductor coil, failed insulation between the anodal and cathodal conductors in a bipolar system, interaction between an active and abandoned pacing electrode(s), and a loose retractable fixation screw.[75–82] There are studies underway at this time to investigate the origin of these signals because there may be other mechanisms operating in addition to the make-break phenomenon.

Oversensing can be confirmed by use of the magnet or reprogramming to the VOO/AOO mode. If the cause of the pauses or slow rate is oversensing, regular pacing resumes during asynchronous pacing. If a lead failure, open circuit, or other cause of no output exists, then this maneuver does not result in asynchronous pacing (Fig. 33–18). The use of intracardiac electrograms and marker telemetry can indicate the presence of oversensing and the culprit electrogram. This is useful for differentiating the causes of oversensing to allow the proper remedy to be used (Fig. 33–19).

Failure of the pulse generator circuit is rare, but it can result in a failure to output (Table 33–10). Complete exhaustion of the power source (battery) also causes this. As the power source begins to fail, slowing of the pacing rate and erratic behavior may occur (Fig. 33–20). The latter may cause apparent mode or rate changes and sensing problems.

There are several problems that may be mistaken for a pulse generator's failure, resulting in a no-output situation. These are generally related to problems at the time of implantation. If the lead is not positioned properly in the connector block of the pacemaker or if an improper lead is used, the electrical connection may not be complete. A transient situation has been reported in unipolar systems following wound closure. It is possible for air to be present in the pocket, especially when a large generator is replaced by a smaller one. The air prevents contact of the anterior anodal surface of the pacemaker's case with the body's tissues. This results in an incomplete circuit until the air is absorbed. Subcutaneous emphysema was also reported to be responsible for loss of anodal contact. A similar pseudofailure occurs when a unipolar pulse generator is out of the pocket.[83, 84]

Remember that, although a pulse generator is bipolar, it may be programmed to function in the unipolar mode. Failure to output may also be seen with bipolar pacemakers that are connected to a unipolar pacing lead. This is more likely with the VS-1 or IS-1 leads because the bipolar and unipolar connectors are similar. Some unipolar leads now have a protective metal band where the anodal screw of the pacemaker connector block might cause damage. This may cause the lead to appear bipolar even though no anodal conductor is present.

FAILURE TO CAPTURE (ARTIFACT IS PRESENT)

With the advent of the newer ECG recording systems and the use of pulse artifact enhancement, the clinician must first be certain that the pace artifact seen is truly from the pacing system. There are many causes of extraneous signals that can cause the enhanced ECG, telemetry system, or Holter recorder to place an erroneous pace artifact on the ECG. EMI (including programmer telemetry), loose ECG electrode connections, and subthreshold pulses associated with normal pacemaker function are examples of situations associated with spurious artifacts (Fig. 33–21). The use of marker telemetry and intracardiac electrograms can often be useful in the identification of the true pacemaker output if the clinician is suspicious of this type of problem.

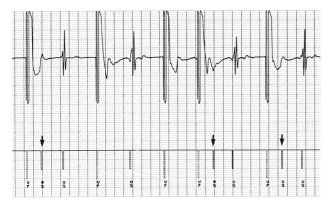

FIGURE 33–15. An electrocardiographic rhythm strip showing oversensing of the polarization artifact with a model 7217B PCD implantable defibrillator (Medtronic, Minneapolis, MN). This was caused by a high-output voltage, high sensitivity, and a short programmed ventricular refractory period. Parameters: 5.4 V, 1.59 msec; sensing, 0.3 mV; ventricular refractory period, 320 msec.

TABLE 33–9. **CAUSES OF POTENTIAL ELECTROMAGNETIC INTERFERENCE**[a]

SOURCE	PACER DAMAGE	TOTAL INHIBITION	ONE BEAT INHIBITION	ASYNCHRONY NOISE	RATE INCREASE	UNIPOLAR/ BIPOLAR
Ablation	Y	Y	N	N	Y	U/B
Antitheft device	N	N	Y	N	N	U
Arc welder	N	Y	Y	Y	N	U/B
Cardiokymography	N	Y	Y	N	Y	U/B
Cardioversion	Y	N	N	N	N	U/B
Citizen's band radio	N	N	Y	N	N	U
Defibrillation	Y	N	N	N	N	U/B
Dental scaler	N	N	Y[b]	Y[b]	Y[e]	U
Diathermy	Y	Y	Y	Y	Y	U/B
Electroconvulsive therapy	N	Y	Y	Y	Y[e]	U
Electric blanket	N	N	N	Y[e]	N	U
Electric power tools	N	N	Y[e]	N	N	U
Electric shaver	N	N	Y[b]	N	N	U
Electric switch	N	N	Y	N	N	U
Electric toothbrush	N	N	Y[b]	N	N	U
Electrocautery	Y	Y	Y	Y	Y[c]	U/B
Electrolysis	N	N	Y	Y	N	U
Electrotome	N	N	Y[b]	N	N	U
Ham radio	N	N	Y	N	N	U
Heating pad	N	N	N	Y	N	U
Lithotripsy	Y[e]	Y[b]	Y[b]	Y[b]	Y[d]	U/B
Magnetic resonance imaging scanner	Y	N	Y	Y	Y[d]	U/B
Positron emission tomographic scanner	Y	N	N	N	N	U/B
Powerline (high voltage)	N	N	N	Y	N	U/B
Pulp tester	N	Y[b]	Y[b]	Y	N	U
Radar	N	N	Y[b]	N	N	U
Radiation (therapeutic)	Y	N	N	N	Y	U/B
Radiotransmission (AM)	N	N	Y[b]	N	N	U
Radiotransmission (FM)	N	N	Y[b]	Y[b]	N	U
Stun gun	N	N	Y	N	N	U/B
Transcutaneous electrical nerve stimulation	N	Y	N	Y	Y[d]	U
Television transmitter	N	Y[b]	Y[b]	Y[b]	N	U
Ultrasound (therapeutic)	Y[e]	Y[b]	Y[b]	N	N	U
Weapon detector	N	N	Y[b]	N	N	U

[a]Adapted from Telectronic, Englewood, CO, technical note.
[b]Remote potential for interference.
[c]Impedance-based sensors.
[d]DDD mode only.
[e]Piezo crystal-based sensors.

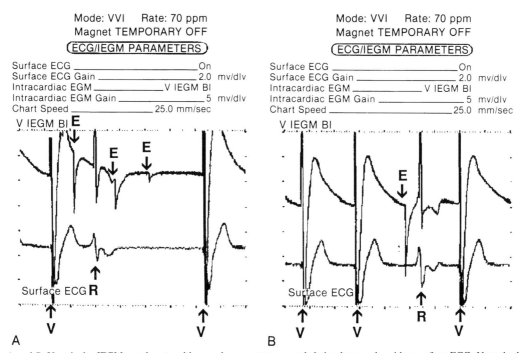

FIGURE 33–17. *A and B,* Ventricular IEGM as telemetered by a pulse generator, recorded simultaneously with a surface ECG. Note the large artifacts (E) on the intracardiac channel seen without ventricular activity (R, native QRS; V, pace output). These were caused by failing insulation in a bipolar coaxial lead system. ECG, electrocardiogram; EGM, electrogram; IEGM, intracardiac EGM.

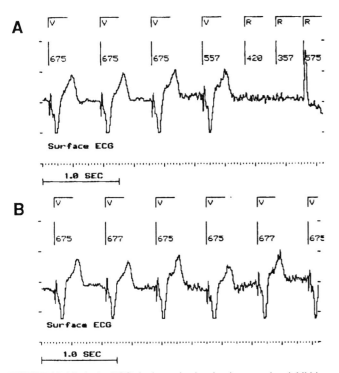

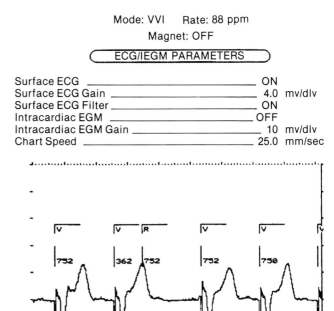

Mode: VVI   Rate: 88 ppm
Magnet: OFF

ECG/IEGM PARAMETERS

Surface ECG	ON	
Surface ECG Gain	4.0	mv/dlv
Surface ECG Filter	ON	
Intracardiac EGM	OFF	
Intracardiac EGM Gain	10	mv/dlv
Chart Speed	25.0	mm/sec

FIGURE 33–18. *A,* An ECG rhythm strip showing inappropriate inhibition caused by myopotential oversensing. *B,* An ECG rhythm strip of the same pacing system with a magnet placed over the pulse generator. If a loss of output was still evident with the magnet on, then the problem is not likely to be oversensing. ECG, electrocardiogram.

FIGURE 33–19. An ECG rhythm strip with pulse identification markers showing oversensing. Note that the pulse generator is identifying a QRS where none exists. This was caused by faulty lead insulation not oversensing of the T wave, as suggested by the timing of the event that was sensed (R). ECG, electrocardiogram; EGM, electrogram; IEGM, intracardiac EGM.

Another common cause of pseudononcapture is undersensing, with a resultant delivery of the pacemaker impulse during the refractory period of the myocardium. Although the output does not elicit a depolarization, the problem in this case is related to sensing, not output, and should be evaluated as such (Fig. 33–22).

After noncapture is documented, the patient's safety must be ensured. If the patient is pacemaker dependent or is intolerant of the subsequent bradycardia associated with complete or intermittent loss of capture, the device should be programmed to its highest output. If consistent capture is still not secured, placement of a temporary pacemaker may be necessary. Some bipolar devices allow programming to the unipolar mode. This may acutely correct the situation so that an invasive intervention is not urgent.

The causes of noncapture are listed in Table 33–11. The onset of noncapture relative to the implant of the device and lead system can be valuable in leading the clinician to the correct cause. If this occurs within 24 to 48 hours of implantation, dislodgement, malposition, or perforation of the heart by the lead should be high on the list of possible problems.

Elevated thresholds occurring during the first several weeks following the implantation are not uncommon. This may occur during the maturation process between the electrode and myocardium. The peak of the early threshold rise is usually from 2 to 6 weeks postimplant. Using a higher output during this "acute" period should prevent noncapture until the threshold improves to its "chronic" level. With the introduction of modern electrode technology and steroid-eluting leads, this threshold rise is now minimal and frequently nonexistent (see Chapter 3).

A rise in threshold occurring after the 6th week is usually considered to be in the chronic phase of the lead maturation process. The threshold may rise steadily over time until noncapture occurs or until the threshold exceeds the pacemaker's maximum output. This is commonly referred to as "exit block."[85–91] Older lead models and some epicardial leads are more likely to develop this condition.[92–95] Some patients demonstrate repeated episodes of this phenomenon and have required multiple lead revisions and/or replacements. Pediatric epicardial implants are especially prone to develop this condition.[96] The use of steroid-eluting leads is useful to prevent

FIGURE 33–20. This is a rhythm strip from a patient whose pulse generator is beyond the elective replacement interval. Not only is the pacing rate below the programmed rate of 70 bpm, the device is not sensing properly. The leads were found to function normally when the device was replaced.

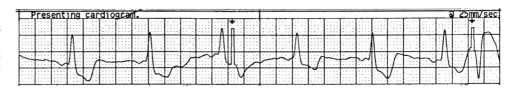

TABLE 33–10. **POTENTIAL CAUSES OF PULSE GENERATOR FAILURE**

Electrocautery
Defibrillation
Therapeutic radiation
Lithotripsy
Direct trauma or loss of hermetic seal
General circuitry failure

exit block.[97–105] There have been some anecdotes on the use of high-dose systemic steroids to lower high thresholds, but thresholds usually rise when the steroids are discontinued.[106–108]

There are many causes of threshold rises in both the acute and chronic phases. Any severe metabolic or electrolyte derangement can lead to acute threshold changes (Table 33–12).[109–118] These are not uncommon in critically ill patients, during and immediately following a cardiac arrest. Thus, noncapture may be secondary to the hypoxemia, acidemia, or hyperkalemia rather than the primary event leading to the arrest. In addition, some medications may affect capture thresholds, resulting in significant changes from the patient's baseline (Table 33–13).[94, 113, 117–124]

Although the clinician might expect a fracture of a lead to present as the absence of any visible pacing artifact, this is frequently not the case. The ECG may display failure to capture, especially in unipolar systems. This occurs because of the current passing across the gap in the conductor coil through the fluid in the lead. Unipolar systems virtually always have the anode intact (the pulse generator surface), which provides enough of an electrical transient to trigger the artificial pace artifact circuitry of many monitoring systems.

Although modern pulse generators attempt to maintain the programmed output until the battery is exhausted, a reduction in the delivered voltage may occur prior to the elective replacement indicator. At advanced stages of depletion of the battery, this may result in an ineffective pacing stimulus.

Latency is a finding that may be mistaken for failure to capture. This is defined as the delay between the delivery of the pacing impulse until the onset of electrical systole.[125] Some antiarrhythmic agents or severe electrolyte distur-

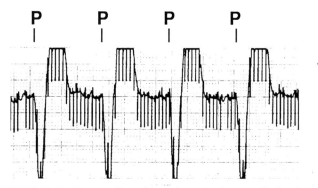

FIGURE 33–21. Electrocardiographic rhythm strip of a normally functioning VVIR pacing system. The multiple artifacts were caused by minute ventilation sensing technology that delivers subthreshold stimuli every 50 msec. The signals were misinterpreted by the monitor as pacing outputs and displayed as such. P, actual paced event.

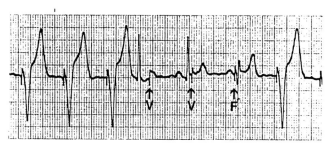

FIGURE 33–22. This electrocardiographic rhythm strip showing physiologic noncapture. The problem in this case is the pacing system's failure to sense the QRS. A pace output (V) then occurs during the myocardial refractory period and should not be expected to capture. The second to last QRS represents fusion (F) between the pace artifact and the native QRS.

bances, such as hyperkalemia, may cause latency and even a Wenckebach type of prolongation, leading to a noncaptured stimulus and a repeat of the cycle (Fig. 33–23).

FAILURE TO SENSE

To understand why undersensing occurs, the clinician must understand how the sensing amplifier works, when in the cardiac cycle the sensing occurs, and when the sensing cannot occur (see Chapter 2). Remember that the electrogram must possess both an adequate amplitude and frequency content (slew rate) to be sensed properly. A signal of apparent adequate peak-to-peak amplitude may be markedly attenuated by the sense amplifier because of its poor slew rate.

TABLE 33–11. **CAUSES OF LOSS OF CAPTURE (PULSE ARTIFACT IS PRESENT BUT NO COMPLEX FOLLOWS)**

AAI mode programmed when looking for ventricular complex
Latency
Lead movement
"Microdislodgement"
"Macrodislodgement"
Elevated threshold
Acute postoperative
Early
Late
Myocardial infarction
Metabolic
Electrolyte
Drugs
Defibrillation (capacitive coupling)
Electrocautery
Exit block
Perforation
Inappropriate placement of lead (superior vena cava, gastric vein, coronary sinus)
Lead fracture
Poor/failed connection at connector block
Improper pin insertion
Incompatible connectors
Poor setscrew tension
Insulation failure (internal, external, or unipolar)
Battery failure
Circuit failure
Air in pacer pocket (unipolar)
Pseudomalfunction
Recording artifact
Pace during ventricular or atrial refractory period
Metabolic factors
Drug therapy

TABLE 33–12. **METABOLIC FACTORS THAT MAY CAUSE AN INCREASE IN CAPTURE THRESHOLD**

MAJOR CHANGES	MINOR CHANGES
Acidosis	Sleep
Alkalosis	Viral infection
Hypercarbia	Eating
Hyperkalemia	
Severe hyperglycemia	
Hypoxemia	
Myxedema	

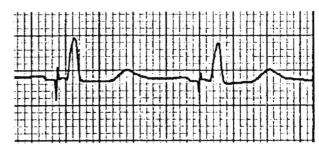

FIGURE 33–23. This electrocardiographic rhythm strip showing latency. Note the prolonged period from the pace artifact until the evoked QRS. This patient had a serum potassium concentration of 7.1 mEq because of renal failure.

The resultant "filtered" signal may be of insufficient size to be recognized as a valid event.[126–131] Table 33–14 lists the causes of sensing failure.

It is often assumed that the pacemaker senses a cardiac event at the beginning of the P wave or QRS complex, as seen on the surface ECG. This is not the case. The clinician must recognize that the surface P wave or QRS is a summation of all events occurring at the cellular level over time. If the clinician looks at the intracardiac electrogram as recorded from a pacing electrode, it appears as a spike (Fig. 33–24). This event is generated as the wave of depolarization passes by the electrode. An excellent example of this "delayed sensing" is the patient who has right bundle branch block and a pacing electrode in the right ventricle. A nonpaced depolarization occurs late in the right ventricle because of the conduction delay, and thus, the pacemaker does not sense this event until late in the ECG complex. By assuming that sensing occurred earlier, the clinician might misinterpret the timing cycle by more than 100 msec. Thus, an ECG with a pacing artifact in the QRS (pseudofusion) can occur, although sensing is entirely normal (Fig. 33–25).[132, 133]

The programmed refractory period is important when determining whether sensing should occur at any given time. Long refractory periods may cause undersensing of events occurring during this time of nonsensing (Fig. 33–26). This might occur in the case of a closely coupled PVC or PAC. Again, this is not a device malfunction but is a result of a the programmed parameters interacting with the patient's intrinsic rhythm.

As in noncapture, the onset of undersensing relative to the

implantation of the pacemaker and lead system may direct the clinician to the correct diagnosis of the malfunction. The undersensing that occurs in close proximity to the implant should lead the physician to suspect dislodgement, malposition, or perforation of the electrode. Problems occurring in chronic systems are frequently caused by insulation or conductor failure and programming errors. The latter is not uncommon, especially when sensitivity threshold testing has been performed during follow-up. The clinician may forget to return the sensitivity to the appropriate setting and leave it at or above the threshold setting. Occasionally, the sensing threshold may show a slow decline as the lead-tissue interface changes over time.[134]

The vector of depolarization can affect the amplitude and the slew rate of the intracardiac electrogram. Any change in the vector may result in significant changes in the sensing threshold. Should the patient with a ventricular pacemaker have a myocardial infarction, develop a bundle branch block, or have PVCs, the intracardiac signal may be insufficient to

TABLE 33–13. **EFFECT OF SPECIFIC DRUGS ON PACING THRESHOLDS**

INCREASE THRESHOLD
Bretylium
Encainide
Flecainide
Moricizine
Propafenone
Sotalol
POSSIBLY INCREASE THRESHOLD
Beta-blockers
Bretylium
Lidocaine
Procainamide
Quinidine
DECREASE THRESHOLD
Atropine
Epinephrine
Isoproterenol
Corticosteroids

TABLE 33–14. **CAUSES OF UNDERSENSING**

Change of intrinsic complex
    Bundle branch blocks
    Ventricular fibrillation or tachycardia
    Atrial fibrillation or flutter
    Respiratory variation
Myocardial infarction
Poor or inappropriate lead positioning
Lead dislodgement (micro or macro)
Device failure
Magnet application
Sticking reed switch
Elective replacement indicator
Electromagnetic interference (with interference mode)
Poor slew rate
Poor peak-to-peak signal
Inappropriate pacing system analyzer filters relative to device filters
Intrinsic beat falling in device refractory period
Pacemaker-mediated tachycardia prevention (DVI on premature ventricular contraction or postventricular atrial refractory period extension)
Fusion and pseudofusion (especially with right bundle branch block morphologies)
Upper rate behavior
    Wenckebach
    Multiblock
VVT mode
Defibrillation (capacitive coupling)
Device idiosyncrasy (Meta at implant)

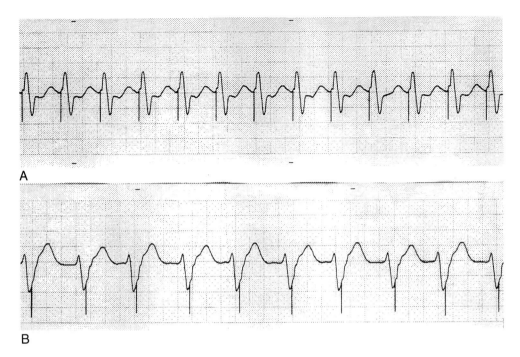

A

B

FIGURE 33–24. Electrocardiographic rhythm strip from a patient in VVT mode with a demand rate of 60 bpm and slow ventricular tachycardia of two different morphologies. *A,* This ventricular tachycardia had a left bundle branch block morphology. The pacemaker is sensing this QRS at the beginning of the complex and triggering an output there. The early site of activation is likely near the right ventricular apex. *B,* This is from the same patient after an attempt at overdrive pacing. The morphology of the QRS changed to a right bundle branch block, and now the device is sensing and triggering much later in the complex.

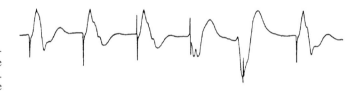

FIGURE 33–25. An electrocardiographic rhythm strip showing pseudofusion beats. The premature ventricular contractions have a right bundle branch block morphology; thus right ventricular depolarization occurs late. The QRS complexes cannot be sensed by the pacemaker until late into the surface QRS, resulting in pseudofusion.

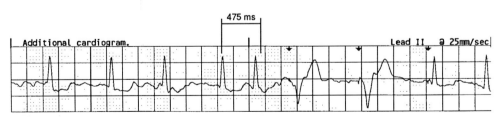

FIGURE 33–26. This electrocardiographic rhythm strip showing undersensing of the QRS complexes in a patient with atrial fibrillation. The device is programmed to VVI with a demand rate of 70 bpm and a refractory period of 475 msec. Because of a long programmed ventricular refractory period, this does not represent a pacemaker malfunction. The pacemaker will not respond to intrinsic events during the refractory period.

allow sensing at the previous appropriate setting (Fig. 33–27).[135–137] The same may be seen with atrial implants and PACs. Another cause of vector change is movement of the lead's position with respiratory movements. Marked changes in the intracardiac signal can be documented in some patients as the angle of the lead relative to the heart changes with body position or diaphragmatic motion (Fig. 33–28).[138–141]

As the pacemaker's battery begins to deplete, erratic behavior may occur, including failure to sense or intermittent undersensing. Failure of a circuit component may also cause sensing failure. Rarely, the reed switch that activates the magnet mode may stick in the closed position, causing (in most cases) asynchronous pacing. For the same reason, when reviewing a rhythm strip, the clinician must be certain whether or not the magnet was over the device when the recording was made. Asynchronous pacing may also be seen during the interference mode function of the device. The latter obligates pacing when the presence of electrical noise is sensed by the pulse generator. Typically, this is defined as multiple sensed events occurring within the ventricular refractory period. The device then paces asynchronously to protect the pacemaker-dependent patient against inappropriate device inhibition.[142, 143]

One frequently misinterpreted reason for failure to sense involves pacemakers that use impedance plethysmography as a rate-modulation sensor. This applies primarily to minute-ventilation sensors. Because the system uses the pacemaker's

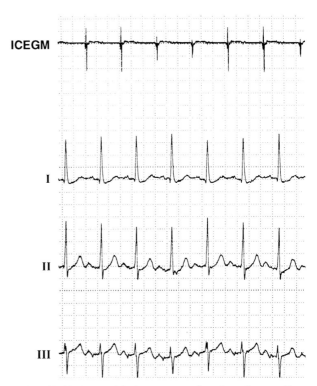

FIGURE 33–28. Intra-atrial electrogram and surface electrocardiogram. Note the profound variation of the intracardiac signal without apparent change of the surface P-wave morphology. This was synchronous with respiratory movements. This may be seen in either the atrium or the ventricle. ICEGM, intracardiac electrogram.

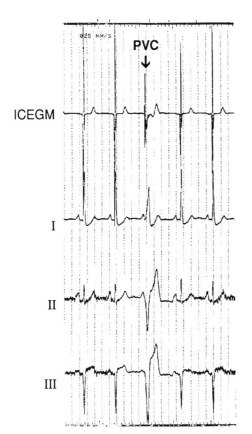

FIGURE 33–27. The ICEGM and surface electrocardiogram (I,II,III) of intrinsic beats and a PVC. In this example, the PVC electrogram has a significantly lower amplitude than the normal beats and may lead to undersensing. PVC, premature ventricular contractions; ICEGM, intracardiac electrogram.

case as the anode for the impedance sensing impulses, when the case is out of the pocket, a great deal of electrical noise is generated because the system is not grounded. This results in asynchronous pacing until the device is placed into the pocket. If the clinician is not aware of this idiosyncrasy, a malfunction of the pulse generator might be inappropriately diagnosed.

Finally, the use of either external or internal defibrillation may cause temporary or permanent loss of the sensing function. This may be caused by transient saturation of the sensing amplifier or circuit damage. This phenomenon is caused when the large electrical current delivered by the defibrillator is diverted from the pacemaker's circuitry to the pacing lead. The result may cauterize the myocardium and thus reduce or eliminate the local electrogram. It may also cause a marked elevation in the capture threshold or result in exit block. Capacitive coupling is another mechanism that may allow a current to be induced into the pacing lead by nearby electrocautery use.[144]

DUAL-CHAMBER PACEMAKER ISSUES

CROSSTALK INHIBITION

Crosstalk is a potentially catastrophic form of ventricular oversensing that can occur in any dual-chamber mode in which the atrium is paced and the ventricle is sensed and paced. Consider the fact that the common output voltages for the atrial channel range from 2.5 to 5.0 V. This is the same as 2500 to 5000 mV. The ventricular lead is just several centimeters away from this atrial lead and is "looking" for

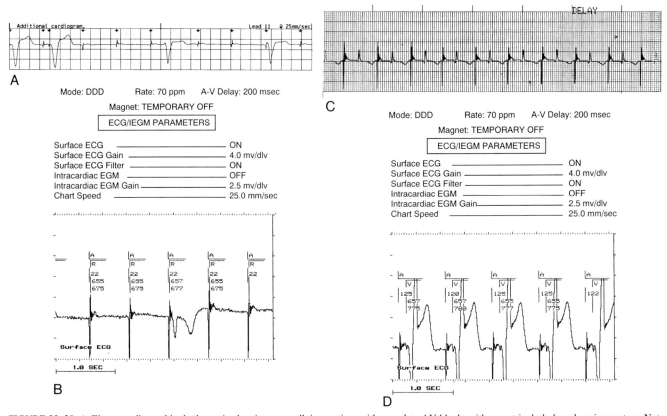

Mode: DDD   Rate: 70 ppm   A-V Delay: 200 msec

Magnet: TEMPORARY OFF

ECG/IEGM PARAMETERS

Surface ECG	ON
Surface ECG Gain	4.0 mv/dlv
Surface ECG Filter	ON
Intracardiac EGM	OFF
Intracardiac EGM Gain	2.5 mv/dlv
Chart Speed	25.0 mm/sec

FIGURE 33–29. *A*, Electrocardiographic rhythm strip showing crosstalk in a patient with complete AV block, with a ventricularly based pacing system. Note the presence of an atrial output without a ventricular output. A comparison of the interval from the first atrial pulse until the second with the second until the third demonstrates that the pacing interval is shortened by the AV interval minus the blanking period (120 msec). *B*, Electrocardiographic strip with event markers during crosstalk. Note that the ventricular sensing (R) occurs immediately after the atrial output pulse (A). Safety pacing was turned off. *C*, Electrocardiographic rhythm strip showing crosstalk in a patient with intact AV conduction. Because this pacemaker operates with ventricular-based timing, the atrial escape interval resets with each atrial output, elevating the frequency of atrial stimulation. *D*, Electrocardiographic rhythm strip and event markers during crosstalk and ventricular safety pacing. Note that despite the AV interval being set to 200 msec, the event markers demonstrate the ventricular stimulus at 125 msec after the atrial output pulses. ECG, electrocardiogram; EGM, electrogram; IEGM, intracardiac EGM; AV, atrioventricular.

an electrical event of approximately 2 mV, which would represent a ventricular depolarization. If the ventricular channel senses the pacing impulse delivered to the atrium, it interprets the event as a R wave. The ventricular output is inhibited, and the patient is left without pacing support. Should crosstalk occur in a patient with complete AV block, ventricular asystole could result, with only paced P waves visible. Conversely, crosstalk is more difficult to detect when AV nodal conduction is intact.

As demonstrated in Figure 33–29, crosstalk can be recognized by an acceleration of the atrial paced rate in a nonsensor-driven dual-chamber system incorporating ventricular-based timing. Note that ventricular sensing occurs simultaneously with atrial output. The AV delay is immediately terminated with ventricular sensing, and the atrial escape interval is started. Thus, the pacing interval with this type of timing is equal to the atrial escape interval (programmed pacing interval minus the AV delay) plus the ventricular blanking period.

Pacing systems that use atrial-based timing do not exhibit this rate increase. Although ventricular sensing of the atrial output inhibits the ventricular output, the AV interval is added to the atrial escape interval, maintaining atrial pacing at the programmed interval (Fig. 33–30). Modulated-rate

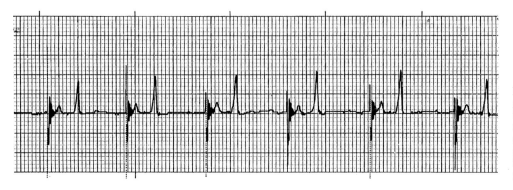

FIGURE 33–30. Electrocardiographic rhythm strip showing crosstalk with a pacemaker operating with atrial-based timing. Note that the atrial pacing rate remains at the programmed rate of 70 bpm. The AV interval was programmed to 175 msec.

TABLE 33–15. **FACTORS INCREASING THE CHANCE OF CROSSTALK**

High atrial amplitude setting
Wide atrial pulse width setting
High ventricular sensitivity setting
Short ventricular blanking period

pacing systems that use ventricular-based timing have this rate acceleration documented at rest. Crosstalk may not be readily diagnosed in patients with modulated-rate pacing systems and intact AV nodal conduction because the increased atrial pacing rate may be thought to be caused by the sensor. Even so, the shortening of the AV delay as a result of crosstalk, during rate-modulated upper rate pacing, can significantly increase the paced rate above the upper rate limit.

There are several factors that increase the likelihood of crosstalk (Table 33–15). Programmed settings that increase the ventricular sensitivity or the atrial energy output predispose to this problem. Insulation failure on the atrial lead also increases the chances of crosstalk. The clinician must be aware that certain pacemaker models are more prone to this phenomenon than are others. This is related to differences in circuit designs and the degree of isolation between the two channels within the pulse generator.[145] Crosstalk may occur within the circuitry of the pulse generator rather than between the pacing leads. Unipolar systems are also significantly more prone to crosstalk because of the larger electrical signal, as sensed by the ventricular channel.[146]

There are two approaches to the problem of crosstalk:

1. Prevention of crosstalk.
2. Prevention of the consequences of crosstalk.

PREVENTION OF CROSSTALK. Prevention of crosstalk is approached by proper programming of the device and proper lead placement. Atrial amplitude and pulse width settings that provide an appropriate safety margin without being excessive and ventricular sensitivity settings that are not unnecessarily sensitive are helpful. Newer circuit designs are much more resistant to this problem. However, even under "ideal" circumstances, crosstalk may still occur.

The use of an additional ventricular refractory period, known as the "blanking period," is fundamental to prevention.[147] The blanking period begins with the atrial output and usually lasts 20 to 50 msec. During this time, nothing (including the atrial output) can be sensed on the ventricular channel. Short blanking periods help to prevent the undersen-

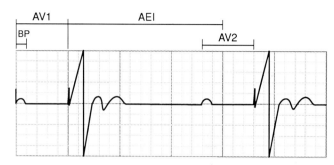

FIGURE 33–31. Timing diagram of the ventricular blanking period. This represents an absolute refractory period to prevent crosstalk by preventing ventricular oversensing of the atrial output pulse. Note that a blanking period is not inserted after a sensed atrial event.

sing of intrinsic ventricular activity but may allow crosstalk to occur. Long blanking periods virtually ensure the prevention of crosstalk but may cause intrinsic events to be undersensed (Fig. 33–31). If the AV interval is programmed to a long length, an undersensed PVC may be followed by a ventricular output beyond the myocardial refractory period. This might result in the induction of a ventricular arrhythmia, which may also occur with atrial undersensing when a normally conducted QRS falls into the blanking period. The latter event would not be detected, and an inappropriate stimulus would be delivered (Fig. 33–32).

PREVENTION OF CROSSTALK SEQUELAE. The earliest approach to the prevention of ventricular output loss as a result of crosstalk was the introduction of the DVI-committed mode (DVI-C). In this version of DVI, ventricular sensing is completely disabled during the AV interval that follows an atrial output pulse. Following the termination of the AV interval, a ventricular output pulse is committed whether or not an intrinsic ventricular event has occurred (Fig. 33–33). Thus, with DVI-C, there can never be an inhibition of the ventricular output by an atrial output. Although this approach works, it results in confusing ECGs and wastes energy because of the delivery of unnecessary pacing impulses.[132, 148] It is also not practical for DDD devices for the same reasons.

The most common approach is the use of a "safety output pulse." This is referred to by multiple names, depending on the manufacturer of the device (safety pacing, nonphysiologic AV delay, or ventricular safety standby). This method uses a brief sensing period ("crosstalk sensing window") following the blanking period. Any electrical event sensed during this crosstalk sensing period is assumed to be cross-

FIGURE 33–32. Electrocardiographic rhythm strip showing undersensing of native QRS. The device was programmed to the DVI mode; thus there is no atrial sensing. When the atrial escape interval expires, the atrial output coincidentally occurs just before the native QRS. As the ventricular blanking period occurs, turning off ventricular sensing for 38 msec with the atrial output, the native QRS is not sensed, and a ventricular output occurs at the end of the AV interval.

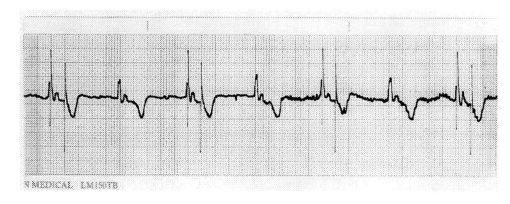

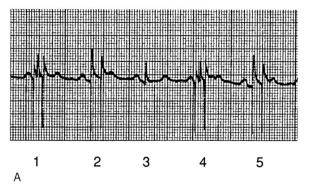

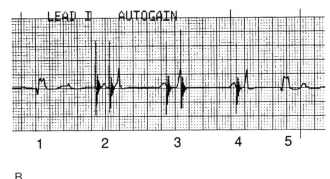

A   B

FIGURE 33–33. *A*, Electrocardiographic rhythm strip of committed DVI pacing. Note that, after any atrial output, ventricular sensing is disabled during the AV interval. As a ventricular output is "committed" after any atrial pace, ventricular inhibition as a result of crosstalk is not possible. *B*, Electrocardiographic rhythm strip of noncommitted DVI pacing. In this version of DVI, sensing occurs as expected after the blanking period terminates (complex 4). This allows inhibition by intrinsic ventricular activity. Complex 1 results in the complete inhibition of the device.

talk. A ventricular output is then committed after a shortened AV delay (Fig. 33–34). Other events may cause a safety output pulse to occur. These include premature ventricular beats, premature junctional beats, and normally conducted ventricular events that may occur following undersensed intrinsic atrial beats (Fig. 33–35). Following one of the latter events, if the safety output pulse were delivered using a long AV interval, there would be a potential for delivering a tightly coupled and potentially arrhythmogenic stimulus to the ventricle. Therefore, a shortened AV interval is used (typically, about 120 msec) to deliver the stimulus harmlessly into the depolarizing ventricle while maintaining the ability to rescue the patient in the presence of actual crosstalk.

As in crosstalk, the delivery of the safety output pulse causes a shortening of the base pacing interval because of the shortening of the AV interval (see Fig. 33–29*B*). However, if the baseline AV interval is programmed to the same duration as that of the safety output pulse, or if a rate-modulated or differential AV interval is present, the presence of safety pacing (thus, crosstalk) may be difficult, if not impossible, to discern on the standard ECG. The use of event marker telemetry documents the presence of crosstalk or safety output pulses in these situations (Fig. 33–36).

Finally, delivery of a safety output pulse does not prevent crosstalk. It is designed to prevent the sequelae of crosstalk by preventing ventricular asystole. It is unwise to allow a patient to use this backup mechanism continually. If crosstalk is suspected or documented, the clinician should pursue the potential causes and make the necessary adjustments to terminate this condition. In some situations such as failure of the lead's insulation, programming changes may not be adequate, and surgical intervention may be required.

PACEMAKER-MEDIATED TACHYCARDIA

Any undesired rapid pacing rate caused by the pulse generator or an interaction of the pacing system with the patient may be termed pacemaker-mediated tachycardia (PMT). This has classically been associated with the endless loop tachycardia (ELT) seen in dual-chamber devices. However, PMT should be assumed to be a more general term. The following are several conditions that are well documented to cause PMT.

RUNAWAY PACEMAKER. The runaway pacemaker is a pacemaker malfunction that may occur in single- or dual-chamber pacing systems. It is usually the result of a significant component failure within the pulse generator. The result is the rapid delivery of pacing stimuli to the heart with the potential for inducing lethal arrhythmias, such as ventricular tachycardia or fibrillation. Newer devices incorporate a runaway protect circuit that prevents stimulation above a preset rate, typically around 180 beats per minute (bpm). Although extremely rare with modern pacing devices, this represents a medical emergency. Emergent surgical intervention to cut the pacing electrode or to exchange the device must be performed. Obviously, a patient who is pacemaker dependent presents a new challenge as soon as the defective pacing system is disabled.[149, 150]

SENSOR-DRIVEN TACHYCARDIA. Sensor-driven tachycardia is a rapid heart rate occurring in modulated-rate pacemakers. This can occur with any type of sensor-driven pacing system (Table 33–16). Interaction between the patient and external stimuli may cause the rate-modulation system to overreact and pace at high rates. The most common cause of this PMT type is inappropriate programming of the sensor parameters.

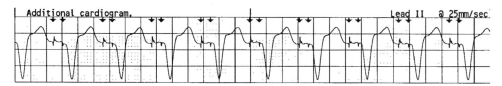

FIGURE 33–34. Electrocardiographic rhythm strip of safety pacing. Sensing is occurring on the ventricular channel during the crosstalk sensing window. This causes a ventricular output to be committed as a shortened AV interval. Note that the pacing interval is shortened by the difference between the programmed AV interval and the safety paced AV interval. This results in a paced rate of 93 bpm, even though the device is programmed DDD at 75 bpm.

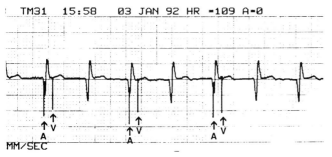

TM31   15:58   03 JAN 92 HR =109 A=0

MM/SEC

FIGURE 33–35. Electrocardiographic rhythm strip of safety pacing caused by accelerated junctional beats falling within the crosstalk sensing window. Atrial pacing (A) occurs coincidentally with the junctional beat. The junctional beat is sensed by the ventricular channel during the crosstalk sensing window, with the subsequent delivery of a safety pace. The pacemaker cannot differentiate between an intrinsic beat and actual crosstalk; thus safety pacing occurs.

TABLE 33–16. **CAUSES OF SENSOR-DRIVEN PACEMAKER TACHYCARDIA**

VIBRATION SENSORS
    Sleeping on ipsilateral side from device
    Submuscular implantation
    Loud music
    Riding in a car, tractor, or mower
    Use of vibration-generating tools
TEMPERATURE SENSORS
    Fever
CHEST WALL IMPEDANCE BASED (RESPIRATORY AND MINUTE VENTILATION)
    Hyperventilation
    Electrocautery
    Proximity to strong alternating current power sources
EVOKED QT INTERVAL
    Rate-dependent QT shortening spiral

In piezoelectric devices, a threshold setting that is too low and/or a slope setting that is too high results in high pacing rates for low levels of activity. It also exposes the patient to increased pacing rates for nonphysiologic events, such as riding in a car, exposure to loud noise or music, and sleeping on the ipsilateral side as the device implant.[151–157]

One unpublished incident concerns a patient with a bipolar piezoelectric VVIR device. The emergency medical squad had been summoned to treat an unconscious patient. They arrived to find the patient with tonic seizure activity. On viewing the ECG, the patient's condition was found to be wide complex tachycardia at 150 bpm. The patient received repeated direct current cardioversion for this tachycardia without reversion to sinus rhythm. In this case, the seizures were caused by epilepsy, and the vibration-based sensor responded to the seizure by pacing at its upper rate. No spikes had been noted on the ECG because the pacemaker's polarity was bipolar, which resulted in a diminutive artifact (Fig. 33–37).

Patients with pacing systems responsive to central venous temperature changes may respond to a fever with upper rate pacing. This requires a nulling feature to restore a more appropriate pacing rate after a specified time at the upper rate has occurred. In a similar fashion, devices that respond to changes in the evoked QT interval use this nulling feature, although for different reasons. As the QT interval shortens because of catecholamine increases and changes in the autonomic nervous system, the pacing rate is increased by the device. However, this may cause further shortening of the QT interval by a rate-dependent mechanism. The latter further increases the pacing rate, which may then spiral to the upper rate limit.[158, 159]

Devices that use thoracic impedance plethysmography to determine changes in minute ventilation may pace at the upper rate during marked hyperventilation, use of electrocautery, hyperventilation during anesthesia induction, and when in close proximity to an electrical power supply. Thus, it is highly recommended that any patient undergoing a surgical

2:1 Block Rate at 122 ppm

Mode: DDD   Rate: 80 ppm   A–V Delay: 250 msec
Magnet: TEMPORARY OFF

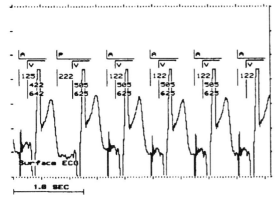

ECG/EGM PARAMETERS

Surface ECG _____ ON
Surface ECG Gain _____ 4.0 mv/dIv
Surface ECG Filter _____ ON
Intracardiac EGM _____ OFF
Intracardiac EGM Gain _____ 2.5 mv/dIv
Chart Speed _____ 25.0 mm/sec

FIGURE 33–36. Electrocardiographic rhythm strip with event marker telemetry showing the presence of safety pacing. The device is programmed to DDD with an AV interval of 250 msec after an atrial pace and 225 msec after an atrial sensed event. Note that, after each atrial paced event (A), a ventricular pace (V) occurs after about 120 msec. A sensed atrial event (P) occurs inhibiting the atrial output on the second event. Note the appropriate AV interval that follows. ECG, electrocardiogram; EGM, electrogram; IEGM, intracardiac EGM; AV, atrioventricular.

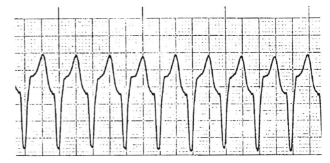

FIGURE 33–37. Electrocardiographic rhythm strip of "pseudoventricular tachycardia" caused by rapid ventricular pacing using a bipolar device. Note that the pace artifact is not well seen, leading to this potential misdiagnosis.

procedure, treatment with a mechanical ventilator, or a critical care therapy have the rate-modulation feature disabled.[160]

MAGNETIC RESONANCE IMAGING. Exposure to magnetic resonance imaging scanners has been reported to cause inappropriately high pacing rates when tested in animals. Some pacemakers have been noted to pace at the pulse rate of the scanner. This situation resolves immediately with the cessation of the radiofrequency output by the scanner.[161-163] Magnetic resonance imaging may also result in the inhibition of the pacing output during the scanning process. Because of these issues, such scanning has been cautioned against by all manufacturers of pacemakers. This is true even though some patients have inadvertently or intentionally undergone magnetic resonance imaging without sequelae. Some physicians have programmed nonpacemaker-dependent patients to the OOO mode or to a subthreshold voltage output and/or pulse width. Although this may help, the induced current from having a wire in a moving magnetic field can theoretically stimulate the heart without being connected to the generator.

MYOPOTENTIAL TRACKING. Myopotential tracking is caused by oversensing of the atrial channel in a dual-chamber pacing system capable of P-wave tracking. This has become far less common with the use of bipolar sensing, which is increasingly preferred by implanting physicians. Myopotential tracking occurs when the atrial channel senses the electrical activity of the muscle underlying the pulse generator, as in myopotential inhibition. Because the atrial sensitivity setting is usually higher (more sensitive) than that in the ventricular channel, atrial output is inhibited. However, although the atrial output is inhibited, the AV interval is continuously triggered by this oversensing, and ventricular pacing may occur up to the programmed maximum P-wave tracking rate (Fig. 33–38). If the myopotentials are of large enough amplitude, ventricular inhibition may also occur.[48-54]

ENDLESS LOOP TACHYCARDIA. The most classic form of PMT is ELT, which can occur in dual-chamber pacemakers that are capable of atrial tracking modes, most commonly DDD or VDD. Only patients who are capable of retrograde ventriculoatrial conduction through the AV node or an AV accessory pathway are capable of sustaining this rhythm. The mechanism is identical to any macroreentrant tachycardia seen in the heart in which two electrical pathways exist between the atria and ventricles. Pacemaker ELT is classically initiated by a PVC. The depolarization is then conducted retrogradely to the atria. If the postventricular atrial refractory period (PVARP) has ended and the retrograde complex is of sufficient amplitude, the atrial channel senses the event and triggers an AV interval. At the end of the AV interval, the pacemaker then delivers a stimulus to the ventricle, and the loop is reinitiated (Fig. 33–39). Although a PVC

is the classic cause of PMT initiation, any situation that leads to a ventricular depolarization without a normally coupled atrial paced or sensed event may begin the loop (Table 33–17). The latter includes atrial noncapture, oversensing, and undersensing. In addition, if the programmed AV interval is long (some units allow programming of up to a 300-msec interval), it may be possible for the AV node to recover in time to conduct the subsequent ventricular event retrogradely and cause ELT (Fig. 33–40). The absence of antegrade AV nodal conduction does not rule out retrograde conduction over the AV node or a concealed AV accessory pathway. Patients may also exhibit intermittent retrograde conduction or have variations in the retrograde conduction time relative to their sympathetic tone and catecholamine status.[164-171]

The rate of ELT depends on the conduction velocity and refractory period of the retrograde AV pathway. If the retrograde AV conduction is the same or shorter than the upper rate interval (but not shorter than the PVARP), then the tachycardia rate is at the programmed upper rate. However, if the retrograde AV conduction time is slower than the upper rate interval, the tachycardia rate is below the upper programmed rate (Fig. 33–41). Thus, the rate of the ELT never exceeds the upper rate programming of the pacemaker; however, it may be lower.[172-174]

As with crosstalk, there are two approaches to ELT:

1. Prevention of ELT initiation.
2. Termination of ELT once it occurs.

PREVENTION OF ENDLESS LOOP TACHYCARDIA. The main defense against ELT is the use of an appropriate PVARP interval. During the PVARP, the atrial channel cannot sense the retrograde depolarization that initiates ELT no matter what the source of that event. If retrograde conduction is present during implant or follow-up, it is a simple matter to measure the ventriculoatrial time and program PVARP to an interval that is longer. However, many patients exhibit only intermittent ventriculoatrial conduction, making an accurate assessment difficult. The major limitation of using a long PVARP is that it limits the upper tracking rate of the device (2:1 blocking rate). Some patients in our clinics have ventriculoatrial times in excess of 430 msec. Thus, using a PVARP of 450 msec and an AV interval of 150 msec, the total atrial refractory period is 600 msec. This causes 2:1 blocking at an atrial rate of 100 bpm, which is far too low for an active patient.

One solution to this problem is the use of ELT prevention algorithms.[175, 176] The most common algorithm is PVARP extension on premature ventricular event (PVE) detection. A PVE is defined as a ventricular sensed event that is not

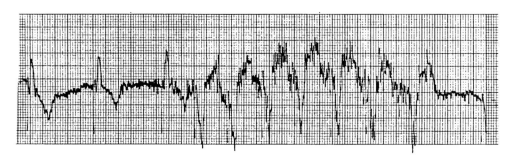

FIGURE 33–38. Electrocardiographic rhythm strip of myopotential tracking. The electrical activity of the muscle adjacent to the pacemaker case in a unipolar system is oversensed by the atrial channel. This causes repeated initiation of the AV interval up to the maximum tracking rate. Higher amplitude myopotentials may also cause the inhibition of the ventricular channel.

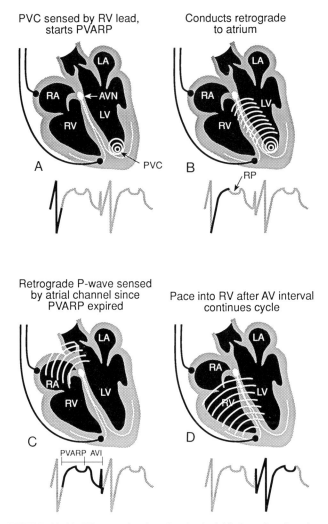

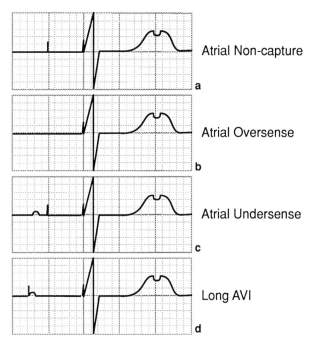

FIGURE 33–40. Diagram of different initiating events leading to retrograde P-wave conduction and the potential for endless loop tachycardia. *A,* Atrial noncapture causes ventricular stimulation without the AV node being blocked by an antegrade event. *B,* Atrial oversensing inhibits atrial output and provides just a ventricular output with the same results as in *A. C,* Atrial undersensing allows a long AV interval, allowing the AV node time to recover and conduct retrograde. *D,* A long programmed AV interval may also allow the AV node to recover. AV, atrioventricular.

FIGURE 33–39. Diagram showing the classic initiation of endless loop tachycardia by a PVC in a patient with retrograde AV conduction. *A,* A PVC occurs. *B,* The event is conducted in a retrograde fashion to the atrium, as seen by the inverted (retrograde) P wave. *C,* The retrograde event is sensed by the atrial channel, which causes an AV interval to be started. *D,* At the end of the AV interval, a stimulus is delivered to the ventricle if or when the maximum rate limit is not violated, resulting in retrograde conduction and the perpetuation of this cycle. PVC, premature ventricular contractions; RV, right ventricle; RA, right atrium; LA, left atrium; LV, left ventricle; AVN, atrioventricular node; PVARP, postventricular atrial refractory period; AVI, atrioventricular interval.

Newer approaches have been made possible by the advent of sensor-driven pacing systems. With a DDDR system, even though the maximum tracking rate may be limited by a long PVARP, faster AV sequentially paced rates may be possible through the sensor. Even though atrial sensing does not occur during the PVARP, sensor-driven atrial pacing may occur. Another alternative in some DDDR pulse generators is to use an adaptive PVARP that is long when the sensor determines

preceded by an atrial paced or sensed event. When a PVE is detected, the device prolongs PVARP by a fixed or programmable value for the following cycle (Fig. 33–42*A*). It allows a shorter baseline PVARP to be used, with associated higher 2:1 blocking rates. A variation on this technique is to proceed with one DVI cycle following the PVE. This is the ultimate PVARP extension because the atrial channel remains refractory to sensing throughout the entire atrial escape interval (Fig. 33–42*B*). One problem with PVARP extension algorithms is that situations, such as atrial noncapture, are not prevented from causing ELT. In the latter case, the pacemaker does not define a PVE because it has delivered an atrial stimulus (although ineffective) prior to a ventricular event. The subsequent ventricular paced event then leads to ELT (Fig. 33–43).

TABLE 33–17. **ENDLESS LOOP TACHYCARDIA SUMMARY**

INITIATION
PVC
Atrial undersensing
Long programmed AV interval
Myopotential sensing
PREVENTION
PVARP
PVARP extension of PVE detection
DVI cycle on PVE detection
Differential atrial sensing
Adaptive PVARP
DETECTION
P-wave tracking at upper rate
P-wave tracking at intermediate rate
AV-interval modulation
TERMINATION
PVARP extension
DVI mode change
Failure to track after X beats

Abbreviations: PVC, premature ventricular contractions; PVE, premature ventricular event; AV, atrioventricular; PVARP, postventricular atrial refractory period.

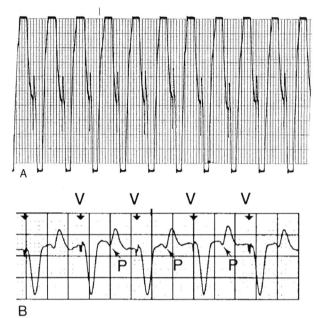

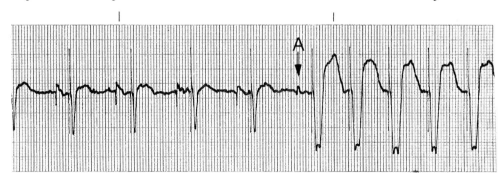

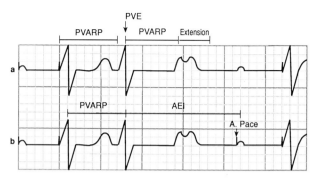

FIGURE 33–42. Diagram of endless loop tachycardia prevention algorithms. *A,* PVARP extension following PVE detection adds an additional period to PVARP, causing the retrograde P wave to fall within the refractory period. *B,* DVI cycle following PVE detection does the same as PVARP extension; however, atrial sensing remains off for the entire AEI. PVARP, postventricular atrial refractory period; PVE, premature ventricular event; AEI, atrial escape interval; A., atrial.

FIGURE 33–41. *A,* Electrocardiographic rhythm strip of ELT with fast VA conduction, resulting in a rapid ELT at the upper programmed rate of 155 bpm. Lower rate, 60 ppm; sensed AV interval, 150 msec; PVARP, 275 msec; VA time, 300 msec. *B,* Electrocardiographic rhythm strip of ELT with slow VA conduction, resulting in ELT below the programmed upper rate. As a result of the slow retrograde conduction, the ELT rate is significantly slower than the programmed upper rates. Retrograde P wave (P); ventricular output (V); lower rate, 60; upper rate, 145; AV interval, 165 msec; PVARP, 250 msec). ELT, endless loop tachycardia; VA, ventriculoatrial; AV, atrioventricular; PVARP, postventricular atrial refractory period.

TERMINATION OF ENDLESS LOOP TACHYCARDIA. The most difficult aspect of applying an ELT termination protocol is having the device determine whether ELT is present or not. This has been approached by several different criteria by different manufacturers. Some of these are simple; others are more complex. The following are some of the most common techniques for identifying the presence of ELT.

The first is sustained P-wave tracking at the upper rate. This is the most common method of ELT detection. If the pacemaker P wave tracks at the upper rate for a specific number of intervals, PVARP is prolonged for one cycle or DVI is used for one cycle. The number of events at the upper rate that trigger an ELT termination attempt depend on the particular pulse generator. Some algorithms use a fixed number of beats, and others may be programmable. The method of ELT termination may also be programmable (PVARP extension or DVI cycle).[184, 185]

The second is sustained P-wave tracking at a specific rate that is lower than the upper rate. As previously noted, not all ELTs occur at the upper programmed tracking rate. An ELT rate is always limited by the slowest point in the loop. If the patient has a ventriculoatrial conduction time that is longer than the upper tracking interval, then the resulting ELT is slower than the upper tracking rate that is programmed. This presentation of ELT is not identified by the sustained upper rate method. Some devices allow an initiation of the ELT termination algorithm at a P-wave tracking rate that is lower than the upper tracking rate. This lower rate is typically a programmable option to provide for the termination of ELT in this subset of patients.

that the patient is at rest. When the patient's sensor-indicated rate increases along with the need for higher heart rates, the PVARP is shortened proportionately, allowing higher rates before a 2:1 block occurs. This approach allows the device to discriminate between early atrial depolarizations at rest (possibly retrograde beats or PACs) versus sinus tachycardia with exertion.[177, 178]

A comparison of P-wave morphology can allow discrimination between sinus and retrograde atrial depolarizations in some cases. This was referred to as differential atrial sensing.[179–183] Mapping of the atrium may allow positioning of the lead at a site that has a large P wave when generated by the sinus node, although the retrograde P waves appear small in comparison. The pacemaker may be programmed to be sensitive enough to allow sensing of the antegrade P wave but be insensitive enough to undersense the retrograde P wave. Thus, ELT cannot be initiated or sustained because the loop cannot be completed.

FIGURE 33–43. Device programmed with PVARP extension on PVE detection. An atrial output occurred (A) with a loss of atrial capture. The ventricular output captures the ventricle, resulting in VA conduction and endless loop tachycardia. The prevention algorithm failed because this was not caused by a PVE. PVARP, postventricular atrial refractory period; PVE, premature ventricular event.

The third is a modulation of the AV interval during sustained P-wave tracking at the upper rate. One company introduced a unique method of discriminating between sinus rates at the upper rate and ELT. The technique used is based on the observation that the ventriculoatrial conduction time in any individual is relatively constant. When the device is P-wave tracking with a V-pace to P-sense interval less than 450 msec, it slightly shortens the AV interval every other cycle. If ELT is present, the V-pace to P-sense interval remains constant (the atrial cycle length is shortened by the shortening of the AV interval), the device confirms ELT and initiates a termination algorithm (Fig. 33–44*A*). However, if the V-pace to A-sense interval lengthens (the atrial cycle length is not affected by the AV interval shortening), then ELT is not confirmed, and the device continues to track the atrium normally (Fig. 33–44*B*).

CROSS STIMULATION

Cross stimulation may be defined as stimulation of one cardiac chamber when stimulation of the other is expected (Fig. 33–45). An embarrassing cause of this phenomenon is the inadvertent placement of the ventricular lead into the atrial connector and the atrial lead into the ventricular connector of the pulse generator. Dislodgement of either lead into the other chamber may also be a cause. Coronary sinus placement of either lead, either intentionally or accidentally, may cause continued or intermittent cross stimulation. For all of the latter, surgical revision of the pacing system is the only option for correction. Several reports of cross stimulation have been reported, which are not related to the latter situations.[186–189] This seems to be caused by an internal crossover within the pulse generator. In all cases, this resolved after several weeks. It has been suggested that low imped-

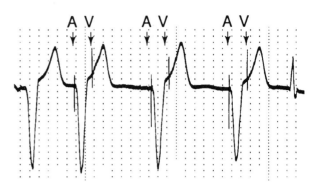

FIGURE 33–45. Electrocardiographic rhythm strip showing cross-stimulation as a result of lead reversal. The atrial lead was placed into the ventricular connector, and the ventricular lead was placed into the atrial connector. Note that the first output delivered stimulated the ventricle, and the second falls into the ST segment when it is delivered into the atrium at the end of the AV interval.

ance in the lead system allows a higher current on each channel. As the impedance rises with lead maturation, the current load falls, and the problem resolves.

Conclusion

Pacemaker dysfunction, although seemingly difficult to assess, can be categorized in relation to the dysfunction of the leads or the generator and apparent dysfunction related to the idiosyncratic characteristics of the pacemaker's timing algorithms. Although lead failure, either as a result of implantation error or deterioration of the lead materials, is common, malfunction of the pulse generator is rare. Consequently, the key to unlocking the understanding of unexpected pacemaker behavior is related to verification of the integrity of the leads and an understanding of the timing cycles of the specific pacemaker. The clues are in the patient's history of symptoms, physical examination, and pacemaker telemetry. However, the answer is usually lead dysfunction or may be found in the pacemaker's physician manual.

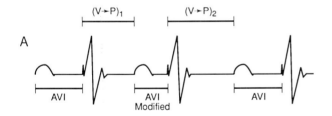

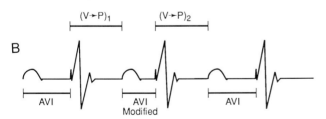

FIGURE 33–44. Diagram of Ela (Paris, France) ELT detection scheme. *A,* Rapid tracking of sinus tachycardia. The device causes the AV interval to be varied. When the AV interval is shortened (AVI modified), there is a prolongation of the P-to-P interval (V-P2 is longer than V-P1) because the sinus node rate is not affected. *B,* ELT caused by tracking of retrograde P waves. The device again causes the AV interval to be varied. In this case, shortening of the AV interval has no effect on the next retrograde event (V-P2 is the same as V-P1). This is defined by the device as an ELT, and a termination algorithm is activated. AVI, atrioventricular interval; ELT, endless loop tachycardia.

REFERENCES

1. Garson A Jr: Stepwise approach to the unknown pacemaker ECG. Am Heart J 119:924, 1990.
2. Furman S: Cardiac pacing and pacemakers VI: Analysis of pacemaker malfunction. Am Heart J 94:378, 1977.
3. Mond HG: The Cardiac Pacemaker, Function and Malfunction. New York, Grune & Stratton, 1983.
4. Barold SS: Modern Cardiac Pacing. Mt Kisco, NY, Futura Publishing, 1983.
5. Levine PA: Pacing system malfunction. *In* Ellenbogen KA (ed): Cardiac Pacing. Boston, Blackwell Scientific Publications, 1992, pp 309–382.
6. Morse DP, Steiner RM, Parsonnet V: A Guide to Cardiac Pacemakers. Philadelphia, FA Davis, 1983.
7. Morse DP, Steiner RM, Parsonnet V: A Guide to Cardiac Pacemakers: Supplement 1986–1987. Philadelphia, FA Davis, 1986.
8. Morse DP, Parsonnet V, Gessment LJ, et al: A Guide to Cardiac Pacemaker, Defibrillator and Related Produces. Durham, NC, Droege Computing Services, 1991.
9. Van Gelder LM, El Gamal MIH: Myopotential interference inducing pacemaker tachycardia in a DVI programmed pacemaker. PACE Pacing Clin Electrophysiol 7:970, 1984.
10. Lindenberg BS, Hagan CA, Levine PA: Design dependent loss of

telemetry: Uplink telemetry hold. PACE Pacing Clin Electrophysiol 12:823, 1989.

11. Levine PA, Lindenberg BS: Upper rate limit circuit-induced rate slowing. PACE Pacing Clin Electrophysiol 10:310, 1987.

12. Levine PA, Lindenberg BS, Mace RC: Analysis of AV universal (DDD) pacemaker rhythms. Clin Prog Pacing Electrophysiol 2:54, 1984.

13. Bertuso J, Kapoor A, Schafer J: A case of ventricular undersensing in the DDI mode: Cause and correction. PACE Pacing Clin Electrophysiol 9:685, 1986.

14. Erlbacher JA, Stelzer P: Inappropriate ventricular blanking in a DDI pacemaker. PACE Pacing Clin Electrophysiol 9:519, 1986.

15. Ajiki K, Sagara K, Namiki T, et al: A case of a pseudomalfunction of a DDD pacemaker. PACE Pacing Clin Electrophysiol 14:1456, 1991.

16. Meyer JA, Fruehan CT, Delmonico JE: The pacemaker twiddler's syndrome, a further note. J Thorac Cardiovasc Surg 67:903, 1974.

17. Veltri EP, Mower MM, Reid PR: Twiddler's syndrome: A new twist. PACE Pacing Clin Electrophysiol 7:1004, 1984.

18. Lal RB, Avery RD: Aggressive pacemaker twiddler's syndrome, dislodgement of an active fixation ventricular pacing electrode. Chest 97:756, 1990.

19. Roberts JS, Wenger NK: Pacemaker twiddler's syndrome. Am J Cardiol 63:1013, 1989.

20. Ellis GL: Pacemaker twiddler's syndrome: A case report. Am J Emerg Med 8:48, 1990.

21. Ekbom K, Nilsson BY, Edhag O: Rhythmic shoulder girdle muscle contractions as a complication in pacemaker treatment. Chest 66:599, 1974.

22. Gelleri D: Retrograde (ventriculo-atrial) conduction, premature beats, pseudotricuspid regurgitation, systolic atrial sounds, and pacemaker sounds observed together in two patients with ventricular pacing. Acta Med Hung 48:157, 1991.

23. Flickinger AL, Peller PA, Deran BP, et al: Pacemaker-induced friction rub and apical thrill. Chest 102:323, 1992.

24. Jalin P, Kaul U, Wasir HS: Myopotential inhibition of unipolar demand pacemakers: Utility of provocative manoeuvres in assessment and management. Int J Cardiol 34:33, 1992.

25. Levine PA: Electrocardiography of bipolar single- and dual-chamber pacing systems. Herzschrittmacher 8:86, 1988.

26. Cherry R, Sactuary C, Kennedy HL: The question of frequency response. Ambulatory Electrocardiol 1:13, 1977.

27. Sheffield LT, Berson AL, Bragg-Remschel D, et al: AHA special report, recommendation for standards of instrumentation and practice in the use of ambulatory electrocardiography. Circulation 71:626A, 1985.

28. Schuller H, Fahraeus T: Pacemaker EKG: A Clinical Approach. Solna, Sweden, Siemens-Elema, 1980.

29. Levine PA, Schuller H, Lindgren A: Pacemaker ECG: An Introduction and Approach to Interpretation. Solna, Sweden, Siemens-Pacesetter, 1986.

30. Sholder J, Levine PA, Mann BM, et al: Bidirectional telemetry and interrogation in cardiac pacing. In Barold SS, Mugica J (eds): The Third Decade of Cardiac Pacing, Advances in Technology and Clinical Application. Mt Kisco, NY, Futura Publishing, 1982, pp 145–171.

31. Levine PA: The complementary role of electrogram, event marker, and measured data telemetry in the assessment of pacing system function. J Electrophysiol 1:404, 1987.

32. Kruse I, Markoviwtz T, Ryden L: Timing markers showing pacemaker behavior to aid in the follow-up of a physiologic pacemaker. PACE Pacing Clin Electrophysiol 6:801, 1983.

33. Wilkoff BL, Firstenberg MS, Moore S, Ching B: Lead impedance velocity as a predictor of pacing lead instability. PACE Pacing Clin Electrophysiol 16:930, 1993.

34. Levine PA: Clinical manifestations of lead insulation defects. J Electrophysiol 1:144, 1987.

35. Karis JP, Ravin CE: Counterclockwise exit of cardiac pacemaker leads: Sign of pulse-generator flip. Radiology 174:711, 1990.

36. Suzuki Y, Fujimori S, Sakai M, et al: A case of pacemaker lead fracture associated with thoracic outlet syndrome. PACE Pacing Clin Electrophysiol 11:326, 1988.

37. Stokes K, Staffenson D, Lessar J, et al: A possible new complication of subclavian stick: Conductor fracture. PACE Pacing Clin Electrophysiol 10:748, 1987.

38. Anonymous: Subclavian puncture procedure may result in lead conductor fracture. Medtronic News Winter 16(2):27, 1986/87.

39. Magney JE, Flynn DM, Parsons JA, et al: Anatomical mechanisms

explaining damage to pacemaker leads, defibrillator leads, and failure of central venous catheters adjacent to the sternoclavicular joint. PACE Pacing Clin Electrophysiol 16:445, 1993.

40. Jacobs DM, Fink AS, Miller RP, et al: Anatomical and morphological evaluation of pacemaker lead compression. PACE Pacing Clin Electrophysiol 16:434, 1993.

41. Arakawa M, Kambara K, Ito HA, et al: Intermittent oversensing due to internal insulation damage of temperature sensing rate-responsive pacemaker lead in subclavian venipuncture method. PACE Pacing Clin Electrophysiol 12:1312, 1989.

42. Fyke FE: Simultaneous insulation deterioration associated with side-by-side subclavian placement of two polyurethane leads. PACE Pacing Clin Electrophysiol 11:1571, 1988.

43. Kranz J, Crystal DK, Wagner CL, et al: Thoracic outlet compression syndrome, the first rib. Northwest Med 68:646, 1969.

44. Witte A: Pseudo-fracture of pacemaker lead due to securing suture: A case report. PACE Pacing Clin Electrophysiol 4:716, 1981.

45. Deering JA, Pederson DN: A case of pacemaker lead fracture associated with weightlifting. PACE Pacing Clin Electrophysiol 15:1354, 1992.

46. Schuger CD, Mittleman R, Habbal B, et al: Ventricular lead transection and atrial lead damage in a young softball player shortly after the insertion of a permanent pacemaker. PACE Pacing Clin Electrophysiol 15:1236, 1992.

47. Widlansky S, Zipes DP: Suppression of a ventricular inhibited bipolar pacemaker by skeletal muscle activity. J Electrocardiol 7:371, 1974.

48. Fetter J, Bobeldyk GL, Engman FJ: The clinical incidence and significance of myopotential sensing with unipolar pacemakers. PACE Pacing Clin Electrophysiol 7:871, 1984.

49. Halperin JL, Camunas JL, Stern EH, et al: Myopotential interference with DDD pacemakers: Endocardial electrographic telemetry in the diagnosis of pacemaker-related arrhythmias. Am J Cardiol 54:97, 1984.

50. Williams DO, Thomas DJ: Muscle potentials simulating pacemaker malfunction. Br Heart J 38:1096, 1976.

51. Ohm OJ, Morkrid L, Hammer E: Amplitude-frequency characteristics of myopotentials and endocardial potentials as seen by a pacemaker system. Scand J Thorac Cardiovasc Surg Suppl (22):41–6, 1978.

52. Levine PA, Caplan CH, Klein MD, et al: Myopotential inhibition of unipolar lithium pacemakers. Chest 82:461, 1982.

53. Ohm OJ, Bruland H, Pedersen OM, et al: Interference effect of myopotentials on function of unipolar demand pacemakers. Br Heart J 35:77, 1974.

54. Gabry MD, Behrens M, Andrews C, et al: Comparison of myopotential interference in unipolar-bipolar programmable DDD pacemakers. PACE Pacing Clin Electrophysiol 10:1322, 1987.

55. Gross JN, Platt S, Ritacco R, et al: The clinical relevance of electromyopotential oversensing in current unipolar devices. PACE Pacing Clin Electrophysiol 15:2023, 1992.

56. Volosin KJ, Rudderow R, Waxman HL: VOOR—nondemand rate-modulated pacing necessitated by myopotential inhibition. PACE Pacing Clin Electrophysiol 12:421, 1989.

57. Dodinot B, Godenir JP, Costa AB: Electronic article surveillance: A possible danger for pacemaker patients. PACE Pacing Clin Electrophysiol 16:46, 1993.

58. Inbar S, Larson J, Burt T, et al: Case report: Nuclear magnetic resonance imaging in a patient with a pacemaker. Am J Med Sci 305:174, 1993.

59. Marco D, Eisinger G, Hayes DL: Testing of work environments for electromagnetic interference. PACE Pacing Clin Electrophysiol 15:2016, 1992.

60. Toivonen L, Valjus J, Hongisto M, et al: The influence of elevated 50 Hz electric and magnetic fields on implanted pacemakers: The role of the lead configuration and programming of the sensitivity. PACE Pacing Clin Electrophysiol 14:2114, 1991.

61. Mellenberg DE Jr: A policy for radiotherapy in patients with implanted pacemakers. Med Dosim 16:221, 1991.

62. Mangar D, Atlas GM, Kane PB: Electrocautery-induced pacemaker malfunction during surgery. Can J Anaesth 38:616, 1991.

63. Teskey RJ, Whelan I, Akyurekli Y, et al: Therapeutic irradiation over a permanent pacemaker. PACE Pacing Clin Electrophysiol 14:143, 1991.

64. Salmi J, Eskola HJ, Pitkanen MA, et al: The influence of electromagnetic interference and ionizing radiation on cardiac pacemakers. Strahlenther Onkol 166:153, 1990.

65. Chin MC, Rosenqvist M, Lee MA, et al: The effect of radiofrequency

catheter ablation on permanent pacemakers: An experimental study. PACE Pacing Clin Electrophysiol 13:23, 1990.

66. McDeller AG, Toff WD, Hobbs RA, et al: The development of a system for the evaluation of electromagnetic interference with pacemaker function: Hazards in the aircraft environment. J Med Eng Technol 13:161, 1989.

67. Godin JF, Petitot JC: STIMAREC report. Pacemaker failures due to electrocautery and external electric shock. PACE Pacing Clin Electrophysiol 12:1011, 1989.

68. Belott P, Sands S, Warren J, et al: Resetting of DDD pacemakers due to EMI. PACE Pacing Clin Electrophysiol 7:169, 1984.

69. Erdman S, Levinsky L, Strasberg B, et al: Use of the new Shaw scalpel in pacemaker operations. J Thorac Cardiovasc Surg 89:304, 1985.

70. Gascho JA, Newton MC: Electromagnetic interference in dynamic electrocardiography caused by an electric blanket. Am Heart J 95:408, 1978.

71. Irnich W: Interference in pacemakers. PACE Pacing Clin Electrophysiol 7:1021, 1984.

72. Kuan P, Kozlowski J, Castellanet MJ, et al: Interference with pacemaker function by cardiokymographic testing. Am J Cardiol 58:362, 1986.

73. Leeds CJ, Akhtar M, Damato AN, et al: Fluoroscope-generated electromagnetic interference in an external demand pacemaker. Circulation 55:548, 1977.

74. Warnowicz-Papp M: The pacemaker patient and the electromagnetic environment. Clin Prog Pacing Electrophysiol 1:166, 1983.

75. Van Gelder LM, El Gamal MIH: False inhibition of an atrial demand pacemaker caused by insulation defect in a polyurethane lead. PACE Pacing Clin Electrophysiol 6:834, 1983.

76. Sanford CF: Self-inhibition of an AV sequential demand pulse generator due to polyurethane lead insulation disruption. PACE Pacing Clin Electrophysiol 6:840, 1983.

77. Salem DN, Bornstein A, Levine PA, et al: Fracture of pacing electrode mimicking failure of pulse generator. Chest 74:673, 1978.

78. Coumel P, Mujica J, Barold SS: Demand pacemaker arrhythmias caused by intermittent incomplete electrode fracture. Am J Cardiol 36:105, 1975.

79. Barold SS, Scovil J, Ong LS, et al: Periodic pacemaker spike attenuation with preservation of capture: An unusual electrocardiographic manifestation of partial pacing electrode fracture. PACE Pacing Clin Electrophysiol 1:375, 1978.

80. Sarmiento JJ: Clinical utility of telemetered intracardiac electrograms in diagnosing a design dependent lead malfunction. PACE Pacing Clin Electrophysiol 13:188, 1990.

81. Nalos PC, Nyitray W: Benefits of intracardiac electrograms and programmable sensing polarity in preventing pacemaker inhibition due to spurious screw-in lead signals. PACE Pacing Clin Electrophysiol 13:1101, 1990.

82. Chew PH, Brinker JA: Oversensing from electrode ''chatter'' in a bipolar pacing lead: A case report. PACE Pacing Clin Electrophysiol 13:808, 1990.

83. Santomauro M, Ferraro S, Maddalena G, et al: Pacemaker malfunction due to subcutaneous emphysema: A case report. Angiology 43:873, 1992.

84. Giroud D, Goy JJ: Pacemaker malfunction due to subcutaneous emphysema. Int J Cardiol 26:234, 1990.

85. Shepard RB, Kim J, Colvin HC, et al: Pacing threshold spikes months and years after implant. PACE Pacing Clin Electrophysiol 14:1835, 1991.

86. Trautwein W: Electrophysiological aspects of cardiac stimulation. In Schaldach M, Furman S (eds): Advances in Pacemaker Technology. New York, Springer-Verlag, 1975, pp 11–23.

87. Siddons H, Sowton E: Threshold for stimulation. In Cardiac Pacemakers. Springfield, IL, Charles C Thomas, 1967, pp 145–174.

88. Ohm OJ, Breivik K, Anderssen KS: Strength-duration curves in cardiac pacing. In Meere C (ed): Proceedings of the Sixth World Symposium on Cardiac Pacing, Montreal, January 1979, Chap. 20.

89. Irnich W: The chronaxie time and its practical importance. PACE Pacing Clin Electrophysiol 3:292, 1980.

90. Davies JG, Sowton E: Electrical threshold of the human heart. Br Heart J 28:231, 1966.

91. Furman S, Hurzeler P, Mehra R: Cardiac pacing and pacemakers. IV. Threshold of cardiac stimulation. Am Heart J 94:115, 1977.

92. Helguera ME, Maloney JD, Woscoboinik JR, et al: Long-term performance of epimyocardial pacing leads in adults: Comparison with endocardial leads. PACE Pacing Clin Electrophysiol 16:412, 1993.

93. Esperper HD, Mahmoud PO, von der Emde J: Is epicardial dual-chamber pacing a realistic alternative to endocardial DDD pacing? Initial results of a prospective study. PACE Pacing Clin Electrophysiol 15:155, 1992.

94. Bianconi L, Boccadamo R, Toscano S, et al: Effects of oral propafenone therapy on chronic myocardial pacing threshold. PACE Pacing Clin Electrophysiol 15:148, 1992.

95. Szabo Z, Solti F: The significance of the tissue reaction around the electrode on the late myocardial threshold. In Schaldach M, Furman S (eds): Advances in Pacemaker Technology. New York, Springer-Verlag, 1975, pp 273–287.

96. DeLeon SY, Ilbawi MN, Backer CL, et al: Exit block in pediatric cardiac pacing. Comparison of the suture-type and fishhook epicardial electrodes. J Thorac Cardiovasc Surg 99:905, 1990.

97. Stojanov P, Djordjevic M, Velimirovic D, et al: Assessment of long-term stability of chronic ventricular pacing thresholds in steroid-eluting electrodes. PACE Pacing Clin Electrophysiol 15:1417, 1992.

98. Karpawich PP, Hakimi M, Arciniegas E, et al: Improved epicardial pacing in children: Steroid contribution to porous platinized electrodes. PACE Pacing Clin Electrophysiol 15:1551, 1992.

99. Johns JA, Fish FA, Burger JD, et al: Steroid-eluting epicardial pacing leads in pediatric patients encouraging early results. J Am Coll Cardiol 20:395, 1992.

100. Stamato NJ, O'Tolle MF, Petter JG, et al: The safety and efficacy of chronic ventricular pacing at 1.6 volts using a steroid-eluting lead. PACE Pacing Clin Electrophysiol 15:248, 1992.

101. Hamilton R, Gow R, Bahoric B, et al: Steroid-eluting epicardial leads in pediatrics: Improved epicardial threshold in the first year. PACE Pacing Clin Electrophysiol 14:2066, 1991.

102. Anderson N, Mathivanar R, Skalsky M, et al: Active fixation leads: Long-term threshold reduction using a drug-infused ceramic collar. PACE Pacing Clin Electrophysiol 14:1767, 1991.

103. Kruse IM, Terpstra B: Acute and long-term atrial and ventricular stimulation thresholds with a steroid-eluting electrode. PACE Pacing Clin Electrophysiol 8:45, 1985.

104. Mond H, Stokes K, Helland J, et al: The porous titanium steroid-eluting electrode: A double-blind study assessing the stimulation threshold effects of steroid. PACE Pacing Clin Electrophysiol 11:214, 1988.

105. Klein HH, Steinberger J, Knake W: Stimulation characteristics of a steroid-eluting electrode compared with three conventional electrodes. PACE Pacing Clin Electrophysiol 13:134, 1990.

106. Beanlands DS, Akyurekli Y, Keon WJ: Prednisone in the management of exit block. In Meere C (ed): Proceedings of the Sixth World Symposium on Cardiac Pacing, Montreal, January 1979, Chap. 18.

107. Nagatomo Y, Ogawa T, Kumagae H, et al: Pacing failure due to markedly increased stimulation threshold two years after implantation: Successful management with oral prednisolone, a case report. PACE Pacing Clin Electrophysiol 12:1034, 1989.

108. Preston TA, Judge RD, Lucchesi BR, et al: Myocardial threshold in patients with artificial pacemakers. Am J Cardiol 18:83, 1966.

109. Schlesinger Z, Rosenberg T, Stryjer D, et al: Exit block in myxedema, treated effectively with thyroid hormone therapy. PACE Pacing Clin Electrophysiol 3:737, 1980.

110. Lee D, Greenspan K, Edmands RE, Fisch C: The effect of electrolyte alteration on stimulus requirement of cardiac pacemakers. Circulation 38:VI-124, 1968.

111. Gettes LS, Shabetai R, Downs TA, et al: Effect of changes in potassium and calcium concentrations on diastolic threshold and strength-interval relationships of the human heart. Ann NY Acad Sci 167:693, 1969.

112. O'Reilly MV, Murnaghan DP, Williams MB: Transvenous pacemaker failure induced by hyperkalemia. JAMA 228:336, 1974.

113. Dohrmann ML, Godschlager N: Metabolic and pharmacologic effects on myocardial stimulation threshold in patients with cardiac pacemakers. In Barold SS (ed): Modern Cardiac Pacing. Mt Kisco, NY, Futura Publishing, 1985, pp 161–170.

114. Sowton E, Barr I: Physiologic changes in threshold. Ann NY Acad Sci 167:679, 1969.

115. Finfer SR: Pacemaker failure on induction of anaesthesia. Br J Anaesth 66:509, 1991.

116. Hughes JC Jr, Tyers GFO, Torman HA: Effects of acid-base imbalance on myocardial pacing thresholds. J Thorac Cardiovasc Surg 69:743, 1975.

117. Preston TA, Judge RD: Alteration of pacemaker threshold by drug and physiologic factors. Ann NY Acad Sci 167:686, 1969.

118. Preston TA, Fletcher RD, Lucchesi BR, et al: Changes in myocardial threshold: Physiologic and pharmacologic factors in patients with implanted pacemakers. Am Heart J 74:235, 1967.

119. Hellestrand KJ, Burnett PJ, Milne JR, et al: Effect of the antiarrhythmic agent flecainide acetate on acute and chronic pacing thresholds. PACE Pacing Clin Electrophysiol 6:892, 1983.

120. Levick CE, Mizgala HF, Kerr CR: Failure to pace following high-dose antiarrhythmic therapy: Reversal with isoproterenol. PACE Pacing Clin Electrophysiol 7:252, 1984.

121. Nielsen AP, Griffin JC, Herre JM, et al: Effect of amiodarone on acute and chronic pacing thresholds. PACE Pacing Clin Electrophysiol 7:462, 1984.

122. Montefoschi N, Boccadamo R: Propafenone-induced acute variation of chronic atrial pacing threshold: A case report. PACE Pacing Clin Electrophysiol 13:480, 1990.

123. Salel AF, Seagren SC, Pool PE: Effects of encainide on the function of implanted pacemakers. PACE Pacing Clin Electrophysiol 12:1439, 1989.

124. Guarnieri T, Datorre SD, Bondke H, et al: Increased pacing threshold after an automatic defibrillatory shock in dogs: Effects of class I and class II antiarrhythmic drugs. PACE Pacing Clin Electrophysiol 11:1324, 1988.

125. Grant SC, Bennett DH: Atrial latency in a dual-chambered pacing system causing inappropriate sequence of cardiac chamber activation. PACE Pacing Clin Electrophysiol 15:116, 1992.

126. Furman S, Hurzeler P, DeCaprio V: Cardiac pacing and pacemakers III: Sensing the cardiac electrogram. Am Heart J 93:794, 1977.

127. Ohm OJ: The interdependence between electrogram, total electrode impedance, and pacemaker input impedance necessary to obtain adequate functioning demand pacemakers. PACE Pacing Clin Electrophysiol 2:465, 1979.

128. Kleinert M, Elmqvist H, Strandberg H: Spectral properties of atrial and ventricular endocardial signals. PACE Pacing Clin Electrophysiol 2:11, 1979.

129. Myers GH, Kresh YM, Parsonnet V: Characteristics of intracardiac electrograms. PACE Pacing Clin Electrophysiol 1:90, 1978.

130. Evans GL, Glasser SP: Intracardiac electrocardiography as a guide to pacemaker positioning. JAMA 216:483, 1971.

131. Levine PA, Klein MD: Discrepant electrocardiographic and pulse analyzer endocardial potentials, a possible source of pacemaker sensing failure. In Meere C (ed): Proceedings of the Sixth World Symposium on Cardiac Pacing, Montreal, January 1979, Chap. 34.

132. Levine PA, Seltzer JP: Fusion, pseudofusion, pseudo-pseudofusion and confusion: Normal rhythms associated with atrioventricular sequential "DVI" pacing. Clin Prog Pacing Electrophysiol 1:70, 1983.

133. Barold SS, Falkoff MD, Ong LS, et al: Characterization of pacemaker arrhythmias due to normally functioning AV demand (DVI) pulse generators. PACE Pacing Clin Electrophysiol 3:712, 1980.

134. Breivik K, Ohm OJ, Engedal H: Long-term comparison of unipolar and bipolar pacing and sensing, using a new multiprogrammable pacemaker system. PACE Pacing Clin Electrophysiol 6:592, 1983.

135. Ohm OJ: Demand failures occurring during permanent pacing in patients with serious heart disease. PACE Pacing Clin Electrophysiol 3:44, 1980.

136. Griffin JC, Finke WL: Analysis of the endocardial electrogram morphology of isolated ventricular beats. PACE Pacing Clin Electrophysiol 6:315, 1983.

137. Barold SS, Gaidula JJ: Failure of demand pacemaker from low-voltage bipolar ventricular electrograms. JAMA 215:923, 1971.

138. Van Mechelen R, Hart CT, De Boer H: Failure to sense P waves during DDD pacing. PACE Pacing Clin Electrophysiol 9:498, 1986.

139. Bricker JT, Ward KA, Zinner A, Gillette PC: Decrease in canine endocardial and epicardial electrogram voltage with exercise: Implications for pacemaker sensing. PACE Pacing Clin Electrophysiol 11:460, 1988.

140. Frohlig G, Schwerdt H, Schieffer H, et al: Atrial signal variations and pacemaker malsensing during exercise: A study in the time and frequency domain. J Am Coll Cardiol 11:806, 1988.

141. van Gelder BM, van Mechelen R, den Dulk, et al: Apparent P-wave undersensing in a DDD pacemaker post exercise. PACE Pacing Clin Electrophysiol 15:1651, 1992.

142. Warnowicz-Papp MA: The pacemaker patient and the electromagnetic environment. Clin Prog Pacing Electrophysiol 1:166, 1983.

143. Sager DP: Current facts on pacemaker electromagnetic interference and their application to clinical care. Heart Lung 16:211, 1987.

144. Lau FYK, Bilitch M, Wintroub HJ: Protection of implanted pacemakers from excessive electrical energy of D.C. shock. Am J Cardiol 23:244, 1969.

145. De Keyser F, Vanhaecke J, Janssens L, et al: Crosstalk with external bipolar DVI pacing: A case report. PACE Pacing Clin Electrophysiol 14:1320, 1991.

146. Sweesy MW, Batey RL, Forney RC: Crosstalk during bipolar pacing. PACE Pacing Clin Electrophysiol 11:1512, 1988.

147. Batey FL, Calabria DA, Sweesy MW, et al: Crosstalk and blanking periods in a dual-chamber pacemaker. Clin Prog Pacing Electrophysiol 3:314, 1985.

148. Barold SS, Falkoff MD, Ong LS, et al: Interpretation of electrocardiograms produced by a new unipolar multiprogrammable "committed" AV sequential demand (DVI) pacemaker. PACE Pacing Clin Electrophysiol 4:692, 1981.

149. Heller LI: Surgical electrocautery and the runaway pacemaker syndrome. PACE Pacing Clin Electrophysiol 13:1084, 1990.

150. Mickley H, Andersen C, Nielsen LH: Runaway pacemaker: A still existing complication and therapeutic guidelines. Clin Cardiol 12:412, 1989.

151. Snoeck J, Beerkhof M, Claeys M, et al: External vibration interference of activity based rate-responsive pacemakers. PACE Pacing Clin Electrophysiol 15:1841, 1992.

152. Lamb LS Jr, Judosn EB: Maximal rate response in a permanent pacemaker during chest physiotherapy. Heart Lung 21:390, 1992.

153. Lau CP, Tai YT, Fong PC, et al: Pacemaker-mediated tachycardias in single-chamber rate-responsive pacing. PACE Pacing Clin Electrophysiol 13:1575, 1990.

154. Madsen GM, Andersen C: Pacemaker-induced tachycardia during general anaesthesia: A case report. Br J Anaesth 63:360, 1989.

155. Fetter J, Patterson D, Aram G, et al: Effects of extracorporeal shock wave lithotripsy on single-chamber rate-response and dual-chamber pacemakers. PACE Pacing Clin Electrophysiol 12:1494, 1989.

156. Lau CP, Linker NJ, Butrous GS, et al: Myopotential interference in unipolar rate-responsive pacemakers. PACE Pacing Clin Electrophysiol 12:1324, 1989.

157. French RS, Tillman JG: Pacemaker function during helicopter transport. Ann Emerg Med 18:305, 1989.

158. Volosin KJ, O'Connor WH, Fabiszewski R, et al: Pacemaker-mediated tachycardia from a single-chamber temperature-sensitive pacemaker. PACE Pacing Clin Electrophysiol 12:1596, 1989.

159. Fearnot NE, Kitoh O, Fujita T, et al: Case studies on the effect of exercise and hot water submersion on intracardiac temperature and the performance of a pacemaker which varies pacing rate based on temperature. Jpn Heart J 30:353, 1989.

160. Seeger W, Kleinert M: An unexpected rate response of a minute ventilation dependent pacemaker (letter). PACE Pacing Clin Electrophysiol 12:1707, 1989.

161. Holmes DR, Hayes DL, Gray JE, Merideth J: The effects of magnetic resonance imaging on implantable pulse generators. PACE Pacing Clin Electrophysiol 9:360, 1986.

162. Hayes DL, Holmes DR, Gray JE: Effect of 1.5 Telsa nuclear magnetic resonance imaging scanner on implanted permanent pacemakers. J Am Coll Cardiol 10:782, 1987.

163. Erlebacher JA, Cahill PT, Pannizzo F, Knowles RJR: Effect of magnetic resonance imaging on DDD pacemakers. Am J Cardiol 57:347, 1986.

164. Levine PA, Selznick L: Prospective Management of the Patient with Retrograde Ventriculoatrial Conduction: Prevention and Management of Pacemaker Mediated Endless Loop Tachycardias. Sylmar, CA, Pacesetter Systems, 1990.

165. Limousin M, Bonnett JL: A multi-centric study of 1816 endless loop tachycardia (ELT) responses. PACE Pacing Clin Electrophysiol 13:555, 1990.

166. Oseran D, Ausubel K, Klementowicz PT, et al: Spontaneous endless loop tachycardia. PACE Pacing Clin Electrophysiol 9:379, 1986.

167. Rubin JW, Frank MJ, Boineau JP, et al: Current physiologic pacemakers: A serious problem with a new device. Am J Cardiol 52:88, 1983.

168. Levine PA: Postventricular atrial refractory periods and pacemaker-mediated tachycardias. Clin Prog Pacing Electrophysiol 1:394, 1983.

169. Furman S, Fisher JD: Endless loop tachycardia in an AV universal (DDD) pacemaker. PACE Pacing Clin Electrophysiol 5:486, 1982.

170. Den Dulk K, Lindemans FW, Bar FW, et al: Pacemaker-related tachycardias. PACE Pacing Clin Electrophysiol 5:476, 1982.

171. Luceri RM, Castellanos A, Zaman L, et al: The arrhythmias of dual-chamber cardiac pacemakers and their management. Ann Intern Med 99:354, 1983.

172. Ausubel K, Gabry MD, Klementowicz PT, et al: Pacemaker-mediated endless loop tachycardia at rates below the upper rate limit. Am J Cardiol 61:465, 1988.

173. Denes P, Wu D, Dhingra R, et al: The effects of cycle length on cardiac refractory periods in man. Circulation 49:32, 1974.

174. Amikam S, Furman S: Programmed upper rate limit dependent endless loop tachycardia. Chest 85:286, 1984.

175. Haffejee C, Murphy J, Gold R, et al: Automatic extension vs. programmability of the atrial refractory period in the prevention of pacemaker-mediated tachycardia. PACE Pacing Clin Electrophysiol 8:A-56, 1985.

176. Den Dulk K, Hamersa M, Wellens HJJ: Role of an adaptable atrial refractory period for DDD pacemakers. PACE Pacing Clin Electrophysiol 10:425, 1987.

177. Rognoni G, Occhetta E, Perucca A, et al: A new approach to the prevention of endless loop tachycardia in DDD and VDD pacing. PACE Pacing Clin Electrophysiol 14:1828, 1991.

178. Nitzsche R, Gueunoun M, Lamaison D, et al: Endless-loop tachycardias: Description and first clinical results of a new fully automatic protection algorithm. PACE Pacing Clin Electrophysiol 13:1711, 1990.

179. Klementowicz PT, Furman S: Selective atrial sensing in dual-chamber pacemakers eliminates endless loop tachycardias. J Am Coll Cardiol 7:590, 1986.

180. Pannizzo F, Amikam S, Bagwell P, et al: Discrimination of antegrade and retrograde atrial depolarization by electrogram analysis. Am Heart J 112:780, 1986.

181. McAlister HF, Klementowicz PT, Calderon EM, et al: Atrial electrogram analysis: Antegrade versus retrograde. PACE Pacing Clin Electrophysiol 11:1703, 1988.

182. Bernheim C, Markewitz A, Kemkes BM: Can reprogramming of atrial sensitivity avoid endless loop tachycardia? PACE Pacing Clin Electrophysiol 9:293, 1986.

183. Throne RD, Jenkins JM, Winston SA, et al: Discrimination of retrograde from anterograde atrial activation using intracardiac electrogram waveform analysis. PACE Pacing Clin Electrophysiol 12:1622, 1989.

184. Van Gelder LM, El Gamal MIH, Sanders RS: Tachycardia-termination algorithm: A valuable feature for interruption of pacemaker-mediated tachycardia. PACE Pacing Clin Electrophysiol 7:283, 1984.

185. Duncan JL, Clark MF: Prevention and termination of pacemaker-mediated tachycardia in a new DDD pacing system (Siemens Pacesetter model 2010T). PACE Pacing Clin Electrophysiol 11:1679, 1988.

186. Puglisi A, Ricci R, Azzolini P, et al: Ventricular cross stimulation in a dual-chamber pacing system: Phenomenon analysis. PACE Pacing Clin Electrophysiol 13:993, 1990.

187. Goldschlager N, Francoz R: Ventricular cross stimulation using a pacing system analyzer. PACE Pacing Clin Electrophysiol 13:986, 1990.

188. Doi Y, Takada K, Nakagaki O, et al: A case of cross stimulation. PACE Pacing Clin Electrophysiol 12:569, 1989.

189. Levine PA, Rihanek BD, Sanders R, et al: Cross-stimulation: The unexpected stimulation of the unpaced chamber. PACE Pacing Clin Electrophysiol 8:600, 1985.

RELATED ISSUES

CHAPTER 34

TEMPORARY CARDIAC PACING

Mark A. Wood

Temporary cardiac pacing may serve as definitive therapy for transient bradyarrhythmias or to support patients with sustained bradycardia until a permanent pacemaker system is implanted. Currently several modalities of temporary pacing are in clinical practice, and a variety of indications exist for their use. This chapter reviews the indications for temporary cardiac pacing as well as the clinically important aspects of transvenous, transcutaneous, and transthoracic pacing.

Indications for Temporary Pacing

Temporary cardiac pacing may be used for therapeutic or prophylactic indications. Therapeutic cardiac pacing is warranted in virtually any instance of sustained symptomatic or hemodynamically compromising bradyarrhythmia that is unresponsive to medical therapy or in which medical therapy is not tolerated. Prophylactic pacing is warranted when there is the potential for significant bradycardia. Specific indications for temporary pacing vary with different clinical situations (Table 34–1). In the absence of acute myocardial infarction, temporary pacing is indicated in the setting of symptomatic high-grade (second- or three-degree) atrioventricular (AV) block that is not responsive to medical management. Minimally symptomatic patients with slow (<50 beats per minute [bpm]), wide complex escape rhythms or those who require medical therapy likely to suppress an escape focus should also be considered candidates. Therapeutic temporary pacing may also be useful in the termination of recurrent supraventricular and ventricular tachycardias, suppression of bradycardia-related ventricular tachyarrhythmias, and suppression of torsade de pointes. The indications for cardiac pacing in the setting of acute myocardial infarction are complex and are covered in detail in Chapter 20.

Prophylactic pacing is indicated in situations or procedures likely to precipitate bradyarrhythmias. Trauma to the right bundle branch during Swan-Ganz catheterization or endo-myocardial biopsy in patients with preexisting left bundle branch block may result in complete heart block. Right bundle branch block may develop in 3% or less of patients undergoing pulmonary artery catheterization.[1, 2] Others have reported no occurrence of heart block in patients with chronic left bundle branch block undergoing repeated cardiac catheterization procedures, and the need for prophylactic pacing in this circumstance has been questioned.[2] Recent studies have shown that prophylactic temporary pacing has no significant impact on morbidity or mortality in patients undergoing cardiac catheterization or angioplasty. Cardioversion of atrial arrhythmias in patients with sick sinus syndrome may result in prolonged sinus arrest, and prophylactic pacing is often needed.[3, 4] Prophylactic pacing should also be considered when pharmacologic therapy is needed that may exacerbate bradycardia or conduction disturbances or suppress escape foci. Examples would include beta-blocker therapy for acute myocardial infarction complicated by sinus bradycardia or the need for antiarrhythmic therapy (e.g., procainamide) in patients with severe His-Purkinje system disease. Prophylactic temporary pacing is warranted because of the high incidence of new AV block or new bundle branch block in the setting of acute endocarditis.[5] Up to 22% of patients with aortic valve endocarditis and new first-degree AV block may progress to complete heart block. AV block is the most common cardiac manifestation of Lyme disease and may produce prolonged asystole. Patients in whom second-degree AV block develops or patients whose PR intervals are longer than 0.3 second are at greatest risk for complete heart block.[6] Complete AV block may last up to 10 days, but only rarely is permanent pacing required. Prophylactic temporary pacing is not indicated in patients with chronic bifascicular block undergoing general anesthesia and surgery, unless there is a history of syncope. Bellocci and associates reported no occurrence of complete heart block in 98 patients with bifascicular block undergoing general anesthesia, even though 14% had preoperative H-V intervals greater than 75 msec.[7] H-V

TABLE 34-1. **INDICATIONS FOR TEMPORARY PACING**

GENERAL
Medically refractory symptomatic bradyarrhythmia in absence of contraindications

IN ABSENCE OF ACUTE MYOCARDIAL INFARCTION
Medically refractory sinus node dysfunction with symptomatic or hemodynamically compromising bradycardia
Medically refractory second- or third-degree AV block with symptoms
Third-degree AV block with wide QRS escape rhythm or ventricular response <50 bpm

IN SETTING OF ACUTE MYOCARDIAL INFARCTION
Medically refractory symptomatic sinus node dysfunction
Mobitz II second-degree AV block with anterior myocardial infarction
Third-degree AV block with anterior myocardial infarction
New bifascicular block
Alternating bundle branch block
Alternating Wenckebach block
New bundle branch block with anterior myocardial infarction
Bilateral bundle branch block of indeterminate age with anterior or indeterminate infarction
Bilateral bundle branch block and first-degree AV block
AV block (regardless of site of infarction) associated with marked bradycardia and symptoms (e.g., hypotension, heart failure, low cardiac output)

TREATMENT OF TACHYCARDIAS
Termination of recurrent supraventricular tachycardias
Termination of recurrent ventricular tachycardia
Suppression of bradycardia-related ventricular tachycardia
Suppression of torsade de pointes

PROPHYLACTIC
Swan-Ganz catheterization or right-sided heart biopsy in setting of left bundle branch block
Cardioversion in setting of sick sinus syndrome
New AV block or new bundle branch block in acute endocarditis (especially aortic valve endocarditis)
To allow pharmacologic treatment with agents that may exacerbate bradycardias (e.g., beta-blockers in acute myocardial infarction or antiarrhythmic agents that suppress escape foci)

Abbreviations: AV, atrioventricular.

prolongation was associated with a high overall complication rate, however, including deaths from ventricular fibrillation. The occurrence of new bifascicular block in the immediate perioperative period is suspicious for perioperative myocardial infarction, and temporary pacing may be required. Benign and malignant neck and carotid sinus tumors may give rise to bradyarrhythmias, and temporary cardiac pacing may be required during surgical treatment or irradiation of the neoplasm.

Contraindications to Temporary Pacing

Cardiac pacing by any method is absolutely contraindicated in the setting of severe hypothermia despite profound bradycardia and hypotension. In this situation, cardiac pacing may induce refractory ventricular fibrillation or alter compensatory physiologic mechanisms to the hypothermia. Bradycardic or asystolic arrest of greater than 20 minutes' duration represents a relative contraindication to pacing because of an extremely poor prognosis for survival. Relative contraindications to transvenous pacing include impassible tricuspid valve prostheses, digitalis toxicity with recurrent

ventricular tachycardia, and a bleeding diathesis. Contraindications to transvenous atrial pacing include the presence of multifocal atrial tachycardia, atrial fibrillation, and significant AV conduction system disease. AV conduction may be considered intact if 1:1 AV conduction is present at rates up to 125 bpm.

Methods of Temporary Pacing

TRANSVENOUS TEMPORARY CARDIAC PACING

Transvenous cardiac pacing provides the most reliable means of temporary pacing in clinical practice. The technique offers the advantages of atrial or ventricular pacing, or both, excellent patient tolerance, and high dependability. Disadvantages include the time and operator experience needed to implement the procedure and a variety of potential complications.

Transvenous pacing may be performed in the bipolar or unipolar configurations using a variety of commercially available temporary pacing leads (Fig. 34–1). These leads are typically 3 to 6 F in diameter and are constructed of relatively rigid woven polyester (Dacron) or flexible plastic. Plastic catheters may be flaccid and balloon flow–directed or semirigid without balloons for more responsive handling. Preformed distal curvatures and rigid and semirigid designs may facilitate catheter manipulation and stability. Specialized electrodes include the J tip for atrial pacing, the winged J electrode for atrial pacing without fluoroscopic guidance, single-pass, dual-chamber pacing catheters, and pulmonary artery pressure catheters with one to five pacing electrodes for ventricular or atrial pacing, or both (Fig. 34–2). Lead stability has been problematic with many pacing pulmonary

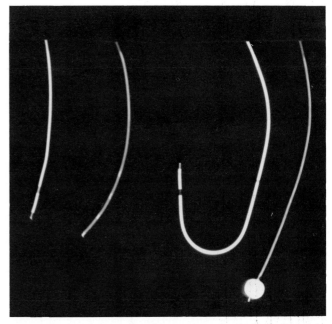

FIGURE 34–1. Single-chamber transvenous pacing leads. *Left to right,* Semifloating plastic bipolar catheter, "stiff" woven polyester (Dacron) quadripolar catheter, semifloating bipolar catheter with preformed distal J tip, and floating flow-directed bipolar catheter with distal inflatable balloon. (Reprinted by permission of Ellenbogen KA [ed]: Cardiac Pacing. Oxford, Blackwell Scientific Publications, Inc., 1992, pp 162–210.)

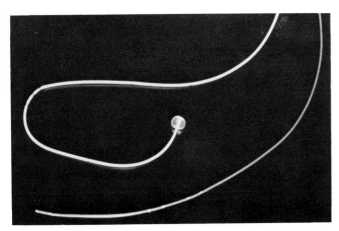

FIGURE 34–2. Single-pass dual-chamber transvenous pacing leads. *Top*, Pulmonary artery pressure catheter with distal inflatable balloon, three proximal atrial ring electrodes, and two distal ventricular ring electrodes 20 cm from catheter tip. *Bottom*, Hexapolar woven polyester catheter with four proximal atrial ring electrodes and distal ventricular tip and ring electrodes. (Reprinted by permission of Ellenbogen KA [ed]: Cardiac Pacing. Oxford, Blackwell Scientific Publications, Inc., 1992, pp 162–210.)

artery catheters; however, new designs may represent improvements.[8] Unipolar cardiac pacing has been accomplished using standard angioplasty guidewires positioned in the coronary arteries and distal uninsulated 0.035-mm guidewires in contact with the left ventricle.[9]

Commonly available temporary pacing pulse generators are usually constant current output devices powered by disposable commercial 9 V batteries and provide up to 12 to 15 V of output. These generators are designed to function against impedance loads of 300 to 1000 ohms. Until recently, external generators were capable of only SOO, SSI, DVI, and DOO modes. These generators typically have programmable rates (30–180 bpm), sensitivity (0.1 mV–asynchronous), current output (0.1–20 mA), and AV delays (0–300 msec). Specialized rapid atrial pacing generators provide rates up to 800 bpm for termination of atrial tachycardias. External temporary DDD generators have recently become commercially available. These units feature extensive programmability of operating modes (DDD, DVI, DDI, DOO, SOO, SSI, SST), outputs, and sensitivities and may also allow high-rate pacing (Fig. 34–3).

The site of venous access for pacing should account for the urgency to initiate pacing, the desired lead stability, the anticipated duration of pacing, and the need to avoid specific complications. Satisfactory catheter position is most rapidly obtained from the right internal jugular vein approach, even without fluoroscopy.[10] The left subclavian vein is also easily cannulated and coursed in emergent situations. The external jugular, brachial, cephalic, and femoral routes, although accessible, may be virtually impassable without fluoroscopic guidance. Catheter stability is best preserved using the internal jugular or subclavian access, whereas brachial and femoral routes may allow for lead dislodgments of several centimeters with motion of the extremities. Peripheral access does, however, avoid inadvertent trauma to the central arteries and pneumothorax and allows greatest control of bleeding complications. Femoral access requires changes of venipuncture sites every 24 hours to avoid the high risk of thrombosis, phlebitis, and infection. Subclavian vein trauma may preclude future use of this vessel for permanent pacing if needed.

Once access to the central circulation has been gained, the catheters may be directed to the desired intracardiac positions by fluoroscopic or, less desirably, electrocardiographic guidance. A working defibrillator should *always* be available to treat ventricular tachyarrhythmias induced by lead manipulation. The right atrial appendage and right ventricular apex provide the most stable catheter positions; however, following cardiac surgery the atrial appendage may be deformed or excised and alternate positions are necessary. Similarly, the right ventricular apex may provide unacceptably high pacing thresholds because of apical scarring following infarction. In these situations, the ventricular lead may be positioned in the right ventricular inflow tract or against the ventricular septum. Methods for gaining access to the atrial appendage and ventricular apex under fluoroscopy are outlined elsewhere.[11]

When fluoroscopy is unavailable or in urgent situations, flow-directed or semifloating catheters may be positioned by electrocardiographic guidance. By connecting the distalmost catheter electrode to lead V_1 of a standard electrocardiogram (ECG) recorder, the catheter position is known by the char-

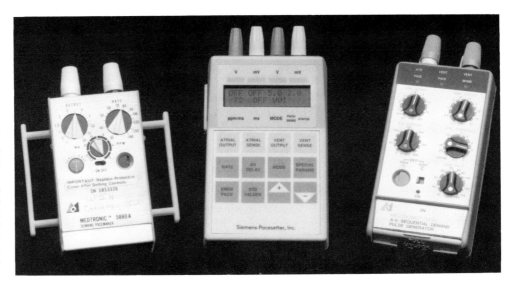

FIGURE 34–3. Temporary transvenous pacemaker generators. *Left*, Temporary single-chamber generator with adjustable current output, rate, and sensitivity. *Center*, Temporary dual-chamber generator capable of DDD, DVI, DDI, SSI, SOO, and SST pacing modes. Atrial and ventricular outputs and sensitivities are separately programmable. High-rate SSI pacing is also available. *Right*, Temporary DVI generator with adjustable rate, atrioventricular (AV) delay, and atrial and ventricular output. Ventricular sensitivity is also adjustable.

acteristic unipolar electrograms recorded in each intravascular location (Fig. 34–4). Once the right ventricle is entered, balloons are deflated, if used, and catheters are advanced gently until marked ST segment elevation (injury pattern) indicates contact with the ventricular myocardium. For emergent situations or asystole, catheters may be advanced blindly during asynchronous pacing at maximal output until ventricular capture is documented. Flow-directed catheters and a right internal jugular venous access site provide the shortest insertion times.[12] Failure to reach the ventricle in these situations often results from the catheter coiling in the atrium. J-tipped atrial catheters advanced from subclavian access may readily enter the ventricle without coiling.[13] The reported incidence of ventricular capture without fluoroscopy in urgent situations ranges from 30% to 90%.[10, 14, 15]

Once catheters are positioned, pacing is initiated using the distal electrode as the cathode (negative pole) and the proximal electrode as the anode (positive pole). For unipolar pacing, cathodal intracardiac stimulation minimizes thresholds and pacing-induced tachyarrhythmias.[16] The unipolar anode may be a surface patch electrode with a surface area greater than 50 mm^2 to reduce thresholds or a subcutaneous wire electrode. Ideally, the atrial and ventricular capture thresholds are less than 1 mA (or 1 V) and sensing thresholds are greater than 1 mV and greater than 6 mV, respectively. Pacing output should be maintained at three to five times threshold values to overcome expected acute rises in threshold and to compensate for changes in lead position, physio-

logic alterations, and pharmacologic interventions. Likewise, sensitivity settings are maintained at 25% to 50% of threshold values. For dual-chamber pacing, AV delays of 100 to 200 msec are usually programmed empirically; however, patients dependent on atrial contribution to ventricular filling may be hemodynamically sensitive to adjustments in this parameter.

Final catheter positions should be confirmed by anteroposterior and lateral chest x-ray films *and* by electrocardiographic evaluation. On chest x-ray studies, a catheter in the right ventricular apex should cross to the left of the spine near the lateral cardiac border and the tip should point inferiorly and anteriorly. Paucity or redundancy of the intravascular lead should be noted and corrected. J leads in the right atrial appendage orient the tip of the curve superiorly, anteriorly, and slightly medially. Nevertheless, chest x-ray studies cannot completely exclude lead malposition into the coronary sinus, cardiac veins, left ventricle, or pericardial space.[17] Electrocardiography can, however, greatly assist in localizing lead positions by analysis of unipolar electrograms and paced QRS complex morphology. Paced QRS complexes arising from the right ventricular apex should demonstrate a left bundle branch block pattern with a superior axis. Paced complexes with a right bundle branch block pattern usually indicate coronary sinus pacing or lead penetration into the left ventricle or pericardial space. Rarely, right bundle branch patterns result from right ventricular pacing because of preferential activation of the interventricular septum and left ventricle.[18] In this circumstance, however, the axis of the QRS complex remains oriented superiorly. Unipolar electrograms of intrinsic cardiac depolarizations may also document intracardiac versus extracardiac lead positions. When recorded through lead V$_1$ of standard ECG recorders, the distal unipolar ventricular endocardial electrogram should demonstrate ST segment elevation acutely and a predominantly negative complex regardless of the origin of the intrinsic beats (see Fig. 34–4). Predominantly positive or biphasic unipolar electrograms and lack of ST segment elevation strongly suggest a lead position in the coronary sinus or cardiac vein, penetration into the myocardium, or perforation into the pericardial space. Coronary sinus pacing is also suggested by high pacing thresholds, a posterior course of the catheter as seen on lateral chest x-ray film, simultaneous atrial and ventricular pacing, and recording both atrial and ventricular electrograms from the lead. Coronary sinus pacing is generally unreliable but may permit ventricular capture in the presence of impassable tricuspid valve anatomy.

Maintenance of the transvenous lead requires secure anchoring to the skin. Changes of protective dressings, evaluation for infection, determination of pacing and sensing thresholds, and paced 12-lead ECGs should be performed daily.

Although most patients without underlying heart disease demonstrate similar hemodynamic responses to atrial and ventricular pacing, AV sequential pacing is clearly beneficial to those patients with ventricular systolic or diastolic dysfunction, or both.[19, 20] Patients with acute myocardial infarction, especially right ventricular infarction; hypertensive or hypertrophic heart disease; dilated cardiomyopathies; valvular heart disease, such as aortic stenosis or mitral stenosis; or recent cardiac surgery are known to benefit from maintenance of AV synchrony.[21, 22] Patients with inadequate re-

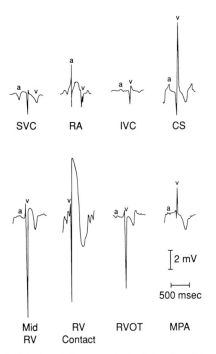

FIGURE 34–4. Unipolar electrograms obtained at various intravascular positions from the distal electrode of a temporary pacing catheter connected to lead V$_1$ of a standard ECG recorder. a, atrial electrogram; v, ventricular electrogram; SVC, superior vena cava; RA, right atrium; IVC, inferior vena cava; CS, coronary sinus; mid-RV, middle right ventricle; RV Contact, electrode contact with the right ventricular wall; RVOT, right ventricular outflow tract; MPA, main pulmonary artery. Note the marked ST segment elevation on contact with the right ventricular wall and the predominantly upright ventricular electrogram morphology of the CS and MPA recordings. (Reprinted by permission of Ellenbogen KA [ed]: Cardiac Pacing. Oxford, Blackwell Scientific Publications, Inc., 1992, pp 162–210.)

TABLE 34–2. **LOSS OF CAPTURE DURING TRANSVENOUS PACING**

ETIOLOGY	DIAGNOSTICS	SOLUTION
Catheter dislodgment	Change in lead position on chest x-ray	Increase output
	Change in paced QRS morphology or unipolar electrograms	Stabilize under fluoroscopy
Local myocardial necrosis-fibrosis	Check unipolar electrograms	Increase output
	Evaluate for infarction	Reposition lead
Local myocardial inflammation	Check lead position on chest x-ray	Increase output
	Evaluate unipolar electrograms	Reposition lead
		Glucocorticoid administration
Metabolic disturbance, drug effects	Confirm lead position	Increase output
	Check laboratory values and drug levels	Correct metabolic disturbance
		Reduce drug level
Electrocautery, DC cardioversion	Recent exposure to current source	Increase output
		Reposition lead
		Replace lead or generator, or both
Lead conductor or insulation fracture	Check unipolar pacing	Unipolarize functional electrode
	Check unipolar resistance	Replace lead
Unstable electric connections	Check connections and connectors	Secure or replace connectors
Generator malfunction, battery depletion	Check connections and lead positions	Replace battery or generator
	Check battery reserve	

Abbreviations: DC, direct current.

sponses to ventricular pacing alone or those who exhibit signs of pacemaker syndrome are also candidates for AV sequential pacing. In such patients, AV sequential pacing may significantly enhance systemic arterial pressure and ventricular end-diastolic filling and lower left atrial and pulmonary artery pressures. Cardiac output may increase by 20% to 30% over ventricular pacing. In patients with acute myocardial infarction complicated by bradycardia or heart block, ventricular pacing alone may fail to improve hemodynamics over the intrinsic rhythm.[22] In these patients, temporary DDD pacing may augment cardiac output by 29%, raise mean systemic arterial pressure by 21%, and reduce atrial filling pressures by 10% to 24% through maintenance of AV synchrony.

Initiating and maintaining myocardial capture depends on the electrical integrity of the pacing system and viability of the myocardium-electrode interface. Ventricular excitability and capture thresholds are compromised in the setting of hypoxia, myocardial ischemia and infarction, acidosis, alka-losis, severe hyperglycemia, and hypercapnia. Beta-blockers; verapamil; class Ia, Ic, and III antiarrhythmics; hypertonic saline; glucose and insulin; mineralocorticoids; and sleep may increase ventricular capture thresholds by up to 60%.[23, 24] Pacing thresholds may be reduced by epinephrine, ephedrine, glucocorticoids, and hyperkalemia. Isoproterenol may initially decrease and then increase thresholds up to 80%.[23] Digitalis, calcium gluconate, morphine, lidocaine, and atropine have minimal effects on ventricular pacing thresholds. Current from external cardioversion or electrosurgical cautery may damage the electrode-tissue interface and elevate pacing thresholds.

Pacing system malfunction manifesting as inconsistent pacing or sensing may occur in 14% to 43% of patients following successful initiation of temporary transvenous pacing.[25–27] Potential causes and remedies for loss of capture, loss of sensing, and oversensing are listed in Tables 34–2 to 34–4. The most common cause for loss of capture or sensing is catheter dislodgment. Catheter instability is most problem-

TABLE 34–3. **LOSS OF SENSING DURING TRANSVENOUS PACING**

ETIOLOGY	DIAGNOSTICS	SOLUTION
Lead dislodgment	Change in lead position on chest x-ray, paced QRS morphology, or unipolar electrograms	Increase sensitivity
		Stabilize lead under fluoroscopy
Local myocardial necrosis-fibrosis	Check unipolar or bipolar electrograms	Increase sensitivity
		Reposition lead
Electrodes perpendicular to depolarization wave-front or low dV/dt	Check unipolar or bipolar electrograms	Unipolarize lead or reposition
Lead fracture	Check unipolar electrograms	Unipolarize functional electrode
		Replace lead
Electrocautery, DC cardioversion	Exposure to current source	Increase sensitivity
	Check electrograms	Reposition lead
		Replace lead or generator, or both
Intrinsic complexes during refractory period	Analyze appropriate ECG recordings	No intervention
		Reprogram refractory periods if possible
Inappropriate-asynchronous programming	Check sensitivity settings	Increase sensitivity
Unstable electric connections	Check connections	Secure connections
	Confirm adequate electrograms	
Generator malfunction	Confirm adequate electrograms	Replace generator
	Confirm appropriate sensitivity settings	

Abbreviations: DC, direct current; ECG, electrocardiogram.

TABLE 34–4. OVERSENSING DURING TRANSVENOUS PACING

ETIOLOGY	DIAGNOSTICS	SOLUTION
Far-field sensing of P wave, QRS, pacemaker output	Catheter tip near tricuspid annulus on chest x-ray	Reposition lead
		Reduce sensitivity
	Time electrograms to electrocardiographic events	Reduce output
		Asynchronous pacing
	High generator outputs	
T-wave sensing	Time electrograms to electrocardiographic events	Reduce sensitivity
		Reposition lead
		Extend refractory period if possible
Myopotential sensing	Check electrograms during provocative maneuvers	If unipolar replace with bipolar system
		Reduce sensitivity
Electromagnetic interference	Check electric grounding and isolation of patient-pacemaker	Remove source (e.g., TENS unit)
		Ground equipment
	Check electrograms	Reduce sensitivity or asynchronous pacing
Competing permanent pacemaker with subthreshold output	Check output-sensitivity permanent pacer	Reprogram permanent pacer
		Reduce sensitivity
Unstable electric connections	Monitor sensing during manipulation of connections	Secure connections

Abbreviations: TENS, transcutaneous electric nerve stimulation.

atic with brachial or femoral pacing sites and is not consistently influenced by catheter size or stiffness. Most failures occur within 48 hours of initiation of pacing and can usually be overcome by adjusting the generator output or sensitivity. Up to 38% of malfunctions may require repositioning or replacement of the lead.[26] As mentioned, many pharmacologic and physiologic changes may influence consistent pacing and sensing and should be considered during pacemaker troubleshooting.

The reported frequency of complications associated with transvenous pacing is somewhat variable and is related to the setting in which pacing is implemented. Prophylactic lead placement in the cardiac catheterization laboratory may carry negligible risk, whereas placement in the intensive care setting carries a 20% risk of complications in some series.[26] Induction of ventricular tachycardia or fibrillation is one of the most common complications of transvenous pacing (incidence of up to 20%).[28] Ventricular tachycardia is common with lead manipulation in the setting of myocardial ischemia, infarction, hypoxia, general anesthesia, vagal stimulation, catecholamine administration, and coronary artery catheterization. Ventricular fibrillation during lead insertion may complicate up to 14% of acute myocardial infarctions requiring transvenous pacing and is more common during the first 24 hours following infarction and with inferior infarction.[29]

Myocardial perforation is probably underrecognized clinically but has been reported in 2% to 20% of cases.[30–32] Perforation is more likely with femoral or brachial access and possibly with more rigid catheters. Loss of pacing or sensing, changes in paced QRS morphology, and diaphragmatic or skeletal muscle pacing are the most common signs, although even extracardiac lead migration can be clinically silent. Pericardial tamponade can occur in about 1% of perforations.[33] The diagnostic features of myocardial perforation by pacing catheters are listed in Table 34–5. In the absence of hemodynamically significant pericardial effusion or anticoagulation, perforation is managed by repositioning the catheter, followed by careful patient monitoring. Unipolar electrograms recorded from the tip of the catheter will demonstrate a pathognomonic transition from R to S wave morphology on withdrawal from extracardiac locations (Fig. 34–5).[33]

Thromboembolic events associated with temporary pacing are also more frequent than clinically appreciated. Femoral pacing sites may produce silent venous thrombosis in approximately 30% of patients, and of these more than half may exhibit evidence of pulmonary embolism despite subcutaneous heparin prophylaxis.[34] The incidence of thrombosis with other pacing sites remains uncertain. Bacteremia may be demonstrated in 50% of patients by the third day of temporary pacing, although sepsis is much less common.[32] Clinical infection or phlebitis may occur in 3% to 5% of patients and is more likely with femoral pacing sites.[26] Generally, femoral pacing sites should be changed every 24 hours and other sites rotated every 72 hours to minimize the risk of infection. Other complications of transvenous pacing include arterial trauma, air embolism, or pneumothorax (1%–2%), bleeding complications (4%), right bundle branch block (1%), and diaphragmatic or phrenic nerve pacing (10%).[26, 32] A summarization of temporary transvenous pacemaker complications by site of venous access is shown in Table 34–6.

TABLE 34–5. DIAGNOSTIC FEATURES OF MYOCARDIAL PERFORATION BY A TEMPORARY PACING CATHETER

Symptoms: pericardial chest pain, skeletal muscle stimulation, dyspnea (with tamponade), shoulder pain

Signs: pericardial rub, intercostal or diaphragmatic pacing, presystolic pacemaker ''click'' on cardiac auscultation, failure to pace or sense, or both, evidence of pericardial tamponade: hypotension, pulsus paradoxus

ECG: change in paced QRS axis or morphology, or both, pericarditis pattern

Chest x-ray study: change in lead position, extracardiac location of lead tip[a], new pericardial effusion

Echocardiography: extracardiac position of lead tip[a], pericardial effusion, loss of paradoxical anterior septal motion or rapid initial left posterior septal motion characteristic of right ventricular apical stimulation

Intracardiac electrograms: biphasic or predominantly positive unipolar ventricular electrogram recorded from lead tip, change in unipolar electrogram morphology from biphasic, R or Rs pattern to rS or S with ST elevation during catheter withdrawal[a]

Abbreviations: ECG, electrocardiogram.
[a]Pathognomonic of perforation.

FIGURE 34–5. Continuous unipolar recording from the distal electrode of a catheter perforating the right ventricle. As the catheter is withdrawn from the pericardial space (P), intramyocardially (M), and into the ventricular cavity (E), there is the characteristic transition from a biphasic or primarily upright ventricular electrogram to a negative electrogram morphology with ST segment elevation. (From Van Durme JP, Heyndrickx G, Snoeck J, et al: Diagnosis of myocardial perforation by intracardiac electrograms recorded from the indwelling catheter. J Electrocardiol 6:97, 1973. Reprinted by permission of Churchill Livingstone, New York.)

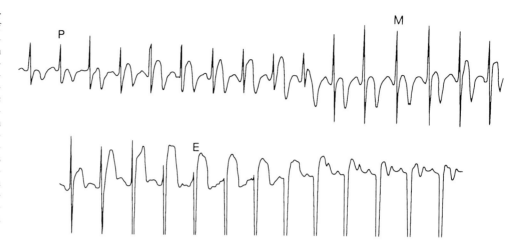

TRANSCUTANEOUS PACING

Transcutaneous external pacing provides a means of noninvasive cardiac stimulation with great safety, speed, and ease of initiation. Despite a somewhat variable incidence of cardiac capture, this technique is now considered by many to be the method of choice for prophylactic and emergent applications.[35]

Transcutaneous external pacing activates excitable myocardium contained in the current path between surface patch electrodes on the chest wall. These electrodes are typically self-adhesive, large (8-cm diameter), nonmetallic, and impregnated with a high-impedance conductive gel. This high-impedance system is unsuitable for external cardioversion-defibrillation. External pacing requires delivery of high current (up to 200 mA) at long pulse durations of 20 to 40 msec to achieve effective capture and minimize patient discomfort, respectively. External pacing generators provide output as rectangular or truncated exponential pulses and also feature built-in oscilloscope displays that electronically filter or blank the large pacing artifact that obscures conventional monitors. A blanking time of approximately 70 to 80 msec may be required for artifact-free QRS recordings; however, the blanking period must be extended as the pacing threshold increases.[36]

Attention to proper placement of the pacing electrodes is important for effective capture and patient comfort (Fig. 34–6). It is essential that the negative electrode (cathode) be placed anteriorly on the chest, otherwise pacing thresholds may be extremely high or unobtainable. Placement of the cathode over the palpable cardiac impulse or centered over the chest lead V_3 position is recommended to minimize capture threshold. The positive electrode (anode) is typically positioned on the posterior portion of the chest, although in healthy volunteers placement over the upper right anterior portion of the chest may be equally effective.[37] For posterior placement, the electrode should be centered between the thoracic spinous processes and the inferior aspect of either the right or left scapula. Placement directly over bony prominences such as the spine or scapulae may elevate pacing thresholds, however. Before application of the patches, the skin should be thoroughly cleansed with alcohol to remove salt deposits and skin debris, which contribute to painful pacing or elevate thresholds, or both. Shaving directly beneath the electrode site abrades the skin and may significantly worsen discomfort during pacing.

Once initiated, cardiac capture must be documented. On filtered electrocardiographic displays, capture is suggested by the appearance of depolarization or repolarization artifacts after each pacing stimulus artifact (Fig. 34–7). Capture should also be confirmed by palpation of a pulse or by Doppler auscultation. Once capture is achieved, pacing thresholds are determined and the desired rate and mode of pacing (demand vs. asynchronous) set. Maintenance current output is set 5 to 10 mA above threshold if patient tolerance permits.

Pacing thresholds appear to be lowest in healthy volunteers, in patients with minimal hemodynamic compromise,

TABLE 34–6. **INCIDENCE OF COMPLICATIONS FOR TRANSVENOUS CARDIAC PACING BY VENOUS INSERTION SITE**

COMPLICATION	ANTECUBITAL (N = 606)	SUBCLAVIAN (N = 177)	INTERNAL JUGULAR (N = 111)	FEMORAL (N = 48)	TOTAL
Pericardial friction rub	43	6	5	0	54
Dysrhythmia*	18	5	0	1	24
Right ventricular perforation	17	3	0	1	21
Local infection	6	3	1	2	12
Inadvertent arterial puncture	5	5	1	0	11
Diaphragmatic stimulation	8	0	2	0	10
Phlebitis	6	0	0	0	6
Pneumothorax	0	1	0	0	1
Cardiac tamponade	1	0	0	0	1
Total	104 (17.2%)	23 (13.0%)	9 (8.1%)	4 (8.3%)	140

*Catheter-induced ventricular flutter or fibrillation that necessitated direct-current cardioversion.
From Hynes JK, Holmes DR, Harrison CE, et al: Five-year experience with temporary pacemaker therapy in the coronary care unit. Mayo Clin Proc 58:122, 1983.

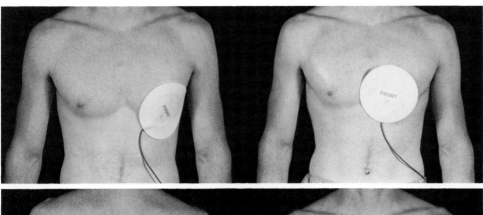

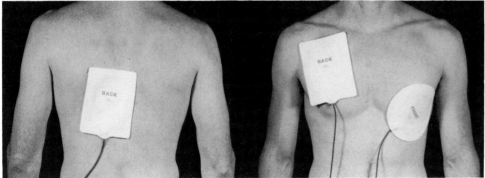

FIGURE 34–6. Proper positions for transcutaneous pacing electrodes. *Upper Panel*, Anterior cathodal electrode placement over the cardiac apex *(left)* or chest lead V_3 position *(right)*. *Lower Panel*, The anodal electrode is typically positioned posteriorly between the spine and either the left or the right scapula *(left)*. Anterior placement of the anodal electrode on the right side of the chest may also be effective *(right)*. Note that the cathodal (negative) electrode must be positioned anteriorly. (Reprinted by permission of Ellenbogen KA [ed]: Cardiac Pacing. Oxford, Blackwell Scientific Publications, Inc., 1992, pp 162–210.)

and with prophylactic use. In these circumstances, thresholds usually average 40 to 80 mA.[38–41] In clinical use, thresholds of 20 to 140 mA may be encountered. Biphasic external stimulation pulses do not appear to reduce thresholds.[42] No clear correlation has been established between pacing threshold and age, body weight, body surface area, chest diameter,

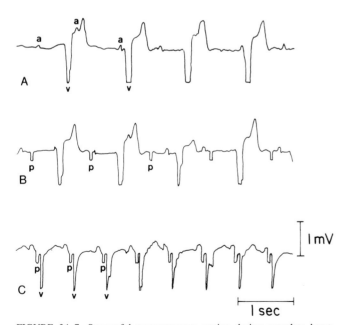

FIGURE 34–7. Successful transcutaneous pacing during complete heart block. a, atrial depolarization; v, ventricular escape complex; p, filtered pacing stimulus artifact. *A*, Complete heart block with slow ventricular escape rhythm. *B*, Subthreshold pacing stimuli at 20 mA fail to capture the ventricles. *C*, One-to-one ventricular capture at 60-mA generator output. (Reprinted by permission of Ellenbogen KA [ed]: Cardiac Pacing. Oxford, Blackwell Scientific Publications, Inc., 1992, pp 162–210.)

underlying heart disease, or cardiac drug therapy.[39, 40, 42] Thresholds may, however, be elevated in the 24 hours following cardiac surgery possibly because of incomplete rewarming, transient myocardial ischemia, or entrapped mediastinal air.[43] Pacing thresholds may also be higher in the setting of emphysema, pericardial effusion, or positive pressure ventilation, or when used to terminate ventricular tachycardias.[40, 44, 45] As with all forms of pacing, ventricular capture may be compromised in the setting of myocardial ischemia or severe metabolic derangements or during prolonged resuscitation efforts. Failure to capture most frequently results from suboptimal lead positions, severe underlying metabolic derangements, or patient intolerance to pain.

The incidence of ventricular capture with transcutaneous pacing is highly variable and greatly influenced by the situations requiring its use. The incidence of ventricular capture in healthy volunteers is generally high but ranges from 50% to 100%.[40, 45, 46] Clinically, success rates may exceed 90% when initiated prophylactically or early (less than 5 minutes) into bradycardic arrests.[40] With emergent use, successful capture is generally lower but ranges from 10% to 93%.[41, 47, 48] In a large series of 134 patients in diverse clinical situations, capture was achieved in 78% of cases overall.[40] In this series, capture was achieved in 95% of cases of stand-by use but only 58% of cardiac arrests. Despite electrocardiographic capture during arrest in 52% to 93% of patients, palpable pulses may be documented in only 8% to 20% when implemented for out-of-hospital arrests.[49, 50] Inclusion of transcutaneous pacing in out-of-hospital or emergency room resuscitation protocols has not improved the dire outcome in these patients even in prospective and controlled studies.[50] More recently, a 3-year study of transcutaneous cardiac pacing in 112 of 278 patients with asystolic cardiac arrest showed no difference in survival or rate of hospital admission for the group who received early transcutaneous pacing compared with the group who received basic cardiopulmonary resuscitation (CPR) without transcutaneous pacing.[51] Similarly, early use during in-hospital arrests may not alter long-term survival.[52] It is unclear if these shortcomings represent primary failure of transcutaneous pacing to restore hemodynamics or merely the unsalvageable situation that precipitates or soon follows bradycardic-asystolic arrests. Transcutaneous pacing has also been used to terminate ventricular tachycardia, AV nodal reentrant tachycardia, and AV reciprocating tachycardia.[53]

Transcutaneous pacing effects ventricular capture in humans. The threshold for atrial capture exceeds 100 mA and may be possible in only about 50% of patients with outputs to 150 mA.[54] Simultaneous atrial and ventricular capture in humans at ventricular threshold outputs has been reported, however.[48] Retrograde atrial activation may occur with ventricular capture. Current evidence suggests focal rather than simultaneous global ventricular excitation based on discordant right and left ventricular pressure profiles, sequential ventricular activation by catheter mapping, different paced QRS morphologies with different external patch positions, and induction of bundle branch reentry with single pacing extrastimuli.[55] Recent data suggest that the focus of cardiac excitation may be either the right or left ventricle, depending on patch positions. Cathodal patch placement at the cardiac apex and upper left sternal border appear to activate the right ventricular apex and outflow tracts, respectively.[55]

The hemodynamic responses to transcutaneous pacing are similar to endocardial VVI pacing. Both methods may induce modest reductions in left ventricular systolic pressure with up to 24% reduction in stroke volume and elevation of right-sided heart pressures presumably due to loss of atrioventricular synchrony.[40, 56] Reductions in cardiac output may be partially offset by faster pacing rates. Not surprisingly, hemodynamic responses consistent with pacemaker syndrome have been described with transcutaneous pacing. Compared with rapid atrial or ventricular endocardial pacing, transcutaneous pacing at similar rates has been associated with enhanced cardiac output.[57] This response may result from concomitant skeletal muscle stimulation that increases regional blood flow or from synchronous chest, abdominal, and diaphragmatic contractions that simulate cough CPR.

Complications from transcutaneous pacing are extraordinarily rare in the clinical setting. The most frequent problems are the induction of coughing and severe pain during pacing. Pain results from activation of cutaneous nerves and intense skeletal muscle contraction. The degree of discomfort appears directly related to the stimulus amplitude and mass of muscle activated.[55] Painful pacing may also be worsened by salt deposits, skin abrasions, foreign bodies, or dried gel beneath the electrodes. The current necessary to produce severe pain is highly variable among patients, but most patients can be paced at least briefly at tolerable levels of discomfort. There have been no reports of significant damage to skin, lung, skeletal muscle, or cardiac muscle in humans despite continuous transcutaneous pacing for up to 108 hours and intermittent pacing for 17 days.[40, 55, 58] There is only one report of ventricular tachycardia induction from therapeutic transcutaneous pacing.[59] Near threshold outputs, transcutaneous pacing may prolong ventricular effective refractory periods when compared with endocardial pacing, thereby minimizing arrhythmogenicity.[39] In animal studies, ventricular fibrillation thresholds average 12.6 times the pacing threshold and thus exceed the current output of most clinical generators.[60]

TRANSTHORACIC PACING

Transthoracic cardiac pacing remains a controversial procedure despite more than 30 years of clinical use. The technique is rapid and simple to initiate and requires no venous access, fluoroscopy, blood flow, or electrocardiography for guidance. These attributes are offset by a high potential for complication and scores of studies demonstrating no beneficial effects on survival. The procedure may be largely supplanted by noninvasive external transcutaneous pacing in all but the most dire of situations.

Transthoracic pacing requires direct introduction of a unipolar or bipolar pacing electrode through the thorax into the ventricular cavity. Commercially available transthoracic pacing kits provide a 15-cm 18-gauge steel introducing cannula and trocar, 32-cm bipolar J pacing wire, and an adapter for connecting the pacing wire to standard temporary transvenous pacing generators (Fig. 34–8). To implement, access to the right ventricle may be gained through subxiphoid or left parasternal approaches (Fig. 34–9). The right ventricular cavity is the desired location; however, left ventricular puncture may also permit successful pacing. Atrial capture is theoretically possible with widely misdirected wires but has not been reported. Using human cadavers, the left parasternal approaches appear to provide the most accurate lead placement with the fewest "injuries" (see further on).[61] Clinically, the subxiphoid approach is favored and involves advancing the trocar from the left xiphochondral notch toward the left shoulder or sternal notch at an angle of 30 to 45 degrees to the skin. The introducer is advanced to approximately 75% of its length. Chest compressions should be discontinued during manipulation of the introducer. On free blood return with removal of the trocar, the pacing wire is advanced through the cannula as far as possible. The cannula is removed from around the wire and pacing is attempted. Failure to capture necessitates manipulation and gradual withdrawal of the wire. Ideally the distalmost electrode (cathode) is in an intraventricular position, whereas the proximal electrode (anode) is in an intramyocardial or epicardial location. The intracavitary distal electrode need not contact myocardium for capture. Unipolar pacing configurations may be used with the intracardiac electrode as the cathode. In human studies, capture thresholds ranged from 1 to 6 mA.[61] During subxiphoid introduction of the cannula, chest compressions should be discontinued and the lungs fully inflated to depress the diaphragm and abdominal viscera from the needle path. For left parasternal access, the cannula is advanced at 30 degrees to the skin from a site immediately adjacent or 6 cm lateral to the sternum in the left fifth intercostal space and toward the right second costochondral joint. Using this approach, the lungs should be fully deflated to reduce the risk of pneumothorax. In skilled hands using preassembled pacing kits, transthoracic wires may be positioned in 10 to 60 seconds.[62] Following capture and stabilization of the wire to the skin, a chest x-ray film is obtained to rule out pneumothorax and evaluate lead position. Replacement with a transvenous pacing system is recommended as soon as possible because of the undocumented stability of transthoracic leads.

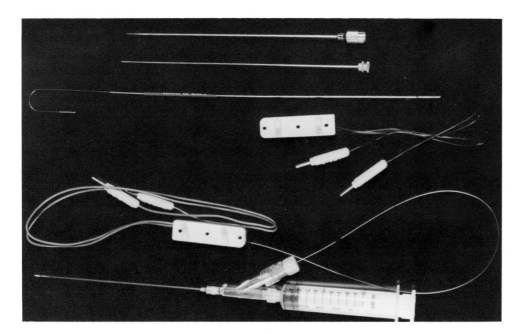

FIGURE 34–8. Transthoracic pacing apparatus. *Top*, Kit containing separate introducing needle and trocar, distal J bipolar wire electrode, and adapter for connecting wire electrode to transvenous pacing generator. *Bottom*, Completely preassembled transthoracic pacing kit. When blood return into the syringe is obtained, the wire electrode is advanced through the side-arm of the needle. Pacing may begin immediately.

The incidence of successful ventricular capture in emergent cardiac arrest situations using transthoracic pacing varies from 4% to 100%.[62–65] Survival rates invariably are dismally low, often 0% in large series.[63, 65] Nevertheless, anecdotal reports of successful transthoracic pacing for 3 weeks in an individual patient and successful transthoracic pacing despite failure of transvenous attempts suggest benefit in isolated cases.[64] Although frequently successful in animal models and human patients who have not experienced cardiac arrest (in early literature), contemporary failure of the procedure may arise from delayed application in cardiac arrest situations, traditionally waiting until after the failure of medical therapy and conventional pacing techniques.[63] No controlled prospective studies comparing early use of transthoracic pacing to other pacing modalities are available.

The analysis of complications from transthoracic pacing is greatly limited by the infrequency of even short-term survivors and the lack of pathologic evaluation of nonsurvivors in most studies. Potential complications are those related to vascular and visceral trauma from misdirected leads. Laceration of epicardial coronary arteries is possible even with accurate placement. Hemopericardium up to 100 ml in volume is a common finding in autopsy studies, and cardiac tamponade has been reported.[63, 66] Tension pneumothorax is possible in patients receiving positive pressure ventilation, and puncture of ventricular aneurysms may theoretically result in ventricular noncapture, extensive bleeding, or mobilization of mural thrombi. Nevertheless, a review found no evidence of death directly attributable to complications of transthoracic pacing.[67]

TEMPORARY EPICARDIAL PACING

Epicardial pacing uses thin polytetrafluoroethylene (Teflon)-coated unipolar wires sutured to the atria and ventricles at the time of cardiac surgery to pace and sense the heart. These leads are typically sutured in pairs to the right atrium and ventricular apex and externalized in the epigastrium for use with standard transvenous temporary pacing generators. A fifth wire terminating subcutaneously is sometimes implanted for unipolar pacing. Atrial wires are typically exposed on the patient's right side and ventricular wires on the

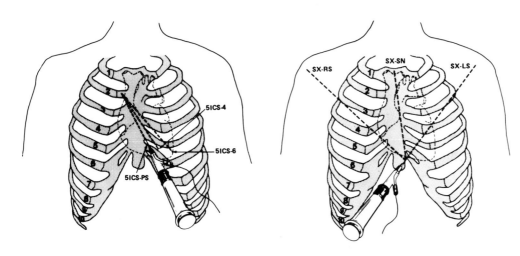

FIGURE 34–9. Approaches to the right ventricular cavity for transthoracic pacing. *Left*, Parasternal approach: 5ICS-PS = fifth intercostal space parasternally; 5ICS-4 and 5ICS-6 = fifth intercostal space 4 and 6 cm lateral to the sternum, respectively. *Right*, Subxiphoid approach: SX-RS, SX-SN, SX-LS = subxiphoid directed toward the right shoulder, sternal notch, and left shoulder, respectively. See text for details. (From Brown CG, Hutchins GM, Gurley HT, et al: Placement accuracy of percutaneous transthoracic pacemakers. Am J Emerg Med 3:193, 1985.)

left side. When no longer needed, the wires are removed percutaneously by gentle traction. Complications resulting from the implantation and removal of these wires are exceptionally rare.[68]

These wires have therapeutic and diagnostic utility in the postoperative period by allowing single- or dual-chamber bradycardia support pacing, pace termination of some atrial tachyarrhythmias, and recording of intracardiac electrograms for differential diagnosis of postoperative arrhythmias. In one study, the wires were used therapeutically or diagnostically, or both, in 81% of patients.[69] Unipolar or bipolar atrial pacing incorporating one wire at the lateral right atrium above the sinoatrial node may provide the lowest pacing thresholds.[70] Both atrial and ventricular sensing and pacing thresholds are quite variable among patients and tend to deteriorate in the days following surgery. Unipolarization of individual leads or reversing polarity of bipolar configurations may identify the lowest pacing thresholds.

MECHANICAL PACING

The ventricular myocardium may be activated mechanically by direct percussion of the chest wall. These "chest thumps" are administered as sharp blows with the ulnar aspect of the fist to the middle to lower two thirds of the patient's sternum. The blows are delivered from a height of 15 to 20 cm above the sternum and repeated serially at approximately 60 to 90 per minute depending on the duration of bradycardia. True cardiac contraction must be documented by palpation of a pulse because percussion artifacts may simulate QRS complexes on the ECG.

The electromechanical transduction mechanism by which percussion activates myocardium is not understood. Using a calibrated external mechanical stimulator, Zoll and colleagues determined the threshold for percussion pacing to be 0.04 to 1.5 J in 10 human subjects.[71] The ventricles are stimulated by percussion, and coupled stimuli demonstrate

absolute and relative refractory periods and supranormal response periods.[71]

In animal studies, mechanical pacing maintains cardiac output and blood pressure at levels twofold greater than conventional chest compressions.[72] The hemodynamic responses in humans have not been fully characterized, but percussion pacing has sustained patients for up to 1 hour as the sole mechanism of cardiac stimulation.[73] Percussion pacing is most successful early in bradycardic arrests, at which time single ventricular depolarizations usually follow each blow (Fig. 34–10). As myocardial ischemia progresses, the evoked QRS complexes widen and occur in salvos, and eventually loss of QRS voltage and appearance of injury patterns are noted. Finally, ventricular fibrillation may be induced or electric response is lost.

The incidence of myocardial "capture" during percussion pacing is unknown and the published literature tends to be anecdotal. The maneuver appears useful in witnessed, transient bradyarrhythmias and has also been used to terminate ventricular tachycardia.[74] Percussion pacing may precipitate ventricular fibrillation but is otherwise free from reported complications. Unstable chest wall lesions or recent sternotomy may be contraindications to this technique.

Cough CPR appears to generate cardiac output by compression of intrathoracic structures with up to 250 to 450 mm Hg of pressure produced by the cough.[75] To perform the maneuver, the conscious patient must cough *forcefully* every 3 seconds until the intrinsic rhythm recovers. Paroxysms of coughing are ineffective. Cough CPR has maintained aortic systolic pressures greater than 130 mm Hg during ventricular fibrillation as compared with 60 mm Hg during conventional chest compressions in the same patients.[76] Consciousness has been maintained for up to 92 seconds during ventricular fibrillation using cough CPR.[76] Cough-induced termination of ventricular tachycardia has also been reported.[76] This technique is most effective in patients previously instructed in the maneuver (such as in the cardiac catheterization labora-

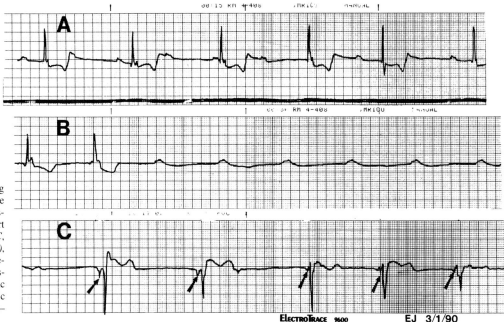

FIGURE 34–10. Percussion pacing during asystolic arrest. *A,* High-grade AV block with slow ventricular escape rhythm. *B,* Complete heart block with ventricular asystole. *C,* Percussion pacing artifacts *(arrows),* each eliciting a single ventricular depolarization. (Reprinted by permission of Ellenbogen KA [ed]: Cardiac pacing. Oxford, Blackwell Scientific Publications, Inc., 1992, pp 162–210.)

TABLE 34–7. CLINICAL FEATURES OF PACING MODES

	TRANS-VENOUS	TRANS-CUTANEOUS	TRANS-THORACIC	TRANS-ESOPHAGEAL	EPICARDIAL	PERCUSSION	COUGH CPR
Time to initiate	3–10 min	<1 min	10–60 sec	Minutes	<1 min	Instantaneous	Instantaneous
Training required	+ + +	+	+ +	+ +	+	+	+
Chambers paced	A, V	V	V	A, ± V	A, V	V	None
Emergency use	+	+	+	–	+	+	+
Prophylactic use	+	+	–	–	+	+	+
Prolonged use	+	–	–	–	+	–	–
Treat VT	+	+	–	–	+	±	±
Treat SVT	+	–	–	+	+	–	–
Vascular trauma	+	–	+	–	–	–	–
Arrhythmias	+	–	+	–	–	+	–
Visceral trauma	+	–	+	–	–	–	–
Infection	+	–	+	–	±	–	–
Discomfort	–	+	+	+	–	+	–
Comments	Most versatile and reliable	Fast and easy	Emergent use only	Primarily atrial pacing	Postoperative only, early lead failure	Witnessed bradycardia	Cooperative patient, supports VF

Abbreviations: A, atria; CPR, cardiopulmonary resuscitation; SVT, supraventricular tachycardia; V, ventricles; VF, ventricular fibrillation; VT, ventricular tachycardia.

tory) and must be used 5 to 10 seconds into the arrest. As mentioned, the technique can be effective in brady- or tachy-arrhythmias but requires a cooperative, conscious patient able to generate a forceful cough.

Selection of Pacing Modality

In emergent situations, the time required to initiate effective cardiac pacing assumes paramount importance. In bradycardic-asystolic arrests, delays of greater than 5 minutes in restoring a pulse virtually preclude successful resuscitation.[77] In these situations, external transcutaneous pacing is regarded by many as the pacing modality of choice given its speed, safety, and ease of initiation. Cardiac capture may not be achieved in all cases, however. Transvenous pacing has traditionally served as the mainstay of temporary pacing and may be attempted if transcutaneous pacing fails or is unavailable. Frequently, transcutaneous pacing can be attempted by ancillary personnel while the staff and materials needed for transvenous pacing are being assembled. The role of transthoracic pacing when other modalities are available remains undefined. Although highly invasive, the speed of initiation may rival that of transcutaneous pacing. The efficacy of transcutaneous pacing has not been adequately proved or disproved given its delayed use in most studies. The urgency of the situation should justify its use in the face of these uncertainties. Currently, no prospective studies comparing the safety and efficacy of these emergent pacing modes exist. Given the narrow therapeutic time window for successful resuscitation from asystolic arrest, it is advisable to proceed with the mode of emergent pacing that is most readily available and that will attain ventricular pacing *most rapidly*.

In selecting prophylactic or nonemergent pacing modalities, the anticipated duration of pacing, patient comfort, and the desire to avoid specific complications become important. For brief prophylactic use, transcutaneous pacing would appear the method of choice given its high degree of efficacy and remarkable safety. For example, this technique may be well suited for use in right-sided heart catheterization in patients with preexisting left bundle branch block or in cardioversion of patients with tachycardia-bradycardia syndrome. Effective capture must be demonstrated before relying on this technique, however. Anticipated transient brady-arrhythmias may be managed by instructing the patient to perform cough CPR on command. Such a situation is common during coronary artery injections in the cardiac catheterization lab. Similarly, percussion pacing may interrupt prolonged, albeit transient, asystole. For protracted pacing requirements or the need for dual-chamber stimulation, transvenous pacing is necessary. Following cardiac surgery, epicardial pacing wires may be used in place of transvenous leads for single- or dual-chamber pacing. Esophageal pacing may permit atrial capture in most patients; however, ventricular capture frequently requires specialized esophageal balloon electrodes or very high output generators.[78] Table 34–7 compares the clinical features of the various pacing modes.

REFERENCES

1. Sprung CL, Elser B, Schein RMH, et al: Risk of right bundle-branch block and complete heart block during pulmonary artery catheterization. Crit Care Med 17:1, 1989.
2. Morris D, Mulvihill D, Lew WYW, et al: Risk of developing complete heart block during bedside pulmonary artery catheterization in patients with left bundle branch block. Arch Intern Med 147:2005, 1987.
3. Mancini GBJ, Goldberger AL: Cardioversion of atrial fibrillation: Consideration of embolization, anticoagulation, prophylactic pacemaker, and long-term success. Am Heart J 104:617, 1982.
4. Sharkey SW, Chaffee V, Kapsner S: Prophylactic external pacing during cardioversion of atrial tachyarrhythmias. Am J Cardiol 55:1632, 1985.
5. Roberts NK, Somerville J: Pathological significance of electrocardiographic changes in aortic valve endocarditis. Br Heart J 31:395, 1971.
6. Steere AC, Batsford WP, Weinberg M, et al: Lyme carditis: Cardiac abnormalities of Lyme disease. Ann Intern Med 93(Pt I):8, 1980.
7. Bellocci F, Santarelli P, Di Gennaro M, et al: The risk of cardiac complications in surgical patients with bifascicular block. Chest 77:343, 1980.
8. Trankina MF, White RD: Perioperative cardiac pacing using an atrioventricular pacing pulmonary artery catheter. J Cardiothorac Anesth 3:154, 1989.
9. Meier B, Rutihauser W: Coronary pacing during percutaneous transluminal coronary angioplasty. Circulation 71:557, 1985.

10. Syverud SA, Dalsey WC, Hedges JR, et al: Radiologic assessment of transvenous pacemaker placement during CPR. Ann Emerg Med 15:131, 1986.
11. Wood M, Ellenbogen K, Haines D: Temporary cardiac pacing. *In* Ellenbogen K (ed): Cardiac Pacing. Oxford, Blackwell Scientific, 1992, pp 162–210.
12. Lang R, David D, Klein HO, et al: The use of the balloon-tipped floating catheter in temporary transvenous cardiac pacing. PACE 4:491, 1981.
13. Davis MJE: Emergency ventricular pacing using a J-electrode without fluoroscopy. Med J Aust 152:194, 1990.
14. Hazard PB, Benton C, Milnar JP: Transvenous cardiac pacing in cardiopulmonary resuscitation. Crit Care Med 9:666, 1981.
15. Phillips SJ, Butner AN: Percutaneous transvenous cardiac pacing initiated at bedside: Results in 40 cases. J Thorac Cardiovasc Surg 59:855, 1970.
16. Furman S, Hurzeler P, Mehra R: Cardiac pacing and pacemakers. IV. Threshold of cardiac stimulation. Am Heart J 94:115, 1977.
17. Gulotta SJ: Transvenous cardiac pacing: Techniques for optimal electrode positioning and prevention of coronary sinus placement. Circulation 42:701, 1970.
18. Castellanos A, Maytin O, Lemberg L, et al: Unusual QRS complexes produced by pacemaker stimuli with special reference to myocardial tunneling and coronary sinus stimulation. Am Heart J 77:732, 1969.
19. Befeler B, Hildner FJ, Javier RP, et al: Cardiovascular dynamics during coronary sinus, right atrial, and right ventricular pacing. Am Heart J 81:372, 1971.
20. Benchimol A, Ells JG, Dimond EG: Hemodynamic consequences of atrial and ventricular pacing in patients with normal and abnormal hearts. Am J Med 39:911, 1965.
21. Hartzler GO, Maloney JD, Curtis JJ, et al: Hemodynamic benefits of atrioventricular sequential pacing after cardiac surgery. Am J Cardiol 40:232, 1977.
22. Murphy P, Morton P, Murtach JG, et al: Hemodynamic effects of different temporary pacing modes for the management of bradycardias complicating acute myocardial infarction. PACE 15:391, 1992.
23. Preston TA, Fletcher RD, Luccesi BR, et al: Changes in myocardial threshold: Physiologic and pharmacologic factors in patients with implanted pacemakers. Am Heart J 74:235, 1967.
24. Sowton E, Ban I: Physiologic changes in threshold. Ann NY Acad Sci 167:678, 1969.
25. Krueger SK, Rakes S, Wilkerson J, et al: Temporary pacing by general internists. Arch Intern Med 143:1531, 1983.
26. Austin JL, Preis LK, Crampton RS, et al: Analysis of pacemaker malfunction and complications of temporary pacing in the coronary care unit. Am J Cardiol 49:301, 1982.
27. Lumia FJ, Rios JC: Temporary transvenous pacemaker therapy: An analysis of complications. Chest 64:604, 1973.
28. Paulk EA, Hunst JW: Complete heart block in acute myocardial infarction. Am J Cardiol 17:695, 1966.
29. Mooss AN, Ross WB, Esterbrooks DJ, et al: Ventricular fibrillation complicating pacemaker insertion in acute myocardial infarction. Cathet Cardiovasc Diagn 8:253, 1982.
30. Weinstein J, Gnoj J, Mazzara JT, et al: Temporary transvenous pacing via the percutaneous femoral vein approach. Am Heart J 85:695, 1973.
31. Nathan DA, Center S, Pina RE, et al: Perforation during indwelling catheter pacing. Circulation 33:128, 1966.
32. Silver MD, Goldschlager N: Temporary transvenous pacing in the critical care setting. Chest 93:607, 1988.
33. Van Durme JP, Heyndrickx G, Snoeck J, et al: Diagnosis of myocardial perforation by intracardiac electrograms recorded from the indwelling catheter. J Electrocardiol 6:97, 1973.
34. Nolewajka AJ, Goddard MD, Broun TC: Temporary transvenous pacing and femoral vein thrombosis. Circulation 62:646, 1980.
35. Zoll PM: Noninvasive cardiac stimulation revisited. PACE 13:2014, 1990.
36. Prochaczek F, Galecka J: The effect of suppression of the distortion artifact during transcutaneous pacing on the shape of the QRS complex. PACE 13:2022, 1990.
37. Falk RH, Ngai STA: External cardiac pacing: Influence of electrode placement on pacing threshold. Crit Care Med 14:931, 1986.
38. Madsen JK, Pedersen F, Grande P, et al: Normal myocardial enzymes and normal echocardiographic findings during noninvasive transcutaneous pacing. PACE 11:1188, 1988.
39. Klein LS, Miles WM, Heger JJ, et al: Transcutaneous pacing: Patient tolerance, strength-interval relations, and feasibility for programmed electrical stimulation. Am J Cardiol 62:1126, 1988.
40. Zoll PM, Zoll RH, Falk RH, et al: External noninvasive temporary cardiac pacing: Clinical trials. Circulation 71:937, 1985.
41. Falk RH, Ngai STA: Cardiac activation during external cardiac pacing. PACE 10:503, 1987.
42. Zoll PM, Linenthal AJ, Normal CR, et al: External electrical stimulation of the heart in cardiac arrest. Arch Intern Med 96:639, 1955.
43. Kelly IS, Royster RL, Angert KC, et al: Efficacy of noninvasive transcutaneous cardiac pacing in patients undergoing cardiac surgery. Anesthesiology 70:747, 1989.
44. Luck JC, Grubb BP, Artman SE, et al: Termination of sustained ventricular tachycardia by external noninvasive pacing. Am J Cardiol 61:574, 1988.
45. Hedges JR, Syverud SA, Dalsey WC, et al: Threshold, enzymatic, and pathologic changes associated with prolonged transcutaneous pacing in a chronic heart block model. J Emerg Med 7:1, 1989.
46. Falk RH, Zoll PM, Zoll RH: Safety and efficacy of noninvasive cardiac pacing: A preliminary report. N Engl J Med 17:279, 1988.
47. Kelly JS, Royster RL: Noninvasive transcutaneous cardiac pacing. Anesth Analg 69:229, 1989.
48. Altamura G, Bianconi L, Boccadamo R, et al: Treatment of ventricular and supraventricular tachyarrhythmias by transcutaneous cardiac pacing. PACE 12:331, 1989.
49. Paris PM, Stewart RD, Kaplan RM, et al: Transcutaneous pacing for bradysystolic cardiac arrests in prehospital care. Ann Emerg Med 14:320, 1985.
50. Hedge JR, Syverud SA, Dalsey WC, et al: Prehospital trial of emergency transcutaneous cardiac pacing. Circulation 876:1337, 1987.
51. Cummins RO, Graves JR, Larsen MP, et al: Out-of-hospital transcutaneous pacing by emergency medical technicians in patients with asystolic cardiac arrest. N Engl J Med 328:1377, 1993.
52. Knowlton AA, Falk RH: External cardiac pacing during in-hospital cardiac arrest. Am J Cardiol 57:1295, 1986.
53. Altamura G, Bianconi L, Toscano S, et al: Transcutaneous cardiac pacing for termination of tachyarrhythmias. PACE 13:2026, 1990.
54. Altamura G, Toscano S, Bianconi L, et al: Transcutaneous cardiac pacing: Evaluation of cardiac activation. PACE 13:2017, 1990.
55. Luck JC, Markel ML: Clinical applications of external pacing: A renaissance? PACE 14:1299, 1991.
56. Talit U, Leach CN, Werner MS, et al: The effect of external cardiac pacing on stroke volume. PACE 13:598, 1990.
57. Feldman MD, Zoll PM, Aroesty JM, et al: Hemodynamic responses to noninvasive external cardiac pacing. Am J Med 84:395, 1988.
58. Zoll PM: Resuscitation of the heart in ventricular standstill by external stimulation. N Engl J Med 247:768, 1952.
59. Béland MJ, Hesslein PS, Rowe RD: Ventricular tachycardia related to transcutaneous pacing. Ann Emerg Med 17:279, 1988.
60. Voorhees WD III, Foster KS, Geddes LA, et al: Safety factor for precordial pacing. Minimum current thresholds for pacing and for ventricular fibrillation by vulnerable-period stimulation. PACE 7:356, 1984.
61. Brown CG, Hutchins GM, Gurley HT, et al: Placement accuracy of percutaneous transthoracic pacemakers. Am J Emerg Med 3:193, 1985.
62. Gessman LJ, Wertheimer JH, Davison J, et al: A new device and method for rapid emergency pacing: Clinical use in 10 patients. PACE 5:929, 1982.
63. Tintanalli JE, White BC: Transthoracic pacing during CPR. Ann Emerg Med 10:113, 1981.
64. Kodjababian GH, Gray RE, Keenan RL, et al: Percutaneous implantation of cardiac pacemaker electrodes. Am J Cardiol 19:372, 1967.
65. White JD: Transthoracic pacing in cardiac asystole. Am J Emerg Med 3:264, 1983.
66. Roberts JR, Greenburg MI, Crisant JW, et al: Successful use of emergency transthoracic pacing in bradysystolic cardiac arrest. Am J Emerg Med 13:277, 1984.
67. Roberts JR, Greenburg MI: Emergency transthoracic pacemaker. Ann Emerg Med 10:600, 1981.
68. Waldo AL, MacLean WAH: Diagnosis and Treatment of Cardiac Arrhythmias Following Open Heart Surgery: Emphasis on the Use of Atrial and Ventricular Epicardial Wire Electrodes. Mt Kisco, NY, Futura Publishing, 1980.
69. Waldo AL, MacLean WAH, Cooper TB, et al: Use of temporarily placed epicardial atrial wire electrodes in the diagnosis and treatment of

cardiac arrhythmias following open-heart surgery. J Thorac Cardiovasc Surg 76:500, 1978.

70. Almassi GH, Wetherbee JN, Hoffman RG, et al: Optimal lead positioning for postoperative atrial pacing. Chest 101:1194, 1992.

71. Zoll PM, Belgard AH, Weintraub MJ, et al: External mechanical cardiac stimulation. N Engl J Med 294:1274, 1976.

72. Iseri LT, Allen BJ, Baron K, et al: Fist pacing, a forgotten procedure in bradysystolic cardiac arrest. Am Heart J 113:1545, 1987.

73. Scherf D, Bornemann C: Thumping of the precordium in ventricular standstill. Am J Cardiol 5:30, 1960.

74. Caldwell G, Miller G, Quinn E, et al: Simple mechanical methods for cardioversion: Defences of the precordial thump and cough version. Br Med J 291:627, 1985.

75. Wei JY, Greene HL, Weisfeldt ML: Cough-facilitated conversion of ventricular tachycardia. Am J Cardiol 45:174, 1980.

76. Criley JM, Blausfuss AH, Kissel GL: Cough-induced cardiac compression: Self-administered form of cardiopulmonary resuscitation. JAMA 236:1246, 1976.

77. Burack B, Furman S: Transesophageal cardiac pacing. Am J Cardiol 23:469, 1969.

78. Touborg P, Andersen HR, Pless P: Low-current bedside emergency atrial and ventricular pacing from the esophagus. Lancet 16:166, 1982.

CHAPTER 35

ESOPHAGEAL PACING

Barbara J. Deal

Several decades elapsed between the earliest report of successful recording of an esophageal electrocardiogram (ECG) by Cremer in 1906 and the recognition of the potential clinical applications of this technique.[1] In 1936 the clinical value of the esophageal ECG in evaluating rhythm and conduction disorders was reported by Brown.[2, 3] The first successful cardiac pacing in humans using the transesophageal route was reported by Shafiroff and Linder in 1957.[4] Emergency transesophageal cardiac pacing was first reported by Burack and Furman[5] in 1969, when they successfully performed chronic atrial pacing for a period of 36 hours in a critically ill patient. Limited reports of the use of transesophageal pacing appeared during the next decade.[6–8] More widespread interest in the diagnostic and therapeutic utility of the technique dates from the report by Gallagher and colleagues[9] in 1980, when they demonstrated the use of the esophageal ECG in distinguishing between the different mechanisms of supraventricular tachycardia (SVT). Currently, recording the esophageal ECG and performing atrial pacing are accepted as simple and noninvasive means of diagnosing the mechanism of rhythm disturbances, rapidly performing antibradycardia pacing, and terminating episodes of tachycardia.

The basis of esophageal electrophysiologic evaluation is the ability to record a discrete atrial electrogram and successfully pace the atria, using a technique that allows easy access and is relatively noninvasive. The major clinical applications of this technique include (1) interpretation of the mechanism of arrhythmias based on an analysis of the relative timing of atrial and ventricular depolarization, (2) performance of atrial pacing in patients with bradycardia or when overdrive atrial pacing would be useful, (3) termination of acute episodes of SVT, and (4) initiation of supraventricular arrhythmias, allowing an assessment of the functional characteristics of the tachycardia circuit and the testing of drug efficacy. In this discussion the technical aspects of pacing are described first, and a summary of the diagnostic and therapeutic applications follows.

Methodology

ANATOMY

The initial application of esophageal pacing was hampered by the lack of a suitable animal model with an esophageal-cardiac anatomy similar to that of humans. In the dog, the esophagus is not in close proximity to the epicardial surface, and successful transesophageal cardiac pacing required suturing the esophagus directly to the heart.[5] In humans the esophagus lies in close proximity to the posterior atrial surface; the ventricles are separated from the esophagus by several centimeters. Early attempts to accomplish ventricular pacing were thus difficult, and the use of unipolar pacing resulted in chest muscle and diaphragmatic pacing, discouraging its application.

Reports of successful conversion of SVT using transesophageal pacing in 1973 by Montoyo and colleagues[10] rekindled interest in atrial pacing through the esophagus. Because of the proximity of the esophagus to the left atrium, it was assumed that the esophageal electrogram reflected left atrial activity. In 1980 Prystowsky and colleagues[11] demonstrated that the origin of the atrial electrogram as recorded from the esophagus reflects posterior paraseptal depolarization. Subsequent work by Binkley and coworkers[12] suggested that the electrogram reflected left atrial electrical activity at a site 1 cm to the left of the interatrial septum. Subsequently, much work centered on the factors necessary to minimize pacing thresholds to allow the technique to be useful clinically.

ELECTRODE PLACEMENT

There is now a wide variety of catheters available for esophageal use (Fig. 35–1). In early studies a silicone-coated, bipolar permanent pacing lead was used; this was followed by the introduction of an esophageal ''pill'' electrode that facilitated placement by allowing the patient to swallow the

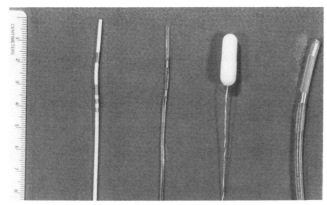

FIGURE 35–1. Esophageal pacing catheters commonly used are shown above. *From Left*, A no. 5 French quadripolar catheter (Elecath); a no. 4 French bipolar catheter (Arzco, Inc.); a bipolar pill electrode (Arzco, Inc.); a no. 10 French silicone-coated bipolar implantable coronary sinus catheter (Medtronics Inc., Minneapolis, MN).

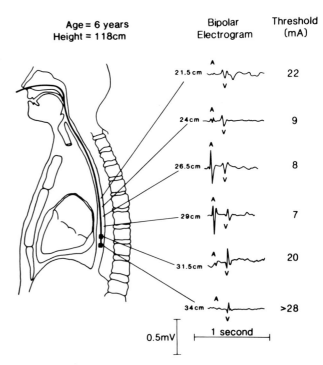

FIGURE 35–2. Schematic of sagittal section of torso during transesophageal recording and stimulation at six sites, each separated by 2.5 cm. Pacing thresholds were determined with stimuli of 9.9 msec. (From Benson DW Jr, Sanford M, Dunnigan A, Benditt DG: Transesophageal atrial pacing threshold: Role of interelectrode spacing, pulse width, and catheter insertion depth. Am J Cardiol 53:63, 1984.)

capsule.[7] The use of the pill electrode requires an alert, cooperative patient, and contact with the esophagus varies with peristalsis, sometimes requiring higher energy output to maintain capture. Newer catheters have been designed in smaller French sizes (4 and 5 Fr) and incorporate four poles to allow simultaneous pacing and recording for diagnostic studies. The smaller, more flexible catheters are tolerated well by patients and are suitable for use in pediatric patients, including neonates.

The technique of electrode placement is similar to that used for nasogastric tube placement. The catheter is inserted through the nares and positioned to a depth determined by the patient's height, usually 40 cm in the adult. Benson and coworkers[13] observed that the sites of maximal atrial electrogram recordings were located 0 to 3 cm from the site of the minimal pacing threshold, and that the site of the minimum pacing threshold could be estimated from the patient's height (Figs. 35–2 and 35–3). In smaller patients, use of this chart for estimation of the appropriate insertion depth minimizes the time necessary to obtain optimal recordings and pacing thresholds.

A standard ECG machine may be used to obtain recordings, allowing performance of the technique at the bedside. Bipolar ECG recordings are obtained by connecting the proximal and distal catheter electrodes to the right and left arm leads, as illustrated in Figure 35–4. The use of a preamplifier unit with low-frequency filters limits motion artifact and improves the quality of recordings. Optimal recordings are obtained with filter settings of between 30 and 500 Hz; the low-frequency cut-off on standard ECG machines is 0.5 Hz. To perform pacing, the catheter electrodes may be directly connected to the stimulator, or a commercially available preamplifier with a switching device may be employed (Arzco Medical Systems, Inc., Vernon Hills, IL).

PACING THRESHOLD

The determinants of the pacing threshold include the site of stimulation, the stimulus duration, and the interelectrode spacing. The site of minimal pacing threshold closely approximates that of maximal recorded atrial electrograms.[14–16] A prolonged stimulus duration is essential to reduce the cur-

rent strength necessary for esophageal capture, in contrast to intracardiac stimulation. For direct stimulation of human cardiac tissue, there is little decrease in pacing threshold as the stimulus duration is increased beyond 1 msec. However, several investigators have demonstrated a significant decrease in esophageal pacing threshold as the pulse width is increased from 5 to 10 msec.[13, 14] A pulse width of 10 msec is most commonly used except in certain patients with pacing thresholds of greater than 14 mA, in whom increasing the pulse

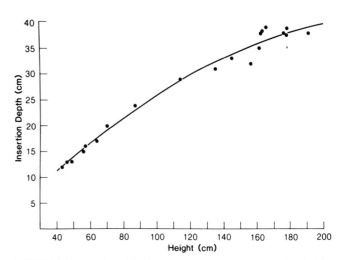

FIGURE 35–3. Esophageal catheter insertion depth versus patient height. (From Benson DW Jr: Transesophageal electrocardiography and cardiac pacing: State of the art. Circulation 75[4 Pt. 2]:III86, 1987.)

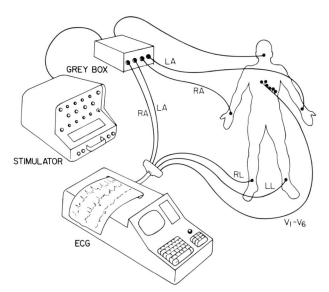

FIGURE 35–4. Schematic of patient hook-up for esophageal recording and pacing using a standard ECG machine.

width to 15 to 20 msec may reduce the pacing threshold significantly.[13] Variations in interelectrode spacing in the range of 15 to 30 mm have only a minor effect on pacing threshold.[13, 14, 16] Based on these considerations, the transesophageal pacing generator must be capable of delivering up to 30 mA of current with a pulse width of 10 msec.

Applications

CARDIAC PACING

ATRIAL PACING. Transesophageal atrial pacing is ideally suited for temporary pacing in patients with sinus bradycardia with intact atrioventricular conduction. Several studies of large numbers of patients have demonstrated uniform success in transesophageal atrial pacing using pulse width durations of 7 to 12 msec.[13–16] In patients with sinus bradycardia who require general anesthesia, this technique has the advantages of rapid institution of pacing, avoidance of intravascular instrumentation, and avoidance of the side effects of drug therapy. Backofen and colleagues[17] reported the successful use of this technique in 37 patients with sinus bradycardia undergoing surgical procedures, demonstrating its usefulness in achieving a predetermined heart rate without the hemodynamic consequences and proarrhythmic potential of pharmacologic measures. Subsequently, Pattison and colleagues[18] used an esophageal stethoscope modified for pacing in 100 patients undergoing surgery with general anesthesia, and demonstrated an average increase of 13 to 16 mm Hg in blood pressure with esophageal pacing for sinus bradycardia or junctional rhythm. Greeley and Reves[19] reported the use of transesophageal pacing during surgery in pediatric patients with congenital heart disease for both emergency pacing for bradycardia and conversion of repeated episodes of SVT.

VENTRICULAR PACING. The high output requirements necessary to achieve successful ventricular pacing using a standard electrode catheter have limited the utility of the transesophageal route in the nonanesthetized patient. Because of the

distance of the ventricles from the esophagus, the ventricles receive only 20% of the current density achieved at the left atrium during transesophageal stimulation. Using a standard generator, successful transesophageal ventricular capture has been reported in 3% to 60% of patients;[14, 20] with a high-output generator, one study reported successful ventricular capture in 88% of patients during cardiac arrest.[21] Using specially designed balloon catheters, successful ventricular capture was reported in 100% of patients evaluated by Anderson and Pless.[22] The lack of uniformly reliable ventricular capture limits the widespread application of transesophageal ventricular pacing using currently available technology.

TERMINATION AND INITIATION OF SUPRAVENTRICULAR TACHYCARDIA. Transesophageal atrial pacing has been shown to be a highly successful means of terminating SVT, including atrial flutter, orthodromic reciprocating tachycardia, and atrioventricular (AV) nodal reentry tachycardia. The reported success rates for conversion of atrial flutter using this technique vary between 65% and 90%,[15, 23] and the technique is effective in patients of all ages and following open-heart surgery (Fig. 35–5). This technique for the conversion of atrial flutter has the major advantages of avoiding direct-current electrical cardioversion, with its attendant risks of general anesthesia, and is readily performed as an outpatient procedure requiring 30 to 45 minutes of time (see Fig. 35–5). Butto and colleagues[24] reported the successful conversion of 48 of 51 episodes of atrial tachycardia in patients who had undergone atrial baffle procedures for transposition of the great arteries. In a prospective evaluation of transesophageal conversion of spontaneous episodes of atrial flutter in patients receiving antiarrhythmic medications, Crawford and colleagues[25] reported successful conversion in 82% of patients. In that study, efficacy was not affected by the patients' age, underlying cardiac disease, atrial size, atrial cycle length, or duration of atrial flutter. Rapid atrial stimulation protocols result in conversion of atrial flutter to fibrillation in up to 44% of patients,[23–25] with later spontaneous conversion to sinus rhythm occurring in a significant number of patients. The use of a minimum stimulus algorithm as reported by Butto and colleagues[24] may minimize both the development of fibrillation and patient discomfort by limiting the duration of pacing bursts.

TERMINATION OF ATRIAL TACHYCARDIA

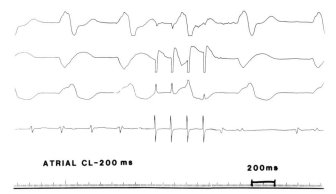

ATRIAL CL–200 ms   **200ms**

FIGURE 35–5. Transesophageal pacing conversion of atrial flutter in patient following atrial baffle repair for transposition of the great arteries. Atrial tachycardia, CL 200 msec, is converted with four extrastimuli at 140 msec.

The success rate for transesophageal conversion of paroxysmal SVT is higher than that for atrial flutter, approximating 87% to 100%.[10, 14, 26] Successful conversion of reciprocating tachycardia has been reported by Gallagher and associates[14] in 33 of 38 adult patients, and by Dick and colleagues[27] in 42 of 46 episodes in children. Benson and coworkers[26] reported their findings in 14 infants who underwent successful pacing conversion of tachycardia; they used the ventriculoatrial (VA) intervals to diagnose the mechanism of SVT. Transesophageal pacing conversion of SVT is particularly useful in patients with frequent recurrences of tachycardia while oral drug loading is being performed.

DIAGNOSTIC USES

MECHANISM OF TACHYCARDIA. During episodes of tachycardia in which the P wave is not clearly defined, recording the atrial electrogram through the esophagus provides a rapid means of establishing the AV relationship. This technique is frequently useful in the postoperative cardiac patient to distinguish sinus tachycardia from accelerated junctional rhythms or other forms of SVT, and in patients who have undergone atrial surgery, in whom the P-wave amplitude is often diminished. In patients with SVT, Gallagher and colleagues[9] established the utility of recording VA intervals to distinguish the mechanism of tachycardia. Tachycardia due to reentry within the AV node is characterized by VA intervals of less than 70 msec, whereas reentry using an accessory connection has VA intervals of greater than 70 msec, typically ranging from 100 to 110 msec. Using atrial incremental pacing and extrastimulus testing in the baseline state and with isoproterenol infusion, transesophageal studies can reproduce clinical episodes of SVT in close to 100% of patients with ECG-documented episodes of tachycardia.[28] In patients with unexplained episodes of palpitations suggestive of SVT, Pongiglione and associates[29] reported the successful initiation of SVT in 71% of young patients using a similar protocol.

DRUG TESTING. In patients with reentrant forms of SVT, esophageal pacing may be used to test the efficacy of antiarrhythmic medications. Benson and associates[30] reported the outcome of quinidine therapy to prevent SVT and found an excellent correlation between the results of acute drug testing and the clinical recurrence of tachycardia. Transesophageal pacing has been used to predict the outcome of digoxin therapy for SVT in infants, with similar results.[31]

RISK STRATIFICATION IN WOLFF-PARKINSON-WHITE SYNDROME. In asymptomatic patients with Wolff-Parkinson-White syndrome, transesophageal pacing has been successfully used as a screening test to assess the risk of developing tachycardia as well as a means of determining antegrade conduction characteristics of the accessory connection. Similarly, the ventricular response during atrial fibrillation and the effects of drug therapy may be easily assessed using this technique.[32–34] With the widespread availability of catheter ablation techniques, a transesophageal pacing study may help select asymptomatic patients at risk for developing tachycardia who might benefit from ablation.[35]

STRESS ECHOCARDIOGRAPHY. Noninvasive detection of coronary artery disease in patients who are unable to exercise may be facilitated by the use of rapid atrial pacing combined with either transthoracic or transesophageal echocardiography. This technique avoids motion artifacts and radiation exposure and permits high-quality image acquisition in most patients.[36–38]

Complications

Transesophageal pacing may be performed rapidly at the bedside, avoiding the need for fluoroscopy and vascular access. Most patients experience relatively minor degrees of discomfort, which can be minimized by optimal catheter placement to achieve lower pacing thresholds (less than 15 mA). Although pacing-induced damage to the esophagus is a potential concern, no significant damage has been reported. Burack and Furman[5] reported the autopsy findings after long-term esophageal pacing and found only areas of mild pressure necrosis. McNally and colleagues[39] reported the results of high-energy countershock delivered through the esophagus in anesthetized subjects; no significant lesions were noted.

Immediate complications of transesophageal pacing are rarely encountered and usually minor. Phrenic nerve and brachial plexus stimulation have been reported.[14, 26] Ventricular tachycardia was induced with atrial stimulation in two patients, and atrial fibrillation may be induced during attempts to convert atrial flutter.[14] Rarely, ventricular fibrillation has been reported during attempted conversion of SVT in patients with Wolff-Parkinson-White syndrome.[40]

Summary

Presently, transesophageal pacing is a simple and easily accessible technique that is used not only for providing emergency antibradycardia pacing but also for diagnosing the mechanisms of tachycardia, terminating episodes of SVT, and performing drug testing. As familiarity with the technique is gained, its application will become more widespread, and other applications, such as stress echocardiography, will become more common.

REFERENCES

1. Cremer M: Ueber die direkte Ableiting der Aktionsstrome des menschlichen Herzens vom Oesophagus und über das Elektrokardiogram des Foetus. München Med Wochenschr 53:811, 1906.
2. Brown WH: A study of the esophageal lead in clinical electrocardiography: Part I. The application of the esophageal lead to the human subject with observations on the Ta-wave, extrasystoles, and bundle branch block. Am Heart J 12:1, 1936.
3. Brown WH: A study of the esophageal lead in clinical electrocardiography: Part II. An electrocardiographic study of auricular disorders in the human subject by means of the esophageal lead. Am Heart J 12:307, 1936.
4. Shafiroff BFP, Linder J: Effects of external electrical pacemaker stimuli on the human heart. J Thorac Cardiovasc Surg 33:544, 1957.
5. Burack B, Furman S: Transesophageal cardiac pacing. Am J Cardiol 23:469, 1969.
6. Barold SS: Filtered bipolar esophageal electrocardiography. Am Heart J 83:431, 1972.
7. Arzbaecher R: A pill electrode for the study of cardiac arrhythmia. Med Instrum 12:277, 1978.
8. Jenkins JM, Wu D, Arzbaecher RC: Computer diagnosis of supraventricular and ventricular arrhythmia: A new esophageal technique. Circulation 60:977, 1979.
9. Gallagher JJ, Smith WM, Kasell J, et al: Use of the esophageal lead in

the diagnosis of mechanisms of reciprocating tachycardia. PACE 3:440, 1980.

10. Montoyo JV, Angel J, Valle V, et al: Cardioversion of tachycardias by transesophageal atrial pacing. Am J Cardiol 32:85, 1973.

11. Prystowsky EN, Pritchett ELC, Gallagher JJ: Origin of the atrial electrogram recorded from the esophagus. Circulation 61:1017, 1980.

12. Binkley PF, Bush CA, Fleishman BL, et al: In vivo validation of the origin of the esophageal electrocardiogram. J Am Coll Cardiol 7:813, 1986.

13. Benson DW Jr, Sanford M, Dunnigan A, Benditt DG: Transesophageal atrial pacing threshold: Role of interelectrode spacing, pulse width, and catheter insertion depth. Am J Cardiol 53:63, 1984.

14. Gallagher JJ, Smith WM, Kerr CR, et al: Esophageal pacing: A diagnostic and therapeutic tool. Circulation 65:336, 1982.

15. Kerr C, Gallagher JJ, Smith WM, et al: The induction of atrial flutter and fibrillation and termination of atrial flutter by esophageal pacing. PACE 6:60, 1983.

16. Nishimura M, Katoh T, Hanai S, Watanabe Y: Optimal mode of transesophageal atrial pacing. Am J Cardiol 57:791, 1986.

17. Backofen J, Schauble J, Rogers M: Transesophageal pacing for bradycardia. Anesthesiology 61:777, 1984.

18. Pattison C, Atlee J, Mathews E, et al: Atrial pacing thresholds measured in anesthetized patients with the use of an esophageal stethoscope modified for pacing. Anesthesiology 74:854, 1991.

19. Greeley W, Reves J: Transesophageal atrial pacing for the treatment of dysrhythmias in pediatric surgical patients. Anesthesiology 68:282, 1988.

20. Lubell DL: Cardiac pacing from the esophagus. Am J Cardiol 27:641, 1971.

21. Sadowski Z, Szwed H: The effectiveness of transesophageal ventricular pacing in resuscitation procedure of adults. [Abstract]. PACE 6:132, 1983.

22. Anderson JR, Pless P: Trans-oesophageal dual-chamber pacing. Int J Cardiol 5:745, 1984.

23. Guarnerio M, Furlanello F, Del Greco M, et al: Transesophageal atrial pacing: A first-choice technique in atrial flutter therapy. Am Heart J 117:1241, 1989.

24. Butto F, Dunnigan A, Overholt E, et al: Transesophageal study of recurrent atrial tachycardia after atrial baffle procedures for complete transposition of the great arteries. Am J Cardiol 57:1356, 1986.

25. Crawford W, Plumb V, Epstein A, Kay G: Prospective evaluation of transesophageal pacing for the interruption of atrial flutter. Am J Med 86:663, 1989.

26. Benson DW Jr, Dunnigan A, Benditt DG, et al: Transesophageal study of infant supraventricular tachycardia: Electrophysiologic characteristics. Am J Cardiol 52:1002, 1983.

27. Dick M, Scott W, Serwer G, et al: Acute termination of supraventricular tachyarrhythmias in children by transesophageal atrial pacing. Am J Cardiol 61:925, 1988.

28. Brembilla-Perrot B, Spatz F, Khaldi E, et al: Value of esophageal pacing in evaluation of supraventricular tachycardia. Am J Cardiol 65:322, 1990.

29. Pongiglione G, Saul P, Dunnigan A, et al: Role of transesophageal pacing in evaluation of palpitations in children and adolescents. Am J Cardiol 62:566, 1988.

30. Benson DW Jr, Dunnigan A, Sterba R, Benditt D: Atrial pacing from the esophagus in the diagnosis and management of tachycardia and palpitations. J Pediatr 102:40, 1983.

31. Benson DW Jr, Dunnigan A, Benditt D, et al: Prediction of digoxin treatment failure in infants with supraventricular tachycardia: Role of transesophageal pacing. Pediatrics 75:288, 1985.

32. Critelli G, Grassi G, Perticone F, et al: Transesophageal pacing for prognostic evaluation of preexcitation syndrome and assessment of protective therapy. Am J Cardiol 51:513, 1983.

33. Gonzalez M, Guillen R, Pellizzon O, Raimondi E: Study of Wolff-Parkinson-White syndrome by transesophageal pacing and assessment of long-term amiodarone therapy. Am J Cardiol 55:852, 1985.

34. Chung DC, Kerr C: Transesophageal recording and pacing techniques for evaluation of patients with preexcitation. *In* Benditt DG, Benson DW Jr (eds): Cardiac Preexcitation Syndromes: Origins and Evaluation and Treatment. Boston, Martinus Nijhoff, 1986, p 321.

35. Drago F, Turchetta A, Calzolari A, et al: Detection of atrial tachyarrhythmias by transesophageal pacing and recording at rest and during exercise in children with ventricular preexcitation. Am J Cardiol 69:1098, 1992.

36. Chapman P, Doyle T, Troup P, et al: Stress echocardiography with transesophageal atrial pacing: Preliminary report of a new method for detection of ischemic wall motion abnormalities. Circulation 70:445, 1984.

37. Matthews R, Haskell R, Ginzton L, Laks M: Usefulness of esophageal pill electrode atrial pacing with quantitative two-dimensional echocardiography for diagnosing coronary artery disease. Am J Cardiol 64:730, 1989.

38. Lambertz H, Kreis A, Trumper H, Hanrath P: Simultaneous transesophageal atrial pacing and transesophageal two-dimensional echocardiography: A new method of stress echocardiography. J Am Coll Cardiol 16:1143, 1990.

39. McNally EM, Meyer EC, Langendorf R: Elective countershock in un-anesthetized patients with use of an esophageal electrode. Circulation 33:124, 1966.

40. Kugler J, Danford D, Gumbiner C: Ventricular fibrillation during transesophageal atrial pacing in an infant with Wolff-Parkinson-White syndrome. Pediatr Cardiol 12:36, 1991.

CHAPTER 36

PEDIATRIC PACING

Gerald A. Serwer
Parvin C. Dorostkar

Permanent cardiac pacemakers have been used in pediatric patients for more than 30 years.[1] Through advances in pacemaker technology, permitting greater customization of the pacemaker to the patient and a smaller generator size coupled with increased generator longevity, their use in pediatric patients has been expanded. Although many aspects of pediatric pacing are similar to their counterparts in adult pacing, major differences exist. Not only are children physically smaller than adult patients, but their underlying cardiac diseases are different. Their expected longevity, together with the lifestyle that these children lead, is often different. As a consequence of this, differences exist, not only in selection of the optimal pacing system, but also in implantation techniques, programming considerations, and follow-up methods.

No pacemaker and only a limited number of electrodes are designed specifically with the pediatric patient in mind. As a consequence, the manner in which these devices are used often requires modifications from the standard practice employed in the adult patient. In this chapter, we discuss the unique aspects of pediatric pacing, specifically focusing on pacing indications, electrode and generator selection, implantation techniques, follow-up considerations and methods, and adjustments to the child's lifestyle that are necessitated by pacemaker implantation. Much of the material presented in other chapters is equally applicable to children, and therefore, this chapter is intended as a supplement rather than a replacement for chapters dealing with similar material.

Midwest Pediatric Pacemaker Registry

Because the number of children requiring pacemakers is small, one difficulty plaguing research into pediatric pacing has been the lack of a large experience in any one center. This has led to conclusions based on limited experience that are susceptible to statistical inaccuracies. To address this problem, the Midwest Pediatric Pacemaker Registry was formed as a voluntary project of the members of the Midwest Pediatric Cardiology Society in 1980. Member institutions of this society submit data on patients requiring pacemaker implantation, consisting of patient demographics, pacing indication, associated structural cardiac disease, type of generator, type of electrode and threshold data at implant, and device explant data. No chronic follow-up data is provided. To promote the submission and validity of the data, annual reports are presented to the Midwest Pediatric Cardiology Society at its annual meeting. Concerns about the type of data collected and the method of data acquisition are discussed to ensure uniformity among participating institutions.

To date, the registry contains information on 608 patients who have had implantations of 812 pulse generators and 863 electrodes. These data present a representative sample of current pacing practice among pediatric cardiologists and avoid the bias inherent in data obtained from a single institution. The data are obtained at the time of implantation and subsequent invasive electrode evaluation. Figure 36–1 presents a summary of the data collected. Chronic follow-up data are confined to the date and reason that a generator or electrode was removed from service. Noninvasive electrode threshold data and reprogramming information following the implant are not collected. Throughout this chapter, much of the information presented on pacing indications, device selection, and acute thresholds was obtained from this source.

Indications for Permanent Pacemaker Implantation

SURGICALLY INDUCED HEART BLOCK

The single largest cause for pacemaker implantation in children remains surgically induced heart block. Approxi-

Patient Demographics

- ID number and institution
- Birthdate
- Date of initial implant
- Pacing indication
- Associated structural cardiac disease

Generator Information

- Manufacturer and model
- Implant date
- Programming at implant
- Explant date
- Programming at explant

Electrode Information

- Manufacturer and model
- Implant site and route
- Pacing thresholds (multiple pulse widths)
- Sensing values (RMS amplitude, slew rate)

FIGURE 36–1. Information collected by the Midwest Pediatric Pacemaker Registry. The data are collected on all new patients entered in the registry; all generators implanted and explanted; and all electrodes implanted, explanted, or invasively tested. ID, identification; RMS, mean spontaneous waveform amplitude.

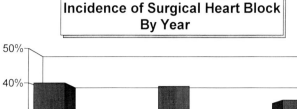
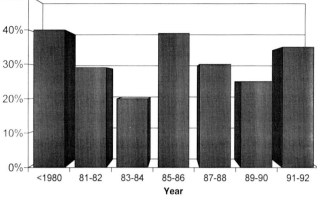

FIGURE 36–2. The percentage of all children undergoing initial pacemaker implantation in a given period, whose indication was surgically induced complete heart block. During the last 12 years, there has been no significant change in this percentage. (Data from the Midwest Pediatric Pacemaker Registry.)

mately 30% to 60% of children undergoing pacemaker implantation do so as a consequence of this.[2-7] Data from the Midwest Pediatric Pacemaker Registry show the indication for initial pacemaker placement to be surgically induced heart block in an average of 32% of patients (Fig. 36–2). The percentage varies from year to year; it reached a low of 20% in 1983 to 1984. However, there has been no definite downward trend during the last 10 years, but the underlying structural cardiac disease in patients with surgically induced heart block has changed dramatically. The majority of children acquiring surgical heart block in the last 5 years have complex disease and undergo complex surgical repairs. The surgical procedure resulting in the greatest incidence of heart block is the repair of an atrioventricular (AV) septal defect, which accounted for 17% of patients with surgical heart block since 1988. The other common diagnoses associated with surgical heart block during the last 5 years are listed in Figure 36–3.

It is unusual currently for a child with an isolated ventricular septal defect (VSD) to acquire heart block. This was not the case previously. During the 5-year period, VSDs ac-

counted for 14% of implants; atrial switch procedures (Mustard or Senning procedure) for the correction of dextrotransposition of the great arteries accounted for 12%. Other common lesions associated with surgical heart block are levotransposition of the great arteries, repair of the tetralogy of Fallot, and aortic valvular replacement, usually associated with the resection of a subaortic obstruction.

Surgical heart block can develop at the time of the initial cardiac repair or at some later point. In addition, the heart block acquired at the time of the repair may be temporary, with return of reliable AV conduction. For this reason, our current practice is to implant only temporary pacing electrodes at the time of the initial surgery and to defer permanent pacemaker implantation for 1 to 2 weeks in hopes of a return of AV conduction. However, ventricular escape rhythms are unstable, and no child with a permanent surgically acquired complete heart block is discharged without a permanent pacemaker. Even in the hospital, all children are supported with an external pacemaker through temporary pacing wires placed at the time of surgery until consistent AV conduction returns or a permanent pacemaker is inserted. Monitoring should consist of both electrocardiographic

Most Prevalent Structural Cardiac Defects Associated with Surgical Complete Heart Block	
Atrioventricular Septal Defects	17%
Isolated Ventricular Septal Defect	14%
D-Transposition of the Great Arteries	12%
L-Transposition of the Great Arteries	12%
Tetralogy of Fallot	7%
Aortic Valve Replacement	3%

FIGURE 36–3. The most common structural cardiac lesions associated with surgically induced heart block at the time of complete repair for children undergoing initial implantation since 1988. D, dextro; L, levo. (Data from the Midwest Pediatric Pacemaker Registry.)

(ECG) monitoring and non-ECG monitoring, such as arterial pressure measurements or pulse oximetry. Many ECG monitors detect the pacing artifact and do not recognize the lack of capture with subsequent bradycardia or asystole. This is avoided by the use of a non-ECG method of detecting cardiac ejection.[8]

CONGENITAL COMPLETE HEART BLOCK

The second most common indication for pacemaker implantation is congenital complete heart block. The cause of congenital heart block is variable. In many cases, an autoimmune mechanism can be implicated, with clinical and/or laboratory evidence of connective tissue disease in the mother.[9] Congenital block is also associated with specific forms of structural disease, particularly those involving abnormalities of the AV junction, such as levotransposition of the great arteries with AV discordance and atrial situs ambiguous.[10] It is common for fetal heart block to ''develop'' in utero with intact conduction present in the young fetus and heart block developing at 20 to 30 weeks of gestation.

Data from the Midwest Pediatric Pacemaker Registry indicate that approximately 25% of patients have congenital heart block as the primary indication for permanent pacing. The age at which the pacing system is implanted is quite variable, ranging from a few hours of age to older than 20 years of age. The majority of children with associated structural cardiac disease who require pacing prior to 1 year of age have congestive heart failure requiring an increased heart rate for adequate therapy. The mortality rate in such children is also high, with 43% dying by 2 years of age.[11] Death was the result of intractable congestive heart failure in spite of pacing. There was no sudden death. In children with no structural heart disease, 14% required pacing by age 6 months, and 74% required pacing by 20 years of age (Fig. 36–4). Death is rare in children with no structural cardiac disease (only 5% by 20 years of age), but it can occur suddenly.

Current recommendations call for the implantation of a

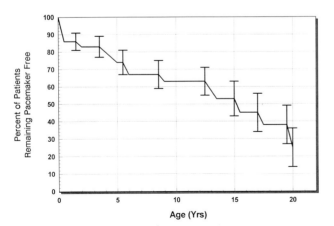

Actuarial Analysis of Years Pacemaker Free

FIGURE 36–4. Actuarial analysis of months free from pacemaker need for children with congenital complete heart block and structurally normal hearts. By age 20 years, fewer than 30% of patients are pacemaker free. The brackets represent 1 standard error around the mean. (Data from Dorostkar and coworkers.[11])

permanent pacemaker system whenever congestive heart failure is present. In addition, implantation is recommended when the average heart rate is less than 50 beats per minute (bpm) in the awake young infant, there is a history of a syncopal or presyncopal event, there is significant ventricular ectopy present, or there is exercise intolerance.[12, 13] However, symptoms of exercise intolerance can be difficult to elicit. Many children deny such symptoms as do their parents, when in fact their exercise tolerance would be improved with permanent pacing. Many parents return following pacemaker implantation to relate that the activity level of their child has markedly increased. They are amazed at this change because they did not believe that the child was significantly hindered prior to pacemaker implantation. Exercise testing is often useful as an indicator of the child's exercise capabilities compared with those of a normal child. The physician should also periodically assess the child for increasing cardiac size by chest roentgenography and decreasing cardiac function by echocardiography. The presence of either of these should be considered an indication for permanent pacemaker placement.

Finally, some children with congenital complete heart block do develop tachydysrhythmias, specifically ventricular tachycardia, which can only be controlled with permanent pacing.[14] The maintenance of a minimal heart rate often suppresses the tendency toward ventricular ectopy, particularly during exercise. The development of tachyarrhythmias with the stress of exercise, even in the otherwise asymptomatic child, would necessitate pacemaker implantation.

Controversy exists as to the need for pacing in the asymptomatic child with bradycardia of less than 50 bpm while asleep. This is not an absolute indication for pacemaker implantation. However, when bradycardias below 50 bpm are present, detailed histories and close follow-up are required to determine the need for pacemaker implantation.

SICK SINUS SYNDROME

The next most common indication is sick sinus syndrome. This indication is listed for approximately 15% of the patients in the Midwest Pediatric Pacemaker Registry. The majority of these patients have undergone cardiac surgery, specifically extensive atrial procedures. The single most common surgical procedure is the atrial switch operation for transposition of the great arteries.[15] The likelihood of needing permanent pacing in this situation increases with the time from surgery.[16] The indications are similar to those for congenital complete heart block. In addition, the presence of tachyarrhythmias, with the subsequent risk of prolonged asystole following acute termination of the tachycardia, also is an indication for pacemaker implantation (Fig. 36–5). In patients with sick sinus syndrome following an atrial switch operation, our practice is to recommend pacemaker implantation in all patients with sleeping heart rates less than 30 bpm even in the absence of symptoms. The need for drugs known to affect AV conduction for the control of tachyarrhythmias in these patients would also necessitate pacemaker placement.[16]

OTHER INDICATIONS

Patients with intermittent complete heart block secondary to lesions such as cardiac rhabdomyomas associated with

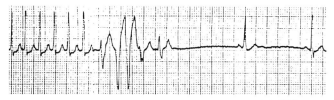

FIGURE 36–5. Electrocardiogram from a patient with sick sinus syndrome, demonstrating a 1.5-second period of asystole following acute termination of a tachyarrhythmia. Long pauses can result in syncope and are indications for pacemaker implantation. The paper speed is 25 mm/sec.

tuberous sclerosis (Fig. 36–6) and those with long QT syndrome and uncontrollable ventricular tachycardia may also benefit from pacemaker placement.[17] A chronic increase in heart rate shortens the QT interval and decreases the occurrence of ventricular tachycardia. The combined use of pacing and an implantable cardioverter-defibrillator may be even more efficacious, but there has been little experience with such therapy in pediatric patients. Other indications for pacemaker placement reported in the Midwest Pediatric Pacemaker Registry include the control of atrial tachyarrhythmias unresponsive to pharmacologic therapy, second-degree heart block associated with symptoms, and concern about a sudden loss of AV conduction in patients receiving certain antiarrhythmic therapy known to interfere with AV conduction. Although such indications are rare, the clinician should not restrict pacemaker use only to those children with complete heart block. First-degree heart block and trifascicular block with no documented loss of AV conduction are not considered indications for pacemaker implantation.[18]

Categorization of pacing indications is helpful only as a general guide. Each patient must be carefully evaluated to determine the benefits from permanent pacing versus the risks of the implant and the burden placed on the family and child for the subsequent care needed.

Selection of the Appropriate Pacemaker System

Many factors must be considered in the selection of the most appropriate pacemaker generator and electrode system for an individual child. Unlike the rate in the adult patient, the 5-year survival rate following pacemaker implantation exceeds 70% in children (Fig. 36–7), and death is usually related to the underlying structural heart defect.[6, 19] Thus, pacing may be needed for more than 50 years in the average child. This affects pacing choices because the number of replacement generators and electrodes may be high. The av-

erage longevity of the currently available lithium-powered pulse generators is only 5 years, although this has improved from that found in earlier generators (Fig. 36–8). The average epicardial electrode lasts 7 years.[20] Although the average endocardial electrode's longevity in the child is significantly increased, it is still only slightly more than 10 years (Fig. 36–9).[21] In the child undergoing an initial implantation at age 1 year, a minimum of nine electrode changes and 17 generator changes can be expected. The fact that multiple procedures will be needed and the effect of one procedure on subsequent procedures must be considered.

GENERATOR SELECTION

The major factors to be considered must be the features of the generator that are of significant benefit to the individual child, a battery capacity coupled with a projected generator's longevity, and the size of the generator. Newer generators are smaller than prior ones; therefore, size is becoming less of a factor; yet, all are not the same size. Large generators not only create unsightly protuberances that can have negative psychological consequences but also increase the risk of skin breakdown over the generator because of erosion of the generator or trauma to the skin over the generator, especially in the active child, with a subsequent infection leading to pacing system removal.

GENERATOR MODE SELECTION. The choices concerning the pacing mode to use are related to single-chamber versus dual-chamber pacing and fixed-rate versus rate-variable pacing. In general, it has been our policy to avoid the use of fixed-rate pacemakers, except in situations in which sinus and AV node function are intact for most of the time with the pacemaker serving only as a backup for those times when such function is not adequate. This is often the situation when sinoatrial (SA) and AV node function is marginal and antiarrhythmic drugs are required. Even in these cases, generators capable of rate-variable operation are preferable because the electrophysiologic state may change, and this allows for a change in mode without replacement of the generator. This situation may occur in children because the cardiovascular state may show constant evolution with time. There is no difference in the size or capacity of the battery between fixed-rate and rate-variable units, and the difference in cost is minimal.

Although cardiac output increases with exercise, even during fixed-rate pacing (Fig. 36–10), this occurs as a result of a large increase in stroke volume (Fig. 36–11), with presumed increased wall stress and potentially increased myocardial work compared with the same change in cardiac output when a heart rate increase is possible.[22] However,

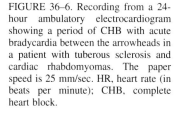

FIGURE 36–6. Recording from a 24-hour ambulatory electrocardiogram showing a period of CHB with acute bradycardia between the arrowheads in a patient with tuberous sclerosis and cardiac rhabdomyomas. The paper speed is 25 mm/sec. HR, heart rate (in beats per minute); CHB, complete heart block.

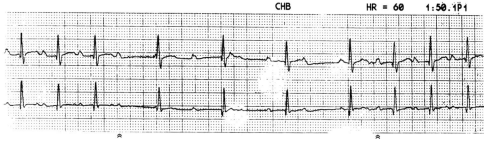

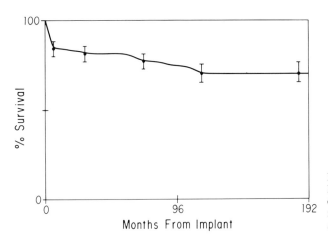

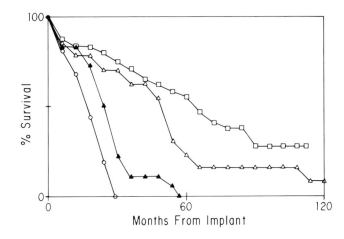

FIGURE 36–7. Actuarial survival for patients following pacemaker implantation. Excellent patient longevity is demonstrated. The brackets represent 1 standard error around the estimate. (From Serwer GA, Mericle JM: Evaluation of pacemaker pulse generator and patient longevity in patients aged 1 day to 20 years. Am J Cardiol 59:824, 1987.)

FIGURE 36–8. Actuarial survival curve for generators using various battery types. Even for lithium-powered generators, only 50% of generators survive 5 years. □, current models using lithium batteries; ○, models using mercury-zinc batteries; ▲, models using mercury-silver batteries; △, models using rechargeable batteries. (From Serwer GA, Mericle JM: Evaluation of pacemaker pulse generator and patient longevity in patients aged 1 day to 20 years. Am J Cardiol 59:824, 1987.)

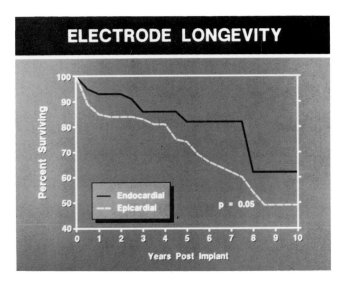

FIGURE 36–9. Actuarial analysis of endocardial *(solid line)* and epicardial *(dashed line)* electrode survival. Fifty per cent of epicardial electrodes last approximately 8 years; for endocardial electrodes, the 50% survival is greater than 10 years. The curves are significantly different (*p* = .05). (Epicardial electrode data from Serwer and colleagues.[19] Endocardial electrode data from Serwer and associates.[20])

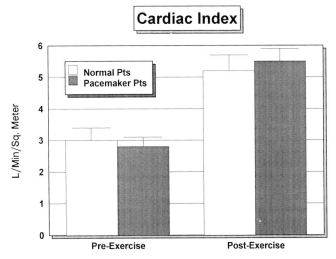

Cardiac Index

FIGURE 36–10. Changes in cardiac index as measured by acetylene rebreathing from rest to maximal exercise in normal children and those with fixed-rate ventricular pacing. The cardiac index was identical at rest and maximal exercise. The brackets represent 1 standard error about the mean. Pts, patients. (Data from Serwer and coworkers.[21])

enhanced exercise tolerance is achieved when rate-variable pacing is used.[23] This suggests an advantage to rate-variable pacing in the child expected to lead an active life. The rate-responsive mode should always be used unless the patient can demonstrate an adequate intrinsic rate response to exercise by exercise testing or ambulatory ECG.

Single-chamber pacing in either the atrium or the ventricle has been advocated for the treatment of sick sinus syndrome.[12] When atrial pacing is chosen, the presence of normal AV node function must be established by provocative electrophysiologic testing prior to the implant, especially in the postsurgical patient, because AV nodal disease can accompany SA nodal disease and may not be apparent in the

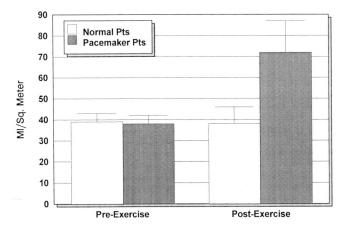

Stroke Index

FIGURE 36–11. Stroke index changes from rest to maximal exercise in normal children and those with fixed-rate ventricular pacemakers. Preexercise values were similar; the stroke index increased significantly in the patients with pacemakers to provide an increased output in the face of a fixed heart rate. The brackets represent 1 standard error about the mean. Pts, patients. (Data from Serwer and colleagues.[21])

resting nonprovoked state. AAI(R) pacing has the advantage of preserving the normal ventricular activation sequence with potentially better cardiovascular function. In addition, some evidence in animals points toward the long-term development of myocardial changes when an abnormal pattern of myocardial activation is present.[24]

A comparison of cardiac myocyte changes between ventricular free wall pacing and high septal pacing near the bundle of His with a subsequently narrower QRS morphology is striking. However, the clinical implication of these changes is unknown.

Atrial electrodes are less reliable than ventricular electrodes, even when placed endocardially. As such, conditions associated with early atrial electrode failure should serve as a contraindication to AAI pacing. Such conditions include prior extensive atrial surgery in which extensive atrial fibrosis is likely, small atrial size, and prior placement of a large intra-atrial baffle, limiting venous access to viable atrial tissue. Following Fontan's procedure (right atrial to pulmonary artery connection), patients also have a low-flow velocity present within the atrium, increasing the risk for venous thrombosis when endocardial electrodes are placed. This is one situation in which long-term anticoagulation may be indicated.

Single-chamber ventricular pacing—VVI(R)—allows the use of more stable electrode systems and, in the rate-responsive mode, still allows rate variability to be maintained. The importance of atrial systole toward the maintenance of the cardiac output is debatable and variable from child to child. Because most children have good myocardial function, the atrial contribution is probably minimal. The cardiac output increase with exercise is improved in children with DDD versus VVI pacing. It is unclear, however, whether this increase is the result of atrial synchrony or rate variability. The pacemaker syndrome from VVIR pacing is rare in children and is generally not a concern in choosing between single- and dual-chamber pacing. The major factor to be considered in such a choice is the difficulty in placing an adequate atrial electrode. If prior surgery or underlying structural disease precludes atrial electrode placement, single-chamber pacing is an acceptable alternative. However, dual-chamber pacing should be considered for all patients, with single-chamber pacing used only if contraindications to dual-chamber pacing (as discussed later) exist. Even in sick sinus syndrome, dual-chamber pacing should be considered, especially if AV nodal function is suspect.

We now consider dual-chamber pacing to be the mode of choice in children and use single-chamber pacing only when a contraindication to dual-chamber pacing exists. The major contraindications to the use of dual-chamber pacing include (1) persistent atrial tachyarrhythmias; (2) changing AV nodal status, making numerous programming changes necessary; and (3) inability to place reliable atrial and ventricular electrodes. Examples of this last contraindication would be (1) the small child in whom endocardial pacing is preferred, but the presence of two electrodes in the superior vena cava might present a high risk for thrombosis, or (2) the child requiring epicardial electrode placement in whom atrial electrode placement would necessitate a greatly enhanced surgical procedure. This is of particular concern in the child who has undergone a median sternotomy with resultant severe mediastinal fibrosis. If the durability of the atrial elec-

---

Contraindications to Dual Chamber Pacing

* Inability to place both an atrial and ventricular electrode
    Small patient size
    Limited venous access
    Extensive epicardial fibrosis

* Persistent atrial tachyarrhythmia
    Uncontrolled atrial flutter
    Arrhythmia easily triggered by atrial pacing
    Pacemaker inability to detect atrial arrhythmia
    and limit ventricular rate

* Changing electrophysiologic status of AV conduction

FIGURE 36–12. Contraindications to dual-chamber pacing in children. AV, atrioventricular.

trode is a concern, the approach commonly used is to implant a unit with the ability to be programmed to the VVIR mode should the atrial electrode fail. The generator's size and functionality is no longer a consideration because dual- and single-chamber pacemakers are comparable in both regards. Figure 36–12 relates the most common reasons for not implanting a dual-chamber system.

Dual-chamber pacing in children has previously been underused. Midwest Pediatric Pacemaker Registry data show a significant increase in dual-chamber pacing, with 43% of generators implanted in 1991 to 1992 using the DDD or DDDR mode. This is in marked contrast to the years prior to 1983 when less than 10% of generators were in the DDD mode (Fig. 36–13). This increase in dual-chamber pacing has been the result of improvements in atrial epicardial electrodes, increased experience with endocardial pacing in children, the smaller size of dual-chamber generators, and a better understanding of the benefits of dual-chamber pacing.

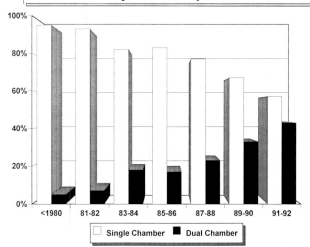

FIGURE 36–13. Comparison of the percentage of dual-chamber versus single-chamber generators implanted by year. Note the gradual shift from single-chamber to dual-chamber use. (Data from the Midwest Pediatric Pacemaker Registry.)

DESIRABLE GENERATOR FEATURES

Current pacemakers permit an almost infinite number of possible programming combinations, allowing far more programming possibilities than will ever be used in any given patient. However, because of the diversity among pediatric patients, such programmability is necessary. There are certain features that are more important for children than for adults. In this section, we discuss those programming features considered to be essential in the pediatric patient, which should influence the choice of the most appropriate pacing generator for a given patient. We begin with a discussion of those features applicable to all generators, both single and dual chamber, and then expand to encompass features unique to rate-responsive pacemakers and dual-chamber pacemakers.

GENERAL CHARACTERISTICS. The most important consideration is related to the range of energy output available, which includes both the pulse width and the pulse amplitude programmability. Although most pacemakers are chronically programmed to have either 2.5 or 5 V of amplitude, the presence of other amplitudes is of key importance. Specifically, when a generator is used with an epicardial electrode, high-output features are mandatory. Although only a minority of children require chronic pacing at outputs greater than 5.0 V, many children have an initial threshold rise and temporarily require such high outputs. Even with endocardial implants, acute increases in thresholds can occur, and the ability to increase the pacemaker amplitude to 8 V may avert the necessity for emergent electrode replacement. In addition, threshold testing at multiple low-pulse amplitudes allows a more accurate determination of the characteristics of the strength-duration curve. This is mandatory to determine the lowest, but still safe, pulse amplitude and width settings. The strength-duration curve characteristics are not constant and vary not only with time but also in relationship to activity and the time of day.[25] Such changes are discussed more fully in relation to appropriate follow-up. Knowing where the steep part of the strength-duration curve begins is critical in appropriate programming in which the clinician wants to ensure an adequate safety margin but, at the same time, minimize the energy output to maximize the generator's longevity. The ability to determine thresholds at a multitude of pulse amplitudes is a necessity.

The same argument also applies to the ability to vary duration of the pulse width. Again, although the pacemakers in the majority of children are programmed to a relatively small number of pulse durations, the ability to have a much larger number of such settings available increases the accuracy with which the clinician can characterize the strength-duration curve.

The third universal parameter of key importance to children is the rate. Although the use of fixed-rate pacemakers is becoming less frequent, the availability of a wide range of both lower and upper pacing rate limits is important in meeting the varying metabolic demands of the pediatric patient. Programming the upper rate limit of dual-chamber or rate-responsive pacemakers to values less than 150 bpm is inadequate, particularly in the small child. Even older patients can raise their heart rates above this value when exercising maximally in the absence of heart block, and therefore pulse generators must provide an upper rate limit of at least 180

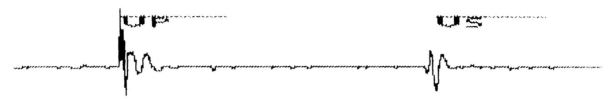

FIGURE 36–14. Intracardiac electrogram on a patient with VVI pacing showing the duration of the ventricular refractory period represented by the dashed line following either ventricular pacing (VP) or sensing (VS). In this example, it extends well beyond the termination of electric activity seen by the electrode to prevent inappropriate T-wave sensing.

bpm and preferably higher. The lower rate limit needs are also variable. In the child immediately after surgery, greater lower rate limits are often necessary to maintain an adequate cardiac output. This is especially important in the patient following atrial surgery in whom SA nodal function may be impaired. In our opinion, lower rates must be programmable from at least 50 to 120 bpm.

Another parameter often overlooked is the refractory period. In single-chamber pacing, this is often fixed to an arbitrary value of 325 msec without much thought being given to whether or not this is appropriate. For the ventricular channel, this value must be of sufficient duration to prevent inappropriate T-wave sensing and yet not prevent sensing of spontaneous ventricular depolarizations. The measurement of the pace or sensing point to the T-wave interval from the intracardiac electrogram is straightforward (Fig. 36–14). In the normal child the QT interval decreases with an increasing heart rate. When rate-variable pacing is used, the ventricular refractory period may be appropriate at rest but too long during exercise. Ideally, the ventricular refractory period should vary with the pacing rate, but this is not available in current generators. Thus, this value must be long enough to prevent T-wave sensing at the resting heart rate and short enough not to limit the upper pacing rate. As an example, a ventricular refractory period of 325 msec would limit the upper pacing rate to 185 bpm with no window to sense spontaneous beats. It is not uncommon for children with complete heart block to have spontaneous ventricular beats during the stress of exercise, which must be appropriately sensed. Appropriate programming is discussed later. Again, the wider the range of available refractory periods that is permitted, the more universally applicable the pacemaker generator is to the entire pediatric population.

For AAI(R) pacing, the refractory period must be long enough to prevent sensing of ventricular events but again not be too limiting in terms of the upper rate. Recording of the intracardiac electrogram shows the extent to which ventricu-lar events are seen by the pacemaker and the minimum value to which the atrial refractory period may be safely programmed (Fig. 36–15). Appropriate programming may be difficult and is a problem with AAI(R) pacing.

RATE-RESPONSIVE PACING. For the single-chamber rate-responsive pacemaker, appropriate settings to mimic the pediatric response to exercise are mandatory. During exercise, the normal child's heart rate increases in a linear manner with the increasing intensity of exercise (Fig. 36–16).[26] When normal children are exercised using the Bruce protocol, the heart rate increases an average of 20 bpm with each subsequent increase in exercise stage. This continues throughout the course of the exercise. Following an abrupt increase in exercise intensity (i.e., by advancing from stage I to stage II), the heart rate shows a sudden rather rapid increase, reaching a plateau value. Thus, the pacemaker must not only increase its rate in an appropriate manner with increasing exercise intensity, but such an increase much occur quickly, reaching a plateau value for that level of intensity rapidly. Therefore, not only must the heart rate increase to an appropriate degree, but also it must increase in an appropriate time frame to mimic the normal physiologic response to exercise in the pediatric patient.

Following the termination of exercise, the heart rate decreases in an exponential fashion (Fig. 36–17). Although there is an initial rapid drop, the heart rate does not reach resting levels for at least 10 minutes. Inappropriate rapid declines in the heart rate following exercise termination may not meet the metabolic demands of the body and result in inadequate cardiac output and a syncopal episode.

With these considerations of the normal heart rate response to exercise in children taken into account, the ideal rate-responsive pediatric pacemaker must have the ability to offer a variety of linear increases in heart rate with increasing exercise intensity (rate-response curves). In addition, it should offer a range of acceleration times (the rate of the heart rate increase with increased exercise intensity), with

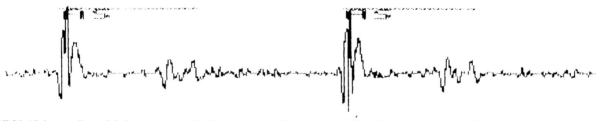

FIGURE 36–15. Intracardiac atrial electrogram recorded from a patient with AAI pacing. The refractory period *(dashed line)* must be long enough to prevent sensing of ventricular events by the atrial electrode. Note the marked increase in refractory period required compared with VVI pacing. When AAIR pacing is used, the length of this refractory period may significantly restrict the upper rate limit of the pacemaker.

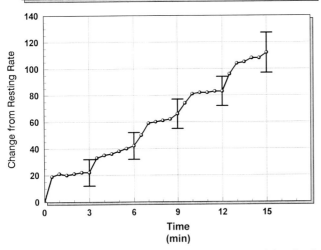

FIGURE 36–16. Normal heart rate increases from the resting value in normal children exercised using the Bruce treadmill protocol. The brackets represent 1 standard error about the estimate. (Data from Serwer and associates.[26])

more rapid acceleration times being preferred. Such increases in heart rate should be independent of resting and maximal rates. Following the termination of exercise, the heart rate decline should be exponential but slow enough so that the lower rate limit is not reached for a minimum of 10 minutes. Finally, the pacemaker must be able to tailor its detection of increasing exercise levels to the individual patient. Several approaches have been used to address this problem by different manufacturers, and it is unclear which approach ultimately will be the best. However, all manufacturers do allow tailoring of exercise detection to the individual patient, realizing that not all patients produce the same characteristics detectable by the pacemaker in response to the same degrees of exercise. Although simplicity in programming is desirable, the clinician must weigh against it the ability to tailor the

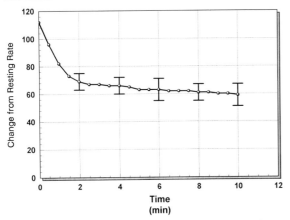

FIGURE 36–17. Normal heart rate decreases following exercise compared with the preexercise value in normal children. Even at 10 minutes after exercise, the heart rate has not reached the resting value. The brackets represent 1 standard error about the estimate. (Data from Serwer and associates.[26])

pacemaker's settings and optimize the pacemaker's performance to a given patient.

Numerous types of sensors have been used, with the most common sensing being either activity (as a function of body vibration), blood temperature, or minute ventilation. Body vibration sensing is the most useful in children because it does not require special electrodes and is not markedly different in the child compared with the adult. Blood temperature and minute-ventilation sensing[27] have been used in children, but to a lesser degree.

DUAL-CHAMBER PACING. Not only do all the considerations discussed previously apply to dual-chamber pacing, but additional programmable features must be considered. The first is the ability to program an appropriate AV interval and to decrease it with increasing atrial rate. Such shortening of the AV interval with increasing atrial rate is clearly desirable in children and should occur, not only with changes in the sensed atrial rate, but also with increases in the paced atrial rate during DDDR pacing. Not only does such a decrease more closely mimic the physiologic response, but also because it provides a shorter total atrial refractory period at higher rates, the multiblock rate is higher. This is probably the most important feature of dual-chamber generator selection because children often reach much higher atrial rates than do adults. If the total atrial refractory period is inappropriately long, multiblock occurs during the course of normal exercise, with a subsequent rapid decline in ventricular rate and the potential for syncope. It is common in children to reach atrial rates in excess of 180 bpm during routine exercise. Should the total atrial refractory period, of which the AV delay is a major part, be abnormally long, problems will occur.

In addition, multiple settings for the postventricular atrial refractory period (PVARP) also are considered desirable because of its contribution to the total atrial refractory period and, ultimately, the multiblock rate. This parameter must have enough programmability to prevent inappropriate ventricular sensing by the atrial electrode and, yet at the same time, allow a multiblock rate of at least 185 bpm (and preferably 200 bpm), particularly in younger children.

One closely allied feature that is mandatory is the ability to control the degree of PVARP extension following a spontaneous ventricular depolarization. An automatic extension of the PVARP following the spontaneous ventricular depolarization is often used to prevent sensing of retrograde atrial activation, thus avoiding pacemaker-mediated tachycardia. This is not necessarily desirable in children because the presence of retrograde-only ventriculoatrial conduction is rare and, therefore, the risk of pacemaker-mediated tachycardia is rare. With exercise, spontaneous ventricular depolarizations do occur, and if an inappropriate PVARP extension occurs, normal atrial depolarizations may not be sensed, with a subsequent sudden overall decline in the heart rate. The ability to disable this feature must be present for the generator to be appropriate for use in children. This concern is discussed later when the use of exercise testing in pacemaker follow-up is discussed.

Other features that must be considered include the ability to lower the upper rate limit in the presence of atrial tachycardia(s). The occurence of such rhythms, particularly atrial flutter, is not uncommon, particularly in the postoperative patient. Another feature that may find utility in children is the ability to decrease the lower rate limit based on the time of day. Children, who tend to have a much more predictable schedule than the adult patients do, can benefit from having their pacemakers programmed to a lower pacing rate during sleep than during the daytime hours when a higher heart rate may be needed. This is particularly useful for the child with SA nodal disease in whom the clinician cannot rely on the intrinsic atrial rate to totally govern the paced ventricular rate. With an intact SA node, one can simply set the pacing rate at an appropriately low level for sleep and rest assured that it will be at an appropriate rate during waking hours. With SA nodal disease, however, this may not be the case, and the ability to vary the lower pacing rate with the time of day may be helpful because this feature can lower the average daily rate and prolong the generator's life. This feature may also be helpful in the single-chamber rate-responsive pacemaker.

Traditional factors that were once important in pediatric pacing, such as the generator's longevity and size, are now less of a concern in the selection of a generator. All generators are much smaller than previous models, and yet longevity has not been sacrificed. This is a consequence of improved circuit efficiency. The difference in size between single-chamber, dual-chamber, and rate-responsive pacemakers often is undetectable. Pediatric patients generally have long life expectancies, and the ability to have a highly programmable pacemaker implanted to meet changing metabolic demands as a consequence of growth, age, or patient desires is indispensable. The relatively minute difference in cost between a highly programmable unit and one with fewer features is minimal, particularly when the cost is spread over the lifetime of the pacemaker. Figure 36–18 summarizes the features that must be considered for the appropriate selection of a generator. Thus, the choice of a pacemaker should be based solely on the features it possesses and its ability to appropriately meet the demands of the given patient.

PACING ELECTRODE SELECTION

There are many aspects to the choice of the appropriate electrode system in children. The first obvious choice is between the placement of an endocardial versus an epicardial system; yet other choices are often equally important and overlooked. Such choices include the selection of a unipolar versus a bipolar system, the type of electrode fixation to be used, and steroid- versus non–steroid-eluting capabilities.

ENDOCARDIAL VERSUS EPICARDIAL PACING

Initially, almost all children had epicardial electrode systems implanted. This was a consequence of the large size of the endocardial electrodes and the pacing generators. With the development of smaller electrodes and generators, this is changing; however, the majority of children still undergo epicardial lead placement as a consequence either of small patient size or other factors that do not permit the placement of an endocardial electrode system. Midwest Pediatric Pacemaker Registry data show a gradual increase in endocardial electrode use, but 60% of patients still receive epicardial electrodes (Fig. 36–19). Our basic approach is to assume that all children should undergo the placement of an endocardial system, and then we evaluate the child for factors that do not

---

Desirable Generator Features in Pediatric Pacing

✴ Highly programmable for mode, output, and AV intervals

✴ Rate responsive mode available

✴ Diagnostic rate counters available

✴ Performance indicators provided (battery voltage, battery current drain, electrode impedance)

✴ Intracardiac electrograms provided

✴ Automatic adjustments to changing status such as a change in the upper rate limit with the onset of atrial tachyarrhythmias

✴ Variable AV interval with increasing heart rate - either atrial or sensor driven

FIGURE 36–18. Generator features desirable in children. AV, atrioventricular.

allow endocardial electrode use. The major factors to be considered, in addition to patient size, are (1) venous access to the ventricle, (2) the presence of intracardiac right-to-left shunting, (3) the presence of increased pulmonary vascular resistance, (4) the presence of right-sided prosthetic valves, and (5) the presence of severe right ventricular dysfunction and/or fibrosis.

Initially, it was believed that children below 15 kg in weight and younger than 4 years of age should not undergo placement of endocardial electrodes.[28] This was based on the concern that the subclavian vein and superior vena cava were too small, leading to a high risk of thrombosis, and the large size of the generators made implantation in the subclavicular area impractical. With increased experience and smaller device sizes, however, many centers now routinely implant endocardial lead systems in children weighing much less than 15 kg.[7, 29, 30] What the lower range for weight is is not yet

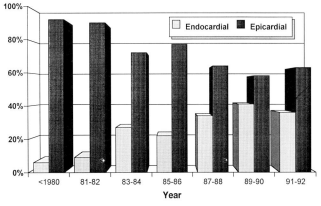

FIGURE 36–19. Comparison of epicardial versus endocardial electrode use during each period in children. Note the gradual increasing use of endocardial electrodes. (Data from the Midwest Pediatric Pacemaker Registry.)

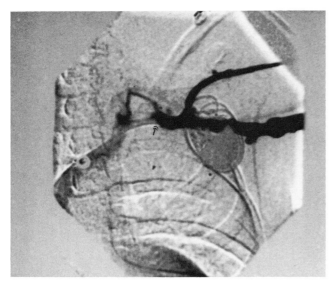

FIGURE 36–20. Venous angiogram in a patient following endocardial pacemaker implantation through the left subclavian vein. Note the complete obstruction of the subclavian vein at the site of electrode entry *(arrow)*, with collateral flow around the obstruction.

known. From a technical standpoint, children as small as 3 kg in weight can undergo endocardial electrode placement, but the follow-up of such children is too limited to know whether this is in their best interest. The risk of vessel thrombosis appears to be less than what was once thought, at least in the short term.[31] Although superior vena caval thrombosis has been reported,[32, 33] the true incidence is unknown because noninvasive methods of detecting thrombosis are not sensitive and angiography is not routinely done unless thrombosis is suspected clinically (Fig. 36–20). Lead displacement secondary to growth remains a concern, although techniques have been proposed to deal with this problem.[7, 30] The placement of large electrode loops within the atrium was proposed to allow for growth, but they may not be as effective as originally thought because they may fibrose to the cardiac wall and not uncoil with growth.

The major objection to endocardial electrode use in the small child is related to long-term problems. Because young children can be expected to require numerous electrodes over their lifetimes, many more than in adult patients, the clinician must consider how many electrodes can be left in place before problems with either vessel obstruction or tricuspid valve dysfunction occur, and the difficulty with which old electrodes can be extracted. Although lead extraction has become more widely used, it still represents a significant problem in children with the potential for damage to the cardiac structures, mainly the tricuspid valve. To commit a child to potentially numerous lead extractions is still a worry. In our institution current guidelines call for the placement of dual-chamber endocardial systems in children weighing 15 kg or more and the placement of single-chamber endocardial systems, when single-chamber pacing is appropriate, in children heavier than 8 kg. These guidelines may change as electrode development continues, and long-term follow-up of children with endocardially placed electrodes becomes available.

The next factor that must be considered is the presence of intracardiac shunting. Newly placed electrodes are potential

sources of small particulate matter, with the risk of subsequent embolization until endothelialization occurs. In general, this does not tend to be a problem when such particulate matter goes only to the lungs where it is filtered out of the circulation and eventually absorbed. However, in the presence of right-to-left shunting, the potential for systemic embolization is great. The general recommendation is to avoid such electrodes in any patient with documented right-to-left shunting and in those with the potential for right-to-left shunting.[28] This also must be considered in patients with the potential for right-to-left shunting, even if their net intracardiac shunt is left to right. Children with atrial septal defects and VSDs can show right-to-left shunting in the setting of elevated right ventricular pressure, even with a net left-to-right shunt.[34, 35] The specific hemodynamic situation of the individual child must be considered before endocardial electrode implantation is performed.

The same concerns apply to the child with elevated pulmonary vascular resistance in whom pulmonary embolization of small matter may further elevate the pulmonary resistance. Whether or not short-term anticoagulation of such patients until lead endothelialization can occur would prevent such concerns and permit transvenous pacemaker placement has yet to be investigated. In the situation in which epicardial pacing is not possible, this may be an acceptable alternative, but given the current lack of knowledge concerning the benefit of anticoagulation in this setting, it should not be general practice.

The presence of an artificial tricuspid valve prosthesis negates the ability of the clinician to use an endocardial pacing system. There have been isolated reports of endocardial electrode placements at the time of open heart surgery through the perivalvular area.[36] This requires cardiopulmonary bypass and can only be done at the time of valvular placement. This is not a technique that can be used in the usual transvenous implantation, and it also prevents lead extraction should that become necessary, except during repeat open heart surgery.

Finally, the physician must consider the state of the right

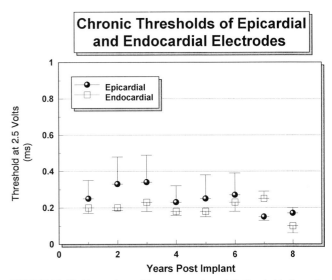

FIGURE 36–21. Comparison of long-term pulse width thresholds for endocardial versus epicardial electrodes measured at a pulse amplitude of 2.5 V. Thresholds for both groups show no significant rise, and they do not differ significantly from each other. The brackets represent 1 standard error of the mean.

FIGURE 36–22. Contraindications to endocardial pacing.

ventricle. Severe right ventricular dysfunction and endocardial fibrosis can occur in children with congenital cardiac disease and may prevent adequate pacing of the right ventricle. This tends to be more prevalent in the older child with long-standing disease. In such children, left ventricular pacing and, therefore, epicardial pacing may become necessary. In the setting of severe right ventricular dysfunction and dilatation, an appropriate endocardial site that permits both adequate sensing and pacing may not be achievable.

In summary, endocardial pacing is generally preferable because of the ease of implantation and the improved longevity of the electrode. Long-term thresholds are as stable as epicardial electrodes and tend to be lower (Fig. 36–21). This permits lower-output programming of the pacing generator, enhancing its longevity. However, there are many situations in which endocardial electrode use is contraindicated (Fig. 36–22). As such, epicardial electrodes still play a significant role in pediatric pacing, which may be reduced in the future but will not be eliminated.

UNIPOLAR VERSUS BIPOLAR PACING

The choice between a unipolar and bipolar electrode configuration only becomes an issue for endocardial implantation. For the epicardial implant, the unipolar configuration is used almost exclusively. To use a bipolar configuration requires that two electrodes be placed on the heart, with an increased risk for electrode failure. The data from the Midwest Pediatric Pacemaker Registry document the finding that 95% of all epicardial implants use a unipolar configuration. Were bipolar electrodes to be developed, they might be beneficial.

For endocardial pacing systems, the choice between unipolar and bipolar pacing becomes more controversial. Again, data from the Midwest Pediatric Pacemaker Registry show that the majority of endocardial systems are bipolar (Fig. 36–23). Initially, it was believed that unipolar pacing was preferable because of the smaller size of the unipolar pacing electrode.[37] However, with recent improvements in electrode design, this difference in size has become negligible. Electrode body diameters are the important factor in determining the risk for venous thrombosis, and there is a minimal difference. For example, the model 4057M unipolar screw-in electrode (Medtronic, Minneapolis, MN) has a body diameter of 2.2 mm; the 4058M bipolar version has a body diameter of 2.4 mm. This same minimal difference in body size is also seen for passive fixation electrodes, such as the 4023 unipolar steroid-eluting electrode (Medtronic), which has a body diameter of 1.2 mm versus 1.9 mm for the bipolar version (model 4024). In all cases, the diameter of the electrode's head is smaller for a unipolar electrode, which may make insertion easier, but once implanted, the size of the head is of little consequence.

A comparison of acute implantation characteristics between unipolar and bipolar electrodes of similar design from the Midwest Pediatric Pacemaker Registry showed no significant difference for threshold values of voltage, current, or resistance (Fig. 36–24). Long-term thresholds have been thought by some to be improved in unipolar pacing.[37] This has been postulated to be the result of the smaller size of the head and its lower weight, creating less tension on the endocardial surface, particularly when active-fixation electrodes are used, therefore leading to less tip fibrosis. However, this appears to be unique only to active-fixation leads and has not been reported to be a problem with passive-fixation tined electrodes.

It was initially thought that sensing using a bipolar electrode was inferior to unipolar sensing because of the close proximity of the two electrodes. However, data from the Midwest Pediatric Pacemaker Registry show this not to be the case. Acute implantation R-wave amplitudes and slew rates show no significant difference between the unipolar and bipolar electrodes (Fig. 36–25). Unipolar sensing, however, is more affected by myopotentials and more prone to oversensing and inappropriate pacemaker inhibition. This has been estimated to be a problem in 31% to 93% of patients, as is discussed later. Bipolar sensing is rarely affected by such myopotential inhibition from the closer proximity of the electrodes. The degree to which such inappropriate inhibition is seen is dependent on the location of the generator, the provocative tests used, and generator model implanted. All series, however, report a significant incidence of this problem, which can be a particular concern in active children.

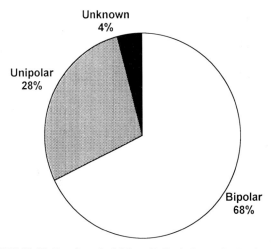

FIGURE 36–23. Data from the Midwest Pediatric Pacemaker Registry indicating the majority of endocardial electrode systems to be bipolar.

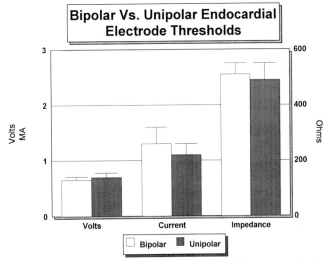

FIGURE 36–24. Acute implantation thresholds for bipolar versus unipolar endocardial electrodes are not significantly different for voltage, current, or electrode impedance. All were measured at a 0.5-msec pulse width. The brackets represent 1 standard error of the mean. (Data from the Midwest Pediatric Pacemaker Registry.)

Thus, it would appear that, in most active children, bipolar pacing is preferred, particularly with the smaller electrode sizes now available. Sensing does not appear to be a problem, and myopotential inhibition is seen less often. In addition, with bipolar pacing, the risk of extracardiac pacing of the surrounding muscle is minimized, particularly in a child in whom it may be difficult to position the generator in a location where all such stimulation of surrounding muscles is avoided. This is particularly relevant to implantations with the pocket placed in the subclavicular region. In many children, the lack of significant subcutaneous tissue requires the placement of the generator in the subpectoralis position where the risk of extracardiac pacing with a unipolar system increases.

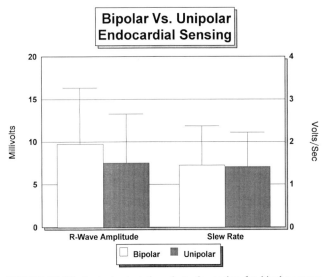

FIGURE 36–25. Acute implantation electrode sensing for bipolar versus unipolar endocardial electrodes demonstrates no significant difference in either R-wave amplitude (millivolts) or slew rate (volts/sec). The brackets indicate 1 standard error about the mean. (Data from the Midwest Pediatric Pacemaker Registry.)

EPICARDIAL ELECTRODE TYPES

Compared with endocardial electrodes, there are relatively few epicardial electrode types from which to choose. Previously, all electrodes were intramyocardial in type, with the intramyocardial portion being either a corkscrew coil, a single wire with a barbed end (fish hook), or an intramyocardial wire drawn through the myocardium (suture type).[38–41]

Recently, a truly epicardial electrode with steroid-eluting capabilities was developed, although, currently, it is available only in clinical trials.[42–44] The most widely used electrodes currently, based on data from the Midwest Pediatric Pacemaker Registry, are the screw-in corkscrew type (6917 [Medtronic], 471 [Intermedics, Angleton, TX], or 4312 [CPI, St. Paul, MN]) and the barbed fish-hook type (4951 or 4951M [Medtronic], Fig. 36–26). The choice of electrode depends on the chamber to be paced and the preference of the implanting physician.

Atrial epicardial implantation requires an electrode that either sits on the epicardial surface or has only a shallow penetration into the atrial myocardium. Should the electrode extend through the chamber wall into the atrial cavity, a low-resistance circuit is established with an inability to pace reliably. Little data can be found concerning the longevity or thresholds of atrial epicardial electrodes. In part, this is related to their limited use and to the fact that constant change

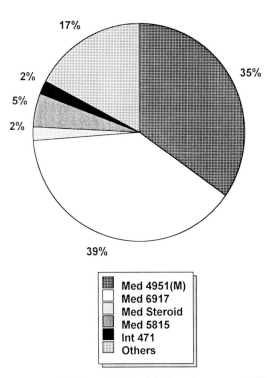

FIGURE 36–26. Distribution of epicardial electrode types used. The two most common epicardial electrodes are the Medtronic 6917 (screw-in) electrode and the Medtronic 4951(M) (fish-hook) electrode (Medtronic, Minneapolis, MN). Med steroid, epicardial steroid-eluting electrode; Med 5815, myocardial stab-in electrode; Int 471, Intermedics screw-in electrode. (Data from the Midwest Pediatric Pacemaker Registry.)

in the electrode design continues, making long-term comparisons difficult. The currently most widely used atrial electrode is the fish-hook or stab-in electrode because it does not penetrate deeply into the myocardium compared with the screw-in or corkscrew type. The newest version (4951M), which has a platinized coating, has resulted in slightly improved thresholds at acute implantation (Fig. 36–27). The average threshold at implantation is approximately 1.05 V and 3.3 mA, measured at a pulse width of 0.5 msec. The average acute electrode impedance is 320 ohms.

Much more diversity exists in the choice of the electrode for ventricular pacing. A comparison of the nonplatinized fish-hook electrode (4951) with the screw-in electrode (6917) reveals essentially no difference in acute implantation thresholds. However, implantation thresholds for the platinized fish-hook electrode (4951M) are improved (Fig. 36–28), and lead survival appears to be longer for the screw-in electrode than for the nonplatinized fish-hook type. At 5 years postimplant, lead survival of the former was found to be approximately 84%, whereas that of the fish-hook electrode was found to be approximately 65%.[40] The majority of such failures were found to be exit block. Whether the same trend will also apply to the platinized version of the fish-hook electrode is not known. Other studies, however, found little difference in longevity between these two types of electrodes.[39] Some of the discrepancy between the results of these studies was believed to be caused by different surgical modes of implantation for the fish-hook electrode. Whether or not the lead was stabilized by being sutured to the myocardium was variable. It has been suggested that a lack of such stabilization leads to more electrode movement within the myocardium and, therefore, greater fibrosis and the risk of exit

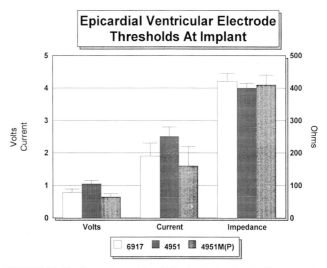

FIGURE 36–28. Comparison of thresholds for the Medtronic 6917 screw-in electrode, the Medtronic 4951 fish-hook electrode, and the Medtronic 4951M(P) platinized fish-hook electrode when implanted on the ventricle shows no significant difference in voltage threshold or impedance, but a slightly lower current at threshold for the 4951M(P) electrode. The brackets represent 1 standard error about the mean. (Data from the Midwest Pediatric Pacemaker Registry.)

block.[40] This is discussed further when implantation techniques are considered.

Others advocated using the suture-type electrode (030-170 [Telectronics, Englewood, CO]).[41] Although implantation thresholds were similar to those of the nonplatinized fish-hook electrode, the incidence of exit block was lower. This may also be related to the better electrode stabilization of the suture-type electrode. Because of its increased surface area, however, the electrode's impedance is lower, with a resultant increased current drain from the generator. Our current epicardial electrode of choice for both the atrium and the ventricle is the 4951M platinized fish-hook electrode. This electrode affords excellent acute thresholds and acceptable long-term performance.

A recent advance in epicardial pacing is the steroid-eluting electrode.[42–44] This electrode consists of a platinized flat electrode that sits atop the epicardial surface with a silicone plug impregnated with dexamethasone to allow elution of the dexamethasone onto the area of myocardium being stimulated. Approximately 1 mg of dexamethasone is present within the electrode. This electrode is affixed to the epicardial surface by sutures, with the active portion of the electrode not extending into the myocardium as with other epicardial electrodes. This is both advantageous and disadvantageous, depending on the individual patient. For patients whose epicardial surfaces are relatively nonfibrotic, this appears to be an advantage because there is less myocardial injury to provoke subsequent fibrotic formation. For patients with markedly fibrotic epicardial surfaces, often present following multiple open heart surgical procedures, however, these electrodes are difficult to use. The physician must find an area of myocardium with a limited epicardial fibrotic reaction or attempt to strip away such a fibrotic reaction to expose the myocardium, which simply leads to further subsequent fibrosis.

Initial experience with this electrode is encouraging.

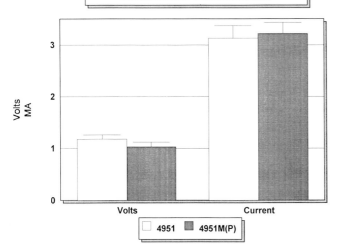

FIGURE 36–27. Acute implantation voltage and current threshold values measured at a 0.5-msec pulse width for the original fish-hook electrode (Medtronic 4951) compared with the newer platinized version (Medtronic 4951M[P]) when implanted on the atrium. When the 4951M values tend to be lower, they do not reach significance. The average voltage threshold was 1.2 V for the 4951 versus 1.05 V for the 4951M. The brackets represent 1 standard error about the mean. (Data from the Midwest Pediatric Pacemaker Registry.)

COMPARATIVE THRESHOLDS
2.5 - 2.7 VOLTS / IMPLANT TIME

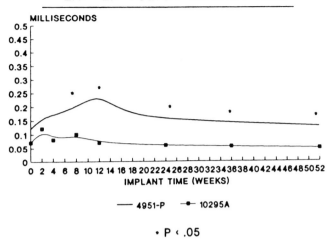

• P ‹ .05

FIGURE 36–29. Comparative thresholds of the Medtronic 4951P platinized fish-hook electrode versus the epicardial steroid-eluting electrode (10295A) showing not only a slight improvement in the initial threshold but also a lack of significant threshold rise in the first 3 months following implantation for the steroid-eluting epicardial electrode with continued threshold improvement at 1 year after implant. (From Karpawich PP, Harkini M, Arciniegas E, Cavitt DL: Improved chronic epicardial pacing in children: Steroid contribution to porous platinized electrodes. PACE Pacing Clin Electrophysiol 15:1152, 1992.)

Lower acute thresholds seem to be present compared with those of other epicardial electrodes, and the threshold rise is less over the first several months following implantation (Fig. 36–29).[43] In selected patients with limited myocardial fibrosis, they appear to be beneficial. However, they are not necessarily ideally suited to all patients, and care must be taken to choose the most appropriate form of ventricular epicardial electrode to fit the individual patient. All three types of ventricular electrodes in current use have advantages and disadvantages, and no one type is ideally suited for all patients.

ENDOCARDIAL ELECTRODE TYPES

Similar to the adult population, there are three general types of endocardial electrodes in use in children: passive-fixation non–steroid-eluting, passive-fixation steroid-eluting, and active-fixation electrodes. The most commonly used endocardial electrode type in children continues to be the active-fixation screw-in electrode (Fig. 36–30). The use of this electrode has been advocated because of its better fixation qualities, given the tremendous range of anatomic variation present in children with congenital heart disease. When implantation is within the morphologic left ventricle in children following an atrial switch repair for the transposition of the great arteries or in those with ventricular inversion, the active-fixation electrode is preferable. Also, in children with markedly dilated right ventricles, such that it is difficult to wedge the electrode into the trabecular recesses of the right ventricle, active-fixation electrodes are preferable.

However, this electrode type is not the best electrode in all children. A comparison of acute threshold data shows that active-fixation electrodes have the highest acute thresholds (Fig. 36–31). Both non–steroid-eluting passive-fixation electrodes and steroid-eluting passive-fixation electrodes have

Endocardial Electrode Usage by Electrode Type

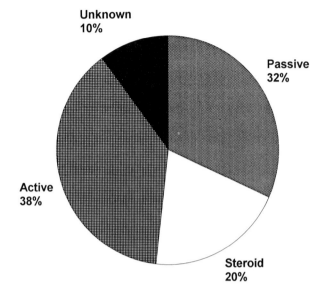

FIGURE 36–30. Distribution of endocardial electrode type use. Active, active-fixation (screw-in) electrode; passive, passive-fixation (tined) non–steroid-eluting electrode; steroid, passive-fixation steroid-eluting electrode. (Data from the Midwest Pediatric Pacemaker Registry.)

lower acute thresholds. However, they do not differ from each other. The presence of the steroid does not influence the acute implantation thresholds, but with increasing electrode age, this is no longer the case. Follow-up data indicate significantly lower electrode thresholds for the steroid-eluting

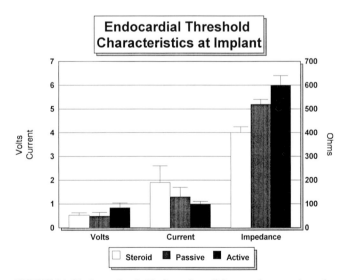

FIGURE 36–31. Acute thresholds for endocardial electrode types showed a tendency toward lower thresholds in the passive-fixation and steroid-eluting electrodes compared with the active-fixation electrodes. However, the difference in voltage threshold is minimal. The changes become more evident in current and impedance values, with steroid electrodes having the lowest impedance and highest current flow. The brackets represent 1 standard error above the mean. (Data from the Midwest Pediatric Pacemaker Registry.)

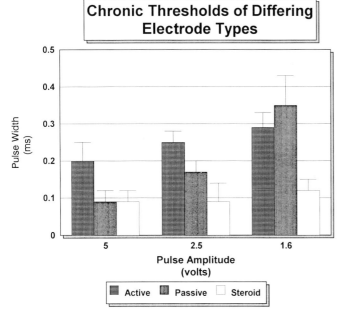

Chronic Thresholds of Differing Electrode Types

FIGURE 36–32. Chronic long-term electrode thresholds are significantly higher for active-fixation electrodes compared with both passive-fixation and steroid-eluting electrodes. At low pulse amplitudes, steroid-eluting electrodes show significantly lower thresholds than the other types. The brackets represent 1 standard error above the mean. (Data from Serwer and associates.[45])

electrode compared with other types.[45] A comparison of steroid- versus non–steroid-eluting electrodes showed no difference in chronic thresholds at 5 V of pulse amplitude but did show significant differences at 2.5 and 1.6 V (Fig. 36–32). Thus, it would appear that the strength-duration curve is significantly shifted leftward for the steroid-eluting electrodes.

Such changes affect generator programming. In one study,[45] only 33% of generators that used non–steroid-eluting electrodes were able to be programmed to 2.5 V of pulse amplitude compared with 77% of generators that used steroid-eluting electrodes. The remainder required a pulse amplitude of 5.0 V or greater. Thus, the use of steroid-eluting passive-fixation electrodes allowed chronically lower output settings for the pulse generator, thereby increasing the generator's longevity. The follow-up averaged 3.3 years (median, 3.6 years).

In summary, we believe that the ideal pacing system in children is a dual-chamber system with the capacity for rate-responsive pacing, using endocardial atrial and ventricular bipolar electrodes with active-fixation electrodes in the atrium and steroid-eluting passive-fixation electrodes in the ventricle. In situations in which the child's size is marginal or it is not thought to be possible to implant an atrial endocardial electrode, we then prefer to use an endocardial single-chamber rate-responsive system. Only in situations in which endocardial pacing is specifically contraindicated do we use epicardial pacing. In such a situation, the currently preferred electrode is the platinized version of the fish-hook electrode because it appears to have lower acute implantation thresholds than does the corkscrew electrode. Long-term data are not yet available to show whether this electrode performs better chronically than the corkscrew electrode does. When

available, the epicardial steroid-eluting electrode may show promise for use in situations in which there is no significant degree of epicardial fibrosis that would require the presence of an intramyocardial electrode.

Implantation Techniques

In many ways, implantation techniques in the child are similar to those used in the adult, but differences do exist. This section does not attempt to describe again those techniques that are similar but focuses on describing the differences that are important in the child and must be considered.

EPICARDIAL IMPLANTATION TECHNIQUES

The approach used for the placement of epicardial electrodes is highly variable, depending on the individual patient's circumstances. Approaches to the epicardial surface that have previously been employed include thoracotomy, sternotomy, and subxiphoid incision. The subxiphoid approach requires the smallest incision, and through the same incision, both the electrode's implantation on the epicardial surface of the heart and the pacemaker's implantation in the abdomen can be accomplished.[46–48] This approach has been used for both ventricular and atrial epicardial electrode implantation. However, the disadvantage to this approach is that it only exposes a limited ventricular epicardial or atrial surface, and in the patient with extensive epicardial fibrosis as a consequence of prior cardiac surgery, finding a suitable location for implantation of the electrode may be difficult. Such an approach requires a 6- to 7-cm skin incision from the xiphoid tip to a point superior to the umbilicus. The dissection is continued as deep as it is thought to be necessary to provide adequate tissue between the pacemaker and the surface of the skin. Depending on the degree of subcutaneous tissue present, the pacemaker can either be implanted above the rectus muscle, below the rectus muscle but above the peritoneum, or in some circumstances, intraperitoneally housed in a Silastic pouch sutured to the underside of the peritoneum and anchored to the rectus fascia.[46] The depth to which the incision is carried should be governed solely by the tissue available to cover the pacemaker. When only minimal tissue is present over the pacemaker, not only does an unsightly bulge result, but more importantly, the skin is more susceptible to traumatic injury, with a resultant risk of pacemaker erosion and infection.

A left thoracotomy approach is often used for the child who has had prior cardiac surgery in whom the risk of significant epicardial fibrosis is high.[49] This affords an increased myocardial surface from which to choose an appropriate pacing site. Implantation of the generator can either be in the abdomen, in the subclavicular region, or in rare settings, intrathoracically. However, for implantation of a dual-chamber system, this approach affords less exposure of the atrium and requires left atrial pacing. Although this has been accomplished, it introduces complexity into the programming because the postpace AV interval must be prolonged enough to afford adequate time for right ventricular filling caused by the time necessary for left atrial to right atrial excitation spread. The postsense AV interval must be short to avoid an excessive AV interval (Fig. 36–33). In this setting, a genera-

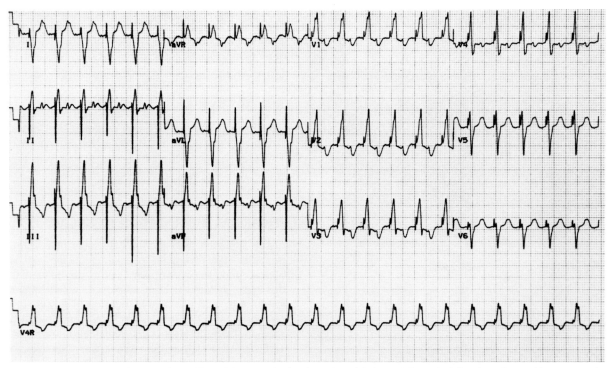

FIGURE 36–33. Electrocardiogram from a patient with a DDD pacemaker in whom the atrial electrode is on the left atrium. To provide an appropriate time for ventricular filling during both atrial pacing and sensing, either a compromise AV interval must be used, or the generator must have the ability to alter the AV interval (dynamic AV delay).

tor with a rate-adaptive AV delay is mandatory. For this reason, we think that right atrial pacing is preferable but use left atrial pacing if right atrial pacing is not possible. When the thoracotomy approach is used with an abdominal placement of the generator, the electrode must be passed subcostally to a pocket created in the abdomen through a separate incision. The electrode must not be passed over a rib because this increases the risk of traumatic electrode fracture.

Finally, a median sternotomy approach can be used, but this creates the largest and most obvious scar. However, it affords the best exposure of the epicardial surface of both the ventricle and right atrium. In the patient with significant epicardial scarring and fibrosis, this affords the best likelihood of finding an appropriate pacing site. Following implantation of the electrode, it can then be pulled through the subxiphoid region to the abdominal wall where, through a separate incision or an extension of the medium sternotomy incision, an appropriate pocket can be created.

Regardless of the electrode type chosen, appropriate anchoring of the electrode to the epicardial surface is critical. Our approach is to insert the electrode into the myocardium and determine the threshold strength-duration curve. If it is acceptable, the electrode is sutured to the epicardial surface, and the thresholds are rechecked. Suturing the electrode to the surface theoretically reduces the movement of the electrode tip within the myocardium with less formation of fibrotic tissue and better long-term performance of the electrode.[40] When the fish-hook electrode is used and there is significant epicardial fibrosis, unbending the barb to permit deeper penetration is often beneficial. The physician should have several types of myocardial electrodes available during implantation to meet whatever situation is encountered.

A gentle loop of the electrode should be left in the thoracic cavity to allow for some growth, but excessive loops should be avoided. Instances of entrapment of vascular structures by pacemaker electrodes have been reported,[50, 51] and thus, excessive length in the thoracic cavity should be avoided. The extra length of the electrode is easily coiled and placed within the generator's pocket; even this may allow for some growth as the electrode wire slowly uncoils with subsequent growth of the patient.

The exact placement of the abdominal pocket is generally left to the discretion of the surgeon. However, it should be placed away from the belt line and not in the upper right quadrant. Placement in the upper right quadrant interferes with subsequent assessment of hepatic size, which may be important in children with structural cardiac disease.

The placement of unused or redundant electrodes is not recommended. It was once believed that the placement of an unused electrode would provide a "spare" electrode that could be used if the primary electrode failed, thus preventing the need for a second thoracotomy. However, it was found that if the primary electrode failed, there was a high likelihood that the redundant electrode was also unusable.[12, 52] Thus, the extra electrode that had been placed provided no benefit to the child.

ENDOCARDIAL IMPLANTATION TECHNIQUES

Prior to any endocardial implantation, echocardiography should be performed to make certain no contraindications to endocardial implantation exist, specifically tricuspid valve dysfunction, right-to-left shunting, or superior vena caval obstruction. Whether the pacemaker is placed under the left or right clavicle is somewhat arbitrary. However, this may be important to some patients, and the location should be discussed with them. Our general policy is to place the pacemaker on the side opposite the patient's handedness (i.e., if the patient is right handed, the pacemaker is placed on the left side).

The endocardial approach used for implantation in children is similar to that in adults. Prior to beginning, transcutaneous pacing electrodes are placed to provide emergency pacing ability if needed. A sudden decrease in the intrinsic heart rate caused by the stress of the procedure or the general anesthesia, if administered, is not unusual. Although placement of a temporary transvenous pacing electrode can be done, the stress of this alone may cause bradycardia. In addition, the risk of infection of the permanent system by the temporary electrode must be considered. Transcutaneous pacing electrodes for all sizes of children are now available and function well.

Whether the electrode is introduced into the vascular system by a direct subclavian vein puncture[29, 53, 54] or by a cephalic vein cut-down procedure[7, 30] is guided by the experience of the implanting physician. In our institution, direct subclavian vein puncture is used exclusively. Our approach is to enter the subclavian vein percutaneously and introduce a guide wire. Using the guide wire's entrance through the skin as the proximal point, an incision is made laterally along the deltopectoralis groove for approximately 4 to 6 cm. The dissection is then carried down to the pectoralis. At this point, the degree of subcutaneous tissue is examined to determine whether there is sufficient tissue to cover the generator. In many children, this tissue is inadequate, and placement of the generator above the pectoralis results, not only in a significant pacemaker bulge, but also in an increased risk of pacemaker erosion and traumatic injury to the tissue above the pacemaker.[53] This is also psychologically important, because many children are self-conscious of a prominent bulge. When the tissue is believed to be inadequate, the dissection is then carried through the pectoralis, using blunt dissection to separate the muscle fibers, with a pocket created in the subpectoralis region. After this pocket is created, a sheath and dilator are introduced into the subclavian vein over the previously positioned guide wire. The electrode is then passed into the right atrium together with a new guide wire. The sheath is then removed. Retention of the guide wire allows for either the introduction of a second electrode, if this is a dual-chamber implant, or the option to remove the prior electrode and replace it without having to again puncture the subclavian vein. After the electrodes have been positioned and tested, the guide wire can be removed. The electrodes are then connected to the generator, and it is placed in the pocket with the noninsulated side placed away from the pectoralis. When the subpectoralis approach is used, it may be difficult to avoid extracardiac pacing with a unipolar system, and for this reason, a bipolar system is preferred.

ACUTE ELECTRODE EVALUATION

Following placement of the electrode, its electrical characteristics must be determined. For active-fixation or intramyocardial electrodes, 15 minutes should be allowed from the introduction of the electrode to electrical testing to permit acute myocardial changes caused by the electrode's entry into the myocardium to subside. All changes do not subside in this amount of time, but this short delay is warranted. Our initial approach is to measure the electrode's impedance and, if possible, intrinsic electrogram amplitudes. The impedance should be between 200 and 600 ohms for the epicardially placed electrode and between 300 and 700 ohms for the endocardially placed electrode. The electrogram's amplitude should be sufficient to allow appropriate sensing by the generator to be implanted. The minimally acceptable signal amplitude varies, depending on the specific generator. If these measurements are found to be acceptable, threshold testing is performed. It is our general practice to set a given pulse width and then determine the minimum pulse amplitude necessary to maintain capture. Multiple threshold determinations are performed to adequately define the strength-duration curve. We think it is important to determine the shape of the strength-duration curve to be certain that the minimum pulse width necessary to pace at any pulse amplitude and the minimum amplitude necessary to pace at any pulse width are sufficiently removed from the proposed generator settings to allow for some movement in the strength-duration curve without the risk of loss of capture (Fig. 36–34). Data from the Midwest Pediatric Pacemaker Registry suggest that the minimum voltage necessary to pace the ventricle at a 0.5 msec pulse width is below 1 V and below 1.5 V for the atrium. Such threshold guidelines apply to both endocardial and epicardial electrodes.

Before the pulse generator is connected to the electrodes, it is advisable to pace the ventricle at the maximal output of the pacing system analyzer. In children, because of the close proximity of the diaphragm to the electrode, diaphragmatic pacing can occur. At the maximal pacing system analyzer output, if diaphragmatic pacing should occur, the electrode must be moved. This is particularly relevant to the child with transposition of the great arteries in whom a ventricular elec-

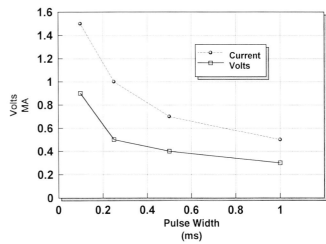

FIGURE 36–34. Example of a strength-duration curve determined at implantation. From this curve, the minimum voltage needed to pace at any pulse width and the minimum pulse width needed to pace at any voltage can be determined.

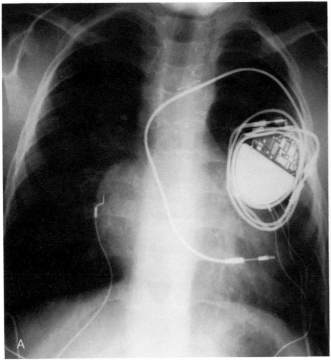
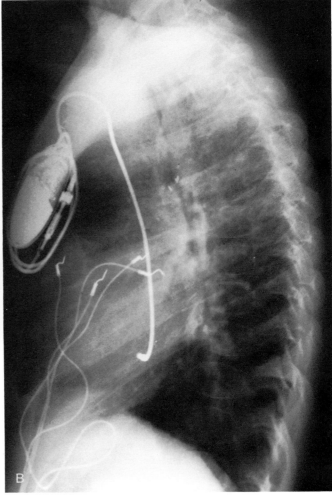

FIGURE 36–35. Posteroanterior *(A)* and lateral *(B)* chest roentgenogram from a patient who underwent endocardial electrode implantation following performance of an atrial switch procedure (Senning) for dextrotransposition of the great arteries. Note the electrode position in the left ventricle away from the ventricular apex and the diaphragm to avoid diaphragmatic stimulation.

trode is positioned within the left ventricle. Positioning the electrode tip at the left ventricular apex puts it in close proximity to the diaphragm, and there is a high incidence of diaphragmatic pacing. To prevent this, we position the electrode on the midposterior free wall at the approximate level of the papillary muscles (Fig. 36–35). This affords acceptable thresholds with a minimal risk of diaphragmatic pacing. This problem is more often seen in endocardial pacing than in epicardial pacing, but it can occur in either setting.

Follow-Up Methods for the Pediatric Patient with a Pacemaker

Proper pacemaker programming and early recognition of inappropriate pacemaker performance require frequent, methodical, and appropriate follow-up. In this section, we discuss the follow-up techniques used and the differences in the follow-up routine with increasing time from the implant.

Pacemaker follow-up can be divided into three periods, based on the length of time from the implant. The two most critical periods are within the first 2 months following the implant (early follow-up) and when the pacemaker approaches its theoretical life expectancy (late follow-up). Between these two periods, the function of the pacemaker and electrode remain fairly stable, and the generator does not require frequent readjustment. However, problems can occur, particularly as a result of electrode breakage in the active child. The major components of pacemaker follow-up (i.e., pacemaker clinic visit, 24-hour ambulatory ECG, and treadmill exercise testing) are discussed, followed by a description of the differences between the three follow-up periods.

PACEMAKER CLINIC VISIT

During a pacemaker clinic visit, all patients undergo a complete history and physical examination, pacemaker interrogation, threshold testing, evaluation of electrode sensing, and routine ECG. When indicated, other tests, such as a chest roentgenogram and echocardiography, are also performed. Specific attention must be paid to obtaining a complete history as it relates to potential pacemaker malfunction. Symptoms suggesting pacemaker malfunction include sudden exercise intolerance, dizziness, nausea, or loss of consciousness. In particular, parents often note that the child has ''less energy'' than previously. One of the more common symptoms in patients with intermittent atrial sensing malfunction is a sudden lack of energy or transient dizziness, which is related to a loss of atrial sensing with a resultant acute drop in the rate to the lower rate limit of the pacemaker. This can often be a subtle finding and must be carefully sought for, not only in the older child from whom a history can be obtained directly, but also from the parents of the younger child who must be asked questions such as have they ever noted sudden changes in the child's activity state or temperament, sudden interruptions of play time, interruptions of eating, or sudden staring episodes suggestive of acute decrease in cardiac output?

The physical examination should relate specifically to complications produced by the presence of pacemaker electrodes, such as AV valve incompetence, the acute appearance of pericardial rubs (suggesting lead perforation), irregular heart rates, pocket infections, or in unusual situations, stenotic lesions (suggesting extracardiac compression of vessels by the epicardial implanted pacemaker electrodes).

Pacemaker interrogation must consist of interrogation of programmed settings and pacemaker performance data, consisting of the electrode's impedance, the generator battery's voltage, the generator's measured pulse amplitude, the electrode's current flow, the energy delivered, the pulse width, and the measured magnet rate. Such parameters can often show early signs of electrode dysfunction or an approaching generator end-of-service. Impedance changes are of particular utility in indicating early exit block (manifested as increasing impedance) and insulation fracture or erosion of the electrode's tip (manifested as a decline in the electrode's impedance).

Following this, interrogation of the pacemaker's diagnostic counters is performed to assess the extent to which the pacemaker is being used and the rate variability the patient is experiencing. Information provided by diagnostic counters is variable, depending on the pacemaker model. The most useful data are those collected over many months to assess the degree to which the pacemaker is providing rate variability and to what extent the patient is dependent on the pacemaker. These can also assess the appropriateness of the lower rate limit in DDD pacing and sinus nodal function. A high percentage of atrial pacing with a low programmed lower rate limit suggests significant sinus nodal dysfunction (Fig. 36–36).

Next, intracardiac electrograms are recorded. The utility of such tracings is discussed later. Sensing thresholds are also performed to determine the least sensitive settings that still maintain appropriate sensing.

Finally, threshold determinations from both atrial and ventricular leads are obtained at all pulse amplitudes, producing 100% capture at any pulse width setting. Pulse width thresholds are generally preferred to pulse amplitude thresholds because the majority of pacemakers have many more pulse width settings than pulse amplitude settings; thus, more accurate thresholds can be determined. All threshold determinations are performed in duplicate. Thresholds are reported as the minimum pulse width that maintains 100% capture at each programmable pulse amplitude. From these data, strength-duration curves are constructed and compared with previously obtained curves to detect shifts. From these data, appropriate programming decisions can be made.

INTRACARDIAC ELECTROGRAM DETERMINATIONS

Intracardiac electrogram(s) should be obtained whenever possible. They are obtained both simultaneously with a surface ECG and with telemetered annotation markers that indicate the point during the electrogram at which sensing

A

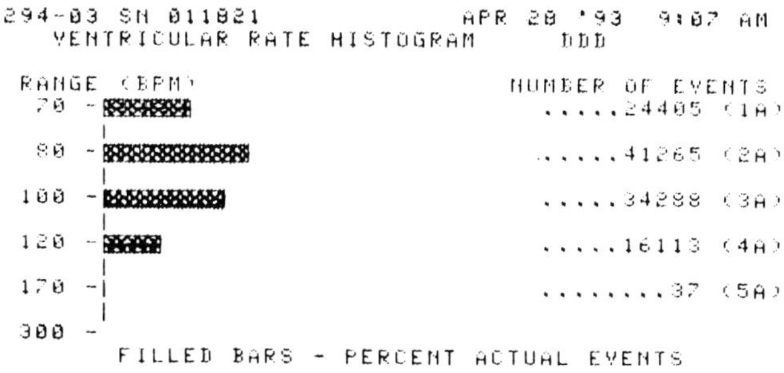

B

RATE BINS (PPM)	TOTAL EVNTS /TERM	% TOTAL EVNTS	% PACED 0	1 TO 24	25 TO 49	50 TO 74	75 TO 99	100
<55	0	0	•					
55-64	0	0	•					
65-74	0	0	•					
75-84	21846	99					•	
85-94	198	1					•	
95-104	0	0	•					
105-114	0	0	•					
>114	0	0	•					
TOTAL	22044							

C

```
DIAGNOSTIC DATA (CARDIAC CYCLES)         DDD MODE
EVENT COUNTERS LAST CLEARED..SEP  9,  1:50 PM
NUMBER OF:
 PREMATURE VENTRICULAR EVENTS.........57      0 %
 ATRIAL PACE EVENTS FOLLOWED
  BY VENTRICULAR SENSE EVENT..........13      0 %
 ATRIAL PACE EVENTS FOLLOWED
  BY VENTRICULAR PACE EVENT.....648,815       4 %
 ATRIAL SENSE EVENTS FOLLOWED
  BY VENTRICULAR SENSE EVENT ........308      0 %
 ATRIAL SENSE EVENTS FOLLOWED
  BY VENTRICULAR PACE EVENT..16,777,215      96 %

PERCENT PACED - ATRIUM ...................    4 %
PERCENT PACED - VENTRICLE ..................100 %
```

FIGURE 36–36. Example of data obtained from generator diagnostic counters showing the number of beats occurring in each rate range. *A*, Data from a patient who had acceptable heart rate variability. *B*, Data from a patient in whom there was minimal heart rate variability and required reprogramming. *C*, Information about the types of atrial and ventricular beats occurring. This patient had predominantly atrial sensing, followed by ventricular pacing, indicating an appropriate lower rate limit.

and/or pacing occurs and the beginning and length of the refractory periods. Thus, the relationship of programmed refractory periods to the waveform is shown. This is particularly useful for the atrial channel to ascertain the appropriateness of the programmed settings. For example, when the atrial electrode has been implanted in the left atrium, a determination of the appropriate AV interval may be difficult because the spontaneous P wave on the body surface significantly precedes the time at which atrial sensing occurs (Fig. 36–37). This results in a prolonged PR interval, as determined from the surface ECG, that could raise concerns about appropriate generator function.

Recording the annotation markers with the intracardiac electrogram also permits minimizing refractory periods as much as possible to maximize the multiblock rate and yet not risk oversensing of ventricular depolarization or repolar-

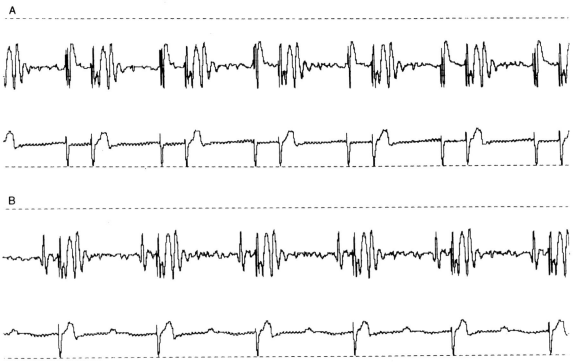

FIGURE 36–37. Example of an intracardiac electrogram from a patient with left atrial pacing. In both panels, the top trace is the atrial electrogram, and the bottom trace is the body surface electrocardiogram. *A* was recorded during atrial pacing. The atrial electrogram and the surface P wave occur close to each other. *B* was recorded during atrial sensing. The P wave now precedes the atrial electrogram by a considerable time.

ization by the atrial channel (crosstalk) (Fig. 36–38). This is of even more concern in young children who experience high atrial rates and are at risk for multiblock, with a subsequent sudden decrease in the ventricular rate and a concomitant decrease in cardiac output. This is demonstrated more fully when the results of exercise testing are discussed.

We also find the intracardiac electrogram to be helpful in determining decreasing atrial amplitudes over time with the potential for loss of atrial sensing. With the electrode's aging and fibrosis of the tip, recorded electrogram amplitudes may decline, and appropriate changes in atrial sensitivity often need to be made. This is particularly relevant to exercise in which atrial amplitudes may further decline, as discussed later.

Finally, the intracardiac electrogram is also useful in the diagnosis of atrial dysrhythmias. In the active child, the presence of a high-paced rate may not be unusual or suggest an atrial tachycardia. An example of such a situation is in the presence of atrial flutter (Fig. 36–39). In the first example, the rapid atrial rate was apparent on the body surface ECG, and the pacemaker is at the upper rate limit. In the second example, the body surface ECG showed an apparently regular rhythm at a rate below the upper rate limit; the atrial electrogram showed atrial flutter.

EXERCISE TESTING

Exercise testing should be an integral part of all pacemaker follow-up in children old enough to undergo treadmill testing. Such testing often pinpoints inappropriate programming,

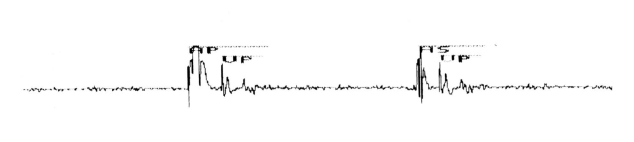

FIGURE 36–38. Intracardiac electrogram recorded while in the DDD mode together with annotation markers showing the time of onset and termination of the various refractory periods. The dashed line following the denotation of AP or AS shows the duration of the TARP and that it is of significant duration to prevent inappropriate sensing by the atrial amplifier of ventricular events. The shorter dashed line following VP shows the duration of the ventricular refractory period but is of little utility in this recording. AP, atrial pacing; AS, atrial sensing; TARP, total atrial refractory period; VP, ventricular pacing.

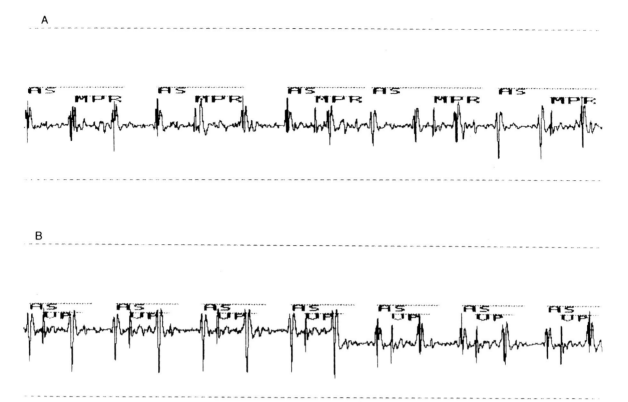

FIGURE 36–39. Atrial electrograms from two patients while in atrial flutter. *A*, The time of AS is variable as is the AV interval because the pacemaker is at the upper rate limit or MPR. Note the changing TARP as a result of to the Wenckebach behavior imposed by the upper rate limit. *B*, There is a definite 2:1 block, and the pacemaker is not at the upper rate limit. The body surface electrocardiogram was suggestive only of atrial flutter in that the heart rate was completely regular. VP, ventricular pacing; AS, atrial sensing; AV, atrioventricular; TARP, total atrial refractory period; MPR, maximal paced rate.

resulting in inappropriate performance. In one series, 43% of patients had clinically significant inappropriate programming while exercising that was not apparent on routine pacemaker testing.[55] Of these patients, 75% showed an inadequate heart rate increase with the stress of exercising. Although the majority were paced in the VVIR mode, one patient in the DDD mode was shown to have an inadequate exercise response indicative of chronotropic incompetence. All such patients underwent reprogramming with subsequent appropriate heart rate increases. Other patients were shown to have spontaneous beats at maximal exercise, causing an automatic extension of the PVARP and acute multiblock with an acute decline in the heart rate (Fig. 36–40). The development of multiblock was also seen with an acute decline in the heart rate from an inappropriately long total atrial refractory period. The multiblock rate was only slightly above the upper rate limit, causing an abrupt decline in the heart rate (Fig. 36–41). If the total atrial refractory period cannot be shortened either by decreasing the AV interval or the PVARP, use of the DDDR or VDDR mode may be helpful. When the multiblock rate is reached during the use of either of these pacing modes, the ventricular rate falls to the sensor rate rather than the inappropriately sensed atrial rate, providing a smaller decline in the heart rate. A loss of capture at the maximal heart rate was also observed, even though there had been 100% capture at rest and programming of the pacemaker was believed to be appropriate, based on resting threshold testing (Fig. 36–42).

Changes in pacing thresholds do occur and can either worsen, as the previous example shows, or improve.[24, 56] For fixed-rate pacing, thresholds decline following exercise, and therefore, resting thresholds are not necessarily indicative of those present during the stress of exercise (Fig. 36–43). However, these findings may not be applicable to the patient whose pacemaker is in the rate-responsive mode, as the example in the patient who developed loss of capture at maximal exercise showed. This is a potentially serious problem that would not have been apparent had evaluation only at rest been performed.

Changes in P-wave amplitude were also documented at maximal exercise.[57–59] A decrease in P-wave amplitude can result in a loss of atrial sensing, and in the DDD mode, this can cause an immediate drop to the lower rate limit of the pacemaker. This can result in syncope from a sudden decrease in the cardiac output. Although DDDR pacing can minimize the magnitude of this heart rate drop, the physician should not rely on this mechanism because the sensor rate may not be the same as the atrial rate, especially during activities such as swimming or cycling. Myopotential sensing by either channel can have similar effects.[60, 61] This is more evident in unipolar systems, but it can occur in bipolar systems.

AMBULATORY ELECTROCARDIOGRAPHIC MONITORING

Ambulatory ECG monitoring is also essential in the appropriate follow-up of pediatric patients with pacemakers. This is particularly true in those patients unable to exercise because this may be the only method to evaluate high-rate

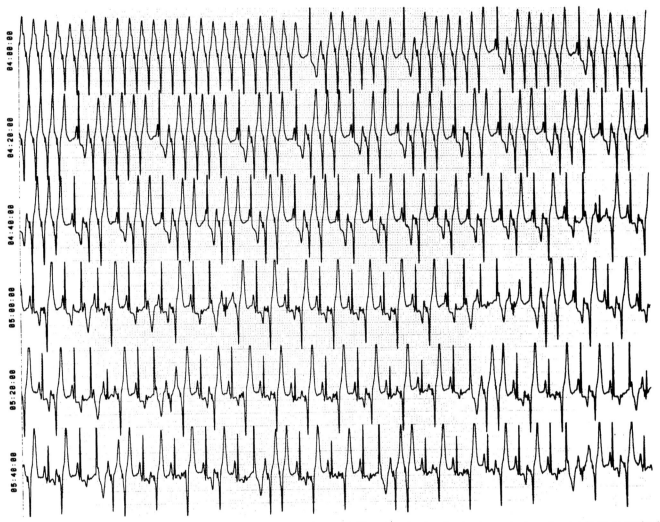

FIGURE 36–40. Continuous electrocardiographic recording during exercise treadmill testing showing the development of spontaneous beats at maximal exercise. This resulted in automatic extension of the postventricular atrial refractory period, with an overall decline in the heart rate from 167 to 141 bpm. This was associated with sudden fatigue and near syncope. This was corrected by the elimination of the automatic postventricular atrial refractory period extension. The paper speed is 12.5 mm/sec, with each row being 20 seconds. The time from the onset of exercise is noted by the numbers in the left margin.

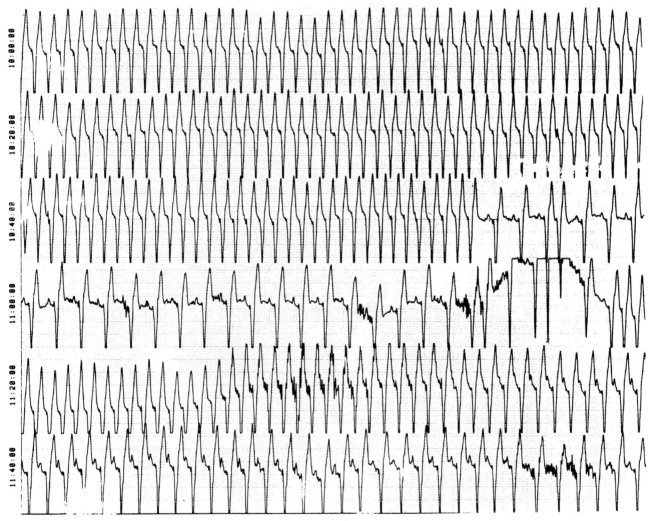

FIGURE 36–41. Example from an exercise test showing the development of multiblock with an acute decline in the heart rate, resulting in syncope. In this example, the patient's upper rate limit was 180 bpm, with a multiblock rate of 187. This lack of difference between the upper rate limit and the multiblock rate provided no gradual heart rate decline but rather an acute decline in heart rate and cardiac output. The multiblock rate was increased by shortening the postventricular atrial refractory period. The paper speed is 12.5 mm/sec, with each row being 20 seconds. The time from the onset of exercise is noted by the numbers in the left margin.

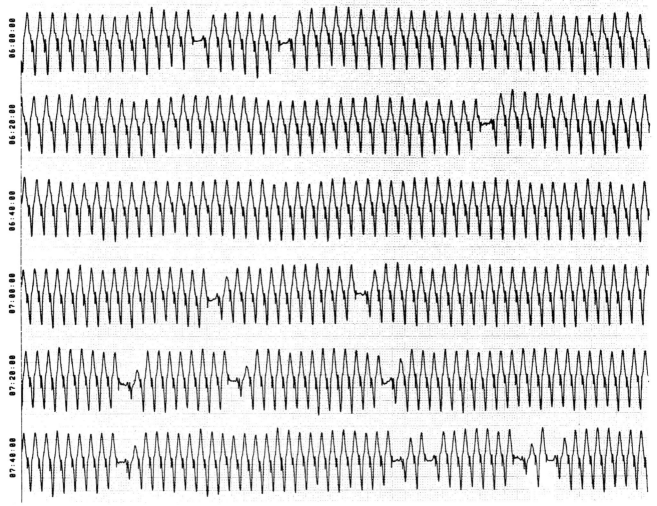

FIGURE 36–42. An example from an exercise test on a patient who developed acute loss of capture at maximal exercise. Threshold testing at rest revealed excellent thresholds with the minimal pulse width necessary to pace being 0.15 msec at a 5.4-V amplitude. The programmed settings were a pulse width of 0.5 msec at a 5.4-V amplitude. At rest and early exercise, there was 100% capture with a loss of capture occurring only at maximal exercise. The pulse width was subsequently increased to 1 msec with no loss of capture on repeat testing. The paper speed is 12.5 mm/sec, with each row being 20 seconds. The time from the onset of exercise is noted by the numbers in the left margin.

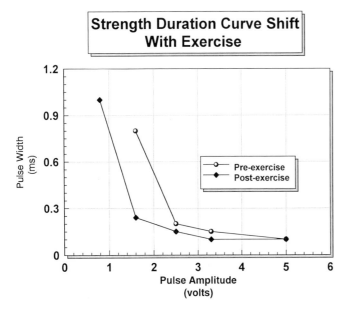

FIGURE 36–43. Data from a patient with fixed rate VVI pacing who demonstrated a decrease in thresholds following termination of exercise compared with preexercise values. At higher pulse amplitudes, there was a minimal change, but marked changes were noted at lower pulse amplitudes. This denotes a shift of the strength-duration curve leftward, implying an increased excitability of the heart with exercise. (Data from Serwer and associates.[56])

performance. In many series, 24-hour ambulatory ECG monitoring was the only means by which pacemaker malfunction was detected.[62–64] Such monitoring is particularly valuable in evaluating atrial and ventricular sensing problems and intermittent lack of capture. This is particularly important because myocardial characteristics and, thereby, appropriate pacemaker programming may vary, depending on the activity state and time of day.[25] Interactions between the patient's intrinsic rhythm and the pacemaker are also more completely evaluated on ambulatory monitoring, which may result in more optimal programming.

TRANSTELEPHONIC ELECTROCARDIOGRAPHIC MONITORING

Transtelephonic ECG monitoring also plays an important role in pacemaker follow-up. In most aspects, its use is similar to that in adults. The major differences relate to the difficulty in performing the test because of the uncooperative nature of some children. We find transmitters in which the phone can be placed in a cradle rather than held to be superior. These units consist of a cradle in which the phone is placed and a small electrode plate that is held against the chest (Fig. 36–44). This leaves the parent with a free hand to calm or hold the child. Also, longer rhythm strips must be run to assess the pacemaker's function if a motion artifact is present. Routinely, 60-second strips are run to be sure adequate data are obtained. Both nonmagnet and magnet strips are obtained, as in adult patients. We allow the parents to choose the best time of day to call. They often vary the time they call, based on nap or school schedules. Reminder notes are sent at the beginning of the month in which a recording is due. Patients are called by the follow-up nurse only if a call has not been received within 3 weeks of the notice's mailing. In general, inadequate recordings are seldom obtained because the parents become adept at sending such ECGs.

EARLY FOLLOW-UP PERIOD

Similar to the adult patient, follow-up during this critical period must be frequent and thorough. This is especially true

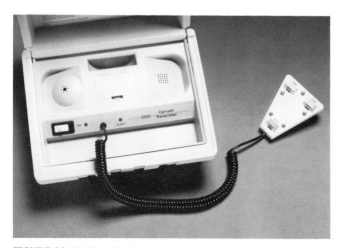

FIGURE 36–44. Example of a transtelephonic transmitter particularly well suited for use in children. It consists of a cradle in which the phone receiver is placed and a small unit that can easily be held against that child's chest with one hand while the other hand is free to steady and calm the child during transmission.

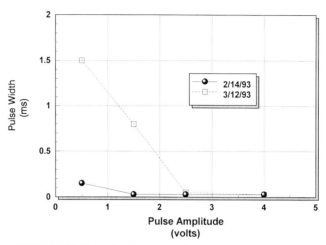

FIGURE 36–45. Example of a change with time of the strength-duration curve of a patient showing changes not necessarily apparent if thresholds had been determined only at pulse amplitudes above 2.5 V.

when a new electrode has been implanted. Our current protocol initially following implant includes both pacemaker interrogation and noninvasive threshold determination at multiple pulse amplitudes performed at 2 days and 2, 4, and 8 weeks following implantation. During this period, thresholds often vary, and the generator's output may also need to be reprogrammed to maintain reliable pacing. Exit block, in particular, is common during this period, with little to no exit block being noted beyond 3 months postimplant.[64] In other series, there appeared to be a slight increase in threshold noted after 3 months, but this occurred only in 24% of patients.[65] It is important to determine thresholds at multiple pulse amplitudes because the strength-duration curve may move only in a horizontal direction, with thresholds at the higher outputs unchanging and thresholds at lower outputs showing marked increases (Fig. 36–45).

In addition, 24-hour ambulatory ECG monitoring is performed within the first week following implantation to assess proper pacemaker function throughout the day, not just for a brief period during pacemaker interrogation. For those children old enough to undergo exercise testing, this is always accomplished within the first 2 weeks following implantation. Transtelephonic ECGs are obtained monthly during this period.

INTERMEDIATE FOLLOW-UP

The next period of time, defined as 3 months to 5 years postimplantation, tends to be a period during which there is a small incidence of electrode or generator malfunction. During this time, pacing systems tend to be more stable and do not require as frequent reevaluations. Our current protocol is to see patients semiannually for pacemaker interrogation and threshold testing and to obtain yearly 24-hour ambulatory ECGs. Transtelephonic ECGs are obtained bimonthly in the absence of complicating features believed to require more frequent monitoring. In addition, patients and their parents are encouraged to send transmissions whenever there is a question about proper pacemaker function.

LATE FOLLOW-UP

From 5 years until the time for the pacemaker's replacement is the period during which generator failure is more likely than electrode failure. Although electrode failure does occur, the thresholds, in general, tend to be stable, and the majority of electrode failures during this period are a consequence of acute lead fracture and not exit block. There tends to be no warning preceding lead fracture, and no follow-up method currently used has been shown to be useful in predicting such events. However, a depletion of the generator's battery can be adequately detected early through the use of monthly transtelephonic ECGs. Ambulatory ECGs are still obtained yearly.

PROPHYLACTIC MEDICATION

There has been significant controversy concerning the need for prophylactic anticoagulants and/or antibiotic agents for the prevention of subacute bacterial endocarditis in children with pacemakers. The current recommendations of the American Heart Association do *not* suggest the use of antibiotics for children with pacemakers.[66] However, most such children have other underlying structural diseases that do require the use of antibiotics for such prophylaxis. Our current practice is to prescribe antibiotics for prophylaxis of subacute bacterial endocarditis for all children who have endocardial electrodes if there is any AV valve regurgitation present by physical examination or echocardiography. Children with epicardial pacing systems without associated structural cardiac lesions do not require such prophylaxis.

Prophylactic anticoagulation has not been shown to be useful in children who have endocardial pacing systems. Only those children with chronic atrial flutter and/or fibrillation are routinely anticoagulated. We believe that the risk to the active child from chronic anticoagulation is significant, with a minimal benefit derived.

Adjustments to Lifestyle

No discussion of pediatric pacing would be complete without a discussion of the psychosocial response of children to having a pacemaker placed. Because the longevity of children with pacemakers is significantly greater than that of adults and we encourage such children to be active and lead "normal" lives, psychological problems are expected. In one series in which 30 patients with pacemakers were evaluated, differences were found.[67] Those with pacemakers are more external in their locus of control orientation, suggesting a diminished sense of self-control and less autonomy. They are more fearful of social rejection than of pacemaker failure and are often sensitive to the physical appearance of the pacemaker's pocket. Many children require their clothing to cover the pacemaker incision at all times. This is particularly relevant to boys who undergo transvenous pacemaker placement because they often refuse to appear in public without a T-shirt. Many often also continue to wear a T-shirt, even while swimming. This is accentuated by the fact that the peers of children with pacemakers often view such children as different, even though the patients themselves may not see themselves as being different. However, on a positive note, no

significant differences in anxiety, self-competence, or self-esteem are found. Children with pacemakers have a significant knowledge of their pacemaker system, and unlike some children with chronic diseases, they do not appear to deny its existence. They appear to cope effectively with their situation. It is postulated that they may experience problems in the development of autonomy and experience social isolation and potentially peer rejection.

As a consequence of these findings, care must be taken to emphasize the positive aspects of the pacemaker to the child and to make certain that the child's level of understanding is adequate to prevent the appearance of excessive fear and excessive loss of self-image. Although the outward appearance of the pacemaker to the child's peers cannot be completely hidden, any steps to minimize such an outward appearance is to the child's psychological benefit. Our current practice is to explain all procedures to children in detail and to allow them to see and ask questions about the pacemaker prior to its implantation and at all subsequent follow-up visits. This must be viewed as any other chronic disease, which requires increased medical supervision throughout children's lives but not to the point that it will severely limit children's lifestyles or cause them to be significantly different from their peers. We try to assure the children that they will be able to participate in almost all activities in which their peers participate, with the only limitation being sports in which there is a high risk of physical contact with potential damage to the pacemaker pocket itself. We do not allow participation in high-contact sports, such as football and hockey, but encourage participation in other sports, such as basketball, baseball, golf, and tennis, assuming the child's underlying cardiac disease will permit this. The current recommendation of the American College of Cardiology is in line with these recommendations.[68] Again, all efforts should be made to allow the child to be as "normal" as possible without placing the child in undue jeopardy. Children must be aware that they will require frequent evaluations and frequent surgical procedures. However, current thought indicates that they should lead normal lives and be able to participate in almost all activities and expect life spans comparable to those of their peers, limited only by other underlying cardiac disease and not by the pacemaker itself. Such children should be expected to lead fairly normal lives and, as technology improves, should expect an increasing time between pacemaker changes and hospitalizations. The outlook of such children has markedly improved over the last 10 years, and we fully expect this trend to continue in the future.

REFERENCES

1. Moquin PM, Vaysse J, Durand M, et al: Implantation d'un stimulateur interne pour correction d'un bloc auriculo-ventriculo-ventriculaire chirurgical chez une enfant de 7 ans. Arch Mal Coeur Vaiss 55:241, 1962.
2. Shearn RPN, Flemming WH: Fourteen years of implanted pacemakers in children. Ann Thorac Surg 25:144, 1978.
3. Simon AB, Dick M II, Stern AM, et al: Ventricular pacing in children. PACE Pacing Clin Electrophysiol 5:836, 1982.
4. Walkens JJS: Cardiac pacemakers in infants and children. Pediatr Cardiol 3:337, 1982.
5. Ector H, Dhooghe G, Daenen W, et al: Pacing in children. Br Heart J 53:541, 1985.
6. Serwer GA, Mericle JM: Evaluation of pacemaker pulse generator and patient longevity in patients aged 1 day to 20 years. Am J Cardiol 59:824, 1987.

7. Walsh CA, McAlister HF, Anders CA, et al: Pacemaker implantation in children: A 21-year experience. PACE Pacing Clin Electrophysiol 11:1940, 1988.

8. Brownlee JR, Serwer GA, Dick M II, et al: Failure of electrocardiographic monitoring to detect cardiac arrest in patients with pacemakers. Am J Dis Child 143:105, 1989.

9. McCue CM, Mantakas ME, Tingelstad JB, Ruddy S: Congenital heart block in newborns of mothers with connective tissue disease. Circulation 56:82, 1977.

10. Kangos JJ, Griffiths SP, Blumenthal S: Congenital complete heart block: A classification and experience with 18 patients. Am J Cardiol 20:632, 1967.

11. Dorostkar P, Serwer GA, LeRoy S, Dick M II: Long-term course of children and young adults with congenital complete heart block. J Am Coll Cardiol 21:295A, 1993.

12. Kugler JD, Danford DA: Pacemakers in children: An update. Am Heart J 117:665, 1989.

13. Karpawich PP, Gillette PC, Garrison A, et al: Congenital complete atrioventricular block: Clinical and electrophysiologic predictors of need for pacemaker insertion. Am J Cardiol 48:1098, 1981.

14. Winkler RB, Freed MD, Nadas AS: Exercise-induced ventricular ectopy in children and young adults with complete heart block. Am Heart J 99:87, 1980.

15. Gillette PC, Wampler DG, Shannon C, Oth D: Use of cardiac pacing after the Mustard operation for transposition of the great arteries. J Am Coll Cardiol 7:138, 1986.

16. El-Said G, Rosenberg HS, Mullins LE, et al: Dysrhythmias after Mustard's operation for transposition of the great arteries. Am J Cardiol 30:526, 1972.

17. Eldor M, Griffin JC, Abbott VA, et al: Permanent cardiac pacing in patients with long QT syndrome. J Am Coll Cardiol 3:600, 1987.

18. Dreifus LS, Fisch C, Griffin VC, et al: Guidelines for implantation of cardiac pacemakers and antiarrhythmic devices. J Am Coll Cardiol 18:1, 1991.

19. McGrath LB, Gonzalez-Lavin L, Morse DP, Levett JM: Pacemaker system failure and other events in children with surgically induced heart block. PACE Pacing Clin Electrophysiol II:1182, 1988.

20. Serwer GA, Mericle JM, Armstrong BE: Epicardial ventricular pacemaker electrode longevity in children. Am J Cardiol 61:104, 1988.

21. Serwer GA, Uzark K, Dick M II: Endocardial pacing electrode longevity in children. J Am Coll Cardiol 15:212A, 1990.

22. Serwer G, Dick M II, Eakin B: Cardiac output response to treadmill exercise in children with fixed-rate pacemakers. Circulation 84:II-514, 1991.

23. Karpawich PP, Perry BL, Farooki ZQ, et al: Pacing in children and young adults in nonsurgical atrioventricular block: Comparison of single-rate ventricular and dual-chamber modes. Am Heart J 113:316, 1987.

24. Karpawich PP, Justice CD, Cavitt DL, Chang CH: Developmental sequelae of fixed-rate ventricular pacing in the immature canine heart: An electrophysiologic, hemodynamic, and histopathologic evaluation. Am Heart J 119:1077, 1990.

25. Preston TA, Fletcher RD, Luechesi BR, et al: Changes in myocardial threshold: Physiologic and pharmacologic factors in patients with implanted pacemakers. Am Heart J 74:235, 1967.

26. Serwer GA, Uzark K, Beekman R, Dick M II: Optimal programming of rate altering parameters in children with rate-responsive pacemakers using graded treadmill exercise testing. PACE Pacing Clin Electrophysiol 13:541, 1990.

27. Yabek SM, Wernly J, Check TW, et al: Rate-adaptive cardiac pacing in children using a minute ventilation biosensor. PACE Pacing Clin Electrophysiol 13:2108, 1990.

28. Gillette PC, Shannon C, Blair H, et al: Transvenous pacing in pediatric patients. Am Heart J 105:843, 1983.

29. Ward DE, Jones S, Shinebourne EA: Long-term transvenous pacing in children weighing ten kilograms or less. Int J Cardiol 15:112, 1982.

30. Spotnitz HM: Transvenous pacing in infants and children with congenital heart disease. Ann Thorac Surg 49:495, 1990.

31. Gillette PC, Zeigler V, Bradhaus GB, Kinsella P: Pediatric transvenous pacing: A concern for venous thrombosis? PACE Pacing Clin Electrophysiol 11:1935, 1988.

32. Yakvevich V, Alogen D, Papo J, Vidne BA: Fibrotic stenosis of the SVC with widespread thrombotic occlusion of its major tributaries. J Thorac Cardiovasc Surg 85:632, 1983.

33. Sunder SK, Ekong EA, Sevalingram K, Kumar A: SVC thrombosis due to pacing electrodes. Am Heart J 123:790, 1992.

34. Levin AR, Spach MS, Boineau JP, et al: Atrial pressure-flow dynamics in atrial septal defects (secundum type). Circulation 37:476, 1968.

35. Serwer GA, Armstrong BE, Anderson PAW, et al: Use of contrast echocardiography for evaluation of right ventricular hemodynamics in the presence of ventricular septal defects. Circulation 58:327, 1978.

36. Westerman GR, Van Revanter SH: Surgical management of difficult pacing problems in patients with congenital heart disease. J Cardiovasc Surg 2:351, 1987.

37. Moak JP, Friedman RA, Moffat D, et al: Dual-chamber pacing in children: The optimal lead configuration—unipolar or bipolar? J Am Coll Cardiol 17:208A, 1991.

38. DeLeon SY, Ilbawi MN, Koster N, Idriss FS: Comparison of the sutureless and suture-type epicardial electrodes in pediatric cardiac pacing. Ann Thorac Surg 33:273, 1982.

39. Michalik RE, Williams WH, Zorn-Chelten S, Hotches CR: Experience with a new epimyocardial pacing lead in children. PACE Pacing Clin Electrophysiol 7:83, 1984.

40. Kugler J, Minsour W, Blodgett C, et al: Comparison of two myoepicardial pacemaker leads: Follow-up in 80 children, adolescents, and young adults. PACE Pacing Clin Electrophysiol 11:2216, 1988.

41. DeLeon SY, Ilbawi MN, Becker CL, et al: Exit block in pediatric cardiac pacing. Thorac Cardiovasc Surg 99:905, 1990.

42. Hamilton R, Gow R, Bahoric B, et al: Steroid-eluting epicardial leads in pediatrics: Improved epicardial thresholds in the first year. PACE Pacing Clin Electrophysiol 14:2066, 1991.

43. Karpawich PP, Harkini M, Arciniegas E, Cavitt DL: Improved chronic epicardial pacing in children: Steroid contribution to porous platinized electrodes. PACE Pacing Clin Electrophysiol 15:1151, 1992.

44. Johns JA, Fuh FA, Burger JD, Hammon JW Jr: Steroid-eluting epicardial pacing leads in pediatric patients: Encouraging early results. J Am Coll Cardiol 20:395, 1992.

45. Serwer GA, Dorostkar PC, LeRoy S, Dick M II: Comparison of chronic thresholds between differing endocardial electrode types in children. Circulation 86:I-43, 1992.

46. Robertson JM, Hillel L: A new technique for permanent pacemaker implantation in infants and children. Ann Thorac Surg 44:209, 1987.

47. Ulicny KS Jr, Detterbeck FC, Starek PJK, Wilcox BR: Conjoined subrectus pocket for permanent pacemaker placement in the neonate. Soc Thorac Surg 53:1130, 1992.

48. Ott DA, Gillette PC, Cooley DA: Atrial pacing via the subxiphoid approach. Tex Heart Inst J 9:149, 1982.

49. Lawrie GM, Seale JP, Morris GC Jr, et al: Results of epicardial pacing by the left subcostal approach. Ann Thorac Surg 28:561, 1979.

50. Brenner JI, Gaines S, Cordier J, et al: Cardiac strangulation: Two-dimensional echo recognition of a rare complication of epicardial pacemaker therapy. Am J Cardiol 61:654, 1988.

51. Perry JC, Nihill MR, Ludomirsky A, et al: The pulmonary artery lasso: Epicardial pacing lead causing right ventricular outflow obstruction. PACE Pacing Clin Electrophysiol 14:1018, 1991.

52. Serwer GA, Dick M II, Uzark K, et al: The value of redundant ventricular epicardial electrode placement in children. PACE Pacing Clin Electrophysiol 9:531, 1988.

53. Gillette PC, Edgerton J, Kratz J, Zeigler V: The subpectoral pocket: The preferred implant site for pediatric pacemakers. PACE Pacing Clin Electrophysiol 14:1089, 1991.

54. Hayes DC, Holmes DR Jr, Maloney JD, et al: Permanent endocardial pacing in pediatric patients. J Thorac Cardiovasc Surg 85:618, 1983.

55. Serwer GA, Dorostkar PC, LeRoy S, et al: Evaluation of rate variable pacemaker function at maximal exertion in children and young adults. PACE Pacing Clin Electrophysiol 16:899, 1993.

56. Serwer GA, Kodali R, Eakin B, et al: Changes in pacemaker threshold with exercise in children and young adults. J Am Coll Cardiol 17:207A, 1991.

57. Gillette PC, Zinner A, Kratz J, et al: Atrial tracking (synchronous) pacing in a pediatric and young adult population. J Am Coll Cardiol 9:811, 1987.

58. Frohlig G, Blank W, Schwerdt H, et al: Atrial sensing performance of AV universal pacemakers during exercise. PACE Pacing Clin Electrophysiol 11:47, 1988.

59. Ross BA, Zeigler V, Zinner A, et al: The effect of exercise on the atrial electrogram voltage in young patients. PACE Pacing Clin Electrophysiol 14:2092, 1991.

60. Bricker JT, Barison A, Traveek MS, et al: The use of exercise testing in children to evaluate abnormalities of pacemaker function not apparent at rest. PACE Pacing Clin Electrophysiol 8:656, 1985.

61. Jain P, Kaul U, Wasir HS: Myopotential inhibition of unipolar demand pacemakers: Utility of provocative manoeuvres in assessment and management. Int J Cardiol 34:33, 1992.

62. Strathmore NF, Mond HG: Noninvasive monitoring and testing of pacemaker function. PACE Pacing Clin Electrophysiol 10:1359, 1987.

63. Kerstjens-Frederikse MWS, Bink-Boelkens MTE, de Jongste MJL, Homan van der Heide JN: Permanent cardiac pacing in children: Morbidity and efficacy of follow-up. Int J Cardiol 33:207, 1991.

64. Jarosik DL, Redd RM, Buckingham TA, et al: Utility of ambulatory electrocardiography in detecting pacemaker dysfunction in the early postimplantation period. Am J Cardiol 60:1030, 1987.

65. Shepard RB, Kam J, Colvin EC, et al: Pacing threshold spikes months and years after implant. PACE 14:1835, 1991.

66. Committee on Rheumatic Fever, Endocarditis, and Kawasaki Disease: Prevention of bacterial endocarditis: Recommendations by the American Heart Association. JAMA 264:2919, 1990.

67. Alpern D, Uzark K, Dick M II: Psychosocial responses of children to cardiac pacemakers. J Pediatr 114:494, 1989.

68. Gutgesell HP, Gessner IH, Vetter VL, et al: Recreational and occupational recommendations for young patients with heart disease. Circulation 74:1195A, 1986.

CHAPTER 37

ANTITACHYCARDIA PACING: CLINICAL CONSIDERATIONS

Karel den Dulk
Hein J. J. Wellens

Tachycardias based on a reentry mechanism are thought to be most suited for pacing therapy. The concept of a circulating impulse was first described and studied by Mayer[1] in his experiments with jellyfish. Mines[2] made decisive contributions to the development of the concept that reentry can cause cardiac arrhythmias. The circuit used by a circulating impulse can be anatomically, as reported by Mines, or functionally determined, as described by Allessie and coworkers.[3] When the circuit is anatomically defined, as in circus movement tachycardia in the Wolff-Parkinson-White syndrome, an excitable gap is usually present between the head and the tail of the circulating wavefront. The tissue constituting this excitable gap is not refractory and can be depolarized. The width of the excitable gap depends on the duration of the refractory period within the circuit, the length of the circuit, and the conduction velocity of the circulating impulse. In the presence of an excitable gap, a correctly timed impulse from outside the circuit is theoretically able to invade and create bidirectional block in the circuit, thereby terminating the arrhythmia. Certain conditions have to be fulfilled before a paced impulse will be able to enter a reentrant circuit. Factors that play an important role in the ability to terminate reentrant tachycardias by pacing are (1) the tachycardia rate, (2) the duration of the refractory period of the components of the reentry circuit and the tissue between the reentry circuit and the pacing site, (3) the distance between the tachycardia circuit and the site of stimulation, and (4) the conduction velocity in the circuit and in the tissue between the reentry circuit and the pacing site.[4]

Any patient with tachycardias that can be terminated by pacing is a potential candidate for an implantable unit.

Indications for Antitachycardia Pacing

Symptomatic paroxysmal reentrant supraventricular tachycardia (SVT) can be treated with drugs, pacing, surgery, or ablation techniques, or a combination of these methods. The usefulness of antitachycardia pacemakers in the management of reentrant SVTs has been well demonstrated.[5–12] Antitachycardia pacing may be the therapy of choice in patients who do not respond to or cannot tolerate drug therapy, in patients who do not take their medication, in patients who are not suited for or refuse surgery or catheter ablation techniques, in patients for whom elective surgery or catheter ablation techniques are not readily available, and in patients who cannot tolerate prolonged episodes of tachycardia because of the development of cardiac failure, angina pectoris, or dizziness.

Antitachycardia pacing is a good form of therapy for drug-resistant atrioventricular (AV) nodal tachycardia. It is safe and effective, and the most physiologic rhythm is preserved (AV synchrony and rate variability). Ablation of the bundle of His has hemodynamic consequences because AV synchrony, heart rate control by the sinus node, and the natural activation sequence of the ventricles by the His-Purkinje system are lost. In addition, ablation of the bundle of His does not prevent AV nodal tachycardias from occurring; it only prevents conduction to the ventricles. Conduction to the atrium during tachycardia can still give rise to troublesome paroxysmal neck vein pulsations. DDD pacing would maintain the paroxysmal palpitations because the device would synchronize ventricular paced complexes to the atrial events during tachycardia unless a DDD pacemaker with appropriate mode switching capabilities is used. In addition, the pacemaker would have to be able to terminate tachycardia. A VVI rate-variable pacemaker could give rise to the pacemaker syndrome if the atrial contribution to ventricular filling is of importance, as is often the case. Because ablation of the bundle of His creates the need for pacemaker implantation anyway, it seems preferable to first investigate if antitachycardia pacing would not be preferable.

Curative surgical and catheter ablation techniques have been developed for AV nodal tachycardias.[13, 14] The initial results in some centers have been encouraging. However, there is a risk of creating AV block during surgery (1%–5%) or catheter ablation (1%–3%), and it remains to be seen if the surgical or ablation scar will not give rise to AV conduction problems in the future, necessitating subsequent pacemaker implantation. Nevertheless, radio-frequency ablation of the slow pathway in AV nodal reentry tachycardia is becoming the mainstay of therapy for these patients.

In young patients seeking a nonpharmacologic cure for symptomatic recurrent episodes of SVT using an accessory pathway, catheter ablation or surgery is the therapy of choice because of its high success rate resulting in cure in more than 90% of patients. Of patients with anterograde conducting pathways, only those with long anterograde refractory periods can be considered for antitachycardia pacing because of the risk of rapidly conducted atrial fibrillation.

Pacing-induced arrhythmias are an undesirable complication of pacemaker treatment of SVT. In a series of 111 consecutive patients undergoing electrophysiologic investigation for SVT at our institution,[15] antitachycardia pacing was contraindicated in 6% of patients, because all pacing modalities attempted either did not interrupt SVT or resulted in the induction of an undesired arrhythmia.

Similarly, in 26% of attempts at terminating ventricular tachycardia (VT), pacing resulted in acceleration of tachycardia or degeneration into ventricular fibrillation.[16] Patients with VT are not considered candidates for antitachycardia pacing unless back-up defibrillation capabilities are available in the implanted unit.

Many patients may prefer treatment of their SVTs with small reliable pacemakers rather than the chronic intake of antiarrhythmic drugs with their possible side effects and accumulating expense over time. In addition, fully automatic pacemakers usually terminate tachycardia so rapidly that the tachycardia is not noticed or is experienced only as a premature beat by the patient.

Electrophysiologic Study

An invasive electrophysiologic study must be performed in all patients being considered for antitachycardia pacing therapy to determine if tachycardias can be terminated safely and reproducibly. Failure to terminate tachycardia reliably or induction of undesirable arrhythmias (e.g., atrial fibrillation, atrial flutter, antidromic tachycardia, or VT) is a contraindication to antitachycardia pacing.

PACING SITE

The electrophysiologic study gives information as to which pacing site is best to use. The closer the stimulating

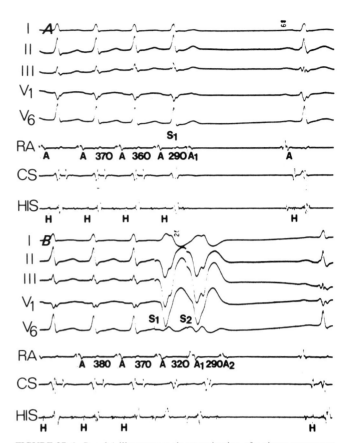

FIGURE 37–1. *Panel A* illustrates pacing termination of a circus movement tachycardia from the coronary sinus with one atrial premature beat. In *panel B* the same circus movement tachycardia is terminated from the right ventricle, but in this situation two premature beats are required to terminate the tachycardia.

electrode is to the site of origin of the tachycardia, the easier it is to terminate. Using a left-sided accessory pathway in patients with circus movement tachycardia, the arrhythmia can usually be terminated by atrial or ventricular stimulation. Tachycardia is, however, more easily terminated by pacing from the coronary sinus, close to the insertion of the accessory pathway and the reentry circuit, than by right atrial stimulation. A greater number of premature stimuli are required from the right ventricular apex to terminate tachycardia when compared with the number of stimuli required from the coronary sinus (Fig. 37–1). Careful evaluation of right atrium, right ventricle, and coronary sinus pacing is the only way to select the best pacing site. Pacing sites or modes that induce undesirable arrhythmias can be identified during the electrophysiologic study and therefore avoided. Easy induction of atrial fibrillation or flutter from the atrium is a reason to evaluate if tachycardias can be terminated safely and reliably from the ventricle. Ventricular stimulation has the risk of inducing VT or ventricular fibrillation especially in patients with ischemia during tachycardia or in patients with an old myocardial infarction.

ATRIAL FIBRILLATION

Atrial fibrillation is a potential problem for antitachycardia pacing in SVT and is the major reason for the discontinuation of antitachycardia pacing therapy. Fisher and colleagues[17] reported that antitachycardia pacing for SVT was discontinued in 3 of 15 patients (follow-up of 68 ± 45 months) because of atrial fibrillation. A careful clinical history can give an indication if paroxysmal atrial fibrillation occurs spontaneously (it should be realized that the patient is not always able to distinguish the reentrant tachycardia from atrial fibrillation). Induction of atrial fibrillation or flutter with one or two premature beats from the atrium during the invasive electrophysiologic study is a good reason to evaluate if right ventricular pacing is a better option for tachycardia termination. Occasionally, atrial fibrillation becomes a clinical problem after pacemaker implantation, as was the case in 3 of 40 patients being paced for SVT in our series.[12] These patients were given antiarrhythmic drug therapy for atrial fibrillation, and antitachycardia pacing modes were programmed to avoid coupling intervals that were too short so that induction of atrial fibrillation did not occur but the tachyarrhythmias for which the pacemakers were implanted were still controlled. A satisfactory situation can be achieved in some of these patients. However, the long-term success in terminating episodes of SVT without inducing atrial fibrillation after the pacemaker is reprogrammed or pharmacologic agents are added, or both, is variable.

RIGHT VENTRICULAR PACING FOR SUPRAVENTRICULAR TACHYCARDIA

Right ventricular pacing is contraindicated if it induces ventricular arrhythmias or if tachycardia induces ischemia in patients with coronary artery disease. Aggressive stimulation protocols should be avoided when using right ventricular stimulation and, if necessary, a drug should be given to slow tachycardia, allowing a less aggressive termination mode. Spurrell and associates[18] reported two cases of sudden death in patients with Wolff-Parkinson-White syndrome and a ventricular antitachycardia pacing system. The role of ventricular pacing or the accessory pathway, or both, in contributing to these deaths remains unknown. To our knowledge there have been no other reports of sudden death that might be attributed to right ventricular pacing for SVT, despite the not infrequent use of right ventricular pacing for termination of SVT.

VENTRICULAR TACHYCARDIA

In 26% of attempts at terminating VT, pacing resulted in acceleration of tachycardia by more than 20 msec or degeneration into ventricular fibrillation.[16]

Patients with VT are not considered candidates for antitachycardia pacing unless back-up defibrillation capabilities are available in the implantable unit.

IMMEDIATE OR BACKUP DIRECT CURRENT SHOCK

The hemodynamic significance of the spontaneously occurring and pacing-induced arrhythmias during the invasive electrophysiologic study allows assessment of the need for immediate or backup direct current (DC) shock in patients with tachycardias. Except for patients with the Wolff-Parkinson-White syndrome who have rapid ventricular rates during atrial fibrillation, syncope or hemodynamic collapse occurs very rarely in patients with SVT who have no organic heart disease. Syncopal VT is, in contrast, a rather frequent clinical observation. Resting ventricular function (most patients with VT have organic heart disease) and the ventricular activation pattern during tachycardia are, together with the rate of the arrhythmia, major determinants of the hemodynamic consequences of tachycardia. In patients with old myocardial infarction, we found that a combination of resting left ventricular function (as assessed from the global ejection fraction) and the rate of VT determine whether VT will present as an arrhythmia, allowing the patient to seek medical assistance, or as sudden death, requiring immediate cardiopulmonary resuscitation and DC shock.[19] During programmed electric stimulation, 25% of induced VT episodes (215 VTs) resulted in syncope and required immediate DC shock.[16] In an additional 12% of patients, pacing-induced acceleration of VT required backup DC shock.[16] The first group of patients are not good candidates for antitachycardia pacing, whereas the second group might be considered for antitachycardia pacing in combination with drugs and an implantable cardioverter defibrillator. Nonsyncopal VT could be terminated safely and reliably by pacing in 61% of the episodes.[16]

Antitachycardia Pacing Techniques

Various pacing techniques are currently being used in implantable devices.

UNDERDRIVE PACING

Asynchronous stimulation at a rate slower than the tachycardia rate is referred to as underdrive pacing. The pacing impulses occur at various times during the tachycardia cycle, as long as the tachycardia rate is not an exact multiple of the pacing rate.[20] As described by Ryan and associates[21] in 1968, underdrive pacing can be achieved with a demand pacemaker by placing a magnet over the pacemaker and converting it to an asynchronous magnet mode. Automatic single- and dual-chamber underdrive pacemakers are available. The effectiveness of AV sequential dual-demand automatic pacemakers has been demonstrated in selected patients.[22, 23] Application of underdrive pacing is limited to tachycardias with rates less than 160 beats per minute (bpm). Rates greater than 160 bpm are rarely terminated by one premature beat unless an accessory pathway is incorporated in the circuit and the pacing catheter is placed close to the reentrant circuit.

OVERDRIVE OR BURST PACING

During overdrive or burst pacing, the heart is stimulated at a rate greater than the tachycardia rate. Addition of a second stimulus facilitates entrance into the reentrant circuit from a distant stimulation site by "peeling back" the refractory period at the site of stimulation and the intervening tissue.[24, 25] By giving more than two premature stimuli, the refractory period of the tissue at the stimulation site and the intervening tissue can be further abbreviated, allowing delivery of earlier stimuli and earlier entrance to the area of slow conduction in the reentrant circuit. This method can be used in patients with atrial flutter, AV nodal tachycardia, circus movement tachycardia using an accessory pathway, and VT. Before implanting such a device for use in the atrium, one must exclude the existence of an accessory pathway with a short antegrade refractory period because of the risk of rapidly conducted atrial fibrillation. Pacing is not without risk if applied to the ventricle because rate acceleration and ventricular fibrillation can be induced in patients with VT. The risk of acceleration is increased by increasing the rate and number of stimuli in the burst. The risk of acceleration may be reduced by late synchronization of the first beat of the burst. The pacing intervals can be determined in milliseconds or as a percentage of the tachycardia cycle length (adaptive-orthorhythmic[26]) to compensate for a change in tachycardia rate.

Various forms of burst pacing modes exist that combine or alter the previously described basic pacing techniques (Fig. 37–2).

SCANNING BURST (CONCERTINA-ACCORDION).[18] In this mode, coupling intervals of all stimuli in the burst are the same and are reduced equally with successive termination attempts. The timing of the first stimulus is programmed separately and is kept constant.

SHIFTING BURST. Coupling intervals of all stimuli in the burst are equal in this mode and remain fixed with successive attempts. The timing of the first stimulus is progressively decreased.

RAMP PACING. In this burst pacing mode, the pacing rate of

the burst gradually accelerates (tune up) or decelerates (tune down), starting at a rate faster than the tachycardia rate.[27, 28]

CHANGING RAMPS. In this mode, the pacing rate of the burst accelerates and then decelerates, or decelerates and then accelerates, in a burst sequence.[27]

SCANNING BURST WITH RAMP PACING. The timing of the first stimulus in this pacing mode is progressively decreased with successive attempts.

SELF-ADAPTING AUTODECREMENTAL OVERDRIVE PACING. The timing of the first stimulus of a burst is equal to the tachycardia cycle length in this mode. Subsequent stimuli of the burst are decreased by a programmable interval. If tachycardia is not terminated by the initial burst, the burst is repeated with one more stimulus, which is also decreased as previously described. This sequence (adding stimuli) is repeated until the tachycardia is terminated or the programmed maximum number of stimuli is reached.[29]

BURST WITH PROGRAMMED EXTRASTIMULI. In this mode, the burst is followed by one or two independently timed extrastimuli.[30, 31]

ULTRARAPID TRAIN STIMULATION. A short burst of pacing is delivered at a very rapid rate (3000–6000 stimuli per minute) in this pacing mode. The train is started in the refractory period and timed to give one or two captures (directly after the refractory period) with the shortest possible coupling intervals regardless of the tachycardia rate. An inherent risk is tachycardia acceleration or the induction of ventricular fibrillation.[32, 33]

PROGRAMMED EXTRASTIMULATION. This technique requires exact and independent timing of one or more extrastimuli to penetrate the reentrant circuit. The coupling can be in milliseconds or can be a percentage of the tachycardia cycle length. If tachycardia has not been terminated after a first attempt, the coupling intervals or number of stimuli of subsequent pacing attempts may be the same or changed.

EXTRASTIMULUS SCAN. This technique consists of sequential incremental or decremental scanning[5] in which the coupling interval is changed by a small value until the interval to be scanned has been covered or tachycardia has been terminated. Scanning can be performed with the first or the last stimulus or with both if two stimuli are given.

CENTRIFUGAL SCAN. In this method, the timing of the first stimulus increases and decreases on successive attempts.[7, 34]

SELF-SEARCHING SCAN. A process of bisection of the interval to be scanned determines that point in the cycle at which stimulation is to occur. This operation is directed by the response of tachycardia to stimulation.[7, 34]

ADAPTIVE MODE USING AN AUTOMATICALLY INCREASING NUMBER OF STIMULI (UNIVERSAL ANTITACHYCARDIA PACING MODE). In this mode, the timing of the first stimulus is a selected percentage of the tachycardia cycle length. If tachycardia persists, a second stimulus is added at a programmable smaller percentage. If tachycardia persists, a third stimulus is added at a programmable smaller percentage of the cycle length. The coupling intervals of subsequent stimuli, if required, will be the same as those of the third stimulus.[35, 36] This is illustrated in Figures 37–2 and 37–3.

Testing of the Pacemaker

After implantation of an antitachycardia pacemaker, the mode selected needs to be tested and tailored under various

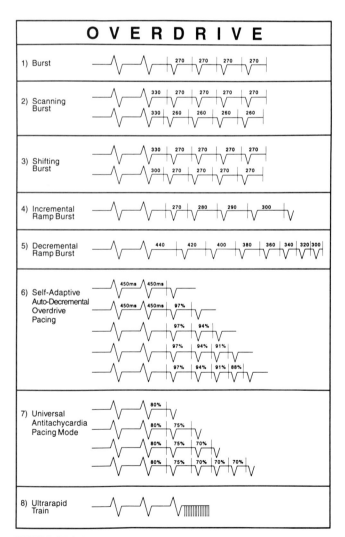

FIGURE 37–2. Schematic representation of various types of overdrive burst pacing.

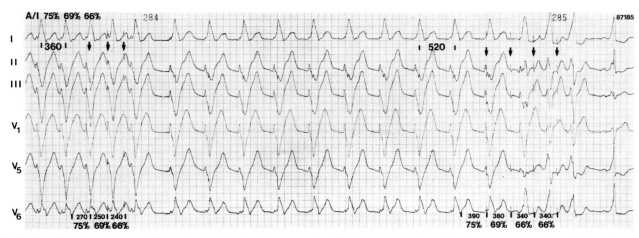

FIGURE 37–3. Six-channel electrocardiographic recording showing conversion with three premature beats of a circus movement tachycardia in a patient with Wolff-Parkinson-White syndrome to an intranodal tachycardia, with subsequent termination with four premature beats with the universal pacing mode. One and two premature beats did not influence the tachycardia. This electrocardiogram (ECG) illustrates an additional tachycardia as well as adaptation of the coupling intervals of the pacing mode to the tachycardia cycle length. (From den Dulk K, Brugada P, Smeets JLRM, Wellens HJJ: Long-term antitachycardia pacing experience for supraventricular tachycardia. PACE 13:1020, 1990.)

circumstances because the number and timing of required stimuli may change with alterations in posture, autonomic tone, tachycardia rate, refractory period, or drug level, or for other reasons. This testing and tailoring takes a long time. An adaptive pacing mode with an increasing number of stimuli adapts to these changes by adjusting the coupling intervals to the tachycardia rate and by delivering the required number of stimuli to terminate tachycardia. This mode represents a universal antitachycardia pacing mode for rapid termination of reentrant SVTs irrespective of rate or site of origin.[35, 36]

We evaluated this mode prospectively in 18 patients[37] with spontaneous atrial flutter. Fourteen of the 18 episodes were terminated with 4 to 16 (mean of 10) premature beats, with coupling intervals of 91%, 81%, and 75%, and 4 to 14 (mean of 9) premature beats, with coupling intervals of 75%, 69%, and 66%. No episodes or only short-lasting (<10 seconds) episodes of atrial fibrillation were seen before termination. The remaining four episodes of atrial flutter degenerated into sustained atrial fibrillation.

Our results support an approach of concentrating on the mechanism of tachycardia and the safety and applicability of antitachycardia pacing and not the reproducibility of termination under various circumstances during the initial invasive electrophysiologic study. Reproducibility of tachycardia termination can be further studied after pacemaker implantation.

Postimplantation Period

The early postimplantation period is an important phase in which to set up the detection and termination parameters correctly and to detect potential problems. This time should be used well. We keep patients on ambulatory monitoring for at least 3 days if possible. Patients are discharged 6 to 7 days following implantation. Pacing and sensing thresholds are checked at least three times before discharge. Sensing thresholds should be determined in sinus rhythm and during tachycardia. Programming and testing of the device should be started on the day of implantation and should be repeated

four or five times. Tachycardias should be initiated and terminated repeatedly with the patient in the supine and upright positions as well as after exercise to ensure safe and reproducible termination with the least number of stimuli and maximal coupling intervals.

DOUBLE SENSING

The presence of double sensing should be checked. Double sensing can, for example, be due to sensing of a far-field QRS complex via an atrial lead. This is more likely to occur with a unipolar sensing configuration and if the electrode is placed close to the AV groove (e.g., a coronary sinus lead). Double sensing can be observed in sinus rhythm or during tachycardia, or both. If atrial and ventricular signals are sensed during sinus rhythm, it could trigger an antitachycardia pacing treatment by sinus rhythm a little faster than half the programmed tachycardia trigger rate. For example, a sinus rhythm of 76 bpm would trigger treatment if the tachycardia detection or trigger interval were programmed to 150 bpm. If atrial and ventricular signals are sensed from an atrial lead during tachycardia, the device could synchronize therapy to the sensed ventricular signal instead of the atrial signal. The triggered mode, if available, could be helpful in evaluating this problem because it serves as a sensing indicator. Figure 37–4 illustrates how the triggered mode was helpful in locating the P wave in a patient with AV nodal tachycardia and atrial tachycardia. The timing of the first coupling interval of a pacing sequence can also help to determine the moment of sensing. Figure 37–5 illustrates this during conversion of an AV nodal reentrant tachycardia to an atrial tachycardia.

Double sensing can usually be resolved by programming. The programming options that can be used alone or in combination are (1) programming a sensitivity value that allows sensing of the desired signal only and (2) programming the refractory period so that the second signal occurs in the refractory period. The refractory period must, however, not be longer than the tachycardia cycle length, otherwise tachycardia will not be sensed. After reprogramming, double sens-

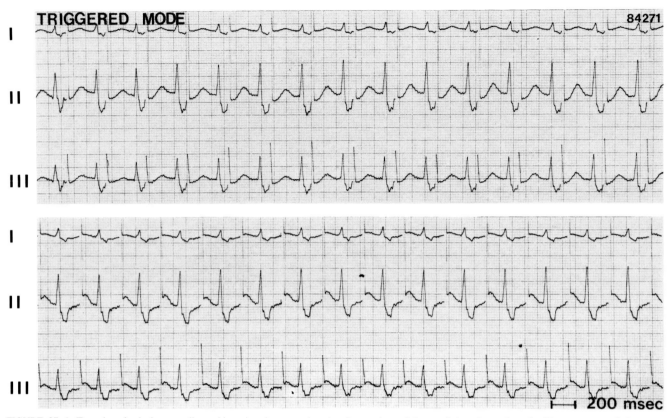

FIGURE 37–4. Two three-lead electrocardiographic strips demonstrating the diagnostic usefulness of the triggered mode. The *upper panel* shows an atrioventricular (AV) nodal reentrant tachycardia. The triggered mode indicates the P waves directly after the QRS complexes. The *lower panel* shows that the patient also had sustained episodes of atrial tachycardia. During the electrophysiologic study, nonsustained episodes of atrial tachycardia were induced during atrial stimulation to terminate AV nodal tachycardia. The presence of an accessory bypass tract was excluded. The rate is similar to that of the AV nodal tachycardia with slight acceleration on the *right side* of the tracing. (From den Dulk K, Brugada P, Waldecker B, et al: Automatic pacemaker termination of two different types of supraventricular tachycardia. J Am Coll Cardiol 6:201, 1985. Reprinted with permission from the American College of Cardiology.)

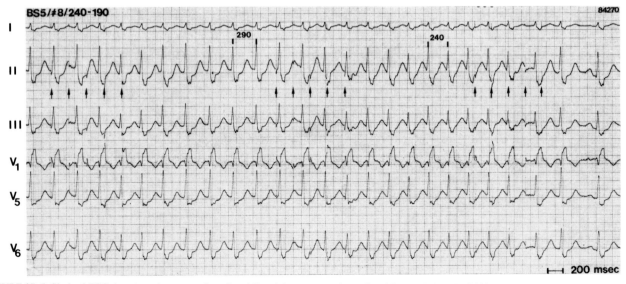

FIGURE 37–5. Six-lead ECG demonstrating conversion of an AV nodal reentrant tachycardia with a cycle length of 290 msec to an atrial tachycardia with a cycle length of 240 msec during a burst scan pacing sequence *(middle)*. The atrial tachycardia was subsequently terminated with the third burst scan stimulation sequence *(right)*. The location of the P waves can be seen in leads II and III. In the AV nodal tachycardia with a cycle length 290 msec, the P wave is located at the end of the QRS complex. In the atrial tachycardia with a cycle length 240 msec, the P wave is located in the peak of the T wave. This is confirmed by the timing of the first coupling interval (R-S₁) to the sensed atrial events. The programmed antitachycardia pacing mode (BS = burst scan), number of stimuli in a burst, scan delta interval (⊕), and maximal and minimal programmed coupling intervals are listed at the *upper left*. (From den Dulk K, Brugada P, Waldecker B, et al: Automatic pacemaker termination of two different types of supraventricular tachycardia. J Am Coll Cardiol 6:201, 1985. Reprinted with permission from the American College of Cardiology.)

ing must be reevaluated in sinus rhythm and during tachycardia.

AUTOMATIC OR MANUAL MODE

Tachycardia detection is usually carried out by detecting a heart rate greater than a programmed rate for a programmed number of consecutive beats. If there is no overlap between the tachycardia rate and the sinus tachycardia rate during exercise, the automatic mode can be programmed. If, however, there is an overlap, this could give rise to induction of tachycardia during exercise when the device attempts to terminate sinus tachycardia greater than the programmed detection rate. In some devices, a sudden-onset parameter can be used to distinguish a slow tachycardia from a sinus tachycardia. This algorithm will recognize the sudden onset of tachycardia if it occurs from a relatively slow sinus rhythm, but it can miss the sudden onset at fast sinus rates because the difference is too small, as shown in Figure 37–6. In some devices, the sudden-onset algorithm is still active after an attempted tachycardia termination. If tachycardia has not been terminated, the sudden-onset criteria are usually not satisfied, preventing further treatment. This has been changed in the newer devices.

An overlap between a slow tachycardia and sinus tachycardia could be a reason to use an external pacemaker activator. In some devices, applying a magnet will enable the rate criteria only, so if sudden-onset criteria are not satisfied, the device can still be activated to treat tachycardia by applying a magnet. The advantage of using an external activator is that the patient is usually able to distinguish a physiologic rhythm from a pathologic one, and a satisfactory situation can be reached because the patient is able to terminate slow, well-tolerated tachycardias quickly without medical assistance.

MEDICATION

We recently reviewed our antitachycardia pacing experience for SVT (40 patients, mean follow-up of 39 months) and found that in 37% of patients, antiarrhythmic drug therapy could be stopped.[12] In 21% of the patients antiarrhythmic drug therapy was not given to control the tachycardia for which the device was implanted, but was given for other reasons, such as paroxysmal atrial fibrillation not induced by pacing, atrial flutter, VT, beta-blockers for hypertension, and beta-blockers for angina, and for symptomatic ventricular premature beats not initiating tachycardia. Forty-two per cent of the patients were receiving antiarrhythmic drug therapy in combination with the antitachycardia pacemaker to control their paroxysmal SVTs (reduce incidence of tachycardia, facilitate termination of tachycardia, improve tachycardia tolerance, lengthen the anterograde refractory period of the accessory pathway, prevent pacing-induced atrial fibrillation). Antiarrhythmic drug therapy was used less in patients with AV nodal tachycardia than in patients with an accessory pathway and could be stopped in 53% of patients with AV nodal reentry versus 13% of patients with AV reciprocating tachycardia.

FOLLOW-UP

We see our patients with antitachycardia pacemakers three to four times a year in the outpatient clinic. The time required for a follow-up visit is 20 to 30 minutes. Follow-up consists of a pacemaker and a cardiac check-up. During the follow-up, a careful history is taken concerning tachycardia epi-

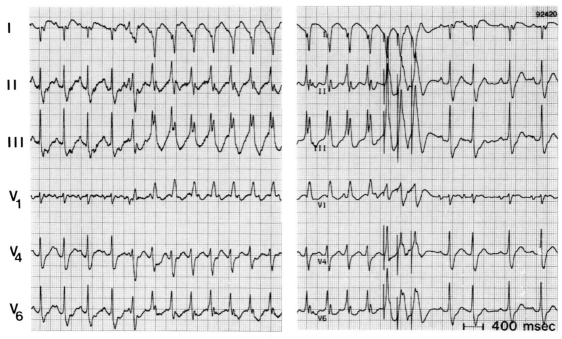

FIGURE 37–6. The six-lead electrocardiographic strip on the left illustrates the onset of a ventricular tachycardia during an exercise test. Antitachycardia pacing was not initiated by the implanted pacemaker cardioverter defibrillator (which was implanted for VT and VF) because the sudden-onset criterion was not met. Cycle length changed from 440 msec during sinus tachycardia to 380 during VT. The strip on the right shows termination of VT with three premature beats after fulfilling the sustained high-rate criterion after exercise.

sodes; pacing and sensing thresholds are tested; and tachycardias are noninvasively induced and terminated once or twice. This is followed by a cardiac check-up.

Careful history taking is important to determine whether the system is functioning properly. Relevant information includes the number of episodes, the duration of episodes, symptoms (e.g., dizziness), and tachycardia tolerance. If tachycardias are not terminated promptly, it is important to ask whether the episode felt similar to previous ones; whether the palpitations were irregular, faster, or slower; or whether there is any suggestion that the episode may have been a sinus tachycardia. Did the episode occur during exercise or emotion and how did it finally stop (abruptly, gradually, during rest, after intake of an antiarrhythmic drug)? If a tachycardia at rest seems to be prolonged but is quickly terminated when the patient gets up and walks around, this suggests that the tachycardia detection rate has been programmed too high and that exercise increases the tachycardia rate to greater than the programmed detection rate with subsequent termination of tachycardia. If the patient is receiving antiarrhythmic drug therapy, was the medication taken at the correct times or was it taken at all? Did another physician change or add medication? Addition of a beta- or calcium-channel blocker for hypertension or angina can slow the tachycardia rate so that it is less than the programmed tachycardia detection rate, and therefore the device will not attempt tachycardia termination.

Induction and termination of tachycardia are often helpful for making minor adjustments, and one can sometimes anticipate problems and correct them. Occasionally it is not possible to induce tachycardias noninvasively from the pacing site chosen for best termination, or it may be that tachycardia is inducible only after intravenous atropine administration. Under these circumstances, induction is limited and is performed only when clinically indicated. If the patient reports a prolonged episode of tachycardia, it is important to try to reproduce the situation and find the cause for the prolonged episode. Once again a careful history during induced episodes can give valuable information. During the induced episode, patients should be asked what they feel, for example, their typical or a different tachycardia, regular or irregular, and so on. This also gives information about the reliability of the symptoms and establishes the opportunity to get a better understanding of what rhythm the patient is describing.

Antitachycardia Pacing Experience for Supraventricular Tachycardia

Our long-term experience (total follow-up of 1503 months) with antitachycardia pacing for drug-resistant SVTs includes an estimated 16,366 episodes of tachycardia that occurred spontaneously; 16,240 (99.2%) of these episodes were terminated promptly by the pacemaker.[12]

The mean number of admissions for termination of tachycardia in the 3 months before implantation was three per patient (range of 0–18). During a total follow-up period of 1503 months (range of 1–82 months), only seven patients were admitted, once each, for termination of tachycardia, and two patients were admitted twice. Hospital admissions for termination of tachycardia decreased from 1 per patient-month to 1 per 137 patient-months.[12]

Long-term results with antitachycardia pacemakers appear to be good. The pacemakers are safe, reliable, and effective in terminating paroxysmal reentrant tachycardias. This mode of therapy has improved the quality of life significantly in these patients by rapidly terminating previously prolonged episodes of tachycardia and by avoiding repeated hospital admissions. Most patients with automatic devices either do not feel the short episodes of pacemaker-terminated tachycardia or experience the episode as a premature beat.

Antitachycardia pacing is an effective form of therapy for patients with paroxysmal SVTs. Versatility and size are no longer a concern for antitachycardia pacing. Device limitations of detection of slow reentrant tachycardias and distinction from atrial fibrillation are aspects that are currently undergoing investigation. New algorithms are being developed, including the use of sensors to differentiate sinus tachycardia from pathologic tachycardias. Monitors are being developed to enable accurate assessment by recording the success or failure of tachycardia termination, as well as discerning the reason for failure. These devices will add new dimensions to antitachycardia pacing.

REFERENCES

1. Mayer AG: Rhythmical pulsations in Scyphomedusae. Carnegie Institution of Washington Publication 47:1, 1906.
2. Mines GR: On dynamic equilibrium in the heart. J Physiol 46:349, 1913.
3. Allessie MA, Bonke FIM, Schopman FJG: Circus movement in rabbit atrial muscle as a mechanism of tachycardia. III. The ''leading circle'' concept. Circ Res 41:9, 1977.
4. Wellens HJJ, den Dulk K, Brugada P: Pacemaker management of cardiac arrhythmias. In Dreifus LS, Brest AN (eds): Pacemaker Therapy. Philadelphia: FA Davis, 1983, pp 165–175.
5. Spurrell RAJ, Nathan AW, Bexton RS, et al: Implantable automatic scanning pacemaker for termination of SVT. Am J Cardiol 49:753, 1982.
6. Griffin JC, Mason JW, Calfee RV: Clinical use of an implantable automatic tachycardia-termination pacemaker. Am Heart J 100:1093, 1980.
7. Sowton E: Clinical results with the tachylog antitachycardia pacemaker. PACE 7:1313, 1984.
8. Barold SS, Falkoff MD, Ong LS, Heinle RA: New pacing techniques for the treatment of tachycardias: The golden age of cardiac pacing. In Barold SS, Mugica JM (eds): The Third Decade of Cardiac Pacing. Mt Kisco, NY, Futura Publishing, 1982, pp 309–332.
9. Fisher JD, Kim SG, Mercando AD: Electrical devices for treatment of arrhythmias. Am J Cardiol 61:45A, 1988.
10. den Dulk K, Bertholet M, Brugada P, et al: A versatile pacemaker system for termination of tachycardias. Am J Cardiol 52:731, 1983.
11. den Dulk K, Bertholet M, Brugada P, et al: Clinical experience with implantable devices for control of tachyarrhythmias. PACE 7:548, 1984.
12. den Dulk K, Brugada P, Smeets JLRM, Wellens HJJ: Long-term antitachycardia pacing experience for supraventricular tachycardia. PACE 13:1020, 1990.
13. Ross DL, Johnson DC, Choong Koo C, et al: Surgical treatment of SVT without the WPW syndrome: Current indications, techniques, and results. In Brugada P, Wellens HJJ (eds): Cardiac Arrhythmias: Where To Go from Here? Mt Kisco, NY, Futura Publishing, 1987, pp 591–603.
14. Jackman WM, Beckman KJ, McClelland JH, et al: Treatment of supraventricular tachycardia due to atrioventricular nodal reentry by radiofrequency catheter ablation of the slow pathway conduction. N Engl J Med 327:313, 1992.
15. Waldecker B, Brugada P, den Dulk K, et al: Arrhythmias induced during termination of SVTs. Am J Cardiol 55:412, 1985.
16. Waldecker B, Brugada P, Zehender M, et al: Importance of modes of electrical termination of ventricular tachycardia for the selection of implantable antitachycardia devices. Am J Cardiol 57:150, 1986.

17. Fisher JD, Johnston DR, Furman S, et al: Long-term efficacy of anti-tachycardia pacing for supraventricular and ventricular tachycardias. Am J Cardiol 60:1311, 1987.
18. Spurrell RAJ, Nathan AW, Camm AJ: Clinical experience with implantable scanning tachycardia reversion pacemakers. PACE 7:1296, 1984.
19. Stevenson WG, Brugada P, Waldecker B, et al: Clinical, angiographic, and electrophysiological findings in patients with aborted sudden death as compared to patients with sustained ventricular tachycardia after myocardial infarction. Circulation 6:1146, 1985.
20. den Dulk K, Lindemans FW, Bär FW, Wellens HJJ: Pacemaker-related tachycardia. PACE 5:476, 1982.
21. Ryan G, Easley RM, Zaroff LI, Goldstein S: Paradoxical use of a demand pacemaker in treatment of supraventricular tachycardia due to the Wolff-Parkinson-White syndrome. Circulation 38:1037, 1968.
22. Castellanos A, Waxman HL, Moleiro F, et al: Preliminary studies with an implantable multimodal A-V pacemaker for reciprocating AV tachycardias. PACE 3:257, 1980.
23. Medina-Ravell V, Maduro C, Portillo B, et al: Follow-up of twenty-five patients with implantable anti-tachycardia DVI, MN pulse generators [abstract]. PACE 6:145, 1983.
24. Moe GK, Cohen W, Vick RL: Experimentally induced paroxysmal AV nodal tachycardia in the dog. Am Heart J 65:87, 1963.
25. Moe GK, Mendez C: The physiologic basis of reciprocal rhythm. Cardiovasc Dis 8:461, 1966.
26. Zacouto F, Guize L, Maurice P, Gerbaux A: Orthorhythmic pacing in cardiac arrhythmias [abstract]. Am J Cardiol 31:165, 1973.
27. Furman S: Therapeutic uses of atrial pacing. Am Heart J 86:835, 1973.
28. Escher DJW, Furman S: Emergency treatment of cardiac arrhythmias: Emphasis on use of electrical pacing. JAMA 214:2028, 1970.
29. Charos GS, Haffajee CI, Gold RL, et al: A theoretically and practically more effective method for interruption of ventricular tachycardia: Self-adapting autodecremental overdrive pacing. Circulation 73:309, 1986.
30. Gardner MJ, Waxman HL, Buxton AE, et al: Termination of tachycardia: Evaluation of a new pacing method. Am J Cardiol 50:1338, 1982.
31. Jantzer JH, Hoffman RM: Acceleration of ventricular tachycardia by rapid overdrive pacing combined with extrastimuli. PACE 7:922, 1984.
32. Fisher JD, Ostrow E, Kim SG, Matos JA: Ultrarapid single-capture train stimulation of termination of ventricular tachycardia. Am J Cardiol 51:1334, 1983.
33. Spurrell RAJ, Sowton E: Pacing techniques in the management of SVT. J Electrocardiol 8:287, 1975.
34. Holt P, Crick JCP, Sowton E: Antitachycardia pacing: A comparison of burst overdrive, self-searching, and adaptive table scanning programs. PACE 9:490, 1986.
35. den Dulk K, Kersschot IE, Brugada P, Wellens HJJ: Is there a universal antitachycardia pacing mode? Am J Cardiol 57:950, 1986.
36. den Dulk K, Della Bella P, Dassen W, et al: Antitachycardia pacing: Is there a universal pacing mode to terminate SVT? In Brugada P, Wellens HJJ (eds): Cardiac Arrhythmias: Where to Go From Here? Mt Kisko, NY, Futura Publishing, 1987, pp 285–295.
37. Smeets JLRM, den Dulk K, Brugada P, Wellens HJJ: Termination of spontaneous atrial flutter using the universal pacing mode [abstract]. Eur J Cardiol 9:348, 1988.

CHAPTER 38

Clinical Experience with Antitachycardia Pacing

Christopher A. Bonnet
Richard N. Fogoros

Although pharmacologic therapy has been the long-standing cornerstone of treatment for both supraventricular and ventricular arrhythmias, the perfect antiarrhythmic medication has yet to be developed. Recurrences of arrhythmias while the patient is receiving therapeutic doses of antiarrhythmic drugs, compliance problems, side effects, and cost have led researchers to explore nonpharmacologic methods to prevent and terminate recurrent tachyarrhythmias. The previous chapter described in detail the numerous pacing modalities that have been developed and the preimplant evaluation of a patient being considered for antitachycardia pacing. In this chapter, the history and clinical results of antitachycardia pacing for both supraventricular tachycardia (SVT) and ventricular tachycardia (VT) are discussed.

Antitachycardia Pacing for Supraventricular Tachycardia

HISTORY

The origin of antitachycardia pacing for the termination of a reentrant rhythm can be traced back to Mines'[1] description of circulating wavefronts in a fish heart preparation in 1914 as follows: ''The wave ran all the way around the ring and then continued to circulate going around about twice a second. After this had continued for 2 minutes extra stimuli were thrown in. After several attempts the wave was stopped. The preparation then remained at rest for 10 minutes. The circulating excitation was again started in the same way as before. This time there was considerable difficulty in stopping the wave. A number of attempts caused slowing of the wave in its passage over part of the course, but failed to

arrest it. Presently a single stimulus was so timed as to arrest the wave. The preparation then remained absolutely quiescent. There was no sign of 'automatic' rhythm throughout this experiment.''

The fact that appropriately timed stimuli could terminate arrhythmias remained a laboratory phenomenon until the first human electrophysiologic studies were performed in the late 1960s. Haft and associates[2] in 1967 reported the termination of atrial flutter by rapid electrical pacing of the atria. Durrer and colleagues[3] in the same year reported the termination of SVT in a patient with Wolff-Parkinson-White (WPW) syndrome by electrically induced atrial or ventricular premature beats.

These observations in the electrophysiology laboratory led to the first permanent antitachycardia pacemaker implant by Ryan and colleagues[4] in 1968. The patient was a 52-year-old woman with WPW syndrome who had experienced recurrent bouts of SVT for 15 years. She had received numerous antiarrhythmics, including procainamide, phenytoin, quinidine, digoxin, and propranolol, without successful suppression of her SVT. During the previous year, the patient had required approximately 20 emergency room visits and 11 hospital admissions for treatment of her SVT. She underwent numerous cardioversions and had become extremely reluctant to undergo further cardioversions. On May 8, 1968, the patient presented with SVT and hypotension refractory to pharmacologic therapy. Two temporary transvenous pacing leads were placed into the right atrium and right ventricle, and a mechanically induced premature ventricular contraction converted the SVT to sinus rhythm. The catheters were removed, and the patient was sent home. However, the patient returned 2 weeks later with another severe episode of SVT associated

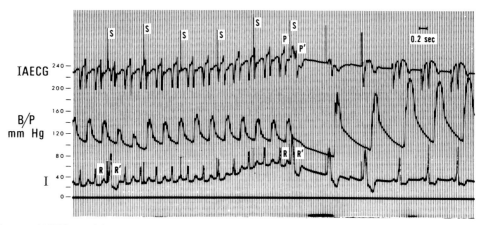

FIGURE 38–1. Simultaneous IAECG, arterial pressure, and lead I illustrating termination of supraventricular tachycardia by the sixth ventricular pacemaker stimulus (S). The first pacemaker stimulus resulted in a paced complex, but the R-R′ interval of 320 msec did not terminate the arrhythmia. However, the sixth pacemaker stimulus resulted in a shorter R-R′ interval of 280 msec and retrograde R′-P′ of 170 msec. This resulted in antegrade block over the AV node, terminating the macroreentrant tachycardia. IAECG, intra-atrial electrocardiogram. (From Ryan GF, Easley RM, Zaroff LI, et al: Paradoxical use of a demand pacemaker in treatment of supraventricular tachycardia due to the Wolff-Parkinson-White Syndrome. Circulation 38:1037, 1968. Reproduced with permission. Copyright 1968 American Heart Association.)

with hypotension. Two transvenous pacing leads were again placed into the right atrium and right ventricle. Using an external pacemaker generator attached to the indwelling lead, pacemaker stimuli were delivered at a rate of 75 beats per minute (bpm) through the right ventricular endocardial lead. This resulted in competitive underdrive ventricular pacing and reverted the SVT back to sinus rhythm (Fig. 38–1).

Subsequently, a permanent endocardial electrode was implanted in the right ventricular apex and attached to a demand pacemaker. This pacemaker had the ability to change from a demand mode to fixed-rate pacing with the application of an external magnet. Thus, whenever SVT recurred, the patient placed a magnet over the pacemaker and caused fixed-rate pacing. Eventually, an appropriately timed stimulus would capture the ventricle and terminate the tachycardia (Fig. 38–2). A follow-up report on this patient was published by Barold and associates[5] in 1989. The patient continued to have frequent recurrent attacks of SVT. She terminated an average of two to three attacks of SVT daily with external application of the magnet over her pulse generator. She did this for 12 years until she eventually died of congestive heart failure.

For the next several years, permanent demand pacemakers were used sporadically in the treatment of SVT. A major problem with this approach was that it required a great deal of input from the patient. The patient had to be able to determine accurately whether the tachycardia had recurred, to tolerate the tachycardia sufficiently and have the presence

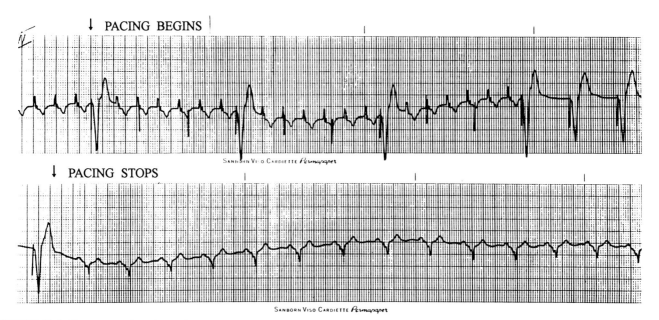

FIGURE 38–2. The upper portion of a continuous lead II recording shows competitive underdrive ventricular pacing at approximately 70 bpm during SVT. The fourth captured ventricular complex results in the termination of the SVT. The magnet was removed after conversion, and sinus rhythm with preexcited complexes can be seen in the lower recording. SVT, supraventricular tachycardia. (From Ryan GF, Easley RM, Zaroff LI, et al: Paradoxical use of a demand pacemaker in treatment of supraventricular tachycardia due to the Wolff-Parkinson-White syndrome. Circulation 38:1037, 1968. Reproduced with permission. Copyright 1968 American Heart Association.)

of mind to apply the magnet to the generator, and to be able to tell when the arrhythmia was terminated so that the magnet could be removed. All these requirements made early attempts at antitachycardia pacing cumbersome.

The early 1970s ushered in the widespread use of electrophysiologic studies to evaluate patients with SVT. It became clear that regular SVTs from entities such as WPW, atrioventricular (AV) node reentry, atrial tachycardia, and atrial flutter could be terminated by appropriately timed electrical extrastimuli delivered near the reentrant circuit (either atrium or ventricle). These observations, coupled with advances in pacemaker design and technology, paved the way for automatic permanent pacemakers that could both sense and terminate tachyarrhythmias without the need for active intervention. The first report of the use of such a device was by Krikler and coworkers[6] in 1976. These authors described two patients with WPW syndrome who had reciprocating AV tachycardia that could be easily and reliably terminated with single premature beats delivered in the right ventricle (patient 1) or coronary sinus (patient 2). Both patients were treated with permanent pacemakers, which had been modified to behave as fixed-rate pacemakers at 70 bpm whenever the sensed heart rate exceeded 150 bpm or fell below 70 bpm. During SVT, asynchronous pacing occurred until an appropriately timed premature stimulus terminated the tachycardia. Such pacemakers, which were labeled "dual-demand" pacemakers, represented the next advance in permanent implantable antitachycardia devices.

In the late 1970s, the widespread use of investigational automatic implantable pacemakers for the treatment of SVT began. The use of programmable antitachycardia pacemakers flourished over the next few years.

POWER SOURCES

Early antitachycardia pacing used one of two basic power sources. The most widely used was an implanted pacemaker that could be either activated by external application of a magnet or programmed to an automatic mode that did not require manual intervention. A second available power source was a hand-held induction coil or radio-frequency unit that would transmit preset stimulation sequences to an implanted receiver attached to an endocardial electrode. The major advantage of this latter system was size, because the implanted receivers were much smaller than the early implanted pacemaker generators. The major disadvantage was that manual intervention was always required.

PROGRAMMABILITY

As previously described, the earliest antitachycardia pacemakers were asynchronous underdrive pacemakers, which operated either manually or automatically. Although asynchronous underdrive pacing was effective in some patients, it was ineffective in many. More effective modes of pacing, such as timed extrastimuli and overdrive pacing with numerous coupled extrastimuli at fixed or decremental intervals, were eventually incorporated into antitachycardia pacemakers. Figure 38–3 shows a burst of rapid atrial pacing terminating an episode of SVT. In addition, newer algorithms allowed the pacemaker to attempt one pacing sequence and, if this was unsuccessful, then to change to a different, often more aggressive sequence. Backup bradycardia pacing was always available, and technologic advances allowed some devices to store in their internal memory information related to sensed events and therapies delivered. An example of programmable parameters used in one antitachycardia pacemaker is shown in Figure 38–4. Using this pacemaker requires programming of a backup bradycardia pacing rate, a tachycardia recognition rate and count (i.e., the number of beats faster than the recognition rate required to initiate antitachycardia pacing), a mechanism of antitachycardia pacing (i.e., timed extrastimuli, burst scanning, etc.), minimum and maximum rapid pacing intervals, the number of impulses to be delivered, the scan delta (i.e., the change in milliseconds between each pacing sequence), the number of ramp steps, and the total number of attempts at overdrive pacing. Obviously, programming of an antitachycardia pacemaker can become complex.

Also shown in Figure 38–4 is a printout of the stored memory from this device listing all tachycardia events for the previous 98 days. In this example, the patient had one episode of a tachyarrhythmia during the last 98 days. The maximum rate of the tachyarrhythmia was 148 bpm, and the duration was 4 seconds. The episode had not occurred during the last 48 hours, as documented by the short-term monitors.

The description cited describes one device from one company. Numerous devices that have been developed and used

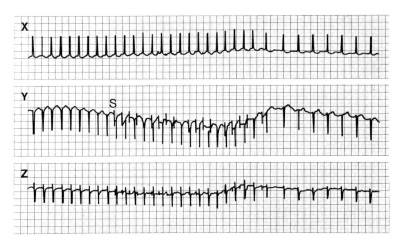

FIGURE 38–3. A simultaneous three-lead electrocardiogram from a patient with recurrent SVT. An automatic pacemaker detects the SVT and delivers a burst of atrial pacing (S) that terminates the arrhythmia and restores sinus rhythm. SVT, supraventricular tachycardia. (From Holmes DR: Pacing for tachycardia. *In* Furman S, Hayes DL, Holmes DR [eds]: A Practice of Cardiac Pacing, 2nd ed. Mt Kisco, NY, Futura Publishing, 1989, p 471.)

PROGRAMMED VALUES

PACING VALUES		ANTI-TACHYCARDIA VALUES	
PACING MODE:	VVI	MECHANISM:	BURST SCANNING
MINIMUM RATE:	50 PPM	MIN. BURST INTERVAL:	220 MSEC
REFRACTORY:	300 MSEC	PRESENT INTERVAL:	240 MSEC
SENSITIVITY:	1.5 MV	MAX. BURST INTERVAL:	320 MSEC
PULSE DURATION:	1.0 MSEC	SCAN DELTA:	8 MSEC
POLARITY:	BIPOLAR	NO. OF PULSES:	8
HYSTERESIS:	0 MSEC	RAMP STEPS:	0 MSEC
MAGNET MODE:	VVT	NO. OF ATTEMPTS:	INFINITE
MAGNET RATE:	30 PPM	**TACHYCARDIA RECOGNITION**	
MAGNET REFRACTORY:	300 MSEC	RATE:	125 BPM
		COUNT:	10

PACING MONITORS
(DATA COLLECTED FROM PACER TELEMETRY)

TIME PERIOD		AVG. RATE (BPM)	PERCENT SENSED	NUMBER OF EPISODES	MAX. DURATION (SECONDS)	MAX. RATE (BPM)
LAST	98 DAY(S)	73	100.0	1	4	148
LAST	161 MIN.	79	100.0	0	0	97
PREVIOUS	4 HOURS	69	100.0	0	0	94
4 -	8 HOURS	69	100.0	0	0	83
8 -	12 HOURS	67	100.0	0	0	86
12 -	16 HOURS	73	100.0	0	0	94
16 -	20 HOURS	75	100.0	0	0	97
20 -	24 HOURS	74	100.0	0	0	107
24 -	28 HOURS	70	100.0	0	0	100
28 -	32 HOURS	72	100.0	0	0	83
32 -	36 HOURS	70	100.0	0	0	87
36 -	40 HOURS	73	100.0	0	0	89
40 -	44 HOURS	73	100.0	0	0	88
44 -	48 HOURS	77	100.0	0	0	93

FIGURE 38–4. A printout from an antitachycardia pacemaker programmer illustrating the numerous programmable parameters and memory for sensed events.

for antitachycardia pacing in SVT are shown in Table 38–1. Many have capabilities similar to the pacemaker described.

CLINICAL RESULTS

As the use of antitachycardia pacemakers became widespread in the late 1970s, reports on the clinical results with these devices began to fill the literature. However, interpreting and comparing the reports from different implanting centers is extremely difficult. The majority of the published reports describe fewer than 10 patients, and many deal with an isolated case report. Preimplant and postimplant evaluations varied widely from center to center, as did the types of SVT treated, the locations of the implanted pacing leads, and concomitant antiarrhythmic therapy. In addition, as described in the last chapter and in an extensive review by Fisher and associates,[8] numerous antitachycardia pacing techniques were used. These include underdrive pacing, programmed extrastimuli (PES) or scanning methods, ultrarapid train stimulation, multiple PES, burst pacing, burst plus PES, ramp pacing, changing ramps, adaptive bursts, shifting bursts, scanning bursts (concertina/accordion), scanning bursts with ramp pacing, incremental-decremental (centrifugal) scan, and adaptive pacing with changes in the number of stimuli. Although some authors[9] have addressed whether any one technique may be a "universal" antitachycardia pacing mode, the preferred pacing method usually varies from patient to patient and center to center. Keeping these significant limitations in mind, Table 38–2 reviews studies in the literature involving at least 10 patients with permanent implanted antitachycardia pacemakers for the treatment of SVT.[10–24]

Generally, most studies report good results with these implanted antitachycardia devices. The initial efficacy appears to be high at approximately 90% at 1 year. The long-term results also appear to be favorable, with one series[18] reporting a 78% efficacy at 5 years. As seen in Table 38–2, from 19% to 66% of the patients required concomitant antiarrhythmic drug therapy. Generally, the results were considered poor in a minority of patients, although a few series reported poor results in as many as 64% of the patients.[20] Poor results were usually considered to be the failure of the implanted pacemaker to quickly and reliably terminate the SVT, or the induction of atrial fibrillation or flutter by rapid atrial pacing. Sudden deaths were relatively rare but were reported.[25] Proposed potential mechanisms for sudden death were the induction of atrial fibrillation in patients with WPW syndrome and an accessory pathway capable of rapid antegrade conduction with degeneration to ventricular fibrillation or the induction of VT or ventricular fibrillation by premature ventricular stimuli if the lead was implanted in the ventricle.

Given the limitations of the published reports, antitachycardia pacing can be considered reasonably safe and effective for the treatment of refractory SVT in a selected patient population.

PACING TO PREVENT SUPRAVENTRICULAR TACHYCARDIA

Our discussion so far has focused on the termination of SVT should it recur. However, investigators have also evaluated pacing methods for preventing SVT. Coumel and co-workers[26] in 1967 documented that simultaneous pacing of

TABLE 38–1. ANTITACHYCARDIA PACEMAKERS

MANUALLY ACTIVATED PACEMAKERS		
MANUFACTURER	MODEL	COMMENTS
Medtronic (Minneapolis, MN)	5842	Underdrive pacing during magnet application
Medtronic	5998	Burst pacing with external radio-frequency transmitter application
Medtronic	SPO500	Burst pacing with external radio-frequency transmitter application
Cordis (Miami, FL)	Omni-Orthocor 234A or 239A	Timed extrastimuli or burst pacing during external overdriver application

AUTOMATIC PACEMAKERS		
MANUFACTURER	MODEL	COMMENTS
Ela (Minnetonka, MN)	Stanium	Dual-demand AAT or VVT
Medtronic	Symbios 7008	Overdrive atrial burst or underdrive atrioventricular dual-demand pacing
Medtronic	DVI, MN	Dual-demand atrioventricular sequential pacing
Intermedics (Angleton, TX)	Cybertach-60 (262-01)	Burst pacing
Intermedics	Intertach 262-12, 262-14	Fixed, adaptive, scanning, and autodecremental burst pacing
Telectronics (Englewood, CO)	PASAR 4151–4171	Timed extrastimuli, fixed or burst scanning modes of pacing
Siemens-Elema (Solna, Sweden)	Tachylog 651B	Timed extrastimuli, burst or scanning modes of pacing
Cordis	Orthocor II 284 A	Timed extrastimuli, burst scanning, and ramp pacing

both the atrium and ventricle (DOO) was effective in preventing AV nodal reentrant tachycardia. In 1976, Spurrell and Sowton[27] showed that AV nodal reentrant SVT could be prevented by an atrial triggered ventricular pacemaker (VAT) with a short AV delay. Sung and associates[28] in 1980 used simultaneous AV sequential pacing (DDT) for the prevention of reentrant supraventricular tachycardia. Portillo and colleagues[29] in 1982 used dual-demand AV sequential (DVI, MN) pacing to suppress SVT. Although these various pacing methods were shown to be effective, the essentially simultaneous AV stimulation can lead to several potential adverse effects. These include hemodynamic compromise, risk of rapid ventricular rates should atrial fibrillation or flutter occur, and the risk of possible VT induction by closely coupled triggered ventricular stimulation. Because of these potential difficulties, dual-chamber pacing to prevent SVT has only rarely been used clinically.

FUTURE CONSIDERATIONS

The major indications for antitachycardia pacing in SVT were for the treatment of AV nodal reentrant and WPW macroreentrant tachycardias. However, recent nonpharmacologic advances, which have resulted in "cures" of these arrhythmias, have largely rendered antitachycardia pacing for SVT an outdated and little used modality. Initially, surgical interruption or cryoablation of the accessory pathways in WPW or AV node reentry led to a high permanent cure rate from SVT, but the use of surgery was limited by the need for a thoracotomy. The recent advent of catheter ablative techniques, initially using direct-current energy and more recently radio-frequency energy, have made catheter ablation the first-line therapy for many reentrant SVTs. The success rates of these procedures are high, and the risk is low, making antitachycardia pacing (which merely treats recurrences and does not prevent or cure an arrhythmia) virtually obsolete.

Antitachycardia pacing also has been used in treating atrial flutter.[30, 31] However, the need for concomitant antiarrhythmic therapy in these patients is very high, and bouts of recurrent atrial flutter are frequent. In addition, reports on ablative techniques resulting in cures of this arrhythmia have also started to surface in the literature. Thus, antitachycardia pacing for atrial flutter is also a treatment of the past.

These advances in curative therapies for SVT led most pacemaker companies to abandon research and product development in this area and to remove most of these investigational devices from clinical trials. At this time, the patient population considered appropriate for antitachycardia pacing to terminate SVT is virtually nonexistent.

Antitachycardia Pacing for Ventricular Tachycardia

The development of antitachycardia pacing for the treatment of VT can be divided into two areas: prevention and termination.

PREVENTION

Using pacing to prevent VT had its beginning in 1960 when Zoll and associates[32] reported on four patients who had been resuscitated from ventricular fibrillation and were supported with external cardiac pacing. At electrically paced heart rates greater than 40 bpm, there were no recurrences of VT, but slowing the external pacemaker to rates of less than 40 bpm resulted in ventricular ectopy, which eventually degenerated to ventricular fibrillation. The use of an implanted permanent ventricular pacemaker to prevent recurrent VT was first reported by Dressler[33] in 1964. In 19 patients who had AV block resulting in VT and syncope, permanent ventricular pacing at rates greater than 60 bpm prevented recurrent VT in 15 of the 19 patients. Thus, permanent pacing can prevent VT if severe underlying bradycardia triggers the VT. Such patients, however, make up only a small percentage of the entire patient population with VT.

Although initial reports suggested that overdrive pacing suppressed spontaneous ventricular ectopy when used in patients with malignant ventricular arrhythmias,[34, 35] long-term

TABLE 38–2. **ANTITACHYCARDIA PACING FOR SUPRAVENTRICULAR TACHYCARDIA**

FIRST AUTHOR (REF. NO.)	NO. OF PATIENTS	PACER MODEL[a]	CONCOMITANT ANTIARRHYTHMIC DRUGS (%)	FOLLOW-UP (MONTHS)	RESULTS		SUDDEN DEATHS
					GOOD	POOR	
Kahn (10)	12	5998	66	15–36	10		
Griffin (11)	91	Cybertach	NS	22	82% alive and using device		
Spurrell (12)	21	PASAR	38	2–40	16		2
Zipes (13)	21	Symbios 7008	NS	NS	21		
Rothman (14)	16	Omni-Orthocor	NS	1–40	14	2	
Sowton (15)	16	Tachylog	19	5–19	14	2	
Peters (16)	10	5998	40	24–60	7	3	
Bertholet (17)	13	PASAR, SPO500	38	5–30	10	3	
Fisher (18)	16	NS	NS	6–177	16		
Moller (19)	13	PASAR	61	4–53	12	1	
Schnittger (20)	11	Cybertach	36	64–108	4	7	
Kappenberger (21)	63	Tachylog	49	30	59	4	
Shandling (22)	17	Intertach	NS	20	17		
Fromer (23)	12	Intertach	33	30	9	2	
den Dulk (24)	40	SPO 500, Orthocor, Intertach	42	38	34	6	

Abbreviation: NS, not stated.
[a]See Table 38–1 for names and addresses of manufacturers.

results using overdrive pacing for suppressing VT were poor.[36, 37] Therefore, overdrive pacing has fallen out of use, except in patients with prolonged QT intervals. Pacing in these patients has been shown to be beneficial, resulting in a marked reduction in recurrent VT.[38]

Several other types of ventricular pacing have been used in an effort to prevent the initiation of VT. These include premature subthreshold stimulation during the effective refractory period,[39] annihilation using critically timed subthreshold or hyperpolarizing stimulation,[40] and high current strength pacing at the site of origin of the tachycardia.[41] To date, none of these techniques has been shown to be reliable enough to be incorporated into the clinical management of VT. Although to prevent an arrhythmia is much more desirable than to treat an arrhythmia after it has occurred, no antitachycardia pacing modality is clinically useful for the prevention of VT, aside from the small subset of patients whose VT is secondary to severe bradycardia or prolonged QT intervals.

TERMINATION

The use of electrical ventricular pacing to terminate VT dates back to the early 1970s. Bennett and Pentecost[42] described four patients with recurrent VT in whom temporary ventricular pacing at rates faster than the VT resulted in the termination of the VT. The work of Wellens and associates[43, 44] further advanced the understanding of reentry as the primary mechanism of recurrent VT. These investigators documented that single or double extrastimuli could reproducibly initiate and terminate VT in patients presenting with VT. The finding that single premature ventricular stimuli could terminate VT was taken from the electrophysiology laboratory and used clinically by Moss and Rivers[45] in 1974. These investigators reported the use of a permanently implanted VVI pacemaker to terminate recurrent VT in a 61-year-old man with a prior anteroseptal myocardial infarction. In 1971, the patient began having recurrent hemodynamically well-tolerated VT, which required repeated hospitalization for pharmacologic or electrical cardioversion. Despite antiarrhythmic therapy, the episodes became more frequent over the next 2 years. In Sep-

tember 1973, an episode of sustained VT was terminated by placing a transvenous pacing electrode in the right ventricle and mechanically inducing premature ventricular beats. Subsequently, a permanent pacemaker was implanted and programmed to the VVI mode at 64 bpm. The patient had a recurrent episode of VT 1 month later and reported to the emergency room. Application of the magnet resulted in the termination of his VT by a single premature ventricular paced beat (Fig. 38–5). The era of implantable devices for the treatment of VT was thus begun.

As was the case with SVT, more aggressive pacing techniques were more effective than asynchronous underdrive pacing for terminating the VT and restoring sinus rhythm. In the electrophysiology laboratory and in acutely ill patients with recurrent VT, various pacing techniques delivered through temporary endocardial electrodes were proven to be both safe and highly efficacious in terminating recurrent VT.[46] These pacing algorithms were then incorporated into automatic implantable devices. An example of using burst ventricular pacing to terminate VT is shown in Figure 38–6.

DEVICES

The devices used for antitachycardia pacing in VT were the same as those used for SVT and are listed in Table 38–1. The earliest antitachycardia pacemakers were nonautomatic and required manual intervention by either the patient or physician to initiate ventricular pacing. Because of concern over the possible acceleration of VT to a more rapid hemodynamically unstable VT or degeneration to ventricular fibrillation, patients initially were always instructed to visit the emergency room where they could be monitored while the pacemaker was activated. However, as clinical experience with antitachycardia pacing in VT grew, antitachycardia pacemakers capable of automatically recognizing and treating VT began to be implanted.

CLINICAL RESULTS

Published reports dealing with antitachycardia pacing for VT usually describe small numbers of patients and only

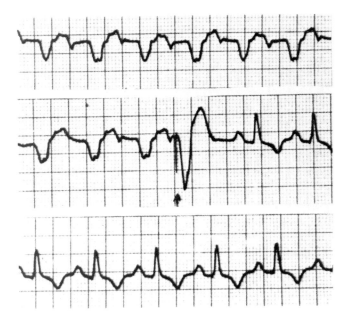

FIGURE 38–5. Lead II rhythm strips illustrating termination of VT by underdrive asynchronous ventricular pacing. *Top*, VT is present at 115 bpm with apparent retrograde P waves. *Middle*, A brief application of an external magnet over the implanted pacemaker results in a single ventricular pacemaker-induced complex *(arrow)*, which terminates the VT and restores sinus rhythm, *Bottom*, Sinus rhythm at 90 bpm. VT, ventricular tachycardia. (From Moss AJ, Rivers RJ: Termination and inhibition of recurrent tachycardias by implanted pervenous pacemakers. Circulation 50:942, 1974. Reproduced with permission. Copyright 1974 American Heart Association.)

poorly document the preimplant and postimplant evaluations of those patients. Furthermore, these reports typically are focused on a particular antitachycardia pacemaker and include patients treated for both SVT and VT. To split out the group treated for VT alone is often difficult. Many of the patients in these reports are receiving concomitant antiarrhythmic therapy. In addition, the pacing sequences used vary widely from center to center, making comparisons difficult. Thus, drawing generally applicable conclusions from these studies is difficult. Table 38–3 lists published studies of antitachycardia pacing for the treatment of VT that include five or more patients.[11, 14–16, 18, 47, 48]

These studies suggest that the use of permanent antitachycardia pacemakers for the management of VT was reasonably effective. Most studies reported poor results in relatively few patients treated with these pacemakers, although Peters and associates[16] reported poor results in five of their six patients (two of whom experienced pacemaker-induced acceleration

of their VT and three of whom were considered to have become refractory to pacing). Early studies only rarely reported sudden death possibly related to the pacemaker, but the two large multicenter studies of Griffin and coworkers[11] and Rothman and colleagues[14] did raise this concern. Griffin's group[11] reported on 52 patients treated with an antitachycardia pacer, and in this series, four sudden deaths occurred. In Rothman's series[14] of 53 patients, three sudden deaths and three documented deaths from VT and ventricular fibrillation occurred. Fisher and associates[49] also raised significant concerns regarding potential acceleration of stable well-tolerated VT to hemodynamically unstable more rapid VT or ventricular fibrillation with stimulation sequences delivered by antitachycardia pacemakers. These studies made it clear that backup defibrillation would be necessary if antitachycardia pacing for VT was to be considered safe and applicable to a large number of patients.

Although our understanding of the mechanisms of VT has progressed rapidly in the last two decades, it is obvious that much is still left to be learned. The following example of a case from our laboratory early in our experience with antitachycardia pacing demonstrates this point. A patient who had suffered numerous recurrences of hemodynamically stable VT refractory to pharmacologic therapy was referred for an antitachycardia pacemaker. After electrophysiologic testing, an antitachycardia pacemaker in combination with an implantable cardioverter-defibrillator (ICD) was recommended, but the patient steadfastly refused to consider a thoracotomy for an ICD and wished to be evaluated for an antitachycardia pacemaker alone. With this goal in mind, further testing was performed during treatment with procainamide, a drug that had slowed the patient's inducible VT. For testing, a temporary right ventricular lead was connected to an external stimulator for the induction of VT and also to an external model of an antitachycardia pacemaker, which could be activated after the VT was induced. On the first day of preimplant testing, 50 episodes of monomorphic VT were induced, with rates of 120 to 140 bpm. Activation of the external pacemaker successfully terminated all 50 episodes with eight beat bursts of ventricular pacing. No episodes of acceleration of VT occurred. The following day the patient was brought back to the laboratory, and another 10 episodes of similar, well-tolerated VT were induced. These were again easily terminated by the external antitachycardia pacemaker. A permanent antitachycardia pacemaker was subsequently implanted without difficulty. The plan was to program the pacemaker to a nonautomatic mode. If VT were to recur, the plan was for the patient to go to the nearest emergency room

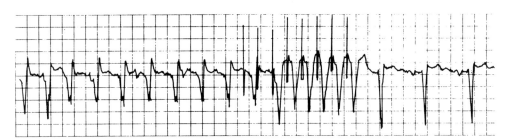

FIGURE 38–6 Monomorphic VT at a rate of 135 bpm is seen on the left. A burst of ventricular pacing results in the termination of the VT. VT, ventricular tachycardia. (From Bonnet CA, Fogoros RN, Elson JJ, et al: Long-term efficacy of an antitachycardia pacemaker and implantable defibrillator combination. PACE 14:814, 1991.)

TABLE 38-3. **ANTITACHYCARDIA PACING FOR VENTRICULAR TACHYCARDIA**

FIRST AUTHOR (REF. NO.)	NO. OF PATIENTS	PACER MODEL[a]	CONCOMITANT ANTIARRHYTHMIC DRUGS (%)	FOLLOW-UP (MONTHS)	RESULTS		
					GOOD	POOR	SUDDEN DEATHS
Griffin (11)	52	Cybertach	NS	13	58% alive with active device		4
Rothman (14)	53	Omni-Orthocor	NS	16	82% tachy termination		6
Sowton (15)	9	Tachylog	33%	10	5		
Peters (16)	6	5998	100%	16	1	5	3
Fisher (18)	20	NS	NS	37	18	2	4
den Dulk (47)	6	SPO 500	83%	15	6		
Herre (48)	28	Omni-Orthocor, 5998	64%	1–25	95% success in 9 patients		1

Abbreviation: NS, not stated.
[a]See Table 38–1 for names and addresses of manufacturers.

to be monitored and then apply an external unit over his pacemaker to deliver preset bursts of ventricular pacing.

Prior to hospital discharge, the patient returned to the electrophysiology laboratory for final testing. Monomorphic VT that was hemodynamically stable was easily induced, and on seven consecutive inductions, the patient was able to place and activate his external unit, resulting in overdrive pacing and termination of his VT (Fig. 38–7). However, on the eighth induction, a much more rapid VT (at approximately 210 bpm) was initiated. This VT had never been seen clinically or in the electrophysiology laboratory previously. The induction of this VT is shown in Figure 38–8. The patient became hypotensive, lightheaded, and presyncopal; yet, he was able to place his external unit over the pacemaker generator and activate it. A burst of ventricular pacing at nearly the identical rate as the tachycardia disrupted the rapid VT and restored sinus rhythm (Fig. 38–9). After experiencing this symptomatic rapid VT, the patient agreed to have a backup ICD, which was subsequently implanted without complication. The postimplant evaluation revealed normal function of both devices, and he was discharged home.

During the next 5 months, the patient had 10 episodes of VT, which were minimally symptomatic and terminated appropriately by the antitachycardia pacemaker. However, 5

months after the implant, he returned to our emergency room with lightheadedness and was found to be in sustained VT at approximately 170 bpm. His serum procainamide levels were therapeutic and similar to those at the time of the initial implant. The antitachycardia pacemaker was sensing the VT appropriately and delivering burst ventricular pacing as programmed, but it could not terminate the VT (Fig. 38–10). The patient's nonprogrammable ICD rate cutoff was 203 bpm. Thus, the VT was under the recognition rate of the ICD, and it would not fire. Reprogramming of the antitachycardia pacemaker to more rapid bursting intervals resulted in a restoration of sinus rhythm. This case illustrates the difficulty often encountered in attempts to use antitachycardia pacing to terminate VT, and the potential need for backup defibrillation despite extensive preimplant testing.

GUIDELINES FOR IMPLANTATION OF AN ANTITACHYCARDIA PACEMAKER

Although ablative techniques have made antitachycardia pacing for SVT virtually obsolete and the risk of VT accel-

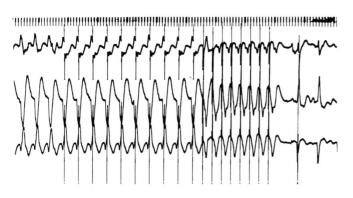

RJ2

FIGURE 38–7. On the left, ventricular tachycardia at approximately 130 bpm is seen. With the application of the external overdriver unit, the pacemaker changes to the VVT mode, and pacemaker stimuli can be seen in each QRS complex. The patient then manually activates the external unit, which results in an eight-beat burst of ventricular pacing, terminating the ventricular tachycardia.

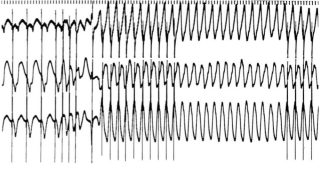

RJ3

FIGURE 38–8. With the external overdriver in place over the implanted pacemaker, programmed stimulation was performed through the device and is shown on the left. Three premature stimuli result in the induction of a very rapid monomorphic ventricular tachycardia at approximately 210 bpm. The patient initially removes the external overdriver from over the pacemaker, causing the pacemaker to revert from the VVT mode to VVI mode (loss of pacemaker stimuli in QRS complexes). This is followed by reapplication on the far right of the monitor strip, reinitiating the VVT mode (pacemaker stimuli are again seen in the QRS complexes) prior to proceeding with burst pacing.

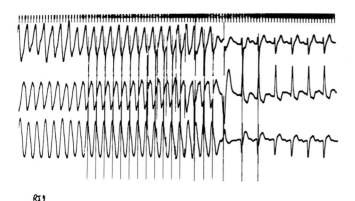

FIGURE 38–9. A continuation of the monitor strip seen in Figure 38–8. With reapplication of the external overdriver, the implanted pacemaker reverts to the VVT mode. The patient then activates the external overdriver, resulting in burst pacing, which terminates the ventricular tachycardia and restores sinus rhythm.

eration has made the use of an antitachycardia pacemaker for VT without backup defibrillation rare, occasional patients can still be considered appropriate candidates for treatment with permanent pacemakers to prevent or terminate tachyarrhythmias. An American College of Cardiology/American Heart Association Task Force[50] published guidelines for the implantation of cardiac pacemakers in the treatment of tachyarrhythmias. They broke down the indications into three classes. Class I indications are ''conditions for which there is general agreement that permanent pacemakers or antitachycardia devices should be implanted.'' Class II indications are ''conditions for which permanent pacemakers or antitachycardia devices are frequently used but there is divergence of opinion with respect to the necessity of their insertion.'' Class III indications are ''conditions for which there is general agreement that pacemakers or antitachycardia devices are unnecessary.''

INDICATIONS FOR PERMANENT PACEMAKERS THAT AUTOMATICALLY DETECT AND PACE TO TERMINATE TACHYCARDIAS

CLASS I

1. Symptomatic recurrent SVT when drugs fail to control the arrhythmia or produce intolerable side effects.

2. Symptomatic recurrent VT after an automatic defibrillator has been implanted or incorporated in the device and recurrence of VT is not prevented by drug therapy or when no other therapy is applicable.

CLASS II

1. Recurrent SVT as an alternative to drug therapy.

CLASS III

1. Tachycardias that are accelerated or converted to fibrillation by pacing.
2. The presence of accessory pathways that have the capacity for rapid anterograde conduction whether or not the pathways participate in the mechanism of the tachycardia.

INDICATIONS FOR EXTERNALLY MANUALLY ACTIVATED ANTITACHYARRHYTHMIA DEVICES THAT ACT TO TERMINATE TACHYCARDIAS

CLASS I

1. Recurrent, symptomatic VT uncontrolled by drugs when surgery, catheter ablation, or the implantation of an automatic ICD is not indicated.

CLASS III

1. Recurrent tachycardia that produces syncope.

INDICATIONS FOR OVERDRIVE OR ATRIAL SYNCHRONOUS VENTRICULAR PACEMAKERS INTENDED TO PREVENT TACHYCARDIA OCCURRENCE

CLASS I

1. AV reentrant or AV node reentrant SVT not responsive to medical therapy.

CLASS II

1. Sustained VT in other conditions when all other therapies are ineffective or inapplicable and the efficacy of pacing is thoroughly documented.
2. Long QT syndrome.

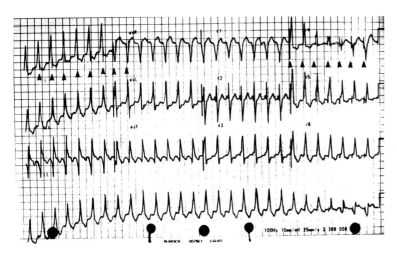

FIGURE 38–10. A 12-lead electrocardiogram reveals monomorphic ventricular tachycardia at approximately 170 bpm. The *arrows* in the top tracing show ventricular stimuli from the antitachycardia pacemaker, which fail to terminate the ventricular tachycardia.

CLASS III

1. Frequent or complex ventricular ectopic activity without sustained VT associated with coronary artery disease, cardiomyopathy, mitral valve prolapse, or a normal heart and in the absence of the long QT syndrome.
2. The long QT syndrome as a result of remediable causes.

ANTITACHYCARDIA PACEMAKERS IN COMBINATION WITH IMPLANTABLE CARDIOVERTER-DEFIBRILLATORS

The first human implantation of an ICD occurred in 1980.[51] During the next few years, the ICD was shown to be effective in terminating recurrent VT and ventricular fibrillation. Although the ICD can easily terminate recurrent hemodynamically stable VT, the shock is discomforting to an awake patient. Thus, the concept of combining an antitachycardia pacemaker that could terminate well-tolerated VT painlessly with a backup ICD at a higher rate cutoff to terminate unstable ventricular arrhythmias was an extremely attractive one.

The use of antitachycardia pacemakers plus ICDs was first reported by Luderitz and associates[52] in 1986. They reported on six patients who, during a follow-up period of 12 months, had 700 episodes of VT terminated with a total of 88 ICD discharges recorded. Greve and colleagues[53] reported their results of combined therapy in 11 patients. Two of the 11 died of congestive heart failure soon after the implantation of their devices. The remaining nine patients experienced an average of seven episodes of VT monthly, and approximately one half of these episodes required termination by an ICD discharge. Newman and associates[54] then described their experiences in eight patients with antitachycardia pacemakers and ICDs followed for a mean of 12 months. Seven of the eight patients used antitachycardia pacing to terminate recurrent VT during the follow-up period (the total number of episodes of VT was not reported). Twenty-three ICD discharges occurred in three patients, but only 2 of the 23 were considered appropriate. One of the eight patients died from congestive heart failure 3 months postimplant. Masterson and coworkers[55] reported on the clinical outcomes of 10 patients who received the antitachycardia pacemaker and ICD combination. During a mean follow-up of 8 months, 1542 episodes of VT were treated, and 179 ICD discharges occurred. Five of the 10 patients died during the follow-up period, three of them suddenly.

These initial reports suggested that the combination of an antitachycardia pacemaker and an ICD could effectively terminate frequent episodes of recurrent VT, but the relatively frequent ICD discharges and significant early mortality rate were of concern. It appeared that many of the patients described in these reports received the antitachycardia pacemaker as a therapy of last resort, only after ICD therapy alone was unsatisfactory, and not as first-line therapy. Our group subsequently reported on 14 patients with recurrent, well-tolerated VT in whom antitachycardia pacing was considered first-line therapy.[56] The pacemaker was intended as primary therapy for VT, and the ICD was intended as a backup should an acceleration of VT occur. Prior to implantation, each patient underwent at least 50 inductions of sustained VT in the electrophysiology laboratory, each of which was terminated by an external model of the antitachycardia pacemaker attached to a temporary indwelling endocardial lead. The patients then underwent a permanent antitachycardia pacemaker and ICD combination implantation only after the external version of the pacemaker was documented to easily and reliably terminate VT, without causing significant acceleration of the VT or degeneration to an unstable arrhythmia. The ICDs implanted had high-rate cutoffs (191 ± 12 bpm) because they were intended to act solely as a backup should unstable arrhythmias occur. During a mean follow-up of 25 months, more than 6000 episodes of VT were treated in these 14 patients. Ten of the 14 patients received a total of 103 discharges from their ICDs during the follow-up period. Despite extensive preimplant testing, acceleration of VT did occur as a result of burst pacing. An example of this is shown in Figure 38–11.

Thus, these studies suggested that, in highly selected patients, an antitachycardia pacemaker and ICD combination could be effective and relatively safe. Although these early studies were promising, implanting two separate electrical devices was often challenging. As discussed in the next chapter, interactions between two electrical devices with individual sensing and energy delivery systems are frequent and require extensive testing during and after implantation to ensure that both systems function appropriately together.

Recognizing these difficulties, several companies began developing devices combining antitachycardia pacing, cardioversion, defibrillation, and bradycardia pacing all in one generator. At this time, several of these systems are undergoing clinical investigation, and the initial results are promising.[57-61] Table 38–4 lists combination antitachycardia pacemakers and defibrillators presently undergoing clinical investigation. Several of these combination devices have recently received approval from the Food and Drug Adminstration and been released to the market.

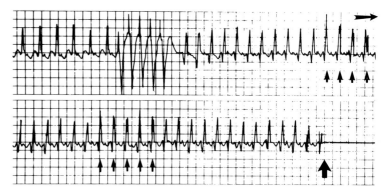

FIGURE 38–11. On the left portion of the upper monitor recording, VT at a rate of 145 bpm is present. A 5-beat burst from the antitachycardia pacemaker at the minimum burst pacing interval accelerates the VT to a rate of 185 bpm. The pacemaker continues to sense VT above its recognition rate and recycles from its minimum burst pacing interval to the maximum burst pacing interval, but repeat bursts of pacing from the pacemaker fail to capture *(small arrows)*. Because the rate of the VT is above the implantable defibrillator rate cutoff, a discharge from the defibrillator is delivered *(large arrow)*. VT, ventricular tachycardia. (From Bonnet CA, Fogoros RN, Elson JJ, et al: Long-term efficacy of an antitachycardia pacemaker and implantable defibrillator combination. PACE 14:814, 1991.)

TABLE 38–4. DEVICES UNDERGOING CLINICAL INVESTIGATION THAT OFFER ANTITACHYCARDIA PACING, BRADYCARDIA PACING, AND LOW- AND HIGH-ENERGY CARDIOVERSION

MANUFACTURER	MODEL
CPI (St. Paul, MN)	PR$_x$[a], PRx II
Intermedics	PCD 7217[a], 7219
Medtronic	PCD[a]
Siemens-Pacesetter	Siecure
Telectronics	Guardian ATP 4210, 4211
Ventritex (Sunnyvale, CA)	Cadence[a]

[a]Approved by the Food and Drug Administration and released to the market.

LIMITATIONS OF ANTITACHYCARDIA PACING

Why antitachycardia pacing can be effective in terminating VT on one occasion but yet result in acceleration to a more unstable VT or degeneration to ventricular fibrillation on another occasion remains unclear. Several factors undoubtedly play a role. The majority of patients with recurrent VT have structural heart disease (i.e., obstructive coronary disease or left ventricular dysfunction), which changes over time, possibly changing the reentrant circuit. Even without ischemia or congestive heart failure, multiple morphologies of VT can be seen clinically and in the electrophysiology laboratory in many patients, suggesting different reentrant pathways. Metabolic changes, including electrolyte shifts, hypoxia, acidosis, alkalosis, or drug toxicity, can change the characteristics of VT. Antiarrhythmic medications alter conduction and refractoriness in the reentrant loop and in the surrounding cardiac tissue, and that can change the ease of induction and termination of VT and alter the rate of the VT. Antiarrhythmic drugs can also be proarrhythmic, leading to arrhythmias that may not be effectively terminated by antitachycardia pacing. Autonomic fluxes cannot only facilitate recurrences of VT but also change the efficacy of antitachycardia pacing in terminating them. Considering the multitude of variables determining the inducibility and terminability of VT, it is surprising that antitachycardia pacing works as well as it does.

Other problems are inherent in the use of mechanical devices. Lead fractures and dislodgments can cause over- or undersensing and failure to deliver therapy. A major problem with all antitachycardia devices is the differentiation of SVT from VT. All existing antitachycardia pacemakers are rate-sensitive devices. Any heart rate above the recognition rate triggers the device. Figure 38–12 shows an example of sinus tachycardia triggering bursts of antitachycardia pacing. Sinus tachycardia, rapid atrial fibrillation or flutter, or other types of SVT can potentially fool these systems and result in unwanted pacing. This problem is especially difficult when treating relatively slow VTs, the rates of which can easily overlap with the patient's sinus rhythm during exercise. Maximal treadmill testing should be considered in all patients with antitachycardia pacemakers to make sure that an intrinsic sinus tachycardia does not exceed the device's recognition rate. If rate overlap is a problem, the recognition rate of the pacemaker should be adjusted upward, or drugs such as beta-blockers can be used to slow the peak sinus rate.

Present investigational devices have addressed this problem by offering programmable functions, such as "sudden onset" and rate variability criteria. The sudden onset function attempts to differentiate the gradual acceleration seen in sinus tachycardia from the sudden onset of most VT. The rate variability criteria are used for differentiating the irregular RR intervals seen in atrial fibrillation from the stable RR intervals seen with most VT. Although these functions have been of help in differentiating SVTs from VTs, they are less than perfect in clinical practice. Future devices may be able to overcome this problem by using sensors that monitor hemodynamics or by independently sensing atrial and ventricular electrograms. However, such features are still in the early stages of investigation.

THE FUTURE OF ANTITACHYCARDIA PACING FOR VENTRICULAR TACHYCARDIA

Although advances are rapidly being made in both surgical and catheter ablation techniques aimed at abolishing the VT circuit, only a small percentage of patients with VT can be cured with these techniques at present. Pharmacologic agents continue to be developed, but it is unlikely that pharmacologic therapy will ever be able to adequately prevent VT in the majority of patients with this arrhythmia. Thus, although antitachycardia pacing in patients with SVT is a technique of

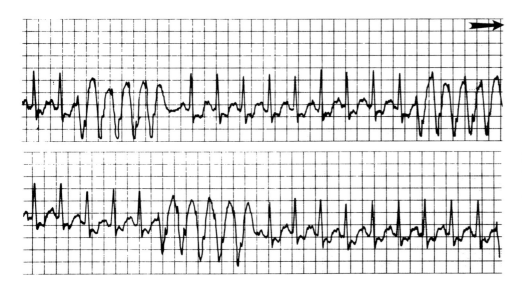

FIGURE 38–12. Sinus tachycardia is present at a rate of 135 bpm, which exceeds the programmed 130-bpm recognition rate of the antitachycardia pacemaker. This results in three episodes of burst ventricular pacing during sinus tachycardia. (From Bonnet CA, Fogoros RN, Elson JJ, et al: Long-term efficacy of an antitachycardia pacemaker and implantable defibrillator combination. PACE 14:814, 1991.)

the past, antitachycardia pacing in combination with backup defibrillation will be an important therapy for VT refractory to pharmacologic therapy in the forseeable future.

However, a word of caution is in order as we enter the era of tiered-therapy devices. Although studies have shown that such devices can be safe and effective in selected patients, the possibility exists that combination therapy could be less effective in preventing sudden cardiac death than the ICD alone. The basic problem is that these devices tempt the clinician to delay a potentially life-saving high-energy shock to deliver "milder" therapies first. Early studies on tiered-therapy devices required rather extensive preimplant and post-implant testing to ensure that, if antitachycardia pacing were used, the pacing sequences would reliably terminate VT. However, after these devices become available for general use and are no longer investigational, the preimplant and postimplant testing may become minimal. Inappropriate pro-gramming of these devices may cause long delays in the delivery of effective therapy. If the delay is long enough, especially if the arrhythmia is hemodynamically unstable, the resultant arrhythmia may be more difficult to terminate with a shock than the original arrhythmia would have been at its onset. Studies[62, 63] show that delaying the time to defibrilla-tion in unstable ventricular arrhythmias can increase defibril-lation thresholds, thus potentially leading to an increased risk of sudden death.

In conclusion, we are entering an era in which antitachy-cardia pacing for VT termination will be an important thera-peutic consideration in every patient undergoing evaluation for an ICD. However, given the complexity of these devices, it is necessary for implanting physicians to have a clear understanding of the principles of antitachycardia pacing, a precise understanding of the devices they are using, and an adequate understanding of their patients' arrhythmias.

REFERENCES

1. Mines GR: On the circulating excitations in heart muscles and their possible relationship to tachycardia and fibrillation. *In* Proceedings and Transactions of the Royal Society of Canada, 3rd series. 1914, p 43.
2. Haft JI, Kosowsky BD, Lau SH, et al: Termination of atrial flutter by rapid electrical pacing of the atrium. Am J Cardiol 20:239, 1967.
3. Durrer D, Schoo L, Schuilenburg RM, et al: Role of premature beats in the initiation and the termination of supraventricular tachycardia in the WPW syndrome. Circulation 36:644, 1967.
4. Ryan GF, Easley RM, Zaroff LI, et al: Paradoxical use of a demand pacemaker in treatment of supraventricular tachycardia due to the Wolff-Parkinson-White syndrome. Circulation 38:1037, 1968.
5. Barold SS, Ryan GF, Goldstein S: The first implanted tachycardia-terminating pacemaker. 12:870, 1989.
6. Krikler D, Curry P, Buffet J: Dual-demand pacing for reciprocating atrioventricular tachycardia. BMJ 1:1114, 1976.
7. Holmes DR: Pacing for tachycardia. *In* Furman S, Hayes DL, Holmes DR (eds): A Practice of Cardiac Pacing, 2nd ed. Mt Kisco, NY, Futura Publishing, 1989, p 471.
8. Fisher JD, Johnston DR, Kim SG, et al: Implantable pacers for tachy-cardia termination: Stimulation techniques and long-term efficacy. PACE Pacing Clin Electrophysiol 9:1325, 1986.
9. den Dulk K, Kersschot IE, Brugada P, et al: Is there a universal anti-tachycardia pacing mode? Am J Cardiol 57:950, 1986.
10. Kahn A, Morris JJ, Citron P: Patient-initiated rapid atrial pacing to manage supraventricular tachycardia. Am J Cardiol 38:200, 1976.
11. Griffin JC, Sweeney M: The management of paroxysmal tachycardias using the Cybertach-60. PACE 7:1291, 1984.
12. Spurrell RAJ, Nathan AW, Camm AJ: Clinical experience with implant-able scanning tachycardia reversion pacemakers. PACE 7:1296, 1984.
13. Zipes DP, Prystowsky EN, Miles WM, et al: Initial experience with Symbios model 7008 pacemaker. PACE 7:1301, 1984.
14. Rothman MT, Keefe JM: Clinical results with Omni-Orthocor^R, an implantable antitachycardia pacing system. PACE 7:1306, 1984.
15. Sowton E: Clinical results with the Tachylog antitachycardia pace-maker. PACE 7:1313, 1984.
16. Peters RW, Scheinman MM, Morady F, et al: Long-term management of recurrent paroxysmal tachycardia by cardiac burst pacing. PACE 8:35, 1985.
17. Bertholet M, Demoulin JC, Waleffe A, et al: Programmable extrastim-ulus pacing for long-term management of supraventricular and ventric-ular tachycardias: Clinical experience in 16 patients. Am Heart J 110:582, 1985.
18. Fisher JD, Johnston DR, Furman S, et al: Long-term efficacy of anti-tachycardia pacing for supraventricular and ventricular tachycardias. Am J Cardiol 60:1311, 1987.
19. Moller M, Simonsen E, Ing PA, et al: Long-term follow-up of patients treated with automatic scanning antitachycardia pacemaker. PACE 12:425, 1989.
20. Schnittger I, Lee JT, Hargis J, et al: Long-term results of antitachycardia pacing in patients with supraventricular tachycardia. PACE 12:936, 1989.
21. Kappenberger L, Valin H, Sowton E: Multicenter long-term results of antitachycardia pacing for supraventricular tachycardias. Am J Cardiol 64:191, 1989.
22. Shandling AH, Li CK, Thomas L: Sustained effectiveness of an atrial antitachycardia pacemaker during follow-up. PACE 13:833, 1990.
23. Fromer M, Gloor H, Kus T, et al: Clinical experience with a new software-based antitachycardia pacemaker for recurrent supraventricular and ventricular tachycardias. PACE 13:890, 1990.
24. den Dulk K, Brugada P, Smeets JL, et al: Long-term antitachycardia pacing experience for supraventricular tachycardia. PACE 13:1020, 1990.
25. Lau CP, Cornu E, Camm AJ: Fatal and nonfatal cardiac arrest in patients with an implanted antitachycardia device for the treatment of supraventricular tachycardia. Am J Cardiol 61:919, 1988.
26. Coumel P, Cabrol C, Fabiato A, et al: Tachycardie permanente par rhythme reciproque. I. Preures du diagnostic par stimulation auriculaire et ventriculaire. II. Traitement par l'implantation intracorporelle d'un stimulateur cardiaque avec entrainement stimulane de l'oreillette et du ventricule. Arch Mal Coeur Vaiss 60:1830, 1967.
27. Spurrell RAT, Sowton E: An implanted atrial synchronous pacemaker with a short atrioventricular delay for the prevention of paroxysmal supraventricular tachycardia. J Electrocardiol 9:89, 1976.
28. Sung RJ, Styperenok JL, Castellanos A: Complete abolition of reentrant supraventricular tachycardia zone using a new modality of cardiac pac-ing with simultaneous atrioventricular stimulation. Am J Cardiol 45:72, 1980.
29. Portillo B, Medina-Ravell V, Portillo-Leon N, et al: Treatment of drug-resistant A-V reciprocating tachycardias with multiprogrammable dual-demand A-V sequential (DVI, MN) pacemakers. PACE 5:814, 1982.
30. Barold SS, Wyndham CRC, Kappenberger LL, et al: Implanted atrial pacemakers for paroxysmal atrial flutter: Long-term efficacy. Ann Intern Med 107:144, 1987.
31. Waldo AL, Olshansky B, Henthorn RW: Use of implanted antitachycar-dia pacemakers to treat paroxysmal atrial flutter. Ann Intern Med 107:247, 1987.
32. Zoll PM, Linenthal AJ, Zarsky LR: Ventricular fibrillation: Treatment and prevention by external electrical currents. N Engl J Med 262:105, 1960.
33. Dressler W: Observations in patients with implanted pacemakers: III. Frequency of ventricular tachycardia as cause of Adams-Stokes attacks and rate of pacing required for its prevention. Am Heart J 68:19, 1964.
34. Sowton E, Leatham A, Carson P: The suppression of arrhythmias by artificial pacemaking. Lancet 2:1098, 1964.
35. Eraklis AJ, Green WJ, Watson CG: Recurrent paroxysms of ventricular tachycardia following mitral valvuloplasty: A case report. Ann Surg 161:63, 1965.
36. Johnson RA, Hoher AM, DeSanctis RW, et al: Chronic overdrive pac-ing in the control of refractory ventricular arrhythmias. Ann Intern Med 80:380, 1974.
37. Fisher JD, Teichman SL, Ferrick A, et al: Antiarrhythmic effects of VVI pacing at physiologic rates: A crossover controlled evaluation. PACE 10:822, 1987.
38. Eldar M, Griffin JC, Abbott JA, et al: Permanent cardiac pacing in patients with the long QT syndrome. J Am Coll Cardiol 10:600, 1987.
39. Stevenson WG, Wiener I, Weiss J, et al: Limitations of bipolar and unipolar conditioning stimuli for inhibition in the human heart. Am Heart J 114:303, 1987.

40. Castellanos A, Luceri R, Moleiro F, et al: Annihilation, entrainment, and modulation of ventricular parasystolic rhythms. Am J Cardiol 54:317, 1984.
41. Marchlinski FE, Buxton AE, Miller JM, et al: Prevention of ventricular tachycardia induction during right ventricular programmed stimulation by high current strength pacing at site of origin. Circulation 76:332, 1987.
42. Bennett MA, Pentecost BL: Reversion of ventricular tachycardia by pacemaker stimulation. Br Heart J 33:922, 1971.
43. Wellens HJ, Schuilenburg RM, Durrer D: Electrical stimulation of the heart in patients with ventricular tachycardia. Circulation 46:216, 1972.
44. Wellens HJJ, Lie KI, Durrer D: Further observations on ventricular tachycardia as studied by electrical stimulation of the heart. Circulation 49:647, 1974.
45. Moss AJ, Rivers RJ: Termination and inhibition of recurrent tachycardias by implanted pervenous pacemakers. Circulation 50:942, 1974.
46. Fisher JD, Mehra R, Furman S: Termination of ventricular tachycardia with bursts of rapid ventricular pacing. Am J Cardiol 41:94, 1978.
47. den Dulk K, Bertholet M, Brugada P, et al: Clinical experience with implantable devices for control of tachyarrhythmias. PACE 7:548, 1984.
48. Herre JM, Griffin JC, Nielsen AP, et al: Permanent triggered antitachycardia pacemakers in the management of recurrent sustained ventricular tachycardia. J Am Coll Cardiol 6:206, 1985.
49. Fisher JD, Kim SG, Matos JA: Pacing for ventricular tachycardia. PACE 7:1278, 1984.
50. Dreifus LS, Fisch C, Griffin JC, et al: Guidelines for implantation of cardiac pacemakers and antiarrhythmia devices: A report of the American College of Cardiology/American Heart Association Task Force on Assessment of Diagnostic and Therapeutic Cardiovascular Procedures (Committee on Pacemaker Implantation). Circulation 84:455, 1991.
51. Mirowski M, Reid PR, Mower MM, et al: Termination of malignant ventricular arrhythmias with an implantable automatic defibrillator in human beings. N Engl J Med 303:322, 1980.
52. Luderitz B, Gerckers U, Manz M: Automatic implantable cardioverter/defibrillator (AICD) and antitachycardia pacemaker (Tachylog): Combined use in ventricular tachyarrhythmias. PACE 9:1356, 1986.
53. Greve H, Koch T, Gulker H, et al: Termination of malignant ventricular tachycardias by use of an automatic defibrillator (AICD) in combination with an antitachycardial pacemaker. PACE 11:2040, 1988.
54. Newman DM, Lee MA, Herre JM, et al: Permanent antitachycardia pacemaker therapy for ventricular tachycardia. PACE 12:1387, 1989.
55. Masterson M, Pinski SL, Wilkoff B, et al: Pacemaker and defibrillator combination therapy for recurrent ventricular tachycardia. Cleve Clin J Med 57:330, 1990.
56. Bonnet CA, Fogoros RN, Elson JJ, et al: Long-term efficacy of an antitachycardia pacemaker and implantable defibrillator combination. PACE 14:814, 1991.
57. Saksena S, Mehta D, Krol RB, et al: Experience with a third-generation implantable cardioverter-defibrillator. Am J Cardiol 67:1375, 1991.
58. Leitch JW, Gillis AM, Wyse DG, et al: Reduction in defibrillator shocks with an implantable device combining antitachycardia pacing and shock therapy. J Am Coll Cardiol 18:145, 1991.
59. Bardy GH, Troutman C, Poole JE, et al: Clinical experience with a tiered-therapy, multiprogrammable antiarrhythmia device. Circulation 85:1689, 1992.
60. Fromer M, Brachmann J, Block M, et al: Efficacy of automatic multimodel device therapy for ventricular tachyarrhythmias as delivered by a new implantable pacing cardioverter-defibrillator: Results of a European multicenter study of 102 implants. Circulation 86:363, 1992.
61. Porterfield JG, Porterfield LM, Smith BA, et al: Conversion rates of induced versus spontaneous ventricular tachycardia by a third generation cardioverter defibrillator. PACE 16:170, 1993.
62. Echt DS, Barbey JT, Black JN: Influence of ventricular fibrillation duration on defibrillation energy in dogs using bidirectional pulse discharges. PACE 11:1315, 1988.
63. Winkle RA, Mead RH, Ruder MA, et al: Effect of duration of ventricular fibrillation on defibrillation efficacy in humans. Circulation 81:1477, 1990.

CHAPTER 39

Pacemaker-Defibrillator Interactions

Andrew E. Epstein
Bruce L. Wilkoff

The first electronic protection against sudden cardiac death was asynchronous ventricular pacing (VOO) to treat Stokes-Adams attacks. Two decades later, the first automatic implantable defibrillators provided unsynchronized shocks,[1] but no bradycardia protection. Ultimately, the capability of synchronized cardioversion was applied to defibrillator devices.[2] Initially, patients who received implantable defibrillators were required to have survived at least two episodes of ventricular tachycardia or ventricular fibrillation that were refractory to drug therapy.[3] Since some patients also needed pacemakers for bradycardia support, two devices were sometimes required.[4, 5] As has been discussed in earlier chapters, when antitachycardia pacing devices became available, pacemakers were also implanted in conjunction with implantable defibrillators for both antitachycardia and antibradycardia pacing indications.[5–9]

Although new generation implantable cardioverter-defibrillators (ICDs) will make some of the interactions described in this chapter obsolete, currently many patients who have combined-device systems and others who have an implantable defibrillator or pacemaker may need a second device for bradycardia or tachyarrhythmia control, respectively. Since pacemakers can affect implantable defibrillators, and vice versa, this chapter will review those interactions and describe methods for combined-device implantation that may help avoid possible problems.

Pacemaker Effects on Implantable Cardioverter-Defibrillators

Pacemakers may affect implantable defibrillators in a variety of ways (Table 39–1). Two of the most important interactions lead to inappropriate arrhythmia detection by defibrillators when no arrhythmia is present and to inhibition of arrhythmia detection when one is occurring. In early clinical trials it was recognized that implantable defibrillators could sense both pacing stimuli and evoked R waves if the interval between the pacing stimulus and the evoked R wave exceeded the 150-msec refractory period of the defibrillator.[10] If both signals were interpreted as ventricular depolarizations, and if the rate of the pacemaker was more than half the tachycardia detection rate, the implantable defibrillator would declare that an arrhythmia was present (Fig. 39–1).

TABLE 39–1. PACEMAKER EFFECTS ON IMPLANTABLE CARDIOVERTER-DEFIBRILLATORS

Counting of the pacemaker stimulus artifacts and evoked R waves may cause inappropriate shocks.

Sensing of pacemaker stimulus artifacts during ventricular tachycardia or fibrillation may inhibit arrhythmia detection.

Changes in autogain can cause oversensing of the pacemaker stimuli after a shock and prevent redetection of the rhythm as a nontachycardia rhythm.

Signals from pacemaker programmers may cause or prevent shocks.

Pacemaker magnet testing may lead to shocks by inducing ventricular arrhythmias or by causing multiple counting during asynchronous pacing.

Esophageal pacing, noninvasive programmed stimulation, and chest wall stimulation at rates greater than the detection rate of an implantable defibrillator may cause shocks owing to sensing of the stimuli or the resultant iatrogenic supraventricular tachycardia.

Rapid pacing due to sensor-indicated rate responses can overlap the tachycardia detection rate and trigger a defibrillator shock.

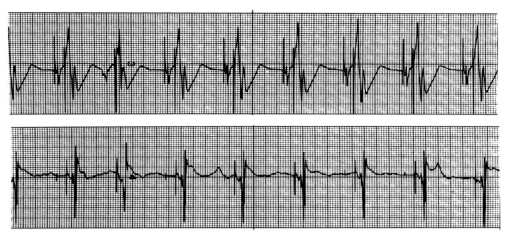

FIGURE 39–1. The figure demonstrates the possibility of double counting. The top tracing shows a transcardiac electrogram recorded from the defibrillating leads, and the bottom tracing shows the bipolar sensing electrogram from the sensing leads of an implanted AID-B system. The interventricular conduction delay separating the pacemaker stimulus artifact from the local evoked R wave in the sensing electrogram may exceed the 150 msec refractory period of the AID-B defibrillator, which could lead to counting both signals. If the measured rate exceeds the detection rate of the defibrillator, a charging cycle would be initiated. See text for discussion. (From Bach SM: AID-B cardioverter-defibrillator possible interaction with pacemakers. Technical Communication, Intec Systems. August 29, 1983.)

For example, consider a patient with an implantable defibrillator having a detection rate of 160 bpm and a pacemaker that delivers stimuli at 80 bpm. If both the pacing stimulus artifacts and the evoked R waves produced by the pacemaker are sensed, the rate detection criterion would be satisfied, and the defibrillator would initiate a charging cycle. In the case of a dual-chamber pacemaker, sensing of the atrial and the ventricular stimulus artifacts, with or without the sensing of the evoked ventricular response, can also lead to incorrect tachyarrhythmia detection. Since unipolar pacing stimuli as seen by the defibrillator are often larger than bipolar stimuli, unipolar pacing has been thought to be contraindicated in patients with implantable defibrillators.[10] Recent observations, however, suggest that an absolute contraindication to pacing in the unipolar mode may not be necessarily correct. Methods for implanting defibrillator sensing leads and pacemaker leads that avoid potential device-to-device interactions are discussed below.

Sensing of pacemaker stimuli can also occur when a tachycardia is present and can lead to inhibition of arrhythmia detection by the defibrillator.[9-11] For implantable defibrillators with an automatic gain sensitivity control that changes according to the amplitude of signals in the sensing electrogram, the sensitivity increases when the signals are small and decreases when the signals are large. Thus, if asynchronous pacing occurs during a ventricular arrhythmia that fails to inhibit the pacemaker because of small R waves (as seen by the pacemaker), and if the pacing stimulus electrograms are large (as seen by the ICD), the automatic gain sensitivity of the implantable defibrillator will decrease. Then, if only the pacing stimulus artifact electrograms but not the arrhythmia R waves are counted, the defibrillator will fail to recognize that an arrhythmia is present (Fig. 39–2).

As was demonstrated in Figure 39–2, bipolar pacing does not always prevent device-to-device interactions. In the same way, unipolar pacing will sometimes allow appropriate function. Implantable defibrillator detection of ventricular fibrillation during DDD unipolar pacing is shown in Figure 39–3. The unipolar pacemaker stimulus electrograms (as seen by the ICD) were small in comparison to the ventricular fibril-

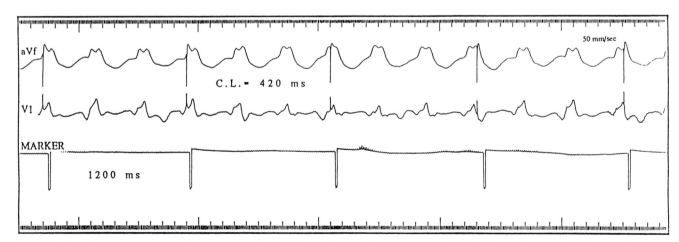

FIGURE 39–2. The surface electrocardiogram (leads aVf and V1) records a ventricular tachycardia (VT) with a cycle length of 420 msec. Because of undersensing by the bipolar VVI pacemaker (lower rate = 50 bpm) of the VT, pacemaker stimuli are emitted at a cycle length of 1200 msec. On the marker channel of the Model 7217 ICD (PCD; Medtronic Inc., Minneapolis, MN), only the pacemaker output is detected. The autogain circuitry detected the large (5 V) pacemaker output instead of the millivolt-level ventricular tachycardia. The result is failure of detection of the VT by the ICD. Note that bipolar pacing does not ensure the absence of pacemaker-ICD adverse interactions.

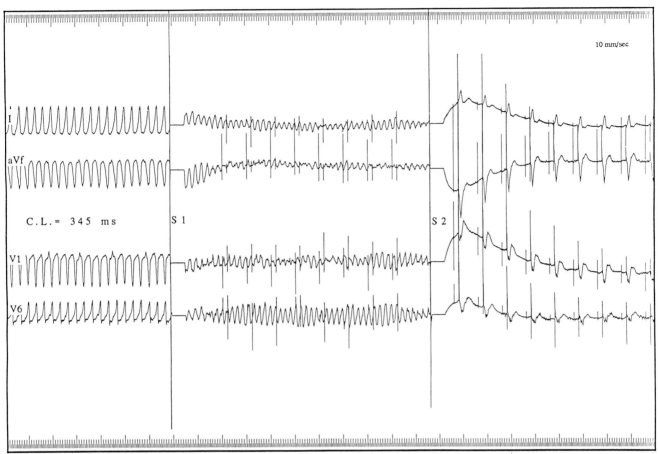

FIGURE 39–3. Surface electrocardiograms (leads I, aVF, V1, and V6) during VF threshold testing of a patient with a Model 1700 ICD (PR$_x$; Cardiac Pacemakers Inc., St. Paul, MN) and Model 2022T DDDR pacemaker (Synchrony II; Pacesetter Systems, Inc.) programmed to unipolar pacing and the DDD mode. Ventricular tachycardia (cycle length = 345 msec) inhibits the pacemaker, is detected by the ICD, but is accelerated by a low-energy shock (S1). The resultant ventricular fibrillation fails to inhibit the unipolar pacemaker stimuli but still is detected by the ICD, which initiates the high-energy shock (S2) that converts the rhythm to an AV paced rhythm.

lation electrograms. This allowed the autogain circuitry of the ICD to detect ventricular fibrillation and initiate the charging of the capacitors. The key to appropriate ICD detection of ventricular tachycardia (VT) or ventricular fibrillation (VF) depends not on unipolar or bipolar stimulation but the geometry (e.g., vector) of the pacemaker stimulation impulse with respect to the ICD sensing electrodes. If the vector of stimulation is perpendicular to the bipole of the sensing electrode, there will be little interference. However, if the two vectors are almost parallel, the ICD will almost certainly detect the pacemaker stimuli that are two orders of magnitude larger than the VT or VF signals. Sometimes this is a moot point, since VT and VF signals (as seen by the pacemaker) may be very large, inhibit the pacemaker, and prevent this type of interaction owing to the appropriate lack of pacemaker stimuli and normal function of the ICD.

In contrast, Ruffy and colleagues[12] reported the implantation of a dual-chamber pacemaker with an implantable defibrillator whereby adverse device-to-device interactions were avoided. The pacemaker electrodes were implanted epicardially near the right atrial appendage and over the lateral right ventricular free wall, whereas the sensing leads of the implantable defibrillator were implanted epicardially on the posterolateral left ventricle. The absence of device-to-device

interaction was confirmed by listening to beeping tones emitted by the defibrillator during AOO and AV sequential pacing, and at postoperative electrophysiologic study when polymorphic ventricular tachycardia was induced and appropriately sensed. These beeping tones represent audible markers of sensed events that can be represented in a graphical fashion with a beep-o-gram (Fig. 39–4).[13] For other devices, similar information is obtained through the defibrillator programmer and is depicted on marker channels or as main timing events. The key to interpretation of marker channels of any sort is to compare the events with a surface electrocardiogram and/or the intracardiac electrogram to determine the clinical appropriateness of the response (Fig. 39–5).

Cohen and associates[4] analyzed and reported other adverse interactions between permanent pacemakers and implantable defibrillators in nine patients with 40 episodes of VF. Asynchronous pacing occurred in 24 of the 40 episodes because of pacemaker failure to sense the induced arrhythmia. In three patients with unipolar pacemakers, inappropriate pacing caused nondetection of the arrhythmia by the defibrillator and subsequent failure to deliver shock therapy. The importance of the relationship between the amplitude of pacemaker stimuli and evoked or spontaneous R waves was highlighted. Two of these patients, who had pacemakers implanted before

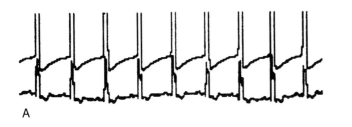
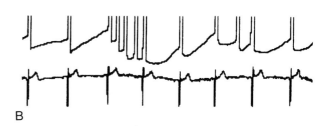

A

B

FIGURE 39–4. *A,* A normal beep-o-gram. The top line demonstrates beep recordings from the implantable defibrillator in the electrophysiologic test mode during normal sinus rhythm. The bottom tracing shows a simultaneous surface electrocardiogram recorded on the second channel of a Holter monitor. *B,* Oversensing from a patient with a documented inappropriate discharge. Further evaluation showed that the O rings had not been attached to the setscrew caps. (From Ballas SL, Rashidi R, McAlister H, et al: The use of beep-o-grams in the assessment of automatic implantable cardioverter-defibrillator sensing function. PACE 12:1737, 1989.)

their defibrillators, demonstrated ratios of the pacemaker stimulus artifact to the evoked R-wave amplitude in the implantable defibrillator sensing electrograms of 3.5 and 2.1, respectively. For patients with bipolar pacemakers and recordable electrograms, the average ratio was 0.2, emphasizing the importance of having small pacemaker stimulus artifacts in the implantable defibrillator sensing electrogram.

Other adverse device-to-device interactions in patients with combined defibrillator-pacemaker systems were reported by Luceri and coworkers.[14] Four important observations were made. First, 25-J defibrillator shocks in one patient with ventricular tachycardia resulted in asystole that required bradycardia pacing support, whereas low-energy shocks did not provoke bradyarrhythmias. Second, the problem of high epicardial pacing thresholds was highlighted in a patient with cardiomyopathy who was receiving amiodarone. Third, routine pacemaker magnet testing in one patient induced ventricular tachycardia. Fortunately, the arrhythmia was detected and converted by the implantable defibrillator. Finally, in one patient, electromechanical dissociation with a wide, paced QRS complex was properly identified and not shocked. The investigators concluded that the documentation and classification of device interactions and terminal events are essential for assessing long-term efficacy of implantable defibrillators and that the observations have implications for new antitachycardia devices. The problem of death due to bradycardia, especially in patients with left ventricular dysfunction, has been well documented.[15–18] High epicardial pacing thresholds have already been problematic with some advanced-generation defibrillator pacing capabilities.[19] Although high-output pacing options are available to handle

high pacing thresholds, their use shortens battery life and narrows the safety margin for patients who depend on pacing for treatment of either bradycardia or tachycardia. Some newer devices have options for high-output pacing both for bradycardia in the immediate postshock period and for antitachycardia pacing that limit the drain on battery longevity and maintain the safety margin when it is most needed. Like Luceri and colleagues,[14] we also have witnessed ventricular tachycardia induction during pacemaker threshold determination.

Not only can appropriate implantable defibrillator shocks be delivered for arrhythmias induced during pacemaker analysis, but also inappropriate defibrillator discharges have been reported to result from signals emitted during programming of implanted pacemakers. Gottlieb and associates[20] reported that during programming of a Cordis Multicor II ventricular demand pacemaker to the stat VVI mode, a concomitantly implanted AID-BR defibrillator (Cardiac Pacemakers Inc., St. Paul, MN) initiated a charging cycle. It was thought that the implantable defibrillator sensed high-frequency electromagnetic signals from the pacemaker programmer. It is important to note that the Multicor II pacemaker employed an older version of telemetry, not transmitted by radio-frequency signals but by an oscillating magnetic field. Signals from pacemaker programmers and other equipment, such as fluoroscopy units, have caused ''noise reversion'' and temporarily prevented appropriate shocks.

Kim and coworkers[21] reported that pacemaker magnet testing in patients with implantable defibrillators may cause inappropriate shock delivery. In an individual with an underlying heart rate of 133 bpm, asynchronous pacing at 70 bpm during a pacemaker magnet test initiated a defibrillator charging cycle, presumably because both the native and the paced R waves, and perhaps the pacing stimulus artifacts, were sensed.

Critelli and colleagues[22] described an unusual case of adverse pacemaker interaction with an implantable defibrillator. During esophageal atrial pacing at a rate just above the implantable defibrillator detection rate, a charging sequence was initiated. Counting of the stimulus artifact was excluded, since the defibrillator discharged only when the ventricular response exceeded the detection rate of the defibrillator. The authors suggested that esophageal pacing could be utilized to assess the potential for inappropriate defibrillator discharges secondary to atrial arrhythmias in patients with implantable defibrillators. This technique for arrhythmia induction will be useful only if the implantable defibrillator is disabled

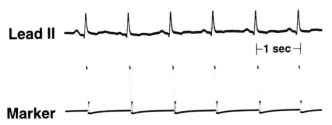

Lead II

⊢1 sec ⊣

Marker

FIGURE 39–5. Marker channel function from a Model 1705 implantable defibrillator (PR$_x$; Cardiac Pacemakers Inc.) is shown on the second line simultaneously with surface electrocardiographic lead II on the first line. The device has separate sensing circuits for tachycardia (*above the line*) and bradycardia detection (*below the line*). The large and small deflections indicate, respectively, that the two circuits are active and functioning properly.

during pacing, and then activated after the termination of pacing. If the implantable defibrillator is not disabled during arrhythmia induction, the defibrillator could be activated not only as a result of the ventricular response of the induced arrhythmia but also by the pacing stimuli or the ventricular response to pacing itself. The same potential for arrhythmia detection (either deliberate or accidental) exists if noninvasive programmed stimulation, available with some pacemakers, is used whether they are implanted or used for chest wall stimulation.[23] Inappropriate antitachycardia pacing for sinus tachycardia can also initiate defibrillator charging cycles.[7] Finally, rate-modulated pacemakers have an unique opportunity to cause tachycardia detection when the sensor-indicated paced heart rate produces, either with or without detection of the pacemaker stimuli, detected rhythms at rates above the rate cutoff.

Despite problems of multiple counting of unipolar pacemaker stimuli by implantable defibrillators, it is possible in some instances to implant a unipolar pacemaker with an implantable defibrillator. As described below, ventricular mapping techniques are available to allow implantation of pacemakers with defibrillators. We believe that it is not so much the mode of pacing that is important but rather the vector at which the pacemaker stimulus is delivered to the implantable defibrillator sensing lead that determines whether the defibrillator will sense the stimulus. Indeed, if a pacemaker lead implantation site is found at which the stimuli are nondetectable in the implantable defibrillator sensing electrogram, it makes no difference whether the pacing mode is unipolar or bipolar. However if a pacemaker has the capacity to be programmed to or revert to the opposite polarity,[24] all possible configurations must be tested. Several programmable polarity pacemakers autoprogram to the unipolar mode when the battery voltage drops to end-of-life levels. Some pacemakers check to see if an electrically intact bipolar lead exists on a beat-to-beat basis and then pace unipolar if the lead impedance is too low or high. All these are safety features, but they provide additional challenges for the physician who chooses to implant two devices in one patient.

Implantable Defibrillator Effects on Permanent Pacemakers

Implantable defibrillator shocks can affect pacemaker function by multiple mechanisms (Table 39–2), including increasing the pacing thresholds following shocks that result

TABLE 39–2. IMPLANTABLE DEFIBRILLATOR EFFECTS ON PERMANENT PACEMAKERS

Increased pacing threshold and pacemaker noncapture following shocks.

Deterioration of the R-wave signal and pacemaker nonsensing caused by shocks.

Pacemakers may be reprogrammed by shocks.

Pacemakers may be injured by shocks.

Pacemakers may be reprogrammed by defibrillator programmers.

Pacemakers may be affected by magnets placed over implantable defibrillators.

in pacemaker loss of capture, deterioration of the R-wave signal with subsequent pacemaker undersensing, reprogramming of the pacemaker, and potential injury to the implanted pulse generator itself. Drugs can compound the problem of these adverse interactions, for example by increasing the pacing threshold.[25-29] Guarnieri and associates[25] reported that following 30-J implantable defibrillator shocks, flecainide makes the duration of capture threshold elevation more pronounced than when flecainide therapy is absent. In addition, radio-frequency signals used for defibrillator programming may lead to pacemaker reprogramming. Finally, placing a magnet over an implantable defibrillator may unintentionally close the reed switch of the implanted pacemaker.

Calkins and coworkers[30] classified interactions between pacemakers and implantable defibrillators into four categories, some of which have already been discussed. First, transient failure to sense or capture immediately following implantable defibrillator discharges occurred in seven patients. Second, oversensing of pacemaker stimulus artifacts by an implantable defibrillator lead to multiple counting in one patient, although no shock therapy resulted. Third, implantable defibrillator therapy was inappropriately inhibited by pacing stimuli sensed by the defibrillator during ventricular fibrillation in three patients, one with a unipolar and two with bipolar pacemakers. Finally, pacemaker reprogramming was shown to occur as a result of implantable defibrillator discharges in three patients. One patient each had a Medtronic 7006 pulse generator and a Cordis 415 pulse generator reprogrammed to the backup mode by defibrillator shocks. The third patient had an Intermedics 262-14 Intertach pulse generator programmed to the ventricular demand pacing mode by a defibrillator discharge. We too have observed an Intermedics 262-14, a Cardiac Pacemakers, Inc., Delta-925, and multiple Medtronic Elite-7074 devices programmed to the backup mode following defibrillator discharges. The Medtronic Elite pacemakers may reprogram to either bipolar or unipolar pacing configurations after transthoracic or implantable defibrillator discharges. A study of the likelihood of other programmable polarity devices being reprogrammed to the unipolar mode was investigated by Ching and colleagues[24] in 56 patients with implantable defibrillators and pacemakers. After 1562 months of combined implant duration and 1009 implantable defibrillator discharges, only one device was reprogrammed to the VVI mode, and none to unipolar stimulation. Even so, the potential for adverse reprogramming and its consequences should be considered whenever two devices are implanted.

The loss of pacemaker capture following defibrillator shocks has been reported by numerous authors.[4, 14, 30-32] One such example from the literature is shown in Figure 39–6. Slepian and associates[31] treated a 78-year-old patient with amiodarone, a ventricular demand pacemaker, and an implantable defibrillator. The authors observed that the time of failure to capture following implantable defibrillator shock delivery was energy related: the greater the shock energy, the longer failure to capture persisted. Reiter and coworkers[32] showed that the longer the duration of ventricular fibrillation, the greater the pacing threshold increased following shock delivery. Thus, both the strength of defibrillator shocks[14, 31] and arrhythmia duration before shock therapy[32] are related to postshock bradycardia[14] and elevation of the pacing threshold following defibrillation.[31, 32] The mechanism for

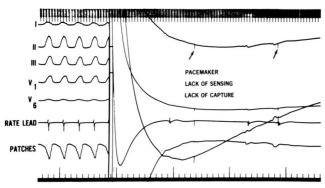

FIGURE 39–6. Pacemaker malfunction following a defibrillator shock is illustrated. Following the shock, two pacemaker stimuli are shown (*arrows*) that occur shortly after intrinsic R waves and demonstrate lack of sensing. The first stimulus occurs after the expected ventricular refractory period and also demonstrates failure to capture. I, II, III, V1, and V6 = surface electrocardiographic leads. (From Cohen AI, Wish MH, Fletcher RD, et al: The use and interaction of permanent pacemakers and the automatic implantable cardioverter defibrillator. PACE 11:704, 1988.)

these changes is uncertain but may be due to cellular injury from the defibrillator shocks.[33–39] However, not all investigators have shown a change in the pacing threshold and loss of pacemaker capture,[40] or myocardial injury following shocks.[41, 42]

A systematic analysis of pacemaker malfunction following implantable defibrillator discharge was provided by Cohen and colleagues.[4] In 11 of 20 episodes of induced ventricular fibrillation, pacemaker nonsensing of ventricular complexes after defibrillation occurred in association with inappropriate pacing. The mean duration of sensing failure was 9.1 ± 11.6 seconds. Failure of ventricular capture was also observed in 8 of 22 analyzable tracings. The mean duration for lack of capture was 4.9 ± 5.1 seconds. One patient had no pacemaker capture for 16 seconds following defibrillator discharge.

Changes in pacing threshold and R-wave amplitude (with implications for nonsensing by the implantable defibrillator)

are related in part to the location of shock delivery relative to the pacing and sensing electrodes, respectively. Yee and associates[43] reported changes in the pacing threshold and R-wave amplitude following transvenous catheter shocks in pigs. Fifteen seconds following shocks, the bipolar R-wave amplitude recorded from the shock delivery catheter decreased from 8.3 ± 1.0 mV to 2.0 ± 0.2 mV ($p < .001$), and the stimulation threshold increased from 1.0 ± 0.1 V to 2.3 ± 0.4 V ($p < .001$). These changes lasted for up to 10 minutes. Since these measurements were made at the shocking catheter tip, a second study was performed in which the site of shock delivery was remote from the recording/pacing site. In these animals no significant change was seen in either the R-wave amplitude or the simulation threshold, suggesting that changes in these parameters following shocks are secondary to local changes at the myocardium-catheter interface.

Methods of Preventing Adverse Device-to-Device Interaction

Pacemakers and defibrillators can be implanted together in the same patient if special precautions are taken to avoid adverse device-to-device interactions (Table 39–3).[5] The pacemaker and defibrillator pulse generators should be implanted as far apart from one another as possible to minimize the potential for interactions between magnets, programmers, and the implanted devices. Since it is frequently impossible to predict which pacemaker patients will require an implantable defibrillator or which implantable defibrillator subjects will require bradycardia support, it is important to be able to understand the physiology of the interactions and how to test for and prevent them during device implantation. Depending on which devices are available, the relative expertise and cooperation of the surgeon and the electrophysiologist, and the needs of the patient, it may be desirable to implant the pacemaker before the implantable defibrillator so R-wave and pacemaker stimulus artifact amplitudes can be assessed

---

TABLE 39–3. **METHODS OF PREVENTING ADVERSE DEVICE-TO-DEVICE INTERACTIONS**

Minimize interaction between pacemakers, defibrillators, programmers, and magnets by implanting the devices as far away from one another as possible, for example on opposite sides of the body.

For thoracotomy ICDs, implant the pacemaker before the defibrillator, if possible, to optimize position of the defibrillator sensing leads. For nonthoracotomy ICDs, implant the ICD first and optimize the position of the pacemaker electrodes.

Defibrillator implantation in patient with previously implanted pacemaker:

A. Use "worst case" scenario in the operating room by programming pacemaker to highest stimulus output, asynchronous pacing, and to unipolar and Bipolar configurations to maximize the possibility of device-device interaction. If interactions are absent under these circumstances, the chances for their ocurrence are low in clinical setting.

B. Map epicardial surface to locate site where pacemaker stimulus artifact amplitude is as small as possible.

C. Maintain electrode tips within 1 cm of each other.

D. When site is located where pacemaker stimulus artifact is minimal and the R-wave amplitude is large during both ventricular paced and spontaneous rhythms, implant the first epicardial lead. Move second epicardial lead circumferentially around the first to find site where pacing stimulus artifact amplitude is the smallest. Implant second electrode at this site.

E. Test sensing of the implantable defibrillator during high-output pacing. If double counting is demonstrated, the sensing leads must be moved.

F. Test combined device system in the operating room to ensure effective defibrillation, and check for pacemaker malfunction after shocks.

Pacemaker implantation in patient with previously implanted defibrillator:

A. Use active fixation leads and a multiprogrammable pacemaker for bradycardia protection.

B. Deactivate tachycardia detection, and advance pacemaker lead to the right ventricle. Use a pacing system analyzer at maximal output and pulse duration to identify a site with acceptable pacing and sensing threshold characteristics.

C. Assess defibrillator sensing by listening to beeping tones from the defibrillator, if the device can emit sounds, or observe real-time electrograms or sensing markers by telemetry during pacing.

D. Implant the pacemaker lead where pacing and sensing are satisfactory, and where there is no detection of pacing stimuli by the defibrillator.

on the defibrillator sensing electrogram. Conversely, the defibrillator could be implanted first for optimal sensing and defibrillation function, followed by implantation of the less finicky pacemaker and leads at a later time.

DEFIBRILLATOR IMPLANTATION IN PATIENTS WITH IMPLANTED PACEMAKERS

One of the most important requirements for successful implantation of a defibrillator in an individual with a previously implanted pacemaker[5] is to ensure that the pacemaker stimulus signal is as small as possible in the defibrillator sensing electrogram. Hence, the observations made here apply to both endocardial and epicardial pacemaker systems. A worst-case scenario is provided in the operating room by programming the pacemaker to its highest stimulus amplitude and pulse duration to maximize the size of the pacemaker stimulus and increase the probability of pacemaker stimulus sensing by the implantable defibrillator. Thus, when the pacemaker is programmed to a lower stimulus amplitude postoperatively, the chances of adverse effects of the pacemaker on the defibrillator are even further decreased.

After signal calibration, the defibrillator sensing leads are implanted to ensure that an adequate R wave is obtained during native conduction, ventricular pacing, and ventricular arrhythmias. The left ventricle is ''mapped'' to locate a site at which a pacemaker stimulus amplitude in the rate sensing electrogram of the implantable defibrillator is as low as possible. This can be accomplished by holding the epicardial sensing leads in their carriers, attaching the leads to monitoring cables, and thereafter moving the leads while held together at various positions on the surface of the heart (Fig. 39–7). The tips should be maintained within 1 cm of each other to keep the R-wave duration of the recorded electro-

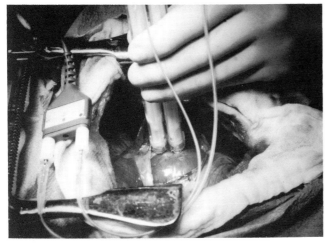

FIGURE 39–7. The surgeon holds the bipolar epicardial electrodes in their lead carriers (*center*) attached to the monitoring cables (*left*). While held together, the electrodes are applied to the surface of the heart during pacing, and the electrogram recordings are analyzed to find a site where the pacemaker stimulus artifact is minimal. At that site the electrodes are implanted. For illustrative purposes this photograph was made in the animal laboratory. See text for further details. (From Epstein AE, Kay GN, Plumb VJ, et al: Combined automatic implantable cardioverter-defibrillator and pacemaker systems: Implantation techniques and follow-up. J Am Coll Cardiol 13:121, 1989. Reprinted with permission from the American College of Cardiology.)

gram as short as possible. In this manner a site is identified where the pacemaker stimulus artifact is minimal and nondetectable and the evoked R waves both in paced and native rhythm can be assessed. In our study, the R-wave amplitude during both paced and native rhythms generally exceeded 7 mV. Similarly, a site where the pacemaker stimulus artifact was less than 0.1 mV could usually be found (Fig. 39–8). Almost always the best site for implantable defibrillator sensing is on the posterior or lateral left ventricle. Epicardial right ventricular placement usually ensures a large pacemaker stimulus on the implantable defibrillator sensing electrogram. If long stimulus–to–R wave intervals are observed, the pacemaker leads should be moved closer to the defibrillator electrodes so that the defibrillator refractory period is not exceeded, leading to potential sensing of both the pacemaker stimulus artifact and the evoked R wave. This minimizes the possibility of double counting if, for example, a drug that prolongs interventricular conduction is administered that lengthens the time from pacing stimulus delivery to ventricular depolarization. To increase the chance of finding an optimal implantable defibrillator sensing lead location, we recommend that sites for sensing lead implantation be mapped before the patches are implanted to avoid placing the patches over a potentially optimal sensing site.

When a site is located where the pacemaker stimulus artifact appears small, one of the sensing leads is permanently implanted. Thereafter, the second lead is moved circumferentially around the first to refine the site where it should be implanted where the pacing stimulus artifact is at truly the lowest amplitude possible (see Fig. 39–8). Indeed, we have found that millimeter movements can greatly change the size of the stimulus artifact. When an optimal site is found, the second electrode is implanted. Following sensing lead implantation, the patches are implanted and defibrillation threshold testing can commence in the usual fashion. If the defibrillation threshold is acceptable, the implantable defibrillator can then be implanted. To assess whether defibrillation shocks cause reprogramming during defibrillation threshold testing, the pacemaker can be programmed to the anticipated mode in which it will be used chronically.

After the defibrillator is implanted, sensing by the implantable defibrillator is assessed. If a Ventak device (Cardiac Pacemakers, Inc., St. Paul, MN) is used, this can be done by placing a magnet over the defibrillator and listening for beeping tones. If during high-output ventricular pacing only one tone is heard for each QRS complex, multiple counting is absent. On the other hand, if more than one beep is heard for every QRS response, multiple counting is then documented, and the sensing leads must be moved. With other implantable defibrillators, the use of marker events instead of beeping tones can be examined with comparison to the surface electrocardiogram.

It is always important to test function of the implantable defibrillator-pacemaker system in the operating room to ensure that defibrillation is effective and to assess whether pacing occurs during ventricular tachycardia or ventricular fibrillation (Figs. 39–9 and 39–10). Electrograms can be easily recorded during the tachyarrhythmias, and the small ratio of pacemaker stimulus to paced and native R-wave amplitudes reconfirmed after the defibrillation testing. By paying attention to these details, later problems can usually be avoided.

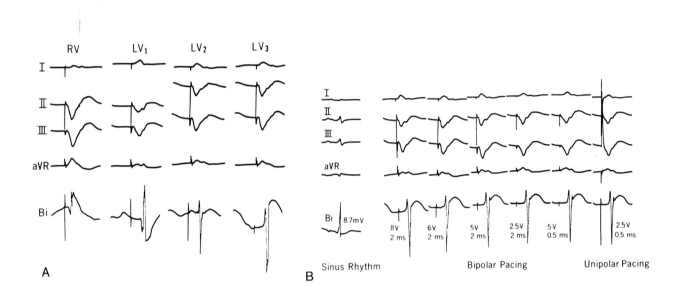

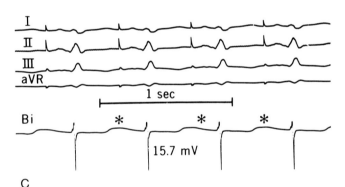

FIGURE 39–8. These recordings are made from a patient with a ventricular demand activity-sensing pacemaker at defibrillator implantation. Surface electrocardiogram leads I, II, III, and aVR are shown on the first four channels. The electrogram recorded from the bipolar sensing leads is labeled Bi. The gain for all recordings is identical. *A*, Epicardial recordings from one right ventricular (RV) and three left ventricular (LV) sites during pacing at an 8-V output and a 1-msec pulse width. The pacemaker stimulus artifact is large close to the apex of the RV, where the pacemaker electrode is implanted, and at LV sites 1 and 2. At LV site 3, the pacemaker stimulus artifact is small compared to the paced R wave, and LV site 3 is the site where the leads were implanted. *B*, Electrograms recorded after the sensing leads were implanted. The R wave during sinus rhythm is 8.7 mV (*left column*). During bipolar pacing (*middle columns*), the pacemaker stimuli amplitudes and pulse widths are shown below the respective stimulus artifacts. As the pacing stimulus amplitude is decreased, the stimulus artifact also decreases. For illustrative purposes to show the hazard of unipolar pacing, the right column shows unipolar pacing at only 2.5 V, which provides a stimulus artifact larger than that at any bipolar output. *C*, Recordings from a patient with an atrial demand pacemaker that have virtually no identifiable pacemaker stimulus artifacts in the bipolar sensing electrogram. See text for discussion. (From Epstein AE, Kay GN, Plumb VJ, et al: Combined automatic implantable cardioverter-defibrillator and pacemaker systems: Implantation techniques and follow-up. J Am Coll Cardiol 13:121, 1989. Reprinted with permission from the American College of Cardiology.)

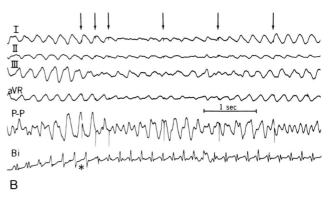

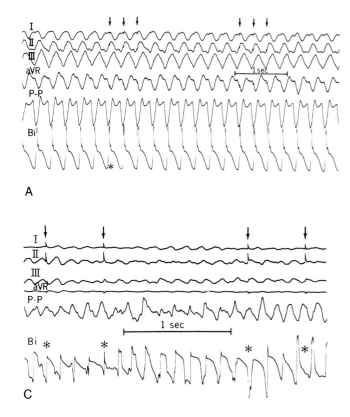

FIGURE 39–9. The recordings were made during defibrillation threshold testing at implantation of an implantable defibrillator. Labels are the same as those in Figure 39–6 except that P-P refers to electrograms recorded from the two defibrillating patch leads. *A and B*, Pacing during ventricular tachycardia and ventricular fibrillation, respectively, in a patient with a previously implanted antitachycardia pacemaker. No pacemaker stimulus artifacts are detectable in the bipolar rate-sensing electrograms (*asterisks*) during pacing (*arrows*). In *B* the fourth through sixth impulses are from the antitachycardia pacemaker functioning in the ventricular demand mode. *C*, Recordings from a patient with an atrial demand pacemaker. Again, no pacemaker stimulus artifact is detectable in the bipolar rate-sensing electrogram (*asterisks*) during pacing (*arrows*). See text for discussion. (From Epstein AE, Kay GN, Plumb VJ, et al: Combined automatic implantable cardioverter-defibrillator and pacemaker systems: Implantation techniques and follow-up. J Am Coll Cardiol 13:121, 1989. Reprinted with permission from the American College of Cardiology.)

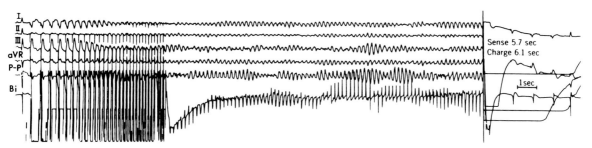

FIGURE 39–10. Intraoperative testing of an implantable defibrillator in a patient with a ventricular demand pacemaker is demonstrated. Surface ECG leads I, II, III, and aVR are shown with electrograms recorded from the defibrillator patch leads (P-P) and bipolar sensing leads (Bi). After 17.0 seconds (standby time 4 seconds, sensing time 5.7 seconds, charging time 6.1 seconds, and synchronization time 1.2 seconds), a 30-J shock restores sinus rhythm. The pacemaker supported postshock bradycardia but did not pace during ventricular fibrillation. (From Epstein AE, Kay GN, Plumb VJ, et al: Combined automatic implantable cardioverter-defibrillator and pacemaker systems: Implantation techniques and follow-up. J Am Coll Cardiol 13:121, 1989. Reprinted with permission from the American College of Cardiology.)

PACEMAKER IMPLANTATION IN PATIENTS WITH A PREVIOUSLY IMPLANTED DEFIBRILLATOR

When a defibrillator is already implanted[5] and the patient requires bradycardia or antitachycardia pacemaker function, either a pacemaker can be implanted later or replacement of the defibrillator with a new-generation device equipped with combined pacing and shock therapy capabilities is possible. Initial defibrillator implantation will become more common, since nonthoracotomy lead systems are less forgiving in where they can be placed. In addition, most new defibrillators universally include VVI bradycardia pacing capabilities. However, since most patients who require defibrillation protection have significantly impaired ventricular function, and since VVI pacing frequently causes hemodynamic deterioration, dual-chamber pacing is often desirable. New-generation implantable defibrillators will undoubtedly incorporate dual-chamber, rate-responsive (DDDR) pacing capability.

In general, it is advisable to use active fixation electrodes, and pacemakers with programmable polarity and other options, to maximize the opportunity to find an acceptable implantation configuration. Usually, atrial lead placement causes little problem and, if the ventricular lead is placed in the right ventricular outflow tract, it also will generally not interfere with the implantable defibrillator function. During pacemaker lead implantation, implantable defibrillator arrhythmia detection should be disabled. The pacemaker lead is advanced to the right ventricle, and acceptable pacing and sensing threshold characteristics are documented through the use of endocardial electrograms and a pacing system analyzer. An initial impression as to whether the lead placement will be adequate can be obtained by using the pacing system analyzer at high outputs representative of those obtainable by the pacemaker in both the unipolar and the bipolar configurations. However, since each pacemaker has a unique pacing stimulus waveform and depolarization vector dependent on the pulse generator placement within the pacemaker pocket, it is essential to test the implantable defibrillator's response to the pacemaker with the pacemaker connected to the leads. Oversensing, defined as more than one sensed event per QRS, can be investigated by audible (beeping) tones or visual markers of sensed events, depending on the model of the implantable defibrillator. If only one tone or marker is seen to be synchronized with the QRS, multiple counting is absent. Conversely, if more than one tone or marker is noticed, multiple counting is present and the pacemaker lead must be moved. An occasional double-counted event is not unusual and is not necessarily a cause for concern. It is theoretically possible to improve the situation by changing the pacing polarity from bipolar to unipolar in this circumstance. If no satisfactory bipolar pacing site can be found, a site where unipolar pacing provides a low stimulus artifact may be identified. If a particular model of pacemaker is known to reprogram to unipolar pacing as a result of pacemaker reset or end-of-life behavior, such as the Model Elite I (Models 7074 and 7076 [Medtronic Inc., Minneapolis, MN]) response to cardioversion, the lack of oversensing and other interactions must be proved in the unipolar and bipolar configurations. A successful implantation requires that the vector of both the atrial and the ventricular pacing stimulus artifacts remains perpendicular to the sensing electrodes of the implantable defibrillator. If the potential unipolar reprogramming related to end of life or reset also reprograms the generator to single-chamber pacing without rate response, then only that degree of compatibility needs to be documented. By assessing the actual pacemaker and lead system during defibrillation testing, both the likelihood of autoreprogramming and its consequences are examined.

In addition to preventing overdetection of tachycardia due to stimulus sensing, one must be certain that during ventricular fibrillation the pacing stimuli do not inhibit arrhythmia detection. Both unipolar and bipolar stimulation at maximum amplitudes and pulse durations should be tested during DOO or VOO pacing, depending on the type of pacing anticipated. High-energy shocks can also reduce the slew rate and amplitude of intrinsic and paced electrograms. Partially related to

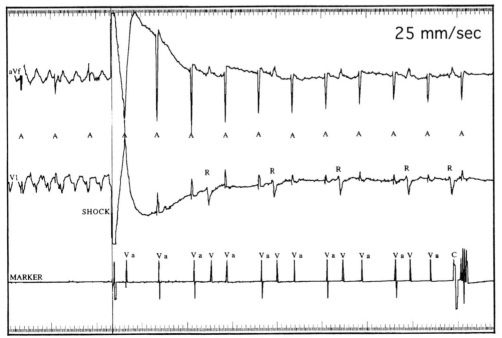

FIGURE 39–11. Intraoperative testing of a Model 1700 implantable defibrillator (PR$_x$; Cardiac Pacemakers, Inc.) during bipolar AOO pacing (A). Ventricular tachycardia is terminated by an ICD discharge (SHOCK). The marker channel indicates sensed events detected by the tachycardia sensing amplifier by upward deflections. Sensed atrial paced events, detected as ventricular events (Va) and conducted ventricular events (V), are seen in triplet groupings at intervals short enough to prevent the detection of the nontachycardia rhythm. The consequence is the initiation of the charging of the capacitors (C), eventuating in a defibrillator shock (*not shown*). This sequence was repeated (*not shown*) and required the deactivation of the pacemaker. Hence, tachycardia detection was normal, but the detection of the return to sinus rhythm was prevented.

this phenomenon, we have seen the autogain circuitry fooled after a shock. The implantable defibrillator sensing function locked in on the dual-chamber paced stimuli only after the initial shock and thus prevented redetection of sinus rhythm after a successful shock, producing additional clinically inappropriate shocks into an AV paced rhythm (Fig. 39–11). Although it is not required, it is comforting to see that ventricular fibrillation inhibits the pacemaker. This observation further reduces the likelihood that ventricular fibrillation will be underdetected. Some newer-generation implantable defibrillators provide real-time electrograms that can also be used to ascertain whether the pacing stimulus artifact is small. Care should be taken when interpreting these electrograms, since the electrogram sensing amplifier is usually separate from the one used for arrhythmia detection.

The use of nonthoracotomy lead system implantable defibrillators increases the likelihood of adverse interactions between the pacemaker and the implantable defibrillator. Since shocking, pacing, and bradycardia and tachycardia sensing occur over leads placed in the right ventricle, the proximity enhances the problems with geometry. Theoretical considerations suggest that as long as the pacemaker and implantable defibrillator shocking electrodes are not touching, damage is unlikely to ensue. This is related to the defibrillation protection circuitry already configured within the pacemaker. Since the endocardial shocking electrode is most likely to give good results in the right ventricular apex, the pacemaker lead will most likely be implanted in the right ventricular outflow tract or along the intraventricular septum. This has been successfully accomplished in many cases despite the technical complexity.

Postoperative Testing

Whether or not postoperative electrophysiologic study is performed before patients are released from the hospital is variable at different centers when only a defibrillator is implanted. However, for patients with combined-device systems, it is always important to test the entire system before the patient is discharged. With the pacemaker programmed to maximum output, ventricular fibrillation should be induced to ensure that pacing during the arrhythmia does not cause inhibition of arrhythmia detection by the defibrillator (Fig. 39–12; see Figs. 39–2 and 39–3). If asynchronous pacing occurs during this test with the largest possible delivered pacing stimuli, the chances for arrhythmia detection to be inhibited by pacing at lower outputs are minimal. If asynchronous pacing did not occur during this test, one may reprogram the pacemaker to the asynchronous mode and repeat the test to be certain that if asynchronous pacing ever occurs, arrhythmia detection will not be inhibited.

Since defibrillator shocks can reprogram pacemakers, postoperative testing is also important to ensure that reprogramming by defibrillator therapy does not occur. Unfortunately, we have observed the first occurrence of reprogramming up to 3 years after initial combined-device implantation even though multiple therapies had been delivered beforehand by the implantable defibrillator. If reprogramming does not occur, the device should still be tested in the reprogrammed mode to ensure that the patient will remain protected. In patients with ventricular tachycardia, arrhythmia conversion should also be tested during antitachycardia pacing and low-energy cardioversion.

Summary

Pacemakers can affect defibrillator function, and defibrillators can affect pacemaker function. Some interactions may not be clinically important, for example, occasional multiple counting. However, many device-device interactions are potentially life-threatening, and it is therefore important to try to minimize the possibility of their occurrence. If careful attention is paid to implantation of the defibrillator and pacing leads, many potentially adverse device-to-device interactions can be avoided by simply minimizing the possibility of defibrillator sensing of pacemaker stimulus artifacts. When two devices are used in the same patient, the possibility that shock therapy may injure or reprogram the pacemaker will always be present. As device technology advances, these problems will be avoided when only one device is used for both pacing and shocking functions.

In general, only bipolar pacemakers should be implanted in conjunction with an implantable defibrillator. During epicardial defibrillator implantation even when a pacemaker is not present or contemplated, the possibility of the future need for bradycardia pacing should always be considered. Thus, bipolar rate-sensing electrodes should be implanted on the left ventricle, far away from the right ventricle, so that if a later pacemaker is required, its leads can be positioned in the right heart with a greater chance for producing small stimulus artifacts as seen by the implantable defibrillator. If defibrillator epicardial sensing electrodes are implanted over the

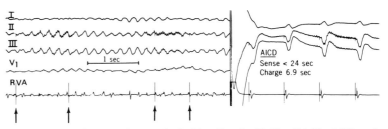

FIGURE 39–12. At postoperative electrophysiologic study in a patient with an implantable defibrillator and an activity-sensing, rate-adaptive ventricular demand pacemaker, conversion of ventricular fibrillation is shown. Surface ECG leads I, II, III, and V1 are shown with electrograms from a temporary transvenous electrode catheter advanced to the right ventricular apex (RVA) for programmed stimulation. The implanted defibrillator was placed in the standby mode, ventricular fibrillation was induced, and then the defibrillator was activated. Despite ventricular pacing during ventricular fibrillation, the arrhythmia was correctly sensed and converted by the defibrillator. Bradycardia is supported by the pacemaker postshock. (From Epstein AE, Kay GN, Plumb VJ, et al: Combined automatic implantable cardioverter-defibrillator and pacemaker systems: Implantation techniques and follow-up. J Am Coll Cardiol 13:121, 1989. Reprinted with permission from the American College of Cardiology.)

right ventricle, the chances of adverse device-to-device interactions are increased if a later pacemaker is implanted in that chamber. Furthermore, since many implantable defibrillators will be upgraded to multiple-function implantable defibrillator-pacemakers, minimal epicardial pacing thresholds and maximum R-wave amplitudes should be obtained. For patients with previously implanted pacemakers, mapping of the left ventricle should be undertaken at the time of defibrillator implantation to find a site where pacemaker stimulus artifacts are minimal even when the pacemaker is programmed to its maximal output.

If dual-device systems are planned, pacemaker implantation should precede thoracotomy defibrillator implantation, since this provides a greater opportunity to find a site for defibrillator lead implantation where the pacemaker stimulus artifact is as small as possible. This will minimize the possibility of pacemaker inhibition of arrhythmia detection by the implantable defibrillator and will avoid multiple counting by the implantable defibrillator of pacing stimulus artifacts and evoked R waves. For transvenous defibrillators, the implantable defibrillator should be implanted first, and the pacemaker positioned to minimize interactions. In either case, testing for overdetection and underdetection of arrhythmias must be performed.

Postoperative testing is always recommended to reverify the absence of adverse device-device interaction. Function of the two devices should always be tested during induced ventricular fibrillation, since if defibrillation is unsuccessful the risk of arrhythmic cardiac death is increased. Antitachycardia pacing and arrhythmia detection during ventricular tachycardia should be similarly tested when appropriate. When attention is paid to these details, the chronic management and excellent outcome of patients with dual-device systems are facilitated.

REFERENCES

1. Mirowski M, Reid PR, Mower MM, et al: Termination of malignant ventricular arrhythmias with an implanted automatic defibrillator in human beings. N Engl J Med 303:322, 1980.
2. Mower MM, Reid PR, Watkins L, et al: Automatic implantable cardioverter-defibrillator structural characteristics. PACE 7:1331, 1984.
3. Mirowski M: The automatic implantable cardioverter-defibrillator: An overview. J Am Coll Cardiol 6:461, 1985.
4. Cohen AI, Wish MH, Fletcher RD, et al: The use and interaction of permanent pacemakers and the automatic implantable cardioverter defibrillator. PACE 11:704, 1988.
5. Epstein AE, Kay GN, Plumb VJ, et al: Combined automatic implantable cardioverter-defibrillator and pacemaker systems: Implantation techniques and follow-up. J Am Coll Cardiol 13:121, 1989.
6. Manz M, Gerckens U, Funke HD, et al: Combination of antitachycardia pacemaker and automatic implantable cardioverter-defibrillator for ventricular tachycardia. PACE 9:676, 1986.
7. Masterson M, Pinski SL, Wilkoff B, et al: Pacemaker and defibrillator combination therapy for recurrent ventricular tachycardia. Cleve Clin J Med 57:330, 1990.
8. Bonnet CA, Forgoros RN, Elson JJ, et al.: Long-term efficacy of an antitachycardia pacemaker and implantable defibrillator combination. PACE 14:814, 1991.
9. Ahern TS, Nydegger C, McCormick DJ, et al: Device interaction—antitachycardia pacemakers and defibrillators for sustained ventricular tachycardia. PACE 14:302, 1991.
10. Bach SM: AID-B cardioverter-defibrillator possible interaction with pacemakers. Technical Communication, Intec Systems. August 29, 1983.
11. Kim SG, Furman S, Waspe LE, et al: Unipolar pacer artifacts induced failure of an automatic implantable cardioverter/defibrillator to detect ventricular fibrillation. Am J Cardiol 57:880, 1986.
12. Ruffy R, Lal R, Kouchoukos NT, et al: Combined bipolar dual-chamber pacing and automatic implantable cardioverter/defibrillator. J Am Coll Cardiol 7:933, 1986.
13. Ballas SL, Rashidi R, McAlister H, et al: The use of beep-o-grams in the assessment of automatic implantable cardioverter-defibrillator sensing function. PACE 12:1737, 1989.
14. Luceri RM, Thurer RJ, Castellanos A, et al: Initial experience with automatic defibrillator-implanted pacemaker interactions [abstract]. PACE 8:296, 1985.
15. Luceri RM, Habal SM, Castellanos A, et al: Mechanism of death in patients with automatic implantable cardioverter defibrillator. PACE 11:2015, 1988.
16. Bayés de Luna A, Coumel P, Leclercq JF: Ambulatory sudden cardiac death: Mechanisms of production of fatal arrhythmias on the basis of data from 157 cases. Am Heart J 117:151, 1989.
17. Luu M, Stevenson WG, Stevenson LW, et al: Diverse mechanisms of unexpected cardiac arrest in advanced heart failure. Circulation 80:1675, 1989.
18. Khastgir T, Aarons D, Veltri E: Sudden bradyarrhythmic death in patients with the implantable cardioverter-defibrillator: Report of two cases. PACE 14:395, 1991.
19. Hurwitz J, Marchlinski F: Epicardial lead location may be inadequate for ventricular tachycardia termination in antitachycardia pacing/implantable cardioverter defibrillators [abstract]. PACE 15:565, 1992.
20. Gottlieb C, Miller JM, Rosenthal ME, et al: Automatic implantable defibrillator discharge resulting from routine pacemaker programming. PACE 11:336, 1988.
21. Kim SG, Furman S, Matos JA, et al: Automatic implantable cardioverter/defibrillator: Inadvertent discharges during permanent pacemaker magnet tests. PACE 10:579, 1987.
22. Critelli G, Monda V, Scherillo M, et al: The automatic implantable cardioverter-defibrillator: Transesophageal atrial pacing discloses the potential for erroneous discharges. PACE 11:419, 1988.
23. Roth JA, Fisher JD, Furman S, et al: Termination of slower ventricular tachycardia using an automatic implantable cardioverter-defibrillator triggered by chest wall stimulation. Am J Cardiol 59:1209, 1987.
24. Ching E, Carlblom D, Wilkoff BL, et al: Risk of pacemaker damage induced by implantable defibrillator shocks [abstract]. PACE 14:629, 1991.
25. Guarnieri T, Datorre SD, Bondke H, et al: Increased pacing threshold after an automatic defibrillator shock in dogs: Effects of Class I and Class II antiarrhythmic drugs. PACE 11:1324, 1988.
26. Salel AF, Seagren SC, Pool PE: Effects of encainide on the function of implanted pacemakers. PACE 12:1439, 1989.
27. Montefoschi N, Boccadamo R: Propafenone induced acute variation of chronic atrial pacing threshold: A case report. PACE 13:480, 1990.
28. Hayes DL: Effects of drugs and devices on permanent pacemakers. Cardio January:70, 1991.
29. Epstein AE, Ellenbogen KA, Kirk KA, et al: Clinical characteristics and outcome of patients with high defibrillation thresholds: A multicenter study. Circulation 86:1206, 1992.
30. Calkins H, Brinker J, Veltri EP, et al: Clinical interactions between pacemakers and automatic implantable cardioverter-defibrillators. J Am Coll Cardiol 16:666, 1990.
31. Slepian M, Levine JH, Watkins L, et al: Automatic implantable cardioverter defibrillator/permanent pacemaker interaction: Loss of pacemaker capture following AICD discharge. PACE 10:1194, 1987.
32. Reiter MJ, Lindenfeld J, Tyndal CM, et al: Effects of ventricular fibrillation and defibrillation pacing threshold in the anesthetized dog. J Am Coll Cardiol 13:180, 1989.
33. Doherty PW, McLaughlin PR, Billingham M, et al: Cardiac damage produced by direct current countershock applied to the heart. Am J Cardiol 43:225, 1979.
34. Koning G, Veefkind AH, Schneider H: Cardiac damage caused by direct application of defibrillator shocks to isolated Langendorff-perfused rabbit heart. Am Heart J 100:473, 1980.
35. Eysmann SB, Marchlinski FE, Buxton AE, et al: Electrocardiographic changes after cardioversion of ventricular arrhythmias. Circulation 73:73, 1986.
36. Leja F, Scanlon PJ, Euler DE: Mechanisms responsible for countershock-induced ventricular tachycardia in the intact canine heart. Am Heart J 113:296, 1987.

37. Marwick TH, McAlister HF, Salcedo EE, et al: Effect of implantable defibrillator patch electrodes on left ventricular filling. J Interven Cardiol 2:161, 1989.
38. Avitall B, Port S, Gal R, et al: Automatic implantable cardioverter/defibrillator discharges and acute myocardial injury. Circulation 81:1482, 1990.
39. Yabe S, Smith WM, Daubert JP, et al: Conduction disturbances caused by high-current density electric fields. Circulation 66:1190, 1990.
40. Khastgir T, Lattuca J, Aarons D, et al: Ventricular pacing threshold and time to capture postdefibrillation in patients undergoing implantable cardioverter-defibrillator implantation. PACE 14:768, 1991.

41. Stoddard MF, Redd RR, Buckingham TA, et al: Effects of electrophysiologic testing of the automatic implantable cardioverter-defibrillator on left ventricular systolic function and diastolic filling. Am Heart J 122:714, 1991.
42. Lucy SD, Jones DL, Klein GJ: Effects of defibrillation shocks delivered directly over a major coronary artery. PACE 15:1711, 1992.
43. Yee R, Jones DL, Jarvis E, et al: Changes in pacing threshold and R wave amplitude after transvenous catheter countershock. J Am Coll Cardiol 4:543, 1984.

CHAPTER 40

INTERFERENCE IN CARDIAC PACEMAKERS

Neil F. Strathmore

Pacemakers as electric sensors are subject to interference from nonbiologic electromagnetic sources.[1-3] In addition, extremes of temperature or irradiation may cause pacemaker malfunction. In general, modern pacemakers are effectively shielded against electromagnetic interference, and the increasing use of bipolar leads has reduced the problem even further. Although formerly there was concern about the electric signals that patients might encounter in their normal environments, it is now recognized that with improved pacemaker protection, these signals rarely cause problems.[1] The principal sources of interference that affect pacemakers are in the medical area and include the previously well-recognized sources of electrocautery and defibrillation, together with the newer technologies of magnetic resonance imaging (MRI), lithotripsy, and transcutaneous nerve stimulation.

The portions of the electromagnetic spectrum that may affect pacemakers are *radio-frequency waves* with frequencies between 0 and 10^9 Hz, including alternating current electricity supplies (50 or 60 Hz) and electrocautery, and *microwaves* with frequencies between 10^9 and 10^{11} Hz, including ultrahigh-frequency radio waves, radar, and microwave ovens (2.45×10^9 Hz). Higher frequency portions of the spectrum, including infrared, visible light, ultraviolet, x-rays, and gamma rays, do not interfere with pacemakers because their wavelength is much shorter than the pacemaker or lead dimensions. However, high-intensity therapeutic x-rays can damage pacemaker circuitry directly.

Electromagnetic interference enters a pacemaker by conduction if the patient is in direct contact with the source or by way of radiation if the patient is in an electromagnetic field with the pacemaker lead acting as an antenna. Pacemakers have been protected from interference by shielding the pacemaker circuitry, reducing the distance between the electrodes to minimize the antenna, and filtering the incoming signal. If interference does enter the pacemaker, noise protection algorithms in the pacemaker timing circuit decrease the effect on the patient.

The modern pacemaker is immune from interference from most sources because the circuitry is shielded inside a stainless steel or titanium case. In addition, the body tissues provide some protection by reflection or absorption of external radiation. Studies of interference on pacemakers in vivo have shown that pacemaker function is not disturbed at field strengths that interfere with pacemakers on a test rig.[4]

Bipolar leads sense less conducted and radiated interference because the electrode distance, and thus the antenna, is smaller than for unipolar leads. Bipolar sensing has effectively eliminated myopotential inhibition and crosstalk as pacemaker problems. In addition, studies have shown that with bipolar sensing there is considerably less sensing of external electric fields[5] and less effect from electrocautery during surgery.[6]

Sensed interference is filtered by narrow bandpass filters to exclude noncardiac signals. However, this still leaves signals in the 5- to 100-Hz range, which overlap the cardiac signal range and are not filtered. These signals can give rise to abnormal pacemaker behavior if they are interpreted as cardiac signals and inhibit or trigger pacemaker output inappropriately.

The possible responses to external interference include inappropriate inhibition or triggering of pacemaker output, asynchronous pacing for the duration of the noise, change in the pacing mode requiring reprogramming to the original mode, and damage to the pacemaker circuitry causing some form of pacemaker failure.

Pacemaker Responses to Noise

ASYNCHRONOUS PACING

In order to protect the patient from inappropriate inhibition of pacemaker output, all modern pacemakers temporarily change to asynchronous pacing if exposed to sufficient interference. This change is usually activated by signals detected during a noise sampling period (NSP) within the pacemaker timing cycle (Fig. 40–1). The NSP occurs immediately after the ventricular refractory period (VRP), which follows a ventricular sensed or paced event. The VRP is an "absolute" refractory period, during which the ventricular sensing channel does not detect any signals and in particular will not sense the ventricular pacing pulse afterpotential or the evoked QRS and T waves. The VRP usually lasts between 200 and 400 msec, and events occurring during this period have no effect on pacemaker timing. The NSP or resettable refractory period lasts between 60 and 200 msec. If an event is sensed during this period, it is interpreted as noise and either the VRP or the NSP is restarted. In addition, in a dual-chamber mode, the postventricular atrial refractory period and the upper rate interval but not the lower rate interval are restarted. If a further noise event is detected in the NSP, the VRP or NSP will again be restarted and the pacemaker will not recognize cardiac signals. Repetitive noise events will eventually cause the lower rate interval to time out, and a pacing pulse will be delivered. Continuous noise will thus result in asynchronous pacing at the lower rate limit.

In some models, rather than timing out the lower rate interval, repetitive detection of noise in the NSP causes temporary switching to a specific "noise reversion mode," which is usually an asynchronous mode (VOO or DOO). In recent Intermedics (Angleton, TX) pacemakers with programmable polarity, the pacing output is unipolar in the noise reversion mode, even if the device is programmed to bipolar pacing.

Whether noise causes inhibition or asynchronous pacing is dependent on the duration and field strength of the signal.[7] At the lowest field strength there is no effect. As the field strength increases, there is a greater tendency to inhibition because the noise may be sensed intermittently and may not be sensed in the NSP but in the alert period between the NSP and the next pacing pulse. At higher field strengths, the noise will be sensed continuously, including in the NSP, and asynchronous pacing will occur. There is considerable variation in pacemaker models in their susceptibility to noise.[7, 8]

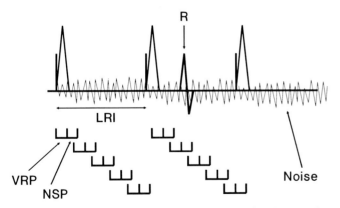

FIGURE 40–1. Response of a VVI pacemaker to noise. There is no sensing during the ventricular refractory period (VRP). Noise is detected in the noise-sampling period (NSP) immediately after the VRP and causes restarting of the VRP. In the next NSP, noise is again detected, and the VRP is again restarted. This continues until the lower rate interval (LRI) times out, and a ventricular pacing pulse is delivered. Because the sensing channel is refractory throughout the LRI, the intrinsic cardiac beat (R) is not sensed, and pacing is asynchronous.

If the entire VRP is restarted by a sensed event in the NSP, cardiac impulses at a cycle length equal to the VRP could cause asynchronous pacing. In most VVI pacemakers, the VRP is on the order of 250 msec, so only cardiac rates greater than 240 min^{-1} will do this. In some DDD pacemakers, however, the VRP may be prolonged after a ventricular premature beat, that is, as defined by the pacemaker logic, a ventricular event not preceded by an atrial event. In some Medtronic pacemakers (e.g., Symbios 7005; Medtronic, Inc., Minneapolis, MN), the VRP is prolonged to 345 msec after a ventricular premature beat, so cardiac rates of greater than 174 minute^{-1} could be interpreted as noise and cause asynchronous pacing. This has been observed during sinus tachycardia, supraventricular tachycardia, and atrial fibrillation.[9–12] If the NSP, rather than the VRP, is restarted by noise, only events at this shorter cycle length will cause asynchronous pacing, that is, if the NSP is 200 msec, only rates of 300 minute^{-1} will cause asynchronous pacing.

It has recently been noted that asynchronous pacing in the noise reversion mode may occur in the absence of noise during implantation of the Telectronics Meta DDDR model 1250 pacemaker (Telectronics, Inc., Englewood, CO). This pulse generator, in all pacing modes, emits small current pulses to determine thoracic impedance changes and so monitor minute volume. Impedance measurement is performed using a tripolar system incorporating the pulse generator casing, so when these pulses are emitted before the pulse generator has been placed in the subcutaneous pocket, they are interpreted as noise and the pacemaker will pace in the noise reversion mode, which is VOO. As soon as the pulse generator casing is in contact with the body tissue, normal pacing function returns.

MODE RESETTING

In addition to the temporary changes already discussed, electric interference can cause a change to another pacing mode that persists after the noise stops. This is usually the pacemaker "backup mode" or "reset mode" and is often the same as the pacemaker elective replacement indicator or end-of-life mode. In pacemakers with an elective replacement indicator or end-of-life flag, this device may be triggered and cause confusion when the pacemaker is subsequently telemetered. Either a pacemaker that has been affected by interference is wrongly assumed to have reached its end of life and is replaced or a pacemaker that has truly reached its end of life may be reprogrammed by an operator believing that the pacemaker has been subject to interference. In both cases, careful attention to the programmer telemetry, when available, will help. If the telemetered cell impedance remains low or the battery voltage is normal, the pacemaker battery is not exhausted and interference is the problem. Another test is to stress the pacemaker power supply by reprogramming to the original pacing mode with maximum output and an increased rate. If the pacemaker battery is truly at the end of its life, the pacemaker will immediately revert to the end-of-life mode.

The backup or reset mode is usually VVI, and if the pulse generator has programmable polarity the backup polarity will be unipolar. This may be significant in patients with implantable defibrillators and will be discussed further on. Some pacemakers, including most Cordis dual-chamber models

(Telectronics, Englewood, CO), reset to VOO mode if subject to interference that can cause pacing to compete with the intrinsic rhythm.

Electromagnetic interference is not the only inappropriate cause of mode resetting in pacemakers. Exposure to low temperatures before implantation causes a rise in the internal battery resistance, with a subsequent fall in the battery voltage causing the end-of-life indicator or reset mode to be activated.[13] This is a frequent occurrence during shipment in cold climates, so all pacemakers should be routinely interrogated before implantation and reprogrammed if necessary.

TRIGGERED MODE

A completely different approach to the interference problem is to program the triggered modes, VVT or AAT. In these modes, sensed signals trigger, rather than inhibit, a pacemaker pulse. Noise will trigger pacing at an upper rate determined by the VRP, so this is usually set to approximately 400 msec, which limits the maximum triggered rate to 150 ppm. The triggered modes are often used to prevent myopotential inhibition in unipolar pacing systems and may be used for patients undergoing surgery to prevent interference by electrocautery.

Environmental Electromagnetic Interference

Electric and magnetic signals are emitted by industrial and domestic sources that the pacemaker patient may come in contact with. Studies of pacemakers in test rigs have shown that they are subject to interference from such environmental interference.[8] However, studies of implanted pacemakers have shown that there are few problems[4, 14] in the domestic area, and problems rarely occur in the industrial area.

Microwave ovens are no longer considered a significant source of interference, partly because they have effective shielding and interlocking circuitry that prevents them being switched on while the door is open. In addition, there is at least one study suggesting that domestic microwaves have little or no effect on pacemakers.[2]

Metal detectors are frequently mentioned as a potential problem, and warning signs are often seen at airport security stations. However, a recent study of patients wearing ambulatory electrocardiographic monitors while passing through metal detector gates set at maximal sensitivity showed no effect on pacing.[15] Asynchronous pacing might occur for one or two beats without ill effect to the patient. The major reason to warn patients about metal detectors is that the detector will be activated by the pacemaker.

There are no reports of other domestic appliances having an effect on modern pacemakers.[1] Potentially an electric shaver moved over a unipolar pacemaker may cause temporary asynchronous pacing. There are no reports of interference from mobile telephones or portable computers, but as this technology expands it is possible that interference may be detected.

In the close vicinity of high-voltage power lines or substations, the electric field may be strong enough to cause transient inhibition or asynchronous pacing in unipolar pacemakers, but it has no effect on bipolar pacemakers with normal sensitivity settings and only a rare effect at maximum sensitivity.[5] At 40 meters (m) from a 400-kV power line, the field strength is less than 1 kV/m and will have no effect on either a unipolar or bipolar pacemaker.[5]

Industrial electrical equipment, such as arc welders, generate large electric fields and can cause interference in unipolar pacemakers but are unlikely to cause interference with bipolar pacemakers.[14] Patients with implanted unipolar devices should be warned not to use arc welders, but patients with bipolar devices can safely use equipment with currents up to 400 amperes (A).[16] Specialized industrial equipment with very heavy current drains, such as high-resistance spot welders, may need to be assessed individually[14] and advice sought from the manufacturer.

Aircraft radio and radar signals are of sufficient strength to interfere with unipolar pacemakers[8] when measured in a testing apparatus but have not been shown to interfere with pacemaker function in implanted pacemakers,[4] either unipolar or bipolar. The vibration associated with helicopter transport will cause an increase in the pacing rate in activity sensing pacemakers,[17] although this could be considered a normal response rather than "interference."

Magnets may cause a change in pacing to the asynchronous magnet mode, but most patients are not in contact with magnets for any significant time. The original automatic implantable cardioverter defibrillator was inactivated by placing a magnet over the device. As the device is in the anterior abdominal wall, there is a much greater chance of the automatic implantable cardioverter defibrillator being accidentally inactivated by a magnet inadvertently or unknowingly placed by a patient. These magnets have included pacemaker magnets, magnetized screws, loudspeakers,[18] and bingo wands.[19]

Electrocautery

Electrocautery continues to be a major problem in patients with implanted pacemakers.[6, 20] Electrocautery or diathermy involves the use of radiofrequency current to cut or coagulate tissues. It is usually applied in a unipolar fashion between the cauterizing instrument (the cathode) and the indifferent plate (the anode) attached at a distance to the patient's skin. Bipolar cautery uses a bipolar instrument for coagulation. The frequency is usually between 300 and 500 kHz (at frequencies less than 200 kHz, muscle and nerve stimulation may occur). Cutting diathermy uses a modulated signal so that bursts of energy are applied, whereas coagulation diathermy uses an unmodulated signal to heat the tissue. Coagulation diathermy is used in radio-frequency ablation of cardiac tissue for the treatment of arrhythmias.

The current generated by electrocautery is related to the distance and orientation of the cautery electrodes relative to the pacemaker and lead.[21] High current is generated if the cautery cathode is close to the pacemaker, and particularly high currents will be generated in the pacemaker if it lies between the two cautery electrodes.

Electrocautery can cause all the standard responses to interference (Table 40–1). The radio-frequency signal may be interpreted as a cardiac impulse and so cause inappropriate inhibition. Prolonged application of the cautery causes repet-

TABLE 40–1. **RESPONSE TO ELECTROCAUTERY**

Inhibition of output
Asynchronous pacing (noise mode)
Reset-backup mode
Elective replacement indicator activation
Pulse generator circuit damage
Myocardial trauma: elevated threshold

itive stimulation in the NSP and thus asynchronous pacing at the lower rate. Pacemaker function will return to normal each time the diathermy is switched off.

Switching to the backup or reset mode may also occur and will not return to normal until reprogramming is performed.[22, 23] This can cause hemodynamic compromise if the mode is VVI and AV synchrony is lost[6] or the rate is slow.[24] If the backup mode is VOO, as in many Cordis pacemakers (Telectronics, Englewood, CO), asynchronous pacing will occur, even after the electrocautery has been switched off.[23]

Pacemaker circuitry can be damaged by the electrocautery in spite of electronic protection, and output failure, pacemaker runaway,[25] or other malfunctions can occur, requiring pacemaker replacement. The electrocautery signal may induce currents in the pacing lead and cause local heating at the electrode, leading to myocardial damage with subsequent elevation of pacing thresholds. This problem is a cause of concern but appears to be infrequently documented.

To prevent inappropriate inhibition of the pacemaker, a magnet is often applied to the chest over the pacemaker during cautery to convert it to the asynchronous mode. This may be successful, although in some pacemakers, including all Medtronic (Minneapolis, MN) models, this may open the pacemaker to reprogramming by the electrocautery signal[26] and is therefore not recommended. Another potential problem is that in certain Siemens (Solna, Sweden) and Telectronics (Englewood, CO) pacemakers, magnet placement triggers the Vario threshold testing sequence, which reduces the output voltage on successive pulses and so may cause transient loss of capture.

Pacemakers with rate-responsive functions may exhibit unexpected responses during surgery. The electrocautery signal may overwhelm the impedance measuring circuit of a minute ventilation rate-responsive pacemaker and cause pacing at the upper rate limit.[27]

Most reported complications of electrocautery are with unipolar pacemakers, and a recent prospective study of pacemaker patients undergoing surgery suggested that bipolar devices are less susceptible to the effects of electrocautery.[6]

Patients with pacemakers who are to undergo surgery in which electrocautery is used should be properly assessed and managed (Table 40–2). Preoperatively, the critical step is to identify the pacemaker so that its response to cautery will be known and so that the appropriate programmer will be available. In particular, the backup mode should be determined from the manufacturer's literature. When the backup mode might compromise the patient because it will reduce AV synchrony, pace asynchronously, or deliver too slow a rate, the programmer must be available in the operating room, the pulse generator must be accessible to the programming head, and someone experienced in programming should be present.

Pacemaker function should be checked with a programmer

preoperatively—the device should be telemetered, programmed settings should be recorded, the underlying rhythm should be determined, and pacing thresholds should be measured. Rate responsiveness and magnet-initiated threshold testing should be turned off. Consideration should be given to programming to an asynchronous mode or triggered mode (VVT), particularly if the patient is pacemaker-dependent.

In the operating room, the indifferent plate of the electrocautery should be placed at a distance from the pacemaker, usually on the thigh, and good contact should be ensured. The effect of the electrocautery may be difficult to assess because it causes interference on the electrocardiogram (ECG) monitor. Other methods of assessing cardiac rhythm should be used—palpation of the pulse or pulse oximetry are the most popular.

Cautery should be used with caution in the vicinity of the pacemaker and its leads. The cathode should be kept as far from the pulse generator as possible, the lowest possible amplitude should be used, and the surgeon should deliver only brief bursts.[20, 28]

During electrocautery, pacemaker function and cardiac rhythm should be carefully assessed. The most likely response will be transient inhibition or asynchronous pacing during electrocautery, which should cause no significant hemodynamic problem. If persistent pacemaker inhibition occurs, a magnet can be applied to the pacemaker during electrocautery application as long as the pacemaker is not one that might be reprogrammed with the magnet in place.

Postoperatively, the pacemaker should be interrogated and, if it is in the reset mode, it should be reprogrammed to the original settings. Threshold testing should be performed. If problems are encountered when interrogating the pacemaker or reprogramming it to its original settings, the manufacturer should be consulted to determine if malfunction has occurred. In some cases, the pacemaker can be reactivated with a special programmer, but if this is not possible, it should be replaced.

TABLE 40–2. **PERIOPERATIVE MANAGEMENT OF PACEMAKERS**

PREOPERATIVE
Identify pacemaker and determine "reset" mode
Check pacemaker program, telemetry, thresholds, battery status
Deactivate rate response, Vario
Consult with anesthesiologist, surgeon

IN THE OPERATING ROOM
Position electrocautery indifferent plate away from pacemaker so that pacemaker will not be between electrocautery electrodes
Monitor pulse or oximeter (ECG will be obscured by artifact)
Pacemaker should be accessible to programmer
Use bipolar cautery when possible
Do not use cautery near pacemaker
Use short bursts
Reprogram if necessary if reset mode hemodynamically unstable
Use VVT mode if necessary
Use magnet with caution (may cause reprogramming)

POSTOPERATIVE
Check pacemaker program, telemetry, thresholds
Reprogram if necessary
Replace if circuit damage has occurred

Abbreviation: ECG, electrocardiogram.

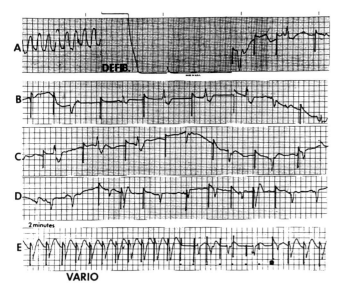

FIGURE 40–2. Serial electrocardiograms (ECGs) showing transient loss of capture after defibrillation (DEFIB.) in a patient. The loss of capture is followed by intermittent capture, first demonstrated in the supernormal zone of the native beats (*strip D*). Sensing function is normal. The refractory period of the pacemaker was programmed to 437 msec. *Strip E* demonstrates stimulation threshold testing using the Vario function of this pacemaker. This is initiated by placing a test magnet over the implanted pulse generator, which starts a test cycle with two phases repeating themselves as long as the magnet is in place. The first part of testing consists of 16 impulses at the magnet rate of 100 beats per minute (bpm) delivered at the full output of the generator. At the end of the first 16 impulses, the Vario mechanism causes pacing at a rate slightly faster than the magnet rate. The output voltage is decreased by a fixed amount successively during the ensuing 16 impulses from the full output to an output of 0 V. The threshold is then calculated by counting the number of ineffective pacing impulses from right to left. At the end of the test cycle, the pacemaker automatically returns to its programmed voltage output. (From Levine PA, Barold SS, Fletcher RD, et al. J Am Coll Cardiol 1:1413, 1983. Reprinted with permission from the American College of Cardiology.)

Defibrillation

External transthoracic defibrillation produces the largest amount of electric energy delivered in the vicinity of a pacemaker and has the potential to damage both the pulse generator and the cardiac tissue in contact with the lead.[29, 30] Internal defibrillation via epicardial or subcutaneous patches or intracardiac defibrillation electrodes delivers smaller amounts of energy but may also interfere with pacemaker function.[31, 32]

The pacemaker is protected from damage from high defibrillation energies by special circuitry incorporating a Zener diode that electronically regulates the voltage entering the pacemaker circuit and should prevent high currents from being conducted via the lead to the myocardium. However, the extremely high energies can overwhelm this protection and cause damage to the pacemaker or the heart. The reports of extensive pacemaker and cardiac damage mostly relate to older unipolar devices, and it is likely that bipolar pacemakers are more resistant[1] (Fig. 40–2).

Most commonly, the backup or reset mode or the elective replacement or end-of-life indicator is activated. It is important to note that in the backup or reset mode, pacemakers with programmable polarity usually deliver unipolar pacing pulses. It is essential that a pacemaker in a patient with an implantable cardioverter defibrillator pace in a bipolar mode to prevent under- and oversensing by the defibrillator, so a dedicated bipolar pacemaker without programmable pacing polarity should be implanted in such patients. Defibrillation may induce high-energy currents in the pacemaker lead, either by capacitive coupling to the defibrillation shock or by shunting in the pacemaker circuit.[30] This energy may be sufficient to cause trauma or burning of the myocardium at the myocardium-electrode interface[29] with chronic threshold elevation,[30] but this has rarely been reported. However, transient loss of capture with elevated capture and sensing thresholds has been frequently reported following both external and internal defibrillation.[30–32] It is likely that unipolar pacing systems are more prone to this form of damage than are bipolar systems,[30] and there are no reports of extensive cardiac damage with bipolar leads. It has also been suggested that the elevation of pacing threshold after defibrillation is related to the duration of ventricular fibrillation rather than to the energy of defibrillation.[33]

The degree of damage seems to be related to the distance of the defibrillation paddles from the pulse generator. It is recommended by all pacemaker manufacturers that the paddles be placed as far as possible from the generator. When possible, an anterior-posterior configuration is preferred (Fig. 40–3). However, in the anterior-anterior configuration, the paddles should be 10 cm away from the pacemaker if possible. Following defibrillation, transient loss of capture or sensing should be anticipated. The pulse amplitude may need to be increased, and this is performed automatically in implanted cardioverter defibrillators with backup bradycardia pacing. The pacemaker should be interrogated and the program checked. Transient threshold rises should be managed by increasing the output energy if necessary. Rarely, pro-

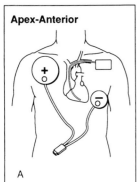
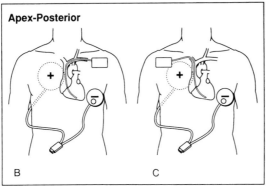

FIGURE 40–3. Schematic representation of positioning of paddles or R2 pads to minimize damage to the pulse generator and pacemaker lead.

TABLE 40–3. **MANAGEMENT OF PATIENTS UNDERGOING CARDIOVERSION AND DEFIBRILLATION**

BEFORE PROCEDURE
Pacemaker programmer should be available for reprogramming
Determine degree of pacemaker dependence if possible prior to cardioversion or by reviewing pacemaker chart
Have transcutaneous external pacemaker available for pacemaker-dependent patients
Use lowest possible energy for cardioversion or defibrillation
Use anteroposterior R2 patches or paddle positioning
Do not put paddles or R2 patches over generator; keep them as far from pulse generator and lead as possible
The vector of energy delivery should be perpendicular to a line joining the pulse generator and ventricular lead; in dual-chamber generators, preference should be given to the ventricular lead

FOLLOWING PROCEDURE
Repeat determination of pacing and sensing thresholds immediately, several hours later, and again in 24 hours
Monitor for 24 hours

longed, severe threshold rises occur that necessitate lead replacement. Our recommendations for management of patients undergoing cardioversion and defibrillation are summarized in Table 40–3.

Catheter Ablation

Catheter ablation of intracardiac structures to control arrhythmias was first performed using direct current (DC)

shock. This technique had a higher tendency to affect pacemakers than does external defibrillation, and 50% to 60% of patients in three series experienced problems, including activation of the backup or reset mode, pacemaker circuit failure, and transient rises in pacing and sensing thresholds.[34–36] DC catheter ablation should be avoided in patients with permanent pacemakers if alternative therapy is available.

Nearly all ablations are now carried out using radio-frequency current, which is the same as coagulation electrocautery, that is, unmodulated radio-frequency current at a frequency of 400 to 500 kHz. Effects similar to those of surgical electrocautery have been reported,[37] including inappropriate inhibition, asynchronous pacing, and resetting to backup mode. An example of oversensing due to sensing of radio-frequency energy during the NSP is shown in Figure 40–4. In addition, high pacing rates (runaway) were observed in an experimental situation with the ablation catheter positioned 1 cm from the pacing electrode,[37] presumably due to current induced in the lead and pacemaker circuit. A preliminary report of radio-frequency ablation in 25 patients reported transient under- or oversensing, noncapture, or runaway pacemaker during radio-frequency energy delivery in almost 80% of patients. Following ablation, all pacemakers were reprogrammed to their preablation settings, with 92% of patients demonstrating proper pacing and sensing. Long-term follow-up at a mean of 308 days did not reveal any further progressive pacemaker damage but required a change in pacing mode or programmed settings in 60% of patients.

The ablation catheter is usually some distance from the pacing lead and radio-frequency ablation has been carried

FIGURE 40–4. Atrial electrograms recorded from a patient with an incessant atrial tachycardia and a Pacesetter Synchrony II generator (Model 2022) (Sylmar, CA) during radiofrequency ablation. During these recordings, the pacemaker was programmed to the AAI mode at 45 bpm with a sensitivity of 0.5 mV and an atrial refractory period of 225 msec. *A*, In the 11:48 AM recording, there is asynchronous atrial pacing due to continuous sensing of noise and refractory period extension. This is seen intermittently during the delivery of the radio-frequency lesion. (A, atrial pacing; P, atrial sensing.) Several minutes later *(B)*, the patient remains in atrial tachycardia (cycle length 550–587 msec), as radio-frequency energy is applied. There is sensing of noise and refractory period extension, which stops several seconds later as the atrial tachycardia is terminated during the radio-frequency lesion.

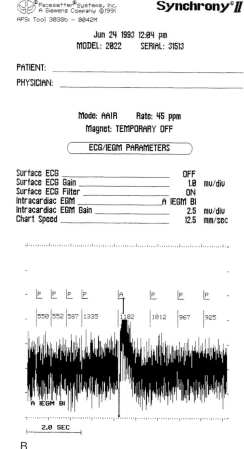

out safely in the presence of implanted pacemakers and does not appear to lead to severe myocardial damage at the site of the pacemaker electrode. Reprogramming of the pulse generator in the clinical setting is uncommon. Prior to performing radio-frequency ablation, however, it is essential to interrogate the pacemaker, record its programmed settings, and measure thresholds. Activity sensing should be switched off. After the procedure, the pacemaker should be checked and reprogrammed if necessary.

Magnetic Resonance Imaging

In magnetic resonance imaging (MRI), formerly called nuclear magnetic resonance scanning, a large magnetic field, generated by an electromagnet is modulated by a radio-frequency electric signal between 30 and 3000 Hz. Ferrous metal objects are attracted by the electromagnet and are not allowed near the scanner. Most recently, manufactured pacemakers contain little ferromagnetic materials. However, there is considerable variability regarding the ferromagnetic content of pacemakers manufactured in the 1980s. Many patients with pacemakers containing ferromagnetic material may experience torque forces when placed near the strong static magnetic field present in the MRI suite.[38, 39] There are no reported instances of pacemaker reprogramming or of permanent component damage by MRI.

The reported problems of pacemakers in MRI scanners include magnet-activated asynchronous pacing, inhibition by the radio-frequency signal, and rapid pacing induced by the radiofrequency signal.[40–42] Other problems reported include conversion of DDD pulse generators to the reset or backup mode and transient reed switch malfunction.

When a pacemaker is brought close to an MRI scanner with the electromagnet on, the reed switch closes, and asynchronous pacing occurs, which may compete with the underlying cardiac rhythm. Measuring the effect of the MRI scanner on pacemakers is made difficult because the radio-frequency pulses cause electrocardiographic artifacts. However, several studies have demonstrated the potential effects using pacemakers connected to resistances and oscilloscopes, and in dogs. In some pacemakers there was no effect except asynchronous pacing.[41] In other pacemakers, however, a signal of approximately 20 V was induced in the lead,[40] which can cause cardiac pacing at the same frequency or a multiple of the frequency of the radio-frequency current.[40–42] Thus, cardiac pacing may occur at the frequency of the pulsed energy, 60 to 300 bpm. In the case of a dual-chamber pacemaker, this may affect the atrial channel or the ventricular channel, or both. The radiofrequency signal is detected by the leads acting as an antenna and is then amplified by the pacemaker circuitry to produce sufficient energy to pace the heart. The lead must be attached to a pacemaker for pacing to occur, so it is not simply related to the radio-frequency energy in the lead.[42] However, the lead does not necessarily have to be in use, as it has been demonstrated that a Cordis dual-chamber pacemaker with both atrial and ventricular leads attached but programmed to the AAI mode will produce rapid ventricular pacing in the presence of an MRI scanner.[42] Asynchronous pacing may occur regardless of the position of the pulse generator with respect to the MRI "tunnel," and it may occur immediately or several seconds after the start of MRI imaging.

Most of the work with MRI interference has been done with unipolar pacemakers, and it is not clear whether bipolar pacemakers will be subject to the same complication. Not all manufacturers and models behave in the same way. Cordis and Telectronics (Englewood, CO) pacemakers are particularly likely to develop rapid pacing,[41, 42] and current Telectronics manuals suggest that MRI should not be used in patients with pacemakers. However, the current manuals of other manufacturers, including Medtronic (Minneapolis, MN), Pacesetter (Sylmar, CA), and Intermedics (Angleton, TX), suggest that MRI may be used with caution. In general, patients with pacemakers should not routinely undergo MRI scanning, and further studies of individual pacemaker models are required.

External pacemakers are also subject to interference from MRI. If operating in the inhibited mode, the radio-frequency signal is sufficient to inhibit the pacemaker output. In the asynchronous mode, however, there does not appear to be any rapid pacing detected or any influence on programmed settings or pacing threshold.

Extracorporeal Shock Wave Lithotripsy

Extracorporeal shock wave lithotripsy (ESWL) is a noninvasive treatment for renal tract calculi that delivers multiple, focused hydraulic shocks, generated by an underwater spark gap, to a patient lying in a water bath. The shock is focused on the calculi by an ellipsoid metal reflector. The shock wave can produce ventricular extrasystoles, so it is synchronized to the R wave. Pacemakers could be subject to electric interference from the spark gap and mechanical damage from the hydraulic shock wave.

Several investigators[41–43] have studied the effect of ESWL on pacemakers suspended in a water bath and on pacemakers strapped to the bodies of patients undergoing ESWL. Pacemaker output was not inhibited by the synchronous shocks, but asynchronous shocks caused inhibition in both unipolar and bipolar devices.[41, 43] The risk of pulse generator inhibition may be lower with single-chamber devices than with dual-chamber devices. Intermittent reversion to magnet mode and rate during lithotripsy has been reported to occur because of transient closure of the reed switch from the high-energy vibration created by the lithotripsy machine. Other responses noted during in vitro testing include an increase in rate of some pulse generators, failure of output (rare), and malfunction of the reed switch. Activity-sensing pacemakers increased their pacing rate to the upper pacing rate within 1 minute of the shock.[43] When a dual-chamber pacemaker was tested, the shock was synchronized to the atrial pacing pulse but was frequently sensed by the ventricular channel, causing either inhibition of the ventricular output if ventricular safety pacing was not enabled or safety pacing at a shortened AV interval when safety pacing was enabled.[42, 43]

ESWL caused no physical damage to the hermetic seal or the internal components of the pacemakers tested,[42, 43] except that when an activity sensing pacemaker was placed at the focal point of the ESWL, the piezoelectric crystal was shattered.[42] Patients with piezoelectric crystal activity rate-adaptive pacemakers can probably undergo lithotripsy safely if the device is implanted in the thorax, but lithotripsy should be avoided in these patients if the device is located in the abdomen.

Subsequent to the these in vitro studies, there are several reports of patients with implanted cardiac pacemakers undergoing ESWL[42, 44, 45] without any ill effects. In addition, no instances of reprogramming of pulse generators or conversion to reset or backup mode have been reported.

ESWL is safe to use with implanted pacemakers, provided that the shock is given synchronously with the ECG and that dual-chamber pacemakers have safety pacing enabled. An activity sensing pacemaker may develop an increase in rate following the shock, and if this is considered clinically undesirable, it should be programmed to the non–rate-responsive mode. Careful pacemaker follow-up should be performed over the next several months to ensure appropriate function of the reed switch. Physicians should contact the pulse generator's manufacturer to ascertain if any clinical experience is available with that particular generator in patients undergoing lithotripsy.

Some investigators recommend that if insufficient experience exists with a particular device, in vitro testing may be helpful. In addition, programming of a DDD pulse generator to the VVI, VOO, or DOO mode will avoid the rare cases in which irregularities of pacing rate may occur, supraventricular arrhythmias that could be tracked are induced, or triggering of the ventricular output by electromechanical interference occurs.

Transcutaneous Electric Nerve Stimulation

Transcutaneous electric nerve stimulation (TENS) is now a popular method for the relief of acute and chronic pain from musculoskeletal and neurologic problems. A TENS unit consists of several electrodes placed on the skin and connected to a pulse generator that applies 20-μsec rectangular pulses of between 1 and 200 V and 0 to 60 mA at a frequency of 20 to 110 Hz. The output and frequency of the unit can be adjusted by the patient to provide maximum relief of pain.

The repetition frequency of the TENS output is similar to the normal range of heart rates, so it would be expected that TENS pulses might cause pacemaker inhibition. However, a study of 51 patients who were monitored for 2 minutes during TENS stimulation showed no inhibition.[46] Cases have been reported of asymptomatic inhibition of pacemaker output by a TENS machine detected by Holter monitoring.[47] These instances took place in unipolar pacemakers and were eliminated by increasing the sensing threshold of the pacemaker (in one case to 5 mV). The effect on dual-chamber pacemakers has not been reported.

It is thought that TENS can be used safely in patients with implanted bipolar pacemakers and in patients with unipolar pacemakers if the sensitivity is reduced.

Dental Equipment

Dental ultrasound scalers may cause inhibition or asynchronous pacing in older pacemakers, but a recent study showed no effect on pacing function.[48] Repetitive activation of other dental equipment may cause inhibition.[49] As would be expected, dental drilling can cause sufficient vibration to increase the pacing rate of an activity sensing pacemaker.[49]

Radiation

Diagnostic radiation has no effect on pacemakers. Therapeutic radiation did not affect the earliest pacemakers but can cause failure in newer pacemakers that incorporate complementary metal oxide semiconductor–integrated circuit technology.[50–52] Radiation causes leakage currents between insulated parts of the circuit, leading to inappropriate charge accumulation in silicon oxide layers, which eventually leads to circuit failure. The degree of susceptibility may be related to the oxide thickness, as the most recent in vitro studies have examined pacemakers incorporating 3-μm complementary metal oxide semiconductor–integrated circuits and have shown less sensitivity to irradiation than the older 8-μm and 5-μm circuits.[52] Recently implanted cardioverter defibrillators have also been shown to fail when exposed to radiation.[52]

The cumulative radiation dose determines whether damage will occur. Therapeutic radiation involves doses of up to 70 Gy (7000 rad) and pacemakers may fail with as little as 10 Gy. Failure is unpredictable and may involve changes in sensitivity, amplitude, or pulse width; loss of telemetry; failure of output; or runaway rates. Pacemaker replacement is usually required, and although some changes may resolve in hours to days, the long-term reliability of the pacemaker is suspect, and it should be replaced. It should be emphasized that radiation therapy to any part of the body away from the site of the pulse generator should not cause a problem with the pulse generator. The dose of radiation used in diagnostic x-ray procedures, including coronary angiography, barium enemas, or cerebral angiography, for example, does not appear to affect pulse generator function either acutely or in a cumulative fashion.

Linear accelerators may cause electromagnetic interference, leading to pacemaker inhibition or reversion to the noise mode in susceptible pacemakers, particularly unipolar models.

Therapeutic radiation centers should have a protocol for patients with pacemakers[53] (Table 40–4). Before commencing radiation, the pacemaker should be identified and evaluated. Shielding should be used to minimize the dose received by the pacemaker. Oblique radiation fields may also reduce the dose. The radiation dose may be measured with dosimeter chips attached to the skin over the pacemaker.[54, 55]

TABLE 40–4. MANAGEMENT OF PACEMAKER PATIENTS UNDERGOING RADIOTHERAPY

Evaluate pacemaker prior to therapy
Avoid direct irradiation of pulse generator
Maximal shielding and distance of pulse generator from radiation beam is desirable; measure radiation to area of pulse generator
Monitor ECG continuously if pacemaker dependent
Testing of pulse generator should be performed frequently during each therapy session
Pulse generator should be moved if it cannot be shielded
Replace pacemaker if evidence of pacemaker failure

Abbreviation: ECG, electrocardiogram.

There may be no alternative but to remove the pacemaker and reimplant it at a distance from the area to be radiated. The pacemaker should be monitored during radiotherapy and should be regularly evaluated by telemetry during and after the course of radiotherapy.

Electroconvulsive Therapy

Electroconvulsive therapy appears safe with respect to pacemaker function, as only a minimal amount of electricity reaches the heart because of the high impedance of body tissues. Electrocardiographic monitoring and interrogation of the pacemaker appears advisable. In unipolar pacemakers, seizure activity may generate sufficient myopotentials to result in inhibition or ventricular tracking.

Diathermy

Short-wave diathermy consists of therapeutic application of current directly to the skin. Diathermy can be a source of interference, and because of its high frequency should be avoided near the implantation site because of its potential to cause pulse generator inhibition or damage to the pulse generator circuitry by excessive heating.[1] Short-wave or microwave diathermy may provide signals of high enough frequency to bypass noise protection mechanisms and directly damage the pacemaker's electronic components.

Electronic Article Surveillance

Antitheft devices in many department stores consist of a tag or marker that is sensed by an electromagnetic field as the individual walks through or by a "gate." Most systems consist of a "deactivator" that a cashier may use to remove or deactivate the tag following the purchase of an item. This allows the individual to purchase an item and leave the store without activating an alarm. These electronic antitheft devices consist of multiple technologies that generate electromagnetic fields in various ranges and include devices using the radio-frequency range of 2 to 10 mHz, magnetic material in the 50 to 10 kHz-range, pulsed systems at various frequencies, and electromagnetic fields in the microwave range. In vitro testing of pulse generators as well as an "in vivo" study of 32 patients with implanted generators was performed to evaluate the safety of these devices. The authors studied 32 volunteers with 26 different pacemaker models and demonstrated that 1 of 22 patients with a single-chamber pacemaker experienced inhibition, whereas 7 of 10 patients with dual-chamber generators experienced inhibition of output, with long pauses being seen in the majority of pacemaker-dependent patients.[57] Inhibition occurred when patients were in regions of low- and high-intensity magnetic fields at 10 kHz and at 300 Hz, or both. Radio-frequency and pulsed electromagnetic fields did not affect pacemaker function. Alterations in pacing thresholds or programmed parameters were not noted. The authors concluded that electronic antitheft devices can be dangerous to pacemaker patients, particularly if a unipolar DDD generator is implanted.

Conclusions

Nearly all patients can be reassured that electric interference will not affect their pacemakers during the course of daily life. Patients in specialized industrial environments should be assessed individually. In the course of medical treatment, patients should be carefully assessed and managed if they are to be exposed to electrocautery or have been subject to defibrillation. MRI scanning should still be regarded with caution, although some pacemaker manufacturers have reduced their warnings. Lithotripsy, TENS, and dental treatment can generally be undertaken without a problem. Therapeutic irradiation in pacemaker patients should be carefully planned to prevent pacemaker circuit destruction.

REFERENCES

1. Barold SS, Falkoff MD, Ong LS, et al: Interference in cardiac pacemakers: Exogenous sources. *In* El-Sherif N, Samet P (eds): Cardiac Pacing and Electrophysiology, 3rd ed. Philadelphia, WB Saunders, 1991, pp 608–632.
2. Irnich W: Interference in pacemakers. PACE 7:1021, 1984.
3. Sager DP: Current facts on pacemaker electromagnetic interference and their application to clinical care. Heart Lung 16:211, 1987.
4. Toff WD, Edhag OK, Camm AJ: Cardiac pacing and aviation. Eur Heart J 13(Suppl H):162, 1992.
5. Toivonen L, Valjus J, Hongisto M, et al: The influence of elevated 50 Hz electric and magnetic fields on implanted cardiac pacemakers: The role of the lead configuration and programming of the sensitivity. PACE 14:2114, 1991.
6. Hayes DL, Trusty J, Christiansen J, et al: A prospective study of electrocautery's effect on pacemaker function. PACE 10:686, 1987.
7. Kaye GC, Butrous GS, Allen A, et al: The effect of 50-Hz external electrical interference on implanted cardiac pacemakers. PACE 11:999, 1988.
8. Toff WD, Camm AJ: Implanted devices and aviation. Eur Heart J 9(Suppl G):133, 1988.
9. Falkoff M, Ong LS, Heinle RA, et al: The noise sampling period: A new cause of apparent sensing malfunction of demand pacemakers. PACE 1:250, 1978.
10. Sudduth BK, Morris DL, Gertz EW: Noise mode response at peak exercise in a DDD pacemaker. PACE 8:746, 1985.
11. Frohlig G, Dyckmans J, Doenecke P, et al: Noise reversion of a dual-chamber pacemaker without noise. PACE 9:690, 1986.
12. Fontaine JM, Alma-Perri C, El-Sherif N: DDD-pacemaker pseudomalfunction during supraventricular tachycardia. PACE 11:1380, 1988.
13. Barold SS, Falkoff MD, Ong LS, et al: Resetting of DDD pulse generators due to cold exposure. PACE 11:736, 1988.
14. Marco D, Eisenger G, Hayes DL: Testing of work environments for electromagnetic interference. PACE 15:2016, 1992.
15. Copperman Y, Zarfati D, Laniado S: The effect of metal detector gates on implanted permanent pacemakers. PACE 11:1386, 1988.
16. Medtronic Inc: Personal communication.
17. French RS, Tillman JG: Pacemaker function during helicopter transport. Ann Emerg Med 18:305, 1989.
18. Schmitt C, Brachman J, Waldecker B, et al: Implantable cardioverter defibrillator: Possible hazards of electromagnetic interference. PACE 14:982, 1991.
19. Ferrick KJ, Johnston D, Kim SG, et al: Inadvertent AICD inactivation while playing bingo. Am Heart J 121:206, 1991.
20. Levine PA, Balady GJ, Lazer HL, et al: Electrocautery and pacemakers: Management of the paced patient subject to electrocautery. Ann Thorac Surg 41:313, 1986.
21. Chauvin M, Crenner F, Brechenmacher C: Interaction between cardiac pacing and electrocautery: The significance of electrode position. PACE 15:2028, 1992.
22. Belott PH, Sands S, Warren J: Resetting of DDD pacemakers due to EMI. PACE 7:169, 1984.
23. Lamas FA, Antman EM, Gold JP, et al: Pacemaker backup-mode reversion and injury during cardiac surgery. Ann Thorac Surg 41:155, 1986.

24. Bailey AG, Lacey SR: Intraoperative pacemaker failure in an infant. Can J Anaesth 38:912, 1991.

25. Heller LI: Surgical electrocautery and the runaway pacemaker syndrome. PACE 13:1084, 1990.

26. Domino KB, Smith TC: Electrocautery-induced reprogramming of a pacemaker using a precordial magnet. Anesth Analg 62:609, 1983.

27. Van Hemel NM, Hamerlijnck RP, Pronk KJ, et al: Upper limit ventricular stimulation in respiratory rate responsive pacing due to electrocautery. PACE 12:1720, 1989.

28. Byrd CL, Schwartz SJ, Byrd CB, et al: Electrocautery and dual-chamber cardiac pacemakers. PACE 11:854, 1988.

29. Aylward P, Blood R, Tonkin A: Complications of defibrillation with permanent pacemaker in situ. PACE 2:462, 1979.

30. Levine PA, Barold SS, Fletcher RD, et al: Adverse acute and chronic effects of electrical defibrillation and cardioversion on implanted cardiac pacing systems. J Am Coll Cardiol 1:413, 1983.

31. Yee R, Jones DL, Klein GJ: Pacing threshold changes after transvenous catheter countershock. Am J Cardiol 53:503, 1984.

32. Calkins H, Brinker J, Veltri EP, et al: Clinical interactions between pacemakers and automatic implantable cardioverter-defibrillators. J Am Coll Cardiol 16:666, 1990.

33. Reiter MJ, Lindenfeld J, Breckinridge S, et al: Does defibrillation raise the ventricular pacing threshold? J Am Coll Cardiol 11:144A, 1988.

34. Bowes R, Benett D: Effect of transvenous atrioventricular nodal ablation on the function of implanted pacemakers. PACE 8:811, 1985.

35. Fontaine G, Lemoine B, Frank R, et al: Effects of fulguration on the permanent pacemaker. *In* Fontaine F (ed): Ablation in Cardiac Arrhythmias. Mt Kisco, NY, Futura Publishing, 1987, p 367.

36. Vaneiro G, Maloney J, Rashidi R, et al: The effects of percutaneous catheter ablation on preexisting permanent pacemakers. PACE 13:1637, 1990.

37. Chin MC, Rosenqvist M, Lee MA, et al: The effect of radio-frequency catheter ablation on permanent pacemakers: An experimental study. PACE 13:23, 1990.

38. Kanal E, Shellock FG, Talagal L: Safety considerations in MR imaging. Radiology 176:593, 1990.

39. Pavlicek W, Geisinger M, Castle L, et al: The effects of nuclear magnetic resonance on patients with cardiac pacemakers. Radiology 147:149, 1983.

40. Fetter J, Aram G, Holmes DR, et al: The effects of nuclear magnetic resonance imagers on external and implantable pulse generators. PACE 7:720, 1984.

41. Holmes DR, Hayes DL, Gray JE, et al: The effects of magnetic resonance imaging on implantable pulse generators. PACE 9:360, 1986.

42. Hayes DL, Holmes DR, Gray JE: Effect of 1.5 tesla nuclear magnetic resonance imaging scanner on implanted permanent pacemakers. J Am Coll Cardiol 10:782, 1987.

43. Langberg J, Abber J, Thuroff JW, et al: The effects of extracorporeal shock wave lithotripsy on pacemaker function. PACE 10:1142, 1987.

44. Cooper D, Wilkoff B, Masterson M, et al: Effects of extracorporeal shock wave lithotripsy on cardiac pacemakers and its safety in patients with implanted cardiac pacemakers. PACE 11:1607, 1988.

45. Fetter J, Patterson D, Aram G, et al: Effects of extracorporeal shock wave lithotripsy on single-chamber rate-response and dual-chamber pacemakers. PACE 12:1494, 1989.

46. Stoller ML, Stack W, Langberg JJ, et al: Extracorporeal shock wave lithotripsy performed on a woman with a cardiac pacemaker. J Urol 140:1510, 1988.

47. Kanazawa T, Kishimoto T, Senju T, et al: A case of stone former with pacemaker treated by extracorporeal shock wave lithotripsy. Acta Urol Jpn 34:1415, 1988.

48. Rasmussen MJ, Hayes DL, Vlietstra RE, et al: Can transcutaneous electrical nerve stimulation be safely used in patients with permanent pacemakers? Mayo Clin Proc 63:443, 1988.

49. Chen D, Philip M, Philip PA, et al: Cardiac pacemaker inhibition by transcutaneous electrical nerve stimulation. Arch Phys Med Rehabil 71:27, 1990.

50. Agarval A, Hewson J, Redding V: Ultrasound dental scalers and demand pacing. PACE 11:853, 1988.

51. Rahn R, Zeglman M: The influence of dental treatment on the Activitrax. PACE 11:852, 1988.

52. Adamec R, Haefliger JM, Killisch JP, et al: Damaging effect of therapeutic radiation on programmable pacemakers. PACE 5:146, 1982.

53. Venselaar JLM, Van Kerkoerle HLJM, Vet AJTM: Radiation damage to pacemakers from radiotherapy. PACE 10:538, 1987.

54. Rodriguez F, Filimonov A, Henning A, et al: Radiation-induced effects in multiprogrammable pacemakers and implantable defibrillators. PACE 14:2143, 1991.

55. Mellenberg DE: A policy for radiotherapy in patients with implanted pacemakers. Med Dosim 16:221, 1991.

56. Muller-Runkel R, Orsolini G, Kalokhe UP: Monitoring the radiation dose to a multiprogrammable pacemaker during radical radiation therapy. PACE 13:1466, 1990.

57. Dodinot B, Godenir JP, Costa AB: Electronic article surveillance: A possible danger for pacemaker patients. PACE 16:46, 1993.

CHAPTER 41

FOLLOW-UP OF THE PACED OUTPATIENT

Nora Goldschlager
Paul Ludmer
Colleen Creamer

In the United States, over 89,000 new permanent pacemaker implants and more than 20,000 replacement procedures are performed annually.[1] Of these patients, only 43% use a pacemaker follow-up clinic for device monitoring and clinical follow-up.[2] Advances in pacemaker technology have increased rapidly in the last 10 years, requiring a greater responsibility for comprehensive surveillance of patients with pacing systems.

Outpatient clinic follow-up of the pacemaker patient allows ongoing clinical evaluation of the patient as well as assessment of pacing system function. The former is achieved by obtaining a thorough yet directed history and performing a focused physical examination each time the patient is seen. The latter is accomplished by chest radiography and electrocardiography, pacemaker generator interrogation, and programming. With the exception of the chest radiograph, these assessments are also undertaken each time the patient is seen, to fully optimize pacing system function, prolong battery longevity, and achieve optimal patient outcomes. Not infrequently, ambulatory electrocardiographic (Holter) recordings and event recorders are necessary to elucidate the nature of a real or potential problem, or to validate an observation or suspicion suggested during a clinic visit. In addition to providing interim pacing system function data, transtelephonic monitoring can also serve to document transient findings. The purpose of this chapter is to review specific features and activities of the pacemaker clinic.

Organization of the Pacemaker Clinic

The recipient of a permanent pacing system must be monitored for the span of his or her life. Pacemaker surveillance is labor-intensive but cost-effective.[2] The pacemaker clinic

provides patient education and reassurance, collects and maintains data, utilizes methods of maximizing battery longevity, and detects pacing system abnormalities. Despite high industry standards in the design and manufacture of pacing systems, the incidence of pacing system malfunction (usually sensing abnormalities correctable by programming) remains significant at 3 to 8% overall.[2]

Additional goals that can be achieved by the pacemaker clinic include the development of a lead and pulse generator database or registry, and creation of a repository of pacemaker hardware information and technical expertise (Table 41-1).

PHYSICAL PLANT

The pacemaker clinic should allow adequate space for all its activities and functions. These include patient reception

TABLE 41-1. **GOALS OF ORGANIZED PACEMAKER FOLLOW-UP**

1. Identification of pacing system abnormalities, allowing prompt diagnosis and corrections; detection and prevention of pacemaker system failure
2. Threshold testing and output programming, to maximize pulse generator longevity
3. Assessment and prediction of battery elective replacement time and end of life, to schedule generator replacement on a nonurgent basis
4. Noninvasive programming utilizing the full range of programmable options, to optimize device function for an individual's specific needs
5. Repository for pulse generator and lead data, to monitor reliability
6. Providing a site for training of medical personnel

and waiting areas; rooms for private history taking and physical examination; a patient exercise area; a multimedia education area containing demonstration pulse generators and leads, heart models, informational videotapes, visual and written materials; cabinets for storage of programmers; transtelephonic and electrocardiographic monitoring areas; and spaces for chart filing and/or computer-assisted data retrieval systems.

STAFF REQUIREMENTS

It is recommended that a board-certified cardiologist, a complement of well-trained registered nursing personnel, and physician assistants and/or certified cardiovascular technologists be available to provide patient care in the pacemaker clinic. Ideally, clerical and computer support for record keeping and data storage and retrieval should be available. The clinic staff should be knowledgeable in clinical and electrocardiography and cardiac physiology, trained in advanced life support and competent at utilizing resuscitative equipment, and comfortable with programming both basic and more advanced pacing systems.

EQUIPMENT

Well-maintained and updated equipment should be available. A page-writing multichannel electrocardiogram (ECG) machine with real-time rhythm strip recording capability is required. Simple, easy-to-use electronic measurement devices for pulse duration and interstimulus interval should be available (Fig. 41–1); ECG technicians can easily notate this measured information directly on the ECG recording. A cardioverter-defibrillator and a transcutaneous pacing system should also be readily accessible. An oscilloscope to visualize pulse wave forms, useful some years ago, is generally no longer necessary since the advent of pulse generator telemetry, which provides battery status information directly. Sterile disposable wound trays and antiseptic solutions should be available for wound evaluation. In the optimal situation, there should be available facilities for radiography, fluoroscopy, head-up tilt-table testing, ambulatory electrocardiography, echocardiography, treadmill or bicycle exercise testing, and electrophysiologic testing. Manufacturer- and product-specific programmers and backup programmers are requisites in a comprehensive and safe clinic. The variety of programmer models and sizes requires a significant amount of storage space, yet ready accessibility and transportation in and out of the clinic area must be ensured. Technical information regarding the behavior of specific pacemakers and programmers should be available, regardless of whether or not they are implanted at one's particular institution. Telephone numbers of local manufacturers' representatives should be prominently displayed. We recommend placing the appropriate Physician's Manual in every patient's pacemaker chart, together with the name and telephone number of the manufacturer's representative.

RECORD KEEPING

The purpose of record keeping is to accurately maintain patient demographic data, and to document pacing system function, symptoms, changes in programmed parameters, potential or real pacemaker-related problems, and the results of evaluation for battery depletion and component failure. Thorough, updated records facilitate patient identification in the event of product advisories and recalls. Ideally, 24-hour availability of the information contained in the data record or pacemaker chart should exist between hospital, following physician, referring physician, house staff when applicable, and the patient.

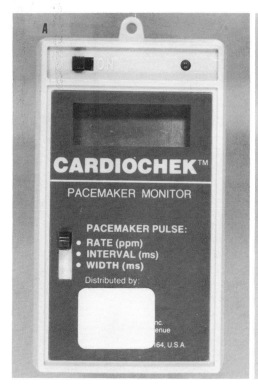
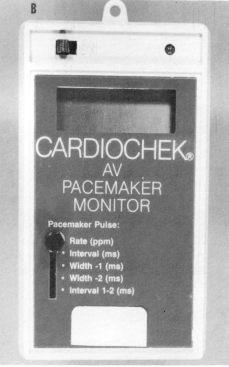

FIGURE 41–1. Pacemaker rate-checking devices for single-chamber (A) and dual-chamber (B) pulse generators. Standby rate in pulses per minute and in millisecond intervals and pulse duration are provided. The device is applied directly to the body surface, and the values read off the digital display. In patients with spontaneous atrial and/or ventricular rhythms, a magnet needs to be in place for the readout to be accurate.

Essential data in the pacemaker chart include the patient's name and address; location and telephone number of the referring physician; a relevant history, physical findings, and ECGs leading to pacing system implantation; the operative note; and model and serial numbers of all previous and currently implanted pacemaker generators, leads, and adapters. Pulse generator and lead specifications, warranties, technical information, including manufacturers' technical notes, advisories, and recall information should also be included. The physician's response to advisories and recalls should be clearly documented. When there is a change in programmed parameters, the reasons for the change should be shared with the patient, the referring physician, and the telephone monitoring service and should be documented in the chart.

A comprehensive pacemaker follow-up clinic should ideally provide 24-hour emergency service, consisting of data retrieval and consultation service for pacemaker troubleshooting and programming. This service can be particularly useful for primary care and emergency room physicians, who may be unfamiliar with rapidly advancing pacemaker technology.

Predischarge Assessment

Immediately after the implantation procedure is concluded, the patient should have a wound and generator pocket assessment; 12-lead ECG with and without magnet to evaluate capture and sensing, and magnet rate and function; and bedside anteroposterior and lateral chest radiographs to confirm lead placement and to screen for pneumothorax, evidence of congestive heart failure, aspiration, and/or other potential complications from the implantation procedure. The ECG is particularly important, since it serves as the baseline to which subsequent tracings are compared.

Paced P waves have mean frontal plane axes that reflect the direction of atrial depolarization and thus the location of the electrode(s). Electrode location itself depends on the type of lead used (passive or active fixation). Because of these considerations, P-wave morphology cannot always be relied on to verify atrial capture, which then must be accomplished by independent means.

Paced QRS complexes are expected to have a superior axis, reflecting ventricular depolarization that proceeds from apex to base, and a left bundle branch block pattern, reflecting right ventricular depolarization initiated in advance of left ventricular depolarization. There have been reports, however, of unusual axes and patterns of intraventricular conduction that have not been accompanied by lead malposition or myocardial penetration or perforation.[3–5] In particular, pacing from a septal or posterior site in the right ventricle can produce unexpected rightward deviation of the frontal plane axis as well as a right bundle branch block pattern of intraventricular conduction. If necessary, two-dimensional echocardiography can be utilized to verify lead position. Patterns of intraventricular conduction that do not meet the classic criteria of left bundle branch block are increasingly common with the use of today's leads and, indeed, should probably no longer be expected.

Prior to hospital discharge, the patient should have an upright posteroanterior chest radiograph of high quality. This film, and not the bedside portable ones obtained earlier, serves as the baseline to which subsequent films are compared; the presence of late-developing, clinically unsuspected pneumothorax can also be evaluated.[6]

The patient should leave the hospital with confirmed arrangements for the initial outpatient assessment at 7 to 10 days after implantation and should be provided with a means of contacting the pacemaker follow-up center, particularly during the first 3 months after implantation, during which the complication rate is greatest.

Goals of Office Visits

The primary goal of office visits after pacemaker implantation is to assess the efficacy of medical intervention and the well-being of the patient. The goals of the first office visit are to evaluate the wound site, assess the cardiac rhythm, assess whether the desired results of pacing have been achieved, and provide patient education. To promote a healthy acceptance of the pacing system, the patient and his family should be educated about the progression of activity, when the patient can return to work, activities of daily living, and any special hazards—real or theoretical—that the patient may encounter (see later).

TIMING OF OFFICE VISITS

Medicare has suggested guidelines for reimbursed follow-up for office visits and transtelephonic checks for implanted cardiac pacemakers[7] (Table 41–2), the adequacy of which

TABLE 41–2. **CURRENT MEDICARE COVERAGE GUIDELINES FOR PACEMAKER FOLLOW-UP**

I. Pacemaker clinic services
  A. Single-chamber pacemakers: twice in the first 6 months following implantation and then once every 12 months
  B. Dual-chamber pacemakers: twice in the first 6 months and then once every 6 months
  C. Transtelephonic monitoring guideline I (applicable to most pacemaker systems):
    1. Single-chamber pacemakers:
      a. First month: every 2 weeks
      b. Second through 36th month: every 8 weeks
      c. Thirty-seventh month through end of life: every 4 weeks
    2. Dual-chamber pacemakers:
      a. First month: every 2 weeks
      b. Second through sixth months: every 4 weeks
      c. Seventh through 36th month: every 8 weeks
      d. Thirty-seventh month through end of life: every 4 weeks
  D. Transtelephonic monitoring guideline II, applicable to pacemaker systems for which sufficient long-term clinical information exists, as established by the International Society Commission for Heart and Disease Resources, to indicate a longevity of greater than 5 years:
    1. 90% cumulative survival at 5 years after implantation
    2. End-of-life decay of less than a 50% drop of output voltage and less than 20% deviation of magnet rate, or a drop of 5 ppm or less over a period of 3 months or more
    3. Single-chamber pacemakers:
      a. First month: every 2 weeks
      b. Second through 48th month: every 12 weeks
      c. Forty-ninth through 72nd month: every 8 weeks
      d. Seventy-third month through end of life: every 4 weeks
    4. Dual-chamber pacemakers:
      a. First month: every 2 weeks
      b. Second through 30th month: every 12 weeks
      c. Thirty-first through 48th month: every 8 weeks
      d. Forty-ninth month through end of life: every 4 weeks

has been questioned.[8] Patients ordinarily visit the clinic twice or three times yearly, whether a single- or dual-chamber device is implanted. Many exceptions exist, however, and include patients who are pacemaker dependent, who have intercurrent changes in their clinical course, and who have devices that have been identified in advisories and recalls. Patients with dual-chamber pacing systems have a greater frequency of problems during the first postimplantation year,[8] and increased surveillance is generally required. The cost of timely pacemaker follow-up visits is likely recovered in reduced numbers of hospitalizations for pacemaker ''malfunction.''

The Clinic Visit

HISTORY TAKING

The history should be directed toward elucidating problems that could be related to the implanted pacing system. The patient should be specifically questioned about symptoms reflecting diminished cardiac output, including those of cerebral hypoperfusion. Such symptoms, while not specific for pacemaker-related difficulties, should nevertheless lead to consideration of a number of diagnoses (Table 41–3), chief among them being rapid paced ventricular rates; pacemaker syndrome; oversensing with either pauses in paced rhythm or, in DDD systems, triggering of ventricular pacing (Table 41–4); undersensing with resulting competitive rhythms; and failure to capture due to threshold elevation, conductor fracture, or insulation break. A more focused history can then be

TABLE 41–3. SOME COMMON SYMPTOMS IN PATIENTS WITH PACING SYSTEMS AND THEIR POSSIBLE CAUSES

SYMPTOMS	ETIOLOGIC CONSIDERATIONS
Palpitations	Rapid paced ventricular rates
	Normal tracking of sinus tachycardia, atrial tachycardia, atrial flutter, atrial fibrillation
	Pacemaker-mediated tachycardia
	Retrograde VA conduction
	Myopotential-triggered
	Electromagnetic-triggered
	Spontaneous tachycardias
	Spontaneous extrasystoles
Weakness, fatigue	Pacemaker syndrome
	Inappropriately programmed rate response parameters
	Underlying cardiopulmonary and systemic disease
	Failure to capture
Breathlessness, orthopnea, paroxysmal nocturnal dyspnea	Pacemaker syndrome
	Underlying cardiac disease
Hiccups	Diaphragmatic stimulation
Muscle twitching	Insulation break
Presyncope, syncope, dizziness	Underlying cardiac disease
	Pacemaker syndrome
	Failure to capture
	Oversensing with pacemaker inhibition

TABLE 41–4. CAUSES OF PACEMAKER OVERSENSING

PHYSIOLOGIC INTRACARDIAC SIGNALS
T-wave sensing (VVI systems)
P-wave sensing (AAI systems)
R-wave sensing (AAI systems)
Concealed extrasystoles

PHYSIOLOGIC EXTRACARDIAC SIGNALS
Muscle potentials (e.g., diaphragm, pectoral)

ELECTROMAGNETIC INTERFERENCE
Power transformers, power lines
Welding equipment
Household appliances (electric razors, microwave ovens, garage door openers) (older generator designs)
Rotating radar detectors
Metal detector gates (older generator designs)
Transcutaneous nerve stimulators
Cardioverting-defibrillating devices
Diathermy
Lithotriptors
Electrocautery, electrocoagulation
Magnetic resonance imaging
Ionizing radiation

SIGNALS GENERATED WITHIN THE PACING SYSTEM
Afterpotential sensing
Autointerference
Inactive leads

obtained, with attention being directed to specific activities that cause the symptoms. (For example, arm movements involving the side ipsilateral to the pacing system that produce symptoms might suggest myopotential inhibition or triggering.) Awareness of pacing might suggest pectoral or diaphragmatic muscle stimulation resulting from lead insulation break, proximity of the ventricular lead tip to the diaphragm, or phrenic nerve stimulation from lateral right atrial lead placement. In the first circumstance, the patient may have observed muscle twitching; in the latter two circumstances, hiccups may be present. Many patients are aware of paced events that are not associated with a pacemaker-related problem; the cause of this awareness is unclear but in our experience may be highly reproducible. It is theoretically possible that an altered sequence of ventricular contraction is perceived by the patient.[9, 10]

Rapid paced ventricular rates can cause palpitations as well as symptoms of cerebral hypoperfusion. The rapid rates may be due to appropriate tracking of sinus tachycardia, atrial tachycardia, or atrial flutter or fibrillation; to pacemaker-mediated tachycardia; or to inappropriately programmed rate response settings in rate-adaptive devices. Electrocardiography, ambulatory ECG (Holter) monitoring, and event recording usually provide the correct diagnosis. Some newer rate-adaptive pulse generators, on detecting a rapid atrial rate unaccompanied by independent sensor-based evidence of increased metabolic need, automatically switch from DDDR to VVIR mode of function until the atrial rate ''normalizes.''

Pacemaker syndrome refers to a constellation of symptoms and signs present in patients in whom the atrial rhythm is dyssynchronous with the ventricular rate or in whom, despite the presence of AV synchrony, an appropriately timed atrial contraction does not precede the paced ventricular event (also see Chapter 25). The prevalence of pacemaker syndrome is

10 to 50%,[11] depending on the diligence with which the history is sought. It is our impression that it is much more common in the elderly, who depend on preload to maintain cardiac output to a much greater extent than do younger patients, owing in part to age-related declines in early diastolic filling capability.[12]

While pacemaker syndrome occurs mainly in patients with VVI pacing systems and sinus rhythm, patients with DDD pacemakers can, under certain circumstances, also develop relative AV dyssynchrony, in which spontaneous P waves do not fall in optimal relationship to paced QRS complexes. Such circumstances can include an inappropriately long programmed AV interval, ''electronic Wenckebach'' occurring either at rest or during exercise, and an inappropriately short programmed AV interval in patients with interatrial conduction delay.[13] In this last instance, the AV valves close because of relatively early ventricular stimulation, before the left atrium has received the stimulus to contract.

Appreciation of the underlying mechanisms of pacemaker syndrome, and thus of the importance of an appropriately timed atrial systole preceding paced ventricular events, requires familiarity with the functions of atrial transport.[14–17] These functions include enhancement of ventricular filling, thus providing adequate preload and obviating the hemodynamic requirement for high filling pressures to exist throughout the entire ventricular diastolic period. Moreover, atrial contraction contributes to AV valve closure in presystole owing to the effects of subvalvular eddy currents.

The symptoms of pacemaker syndrome are varied and not always classic. They include weakness, breathlessness, orthopnea, paroxysmal nocturnal dyspnea, frank pulmonary congestion or edema, presyncope and syncope, and an awareness of neck pulsations.[18–20] Any or all of these symptoms can be exacerbated by effort. Both a suboptimal cardiac output and activation of atrial baroreceptors due to stretch contribute to the weakness and other symptoms of cerebral hypoperfusion. Atrial baroreceptor activation produces reflex peripheral vasodilatation and hypotension through atrial natriuretic peptide secretion.[21–25] Increased pulmonary venous pressure, which has been demonstrated to be due in part to a ''negative atrial kick''[26] that results from AV dyssynchrony or ventriculoatrial (VA) conduction, is the usual underlying cause of breathlessness, orthopnea, and nocturnal dyspnea in patients with pacemaker syndrome, although AV valve regurgitation has been documented[27] and can play a contributing role. Significant tricuspid regurgitation, however, is distinctly unusual.[26] On rare occasions, late-developing pericardial constriction due to either postimplantation Dressler's syndrome or myocardial penetration with pericarditis has been identified as a cause of breathlessness.[28]

The awareness by the patient of neck pulsations, which can be uncomfortable, usually reflects the presence of cannon waves. Symptoms of venous thrombosis should always be sought, as this complication can occur late after pacing system implantation[29] or may be related to retained leads from a prior procedure.[30] Fullness of an extremity and suffusion may have been noticed by the patient; on rare occasions the patient is aware of facial swelling or exophthalmos.[31–33]

PHYSICAL EXAMINATION

During the physical examination, a thorough examination of the wound, pacemaker pocket, and area overlying the lead(s) should be made. The pulse generator should be slightly movable, and the overlying skin nonedematous and of normal color and temperature. The presence of hematoma, related to the implant procedure or to chest trauma, should be noted, and treated conservatively. Signs of infection, such as pain, swelling, and erythema, which usually occur within the first 6 months after implantation, should be sought. In contrast to hematoma formation, if infection is suspected, the wound should be irrigated and cultures performed. To obtain cultures, the skin is cleansed and painted with antiseptic solution (iodine is preferred), and a needle is directed to the pulse generator, taking care to avoid indwelling leads. The passage of the needle will be limited by the generator itself; the needle will lie in a potential space around the generator. To irrigate the pacer site, one should use a syringe filled with normal saline, taken from an intravenous infusion packet rather than from solutions used to dilute medications, since these contain bacteriostatic preservatives and will defeat attempts at culture. The fluid is then cultured for aerobic and anaerobic organisms. Detection of pocket infection mandates immediate antibiotic therapy to avoid explantation of the pulse generator and lead(s).[34, 35]

Manipulation of the pocket and its contents should be performed at each visit. In this way, a tight or loose pocket can be documented, which may prove useful in assessing the causes of erosion or rotation of the pulse generator resulting in lead dislodgment, whether spontaneous or by the patient (''twiddler's syndrome'').[36, 37] During manipulation of the pocket contents, muscle twitching can be observed if there is an underlying insulation break; loss of capture can occur as a manifestation of loose connections. If these diagnoses are to be verified by impedance measurements, the interrogation must be performed during the manipulation that produces the abnormality in pacing system function (Fig. 41–2A through C).

The jugular venous pulsations should be carefully examined for the presence of cannon A waves, which reflect atrial contraction against closed or partially closed AV valves. This is especially important in patients with VVI or VVIR pacing systems. The cannon waves are generally of variable amplitude because of variations in the temporal relationships between atrial and ventricular systole; they should not be mistaken for the C-V waves of tricuspid regurgitation.[26]

Swelling or suffusion of the ipsilateral extremity, shoulder, neck, or face indicates venous obstruction. The subclavian vein is usually involved in this process; however, a superior vena cava syndrome, with edema of the chest wall and dilation of superficial venous collaterals, can occur.[38–41] Symptomatic venous thrombosis requires anticoagulation, usually with heparin followed by Coumadin (sodium warfarin); oral anticoagulation may be required indefinitely. Thrombolysis using streptokinase and urokinase has also been reported,[42] with good results. Balloon angioplasty has also been used to restore lumen patency.[43, 44] Rarely, recurrent pulmonary embolism from thrombosis involving the pacing lead results in the physical findings of pulmonary hypertension.[33] Even more rarely, intracardiac thrombosis around the pacing lead can itself cause inflow obstruction and peripheral signs of right ventricular failure.[45]

Murmurs of hemodynamically significant tricuspid regurgitation are unusual. The mere presence of an endocardial lead crossing the valve does not produce flow disturbances of consequence. Thus, tricuspid regurgitation accompanied

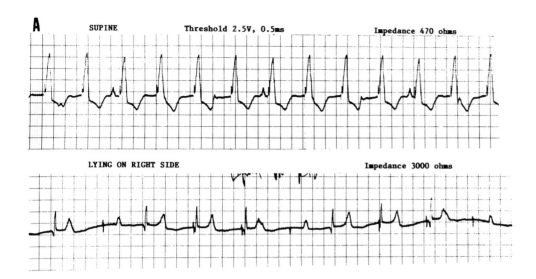

A

SUPINE   Threshold 2.5V, 0.5ms   Impedance 470 ohms

LYING ON RIGHT SIDE   Impedance 3000 ohms

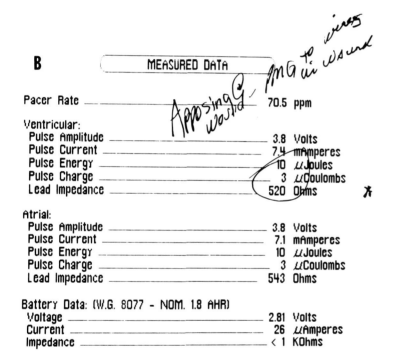

B

MEASURED DATA		

Pacer Rate — 70.5 ppm

Ventricular:
Pulse Amplitude	3.8	Volts
Pulse Current	7.4	mAmperes
Pulse Energy	10	μJoules
Pulse Charge	3	μCoulombs
Lead Impedance	520	Ohms

Atrial:
Pulse Amplitude	3.8	Volts
Pulse Current	7.1	mAmperes
Pulse Energy	10	μJoules
Pulse Charge	3	μCoulombs
Lead Impedance	543	Ohms

Battery Data: (W.G. 8077 - NOM. 1.8 AHR)
Voltage	2.81	Volts
Current	26	μAmperes
Impedance	< 1	KOhms

C

Pacesetter Systems, Inc.
Synchrony II

Feb 19 1991 3:57 pm
MODEL: 2022   SERIAL: 22996

PATIENT: _____
PHYSICIAN: _____

PROGRAMMED PARAMETERS		
	INITIAL	PRESENT
Mode	DDD	DDD
Sensor	PASSIVE	PASSIVE
Rate	70	70 ppm
A-V Delay	200	200 msec
Max Track	110	110 ppm
Vent. Pulse Config.	UNIPOLAR	UNIPOLAR
V. Pulse Width	.4	.4 msec
V. Pulse Amplitude	4.0	4.0 Volts
V. Sense Config.	UNIPOLAR TIP	UNIPOLAR TIP
V. Sensitivity	2.0	2.0 mVolts
V. Refractory	275	275 msec
Atr. Pulse Config.	BIPOLAR	BIPOLAR
A. Pulse Width	.4	.4 msec
A. Pulse Amplitude	4.0	4.0 Volts
A. Sense Config.	BIPOLAR	BIPOLAR
A. Sensitivity	1.5	1.5 mVolts
A. Refractory	300	300 msec
Blanking	25	25 msec
V. Safety Option	ENABLE	ENABLE
PVC Options	+PVARP ON PVC	+PVARP ON PVC
PMT Options	OFF	OFF
Rate Resp. A-V Delay	DISABLE	DISABLE
Magnet	TEMPORARY OFF	TEMPORARY OFF
Threshold	2.0	2.0
Slope	8 (Normal)	8 (Normal)
Maximum Sensor Rate	110	110 ppm
Reaction Time	Fast	Fast
Recovery Time	Medium	Medium

FIGURE 41–2. MCL5 rhythm strips recorded from a patient who had had a VVIR pacing system implanted 6 weeks earlier. She presented to the clinic complaining of intermittent dizziness, which was not clearly related to body position. Ventricular capture threshold with the patient lying supine was less than 2.5 V, 0.5 msec. Manipulation of the pacemaker pocket (first noticed during magnet application) as well as turning the patient on her right side was associated with loss of capture (A). Interrogation during capture (B) and noncapture (C) confirmed an abnormally high impedance only during periods of noncapture, suggesting either conductor break or loose connections. The latter was confirmed at reoperation. These tracings illustrate the relevance of interrogation data measured at the time the abnormality is present, and emphasize the point that interrogated data may be completely normal during periods of normal pacing system function.

MEASURED DATA	

Pacer Rate — 70.5 ppm

Ventricular:
Pulse Amplitude	4.1	Volts
Pulse Current	.6	mAmperes
Pulse Energy	1	μJoules
Pulse Charge	0	μCoulombs
Lead Impedance	>1990	Ohms

Atrial:
Pulse Amplitude	3.9	Volts
Pulse Current	7.2	mAmperes
Pulse Energy	10	μJoules
Pulse Charge	3	μCoulombs
Lead Impedance	534	Ohms

Battery Data: (W.G. 8077 - NOM. 1.8 AHR)
Voltage	2.82	Volts
Current	21	μAmperes
Impedance	< 1	KOhms

by a V wave in the neck and by pulsations in the liver mandates consideration of infective endocarditis; echocardiography is invaluable in this assessment.[46] On rare occasions, adhesions of the lead to the tricuspid valve have resulted in hemodynamically important tricuspid stenosis.[47–49]

Cardiac auscultation occasionally reveals a "pacemaker sound."[50–52] This sound may occur after delivery of the stimulus output and may be caused by intercostal muscle or diaphragmatic contraction or to symptomless myocardial penetration. The first heart sound may be variable, because of the changing relationships of atrial to ventricular systole in patients with VVI and VVIR pacing systems, and to differences in paced or sensed atrial and/or ventricular intervals in patients with dual-chamber pacing systems. The second heart sound is often paradoxically split, owing to right ventricular depolarization occurring in advance of left ventricular depolarization, mimicking left bundle branch block. In patients with left ventricular epicardial leads, a widely, but physiologically split second heart sound during inspiration is due to left ventricular depolarization occurring in advance of right ventricular depolarization, mimicking right bundle branch block. Other auscultatory findings include systolic nonejection clicks, possibly resulting from slapping of the lead against the tricuspid valve; systolic murmurs (due to hemodynamically insignificant tricuspid and mitral valve regurgitation); and systolic "whoops" or musical murmurs, thought to result from movement of the pacing lead within the right ventricular cavity.[52, 53] All of these auscultatory findings are benign and are not unexpected. They must be documented in the medical record, however, and any changes over time noted. A pericardial friction rub developing early after pacing system implantation should suggest myocardial penetration or perforation; however, a friction rub of presumed endocardial origin, with no evidence of myocardial penetration, has been reported.[54] Clinical and echocardiographic evidence of significant pericardial effusion should be sought if a pericardial rub is present. Visible or palpable contractions of the pectoral muscles or diaphragm occurring at the pacing rate should be noted, since they might signify a lead insulation defect, conductor fracture, or an excessively high programmed output.

The presence of the pacemaker syndrome, suspected from the clinical history, can be confirmed by demonstrating fluctuations in systolic blood pressure, including orthostatic changes, visualizing cannon A waves in the jugular venous waves, and hearing the murmurs of AV valve regurgitation, which may be transient. We have occasionally seen patients in whom cannon waves were clearly felt in the enlarged liver. Infrequently, findings of central and pulmonary venous pressure elevation (rales), including tender hepatomegaly, may be present; if they have developed for the first time after pacing system implantation they should be assumed to be due to the pacemaker syndrome.

Evaluation of myopotential inhibition or triggering requires pectoral muscle activity, easily achieved by raising a weight, pulling, and pressing the hands together. These maneuvers should be performed under electrocardiographic monitoring; symptoms may or may not occur or be reproduced. Myopotential inhibition and triggering should be specifically sought in patients with unipolar pacing systems, or in those programmed to unipolar configuration, because of their relatively high prevalence in these circumstances.[55]

TABLE 41–5. CHEST RADIOGRAPH IN PACEMAKER PATIENT FOLLOW-UP

Position of lead(s)
Lead configuration (bipolar, unipolar)
Generator position
Generator identification
Connector block integrity
Faulty connection
Loose setscrew
Lead fracture
Lead insulation defect
Unexplained change in heart size or pulmonary venous pattern suggesting pericardial effusion

CHEST RADIOGRAPH

Highly penetrated posteroanterior and lateral chest x-ray films should be obtained prior to hospital discharge, to assess lead positions, lead integrity, and pulse generator position (Table 41–5). Not infrequently, a large pneumothorax can take up to 24 hours to appear.[6] We have found that after this initial radiographic study, routine follow-up films yield little if any new information. We therefore recommend follow-up radiographs only if a pacemaker-related problem is being evaluated.

INTERROGATION

Interrogation of the implanted device is a mandatory part of the clinic visit. Both programmed data and measured data from the pulse generator itself should be documented in the record. Interrogation should not be attempted unless the particular device the patient has had implanted is known; false programming can result, sometimes with unfortunate consequences (Fig. 41–3).

ELECTROCARDIOGRAM

Twelve-lead ECGs should always be performed without and with the magnet in place. Spontaneous and paced P waves and QRS complexes should be clearly identified when feasible; only by this means can atrial and ventricular fusion and pseudofusion complexes be correctly recognized. If a spontaneous QRS rhythm is not present initially but does develop during rate programming, a 12-lead ECG of the native rhythm should be made at this time. In this manner, the "natural" history of the rhythm for which the pacing system was implanted can be tracked. Native ST and T waves can be markedly abnormal in paced patients[56, 57] (Fig. 41–4); this phenomenon is not well understood, but the explanation appears to have an ionic basis in K⁺ channel physiology.[58, 59] The T-wave abnormalities can suggest nontransmural myocardial infarction; however, serial ECGs, obtained at each clinic visit if possible, serve to confirm the chronic nature of the abnormality. We have also observed marked T-U wave amplitude enhancement during bradycardia, and occasionally patients may develop bradycardia-dependent polymorphic ventricular tachycardia, necessitating rapid programming of a more rapid rate.

The natural history of the bradycardias for which patients receive a permanent pacemaker has not been extensively studied. Observations made in the 1960s and 1970s clearly

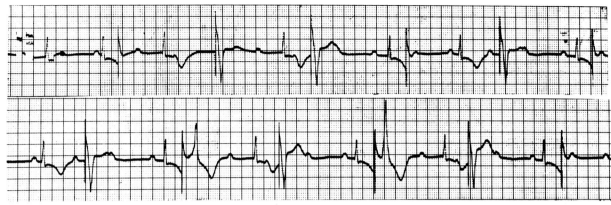

FIGURE 41–3. This continuous lead II rhythm strip was recorded during attempted interrogation of a noninterrogable VVI pulse generator; the patient was thought to have implanted a Cordis model 401 (Multicor) but, in fact, had a Cordis model 337. As a result of repeated attempts to interrogate the generator, asynchronous pacing at a rate of about 37 ppm resulted; the problem was recognized to have been caused by physician error and was resolved by programming.

documented the transient nature of AV block in some paced patients;[60–63] however, because rate programmability was unavailable, the spontaneous QRS rhythm, when AV block was present, could not be ascertained. In a study of 282 patients paced for at least 1 year, Edhag and Rosenqvist[64] observed that 12% were never pacing; 10 of these 33 patients had had prior complete AV block. Another 46% displayed both paced and spontaneous rhythms during the follow-up period. An adequate escape rhythm in patients paced for complete AV block has recently been documented in more than 70% of patients at some time in the follow-up period; however, replication of the escape rhythm did not occur in 13% of patients.[65] Conversely, in a study of 26 patients paced for trifascicular disease and syncope or presyncope, but no documented AV block, Marinato and colleagues[66] showed that 19% developed second- and third-degree AV block during follow-up. Brignole and associates[67] found that evidence of a marked carotid sinus hypersensitivity persisted in 100% of 54 patients paced for this condition. Gwinn and colleagues[68] studied the progression of chronotropic incompetence (defined as inability to achieve an exercise heart rate exceeding

80% of age-predicted maximum) in paced patients undergoing treadmill exercise, and found that the percentage of chronotropically incompetent patients increased with increasing duration of pacing, suggesting progression of this condition over time.

These types of studies enhance our understanding of rhythm disturbances, serve to expand the potential indications for pacing, and allow appropriate device selection to be made early.

APPLICATION OF THE MAGNET

Magnet application is performed to assess capture, evaluate elective battery replacement time and end of life, and, on occasion, treat pacemaker-related arrhythmias (Tables 41–6 and 41–7). Magnet application over the pulse generator eliminates sensing and results in the asynchronous delivery of pacing stimuli. The response to magnet application varies with the manufacturer and the specific pacemaker generator and can be a change in the mode of function (e.g., from DDD to VOO), cyclic functions (e.g., the delivery of three output pulses at a rate faster than that programmed, followed by output pulses delivered at the programmed rate), rates faster than the programmed rate, and "Vario" function in one or two chambers[69] (see Table 41–7). Familiarity with responses to magnet application will avoid mistaken diagnoses of pacing system malfunction or improper positioning of the magnet over the generator (a consideration especially helpful for ECG technicians). Care should be taken to avoid waving the magnet over the pulse generator; in some older-generator models, inhibition of pacer output can result from changing magnetic fields.[69, 70] Newer pulse generators have their magnetic switches located in a part of the circuitry that avoids this problem.

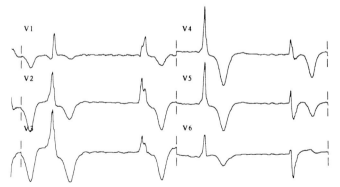

FIGURE 41–4. Spontaneous cardiac rhythm in an asymptomatic patient with a VVIR pacing system, programmed to a temporary standby rate of 30 ppm. The atrial rhythm is fibrillation. The spontaneous QRS complexes presumably originate in the fascicles or ventricular tissue. The marked ST and T wave abnormalities are not expected from the intraventricular conduction delay alone. Comparison tracings recorded at the clinic visits aid in the differential diagnosis of myocardial ischemia and infarction.

TABLE 41–6. **USES OF THE MAGNET**

Assessment of capture
Determination of elective replacement time and end of life
Breaking of pacemaker-mediated tachycardia
Treatment of crosstalk inhibition
Treatment of oversensing

TABLE 41–7. SOME RESPONSES OF PULSE GENERATORS TO MAGNET APPLICATION

SINGLE-CHAMBER PACEMAKERS
AOO or VOO at rate other than that programmed
AOO or VOO at programmed rate
AAT or VVT
Vario function

DUAL-CHAMBER PACEMAKERS
DOO at faster than programmed rate
DOO at faster than programmed rate, shorter than programmed AV interval
DOO at programmed rate and AV interval
Vario function in atrium, followed by ventricle VOO
VOO

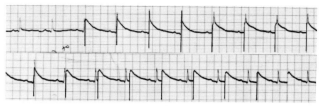

FIGURE 41–5. Magnet application in a patient with a unipolar VVI pacing system. The output stimuli and their associated decay curves essentially obscure the QRS complexes, making assessment of capture impossible. Moreover, T waves, indicating ventricular repolarization (and thus, by inference, the presence of prior depolarization), are not seen. Capture is verified in the latter portion of the lower strip. Prior to the appearance of the paced QRS complexes, eight pacing stimuli fall in the refractory period of ventricular tissue, precluding capture.

Magnet application should be routinely performed at each clinic visit primarily to assess capture (Table 41–8) and to obtain the magnet rate. The magnet rate, rather than the programmed rate, provides the elective replacement and end-of-life indicators for many pulse generators. Knowledge of the specific elective replacement indicators is mandatory for the following physician, as these vary with the manufacturer and the device. Not infrequently, a sudden unexpected failure to capture due to battery depletion occurs only because the appropriate end-of-life indicators have not been recognized.

Assessment of capture is not always easy (Figs. 41–5 to 41–11). Paced complexes must be clearly identified as such, and pseudofusion excluded. True fusion, of course, does indicate capture, but fusion complexes themselves must be clearly shown to be neither purely paced nor purely spontaneous (see Figs. 41–7 and 41–8).

Pacemaker noncapture may occur because of the pacing stimuli falling in the refractory period of atrial or ventricular tissue; this phenomenon represents a "pseudo" noncapture situation. In patients with dual-chamber pacing systems, pseudo noncapture has been referred to as an "AV dyssynchronization arrhythmia."[71] The diagnosis of true failure to capture should be made only when temporal capability to depolarize tissue is present.

An AV dyssynchronization arrhythmia can, on removal of the magnet, result in pacemaker-mediated tachycardia.[72] This rhythm comes about by the retrograde atrial depolarization, itself resulting from magnet-induced AV dyssynchrony, being sensed in the atrial channel and triggering an output in the ventricular channel, with maintenance of the tachycardia due to continued retrograde atrial depolarization. In these instances, reapplication of the magnet is used therapeutically, to break the pacemaker-mediated tachycardia by disallowing sensing of atrial depolarizations. Occasionally, however, reapplication results again in an AV dyssynchronization ar-

rhythmia, followed by pacemaker-mediated tachycardia on magnet removal. Chest wall stimulation (to inhibit ventricular output) and carotid sinus massage (to block VA conduction) have been suggested as maneuvers to abolish the pacemaker-mediated tachycardia in these cases.[71, 73]

Repetitive atrial or ventricular rhythms, or both, resulting from magnet application and asynchronously delivered pacing stimuli are unusual[74, 75] and usually self-limited unless acute myocardial ischemia or infarction, or drug and electrolyte abnormalities, are present. The rarity of life-threatening arrhythmias is attested to by the lack of reported complications among the vast number of patients monitored transtelephonically.

PACEMAKER DEPENDENCY

The phrase "pacemaker dependency" describes a patient who requires rate support to avoid symptoms of cerebral hypoperfusion. Defined thus, a patient may be pacemaker dependent at rates of less than 60 bpm as well as at rates less than 30 bpm. It is important to recognize the former situation, since these patients are often paced at 65 to 70 bpm

BIPOLAR ATRIAL PACING

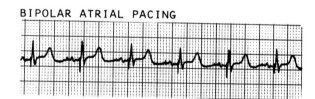

UNIPOLAR ATRIAL PACING

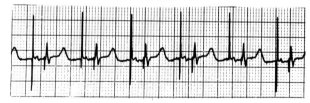

FIGURE 41–6. Lead II rhythm strips recorded during evaluation of atrial capture threshold in a patient with a DDD pacing system. During atrial pacing in bipolar configuration, output pulses are barely discernible, making the diagnosis of atrial capture questionable. Using a polarity programmability feature available in some pacing systems, unipolar atrial pacing can be achieved. The resulting stimulus outputs are readily seen, as are the paced P waves that follow them. In cases in which paced P waves are not clearly seen because of decay curve artifact, simultaneous recording of two or more ECG leads usually solves the problem. Note the varying amplitude of the output pulses in these rhythm strips, which is a function of the digital recording equipment.

TABLE 41–8. CAUSES OF PACEMAKER NONCAPTURE

Refractoriness of tissue
Lead dislodgment
Increase in myocardial stimulation threshold
Lead insulation break
Conductor fracture
Inappropriately low programmed output
Generator end of life
Loose lead-generator connection

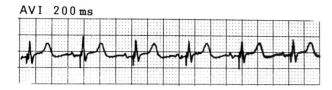

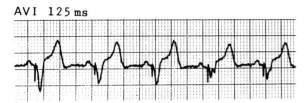

FIGURE 41–7. Lead II rhythm strips recorded during evaluation of ventricular capture threshold in a patient with a DDD pacing system. In the top strip, appropriate ventricular output pulses are delivered after sensing of spontaneous P waves. However, the QRS complexes that follow them are normal-appearing and do not have the expected superior axis. Because of these features, ventricular capture is not confirmed. In the lower strip, the AV interval has been shortened in order to disallow normal AV conduction. The QRS complexes are now purely paced, and thus capture can be confirmed. The QRS complexes in the top strip represent either pseudofusion complexes or true fusion complexes. Without documenting the morphology of purely spontaneous complexes, the differential diagnosis cannot be made with certainty.

minute for hemodynamic purposes and may thus be at some degree of potential risk of earlier-than-expected battery depletion. It should also be borne in mind that symptoms of cerebral hypoperfusion due to decreases in programmed rates, as assessed in the clinic with the patient lying supine, may not be forthcoming because intravascular volume is maximal in the supine position. With the same patient sitting, standing, or ambulating, the same decrease in rate could produce significant symptoms.

Patients who remain asymptomatic despite the absence of spontaneous QRS rhythm at the lowest available program-

mable rate (including any available temporary rate settings) can be considered, for practical purposes, to be pacemaker dependent. Classes or degrees of pacemaker dependency have been suggested,[76] but they rely on rate and origin of the escape rhythm rather than the occurrence of clinical symptoms at a given rate and may thus be misapplied in clinical practice.

The appearance of an escape rhythm is related to both the rate and the duration of overdrive suppression of the escape focus. Thus, we and others have observed that gradual stepwise reduction in pacing rate is more likely to result in an early appearance of an escape rhythm than is sudden cessation of pacing, which can cause a prolonged period of ventricular asystole. In this regard, we recommend that ventricular autothreshold determinations always be performed with continuous external ECG monitoring in addition to surface ECG recording through the programmer, to visualize clearly the first noncapture event. Care must be taken to ensure that the ECG lead being monitored clearly displays the QRS complex (Figs. 41–12 and 41–13).

Evaluation for Ventriculoatrial Conduction and Pacemaker-Mediated Tachycardia

Assessment of VA conduction in patients in whom atrial fibrillation or flutter is not present should be a routine part of the clinic visit. In patients with VVI pacing systems, merely observing the ECG for the presence of retrograde atrial depolarization is usually sufficient. The presence of VA conduction is best evaluated at different paced rates encompassing a reasonable range. Symptoms of palpitations, breathlessness, or chest discomfort should be sought; the presence of signs such as cannon waves in the neck or AV valve regur-

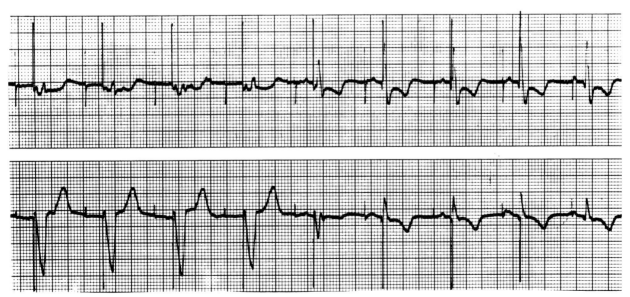

FIGURE 41–8. Simultaneously recorded leads I and II in a patient with a DDD pacing system, illustrating that only by documenting purely paced QRS complexes (complexes 1–4) can ventricular capture be ascertained. QRS complex 5 is a fusion complex, and complexes 6 to 9 are pseudofusion complexes. It is extremely important to recognize that capture is not confirmed if there is a possibility of pseudofusion. Paced QRS complexes are expected to be broad and superiorly directed in the frontal plane; failure to meet these expectations must be addressed and satisfactorily explained.

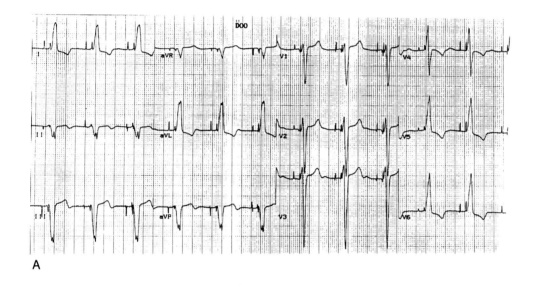

A

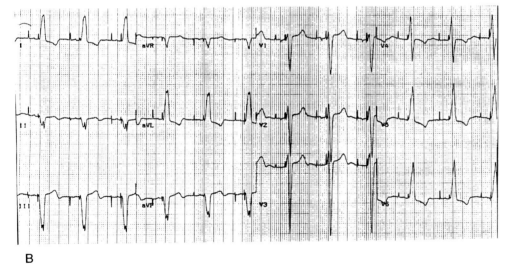

B

FIGURE 41–9. Twelve-lead ECGs performed at different AV intervals in order to assess and confirm atrial capture. In *A*, the AV interval is 120 msec; the atrial output pulse is not clearly followed by a paced P wave. In *B*, the AV interval has been programmed to 200 msec, and broad paced P waves of low voltage are readily seen.

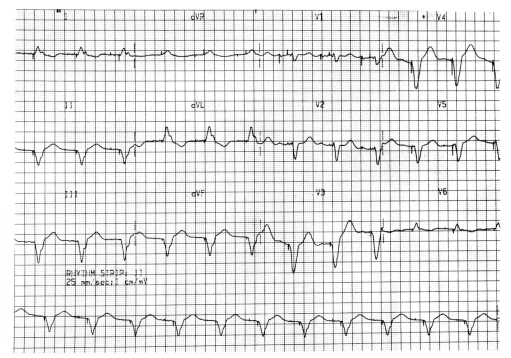

FIGURE 41–10. Twelve-lead ECG and lead II rhythm strip recorded during a routine clinic visit in a patient with a DDD pacing system in which both sensing and pacing are in bipolar configuration. Note that only in leads aVL, II, and V1 are atrial output pulses clearly seen, and that in leads II and aVL atrial capture cannot be confirmed. Only in lead V1 are both atrial and ventricular capture confirmed.

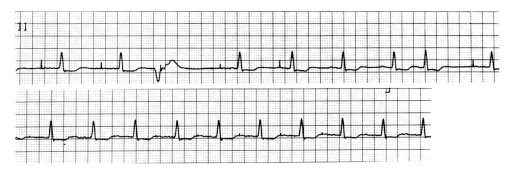

FIGURE 41–11. In cases in which atrial capture is not readily seen from the surface electrocardiographic recordings because of either a low amplitude of the pacing stimulus or low-voltage P waves, varying the paced atrial rate can help confirm capture, provided that AV conduction is present. In this patient with an AAI pacing system, atrial capture is indicated by the QRS rate, which changes with the programmed atrial rate.

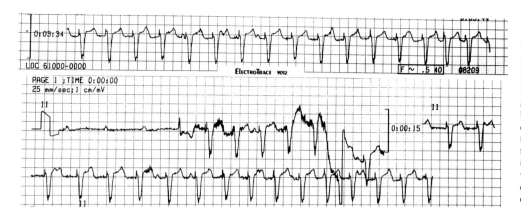

FIGURE 41–12. This lead II rhythm strip was recorded during a ventricular autothreshold determination. The ECG equipment was a digital recorder where signal processing, re-creation, and annotation are accompanied by a brief period of noncontinuous recording. During this period, the patient became asystolic, an occurrence that was unknown to the physician until recording recommenced. Page-writing ECG machines that have this design feature should not be used in clinical pacing.

gitant murmurs should be documented in the record. This information will prove useful in patients in whom upgrading of a VVI system to a DDD system is being contemplated.

In patients with a dual-chamber pacing system, mode programming to VVI will accomplish the purpose of VA conduction assessment. Similarly, AV pacing at a rate high enough to overdrive the spontaneous rate, followed by reduction of atrial energy output to subthreshold levels, will provide, in effect, VVI pacing (Figs. 41–14 and 41–15). Pacemaker-mediated tachycardia, which could occur as the result of this maneuver, can be avoided by programming in advance a long postventricular atrial refractory period. Documentation of VA conduction time at slow, "normal," and faster paced ventricular rates is of value in programming the postventricular atrial refractory period, to avoid occurrence of pacemaker-mediated tachycardia.

The evaluation for pacemaker-mediated tachycardia is an extension of the aforementioned maneuvers and depends on the creation of AV dyssynchrony and temporal opportunity for retrograde atrial depolarization to occur. Loss of AV synchrony can result from subthreshold atrial stimuli, with retrograde VA conduction resulting from the subsequent paced ventricular depolarization; myopotential triggering of ventricular output; magnet application, to eliminate normal tracking, and subsequent magnet removal; and chest wall stimulation-triggered ventricular pacing. All these maneuvers potentially produce ventricular pacing in the absence of an appropriately timed preceding spontaneous or paced atrial depolarization. Because atrial depolarization has not occurred just prior to the paced ventricular event, there is temporal opportunity to depolarize the atria in a retrograde fashion, initiating pacemaker-mediated tachycardia. On occasion in specific individuals, a long AV interval allows an atrial echo beat to occur following the paced ventricular depolarization, initiating pacemaker-mediated tachycardia.

To facilitate the induction of pacemaker-mediated tachycardia in the clinic, a short postventricular atrial refractory period should be programmed. To avoid hemodynamic embarrassment, which could result both from pacing at or near the upper rate limit and from the loss of an appropriately timed preceding atrial systole, the upper rate limit should be programmed to an appropriately low level. Once pacemaker-mediated tachycardia has been created, the steps required to terminate it, such as magnet application or PVARP programming, should be documented. In specific patients whose pulse generators have a tachycardia-terminating algorithm, the efficacy of the algorithm can be validated in this manner.

Whereas it is known that VA conduction assessed at the

V₁

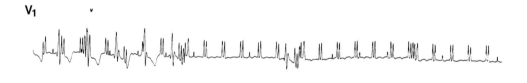

I I

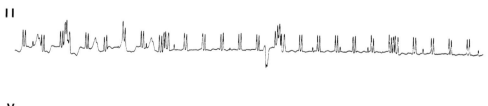

V₅

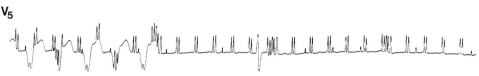

FIGURE 41–13. Simultaneously recorded leads V1, II, and V5 in a patient with a VVIR pacing system, during an autothreshold determination. Note the programming pulses that obscure considerably the paced complex in leads V1 and II. Failure to recognize the loss of capture in this patient due to the programming signals resulted in periods of ventricular asystole, which were accompanied by symptoms of dizziness.

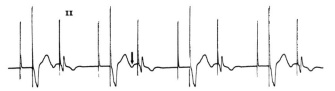

FIGURE 41–14. This lead II rhythm strip illustrates how atrial noncapture, followed by a paced ventricular depolarization, can cause the occurrence of retrograde VA conduction. The retrograde atrial depolarizations (*arrow*) are not sensed and are followed by the delivery of an atrial output pulse. The atrial stimulus occurs at the onset of a spontaneous (sensed) QRS complex (pseudopseudofusion complex), which itself is an "echo" beat.

time of pacing system implantation has little relevance for the outpatient setting, the natural history of VA conduction over time in paced patients is entirely unknown.

Evaluation for Crosstalk

Crosstalk is the sensing of electric signals generated in one cardiac chamber by the sense amplifier in another cardiac chamber. Usually it is the atrial pacing stimulus that is sensed in the ventricular channel, potentially causing inhibition of ventricular output and resetting of the atrial escape interval. Factors that predispose to crosstalk include a high programmed ventricular sensitivity (i.e., low millivolt setting), high programmed atrial output, and/or short ventricular blanking period. The ventricular blanking period is the timing interval that coincides with the release of the atrial output, during which time the ventricular sense amplifier is turned off. The longer the ventricular blanking period, the less likely the chance for crosstalk to occur. If a native R wave (e.g., a premature ventricular depolarization) occurs during the ventricular blanking period, it will not be sensed and, therefore, will not reset the atrial escape interval. It is well to keep the ventricular blanking period as short as possible, in order to sense early-cycle ventricular extrasystoles yet still avoid the occurrence of crosstalk.

To test for crosstalk, the pulse generator is temporarily programmed to the desired high output in the atrial channel and high sensitivity in the ventricular channel. The rate is then programmed to exceed the patient's spontaneous rate. If crosstalk is present, two rhythms can occur: atrial paced rate with inhibition of ventricular output (and consequent native ventricular depolarization from the paced atrial depolariza-

tion, or ventricular asystole), or crosstalk-induced safety pacing, if this feature is available and programmed to "on." Crosstalk-induced safety pacing is recognized by AV sequential pacing at shorter-than-programmed AV interval, equal to the "safety pace" interval. Because of the possibility of ventricular asystole in this setting, establishing the presence of a native QRS rhythm is recommended prior to crosstalk evaluation in pacing systems that do not have a programmable safety pace option.

If crosstalk suddenly develops in a chronic stable pacing system, an atrial lead insulation defect should be suspected. Crosstalk due to atrial lead insulation defect arises from the low lead impedance and resulting high current output traversing the lead.

Summary of Assessment of Pacing and Sensing Functions of DDD Pacing Systems

Sensing threshold is defined as the lowest "sensitivity" setting available in the pacemaker at which sensing of the intracardiac signal is demonstrated. A pacing system that can sense a signal of very small amplitude has a high sensitivity, and one that senses only large-amplitude signals has a low sensitivity. To make the pacing system more sensitive in order to sense smaller signals, the sensing parameter is programmed to a smaller number. To make the system less capable of sensing incoming signals, the sensing parameter is programmed to a higher number.

Sensing threshold is obtained by progressively reducing the sensitivity of the pacemaker (i.e., increasing the programmed sensitivity number) until the native signal is no longer sensed, and an output pulse is therefore delivered. In patients who are paced when first seen, a temporary reduction in paced rate to one below the native rhythm will be required. If the underlying native rhythm is not present or is not stable, sensing threshold cannot be determined. Some pacing systems have a semiautomatic sensing test feature available, using noninvasively obtained intracardiac electrograms or surface ECG recordings to verify the point of loss of sensing.

Capture threshold is the lowest output setting of the pacemaker system that results in depolarization of myocardial tissue. If pacing thresholds are stable, and the pacing system has been in place for longer than 3 months, the output can be programmed to reduce battery current drain and to maxi-

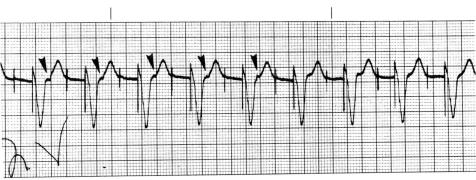

FIGURE 41–15. Atrial noncapture results in ventricular pacing at the end of the AV interval and subsequent intermittent retrograde atrial depolarization (*arrowheads*).

No. ECG 100

mize longevity while preserving an adequate safety margin. The voltage output of the pacemaker is generally programmed at 2.5 times the capture threshold; however, in patients who are pacemaker dependent or who are at risk for periodic or chronic increases in threshold (as might occur in those taking medications such as flecainide or amiodarone or in those in whom the development of renal failure with transient hyperkalemia is possible), a three- to fourfold safety margin is recommended.

If the rhythm is sinus with intact AV conduction ("PR"), sensing thresholds in the atrium and ventricle are easily performed as the first step. Then, AV sequential pacing is accomplished by programming the automatic rate to exceed the spontaneous rate, and the AV interval to one shorter than the native PR interval; this latter step is performed to produce a purely paced complex. (Pseudofusion complexes may be mistaken for paced complexes, and fusion complexes do not allow accurate evaluation of the axis and morphology of paced complexes.) Capture thresholds in atrium and ventricle are then performed, either manually or using an autothreshold function. Since sinus rhythm with intact AV conduction is present, pauses in ventricular rhythm are unexpected and unlikely.

If the atrial rhythm is sinus and the ventricular rhythm is paced (normal tracking function, "PV" pacing), an atrial sensing threshold can be performed as the first step. On loss of atrial sensing, AV stimuli are emitted at the programmed standby rate and interval. The atrial sensing threshold determination can then be followed by atrial capture threshold determination, after the rate has been programmed to exceed the spontaneous atrial rate. Next, it is easiest to program the standby rate to a rate below the spontaneous rate and the AV interval to its maximum duration; should spontaneous AV conduction occur, ventricular sensing threshold can be determined. Should spontaneous AV conduction not occur, it is best and safest to program to VVI mode of function at a low rate. If a spontaneous QRS rhythm develops, ventricular sensing and capture thresholds are determined. If no spontaneous ventricular rate develops, the patient is considered to be pacemaker dependent, and thresholds either are not done or are performed using the autothreshold function of the pulse generator, if available, to avoid prolonged periods of ventricular bradycardia. Thorough familiarity with the autothreshold function and, even more important, its immediate cancellation, is mandatory.

If the atrial rhythm is paced and the ventricular rhythm is conducted from the paced atrial complexes ("AR"), the ventricular sensing threshold is easily performed as the first step. The AV interval is then shortened to produce ventricular capture, and a ventricular capture threshold is performed; in this instance, true fusion (but not pseudofusion) complexes can be used to assess capture because the fusion beats, by definition, are contributed to by the paced depolarizations. The next step is to increase the AV interval and program a low standby rate. If a spontaneous atrial rate develops, the atrial sensing threshold is performed. Because it is now known that a spontaneous atrial rate can occur, thus avoiding ventricular bradycardia, the atrial capture threshold can be assessed once the standby rate has been increased to one exceeding the atrial rate.

Finally, if AV sequential pacing is occurring ("AV"), the easiest first step is atrial capture threshold determination, followed by programming a low standby rate in a stepwise, but rapid fashion. If PV, AR, or PR states develop, the procedure follows the outline recommended above. If AV pacing is still present, we find it expedient and safe to program to VVI mode of function and proceed according to whether or not a spontaneous ventricular rhythm is present. If a ventricular rhythm has been documented to exist, AAI mode of function can be programmed to assess atrial capture and sensing thresholds.

Documentation of the patient's underlying rhythm and rate is important both for optimizing programmed settings and for tracking the history of the rhythm for which the pacemaker was implanted. It is recommended that 12-lead ECGs be performed to document the origin and rate of any spontaneous atrial or ventricular rhythms that emerge during the functional assessment. Similarly, the documentation of the (sometimes marked) ST- and T-wave abnormalities associated with spontaneous QRS rhythms is extremely useful in clinical practice, particularly when comparisons are needed in evaluating the possibility of acute myocardial infarction (see Fig. 41–4).

Telemetry

Through telemetry, data stored in pacemaker memory are transmitted noninvasively to an external receiver through the programmer. In addition to programmed data (functional parameters that can be altered), real-time battery status information is available.[77] These measured data, recorded from the unit itself, indicate pulse generator performance at the time of the interrogation. The free-running and magnet rates, lead impedance and actual stimulus output energy, charge, current, and voltage can be measured. Power source information, including impedance within the battery cell itself, voltage, and current drain, is available. The battery (but not the lead) impedance rises over time and may prove useful, along with rate changes, as an end-of-life indicator. Interpretation of changes in these measurements is extremely helpful in the management or anticipation of pacemaker-related problems.

Recently, rate trending data have been added in appropriate units, to enable optimal programming of rate adaptation parameters.[78, 79] Other stored data, which vary with the manufacturer and the device, can include percentage of time paced in atrial and ventricular channels, percentage of time in which sensing (of spontaneous electrical activity) in atrial and ventricular channels occurs, percentage of time in which atrial pacing is followed by spontaneous QRS complexes and in which ventricular pacing has been preceded by sensed atrial events (tracking), percentage of time in which normal sensing of both atrial and ventricular activity occurs, number of times premature ventricular complexes have been detected, and number of times the tachycardia-terminating algorithm has been activated.

Identification of premature ventricular depolarizations is important in avoiding pacemaker-mediated tachycardias, since they are the most common cause of the retrograde atrial depolarization necessary to initiate such tachycardias. Pulse generators generally define a premature ventricular event as two consecutive ventricular events (sensed or paced) that have no atrial events (sensed or paced) between them. However, it is important to recognize that premature ventricular depolarization detection may be inaccurate. Premature ventricular events may be overcounted if QRS complexes are stimulated by P waves occurring in the postventricular atrial refractory period, if QRS complexes are stimulated by undersensed P waves, and if T-wave or afterpotential oversensing in the ventricular channel is present. Undercounting of premature ventricular depolarizations also occurs, especially in cases of late-diastolic ventricular premature complexes that follow a dissociated P wave.

Activation of the tachycardia-terminating algorithm does not provide a diagnosis of the tachycardia, which should not be assumed to be a pacemaker-mediated tachycardia. The tachycardia may be sinus or atrial in origin and, thus, may require no programming intervention.

Telemetry of intracardiac electrograms is a useful feature in some circumstances (Fig. 41–16),[80, 81] although more often a surface ECG with marker channel information is sufficient for analysis of difficult pacemaker ECGs. Familiarity with the precise meanings of each manufacturer's markers is vital to best utilization of this feature. Intracardiac electrography may be particularly useful during capture autothreshold determinations, in which marker channels supply only stimulus output information but do not indicate whether depolarization of tissue has occurred. The clinician must be familiar with the electrographic appearance of both paced and spontaneous atrial and ventricular complexes in order to avoid unwanted bradycardia. An external ECG is recommended during all autothreshold determinations so that noncapture can be unequivocally seen.

The intracardiac electrogram can indicate the presence of far-field and false signals in atrial and ventricular channels (see Fig. 41–16). Use of telemetered electrograms to display precise depolarization parameters other than signal amplitude (e.g., slew and duration) is much less frequent in clinical practice.

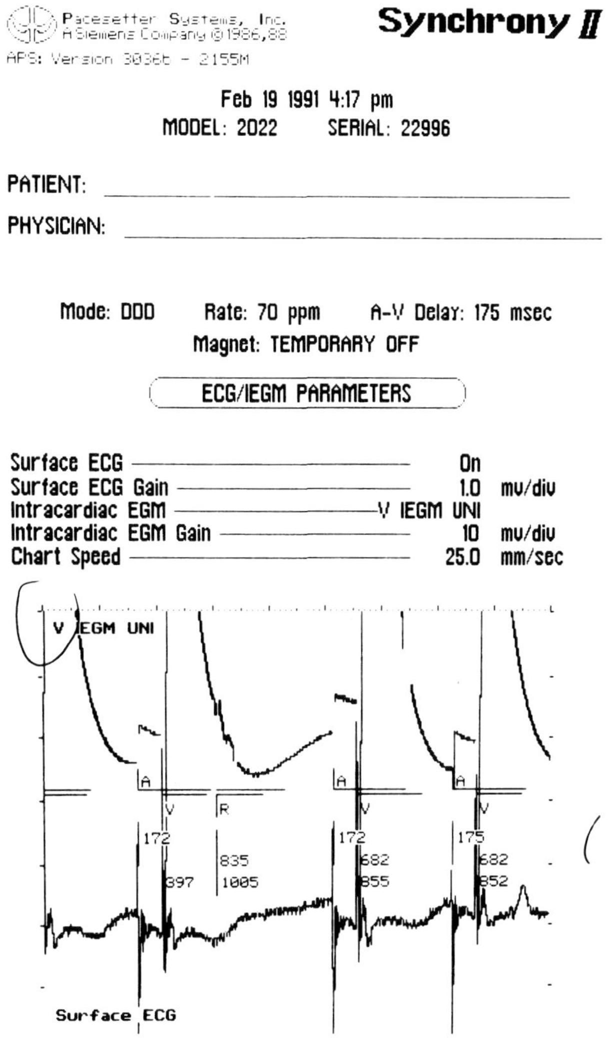

DIAGNOSIS AND MANAGEMENT OF LEAD INSULATION BREAK

A break in lead insulation allows current to flow from the lead through the break. In unipolar leads, the current flows directly into body tissues at the site of the break. If this current flow is in proximity to muscle and is of sufficient strength, the muscle will be stimulated. In addition, if sufficient current is shunted out of the lead at the break site, insufficient current will be available at the lead tip to depolarize myocardium; thus, failure to capture may occur. The ECG can display an increase in pacing artifact amplitude, reflecting the current flow directly into body tissues. The sequelae of insulation breaks depend on their location and the lead configuration. If the insulation between the two wire conductors of a bipolar lead breaks, a short circuit is created; current crossing this circuit will leave insufficient amounts to stimulate myocardium.

Insulation break has important implications for appropriate sensing of the intracardiac signal.[82] If the lead cannot conduct the sensed signal with fidelity, undersensing will result. For example, if a short circuit exists between the two conductors of a bipolar lead, the intracardiac signal, representing the potential difference between the anode and the cathode, will be attenuated in amplitude and thus may not be sensed. If a

FIGURE 41–16. Same patient as in Figure 41–2. Telemetered ventricular unipolar intracardiac electrogram (identified as such in the printout) displayed simultaneously with the surface ECG and marker channels. The surface electrocardiographic recording contains much baseline artifact and, aside from definite QRS complexes (which are not clearly paced), cannot be reliably interpreted. Note the false signal (depicted as a sensed "R" wave, since it is sensed on the ventricular channel), which is unaccompanied by a visible event on the surface ECG. This signal was presumably generated at the loose connection between the ventricular lead and the pacemaker, an assumption that was confirmed at reoperation. This figure and Figure 41–2 illustrate the value of interrogated data and telemetered electrograms in identifying the source of the problem. In this pulse generator design, two consecutive ventricular events without an intervening atrial event is interpreted as a premature ventricular complex, resulting in resetting of the atrial escape interval to exceed the programmed escape interval by 150 msec.

short circuit exists but is intermittent, the false signals generated by the make-break contacts can result in oversensing.

Although the diagnosis of lead insulation break may be suspected on clinical and electrocardiographic grounds, validation is best achieved through telemetered impedance and battery current drain information.[83] As resistance to current flow declines in the presence of insulation break, telemetered impedance will be low, and current drain from the battery will be increased. Until the pacing system can be revised, increasing the pulse generator output is a reasonable temporizing measure; in some systems, lead polarity programming can also be useful.

DIAGNOSIS AND MANAGEMENT OF CONDUCTOR FRACTURE

A break in the lead wire, or loose connections between the lead(s) and the pulse generator, increases the resistance to current flow in the lead. The current reaching the lead tip may therefore be insufficient to stimulate cardiac muscle, resulting in noncapture. The intracardiac signal likewise will not be transmitted through the lead to the pulse generator, resulting in undersensing. If the break is not complete, a potential difference can exist across the break site, resulting in "false signals." These can reach an amplitude sufficient to be sensed, causing clinical oversensing. In a partial conductor fracture, the electrical circuit is sometimes intact and sometimes not intact; this "make-break" circumstance can lead to intermittent failure to capture or to sense, or both.

The diagnosis of conductor fracture or loose connections can be suspected by observing noncapture accompanied by attenuation or absence of pacing artifacts (in analog ECG recording equipment) (Table 41–9). The condition is confirmed by a documented increase in lead impedance during pulse generator interrogation. If the problem is intermittent, interrogation should be performed during times of observed noncapture (see Figs. 41–2 and 42–16). Particular maneuvers, such as arm stretching or change in body position, might be required to elicit the problem, and the patient should be specifically queried about symptoms during these maneuvers. Telemetry of the intracardiac electrogram is generally less helpful in establishing the diagnosis, although the presence of the false signals can be recorded.

Unless the conductor break is readily accessible at operative revision, the lead must be replaced.

Evaluation of Rate-Adaptive Pacing Systems

The evaluation of patients with rate-adaptive devices includes assessment of the continued appropriateness of the programmed rate response settings (see Chapter 7). The availability of event counters and rate histograms facilitates this assessment and, in most circumstances, eliminates the need for repeated ambulatory (Holter) ECGs and treadmill exercise testing. Programmable sensor parameters include the

TABLE 41–9. DIAGNOSIS OF CONDUCTOR WIRE FRACTURE

ELECTROCARDIOGRAM
Absence of stimulus artifacts
Reversal of stimulus artifact polarity (analog ECG machines)
Stimuli delivered at multiples of programmed rate
Voltage transients

INTERROGATION
High impedance

INTRACARDIAC ELECTROGRAMS
Voltage transients sensed as "P" or "R" events

upper and lower sensor-based rate limits and the reaction (rate acceleration) and recovery (deceleration) times. The reaction time (acceleration) refers to the time that the pacemaker takes to accelerate its pacing rate from the programmed low rate to the programmed sensor-based upper rate. The recovery time (deceleration) is the time that it takes the pacing rate to slow from the maximum sensor-based rate to the low sensor-based rate (assuming absence of spontaneous signal input to the sensor). If the patient is deconditioned or has underlying structural heart disease, such as congestive heart failure, the reaction time can be programmed to be fast, to allow for rapid achievement of reasonable heart rates for a given activity. The recovery time is often programmed to be slow, to allow for the maintenance of a faster heart rate for a longer period of time after a period of exercise. A slow recovery time can also be programmed if the pacing system is being used to overdrive an accelerated junctional or ectopic rhythm. During clinic follow-up visits, the patient should be asked to walk at both normal and brisk paces in the office corridor. The event counters during normal and brisk activity can then be telemetered to determine whether the sensor parameters can be expected to respond appropriately to the activities of daily living.

Transtelephonic Monitoring

Transtelephonic monitoring is an important complement to regular outpatient clinic visits and is now standard care. Not only are important data obtained regarding pacing system performance, but also the monitoring personnel can receive and record the cardiac rhythm during symptoms such as dizziness and palpitations. Transtelephonic monitoring is especially useful for patients who live at some distance from the follow-up center and for infirm and immobile patients.

Transtelephonic transmission is accomplished by connecting electrodes, placed on the wrists, ankles, or fingertips, depending on electrode design and configuration of best signal, to a transmitter, over which is held (or placed) the mouthpiece of the telephone. ECG tracings are recorded with and without a magnet in place, for at least 30 seconds each. If available and previously programmed "on," a threshold determination can be performed through a "Vario" function; however, we recommend this only if a stable spontaneous rhythm and rate are known to exist.

Concern is often expressed regarding the potential danger of developing malignant ventricular arrhythmias during application of the magnet to pulse generators during telephone transmissions. Pacemaker-induced premature ventricular depolarizations do occur but are almost never sustained. Only rarely do multiple consecutive extrasystoles require cessation of the use of the magnet.[84] We have never documented an episode of ventricular fibrillation or sustained ventricular tachycardia produced with a magnet in this setting. Transtelephonic monitoring centers, which follow thousands of patients, likewise have not experienced this complication (Hurzeler, P., Cardiac Datacorp Inc., personal communication). Pacemaker-mediated tachycardia is occasionally induced in patients with DDD systems; however, termination is usually easily accomplished by reapplication and removal of the magnet.

High-quality transmission and reception of ECGs is easy

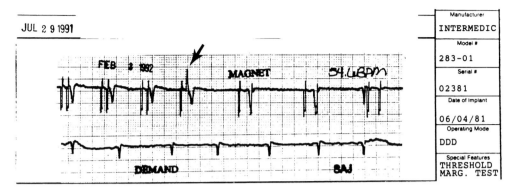

FIGURE 41–17. Transtelephonic transmission of DOO and DDD modes of function in a patient with an Intermedics 283-01 DDD pacing system. Note that the atrial rhythm cannot be discerned (*bottom strip*) and actually appears to be atrial fibrillation with regular ventricular response. This rhythm diagnosis would suggest an abnormality of AV conduction, perhaps due to digitalis toxicity, unless it was known that the patient's rhythm was sinus. Application of the magnet to this pacemaker causes, initially, DOO pacing at a faster than programmed rate (90 ppm) and a short AV interval (100 msec) (to allow the best chance of confirming ventricular capture after atrial pacing), followed by DOO output at the programmed rate and AV interval. After 60 cycles, the programmed mode of function will supervene despite the fact that the magnet is still in place. At the end of the threshold margin test, depicted in this strip (in which the last pacing stimulus is delivered at half the programmed pulse duration), the ventricular pacing artifact is upright (*arrow*), rather than downgoing as it is at all other times. Unless it is known that this is a feature signifying the end of a threshold margin test, mistaken diagnosis of pacemaker malfunction could be made. Unexpected deflections can originate in the pacing system itself, the transmitter, the telephone line, or the writeout equipment.

to achieve even with the most inexpensive equipment. However, transtelephonic ECG transmission can lead to interpretive difficulties and can display artifacts that are similar to those encountered with conventional electrocardiography (Figs. 41–17 and 41–18). A few artifacts are unique to trans-telephonic monitoring. The most potentially serious, in that interpretive errors can be made, is that caused by the use of a single-lead rhythm strip, usually lead I, in which the paced QRS complexes or the pacemaker artifact itself may be iso-electric or otherwise insufficiently diagnostic. Another lead

FIGURE 41–18. *A* to *D*, Examples of the difficulties encountered in interpretation of the electrocardiographic rhythm strips transmitted by telephone. In each case, the top strip is the presenting rhythm, and the bottom strip the rhythm obtained with the magnet in place.

A, A dual-chamber pacing system is in place, but neither atrial nor ventricular capture can be confirmed. In all but the third set of pacing output pulses, the presence of T waves indicates ventricular depolarization (hence, capture), but the paced QRS complexes are not discerned.

B, A VVI pacing system is in place. The spontaneous rhythm is sinus with normal AV conduction. The VOO tracing displays the pacer pulses only; no obvious QRS complex is seen.

C, A VVIR pacing system is in place. Despite the presence of the arrows, which register pacing output pulses, no visible pacing artifacts are seen. During asynchronous pacing, in fact, the precise meaning of the arrows is far from clear, since their intervals are not constant.

D, A DDDR pacing system is in place. Although atrial and ventricular pacing pulses are delivered in the top strip, capture is not seen. In the lower strip, paced QRS complexes can be visualized, but paced P waves are not confirmed.

These tracings, the rule rather than the exception, serve to illustrate how the physician must rely on the personnel responsible for the telephone transmission reports.

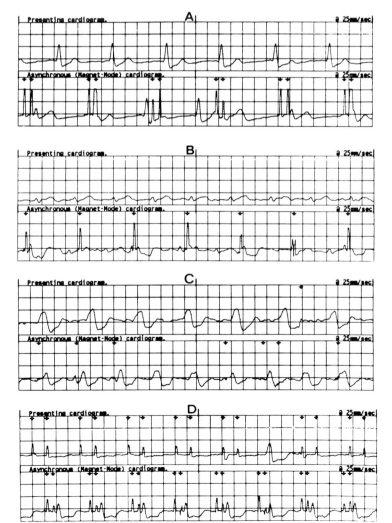

should be selected and the transmission repeated, and this lead system should be used in future transmissions.

Transtelephonic monitoring can be problematic for some patients. The patient needs to be physically able to properly and securely place the electrodes, and to change their placement if so instructed. A high impedance in patients with chronic obstructive pulmonary disease, obese patients, and edematous patients may render the transmitted signals too small to be diagnostically useful. Patients with tremor or who are otherwise unable to hold the telephone steady often transmit a poor signal. Care has to be taken that no environmental interference from, for example, radio or television sets is present. Finally, some patients may place the incorrect end of the telephone over the transmitter. Memory and hearing impairment can contribute to these difficulties. Education of the patient (or friend or relative) by the clinic staff has been extremely useful in eliminating many of these potential problems.

Transtelephonic assessment of rate-adaptive pacing systems to in-place exercise has been described.[79] During this evaluation, the patient wears the electrodes on the wrists, braces the arms and hands on a firm surface on which are placed the transmitter and the telephone mouthpiece, and runs in place. Pacing systems employing rapidly activated sensors programmed to low activity thresholds can be evaluated for rate response to these relatively low levels of effort. The actual clinical use of this maneuver, compared, for instance, to information available from rate histograms, is not clear at the present time.

Symptoms After Pacing System Implantation

Symptoms suggesting cerebral hypoperfusion (syncope and presyncope or dizziness), arrhythmias (potentially including pacemaker-related rhythm disturbances such as pace-maker-mediated tachycardia and tracking of atrial arrhythmias such as flutter and fibrillation), and pacemaker syndrome (weakness, effort breathlessness) can be present in 1% to 30% of patients after pacing system implantation[85–89] (see Table 41–3). Whereas in most patients these symptoms are relatively nonspecific or are more rationally ascribed to underlying heart disease and its progression, or even the medications used to treat it, investigation of pacing system function is warranted because most pacemaker-related problems are correctable, usually noninvasively by programming. To this end, ambulatory ECG (Holter) monitoring and exercise testing may be useful.

Reports of systematic Holter follow-up of paced patients are not plentiful[85, 90–94] and not particularly recent. Early publications[93, 95] suggested that as many as 18% of patients with normal pacing system function in the clinic had abnormalities of function detected by Holter monitoring. In one large study of 570 patients,[85] of whom 8.6% had symptoms after pacing system implantation, Holter monitoring provided the diagnosis in 75%. Importantly, pacemaker-related rhythm disturbances (usually oversensing and failure to capture) were found only about half the time, and spontaneous supraventricular and ventricular arrhythmias unrelated to the pacing system accounted for the remainder.[93]

In another large study of 550 patients with a unipolar single-chamber pacing system,[96] Holter monitoring documented periods of inhibition of pacer output in 57% of 60 patients; 77% of these 60 demonstrated this finding during direct observation of isometric exercise. This study, specifically designed to compare the value of Holter monitoring to directly observed response to isometric stress, suggested that the utility of ambulatory ECG monitoring under these circumstances was minimal and likely to confirm what is already known to the clinician. (Yet it must be acknowledged that Holter monitoring did provide the original data regarding the high prevalence [up to 70%] of myopotential inhibition in unipolar pacing systems.[97, 98])

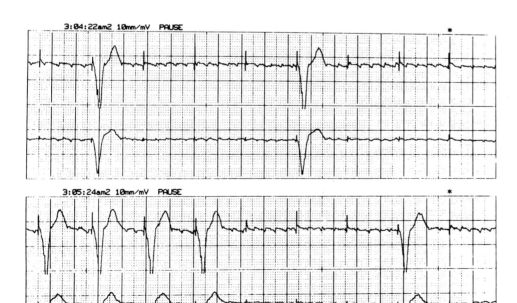

FIGURE 41–19. Holter monitor recording in a patient whose VVIR pacing system was functioning entirely normally during clinic visits, but in whom presyncopal episodes were occurring. The atrial rhythm is flutter. Episodic failure to capture is seen in the early morning hours (3:05 AM in this rhythm strip), suggesting the possibility of a vagally mediated increase in stimulation threshold.

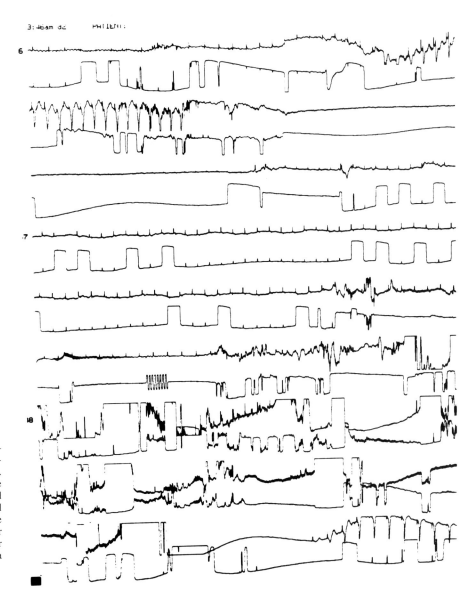

FIGURE 41–20. Same patient as in Figure 41–19. The tracings are a 3-minute recording, illustrating the difficulties occasionally encountered. Failure to capture is clearly demonstrated in the topmost strip; however, recording artifacts and signal attenuation in other strips (especially well seen in the next to last strip) preclude reliable interpretation. Note the patient event marker near the middle of the recording. The pacemaker output was increased, and no further bradycardia episodes were documented.

Our own experience with Holter monitoring in paced patients indicates that truly unsuspected pacemaker-related rhythm disturbances are rare. However, they do occur and can be quite dramatic (Figs. 41–19 and 41–20). Not infrequently, a finding suggested by single-channel ECG recording can be documented or clarified by two-channel recording (Figs. 41–21 and 41–22). More often, Holter findings (e.g., rapid paced ventricular rates causing discomfort) do disclose both the frequency and the duration of pacemaker-related rhythm abnormalities, which in turn suggest the appropriate programming maneuvers that can then be carried out at a subsequent clinic visit. Routine Holter monitoring of asymptomatic paced patients is generally not recommended.

Certain caveats in assessment of Holter recordings should be mentioned. Signal attenuation can mimic pauses in paced rhythm (see Fig. 41–22). Saturation of the recording channel(s) by pacing output pulses can result in absence of recorded complexes (Fig. 41–23). Misalignment of the record-

FIGURE 41–21. Simultaneously recorded modified Holter leads II and V1 in a patient with a VVI pacing system who complained of intermittent palpitations. No pacing system malfunction was found. Note the obscuring of the first paced QRS complex by presumed myopotentials. If only the MCL1 channel had been recorded, myopotential inhibition of pacemaker output would have been incorrectly diagnosed. The rhythm strips illustrate the usefulness of simultaneous two-channel recordings.

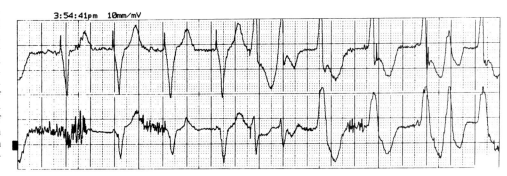

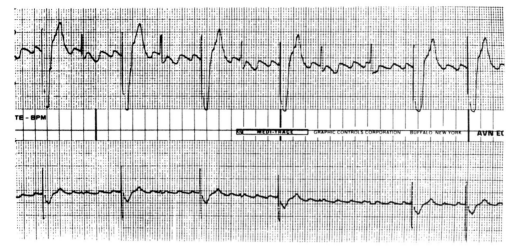

FIGURE 41–22. Simultaneously recorded Holter monitor leads II and MCL1 in a patient with a DDD pacing system, who complained of palpitations; this recording illustrates the value of recording more than a single electrocardiographic lead. The atrial rhythm is flutter. Whereas the lower strip suggests inappropriate pauses in paced ventricular rate, the upper strip demonstrates clearly that the occurrence of spontaneous QRS complexes appropriately inhibits the pulse generator output, and also that some flutter waves are being appropriately tracked, resulting in faster-than-programmed paced ventricular rates.

ing heads has been reported to result in spurious location of pacing stimuli relative to spontaneous complexes in those systems in which the pacing stimulus is recorded separately from the ECG and, in a separate process, added to the ECG channels.[99] In those Holter systems that incorporate a dedicated "pacer channel" that inscribes a deflection on detecting a pacer output pulse from the body surface, delay in depiction of the pacing artifact relative to inscription of the P waves or QRS complexes can lead to incorrect interpretations.[100] Finally, normal capture and sensing functions can be difficult to ascertain with certainty (Fig. 41–24).

Special Considerations in the Paced Patient

DIAGNOSIS OF MYOCARDIAL INFARCTION DURING VENTRICULAR PACING

Since ventricular pacing alters ventricular activation and repolarization, the diagnosis of acute myocardial infarction and/or ischemia during pacing is often difficult. The QRS complex during right ventricular pacing resembles that of a spontaneous left bundle branch block; the diagnosis of myocardial infarction can often be suspected during ventricular pacing by applying the criteria used in complete left bundle branch block. The pacing artifact, particularly during unipolar pacing, frequently distorts the initial part of the QRS complex and makes the presence of Q waves difficult to discern. An extensive anterior wall myocardial infarction may cause an initial Q in leads I, aVL, and V5–6, producing a stimulus-small Q, large R pattern and an initial r in V1, producing a stimulus-small r, large S pattern.[101–104] While the sensitivity of this combined finding is low, the specificity approaches 100%; we have, however, observed this pattern in patients with dilated cardiomyopathy. An underlying inferior myocardial infarction can result in the inscription of a large Q/large R, or large Q/small R complex in leads II, III, and aVF; again, sensitivity is low but specificity better[104, 105] in the relatively small numbers of patients studied.

Cabrera's sign, a late notching of the ascending limb of the QRS complex in the left precordial leads, can be present during an anterior wall myocardial infarction; its development during ventricular pacing suggests the presence of an extensive anterior myocardial infarction. The sensitivity of this sign is low, but its specificity is very high,[101] albeit in small numbers of patients.

Chatterjee and colleagues[56] first described the frequent occurrence of abnormal ST-T waves in the unpaced ECG following the termination of right ventricular endocardial pacing; these abnormalities, sometimes quite pronounced, were noted to persist for varying lengths of time, depending on the duration of pacing. These abnormalities are not specific for acute myocardial infarction. However, new ST-segment elevation in paced QRS complexes can be meaningful. The most useful and potentially diagnostic type of ST elevation is a pronounced primary ST elevation having the same direction as the QRS complex. Inhibition of ventricular pacing by chest wall stimulation, or by reduction of the backup pacing rate or output in non–pacemaker-dependent patients, allows

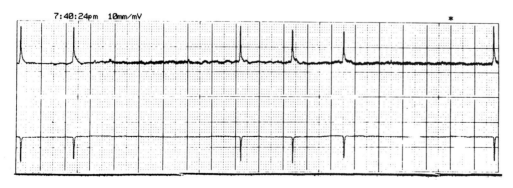

FIGURE 41–23. Signal attenuation in this Holter recording makes the rhythm indiscernible. The deflections are presumably pacemaker output pulses, but this cannot be verified.

FIGURE 41–24. Two continuous sets of simultaneously recorded Holter monitor leads II and MCL1 rhythm strips, illustrating some of the difficulties encountered in assessing pacing system function. The top two strips show atrial and ventricular stimulus outputs; however, atrial capture cannot be confirmed, since paced P waves are not clearly discerned (the deflection following the atrial output pulse might represent a decay curve artifact). The QRS complexes are not especially broad, nor is their axis superior, suggesting that they may represent fusion or pseudofusion complexes. In the lower two strips, however, spontaneous P waves are readily seen, and the third QRS complex is purely spontaneous. The intermediate morphology of the QRS complexes in the top strip indicates that they are ventricular fusions. Purely paced QRS complexes are recognized at the middle and end of the lower strip. The ventricular fusion complexes result from the ventricular pacing stimuli and the (retrospectively recognized) paced P waves. Thus, normal atrial sensing and pacing and normal ventricular sensing and pacing are demonstrated in these strips.

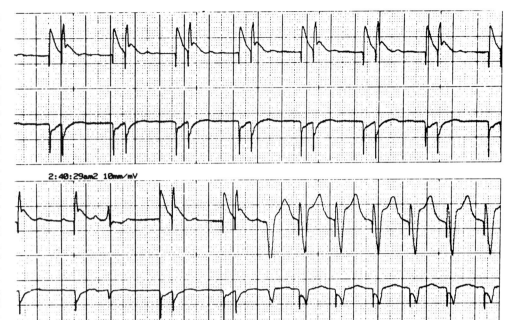

the emergence of the spontaneous QRS rhythm, the morphology of which can aid in the diagnosis of ischemia or infarction. Postpacing abnormalities in ST and T waves will, however, reduce the predictive accuracy of the diagnosis considerably.

CARDIOVERSION AND DEFIBRILLATION

The potentially high transthoracic currents discharged during external (transthoracic) cardioversion and defibrillation can damage an implanted pacing system as a result of the large amount of energy delivered to the heart during a relatively brief period of time.[106–110] The electromagnetic fields associated with these procedures can produce high current flow through the pacing lead to the electrode tip, damaging myocardial tissue and leading to failure to sense, to pace, or both (see Chapter 40). While pulse generators are protected from induced current during defibrillation by a Zener diode that limits the current allowed to enter the pacemaker circuitry through the lead, damage to the pacing and/or sensing circuits or even reprogramming can occur (Table 41–10). Thus, although the pulse generator is expected to withstand without damage a 400-J shock (the maximum energy delivered by transthoracic defibrillators), the pacing system must

TABLE 41–10. EFFECTS OF DEFIBRILLATION, CARDIOVERSION, OR BOTH ON PERMANENT PACEMAKERS

Undersensing
Failure to capture due to stimulation threshold increase
Reprogramming (e.g., lead configuration)
Backup pacing (usually VOO at the backup rate)
Myocardial burns with creatine kinase release
Induction of ventricular fibrillation

be interrogated and temporarily reprogrammed after any defibrillation or cardioversion procedures in order to evaluate the integrity of these functions. The induced current reaching the pacing system can be minimized by avoiding placement of the cardioverting paddles over the pulse generator or along the axis between the generator and the lead electrodes. If the pulse generator is located in the left infraclavicular area, cardioversion can be accomplished with the paddles placed in the usual position. If the pulse generator is located on the patient's right side, anteriorly and posteriorly placed cardioverting electrodes may be best. While most pacemaker malfunctions following DC shock have been described in unipolar pacing systems, bipolar systems, despite a short antenna, are also vulnerable to damage, albeit to a lesser degree.[108, 109]

The discharge of an implanted cardioverting-defibrillating (ICD) device has only rarely been reported to cause any permanent pacemaker malfunction or destruction; however, it is important to be familiar with the interactions between these two implanted devices.[111–114] Shocks from the ICD can occur because of the rate cutoff criterion being satisfied by the sensing of atrial and/or ventricular pacing stimuli and their evoked ventricular potentials (see Chapter 39). An increase in pacing and/or sensing threshold can occur following ICD shock delivery. The ICD discharge can cause reversion or backup pacing and, in some pulse generators, a change in lead polarity from bipolar to unipolar polarity. Finally, failure to detect ventricular fibrillation by the ICD can occur if the pacemaker, undersensing the arrhythmia, continues to deliver pacing stimuli during the ventricular fibrillation, which stimuli are sensed by the ICD and interpreted as a "normal" rhythm. The ICD shock can, in these circumstances, be delayed or suppressed entirely.[112]

Recognizing these device-to-device interactions, some guidelines are prudent. In general, unipolar pacing systems should not be used in patients receiving an ICD. Pacing systems with programmable lead polarity should be carefully tested to ensure that ICD discharges do not reprogram the lead configuration to unipolar. If the ICD senses the larger unipolar spikes, it may not be capable of sensing and treating a potentially lethal arrhythmia. The pacing electrodes should be located as far as possible from the rate-sensing electrodes and/or ICD lead; if epicardial rate-sensing ICD leads are utilized, they should be closely spaced (1 cm or less) in order to minimize sensing of emitted pacing stimuli. The ability of the ICD to sense bipolar pacing stimuli requires ongoing evaluation. When ventricular arrhythmias are induced as part of routine ICD follow-up, the ability of the pacing leads to sense the arrhythmia and inhibit pulse generator output should be evaluated, since failure to inhibit the generator may cause the ICD to undersense the arrhythmia. At the time of ICD implantation, the output of the pacing system should be increased to its maximum in both atrial and ventricular channels, to evaluate the presence of double or triple counting by the ICD. The pacemaker's output should be programmed to the lowest safe value. The sensitivity of the pulse generator should be programmed to a very sensitive setting (i.e., low value) in order to sense ventricular fibrillation and inhibit appropriately.

ELECTROCAUTERY

Several endogenous and exogenous sources of electromagnetic interference can affect pacing system function (Table 41–11; see Chapter 40). Electrocautery is likely the most common exogenous source of this interference. Electrocautery uses radio-frequency current to transect tissue and achieve hemostasis. Coagulation and cutting circuits of electrocautery devices differ in their effects on permanent pacemakers. Bipolar coagulation cautery, in which the current flow is localized between the two poles of the instrument, is not expected to cause problems if it is kept at a distance of

TABLE 41–11. **COMMON SOURCES OF ELECTROMAGNETIC INTERFERENCE**

ENDOGENOUS
Myopotentials
MEDICAL EQUIPMENT
Diathermy
Electrocautery
Magnetic resonance imaging
Cardioversion, defibrillation
Transcutaneous pacing
Electrotherapy
Transcutaneous nerve stimulation
Implanted neuromuscular stimulators
Ionizing radiation
Lithotripsy
AMBIENT
Radio-frequency emissions
Shortwave radio
Mobile radio transmitters
Garage door openers
High-tension lines
Arc welding
Rotating radar detectors
Induction furnaces

more than 6 inches from the pacemaker generator. However, in unipolar electrocautery devices used for cutting, the electric current flow is not restricted to the tissue interposed between two electrodes and thus spreads throughout the body. This conductive electromagnetic interference, as well as the myopotentials resulting from the procedure itself, can result in pulse generator inhibition, electric burns at the myocardial-electrode interface, atrial or ventricular tachycardia and fibrillation, pulse generator component failure, loss of or change in output, or reprogramming of rate, mode, or both.[115–119] Occasionally, electrocautery signals, perceived as "noise" by the pulse generator, can result in reversion mode pacing, which is demand or asynchronous ventricular pacing at a specific rate, both determined by the manufacturer.[117, 119]

Management of pacemaker patients during procedures involving electrocautery includes the following: (1) determination of the presence of pacemaker dependency with hemodynamic inability to tolerate pulse generator inhibition; (2) continuous arterial pressure monitoring, since distortion by the electrocautery of the cardiac rhythm recorded by the ECG machine can make it difficult to determine whether pacemaker inhibition has occurred; (3) avoidance of unipolar electrocautery if the operating field is within 6 inches of the pulse generator or lead; (4) placement of the ground-plate as close as possible to the operating site, and as far away as possible from the pacing system, if unipolar cautery must be used, while attempting to preserve a pathway perpendicular to a line joining the two pacing electrodes; and (5) providing an electrocautery time as short as possible using the lowest amount of energy.

A magnet should not be applied prophylactically in all paced patients, since there is no uniform pulse generator response to this maneuver, and magnet rates and AV intervals may be significantly different from programmed values, resulting in hemodynamic embarrassment. Magnet application may result in initiation of a programming procedure and inappropriate random reprogramming by the electrocautery device, or other device-specific cyclic functions such as Vario pacing. We recommend a preoperative pacing system evaluation, including verification of response to magnet application, prior to any surgical procedure, with appropriate programming changes made if required.

If the electrocautery has resulted in permanent damage to the pacemaker, the generator must be replaced.

DIATHERMY

Short-wave diathermy consists of the application of electric current directly to the skin for relief of musculoskeletal pain. Diathermy should not be used in patients with pacemakers because of the relatively high potential for pulse generator damage, or inhibition, or both, directly from heat or from high-frequency electrical signals that bypass the standard noise protection mechanisms.[120] These complications can occur even if the pacemaker is programmed to an asynchronous mode of operation.

IONIZING RADIATION

Currently available pulse generators with complementary metal oxide semiconductors are more sensitive to the effects of ionizing radiation compared to the semiconductor circuits used in older pulse generators.[121–125] Sources of ionizing radiation include x-rays and cobalt irradiation; therapeutic radiation, if absolutely required, should be accomplished with the pulse generator shielded. If the patient is pacemaker dependent and the pulse generator is situated near or in the radiation field, consideration should be given to relocating the generator to another site. The damage to pacemaker electronic circuitry incurred by ionizing radiation is unpredictable; it can be transient, but is not infrequently permanent, and is cumulative in nature. In pulse generators exposed to radiation, even transient loss of function should be regarded as a precursor of permanent damage.

MAGNETIC RESONANCE IMAGING

Manufacturers of both pacemakers and nuclear magnetic resonance imaging (MRI) scanners have emphasized that MRI scanning is contraindicated in pacemaker patients.[126–132] MRI scanning affects pacemaker function by the development of strong static and time-varying magnetic fields as well as pulsed radio-frequency fields. The changing magnetic fields can result in actual physical movement of the pulse generator's internal components. While damage to the pacemaker reed switch remains a theoretical danger, however improbable, no apparent damage to pacemaker components has been reported in several pulse generators or lead systems.[129]

During MRI scanning, most pacemakers revert to asynchronous mode of function.[131] While asynchronous pacing per se may not cause problems in the stable patient, radio-frequency pulsing can result in induced voltage across the pacemaker electrodes that may be strong enough to stimulate myocardial tissue, leading to rapid rates equal to the MRI pulsing rate; these rates can vary from cycle lengths of 200 msec to 1000 msec.[130] Radio-frequency pulses can also cause inhibition of the pulse generator, with resulting bradycardia and asystole. Resetting of DDD pulse generators to the backup mode can occur as the circuit is activated by high radio-frequency pulse rate.[132]

If MRI scanning is deemed essential for the patient, in vitro tests of the same pulse generator should be performed prior to the actual scanning session to assess that particular pulse generator's behavior. In patients with pulse generators capable of being programmed to "magnet-off" function, consideration should be given to this programming command in order to avoid asynchronous pacing. It has, conversely, also been suggested that pacemaker-dependent patients should be programmed to VOO mode at maximum energy output and at relatively rapid rates (e.g., 100 pulses per minute), in order to avoid arrhythmias.[131] Some workers have recommended that DDD and rate-adaptive pacemakers be programmed to the VVI or VOO mode.[131] Prior to MRI studies, the patient should sign a written consent for anesthesia and revision of the pacemaker system after MRI scanning, should it become necessary. The patient should be clearly informed that MRI-induced pacing system malfunction may necessitate cardiopulmonary resuscitation and/or immediate pacemaker system revision. Equipment must be provided for emergency defibrillation, intubation, artificial ventilation, and central line placement. For the scanning procedure, the patient should be fasting and should have an intravenous access line in place. While the patient is near or in the scanner, his or her rhythm requires telemetric monitoring. If pacing-related difficulties occur during MRI scanning and lead to discontinuation of the procedure, it should be remembered that the patient must be at least 30 feet from the scanner to ensure that there is no interaction between the magnetic field and the pacing system.

LITHOTRIPSY

Extracorporeal shock-wave lithotripsy is a noninvasive treatment for nephrolithiasis and cholelithiasis that has gained worldwide acceptance. The lithotriptor generates electromagnetic and mechanical forces that may influence pacing system function.[133–137] Although this therapy is generally safe in the paced outpatient, published studies of in vitro testing have indicated that about 4% of 144 pacemaker generators of various manufacturers tested failed when exposed to lithotripsy. Pulse generators employing a piezoelectric crystal sensor seem to be the most susceptible to failure,[133] and rate-adaptive generators that utilize this type of sensor should have the activity mode programmed to "off" during lithotripsy; this will avoid an unwanted increase in paced heart rate as well as shatter injury to the piezoelectric element.[133] Whereas patients with rate-adaptive units that employ a piezoelectric crystal implanted in the thorax can probably undergo lithotripsy safely when programmed in the non–rate-responsive mode, patients in whom these devices are implanted in the abdomen should probably not undergo lithotripsy.

Several management guidelines for pacemaker patients undergoing lithotripsy can be offered. First, a model of the implanted pacemaker pulse generator should be tested in vitro prior to the patient's undergoing the procedure, to assess the pulse generator's response. Second, the lithotriptor should be synchronized to the QRS complex or ventricular output pulse to avoid inappropriate inhibition or triggering of the pacemaker by the discharge spark occurring at other portions of the pacing cycle. Third, DDD pacing systems should be programmed to the VVI mode of function to avoid triggering of the shock-wave output by the atrial output pulse. The delay in shock wave delivery (up to 160 msec) can result in detection of the shock wave by the ventricular sensing amplifier, resulting in inhibition of ventricular stimulus output. Fourth, rate-adaptive pacemakers should be programmed to non–rate-responsive mode to avoid alteration in paced heart rate. Fifth, since pacing systems with inherent defects such as loose contacts can be rendered inoperative by lithotripsy, pacing system integrity should be evaluated by preprocedure ECGs and interrogation. Sixth, an external transcutaneous cardiac pacemaker should be available, should unexpected pacemaker malfunction occur; telemetric monitoring of the cardiac rhythm is essential during the procedure. Finally, all pacemakers should be thoroughly checked for proper function immediately following treatment.

TRANSCUTANEOUS ELECTRIC NERVE STIMULATION

Electric stimulating techniques such as transcutaneous electric nerve stimulation (TENS) are often indicated to treat pain related to muscular or neurologic problems. Rasmussen and associates[138] studied the effect of TENS on implanted pacing systems and found no episodes of interference, inhibition, or reprogramming. In this study, however, the TENS electrodes were not placed parallel to the pacemaker electrode vector. Thus, the full range of potential effects of this therapy on pacing system function is not known. Other studies have indicated a low incidence of adverse effects of TENS on older pacemaker models that were more susceptible to electromagnetic interference than are contemporary devices.

Therefore, it appears that electric stimulating techniques are safe to use in pacemaker patients, provided that the electrodes are not placed parallel to the vector of the pacemaker stimulus.

ELECTRICAL AND RADIO-FREQUENCY CATHETER ABLATION IN PATIENTS WITH IMPLANTED PACEMAKERS

Direct-current catheter ablation techniques are less frequently utilized and, in general, are more dangerous than current methods employing radio-frequency energy for ablation. Electrical ablation typically utilizes 150 to 500 J of energy, delivered to the tip of a temporary endocardial electrode. Whereas this technique is seldom utilized for catheter ablation, it may be utilized for intracardiac defibrillation through transvenous leads. The delivery of energy may occur in proximity to the electrodes of a previously implanted pacing system. As a result of temporary increases in stimulation threshold, transient loss of capture can occur.[139] Transient loss of sensing has also been observed[139] and is probably related to injury at the myocardial-electrode interface, causing degradation of the intracardiac electric signal. While chronic pacing and sensing threshold changes may occur, they have not been well described and are therefore presumably not common. Rarely, the pulse generator may be reprogrammed or reset to noise mode or backup mode, or a permanent malfunction can occur, requiring pulse generator replacement. Thus, both pacing and sensing functions of the permanent pacing system require thorough evaluation before and after any electrical catheter ablation.

Radio-frequency energy is now commonly used for catheter ablation of preexcitation syndromes (Wolff-Parkinson-White) with associated tachycardia and for AV node reentry tachycardia, and is being used with increasing frequency for ablation of automatic atrial tachycardia, atrial flutter, and ventricular tachycardia. The consequences of radio-frequency energy delivery in a paced patient include induction of rapid paced rates, inhibition of output, mode resetting in both single- and dual-chamber systems, and transient reed switch malfunction. Rapid pacing at the same rate as the RF modulating pulse has been reported in dogs.[140] Inhibition of output can occur even if the pacemaker generator has been programmed to the asynchronous mode of function.[140] Radio-frequency energy can also cause noise reversion or pacing in backup mode owing to interpretation by the pulse generator of the high pulse repetition rate as interference.

During radio-frequency cardiac catheter ablation procedures, the minimum amount of radio-frequency energy necessary to accomplish the ablation should be utilized in an attempt to minimize permanent pacemaker generator malfunction. Placement of a temporary pacemaker during the electrophysiologic study and ablation procedure may be prudent. The implanted permanent pulse generator can be programmed to the "off" mode if this feature is available, and the patient paced through the temporary pacemaker. Following ablation, the pacemaker can be reprogrammed to its original parameters, after interrogation, to ensure that no permanent effects have occurred.

Psychological Effects of Pacemaker Implantation

The goals of permanent pacemaker implantation are the treatment of symptomatic bradyarrhythmias and the improvement of quality of life. Many factors can influence a patient's psychological recovery from pacing system implantation. These include the effectiveness of the pacing system in achieving rate adaptation to meet the requirements of daily living, the presence and progression of concomitant disease, the availability of social resources, the personality and expectations of the patient, the adjustment to preexisting physical impairment, and communication between the patient, the physician, and the health care team.[141] To improve the psychological adaptation to pacemaker implantation, certain recommendations to foster a positive approach can be made. Health care misinformation may cause falsely low estimates of a patient's concept of his own capabilities, and may engender unrealistic fears regarding activity once a permanent pacemaker has been implanted. Preoperative education of pacemaker patients has been shown to result in a positive outcome in how the patient copes.[142] The challenge of the health care team is to provide a thorough educational program (multimedia-video, demonstration model, and teaching booklet) that begins before pacemaker implantation and extends throughout the postoperative recovery period. A review of the benefits of pacemaker implantation will enhance realistic expectations of the device. Patients usually require concrete guidelines relating to activity, both job-related and recreational. If possible, the skill of pulse monitoring should be taught. Information regarding symptoms related to activity should be provided to the patient so that he or she will be forthright and precise in reporting complaints such as fatigue, dizziness, dyspnea, chest pain, and changes in cognitive function. It has been demonstrated that patients with fixed-rate pacemakers can achieve training effects in exercise programs as demonstrated by increasing work tolerance,[143] although long warm-up periods were required in order to avoid excessive fatigue and shortness of breath. Exercise testing can be used, if necessary, to advise patients regarding the resumption of activities. When limitations in activity are experienced, such as inability to work, fatigue, dyspnea, and sleeplessness, a diminished quality of life exists. Physical functioning, social interaction, psychological state, and somatic sensation all are of importance when one evaluates quality of life of the patient. It has been reported that quality of life and emotional profiles are improved after pacemaker implantation.[144, 145] Improvement in cognitive function has also been observed.[144]

Optimal pacemaker programming, education, exercise evaluation, and rehabilitation all are advisable in order to achieve positive outcomes in pacemaker patients. Optimal function or return to prepacemaker level of function is expected. It should be emphasized that patient coping styles are many and varied. In at least one report, poor adaptation to pacing system implantation resulted in a suicide attempt.[146] Patients who display poor adjustment to permanent pacemaker implantation should be referred to appropriate resource personnel, such as psychologists, social workers, and psychiatrists.

Computerized Follow-Up, Patient Management, and Record Storage

Dramatic rises in health care costs have forced physicians to evaluate the most comprehensive, cost-effective management of pacemaker surveillance. It is now considered a poor utilization of time, labor, and health care dollars for health care personnel to manually retrieve and store pacemaker follow-up data from patient charts. In the 1990s, a computerized data base is the ideal method for maintaining records of patients with permanent pacemakers. Maintenance of these records will aid in identification of potential and actual pacemaker malfunction, provide the actuarial date of pacemaker battery longevity, allow documentation of costs, and provide analysis of trends in device selection and patient population. The data base provides a central communication link among patients, physicians, referring physicians, hospitals, and manufacturers. Essentials for computerized stored data include patient demographic characteristics, implant information, indications for pacing, underlying cardiac rhythm, implant complications and their management, programmed settings, and follow-up measurements. A computer system should be user-friendly, flexible, simple, and able to generate a printed report for the patient, a summary sheet for the referring physician, and a billing charge slip. A focused approach to pacemaker follow-up testing can include a completely computer-based system for transtelephonic and in-office pacemaker follow-up. Using computer-based transtelephonic follow-up, scheduling, ECG editing, and printing of reports can be accomplished with minimal paper clutter. Patient files are easy to access by the computer. ECG transmissions can be adjusted to filter motion artifact and noise. Electronic "cut-and-paste" of ECGs is automatically formatted for report printing. Automated scheduling and an on-screen calendar simplify the management of patient appointments. Since all records are accessed with only a few keystrokes on the computer screen, the physician can avoid sorting through cumbersome paper files and thus have more time for the patient.

Most available computer-based pacemaker follow-up systems are on a 40-megabyte hard drive, which allows storage of approximately 2000 patient files. A centralized data base serves as a tool for management control, checking aspects of implantation regionally, comparing results internationally, calculating pulse generator life expectancy, following the evolution of underlying cardiac rhythm, and assessing lead longevity. Two international centralized data bases exist. One is located at the Chaute in Berlin and was established in 1979 with an IBM under the MS-DOS operating system. Software for file management is D-BASE. As of 1989, data have been collected on 43,000 patients.[147] The second is a "Pacecare," which is IBM compatible under the DOS 3.0 operating system. The program produces files in the format used by D-BASE III, requires 10 megabytes of data storage, and runs from a hard disk drive. It is sophisticated, user-friendly, and fast, and changes in testing parameters can be recognized immediately. Pacecare has two hospitals in Australia with 3600 patients in the data base.[148] In Europe, a pacemaker registry has been established for surveillance of all patients with permanent cardiac pacemakers so that uniform diagnoses, generator and lead models, and information on appropriate management can be rapidly obtained. Patients carry a pacemaker "passport," which lists such pertinent information as date of implant, pulse generator manufacturer and model, lead electrodes manufacturer and model, rate at implantation, thresholds, and other parameters that could be useful in case of emergency or pacemaker malfunction.[148, 149]

At present, there is no uniform method for pacemaker follow-up surveillance in the United States. Two corporations provide surveillance for their own patients. Cardiac Data Corporation is a telephone pacemaker monitoring service that provides services to more than 25,000 recipients of any pacing system. Cardiocare provides pacemaker follow-up through a subsidiary of Medtronic, Inc., but has recently become independent. Five Food and Drug Administration pacemaker contract centers were established in 1980, and data have been reported several times yearly in PACE;[150] unfortunately, however, this "Bilitch Registry" is no longer functional. These data were utilized to identify unexpected pulse generator and lead malfunction. The report has led to discontinuation of the manufacture of some pulse generator models and leads because of unusual or suspicious characteristics of function.[150]

In the future, government, industry, and the medical community must work together to create a national data base or registry modeled after the European example.

REFERENCES

1. Bernstein AD, Parsonnet V: Survey of cardiac pacing in the United States in 1989. Am J Cardiol 69:331, 1992.
2. Griffin JC, Schuenemeyer TD, Hess KR, et al: Pacemaker follow-up: Its role in the detection and correction of pacemaker system malfunction. PACE 9:387, 1986.
3. Saksena S: Mechanism of an unusual QRS pattern associated with right ventricular pacing. Am Heart J 105:337, 1983.
4. Mower MM, Arang CE, Tabatznik B: Unusual patterns of conduction produced by pacemaker stimuli. Am Heart J 74:24, 1967.
5. Castellanos A, Jr, Maytin O, Lemberg L: Unusual QRS complexes produced by pacemaker stimuli. Am Heart J 77:732, 1969.
6. Grier D, Cook PG, Hartnell GG: Chest radiographs after permanent pacing. Are they really necessary? Clin Radiol 42:224, 1990.
7. Medicare. Cardiac pacemaker evaluation services. Effective Oct. 1, 1984. Coverage Issues Manual. HCFA Publication No. 6, section 50–1.
8. Vallario L, Leman R, Gillette P, Kratz J: Pacemaker follow-up and adequacy of medical guidelines. Am Heart J 116:11, 1988.
9. De Nardo D, Antolini M, Pitucco G, et al: Effects of left bundle branch block on left ventricular function in apparently normal subjects. Cardiology 75:365, 1988.
10. Grines CL, Bashore TM, Boudoulas H, et al: Functional abnormalities in isolated left bundle branch block: The effect of interventricular asynchrony. Circulation 79:845, 1989.
11. Ausubel K, Boal BH, Furman S: Pacemaker syndrome: Definition and evaluation. Cardiol Clin 3:587, 1985.
12. Wei JY: Age and the cardiovascular system. N Engl J Med 327:1235, 1992.
13. Wish M, Fletcher RD, Gottdiener JS, et al: Importance of left atrial timing in the programming of dual-chamber pacemaker. Am J Cardiol 60:566, 1987.
14. Benchimol A, Duenas A, Liggett MS, et al: Contribution of atrial systole to the cardiac function at a variable ventricular rate. Am J Cardiol 16:11, 1965.

15. Burchell M: A clinical appraisal of atrial transport function. Lancet 1:775, 1964.
16. Cohen SI, Frank HA: Preservation of active atrial transport: An important clinical consideration in cardiac pacing. Chest 81:51, 1982.
17. Mitchell JH, Gilmore JP, Sarnoff SJ: The transport function of the atrium: Factors influencing the relation between mean left atrial pressure and left ventricular end diastolic pressure. Am J Cardiol 9:237, 1962.
18. Haas JM, Strait GB: Pacemaker-induced cardiovascular failure. Am J Cardiol 33:295, 1974.
19. Alicandri C, Fouad FM, Tarazi RC, et al: Three cases of hypotension and syncope with ventricular pacing: Possible role of atrial reflexes. Am J Cardiol 42:137, 1978.
20. Parsonnet V, Myers M, Perry GY: Paradoxical paroxysmal nocturnal congestive heart failure as a severe manifestation of the pacemaker syndrome. Am J Cardiol 65:683, 1990.
21. Erlebacher JA, Danner RL, Stelzer PE: Hypotension with ventricular pacing: An atrial vasodepressor reflex in human beings. J Am Coll Cardiol 4:550, 1984.
22. Nakaota H, Kitahara Y, Imataka K, et al: Atrial natriuretic peptide with artificial pacemakers. Am J Cardiol 60:384, 1987.
23. Bolli P, Muller FB, Linder L, et al: The vasodilator potency of atrial natriuretic peptide in man. Circulation 75:221, 1987.
24. Stangl K, Weil J, Seitz K, et al: Influence of AV synchrony on the plasma levels of atrial natriuretic peptide (ANP) in patients with total AV block. PACE 11:1176, 1988.
25. Obata K, Yasue H, Horio Y, et al: Increase of human atrial natriuretic polypeptide in response to cardiac pacing. Am Heart J 113:845, 1987.
26. Morgan DE, Norman R, West RO, Burggraf G: Echocardiographic assessment of tricuspid regurgitation during ventricular demand pacing. Am J Cardiol 58:1025, 1986.
27. Reynolds D, Olson E, Burrow R, et al: Mitral regurgitation during atrioventricular and ventriculoatrial pacing. PACE 7:463, 1984.
28. Foster CJ: Constrictive pericarditis complicating an endocardial pacemaker. Br Heart J 47:497, 1982.
29. Spittell PC, Hayes DL: Venous complications after insertion of a transvenous pacemaker. Mayo Clin Proc 67:258, 1992.
30. Zerbe F, Ponizynski A, Dyszkiewicz W, et al: Functionless retained pacing leads in the cardiovascular system: A complication of pacemaker treatment. Br Heart J 54:76, 1985.
31. Deanfield JE, Fox KM, Allison DJ: Facial swelling: A complication of transvenous pacing. Clin Cardiol 5:308, 1982.
32. Blackburn T, Dunn M: Pacemaker-induced superior vena cava syndrome: Consideration of management. Am Heart J 116:893, 1988.
33. Thompson MF, Arnold RM, Bogart DB, et al: Symptomatic upper extremity venous thrombosis associated with permanent transvenous pacemaker electrodes. Chest 83:274, 1983.
34. Choo MH, Holmes DR, Jr, Gersh BJ, et al: Permanent pacemaker infections: Characterization and management. Am J Cardiol 48:559, 1981.
35. Goldman B, MacGregor DC: Management of infected pacemaker systems. Clin Prog Pacing Electrophysiol 2:220, 1989.
36. Bayliss CE, Beanlands DS, Baird RJ: The pacemaker–twiddler's syndrome: A new complication of implantable transvenous pacemakers. Can Med Assoc J 99:371, 1968.
37. Kumar A, McKay CR, Rahimtoola SH: Pacemaker–twiddler's syndrome: An important cause of diaphragmatic pacing. Am J Cardiol 56:797, 1985.
38. Youngson GG, McKenzie TN, Nichol PM: Superior vena cava syndrome: Case report. Am Heart J 99:503, 1980.
39. Yakirevich V, Alagem D, Papo J, Vidne BA: Fibrotic stenosis of the superior vena cava with widespread thrombotic occlusion of its major tributaries: An unusual complication of transvenous cardiac pacing. J Thorac Cardiovasc Surg 85:632, 1983.
40. Montgomery JH, D'Souza VJ, Dyer RB, et al: Nonsurgical treatment of the superior vena cava syndrome. Am J Cardiol 56:829, 1985.
41. Mazzetti H, Dussaut A, Tentori C, et al: Superior vena cava occlusion and/or syndrome related to pacemaker leads. Am Heart J 125:831, 1993.
42. Bradof J, Sands MJ, Lakin PC: Symptomatic venous thrombosis of the upper extremity complicating permanent transvenous pacing: Reversal with streptokinase infusion. Am Heart J 104:1112, 1982.
43. Capek P, Cope C: Percutaneous treatment of superior vena cava syndrome. Am J Radiol 152:183, 1989.
44. Elson JD, Becker GJ, Wholey MH, Ehrman KO: Vena caval and central venous stenoses: Management with Palmaz balloon-expandable intraluminal stents. J Vasc Intervent Radiol 2:215, 1991.
45. Nicolosi GL, Charmet PA, Zanuttini D: Large right atrial thrombosis: Rare complication during permanent transvenous endocardial pacing. Br Heart J 43:199, 1980.
46. Nanda NC, Barold SS: Usefulness of echocardiography in cardiac pacing. PACE 5:222, 1982.
47. Friedberg H, D'Cunha G: Adhesions of pacing catheter to tricuspid valve: Adhesive endocarditis. Thorax 24:498, 1969.
48. Lee M, Chaux A: Unusual complications of endocardial pacing. J Thorac Cardiovasc Surg 80:934, 1980.
49. Old WD, Paulsen W, Lewis SA, Nixon JV: Pacemaker lead-induced tricuspid stenosis: Diagnosis by Doppler echocardiography. Am Heart J 117:1165, 1989.
50. Korn M, Schoenfeld CD, Ghahramani A, Samet P: The pacemaker sound. Am J Med 49:451, 1970.
51. Misra KP, Korn M, Ghahramani AR, et al: Auscultatory findings in patients with cardiac pacemakers. Ann Intern Med 74:245, 1971.
52. Cheng TO, Ertem G, Vera Z: Heart sounds in patients with cardiac pacemakers. Chest 62:66, 1972.
53. Shirato C, Ishikawa K: Newly developed systolic murmur in patients with a transvenous pacemaker. Am Heart J 99(6):111-126, 1981.
54. Glassman RD, Noble RJ, Tavel ME, et al: Pacemaker-induced endocardial friction rub. Am J Cardiol 40:811, 1977.
55. Secemsky SI, Hauser RG, Denes P, Edwards LM: Unipolar sensing abnormalities: Incidence and clinical significance of skeletal muscle interference and undersensing in 228 patients. PACE 5:10, 1982.
56. Chatterjee K, Harris A, Davies G, Leatham A: Electrocardiographic changes subsequent to artificial ventricular depolarization. Br Heart J 31:770, 1969.
57. Gould L, Venkataraman K, Goswami MK, Gomprecht RF: Pacemaker-induced electrocardiographic changes simulating myocardial infarction. Chest 63:829, 1973.
58. Rosenbaum MB, Blanco HH, Elizari MV, et al: Electronic modulation of the T wave and cardiac memory. Am J Cardiol 50:213, 1982.
59. del Balzo U, Rosen MR: T-wave changes persisting after ventricular pacing in canine heart are altered by 4-aminopyridine but not by lidocaine: Implications with respect to phenomenon of cardiac "memory." Circulation 85:1464, 1992.
60. Donato L, Giuntini C, Mariani M, et al: Rhythm evolution during pacing with fixed-rate and ventricular-synchronous pacemakers. Ann NY Acad Sci 167:1060, 1969.
61. Jensen G, Sigurd B, Meibom J, Sandoe E: Adams-Stokes syndrome caused by paroxysmal third-degree atrioventricular block. Br Heart J 35:516, 1973.
62. Sowton E: Artificial pacemaking and sinus rhythm. Br Heart J 27:311, 1965.
63. Johansson BW, Karnell J, Malm A, et al: Electrocardiographic studies in patients with an artificial pacemaker. Br Heart J 25:514, 1963.
64. Edhag O, Rosenqvist M: Heart rhythm during permanent cardiac pacing. Br Heart J 42:182, 1979.
65. Rosenbeck S, Bondy C, Weiss A, Gotsman M: Comparison between patients with and without reliable ventricular escape rhythm in the presence of long-standing complete atrioventricular block. PACE 16:272, 1993.
66. Marinato PG, Bressan M, Buja GF, et al: Programmed chest-wall stimulation to evaluate the progress of A-V block after pacemaker insertion in patients with trifascicular disease. PACE 5:658, 1982.
67. Brignole M, Menozzi C, Lolli G, et al: Long-term outcome of paced and nonpaced patients with severe carotid sinus syndrome. Am J Cardiol 69:1039, 1992.
68. Gwinn N, Leman R, Kratz J, et al: Chronotropic incompetence: A common and progressive finding in pacemaker patients. Am Heart J 123:1216, 1992.
69. Barold SS, Gaidula JJ, Castillo R: Unusual response of demand pacemakers to magnets. Br Heart J 35:353, 1973.
70. Sinnaeve A, Willems R, Stroobandt R: Inhibition of on-demand pacemakers by magnet waving. PACE 5:878, 1982.
71. Barold SS, Falkoff MD, Ong LS, Heinle RA: Magnet-unresponsive pacemaker endless loop tachycardia. Am Heart J 116:726, 1988.
72. Van Gelder LM, El Gamal MIH: Magnet application, a cause of persistent arrhythmias in physiological pacemakers. Report of 2 cases. PACE 5:710, 1982.

73. Friart A: Termination of magnet-unresponsive pacemaker endless loop tachycardia by carotid sinus massage. [To the editor]. Am J Med 87:1, 1989.
74. Cunningham TM: Incessant pacemaker Vario operation. Am J Cardiol 61:656, 1988.
75. Staller BJ: Atrial fibrillation induced by testing magnet applied to VVI pacemaker. PACE 7:293, 1984.
76. Furman S: Pacemaker follow-up. In Furman S, Hayes DL, Holmes DR, Jr (eds): A Practice of Cardiac Pacing. Mt Kisco, NY, Futura Publ Co., 1989, pp 511–544.
77. Castellanet MJ, Garza J, Shaner SP, Messenger JC: Telemetry of programmed and measured data in pacing system evaluation and follow-up. J Electrophysiol 1:360, 1987.
78. Mahaux V, Waleffe A, Kulbertus H: Usefulness and adequacy of sensor data storage and retrieval for rate response simulation. PACE 15:1688, 1992.
79. Hayes DL, Christiansen JR, Vlietstra RE, Osborn MJ: Follow-up of an activity-sensing, rate-modulated pacing device, including transtelephonic exercise assessment. Mayo Clin Proc 64:503, 1989.
80. Clarke M, Allen A: Use of telemetered electrograms in the assessment of normal pacemaker function. J Electrophysiol 1:388, 1987.
81. Levine PA: The complementary role of electrogram, event marker, and measured data telemetry in the assessment of pacing system function. J Electrophysiol 1:404, 1987.
82. Van Beek GJ, Den Dulk K, Lindemans FW, et al: Detection of insulation failure by gradual reduction in noninvasively measured electrogram amplitudes. PACE 9:722, 1986.
83. Levine PA: Clinical manifestations of lead insulation defects. J Electrophysiol 1:144, 1987.
84. Dreifus L, Pennock R, Feldman M: Experience with 3835 pacemakers utilizing transtelephonic surveillance. Am J Cardiol 35:133, 1975.
85. Hoffmann A, Jost M, Pfisterer M, et al: Persisting symptoms despite permanent pacing: Incidence, causes, and follow-up. Chest 85:207, 1984.
86. Famularo MA, Kennedy HL: Ambulatory electrocardiography in the assessment of pacemaker function. Am Heart J 104:1086, 1982.
87. Chokshi DS, Mascarenhas E, Samet P, Center S: Treatment of sinoatrial rhythm disturbances with permanent cardiac pacing. Am J Cardiol 32:215, 1973.
88. Conde CA, Leppo J, Lipski J, et al: Effectiveness of pacemaker treatment in the bradytachycardia syndrome. Am J Cardiol 32:209, 1973.
89. Rockseth R, Hatle L: Prospective study on the occurrence and management of chronic sinoatrial disease, with follow-up. Br Heart J 36:582, 1974.
90. Kelen GJ, Bloomfield DA, Hardage M: Holter monitoring of the patient with an artificial pacemaker—a new approach. Ambulat Electrocardiol 1:1, 1978.
91. Kelen GJ, Bloomfield DA, Hardage M, et al: A clinical evaluation of an improved Holter monitoring technique for artificial pacemaker function. PACE 3:192, 1980.
92. Burckhardt D, Lutold BE, Jost MV, Hoffmann A: Holter monitoring in the evaluation of palpitations, dizziness, and syncope. In Roelandt J, Hugenholtz Ph (eds): Long-term Ambulatory Electrocardiography. The Hague, Martinus Nijhoff, 1982, pp 29–39.
93. Kennedy HL, Caralis DG: Ambulatory electrocardiography: A clinical perspective. Ann Intern Med 87:729, 1977.
94. Murry A, Jordan RS, Gold RG: Pacemaker assessment in the ambulatory patient. Br Heart J 46:531, 1981.
95. Bleifer SB, Bleifer DJ, Hausmann DR, et al: Diagnosis of occult arrhythmias by Holter echocardiography. Prog Cardiovasc Dis 16:569, 1974.
96. Gaita F, Asteggiano R, Bocchiardo M, et al: Holter monitoring and provocative maneuvers in the assessment of unipolar demand pacemaker myopotential inhibition. Am Heart J 107:925, 1984.
97. Breivik K, Ohm OJ: Myopotential inhibition of unipolar QRS inhibited (VVI) pacemakers, assessed by ambulatory Holter monitoring of the electrocardiogram. PACE 3:470, 1980.
98. Ohm OJ, Bruland H, Pedersen OM, Waerness E: Interference effect of myopotentials on the function of unipolar demand pacemakers. Br Heart J 36:77, 1974.
99. van Gelder LM, Bracke FALE, El Gamal MIH: Fusion or confusion on Holter recording. PACE 14:760, 1991.
100. Lesh MD, Langberg JJ, Griffin JC, et al: Pacemaker generator pseudomalfunction: An artifact of Holter monitoring. PACE 14:854, 1991.
101. Barold SS, Falkoff MD, Ong LS, et al: Electrocardiographic diagnosis

102. Castellanos A, Jr, Zoble R, Procacci PM, et al: St-qR pattern: New sign of diagnosis of anterior myocardial infarction during right ventricular pacing. Br Heart J 35:1161, 1973.
103. Dodinot B, Kubler L, Aliot E, et al: Electrocardiographic diagnosis of myocardial infarction and coronary insufficiency in the pacemaker patient. In Thaleuand HJ, Harthorne JW (eds): To Pace or Not to Pace: Controversial Subjects on Cardiac Pacing. The Hague: Martinus Nijhoff, 1978, pp 295–301.
104. Klein HO, Beker B, Disegni E, et al: Pacing electrocardiogram: How important is the QRS complex configuration? Clin Prog Electrophysiol Pacing 4:112, 1986.
105. Barold SS, Ong LS, Banner RL: Diagnosis of inferior wall myocardial infarction during right ventricular apical pacing. Chest 69:232, 1976.
106. Furman S: External defibrillation in implanted cardiac pacemakers. PACE 4:485, 1981.
107. Aylwar DSP, Blood R, Tonkan A: Complications of defibrillation with permanent pacemaker in situ. PACE 2:462, 1979.
108. Barold SS, Ong LS, Scovil J, et al: Reprogramming of implanted pacemaker following external defibrillation. PACE 1:514, 1978.
109. Levine PA, Barold SS, Fletcher RD, et al: Adverse acute and chronic effects of electrical defibrillation and cardioversion on implanted unipolar cardiac pacing system. J Am Coll Cardiol 1:1413, 1983.
110. Yee R, Jones DL, Klein GJ: Pacing threshold changes after transvenous catheter shock. Am J Cardiol 53:503, 1984.
111. Singer I, Guarnieri T, Coopersmith J: Implanted automatic defibrillators: Effects of drugs and pacemakers. PACE 11:2250, 1988.
112. Kim SG, Furman S, Waspe LE, et al: Unipolar pacer artifacts induced failure of an automatic implantable cardioverter-defibrillator to detect ventricular fibrillation. Am J Cardiol 57:880, 1986.
113. Cohen AI, Wish MH, Fletcher RD, et al: The use and interaction of permanent pacemakers and the automatic implantable cardioverter-defibrillator. PACE 11:704, 1988.
114. Ruffy R, Lal R, Kouchoukos NT, et al: Combined bipolar dual-chamber pacing and automatic implantable cardioverter-defibrillator. J Am Coll Cardiol 7:933, 1986.
115. McCormack J: Electrosurgical equipment and pacemakers: A potential hazard (Letter). Br Dent J 139:221, 1975.
116. Titel JH, El Etr AA: Fibrillation resulting from pacemaker electrodes and electrocautery during surgery. Anesthesiology 29:845, 1968.
117. Hayes DL, Trusty J, Christiansen J, et al: A prospective study of electrocautery's effect on pacemaker function. (Abstract.) PACE 10:686, 1987.
118. Erdman S, Levinsky L, Servadio C, et al: Management of pacemaker patients while using electrocautery in surgical procedures. (Abstract.) PACE 10:672, 1987.
119. Lamas GA, Antman EM, Gold JP: Pacemaker backup mode reversion and injury during cardiac surgery. Ann Thorac Surg 41:155, 1986.
120. Feldman RM: The use of diathermy in the presence of metal implants and cardiac pacemakers. Can Med Assoc J 122:276, 1980.
121. Adamac R, Haefliger JM, Killisch JP, et al: Damaging effect of therapeutic radiation on programmable pacemakers. PACE 5:146, 1982.
122. Calfee RF: Therapeutic radiation in pacemakers. PACE 5:160, 1982.
123. Lee RW, Huang SK, Mechling E, et al: Runaway atrial sequential pacemaker after radiation therapy. Am J Med 81:833, 1986.
124. Shehata WM, Daoud GL, Meyer RL: Radiotherapy for patients with cardiac pacemakers: Possible risks. PACE 9:919, 1986.
125. Venselaar JLM, Van Kerkoerle HLMJ, Vet AJTM: Radiation damage to pacemakers from radiotherapy. PACE 10:538, 1987.
126. Fetter J, Aram G, Holmes DR, Jr, et al: The effects of nuclear magnetic resonance imagers on external and implantable pulse generators. PACE 7:720, 1984.
127. Holmes DR, Hayes DL, Gray J, et al: The effects of magnetic resonance imaging on implantable pulse generators. PACE 9:360, 1986.
128. Agarwal A, Hewson J, Redding VJ: Pacemaker patients and NMR imaging. PACE 11:853, 1988.
129. Iberer F, Justich E, Stenzl W, et al: Behavior of the Activitrax pacemaker during nuclear magnetic resonance investigation. First International Symposium on Rate-Responsive Pacing, Munich. PACE 10:1215, 1987.
130. Hayes DL, Holmes DR, Jr, Gray JE: Effect of 1.5 Tesla nuclear magnetic resonance imaging scanner on implanted permanent pacemakers. J Am Coll Cardiol 10:782, 1987.
131. Iberer F, Justich E, Tscheliessnigg KH, Wasler A: Nuclear magnetic

resonance imaging in pacemaker patients. *In* Atlee JL, Gombotz H, Tscheliessnigg KH (eds): Perioperative Management of Pacemaker Patients. Berlin, Springer-Verlag, 1992, pp 86–90.

132. Erlebacher JA, Cahill PT, Pannizzo F, Knowles JR: Effect of magnetic resonance imaging on DDD pacemakers. Am J Cardiol 57:437, 1986.

133. Cooper D, Wilkoff B, Masterson M, et al: Effects of extracorporeal shock-wave lithotripsy on cardiac pacemakers and its safety in patients with implanted cardiac pacemakers. PACE 11:1607, 1988.

134. Langberg J, Arber J, Thuroff JW, Griffin JC: The effects of extracorporeal shock-wave lithotripsy on pacemaker function. PACE 10:1142, 1987.

135. Fetter J, Hayes B, Aram G, et al: Electrohydraulic shock-wave lithotripsy effects on cardiac pulse generators. PACE 10:674, 1987.

136. Steinbeck G, Lehman P, Weber W, et al: Cardiac pacing and induction of arrhythmias by extracorporeal shock-wave lithotripsy. PACE 10(Pt II):711, 1987.

137. Irnich W, Lazica M, Gleissner M: Extracorporeal shock-wave lithotripsy in pacemaker patients. *In* Atlee JL, Gombotz H, Tscheliessnigg KH (eds): Perioperative Management of Pacemaker Patients. Berlin, Springer-Verlag, 1992, pp 98–103.

138. Rasmussen MJ, Hayes DL, Vilestra RE, et al: Can transcutaneous electrical nerve stimulation be safely used in patients with permanent cardiac pacemakers? Mayo Clin Proc 63:433, 1988.

139. Bowes RJ, Bennett DH: Effect of transvenous atrioventricular nodal ablation on the function of implanted pacemakers. PACE 8:811, 1985.

140. Chin MC, Rosenqvist M, Lee MA, et al: The effect of radiofrequency catheter ablation on permanent pacemakers: An experimental study. PACE 13:23, 1990.

141. Wingate S: Levels of pacemaker acceptance by patients. Heart Lung 15:93, 1986.

142. Lanuza D, Marotta SF: Endocrine and psychologic responses of patients to cardiac pacemaker implantation. Heart Lung 16:496, 1987.

143. Superko HR: Effects of cardiac rehabilitation in permanently paced patients with third-degree heart block. J Cardiac Rehab 3:561, 1983.

144. Linde-Edelston C, Nordlander R, Pehrsson K, Ryden L: Quality of life in patients with atrioventricular synchronous pacing compared to rate-modulated ventricular pacing: A long-term, double-blind, crossover study. PACE 15:1467, 1992.

145. Catipovic-Veselica K, Skrinjane S, Mrdenovic S, et al: Emotional profiles and quality of life of paced patients. PACE 13:399, 1990.

146. Simon A, Kleinman P, Janz N: Suicide attempt by pacemaker system abuse: A case report with comments on the psychological adaptation of pacemaker patients. PACE 3:224, 1980.

147. Gunther KH: Databases for prevention, pacemaker, and postoperative treatment. The Charité experience in cardiology. *In* Meester GT, Pinciroli F (eds): Databases for Cardiology. Dordrecht, Kluwer Academic Publishers, 1991, pp 167–177.

148. Strathmore N, Mond H, Hunt D, et al: ''Pacecare''—a computerized database for pacemaker follow-up. PACE 13:1787, 1990.

149. Dreifus L, Ohm O, Pennock R, et al: Long-term monitoring of patients with implanted pacemakers. Heart Lung 11:417, 1982.

150. Bilitch M, Hauser R, Goldman B, et al: Performance of cardiac pacemaker pulse generators. PACE 14:479, 1981.

CHAPTER 42

Pacing: FDA and the Regulatory Environment

Mitchell J. Shein
Jeffrey A. Brinker

There are few physicians who have not formulated an opinion, pro or con, about the United States Food and Drug Administration (FDA). Fewer still understand the FDA's responsibilities under law and how these responsibilities affect the practice of medicine. This chapter is intended to (1) familiarize the reader with some of the history and philosophy of the FDA, (2) demystify how the agency operates and what its goals are, and (3) provide insight into how the regulatory process deals with medical devices in general and cardiac pacing products in particular. Issues addressed include the legal basis for regulation of medical devices, the classification of medical devices, obligations that the manufacturer must meet to commercially distribute a device, and how devices are followed after their approval.

All practicing physicians are influenced by the FDA to some degree. The use of medical devices in accordance with their approved labeling affords the practicing physician a limited degree of protection from litigation should untoward events occur. The FDA also monitors the performance of devices after they have been released onto the market and when warranted may mandate the issuance of warnings or recall of the device should it prove unsafe. Perhaps most importantly, the FDA controls the availability of new technology by requiring a reasonable assurance that the device is safe and effective and has clinical utility prior to allowing its commercial distribution.

The FDA's Mission

The FDA is an agency within the Department of Health and Human Services' Public Health Service (Fig. 42–1). The

FDA, specifically the Center for Devices and Radiologic Health, has been entrusted with the task of ensuring that medical devices are safe and effective when used in accordance with their labeling. To accomplish this mission, the FDA interacts with both the device manufacturers and members of the clinical community. These three parties are interdependent and work together toward the goal of promoting the public health. The FDA can be thought of as a quality assurance–quality control inspector. In short, its mission is to ensure that devices commercially distributed in the United States are reasonably demonstrated to be safe and effective when used in accordance with their labeling. The FDA relies on the manufacturers to provide adequate data to support their claims regarding their devices' use and on the clinical community for feedback on how well the devices actually perform.

The FDA was first empowered to regulate devices on a limited basis under the Federal Food, Drug, and Cosmetic (FFD&C) Act of 1938 (21 USC §301–392), which prohibited the interstate movement of devices that were adulterated or misbranded. The FFD&C Act was significantly amended by the Medical Device Amendments of 1976, which specifically provided for the active premarket review and regulation of medical devices; the Safe Medical Devices Act of 1990; and the Medical Device Amendments of 1992. Before changes were made to the FFD&C Act by these acts, medical devices could be marketed without premarket review by the FDA, except devices that were regulated as drugs. As amended, the FFD&C Act defines a medical device to be:

". . . an instrument, apparatus, implement, machine, contrivance, implant, in vitro reagent, or other similar or related article, including any component, part or accessory, which is:

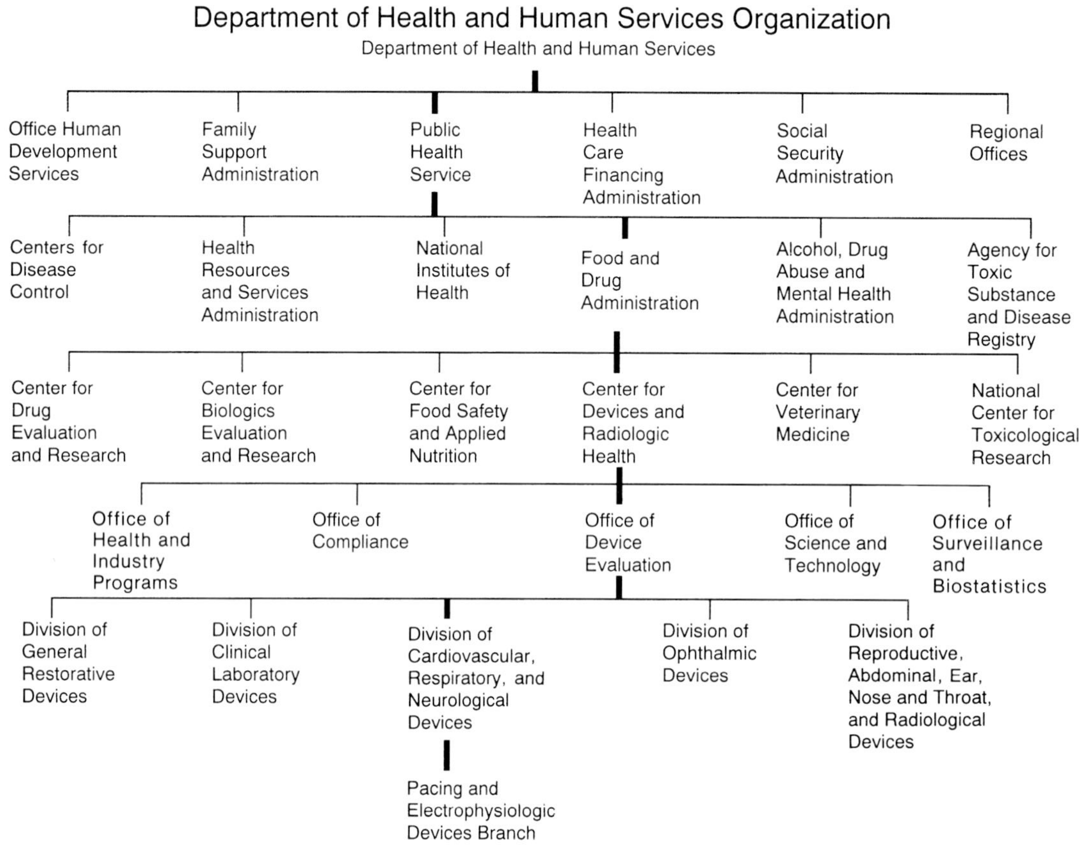

Department of Health and Human Services Organization

FIGURE 42–1. Organizational chart of the Department of Health and Human Services, demonstrating the relationship of the Pacing and Electrophysiologic Devices Branch within the Food and Drug Administration.

TABLE 42–1. **CATEGORIZATION OF MEDICAL DEVICES***

CATEGORY	DESCRIPTION	CLASSIFICATION RULES
Preamendment devices (or old devices)	Devices marketed before May 28, 1976, when the Medical Device Amendments were enacted	Devices are assigned to one of three classes. A presumption exists that preamendment devices should be placed in class I unless their safety and effectiveness cannot be ensured without the greater regulation afforded by classes II and III. A manufacturer may petition the FDA for reclassification.
Postamendment devices (or new devices)	Devices put on the market after May 28, 1976	Unless shown to be substantially equivalent to a device that was on the market before the amendments took effect, these devices are automatically placed in class III. A manufacturer may petition the FDA for reclassification.
Substantially equivalent devices	Postamendment devices that are substantially equivalent to marketed devices	Devices are assigned to the same class as their counterparts and subject to the same requirements. If and when the FDA requires testing and approval of preamendment devices, their substantially equivalent counterparts will also require testing and approval.
Implanted devices	Devices that are inserted into a surgically formed or natural body cavity and intended to remain there for ≥30 days	Devices are assumed to require placement in class III unless a less-regulated class will ensure safety and effectiveness
Investigational devices	Unapproved devices undergoing clinical investigation under the authority of an IDE	Devices are exempt if an IDE has been granted
Transitional devices	Devices that were regulated as drugs before enactment of the statute but are now defined as medical devices	Devices are automatically assigned to class III but may be reclassified in class I or class II.

Abbreviation: IDE, investigational device exemption.

*Implantable devices are classified by law as to what kind of regulatory process will be applied before their commercial release on the basis of whether they were marketed before May 28, 1976 and substantially equivalent to devices marketed before that date or to other devices marketed after that date.

(1) recognized in the National Formulary, or the United States Pharmacopeia, or any supplement to them,

(2) intended for use in the diagnosis of disease or other conditions, or in the cure, mitigation, treatment, or prevention of disease, in man or other animals, or

(3) intended to affect the structure or any function of the body of man or other animals, and which does not achieve its primary intended purposes through chemical action within or on the body of man or animals and which is not dependent upon being metabolized for the achievement of any of its principal purposes."[1]

In accordance with the requirements of the FFD&C Act, medical devices are separated into three distinct classes and six basic overlapping categories (Table 42–1).[2] Specifically, class I includes devices that are regulated only by "general controls." Class II devices are those for which enough information exists to allow the use of "special controls" mandated by the Safe Medical Devices Act of 1990, to protect public health. Such "special controls" include promulgating performance standards, patient registries, guidelines, and other appropriate action. Class III devices are typically unique, new devices or those that potentially pose the greatest hazard to patients and include all implantable and life-sustaining devices. Class III products are required to have FDA approval prior to being commercially distributed, unless the FDA determines that premarket approval is not necessary (e.g., pacemakers determined to be equivalent to marketed devices; see Table 42–1). Implantable cardiac pulse generators and permanent pacing electrodes, that is, "pacemakers" and "leads," as well as implantable defibrillators are class III devices.

How Devices Are Made Commercially Available

The path taken by manufacturers to bring pacemakers and leads into commercial distribution is generally not well understood by those not participating in the effort on a regular basis (Fig. 42–2). The regulatory "process" for devices

Making Devices Commercially Available

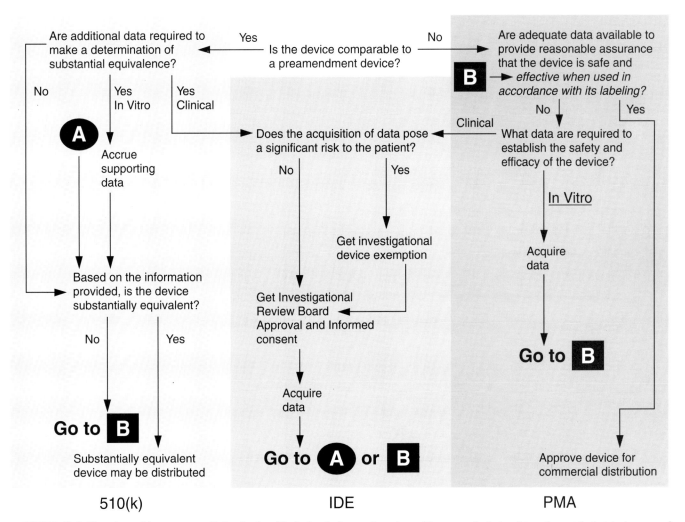

FIGURE 42–2. Flow chart of the process applied to implantable devices before market release. The process is designed to make certain that devices are safe and effective when used in accordance with their labeling. There are three pathways to market release: (1) premarket notification [510(k)], (2) premarket approval (PMA), and (3) investigational device exemptions (IDE).

differs considerably from that for drugs. There are two tracks by which entirely new devices, or new or expanded indications for use for currently marketed devices, may be brought into commercial distribution. The first track is the premarket notification [510(k)][3] route in which devices are evaluated for their equivalence to legally marketed devices in interstate commerce. The second track is the premarket approval (PMA)[4] route in which the manufacturer must provide reasonable assurance that its device is safe and effective when used in accordance with its labeling. A third track is provided by law as an auxiliary to the first two: the investigational device exemption (IDE)[5] route. IDEs provide an exemption to certain requirements of the FFD&C Act, which allows for the limited distribution of a device for the purpose of gathering clinical data on the safety and efficacy of the device to support either a 510(k) or a PMA application.

PREMARKET NOTIFICATION [510(k)]

Section 510(k) of the FFD&C Act requires manufacturers to notify the FDA, at least 90 days in advance, of their intention to market a device. However, it must be made clear that this does not mean a manufacturer is automatically free to market the device on the 91st day. This process is known as premarket notification and represents the easiest way for a manufacturer to get a device to market. Under this process, the FDA is granted the authority to determine if the device to be marketed is ''substantially equivalent'' to a legally marketed classified device that was either in interstate commercial distribution on or before May 28, 1976 or that was itself deemed equivalent to such a device. This process is a grandfather clause for those types of devices in commercial

distribution at the time of the enactment of the Medical Device Amendments Act of 1976. The FDA has considerable discretion in interpreting ''substantial equivalence.'' The general ''litmus test'' for substantial equivalence is, Does the device have a predicate that does not require a PMA application and was labeled and promoted for the same intended use and has the same technologic characteristics, or if it differs in its characteristics can it be demonstrated to be as safe and effective? For those devices deemed by the FDA not to be substantially equivalent, manufacturers must pursue a PMA application to commercially distribute their product (see ensuing section). It should also be noted that all class III devices ultimately are intended either to be brought under the PMA process or reclassified as class I or class II. For devices that are claimed to be substantially equivalent to class III devices, such as pacemakers and leads, the Safe Medical Devices Act sets forth a three-step mandate in which (1) manufacturers must provide, for review, all safety and effectiveness information for a given device; (2) the FDA must evaluate this information and make a determination on whether to reclassify the device; and (3) for those devices not reclassified, the FDA shall require the submission of PMA applications.

Figure 42–3 provides a flow chart for the determination of substantial equivalence. Should a device be found ''not substantially equivalent,'' the only path to commercial distribution is the PMA process.

Of the many devices available to the practitioners of cardiac pacing, only basic single-chamber pulse generators and standard leads can be brought into commercial distribution under section 510(k). Dual-chamber pacemakers, rate-adaptive pacemakers (dual- and single-chamber), steroid eluting

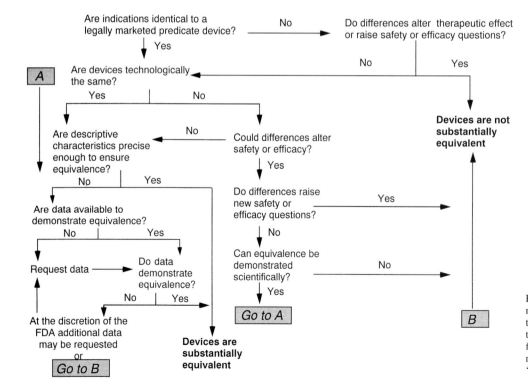

Determining Substantial Equivalence

FIGURE 42–3. The FDA examines new devices to determine whether they are ''substantially equivalent'' to previously marketed devices. This flow chart details the various determinations required in order to prove ''substantial equivalence.''

leads, and leads dedicated to specific pacemakers (single-pass and sensor leads) are evaluated under the PMA process.

PREMARKET APPROVAL

Section 515 of the FFD&C Act provides that a manufacturer must have an approved PMA application before commercially distributing a class III device. An approved PMA can be considered a "license" granted by the FDA allowing the manufacturer to commercially distribute the device described in that PMA. In order to gain this approval, a manufacturer must submit detailed data to provide a reasonable assurance that its device is safe and effective when used in accordance with its labeling. A PMA application includes the following elements:

- A detailed comprehensive summary of the data on which a determination of safety and efficacy is to be based
- All of the preclinical test data including in vitro testing, such as device qualification, software validation, or animal testing
- Clinical data, including data gathered under an approved IDE and foreign studies that are applicable
- Detailed descriptions of the manufacturing process
- All draft labeling for the device

The in vitro data typically provided include the qualification of all discrete device components and the system as a whole. The scope of this chapter prevents a detailed discussion of all testing that would be required for all devices; however, this testing may include any, or all, of the following:

- Electric characterization and qualification of individual discrete circuit elements, as well as the system in which these elements are integrated
- Mechanical qualification
- Software verification and validation
- Biocompatibility
- The effects of environmental influences, for example, electromagnetic interference

For example, for a pacemaker the FDA expects the data to demonstrate that the device is able to perform in accordance with its labeling. Those data would include an evaluation of the effect of electromagnetic interference on the device. We are all exposed in various forms to electromagnetic interference on a daily basis (e.g., security systems, microwave ovens, electric equipment, cellular telephones, and so on). Clinical experience with early pacemakers demonstrated that electromagnetic interference of a specific frequency and amplitude might imitate intrinsic cardiac activity and inappropriately inhibit the device's output.[6–8] Furthermore, some types of extrinsic energy are capable of altering the programming of certain devices.[6, 9] The FDA requires data assuring the mechanical integrity of a pacing lead. For example, the FDA requires that the device be subjected to a simulation of the types of environmental stresses, for example, costoclavicular pinching[10] (simulated by compression and stretching), that it reasonably might be expected to encounter in clinical application.

The results from animal studies or other types of clinical trials involving the device (for example, feasibility or foreign clinical trials, if performed) also must be provided to the agency. These data are generally to support the manufacturer's claim that the device is capable of providing the intended therapy or that the device does not adversely interact with the biologic environment when implanted in a host, for example, that it displays biostability and biocompatibility.

With regard to pacing, examples of preliminary data reported to the FDA include the evaluation of sensor technology in an animal model and in vitro studies of new insulation material for pacing leads. In general, the in vitro and animal studies are performed early in the evolution of a new device and the results are reported to the FDA in the initial review of the IDE for the device. Of course, updates and any additional information that might be deemed pertinent to the PMA review must be provided as they become available.

The first significant decision made during the course of the review of a PMA is whether the application is to be administratively filed. The FDA must conduct a preliminary review within 45 days of submission to determine if all of the required elements are present and adequate to make a decision as to the safety and efficacy of the device.[11] Often the data provided with the initial submission are inadequate to support a favorable determination or additional information or reanalysis is required to allow a detailed review. If the preliminary review is positive, the FDA files the application. In general, if the FDA is unable to perform an in-depth review of the application, it will not file the application. Specifically, a determination not to file under 21 CFR §814.42(e) may be reached if any of the following conditions are met:

1. The application is incomplete because it does not on its face contain all of the information required under §515(c)(1)(A)–(G) of the act.
2. The PMA does not contain each of the items required under 21 CFR §814.20 and justification for the omission of any item is inadequate.
3. The applicant has a pending premarket notification [510(k)] with respect to the same device, and the FDA has not determined whether the device falls within the scope of 21 CFR §814.1(c), which defines the categories of devices requiring PMA review.
4. The PMA contains a false statement of material fact.

Once a PMA has been filed, the FDA undertakes in-depth critical review of the material presented. By statute, the FDA has 180 days to complete its review of a PMA. Any questions, issues, or deficiencies identified during the course of review are presented to the applicant. Deficiencies may require additional bench testing, additional clinical data, or clarification of submitted data. The applicant's responses to questions and additional data are filed as amendments. It should be noted that the 180 days does not include the time spent by the manufacturer responding to requests for additional information. In general, with each request for additional information by the FDA, the 180-day clock stops. On the subsequent submission of the requested information, the clock is restarted. However, if the responses are substantive, for example, provide a major reanalysis of the clinical data, the 180-day period under which PMAs are to be reviewed may be restarted.

The last element to be critically reviewed is the labeling, including promotional material. The labeling for a device must reflect and be supported by the data accumulated and reported as part of the application. The labeling must provide appropriate indications and adequate instructions for use. In general, proper labeling should provide even infrequent users of the device information adequate to allow them to use the device to their patient's greatest benefit. The labeling review, at least for pacemakers, is often an all-day meeting between the FDA and the applicant during which appropriate language is negotiated. This arduous process is particularly important for complex devices such as dual-chamber, rate-adaptive pacemakers and antitachycardia devices.

An important aspect of labeling concerns indications for use. This obviously has an impact on the way a device is marketed because the manufacturer is prevented from making claims for use that are not supported by acceptable scientific data. In some instances, the nature of the evidence obtained during the clinical investigation is inadequate to justify particular indications. For example, with certain DDDR pacemakers, data justifying the DDDR mode as being beneficial for chronotropically incompetent patients was deemed inadequate by the FDA.

When new technology comes under review, the FDA welcomes input from professional organizations (such as the North American Society for Pacing and Electrophysiology) to establish guidelines that would define criteria justifying a clinical indication. In the absence of accepted clinical criteria for efficacy, the FDA may rely on a panel of consultants for opinions pertaining to specific devices and to a general class of devices just as it might for drugs.[12]

The rules governing the use by physicians of an approved device for an unapproved indication are clouded. In the past, as long as a physician or a manufacturer did not promote an unapproved use, there were no repercussions. If the unapproved use represents a research endeavor, the physician or manufacturer should notify the FDA and obtain IDE approval for a formal investigation.

The FDA has taken a proactive view on implied claims. For example, if a sensor-driven pacemaker provides a means of using two different sensors either alone or in combination, there is an implication that the combination of sensors would supply a benefit greater than that achieved by either of the individual sensors acting alone. Therefore, this benefit must be demonstrated in clinical trials. Another example is a vascular stent that is coated with an anticoagulant. The implication is that this stent would offer advantages over a non-coated stent, and these advantages must be demonstrated even if such a claim is not explicitly made by the manufacturer.

After the substantive issues have been resolved, the FDA will generally convene a meeting of an advisory panel, specifically the Circulatory System Devices Panel, although the FDA is no longer required to do so under the FFD&C Act as amended by the Safe Medical Devices Act. This panel consists of physicians, engineers, an industry representative, and a patient advocate, the latter to ensure that the interests of the manufacturers and patients are protected. Although the entire application is open to panel review, the prominent focus is usually on the clinical ramifications of the device. The panel typically is provided the Summary of Safety and Effectiveness Data, the complete clinical study report, and all draft labeling. It is the panel's charge to identify any potential issues that might affect the safety or effectiveness

of the device. Cost-benefit issues, although of obvious importance in many cases (e.g., laser angioplasty), are not intended to be within the scope of the panel's deliberation.

The actual panel review is performed during a public meeting that is announced in the *Federal Register*. At this meeting, the manufacturer may be afforded an opportunity to present a summary of its data and to have consultants (physicians, engineers, and so forth) available to offer information or engage in discussion. The FDA staff representative also presents a summary of his or her findings and specific questions that the agency might want the panel to consider. One panel member usually serves as a primary reviewer and the other members augment that review with questions and comments. The panel discussion is aimed at clarifying information and offering a clinical perspective on the device. After the panel's deliberations, a vote is taken to recommend approval or disapproval of the application for commercial distribution. If approval is recommended, it may be with or without conditions, which might include labeling requirements, postapproval study, or restriction on the use of the device to a specific patient population. If the panel votes to disapprove the application, specific reasons must be given as well as recommendations as to what might be done to gain approval in the future. Panel recommendations are not binding on the FDA, but typically they are respected and accepted. It is important to remember that a favorable panel recommendation is not equivalent to FDA approval. Once the panel's review is complete, other issues may still need resolution prior to the device's release for commercial distribution, including an inspection of the manufacturing facilities to ensure that good manufacturing practice standards are met.

Occasionally, additional information may come to light after the panel has made its recommendation. If the information has a bearing on a concern voiced by the panel or if it raises a significant clinical issue, the panel may be reconsulted concerning the submission. Recognition of dysfunction due to defects in the design or construction may be time-dependent and not obvious prior to panel approval. If the cause can be recognized and easily fixed it may not require representation to the panel.

Once all issues are adequately addressed, an approval package, including an approval order, a notice for publication in the *Federal Register*, and a Summary of Safety and Effectiveness Data, is prepared and issued by the Director of the Center for Devices and Radiologic Health.

In the life of a device's design, particularly a pacemaker's, advances in technology or clinical science, or both, may warrant the modification of an approved device. If a change has a potential effect (either positive or negative) on the safety or efficacy of the device, or both, approval to market the modified device must be granted by the FDA prior to distribution.[13] The appropriate procedure in such cases would be to supplement the original PMA. The content of a PMA supplement obviously depends on the nature of the changes being proposed. In general, it is incumbent on the manufacturer to demonstrate that the device as modified remains safe and effective for use in accordance with its labeling.

For example, the introduction of a new header configuration to afford compatibility with leads having a different pin size would require a demonstration that such a bore size could be accurately reproduced. The amount of testing required becomes slightly more complicated if the manufacturer claims that the new connector size conforms to a voluntary standard, for example, IS-1. Were this the case, the manufacturer would be required to complete all testing prescribed by the referenced standard to demonstrate conformance. If the change were more elaborate, for example, the implementation of a new hybrid circuit design, the manufacturer would be required to provide complete qualification testing of the new components individually, as well as of the pacemaker as modified to demonstrate that the device is still capable of reliably providing safe and effective therapy as outlined in the device's labeling. More complex yet would be the introduction of a new indication for use. In this case, clinical data to support the new indication might be necessary, perhaps requiring an IDE.

Labeling changes also require FDA approval because the labeling represents those indications for which the device has been approved and appropriate directions for use. A labeling change may require test data to support it. For example, if a manufacturer wished to modify the labeled longevity projections for a device, the FDA would require battery drain data to support the new projection. If the ''use before'' date was to be extended, both shelf-life battery drain and sterility data would be required to demonstrate that if a device was implanted at the expiration date, it would be sterile and its longevity would be as described in the labeling.

Investigational Device Exemptions

Section 520(g) of the FFD&C Act provides the FDA with the authority to exempt some devices from some requirements of the act in order to allow their shipment and use in human subjects. IDEs[14] may be granted when it is necessary to gather clinical data on the performance of the device in an effort to establish the safety and efficacy of the device. Clinical data are generally required when bench or animal testing, or both, are insufficient for this purpose. In addition to approval from the FDA, Institutional Review Board (IRB) supervision and appropriate informed consent are required for all studies in which the device presents potential ''significant risk'' to the patient, as is the case with pacemakers and leads. For devices that do not pose a ''significant risk,'' an IDE may not be required. IRB approval and informed patient consent, however, are still necessary to proceed with the study.

There are generally two types of studies performed under IDEs for pacemakers and leads: feasibility studies and studies intended to gather data to support the introduction of devices into commercial distribution. Feasibility studies typically are used when bench testing or animal models, or both, are inadequate to confirm the device's design and operating characteristics.[15] IDEs for feasibility studies must fulfill all of the requirements for investigational studies; however, some latitude is granted in completely qualifying the device prior to human use. In these studies, emphasis is placed on minimizing the risk associated with exposing patients to the device. To this end, the sponsor of such a study, typically the device manufacturer, must establish the lack of unreasonable risk and the expected performance of the device prior to clinical use. A thorough risk-benefit analysis describing the risks, how they will be minimized, and justification that they are reasonable must be provided. Feasibility studies typically include only a single center and approximately 10 devices. A feasibility study might be appropriate, for example, when fine tuning or establishing the feasibility of using a specific sensor, or algorithm for that sensor, in a rate-adaptive pacing system.

In order to obtain an IDE and begin clinical trials with a device, a sponsor-manufacturer must provide the FDA with (1) data demonstrating that patient exposure to the device is not unreasonable and (2) a well-defined protocol, with specific end points, for the evaluation of the device. The data provided in support of an application for an IDE would include the engineering bench data and, when warranted, animal studies or patient studies, or both.

The in vitro and animal testing results to be provided are intended to demonstrate to the FDA, with some level of assurance, that the device is capable of providing the therapy for which it is intended and does not present an unreasonable safety issue. Typically, the information to be submitted is the same as that already described for PMA applications.

In addition to the in vitro and animal studies noted earlier, actual human data, when available, may be submitted in support of a request for an IDE. These data may come from any of the following sources: feasibility study results, foreign clinical trials, dedicated clinical research systems, or other IDEs on the same device. Data from feasibility studies are generally provided to remove concern as to the feasibility and safety of the ''marquee'' features to be studied most intensively during the course of the clinical evaluation of the device. Similarly, data taken from controlled foreign clinical studies are submitted to tilt the balance of the risk-benefit analysis. Finally, many current pacemaker manufacturers have the ability to evaluate features of future devices. This can be accomplished either through ''slaving'' an implanted pacemaker to an external programmer that has the new feature incorporated into its software or by using an external pulse generator with the feature of interest effected through either temporary wires or acute or chronically placed permanent leads during implantation procedures.

It should be noted that devices used strictly as research tools used to acquire basic scientific data generally do not require an IDE use. However, appropriate measures for informed patient consent must be taken, particularly if the patient is being placed at risk, for example, the evaluation of a sensor that might be used in a rate-adaptive pacing system.

In addition to demonstrating that the device has been adequately qualified, sponsors and/or manufacturers must provide a well-structured protocol to govern the clinical evaluation of the device being studied. It is incumbent on the sponsor to design a protocol to answer any questions pertaining to the device's safe and efficacious use. It is quite frequently misunderstood that FDA acceptance of a protocol is not an endorsement of the protocol, nor does it preclude the agency from requiring additional data not acquired by the original protocol should it be found scientifically appropriate and necessary. A considerable amount of thought should go into the design of a human study protocol. The manufacturer would be wise to seek advice from prospective investigators about what is practical to achieve in the patient population to be studied. It is counterproductive to design a protocol that is more demanding than the investigators could comply with. If too many follow-up tests are requested, the potential for noncompliance is increased and ultimately may adversely affect the validity of the data obtained. It is the task of the sponsor to select investigators who are credible and whose work will withstand scrutiny.

The FDA routinely audits investigations. A review of drug study audits shows that deficiencies were found in a high percentage of investigations (54% consent problems, 25% inadequate drug accountability, 26% nonadherence to protocol, 21% inadequate or inaccurate study records, and so on). In 10% of these audits, the deficiencies were of serious magnitude, leading to regulatory action in 100 cases and criminal prosecution in 16! Twenty-three of 49 foreign studies were seriously flawed.[16]

A protocol must provide for the accumulation of audited information that justifies proposed labeling. It has become apparent that metabolic exercise testing provides more valuable information than is obtainable on standard treadmill tests for the evaluation of dual-chamber sensor driven pacemakers. Thus, if the manufacturer seeks approval of such a device with specific labeling for the DDDR mode, metabolic exercise tests should be performed on appropriate patients. Of course, if other testing proves to provide equivalent or better data, such alternative testing would be accepted.

One of the primary goals of any clinical study should be the identification of those patients in whom the device, or specific features available in the device, should be used. This is particularly true in instances in which the standard indications for use deviate from those set forth by professional organizations, for example, the joint American Heart Association–American College of Cardiologists task forces.[17] For instance, the patient population expected to benefit most from the VDD mode consists of those patients with adequate sinus response because they are able to take advantage of the mode's atrial tracking capability. The patient population expected to benefit most from rate adaption typically are those patients with inadequate sinus response, that is, chronotropic incompetence. In what patient population then would a device having the VDDR mode as its feature mode, and no dual-chamber rate-adaptive modes, be expected to be used? Although the answer is not apparent, it is incumbent on the sponsor-manufacturer to design its study to elucidate the answer.

Another essential element to any protocol is the verification that the device will indeed perform as described in its labeling (e.g., the rate response sensor-algorithm provides appropriate graded response to exercise and fails to respond when changes in rate are inappropriate). Traditionally, randomized, controlled trials have not been required for the approval of devices (in contradistinction to new drugs). Devices needed only to demonstrate safety and efficacy equivalent to devices already on the market. More recently, the Circulatory System Devices Panel has pushed for controlled clinical trials in the evaluation of new technology. Randomized trials are not necessary for all devices. If a claim is being made or implied that a device provides an additional benefit compared with preexisting devices, however, it should be substantiated by an appropriate controlled study. It is the responsibility of the study sponsor to appropriately design the study. The FDA merely reviews the protocols and offers recommendations on whether the protocols as designed are likely to develop the data necessary to support applications for commercial distribution.

An issue that has been raised in recent years, and should be addressed in a protocol, is the need to establish the "clinical utility"[18] of the device being studied. Thus, a claim of benefit should be accompanied by evidence that small but statistically significant differences in the parameters examined are advantageous to the patient. For example, is the ability to exercise on a treadmill for 30 seconds longer when programmed to the DDDR compared with the DDD mode a reflection of true benefit? Sponsors and manufacturers clearly have it within their means to adequately study these devices to determine the extent of clinical benefit provided by their devices. In the absence of a clear demonstration of clinical benefit, how can devices appropriately be prescribed? If individual functional modes in devices have not had their clinical benefit demonstrated, should these modes be eliminated from the commercially available product? If not, could the implied benefit of their inclusion in the device be misconstrued? And finally, is it misbranding[19] to sell devices with such modes in the absence of any demonstrated clinical benefit that would define how such modes could safely and appropriately be used? A device is considered "misbranded" if (1) its labeling is false or misleading, (2) its labeling does not bear adequate directions for use and adequate warnings against unsafe use, or (3) it is a restricted device and its advertisements are false or misleading or do not meet the minimum disclosure of product information. Additionally, it is not appropriate to distribute a device and then have the medical community at large establish the appropriate indications for use, for example, electrocardiographic late potential analysis.

An important part of any clinical protocol is the patient informed consent materials. Table 42–2 lists all elements required under 21 CFR §50 for inclusion in patient informed consent forms. Although the consent forms provided to individual investigators in their study materials are not required to be used at their institutions, any deviations determined to be significant, or substantive, by the sponsor must be submitted to the FDA for review. With just cause, it is within the scope of the FDA's authority to preclude the participation of individual centers in studies. Inadequate patient informed consent meets the criteria for such action.

Although the specifics of the protocols for clinical evaluation are at the discretion of the sponsor, the FDA controls the number and pace with which devices are implanted, particularly devices having new technologies. Pacemaker studies typically are designed in four phases. Phase I is an intensive study period during which the basic safety and preliminary efficacy of the device are closely scrutinized. Phase II is also an intensive study period during which the sponsors continue to accrue data, typically focusing on the safety of the device. Phase III may be less intensive and generally runs from the time a PMA has been administratively filed until a favorable recommendation is rendered by the Circulatory System Devices Panel. The intensity of phase III is determined by the nature of the device and the need for either more data or resolution of outstanding issues. Phase IV begins after the panel renders its recommendation and continues until the device is commercially released.

Another area of acute interest to all parties participating in IDE studies is the limit placed on the number of devices available for inclusion in the study. A delicate balance must be struck by the FDA to ensure that studies are not unwar-

TABLE 42–2. INFORMED PATIENT CONSENT REQUIRED ELEMENTS (21 CFR §50)*

REQUIRED ELEMENTS

A statement that the study involves research
An explanation of the purposes of the research
The expected duration of the subject's participation
A description of the procedures to be followed
Identification of any procedures which are experimental
A description of any reasonably forseeable risks or discomforts to the subject
A description of any benefits to the subject or to others
A disclosure of appropriate alternative procedures or courses of treatment that might be advantageous to the subject
A statement describing the extent to which confidentiality of the subject's records will be maintained and that notes FDA may inspect the records
An explanation as to whether any compensation and/or medical treatments are available if injury occurs and, if so, what they consist of or sources of further information
An explanation of whom to contact for answers to questions about the study and the subject's rights and whom to contact in the event of a research-related injury
A statement that participation is voluntary and that subjects may refuse to participate or discontinue participation at any time without penalty or loss of benefits

ADDITIONAL ELEMENTS REQUIRED WHEN APPROPRIATE

A statement that the procedure or treatment may involve unforseeable risks to subject, or to the embryo or fetus should the subject become pregnant
Anticipated circumstances under which the investigator may terminate the subject's participation without regard to the subject's consent
Any additional costs to subject as result of participation consequences of a subject's decision to withdraw and procedures for withdrawal
A statement that significant new findings which may relate to the subject's willingness to participate will be provided to the subject
The approximate number of subjects involved in the study

*Informed consent documents have required elements during supervised clinical studies. This includes, but is not restricted to, the evaluation of implantable pacemakers.

rantedly delayed or prolonged and at the same time limiting patient exposure to devices whose reliability and performance have yet to be adequately established. The current recommended limits for the study of bradycardia devices are listed in Table 42–3.

The preceding limits are merely guidelines and if situations warrant it the FDA may extend or further restrict these limits. It should also be noted that manufacturers are by statute allowed to charge a reasonable sum for devices under an IDE. Sponsors are prohibited from commercializing IDE devices. The regulations provide only for charges to recoup the costs of research and development.

Although the types of data to be collected are at the discretion of the sponsor, the data gathered must reflect the chronic performance of the device. For example, evaluation of pacing thresholds at 1 month (although an important data point) would be inadequate in itself for the assessment of true performance of steroid eluting leads. Similarly, the performance of an oxygen saturation detection lead would have to be evaluated over an extended period to demonstrate that it remains functional despite the potential for fibrin overgrowth.

Although the specifics of each protocol differ, the criteria for expansion of each study generally are similar. Sponsors

must obtain approval to increase the limits placed on a study by the protocol or the FDA, or both. For example, before a bradycardia pacemaker will be granted expansion to phase II, the sponsor must hold a meeting of the primary investigators and gain their recommendation to proceed and present data on a minimum of 30 devices implanted for 30 days each to the FDA along with adequate justification to expand the study. Some of the points considered by the FDA are the safety and efficacy of the device to that point, how recent the data are (reports should have a cutoff date no greater than 4 to 6 weeks prior to their submission), and the adherence to the follow-up schedule (90% adherence or better is expected). Safety is reported in terms of the clinical complications or observations experienced during the course of the study, or both. Clinical complications typically are defined as events requiring intervention beyond simple reprogramming of the device. Observations are defined as events correctable with reprogramming of the device. All such events must be reported, including those typical for the type of device (e.g., oversensing).

Postapproval Requirements and Other Issues

The Safe Medical Devices Act of 1990 (Public Law 101–629) and the Medical Device Amendments of 1992 are intended to correct problems associated with the implementation and enforcement of the Medical Device Amendments of 1976 (Public Law 94–295). Perhaps the most important aspect of the Safe Medical Devices Act for practitioners is the requirement that device user facilities (defined as hospitals, ambulatory surgical facilities, nursing homes, and outpatient treatment facilities that are not physicians' offices) report to the FDA or the manufacturer any death, serious illness, or serious injury to a patient caused or contributed to by a medical device. Facilities should report these incidents within 10 working days of the event. Patient deaths must be reported to the FDA and to the manufacturer, whereas serious illness and injury must be reported only to the manufacturer (or if the manufacturer is not known, to the FDA). The facility also is required to submit to the FDA a semiannual (January and July) summary of the reports it has submitted to the FDA and to the manufacturers.

Under the Medical Device Reporting (MDR) Regulations of 1984 (21 CFR §803), manufacturers and importers of medical devices are required to notify the FDA of any infor-

TABLE 42–3. RECOMMENDED LIMITS FOR BRADYCARDIA DEVICE STUDIES*

	INVESTIGATIONAL CENTERS (NO.)	DEVICES (NO.)
Phase I	15	50
Phase II	50	250
Phase III	100	500
Phase IV	100	1000

*In order to manage the potential risk of exposing patients to new bradycardia devices during IDE clinical trials, limits on the number of investigational centers and implanted devices are placed on the four phases of the trial.

mation reasonably suggesting that a marketed device may have caused or contributed to a death or serious injury, or has malfunctioned such that if the malfunction should recur it would be likely to cause or contribute to death or serious injury. Studies by the Government Accounting Office[20] showed that less than 1% of device problems occurring in hospitals are reported to the FDA and that serious underreporting continued in a second study in 1989 despite implementation of the 1984 MDR regulations. The Safe Medical Devices Act now requires that distributors *and* manufacturers report adverse effects and deficiencies of devices and that manufacturers, importers, and distributors annually certify to the FDA the number of MDR reports they submitted during that year or that no reports were submitted. The additional reporting requirements of the Safe Medical Devices Act should result in earlier detection of problems and the removal of the defective product from the market. Additionally, beginning in August 1993 manufacturers will be required to track certain devices (implants, life-sustaining or life-supporting products) used outside of a facility.

In addition to the preceding required reporting systems, the FDA also has a voluntary reporting system for medical devices, the Product Problem Reporting Program. This system allows device users (clinicians, patients, consumers, and so on) to report hazardous medical device situations through a toll-free hotline number 24 hours a day at 1(800)638–6725.

Product Recalls

The FDA has been criticized for allowing devices on the market that were later found problematic, for example, silicone breast implants. Should problems arise after a device has been placed in commercial distribution, it may be recalled. Recalls generally are initiated by the manufacturer of the device; however, the FDA can initiate a recall. Under the provisions of 21 CFR §518(e), the FDA may order a device recall and under certain conditions may order manufacturers, importers, distributors, or retailers to cease distribution of a product. If there is reason to believe that a device may cause serious risk, the agency may also notify health care professionals and device user facilities to cease using the product or, when appropriate, may require direct patient notification.

Recalls, although usually initiated by the manufacturer, are categorized by the FDA into three classes.[21] Class I recalls comprise situations in which there is a reasonable probability that the use of, or exposure to, a violative product will cause serious adverse health consequences or death. Class II recalls comprise situations in which the use of, or exposure to, a violative product may cause temporary or medically reversible adverse health consequences or in which the probability of serious adverse health consequences is remote. Class III recalls comprise situations in which the use of, or exposure to, a violative product is not likely to cause adverse health consequences. In addition to the three classes of recalls, safety advisories or safety alerts are sometimes designated. These two designations are linguistically equivalent and are less significant than class III recalls. It should be noted that devices used under an IDE typically are not recalled. Although not published as recalls or safety alerts, mechanisms do exist and are routinely used within the IDE regulations to take actions similar to those taken in recall situations. It

should be noted, however, that exportation may constitute commercial distribution and on this basis a recall may be classified.

Facilitation of the Approval of New Devices

The FDA has been taken to task for ''delaying'' new technology from reaching the market. For the fiscal year 1992, the average time elapsed from the filing of the PMA to final approval was 310 days.[22] Table 42–4 lists the significant dates during the approval process for Telectronics' Meta DDDR pacing system (Telectronics, Inc., Englewood, CO) and Intermedics' Relay pacing system (Intermedics, Inc., Angleton, TX). Given the complexity of these systems, 428 and 305 days were required, respectively, to complete the regulatory process. The FDA, manufacturers, and the clinical community should provide a stimulus for new technology to be developed and studied in the United States. The use of expertise of other governmental agencies or consultative panels such as the National Institutes of Health may be helpful in establishing protocol guidelines for specific technology so that the review of PMA and IDE applications may be streamlined.

The most significant way to minimize the administrative time required to make devices commercially available is to eliminate the weaknesses found in applications filed with the FDA. Those most controllable are in protocol design and clinical data quality. The latter can be strengthened by assuring that the requirements set forth in the protocol are closely followed, particularly with respect to patient follow-up visits. The FDA expects that data submitted in support of any application be both current and complete. Although it would be ideal to have 100% follow-up and a report cutoff date of only a few days prior to submission, the FDA understands that this is not realistically possible. Patients lost to follow-up, protocol deviations, and the time necessary to prepare data analyses preclude such lofty goals. However, the FDA as a general rule does not believe it is unreasonable to expect a minimum of 90% follow-up and data cutoff dates no greater than 4 to 6 weeks prior to submission.

Another area in which data quality could be strengthened is the statistical methodology used in the preparation of ap-

TABLE 42–4. SIGNIFICANT DATES IN THE APPROVAL PROCESS*

	META DDDR	RELAY
Date of IDE filing	6/22/89	5/22/90
Date of original PMA submission	11/29/90	4/11/91
Date of PMA administration filing	11/29/90	8/15/91
Date of Circulatory System Devices Panel review	6/03/91	11/26/91
Date of approval	1/30/92	6/15/92

Abbreviations: IDE, investigational device exemption; PMA, premarket approval.
*The approval has several milestones. The preceding examples of two DDDR devices (Meta DDDR [Telectronics, Inc., Englewood, CO] and Relay [Intermedics, Inc., Angleton, TX]) demonstrate the time course of the evaluation procecss.

plications. Although it is generally not for the FDA to specify the type of statistical methodology that would be appropriate for the analysis of a specific set of data, it is imperative that those providing analyses justify their methodology and provide adequate documentation to allow the FDA to assess the validity of the conclusions reached. This includes providing the FDA with the information necessary to retrace the process and confirm the results derived from it.

A recurrent weakness in PMA applications is protocol design. The best time to address protocol issues is early in the design of the study before an IDE is submitted. Failure to clearly identify the end points of the study being designed is common. It is not appropriate for a manufacturer to undertake a study of the device, acquire data, and then "determine" what can be derived from those data. Such "end point shopping" is poor science and should not be expected to be tolerated by the FDA; moreover, it should be prevented by the clinicians serving as investigators in such studies.

Of major concern in designing a protocol is the need to select an appropriate control group. The tradition of simply using historical controls is currently undergoing scrutiny. Manufacturers and their consultants should be able to justify the selection of a specific comparator or to provide justification as to why a randomized control study is unwarranted or inappropriate. Statistical justification when using historical controls is problematic. For example, in the study of dual-chamber, rate-adaptive pacemakers produced by a manufacturer who does not currently market a similar device, would evaluation of the clinical benefit of the rate-adaption capability (DDDR mode) require comparison against a commercially available similar device or is it more appropriate to compare the device against itself, for example, DDDR versus DDD/DDI or VVIR? A more straightforward situation would be one in which a manufacturer currently marketing a DDDR system wishes to introduce a second *alternate* sensor. In this case, comparison of the commercially available sensor versus the new sensor would be acceptable; however the protocol design must account for the need to establish the situations in which either of the available sensors might be more appropriate.

Needless to say, the complexity of these issues does not lend itself to simple solutions. Although the responsibility for providing the information previously noted ultimately falls on the manufacturers submitting these applications, both the FDA and the clinicians consulting and participating in the preparation of these applications must share the burden. It is incumbent on the FDA to provide guidance regarding what is expected and to actively interact with the manufacturers and the investigators as potential problems are identified. Clinical investigators must strive to provide an unbiased assessment of the device, its study protocol, and its actual clinical performance.

Physician Investigators and Their Responsibilities

The objective of the regulatory process for class III devices is to limit the initial patient exposure to the device until adequate knowledge of its risk-benefit ratio has been obtained. It is important that investigators performing the initial

evaluations comply with the protocol so that the data collected can be analyzed and interpreted. There have been a number of new devices that reached the panel and were found unacceptable in terms of safety and efficacy. In some situations this was because the device truly was not on par with other available devices. In other cases, however, the sponsor and his or her investigators did a poor job in accumulating and interpreting data.

There is little to gain by the manufacturers, the clinical community at large, or the patients themselves rushing to get a device through the review process. It is incumbent on participating investigators to provide an unbiased assessment of the performance of the device. Early identification of any problem allows for manufacturers to make revisions to their device during phase I of the investigation, which ultimately saves time and money. Additionally, protocols can be revised so that data that ultimately may be useless are not collected. Most importantly, it may prevent the unnecessary exposure of additional patients to a device that ultimately might not be proved to be safe and efficacious.

A particular area in which clinicians must be extremely cautious is in the use of devices for indications other than those for which they have been approved. Although it is not the intention, nor the mission, of the FDA to regulate medical practice or to stifle innovation or the progress of medical science, federal law requires that devices be safe and effective when used as indicated in accordance with their labeling. Certainly there is benefit in expanding the generally accepted indications for cardiac pacemakers;[23] however, the development of new indications should be a coordinated process. Such a process should include clinicians interested in investigating the appropriateness of the proposed indications, the manufacturers who ultimately may wish to label their products for the proposed indication, and the FDA, which assures that data being accrued are consistent with those necessary to ultimately approve the proposed indication.

An example of the potential chaos that can be created by not following this process is currently being played out in the electrophysiologic community. Specifically, radiofrequency ablation procedures are routinely performed at many clinical centers throughout the United States. In fact, the North American Society for Pacing and Electrophysiology has endorsed the use of this procedure as the therapy of choice for the control of cardiac arrhythmia in drug-intolerant or -resistant patients or in those patients who desire avoidance of life-long drug therapy.[24] Even so, as of the writing of this chapter, no device has been approved for this indication. One system has been reviewed by the Circulatory System Devices Panel.

Finally, there is a tendency among the lay and medical populations alike to regard "new" as synonymous with "better." A manifestation of this is the considerable competition for IDE investigator "slots" for certain new devices because having access to new technology is advantageous to the physician. Some doctors and hospitals subtly "market" new devices either through local news releases or through communications with referring physicians. The nonrandomized nature of many studies provides a mechanism for an investigator to assure a patient or referring physician that the "new" device will be used. There is often the feeling that the investigational device is intuitively better and that the evaluation process is simply to satisfy the FDA. The investigator may acquire a vested interest in seeing the new device succeed. This bias may subtly creep into the selection process of patients or the interpretation of data. The mandate for randomized, controlled trials, closer supervision of investigational device "marketing," and more strict FDA audits at the investigational sites may be beneficial.

Reimbursement

As noted previously, manufacturers may charge patients for devices undergoing clinical investigation. Third-party payers often will pay for such a device if the indication is established. For instance, a patient with heart block requiring a pacemaker probably will have an investigational dual-chamber pacemaker reimbursed by his or her insurer. Conversely, third-party payers generally did not reimburse for initial internal defibrillators because this type of therapy was considered investigational. Further, if a patient requires additional therapy or hospitalization because of participating in an investigational device study, he or she or the insurer, or both, are often liable for additional medical charges. In some cases, the insurer may decline to pay these additional fees resulting from the patient's participation in an investigation of a new device. Thus, the patient may be at risk for expenses solely because he or she participated in a research study. At the least, the patient and the insurer are subsidizing the manufacturer's product. It would seem beneficial if an arrangement were made such that the Health Care Finance Administration or third-party insurers, or both, would cover the costs of medical care surrounding the investigation of a new device. An equal exchange might be that (1) the cost of the investigational device be reduced, (2) the number of devices evaluated would be the minimum allowed for FDA purposes, and (3) a cost-benefit analysis of the device would be performed as part of the investigation and used to determine whether the device will be reimbursed in the future.

Conclusions

The regulatory process has been constructed to protect the public. The FDA endeavors to ensure the safety and efficacy of new devices with as little impediment to patient care and industry as possible. The agency has frequently looked to the medical community for counsel prior to establishing policy; therefore, it is incumbent on the profession to take a proactive role in ensuring that therapy, whether a drug or a device, be proved safe and effective before being widely administered. It is both unreasonable, and unacceptable, to allow the market place alone to determine the safety or efficacy of new technology and its use. If the medical community itself is unwilling to work toward the establishment of standards for approval, the FDA is left with little alternative but to impose them.

REFERENCES

1. Food, Drug, and Cosmetic Act of 1938, 21 USC §321(h).
2. Kessler DA, Pape SM, Sundwall DN: The federal regulation of medical devices. N Engl J Med 317(6):357, 1987.
3. Food, Drug, and Cosmetic Act of 1938, 21 USC §360(k), §510(k).
4. Medical Device Amendments of the Food, Drug, and Cosmetic Act, 21 USC §360e, §515(b) (1976).
5. Medical Device Amendments of the Food, Drug, and Cosmetic Act, 21 USC §360j(g), §520(g) (1976).
6. Sager DP: Current facts on pacemaker electromagnetic interference and their application to clinical care. Heart Lung 16:211, 1987.
7. Irnich W, de Bakker JMT, Bisping H-J: Electromagnetic interference in implantable pacemakers. PACE 1:52, 1978.
8. Chin MC, Rosenquist M, Lee MA, et al: The effect of radiofrequency catheter ablation on permanent pacemakers, an experimental study. PACE 13:23, 1990.
9. Barold SS, Ong LS, Scovil J, et al: Reprogramming of implanted pacemaker following external defibrillation. PACE 1:514, 1978.
10. Suzuki Y, Fujimori S, Sakai M, et al: A case of pacemaker lead fracture associated with thoracic outlet syndrome. PACE 11:326, 1988.
11. Medical Device Amendments of the Food, Drug, and Cosmetic Act, 21 CFR §814.42(a) (1992).
12. Paulus HE: FDA Arthritis Advisory Committee meeting: Guidelines for approving nonsteroidal antiinflammatory drugs for over-the-counter use. Arthritis Rheum 33:1056, 1990.
13. Medical Device Amendments of the Food, Drug, and Cosmetic Act, 21 CFR §814.39 (1992).
14. Medical Device Amendments of the Food, Drug, and Cosmetics Act, 21 CFR §812 (1992).
15. FDA Blue Book Memorandum D89-1, May 17, 1989.
16. Lisook AB: FDA audit of clinical studies: Policy and procedure. J Clin Pharmacol 30:296, 1990.
17. Dreifus LS: Guidelines for implantation of cardiac pacemakers and antiarrhythmia devices. J Am Coll Cardiol 18(1):1, 1991.
18. Medical Device Amendments of the Food, Drug, and Cosmetic Act, 21 CFR §860.7(e)(1) (1992).
19. Food Drug and Cosmetic Act of 1938, 21 USC §352, §502.
20. Government Accounting Office: Fed Reg 56(228):60025, 1991.
21. Medical Device Amendments of the Food, Drug, and Cosmetic Act, 21 CFR §7.3(m) (1992).
22. ODE Annual Report Fiscal Year 1992—Statistical Tables. FDA Division of Small Manufacturers Assistance, released January 1, 1993.
23. Dreifus LS, Fisch C, Griffin JC, et al: ACC/AHA Task Force Report: Guidelines for Implantation of Cardiac Pacemakers and Antiarrhythmia Devices. J Am Coll Cardiol 18(1):1, 1991.
24. Scheinman MM: NASPE Policy Statement: Catheter ablation for cardiac arrhythmias, personnel, and facilities. PACE 15:715, 1992.

INDEX

Note: Page numbers in *italics* refer to illustrations; page numbers followed by t refer to tables.

ISBN 0-7216-5462-2

90038

9 780721 654621